Surgery of Disorders of the Foot and Ankle

Basil Helal

MBChB, MCh (Orth), FRCS, FRCS (Edin)
Emeritus Consultant Orthopaedic Surgeon
The Royal National Orthopaedic Hospital
Honorary Consultant Orthopaedic Surgeon
The Royal London Hospital and
Enfield Group of Hospitals, UK

David I Rowley

MBChB, BMedBiol, MD, FRCS (Edin & Glas)
Professor of Orthopaedic and Trauma Surgery
University of Dundee, UK

Andrea Cracchiolo III

MD
Professor of Orthopaedics
University of California at Los Angeles,
California, USA

Mark S Myerson

MD
Director, Foot and Ankle Services
Union Memorial Hospital,
Baltimore, Maryland, USA

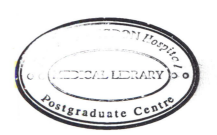

MARTIN DUNITZ

© Martin Dunitz Limited 1996

First published in the United Kingdom in 1996 by
Martin Dunitz Limited, The Livery House, 7–9 Pratt Street,
London NW1 0AE, UK

Portions of this book were originally published in 1988 as
Basil Helal and Derek Wilson, eds, *The Foot*, Churchill
Livingstone, Edinburgh

A CIP record for this book is available from the British
Library.

ISBN 1 85317 212 X

Composition by Scribe Design, Gillingham, Kent, UK
Origination by Imago Publishing Ltd
Manufacture by Imago Publishing Ltd
Printed and bound in Singapore

Contents

Contributors

Rami J Abboud,
BSc, MSc(BioEng)
Foot Pressure Analysis Laboratory
Orthopaedic and Trauma Surgery
Royal Infirmary
Dundee, UK

John Angel, FRCS
Consultant Orthopaedic Surgeon
Royal National Orthopaedic
Hospital
Stanmore, UK

Barbara M Ansell,
CBE, MD, FRCS, FRCP
Retired Head of Rheumatology
Division
Northwick Park Hospital
Harrow, UK

R M Atkins, MA, DM, FRCS
Consultant Orthopaedic Surgeon
Bristol Royal Infirmary
Bristol, UK

Colin G Barnes,
BSc, MBBS, FRCP
Clinical Director
Department of Rheumatology
The Royal London Hospital
London, UK

N Ann Barrington,
MBChB, FRCR
Consultant Radiologist
Northern General Hospital
Honorary Lecturer in
Radiodiagnosis
University of Sheffield
Sheffield, UK

Roderic P Betts, BSc,
MMedSci, PhD, CEng, FIPSM, MIEE
Consultant Clinical Scientist
Central Sheffield University
Hospitals
Medical Physics and Clinical
Engineering
Royal Hallamshire Hospital
Honorary Lecturer
University of Sheffield
Sheffield, UK

Nigel S Broughton,
MBChB(Hons), FRCS(Ed),
FRCS(Eng), FRACS
Consultant Orthopaedic Surgeon
Department of Orthopaedics
Royal Children's Hospital
Victoria, Australia

Nigel Cobb, FRCS
Consultant Orthopaedic Surgeon
St Matthew's Hospital
Northampton, UK

David N Condie, BSc
Rehabilitation Engineering Services
Manager
Dundee Limb Fitting Centre
Dundee, UK

Andrea Cracchiolo III, MD
Professor of Surgery
Department of Orthopaedics
UCLA School of Medicine
Los Angeles
California, USA

H L F Currey, MMed, FRCP
Emeritus Professor of
Rheumatology
The Royal London Hospital
Medical College
Whitechapel
London, UK

B Martina Daly,
MB BCh, BAO NUI, MRCPI
Consultant Dermatologist
Blackburn Royal Infirmary
Blackburn, UK

Piet de Boer, MD, FRCS
Consultant Orthopaedic Surgeon
York District Hospital
York, UK

Nelly De Stoop, MD
Centre de Pathologie et de
Chirurgie du Pied
Clinique du Parc Léopold
Brussels, Belgium

Michael Devas, MChir, FRCS
Chipping Campden, UK

Thomas Duckworth,
MB ChB, BSc, FRCS
Professor of Orthopaedic Surgery
University of Sheffield
Honorary Consultant Orthopaedic
Surgeon
Royal Hallamshire Hospital
Sheffield, UK

John S Early, MD
Assistant Professor of Orthopaedic
Surgery
University of Texas Southwestern
Medical Center
Dallas
Texas, USA

Edward S Forman, DO
Department of Orthopaedic
Surgery
Garden City Hospital
Garden City
Michigan, USA

James D Frame,
MB BS, FRCS, FRCS(Plast)
Consultant Plastic, Reconstructive
and Burns Surgeon
North East Thames Regional Burns
Unit
St Andrew's Hospital
Billericay, UK

Charles S B Galasko,
MSc ChM, FRCS(Eng), FRCS(Ed)
Professor of Orthopaedic Surgery
The University of Manchester
Clinical Sciences Building
Hope Hospital
Manchester, UK

David L Grace,
MB ChB, FRCS
Consultant Orthopaedic Surgeon
Chase Farm Hospitals NHS Trust
The Ridgeway
Enfield, UK

Paul P Griffin, MD
Professor
Department of Orthopaedic Surgery
Medical University of South
Carolina, Charleston
South Carolina, USA

Jeffrey Hallett,
MA, BMBCh, FRCS
Consultant Orthopaedic Surgeon
The Ipswich Hospital NHS Trust
Ipswich, UK

Sigvard T Hansen Jr, MD
Professor of Orthopaedic Surgery
University of Washington
Harborview Medical Center
Seattle
Washington, USA

Douglas H Harrison, FRCS
Consultant Plastic Surgeon
Mount Vernon Hospital
Northwood, UK

Basil Helal,
MCh(Orth), FRCS, FRCS(Ed)
Emeritus Consultant Orthopaedic
Surgeon at the Royal National
Orthopaedic Hospital and
Honorary Consultant at The Royal
London Hospital and Enfield
Group of Hospitals, UK

John A Herring, MD
Chief of Staff
Pediatric Orthopaedics and
Scoliosis Surgery
Texas Scottish Rite Hospital for
Children
Dallas, Texas, USA

Godwin Iwegbu,
MD, MCh(Orth), FRCS(Ed),
FRCS(Glas), FWACS, FICS
Birmingham, UK

Amar S Jain, FRCS(Ed)
Consultant Orthopaedic Surgeon
Orthopaedic and Trauma Surgery
Royal Infirmary
Dundee, UK

John E Jellis,
OBE, FRCS, FRCS(Eng)
Associate Professor of
Orthopaedics
University of Zambia
Lusaka, Zambia

Charles E Johnston II,
MD
Assistant Chief of Staff
Pediatric Orthopaedics and
Scoliosis Surgery
Texas Scottish Rite Hospital for
Children
Dallas
Texas, USA

John Kirkup, FRCS
Consultant Orthopaedic Surgeon
Bath, UK

Marilyn Lord,
PhD, CEng, MBES, FIMechE
Senior Lecturer, Honorary
Consultant Scientist
Medical Engineering and Physics
King's College Hospital (Dulwich)
London, UK

Malcolm F Macnicol,
MCh, FRCSEd(Orth)
Consultant Orthopaedic Surgeon
Princess Margaret Rose
Orthopaedic Hospital
Edinburgh, UK

Bernard F Meggitt,
MA, FRCS
Consultant Orthopaedic Surgeon
Addenbrooke's Hospital NHS Trust
Associate Lecturer
University of Cambridge
Cambridge, UK

Malcolm Menelaus,
MD, FRCS(Eng), FRACS
Senior Orthopaedic Surgeon
Department of Orthopaedics
Royal Children's Hospital
Victoria, Australia

Andrew Milne, DCR, DMS
Superintendent Radiographer,
Trauma/Orthopaedics
Diagnostic Imaging
Northern General Hospital Trust
Sheffield, UK

Mark S Myerson, MD
Director, Foot and Ankle Services
Orthopaedic Surgery
Union Memorial Hospital
Baltimore
Maryland, USA

Sureshwar Pandey,
MBBS(Hons), FICS, MS, FIAMS,
MS(Orth), FACS
Ram Janam Sulakshana Institute of
Orthopaedics
Rameshwaram
Ranchi, India

Nicholas Parkhouse,
DM, MCh, FRCS
Consultant Plastic Surgeon
The Queen Victoria Hospital
East Grinstead, UK

Paul F Plattner, MD
Danville
Illinois, USA

David J Pratt,
BSc, MSc, PhD, CPhys, MInstP,
MBES
Technical Director
Bioengineering Research Centre
Derby Royal Infirmary NHS Trust
Derby, UK

David Prieskorn, DO
Orthopaedic Surgeon
TriCounty Orthopaedics
Farmington Hill
Michigan
Assistant Clinical Professor
Michigan State University
East Lansing, USA

Frank Rand, MD
Orthopaedic Surgeon
Children's Hospital
Boston
Massachusetts, USA

George C Rendall,
BSc, DPodM
Lecturer
Department of Podiatry
Queen Margaret College
Edinburgh
and Podiatrist
Orthopaedics and Trauma Surgery
Royal Infirmary
Dundee, UK

Peter A Revell, PhD,
MRCPath
Professor of Histopathology
The Royal Free Hospital
London, UK

David I Rowley, MBChB,
BMedBiol, MD, FRCS(Ed & Glas)
Head of Department and Clinical
Director
Orthopaedic and Trauma Surgery
Royal Infirmary
Dundee, UK

G James Sammarco,
MD, FACS
The Center for Orthopedic Care
2123 Auburn Avenue, Suite 235
Medical Office Building 2
Cincinnati
Volunteer Professor
Department of Orthopaedic Surgery
University of Cincinnati College of
Medicine
Ohio, USA

Pierce E Scranton Jr, MD
Orthopaedic Surgery
Suite 400
1600 East Jefferson Street
Seattle
Washington, USA

P K Sethi,
MS, FRCS(Ed), FASc, DSc(Hons)
Consultant Orthopaedic Surgeon
SDM Hospital
Emeritus Professor of Orthopaedics
SMS Medical College
Jaipur, India

Brian C Sommerlad, FRCS
St Andrew's Centre for Plastic
Surgery
Billericay and
The Hospital for Sick Children
Great Ormond Street
The Royal London Hospital
London, UK

Kit Song, MD
Assistant Professor of Orthopaedics
University of Washington
Assistant Director,
Pediatric Orthopaedics
Children's Hospital and Medical
Center
Seattle, USA

David Stuart, FRCS
Consultant Orthopaedic Surgeon
Nairobi Hospital
Nairobi, Kenya

Steven I Subotnick,
DPM, MS, ND, CCH
Clinical Professor
Departments of Biomechanics and
Surgery
California College of Podiatric
Medicine
Hayward
California, USA

Malcolm Swann,
MBBS, FRCS
Consultant Orthopaedic Surgeon
Heatherwood and Wexham Park
Hospital Trust
Slough, UK

David B Thordarson, MD
Department of Orthopaedics
University of Southern California
School of Medicine
Los Angeles
California, USA

Karl Tillmann, MD
Chief of Orthopaedic Surgery
Rheumaklinik
Bad Bramstedt, Germany

Antonio Viladot, MD
Professor of Orthopaedic Surgery
Universidad Autónoma de
Barcelona
Past President of the College
International de Podologie
Barcelona, Spain

Michael Ward, CBE
Emeritus Surgeon
St Andrew's Hospital
Bow, UK

Derek W Wilson,
MBBS, FRCS
Oswestry, UK

Isadore Yablon, MD
Professor and Chairman
Department of Orthopaedic
Surgery
Boston University Medical Center
Massachusetts, USA

Preface

In the world of locomotor surgery, the foot moves from strength to strength. When specialty sections are held at meetings, sports-related subjects attract the largest audience, followed closely by the foot and ankle. In the half decade since the first edition of this book, the expansion of knowledge and surgical techniques has been remarkable. Imaging and other investigative methods are more sophisticated, and we have moved into fields such as three-dimensional computerized scanning with subtraction. The computer can isolate a single bone and show you all its aspects on a visual display unit. There is, as a result of basic scientific research, a better understanding of the function and physiology of the foot and its interplay with seemingly remote parts of our central nervous and locomotor systems. Arthroscopy of the ankle and arthroscopic interventions including ankle arthrodesis have enhanced patient care. New methods of fixation of bone, such as metals with a 'shape memory' made pliable by cooling before insertion, new joint implants and tissue manipulation by external fixators (after Ilizarov) have all expanded our clinical armamentarium.

The Editors of this volume are of different ages and come from different fields of experience, and so provide a spectrum of contact with the best in both the traditional and modern aspects of the subject right up to the very forefront of advances in foot and ankle surgery. We believe that this is reflected strongly in this book, which will guide the reader to the best practice in this branch of surgery.

BH
DIR
AC
MSM

I   BASIC SCIENCE

I.1 Anatomy of the Foot

G James Sammarco

Introduction

The anatomy of the foot is the foundation on which is built an understanding of function in the treatment of disabling conditions. The foot is unique. Unlike other parts of the body, it functions by acting on an external surface. In studying the anatomy of the foot and ankle, major consideration must be given to the fact that it is primarily a weight bearing structure and functions to stabilize the body. Its function is fixed at its origin and moves at its insertion. In the foot the insertion is often fixed against a hard surface such as the ground, and the origin in the heel or leg moves in relation to that fixed point.

The requirements of weight bearing in our culture necessitate the need for protection of the foot and ankle (Kelikian 1965), but the foot loses some of its mobility with such protective gear. Boots increase the rigidity of the foot–ankle complex. Ski boots and ice skates are designed to restrict motion into a single plane. The boots of mountaineers stiffen the forefoot to aid in climbing, and cold weather gear restricts motion while insulating the foot. These modifications sacrifice foot mobility and sensitivity in order to aid the body in another way.

Although the foot and ankle primarily stabilize the body, they also have myriad uses demanding flexibility, strength and aesthetics. A large proportion of the world's population goes barefoot. The bare foot, in addition to providing stability, acts as a prehensile limb in some cultures. Where people climb palm trees, for example, there is the obvious necessity to use the shape of the foot in order to hold onto the trunk.

In sport, the foot may be used as a club, as in soccer and American football. Swimming requires increased mobility of the foot for power, locomotion and control. When swim fins are worn, flexibility and control are sacrificed for speed. Highwire artists and gymnasts use a very thin shoe for protection so that strength and balance are not sacrificed. In dance, the foot is used not only for all of its physical qualities of strength and balance, but also for aesthetics. In patients with phocomelia the foot is used extensively as a prehensile limb since the individual substitutes its function for that of rudimentary or absent hands (Swinyard 1969).

Bony anatomy

There are 26 major bones in the foot: seven tarsals, five metatarsals, and 14 phalanges (Fig 1). Each bone has a particular shape, articular surfaces, and appropriate surfaces and orientation to provide a specific function. The hindfoot consists of the talus and calcaneus.

Talus

The talus consists of three parts, the body, the neck, and the head. It is orientated so that it transmits reactive forces from the foot through the ankle joint to the leg. It consists mostly of articular surfaces and has no muscular or tendinous attachments.

Body of the talus
The body of the talus is oriented at 25° medial to the sagittal plane. It has a saddle-shaped trochlear surface, it is narrower posteriorly than anteriorly, and it transmits force through the tibiotalar joint.

The dome of the talus is generally shaped like a portion of a frustum, that is, a portion of a truncated cone. The radius of curvature on the medial ridge is less than that of the lateral ridge. The weight bearing surface has a slight shallow groove in the sagittal plane. The medial and lateral articular surfaces are slightly concave to accept their respective malleolli. At the posterior border, a small groove may be present against which the flexor hallucis longus tendon rides. An apophysis is present on the plantar surface at the posterior extremity of the body. The os trigonum accessory bone, present in 6–8% of specimens, articulates with the tip of the posterior process (Pfitzner 1896). The posterior facet lies on the inferior surface oriented backward at 45° and perpendicular to the sagittal plane.

The blood supply of the body enters through the neck as intraosseous branches of the artery of the sinus tarsi and also through the posterior portion of the dome. Only a small area of the posterior talar dome has a separate arterial supply.

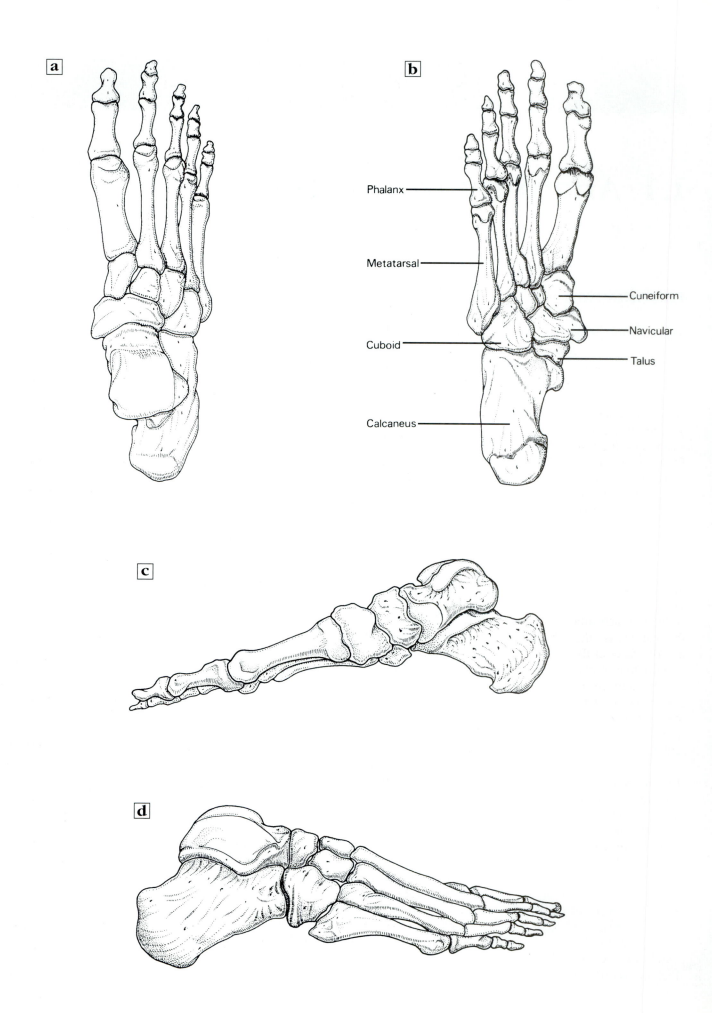

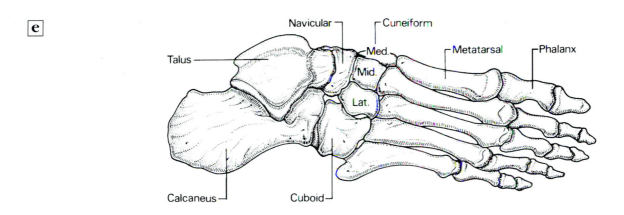

e

Navicular — — Cuneiform
Talus — Med. — Metatarsal — Phalanx
Mid.
Lat.
Calcaneus — Cuboid —

Figure 1

The bones of the foot. (**a**) Dorsal view (**b**) Plantar view (**c**) Medial view (**d**) Lateral view (**e**) Oblique view. Med. = medial, Mid. = middle, Lat. = lateral

Neck of the talus

The talar neck is directed anteriorly, slightly medially and obliquely downward. Articular facets may be present on the dorsal aspect of the neck in those cultures where squatting is the accepted sedentary posture (Charles 1893). Beneath the neck is the sinus tarsi canal, which runs between the talus and calcaneus. The blood supply to the talus enters through the artery of the sinus tarsi from below and from small arteries behind the posterior facet.

Head of the talus

The head of the talus is palpable 1 cm anteromedial to the ankle joint and is convex distally. There are three articulations on its plantar aspect. The posterior plantar medial surface, which articulates with the sustentaculum tali of the calcaneus; the anterior portion forms part of the anterior facet of the subtalar joint, and the medial portion lies on the plantar calcaneal ligament. The distal ovoid articular surface lies in contact with the tarsal navicular.

Most of the talar surface is covered by articular cartilage and its blood supply is mainly through the narrow dorsal and plantar surfaces of the neck; trauma to this area predisposes it to avascular necrosis.

The trabecular pattern of the talus is quite dense because of the high loads that are transferred from the foot through it to the leg. Although there are multiple ligamentous attachments, there are no muscle attachments to the talus. Because of this, the talus functions passively, being held in a sling of tendons connected to adjacent bones by a series of ligament complexes.

Calcaneus

'Calcaneus' derives from the Latin word meaning 'spur'. It is cancellous and quite sturdy and is the largest bone in the foot, occupying the most posterior position. It projects posteriorly, providing a lever arm for the insertion of the tendocalcaneus, Achilles tendon, the largest and strongest tendon in the body, and through which the gastrocnemius and soleus impart powerful plantar flexion forces to the foot. Because of its height and width it permits both high tensile, bending and compressive forces on a regular basis without becoming fatigued. In fact, stress fractures are uncommon in this bone. However, a fall from a height permits extremely high instantaneous loads. Such falls are common and cause fractures in spite of its strong bony structure.

Dorsally, there are three parts to the surface. The dorsal roof lies posteriorly with a fat pad above it. On the anterior portion of the dorsal roof lie attachments of the posterior capsule of the ankle. The mid-portion of the calcaneus contains the convex posterior facet of the subtalar joint and the floor of the sinus tarsi. It also contains the articular surface of the sustentaculum tali, which opposes the talus medially. Anteriorly, the dorsal surface forms the anterior articular facet of the subtalar joint. The anterior surface of the calcaneus contains a concavoconvex surface which articulates with the cuboid. The medial surface of the calcaneus is concave. It contains the sustentaculum tali, which is grooved beneath for the tendon of the flexor hallucis longus. Laterally, a slightly concave surface is present. There is a lateral tuberosity above which the peroneus brevis tendon passes and below which the peroneus longus passes. The inferior tuberosity of the calcaneus accepts the posterior attachment of the plantar aponeurosis.

The calcaneus has a rich blood supply, which promotes healing of fractures. However, the subtalar joints, when misaligned through fracture, can cause persistent, painful arthritis. For this reason accurate alignment of such fractures is important.

Navicular

The tarsal navicular or scaphoid is medial to the cuboid and anterior to the talus. The medial, intermediate and lateral cuneiforms lie distal to it. The tarsal navicular occupies a keystone position at the top of the longitudinal arch of the foot. Its proximal articular surface is concave in shape and articulates with the head of the talus. The distal articular surface has three facets, one to articulate with each cuneiform bone. There is a small facet laterally, which articulates with the cuboid and a medial tuberosity into which the tendon of the tibialis posterior tendon inserts.

In 4–10% of specimens an accessory navicular, os tibiale, is present within the substance of the tibialis posterior tendon. This articulates with a portion of the talar head (Sarrafian & Topouzian 1969).

Cuboid

The cuboid is irregularly shaped. The lateral, dorsal, and plantar sides have a thin cortex; the proximal, distal, and medial surfaces are joints. The cuboid articulates with the calcaneus proximally and the fourth and fifth metatarsals distally. Medially, there is often a small facet which opposes the tarsal navicular; however, this may be only a fibrous attachment. On its inferolateral border there is a groove in which the peroneus longus tendon courses as it passes medially and distally into the fourth muscle layer of the foot.

Cuneiforms

The three cuneiforms are convexly shaped on their broad dorsal aspects. The middle and lateral bones are wedge shaped so that the apex of each bone points inferiorly. The medial cuneiform is convex medially and rounded inferiorly. The plantar surfaces are all concavely shaped. They articulate with the first, second and third metatarsals distally. The medial and lateral cuneiforms project farther distally than the middle cuneiform. This configuration contributes to the stability of the midfoot. A notch is created into which the base of the second metatarsal fits creating a stable 'key-like' configuration of Lisfranc's joint.

Metatarsals

There are five metatarsals. All of the shafts are tapered distally and all articulate with proximal phalanges. The first metatarsal is the shortest and widest. Its base artic-

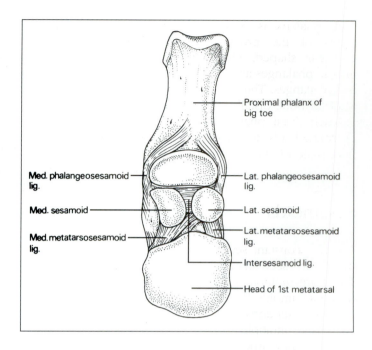

Figure 2

Sesamoids of the hallux. The joint has been opened dorsally so as to expose the head of the metatarsal on end. Lig. = ligament; Lat. = lateral; Med. = medial

ulates through a separate joint with the medial cuneiform. It is somewhat cone shaped. The head of the first metatarsal also articulates with two sesamoids on its plantar articular surface. It has a ridge on its plantar articular surface which rides between the sesamoids.

The second metatarsal extends beyond the first proximally and distally. It articulates with the middle cuneiform as well as with the medial and lateral cuneiforms in a 'key-like' configuration that promotes stability and renders the second ray the stiffest and most stable portion of the foot. Through this bone pass the highest loads within the foot (Manter 1946).

The third, fourth and fifth metatarsals, likewise, are broad at the base, narrow in the shaft and have dome-shaped heads. The plantar aspects of the heads have medial and lateral eminences that protrude downward and assist in weight bearing. The fifth has a prominent styloid, laterally and proximally at its base, onto which the peroneus brevis tendon inserts. A common avulsion (fracture) of the styloid occurs when the foot is inverted against the contracting peroneus brevis muscle.

Phalanges

There are two phalanges for the hallux and three for each lesser toe. Occasionally, the middle and distal phalanges of the fifth toe are fused (Greenfield 1969).

Each phalanx is concave on its plantar surface. The heads of the proximal and middle phalanges are trochlear shaped, allowing for greater stability. The middle phalanges are shorter and broader than the proximal phalanges. The distal phalanges are smaller yet have a tuft of bone distally. These distal expansions at the tip of each distal phalanx anchor the toe pads and also distribute loads during weight bearing, particularly in the final stage of stance.

Sesamoids

The two constant sesamoids present in the foot are the ovoid or 'seed-shaped' tibial and fibular sesamoids. There are multiple variations in the ossification of each of the sesamoids (Kewenter 1936). They lie within their respective tendons of the flexor hallucis brevis muscle and have multiple ligamentous attachments (Fig. 2). Dorsally, they articulate with the inferior surface of the first metatarsal head. The bipartite sesamoid is common and may be confused with fracture.

Occasionally, lateral metatarsals will have sesamoids present at the metatarsophalangeal joint (Fig. 3). The tibialis posterior (os tibiaiae) and the tibialis anterior as well as the peroneus longus tendons (os peroneum) also occasionally have a sesamoid bone within them.

Accessory bones

There are several accessory bones in the foot. The os trigonum is present in 6–8% of specimens. The os vesalianum, at the base of the fifth metatarsal, is uncommon (Dameron 1975). The os tibiale, or accessory navicular, is present in 4–10% of specimens. Other accessory bones include the interphalangeal, intermetatarsal and intercuneiform ossicles. They are significant in that they must be differentiated from fracture and arthritis in order to avoid misdiagnosing an acute condition.

Joints

Ankle joint

The ankle, or talocrural joint, consists of the distal tibia and tibial plafond including its posterolateral border, the posterior malleolus, which articulates with the talar dome, the tibial or medial malleoli, and the fibular or lateral malleolus (Fig. 4). The joint is saddle-shaped. The larger of the circumferences of the dome is lateral and the smaller is medial. The dome itself is somewhat wider anteriorly than posteriorly. As the ankle extends (i.e.

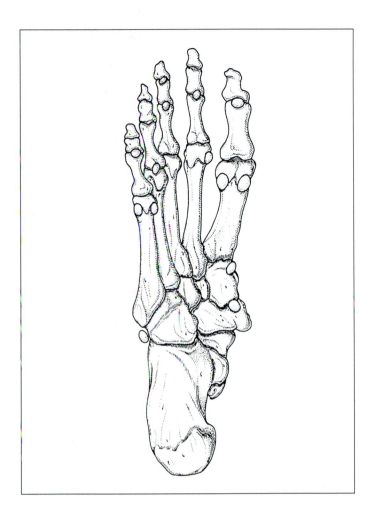

Figure 3
Sesamoids as they appear on the plantar aspect of the foot. Each lies within its respective tendon

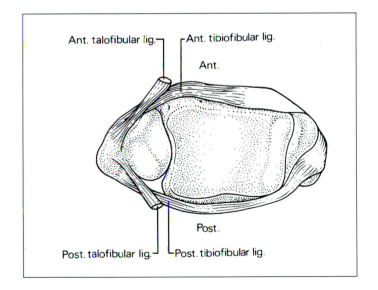

Figure 4
View of the ankle joint from below. Ant. = anterior; Post. = posterior; Lig. = ligament

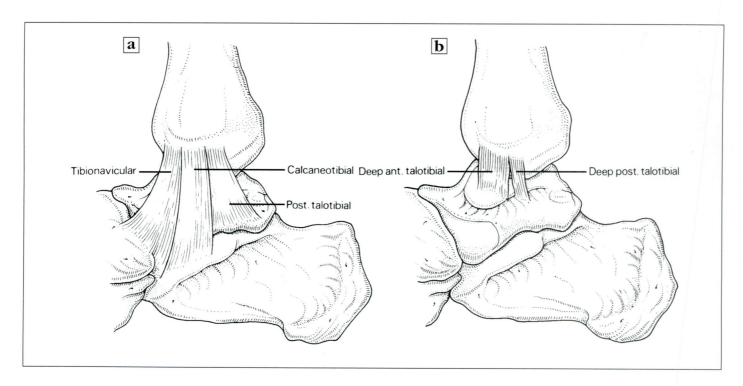

Figure 5

Deltoid ligament showing the two portions. (**a**) Superficial portion (**b**) Deep portion. ant. = anterior; post. = posterior

dorsiflexes), the fibula rotates externally through the tibiofibular syndesmosis to accommodate the widened front edge of the talar dome. The foot also rotates externally.

The ankle achieves its stability both in flexion and extension by means of its saddle shape and its three malleoli. The posterior portion of the posterior malleolus lies along the distal lateral articular surface of the tibia. Additional stability is maintained through the ligaments and capsule which encircle the joint. The capsule itself is thin anteriorly and posteriorly and thickens for medial and lateral support.

Deltoid ligament

The deltoid ligament, or medial collateral ankle ligament, is fan shaped and is divided into a deep and a superficial portion (Fig. 5). The superficial portion has three parts (Spalteholz 1903): the anterior tibionavicular portion, which helps to stabilize the anterior portion of the joint; the tibiocalcaneal portion, which contributes to stability of both the ankle and subtalar joints, and a posterior portion of the superficial ligament, a tibiotalar portion.

The deep portion of the deltoid ligament is short, has two portions, and attaches from beneath the tip of the medial malleolus to the medial talus (Pankovich & Shivram 1979). This, too, contributes to stability of the medial aspect of the joint and is the most common portion of the ligament complex to be injured.

Lateral ligament complex

The lateral ligament complex has three major parts (Fig. 6). The anterior talofibular ligament extends from the anterior portion of the lateral malleolus to the proximal lateral head of the talus. The fibulocalcaneal ligament passes from the inferior tip of the lateral malleolus beneath the peroneus brevis across the subtalar joint to insert and attach to the lateral calcaneus (Laidlaw 1904). The posterior talofibular ligament lies almost horizontal to the ankle joint. These ligaments are prone to rupture through inversion injuries to the foot. The most common ligament to tear is the anterior talofibular ligament. The second most common is the fibulocalcaneal ligament.

The distal tibiofibular syndesmosis is supported by the anterior tibiofibular ligament and the posterior tibiofibular ligament. These broad ligaments may also be disrupted by inversion injuries to the lateral ankle ligaments, the so called high ligament sprain.

Injections into the ankle joint can be performed medially or laterally by palpating where the respective malleoli meet the tibial plafond at the articular border of the tibia. A needle passed into either of these areas will avoid the neurovascular bundle.

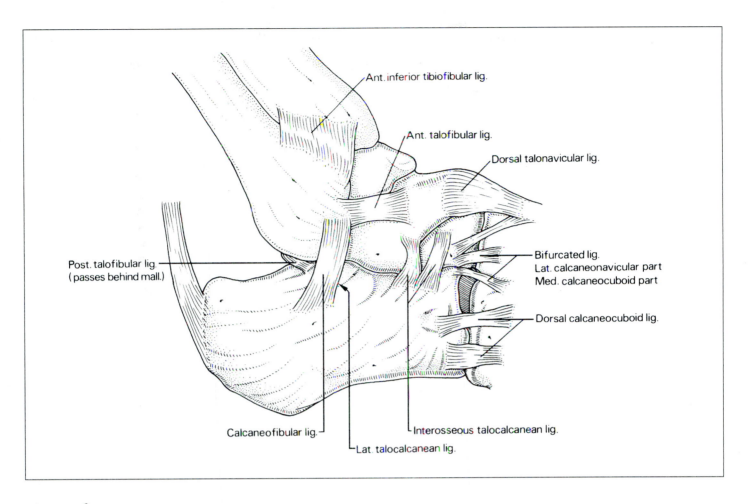

Figure 6
Lateral ankle ligaments. mall. = malleolus; Ant. = anterior; lig. = ligament; Lat. = lateral; Med. = medial

Subtalar joint

The inferior portion of the talus contains two articular surfaces: a large posterior concave surface, which is a true joint in itself, and the smaller talocalcaneonavicular joint (Fig. 7). There is a thin capsule about the posterior facet.

There are three major ligaments of the subtalar joint in the sinus tarsi. These are, in addition to medial and lateral talocalcaneal ligaments, the anterior ligament of the posterior facet, the interosseous talocalcaneal ligament, and the cervical ligament, which covers the lateral aspect of the sinus tarsi. The interosseous talocalcaneal ligament crosses the sinus tarsi and prevents excessive eversion of the foot.

The anterior facet is multiaxial. The convex head of the talus articulates with this facet as well as with the concave proximal navicular. There is a thin talonavicular ligament dorsally. Plantar medial lies the strong plantar calcaneonavicular ligament, the spring ligament. This ligament connects the sustentaculum tali to the inferior navicular. Laterally, the support for this joint is through the bifurcate ligament, which also sends its two limbs from the calcaneus to the navicular. The sustentaculum tali of the calcaneus lies medial and articulates with the rearmost part of the anterior facet of the talus. It supports the medial aspect of the talus beneath the medial talar process.

Calcaneocuboid joint

This joint is saddle-shaped and associated with the talonavicular joint. The combined articulation is called Chopart's joint (Fig. 8). The talocalcaneocuboid joint moves with the subtalar joint during inversion and eversion. Its surface motion is limited, and only a small amount of eversion and inversion is permitted.

Ligaments surrounding the joint include the long plantar ligament, which runs from the calcaneus to the cuboid and also terminates on the third, fourth and occasionally the fifth metatarsals. The short plantar

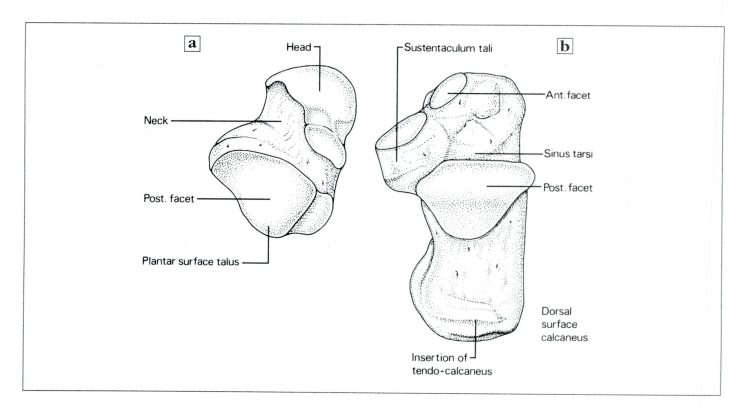

Figure 7

Subtalar joint. The joint is opened so that the medial borders of the joint face each other. (**a**) Plantar surface of talus which articulates with superior surface of calcaneus. (**b**) Dorsal surface of calcaneus. Articular facets are in the anterior portion and support the talus

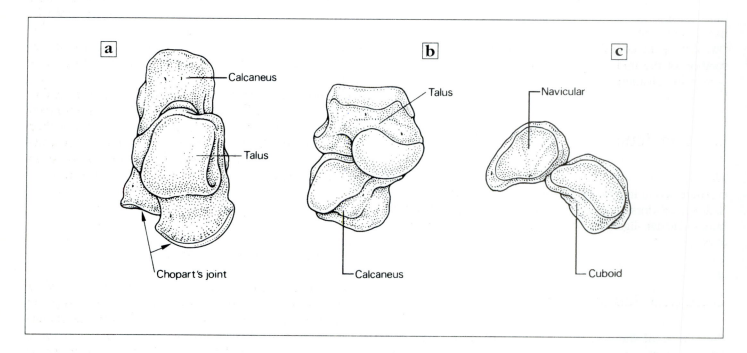

Figure 8

Chopart's joint. (**a**) Dorsal view showing articular surfaces of calcaneus and talar head. (**b**) Anterior facing articular surface of the talus and calcaneus. This articulates with navicular and cuboid. (**c**) Posterior facing articular surfaces of navicular

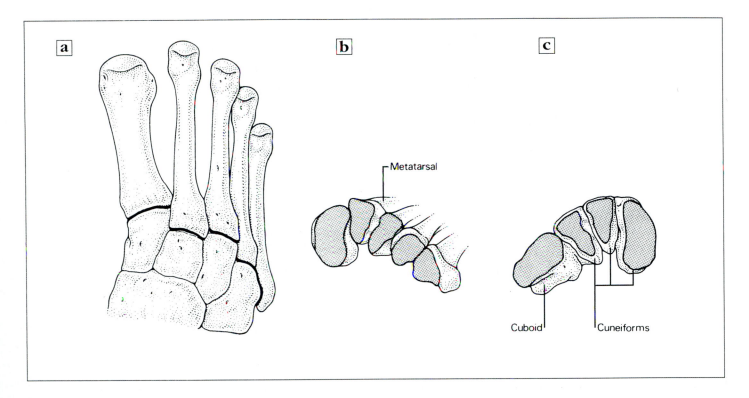

Figure 9

Lisfranc's joint. (**a**) Dorsal view showing Lisfranc's joint (heavy line). (**b**) Posterior facing articular surfaces of the five metatarsals comprising the distal part of the joint. (**c**) Anterior facing articular surfaces of the cuneiforms and cuboid which comprise the proximal part of the joint

ligament connects the calcaneus to the cuboid with deep fibres. Together these ligaments help maintain the longitudinal arch. Dorsolaterally the bifurcate ligament is a major supporter of the joint complex. Motion in the Chopart's joint complex includes flexion, extension and rotation of the mid-foot and forefoot with respect to the talus and calcaneus.

Cubonavicular joint

The cubonavicular joint is considered by some to be a separate joint. It is a syndesmosis with an interosseous ligament, a dorsal cubonavicular ligament and a plantar cubonavicular ligament. Occasionally, it is a synovial joint.

Cuneonavicular joint

The shape of the distal navicular is generally convex, with a facet for each proximal surface of the three cuneiform bones with which it articulates. The proximal cuneiform bones in turn have a concave proximal surface. This joint is a synovial joint but it is also contiguous with the intercuneiform joints, the cuneocuboid joint, the second and third cuneometatarsal joints and the intermetatarsal joints. The significance of this multiple-joint, single-synovial complex is the ease with which a pyarthrosis can spread throughout the tarsal and metatarsal joints beginning in a single articulation.

Motion here includes only a jog of gliding. Some flexion and extension is permitted but this is restricted by interosseous dorsal and plantar ligaments. The limited motion of these joints maintains a longitudinal arch while allowing some accommodation in each joint in order to permit flexibility of the plantar surface of the foot on uneven surfaces.

Tarsometatarsal joints

The first cuneometatarsal joint differs from the other tarsometatarsal joints by having its own separate synovial membrane. The four lateral joints, however, are continuous having a single synovial membrane surrounding them which also contains the intercuneiform joints as well as the cuneonavicular joints. These tarsometatarsal joints are commonly referred to as Lisfranc's joint (Fig. 9).

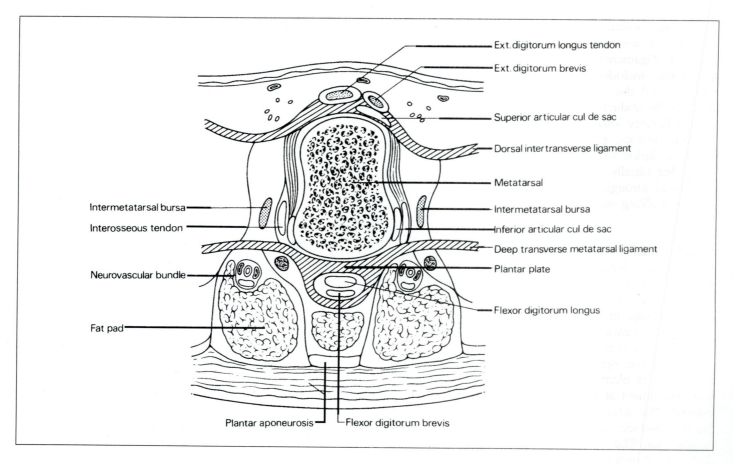

Figure 10

Axial cross section of a portion of the foot at the level of the metatarsal head showing the intermetatarsal ligaments. Note the relationship of adjacent structures. Ext. = extensor

The first cuneometatarsal joint may be round or ovoid. The shape and orientation of the joint may be significant in the development of metatarsus primus varus and bunion, since a more rounded joint permits greater mediolateral motion also. Medial orientation also allows medial rotation of the first metatarsal to occur more easily.

The base of the second metatarsal lies proximal to the base of the first and third metatarsals, articulating with the intermediate cuneiform. In doing so the joint between the tarsal and metatarsal bones is stabilized in a key-like manner. Here, there are strong plantar and dorsal ligaments as well as interosseous cuneometatarsal ligaments. One such ligament is Lisfranc's ligament, which passes from the medial cuneiform to the second metatarsal base. The ligaments aid in passively maintaining the longitudinal arch of the foot. The joints have a small excursion during walking but through their combined motion transfer reactive forces through the bones of the foot from the heel strike to toe-off in the stance phase of gait. There are joints between the metatarsals, intermetatarsal joints, proximally. Extensions of the synovial lining of Lisfranc's joint extend to encompass these joints.

The first and fifth metatarsals are not firmly connected to their adjacent metatarsals, adding an additional flexibility to the middle and fore parts of the foot. The hallux medial cuneiform joint is the most flexible. The fifth, fourth, third, and second joints follow in order of decreasing flexibility.

Metatarsophalangeal joints

Hallux

The metatarsal heads are egg shaped. The first metatarsophalangeal joint of the hallux has a wide dorsal excursion and a range of motion greater than 90° (Sammarco 1985). This accommodates the toe-off part of stance during walking. Plantar flexion of the joint is considerably less, about 40°. There are strong medial and collateral ligaments which are supported by many muscles to maintain power and control over movement. The plantar surface of the metatarsal head has a low ridge centrally and articulates against two sesamoids, each imbedded in a tendon of the flexor hallucis brevis (see Fig. 2).

A strong plantar ligament bridges the two tendons between the sesamoids and includes the intersesamoid ligament. Ligaments that align the sesamoids to the metatarsals include the medial metatarsal sesamoid ligament and the lateral metatarsal sesamoid ligament. Medially the abductor hallucis and laterally the adductor hallucis balance forces at the joint and also help to stabilize the position of the sesamoids. As the hallux is extended during the stance phase of gait, the sesamoids are pulled distally so that weight bearing continues to be aligned through the metatarsal head, the sesamoids and the walking surface.

Smaller toes

The metatarsophalangeal joints of the second to fifth toes also have stabilizing collateral ligaments. The plantar plate of each toe is strong and limits joint extension as well as aiding in the transfer of forces between the plantar pad, flexor tendons and metatarsal heads. The small toes also dorsiflex to 90°. The metatarsal heads are ovoid and the opposing proximal phalanx is deeply concave. The plantar aspect of the metatarsal heads is more prominent and has a medial and lateral eminence present. The lateral eminence is slightly larger. Their function includes the transfer of loads through the ball of the foot. The dorsal capsule is thin. The extensor digitorum longus and the flexor digitorum brevis join at the metatarsophalangeal joint to protect and reinforce it dorsally. Intermetatarsal ligaments maintain the alignment of all the metatarsal rays (Fig. 10).

Interphalangeal joints

The heads of the proximal and middle phalanges have a medial and a lateral condyle. These in turn articulate with the proximal portion of the middle and distal phalanges respectively, which are shaped to accommodate these condylar surfaces.

Strong collateral ligaments maintain medial and lateral stability, while a thick plantar plate prevents hyperextension of the joint. The proximal interphalangeal joints flex more than the distal interphalangeal joints. The significance of these joints becomes apparent in hammer toe, mallet toe and claw toe deformity, particularly when the deformity becomes fixed through fibrosis with ligament and muscle contracture. Such deformity must be corrected by resection of part or all of the joint with or without associated tenotomy.

Retinacula and aponeuroses

The retinacula serve as retainers and as protection so that appropriate vital structures including neurovascular

bundles and tendons can be guided to their areas of function without losing efficiency or being exposed to injury. They also hold these structures in a position to allow adjacent structures to function. The anterior aspect of the ankle contains two retinacula.

Extensor retinacula

Superior extensor retinaculum

The superior retinaculum has attachments on the anterior lateral malleolus and on the anterior tibia. It is attached to the deep fascia of the leg proximally. It holds within it the tendons of the tibialis anterior, extensor hallucis longus, extensor digitorum longus, and the peroneus tertius anterior to the ankle. The neurovascular bundle consisting of the anterior tibial artery and deep branches of the peroneal nerve also run beneath it. There may be a separate tunnel for the tibialis anterior tendon.

Inferior extensor retinaculum

The inferior extensor retinaculum is shaped like an 'X' or a 'Y'. It has two lateral attachments on the calcaneus and two medial attachments, one to the medial malleolus and one to the plantar aponeurosis.

Peroneal retinacula

Superior peroneal retinaculum

Laterally, the superior peroneal retinaculum contains both the peroneal tendons. It is attached to the lateral malleolus and to the lower portion of the tendocalcaneus and lateral calcaneus.

Inferior peroneal retinaculum

The inferior peroneal retinaculum is a continuation of the inferior extensor retinaculum. It has both a superficial and a deep portion and attaches to the trochlear process on the lateral calcaneus, forming portions of the roof of tunnels through which the peroneal tendons pass. Its inferior attachment is on the lateral aspect of the calcaneus.

Upper tibiotalar tunnel

Located at the posteromedial ankle, the upper tibiotalar tunnel has a deep and a superficial portion, which are continuations of the aponeurosis of the leg. It retains the tibialis posterior and flexor digitorum longus tendons

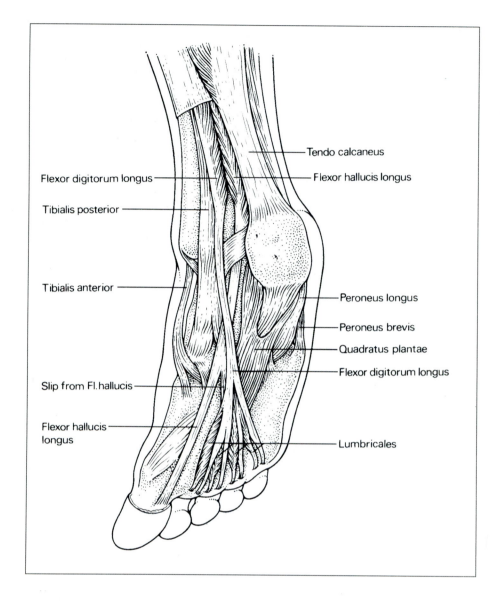

Figure 11

View of the tendons of the tarsal tunnel as they pass into the foot. Note multiple muscles and tendons which attach to the flexor digitorum longus tendons in the foot. Fl. = Flexor

and flexor hallucis longus muscle as well as the posterior tibialis artery and tibial nerve (Fig. 11).

Flexor reticulum and talocalcaneal tunnel

Flexor retinaculum

The triangular-shaped flexor retinaculum, or laciniate ligament, is attached at the medial malleolus, and its base covers the abductor hallucis muscle medially. Anteriorly, its superficial fibres pass over the tibialis anterior tendon and attach to the extensor retinaculum. Its lower, deep fibres pass beneath the tibialis anterior tendon to attach to the anterior tibia. Its base reaches from the calcaneus forward, covering the abductor hallucis muscle.

The talocalcanel tunnel houses the posterior tibial tendon. It passes medial to the talus, posterior to the talotibial portion of the deltoid ligament, and superomedial to the calcaneonavicular ligament and the inferior calcaneonavicular ligament beneath the flexor retinaculum.

The tunnel for the flexor digitorum longus is separate, and its posterior portion is anterior to the posterior tibial artery behind the ankle. It joins the tunnel of the flexor hallucis longus distally. The neurovascular tunnel containing the posterior tibial artery and tibial nerve as well as venae comitantes lies between the flexor digitorum longus and flexor hallucis longus at the posterior tibia. It then courses slightly posterior to the flexor digitorum longus against the medial calcaneus. The positions of the tendons and arteries in this posteromedial compartment are easily remembered by the phrase: Tom, Dick And Harry, i.e. *t*ibialis posterior, flexor *d*igitorum longus, tibialis posterior *a*rtery, flexor *h*allucis longus.

Aponeuroses

Superficial dorsal aponeurosis

On the dorsal aspect of the foot, just beneath the skin, superficial vessels and nerves, lies the superficial dorsal aponeurosis. There are three translucent layers dorsally. The first invests the tendons and is the superficial tendo-connective layer. A second layer encompasses the extensor digitorum brevis. The third layer is an adipoconnective layer in which lie the dorsalis pedis artery, veins and the deep peroneal nerve. These layers permit looseness of the skin over the bone and other structures on the dorsum of the foot, providing flexibility between the bone and the skin during motion of the foot and ankle.

Plantar aponeurosis

The plantar aponeurosis has three parts: a central portion, which is thick and strong, a medial thin portion, and lateral thin portion (Fig. 12). The central portion is the major part and is important in maintaining the longitudinal arch of the foot. It is triangular shaped and attached proximally at the posterior medial calcaneal tuberosity. It passes distally as a heavy structure, dividing and spreading into five slips in the sole. Distally, long sagittal septae are attached from the deep portion into the sole of the foot creating tunnels through which the long flexor tendons pass (see Fig. 10).

The distal attachment of the central plantar aponeurosis inserts through the longitudinal septa into the proximal phalanges as well as into the skin and natatory ligaments. Through these deep connections to the proximal phalanges, the aponeurosis tightens as the toes are extended.

The medial and lateral portions are thinner and may even be incomplete. The medial portion covers the abductor hallucis. The long sagittal septae lie on each side of the long flexor tendons and insert into the interosseous fascia deep in the foot. The special attachments that lie between the calcaneus proximally and ligaments and skin distally allow the plantar aponeurosis to perform an important function through a 'windlass' mechanism. When the toes are dorsiflexed, as in the last portion of stance prior to toe-off, the aponeurosis is pulled distally. This has a tethering effect on the posterior and anterior aspects of the foot, drawing them together. When this occurs, the bones of the foot are held tightly and the foot functions as a single unit rather than as multiple separate bones.

Longitudinal septa pass between the medial and central portions, and the central and lateral portions of the plantar aponeurosis to the interosseous ligaments along the lateral side of the first metatarsal and medial portion of the fifth metatarsal respectively. These create compartments within the foot: a central compartment, an interosseous compartment, peroneal compartment and a tibial compartment (Fig. 13). These are significant, since

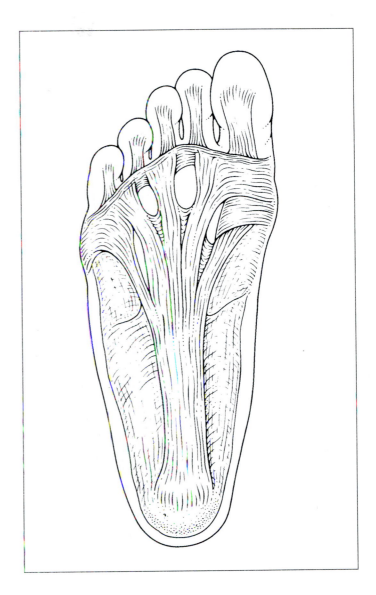

Figure 12

The plantar aponeurosis

a penetrating wound to the medial aspect of the foot may infect the compartments surrounding one of the short muscles of the hallux and yet not spread to other compartments. Infection in the central compartment, however, may pass from the toes up into the leg without involving the other compartments.

Muscles

Extrinsic muscles of the foot

The muscles in the foot can be divided into those muscles of extrinsic origin and those that arise within the foot, of intrinsic origin. Many muscles in the foot span more than

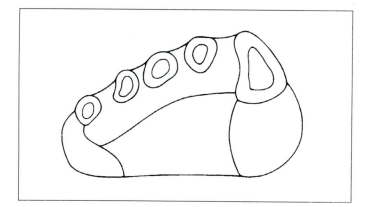

Figure 13

Compartments of the foot

a single joint and in some cases span several joints (Fig. 14). The polyarthrodial characteristics of such muscles allow the muscle belly to shift along with the changing position of one or more of the joints that it spans. This allows the resting length of the muscle to be in its most efficient position for any given position of the foot and ankle so that the most powerful portion of muscle contraction may be used during a particular activity. This aids the muscle's efficiency during standing and walking.

There are four compartments for muscles in the leg. Two compartments are in the posterior calf, the superficial and deep posterior compartments. The peroneal compartment, laterally, contains the peroneal muscles, and the anterior compartment contains the extensors of the foot and ankle. Muscles of the anterior and lateral compartments are innervated by branches of the common peroneal nerve.

Superficial posterior compartment

The superficial posterior compartment for the flexors of the ankle lies posterior to the deep compartment. Two of the three muscles begin on the femur and one on the proximal tibia. The femoral component includes the origins of the two heads of the gastrocnemius, one from each condyle, and the plantaris muscle from the lateral femoral condyle. The soleus arises below the knee from the posterior aspect of the tibia and fibula proximally and completes the triceps surae. These muscles are innervated by branches of the tibial nerve and function to flex the ankle and foot. The plantaris and gastrocnemius muscles aid in knee flexion.

Plantaris

The plantaris arises from the lateral femoral condyle. It is a small muscle immediately forming a tendon which

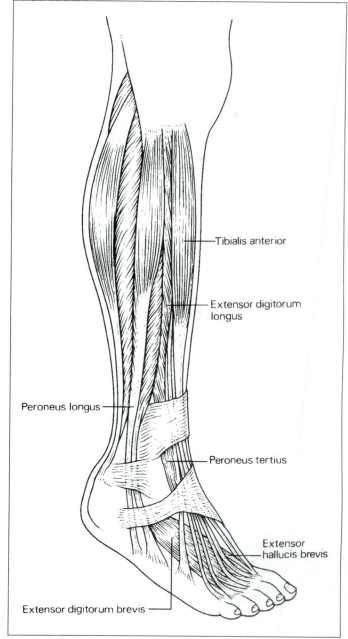

Figure 14

Extrinsic muscles of the foot

then courses between the soleus and gastrocnemius medially to insert distally on the medial portion of the calcaneal tendon of the soleus and gastrocnemius.

It functions with the triceps and has a variable insertion. It is often harvested to be used as a tendon graft. The tendon is absent in 7% of cadaver specimens (Cummins et al 1946).

Achilles tendon

The largest and strongest tendon in the body is the Achilles tendon (tendo Achillis) or tendo calcaneus. It is

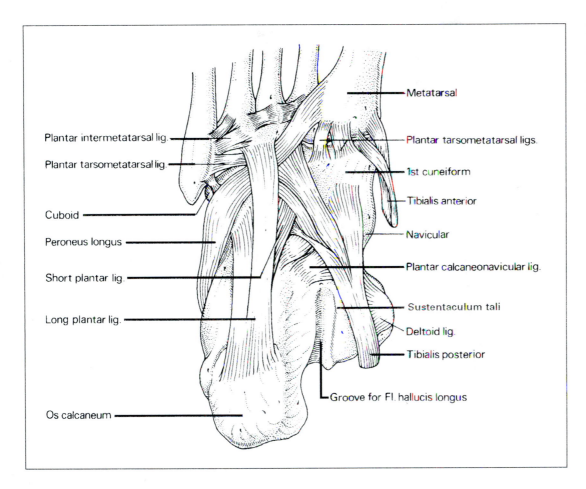

Plantar intermetatarsal lig.

Plantar tarsometatarsal lig.

Cuboid

Peroneus longus

Short plantar lig.

Long plantar lig.

Os calcaneum

Metatarsal

Plantar tarsometatarsal ligs.

1st cuneiform

Tibialis anterior

Navicular

Plantar calcaneonavicular lig.

Sustentaculum tali

Deltoid lig.

Tibialis posterior

Groove for Fl. hallucis longus

Figure 15

Plantar ligaments and tendon insertions of the tarsals and metatarsals. Fl. = Flexor; lig. = ligament

formed proximally by the union of the soleus muscle from deep in the calf and the gastrocnemius muscle arising from the distal femur. A long musculotendinous junction forms posteriorly. Tendon fibres from the soleus tend to be situated somewhat anteriorly in the proximal portion of the tendon while the tendon fibres from the gastrocnemius are situated posteriorly. In its path to the insertion on the posterior portion of the calcaneus, the fibres rotate so that those fibres originally situated in the proximal medial aspect of the tendon terminate distally at an anterior insertion. The significance of the orientation of these fibres during certain types of tendon lengthenings can be remembered by the mnemonic 'Poor Man's District Attorney', i.e. fibre orientation is *p*roximally *m*edial to *d*istally *a*nterior. The surgeon is able, therefore, to orientate the incisions for Z-plasty or percutaneous lengthenings with respect to the position of the tendon fibres.

Deep posterior compartment

Tibialis posterior

The tibialis posterior originates on the posterior tibia and a large portion of the interosseous membrane. At the ankle it passes through a shallow groove just posterior to the medial malleolus bounded by a fibrous tunnel. It courses over the medial aspect of the posterior talus and talar neck, passing beneath the inferior calcaneonavicular ligament or 'spring ligament'. At this point, it lies superficial to the deltoid ligament above the level of the sustentaculum tali.

It has three major insertions (Fig. 15). There is a major broad insertion on the anterior aspect of the tuberosity of the navicular, the navicular–cuneiform joint and the first cuneiform. The middle insertion of the tendon is deep and inserts on the plantar aspect of the second and third cuneiforms and a portion of the cuboid as well as the second, third, fourth and sometimes fifth metatarsals. The posterior portion of its insertion is at the anterior part of the sustentaculum tali. The function of the tibialis posterior is to invert and adduct the foot and flex the ankle. Along with the peroneus longus tendon it acts as a sling which supports the longitudinal arch in both static and dynamic functions.

Injury to or paralysis of this muscle permits acquired flatfoot to occur. Chronic tears of the tendons lead to slow development of this entity (Mann 1984). It is a major portion of the strength and stability of the foot. Because of its strength, it may be used as a transfer either through the interosseous membrane or redirected medially around the tibia to substitute as a dorsiflexor of the foot and ankle.

Flexor digitorum longus

The flexor digitorum longus arises from the middle three fifths of the posterior tibial interosseous membrane, passes with its common tendon into its own canal at the posterior aspect of the ankle and lies adjacent to the tibialis posterior at the medial talus (see Fig. 11). The tendon then passes medial to the sustentaculum tali in its own canal, and crosses plantar to the flexor hallucis longus, beneath the talus. It then divides into four slips. Several tendons and muscles attach to these tendons in the foot. The flexor hallucis longus sends a tendinous slip to the flexor digitorum longus. Each tendon slip also receives a part of the insertion of the quadratus plantae muscle on its deep surface. In addition, the four lumbricals arise from the medial side of each tendinous slip. Each tendon slip courses with the more superficial flexor digitorum brevis tendon through the individual arches of the deep septa of the plantar aponeurosis. Each flexor digitorum longus tendon then passes through the bifurcation of the flexor digitorum brevis tendon at the proximal phalanx of the toe to insert on the plantar aspect of the distal phalanx.

The function of the flexor digitorum longus is to flex the ankle, actively elevate the arch, and flex the toes. It aids significantly in the final stages of gait.

The attachment of the flexor hallucis longus tendon to the flexor digitorum longus tendon is significant in that a deformity which includes contracture of the flexor hallucis longus and great toe can affect position of the lesser toes. Contracture of this muscle secondary to deep compartment syndrome in the calf causes some clawing of the lesser toes. Deep compartment syndrome or spastic paralysis of this muscle can also lead to clawfoot.

Flexor hallucis longus

The flexor hallucis longus has its origin on the interosseous membrane and the posterior portion of the tibia and tibialis posterior and peroneal muscles. It is the most lateral of the muscles in the posterior deep compartment of the calf. The muscle fibres have the lowest origin in the leg, some of them arising almost at the ankle. This aids in its identification at time of surgery. The tendon lies most lateral in the upper tibiotalar tunnel at the posterior talus. It passes in its own tunnel beneath the sustentaculum tali and then crosses deep to the flexor digitorum longus tendon into the medial compartment of the foot. It passes through the arch of the plantar aponeurosis toward the hallux and penetrates the fibrous flexor tunnel at the level of the sesamoids to insert on the plantar aspect of the distal phalanx. A sesamoid may be present at its insertion.

Its function includes ankle flexion, maintaining stability of the foot, elevating the arch, and flexing the great toe. During gait, the flexor hallucis longus functions in the terminal portion of the stance phase. This is important in normal gait as well as in all sports activities. Tendon tears usually occur at the ankle and may cause triggering of the great toe. Deep compartment syndrome usually affects this muscle.

Lateral compartment

Peroneus longus

The peroneus longus muscle located superficial to the peroneus brevis muscle arises from the upper two thirds of the lateral fibula, anterior and posterior intermuscular septa and fascia overlying it. The course of the tendon is from lateral to posterior with relation to the peroneus brevis tendon as it passes the tip of the lateral malleolus. It is retained in the common peroneal tunnel at the posterior ankle along with the peroneus brevis tendon. Inferior to the malleolus, it separates from the peroneus brevis, passing into its own tunnel beneath the processus trochlearis, i.e. lateral process of the calcaneus. At the lateral border of the cuboid, a third tunnel is present through which the tendon courses medially in a groove beneath the cuboid to insert on the lateral tubercle of the first metatarsal and the first cuneiform. This important muscle functions to plantarflex the first metatarsal and also to flex the ankle as well as abduct the foot. Occasionally a sesamoid (the os peroneum) forms within the tendon at the lateral cuboid. A sesamoid is occasionally present in the tendon at the lateral malleolus.

The peroneus longus is an important muscle of the foot inasmuch as it controls the position of the first ray. Isolated paralysis or undiagnosed laceration of the tendon may be responsible for the development of a dorsal bunion. Along with the tibialis posterior tendon a sling is formed beneath the foot which supports the longitudinal arch. These two tendons are important in controlling both static and dynamic foot and ankle function.

Peroneus brevis

The peroneus brevis muscle arises from the lower two-thirds of the fibula and anterior and posterior intermuscular septa above the ankle. It courses posteriorly against the surface of the lateral malleolus and, at that point, lies in the common tunnel with the peroneus longus tendon. It then passes into its own tunnel above the processus trochlearis (the lateral process of the calcaneus). It lies superficial to the calcaneofibular ligament and inserts onto the styloid process of the fifth metatarsal. It functions to flex the ankle and evert the foot. Thirteen per cent of specimens will yield a variation of insertion, some as far distal as the fifth metatarsal head along the medial border (Hecker 1924).

Part or all of the peroneus brevis may be used as a donor tendon for reconstruction of the lateral ligaments of the ankle.

Anterior compartment

Tibialis anterior

The tibialis anterior muscle takes its origin from the lateral condyle and upper one-half of the anterior tibia, interosseous membrane and interosseous septum. It courses beneath the superior extensor retinaculum at the anteromedial aspect of the ankle. It then passes beneath the inferior extensor retinaculum, often within its own tunnel, to insert at the medial border of the foot on the first metatarsal and first cuneiform.

This muscle functions to extend and dorsiflex the ankle, invert the foot and actively support the arch. It can be significant in disease in that flaccid paralysis from peroneal nerve palsy leads to a dropfoot. It is also significant, for stroke victims with spastic paralysis of the lower extremity have this muscle overpowered by the stronger flexors of the ankle and require bracing to avoid spastic equinus deformity from the weakened tibialis anterior muscle. Isolated tendon rupture necessitates the use of the other extensors to dorsiflex the ankle.

Extensor hallucis longus

The extensor hallucis longus muscle takes its origin from the middle two-thirds of the anterior fibula and interosseous membrane, passing distally beneath the superior extensor retinaculum. The anterior tibial artery and deep peroneal nerve lie between it and the tibialis anterior muscle. The muscle then passes anterior to the ankle beneath the inferior extensor retinaculum, occasionally within its own tunnel. Here it lies medial to the anterior neurovascular bundle. The muscle fibres insert low on the lateral aspect of the tendon just above the ankle. The tendon passes along the dorsal aspect of the first metatarsal to insert on the dorsal aspect at the base of the distal phalanx of the hallux. Variations are common in the insertion. Often portions of the tendon insert on the proximal phalanx of the hallux.

The extensor hallucis longus muscle functions to extend the ankle and great toe, and to invert the foot. It is used in transfers for the surgical correction of dropfoot and to control paralytic cavus deformity.

Extensor digitorum longus

The extensor digitorum longus muscle takes its origin from the lateral tibial condyle, interosseous membrane and intermuscular septa. Its tendon is laterally placed and splits into several slips approximately 1 cm above the inferior extensor retinaculum. It passes over the dorsal aspect of the foot to form an extensor hood at each lesser metatarsal phalangeal joint. Here it is joined on its fibular side by the tendons of the extensor digitorum brevis at the second, third and fourth toes. Each tendon divides at its insertion into a central and two lateral slips. The central slip inserts on the base of the middle phalanx. Each lateral tendon slip on the tibial side of the joint receives the insertion of a lumbrical muscle, also on the tibial side of the joint. The extensor hood formed from these tendons then passes over the middle phalanx to insert on the dorsal aspect of the distal phalanx.

The extensor digitorum longus functions to extend the metatarsophalangeal joints through direct attachment on the joint capsule and its extensor sling. It also extends the proximal interphalangeal and distal interphalangeal joints by means of the dorsal hood along with those intrinsic muscles which attach to the hood (Sarrafian & Topouzian 1969). This important foot stabilizer also functions in the swing phase of gait to aid in dorsiflexion of the ankle and foot before heel strike and to decelerate the foot after heel strike.

Peroneus tertius

The peroneus tertius muscle is often considered part of the extensor digitorum longus muscle. It is the most lateral muscle in the anterior compartment and takes its origin from the distal one-third fibular interosseous membrane. Its tendon lies lateral to the extensor digitorum longus. The tendon courses laterally to insert on the base of the lateral aspect of the fifth metatarsal.

It functions to extend the ankle and evert the foot, and is absent in 9% of anatomical specimens.

Intrinsic muscles of the foot

The dorsal foot

The single muscle on the dorsal aspect of the foot is the extensor digitorum brevis muscle. It takes its origin partly from the superolateral aspect of the calcaneus anteriorly and the anterior portion of the sinus tarsi. Its muscle bulk lies in the dorsolateral aspect of the midfoot. The lateral three tendons pass medially and insert on the lateral side of the second, third and fourth tendons of the extensor digitorum longus muscle. The first and most medial tendon courses over the neurovascular bundle and inserts on the dorsolateral aspect of the base of the proximal phalanx of the hallux. It is often called the extensor hallucis brevis. This muscle is innervated by a lateral branch of the deep peroneal nerve.

In the correction of hammer toe, this tendon, along with the extensor digitorum longus tendon, is often divided to permit correction of the extended metatarsophalangeal joint. On occasion, its hypertrophied muscle belly has been mistaken for a cyst or soft tissue tumour.

Plantar intrinsic muscles

There are four layers of muscles on the plantar aspect of the foot. These layers differ from the compartments of the foot which are separated from one another by interosseous and intermuscular membranes. The muscle layers are related to their position with respect to the sole.

First layer

The first layer is unique. All muscles arise from the calcaneus and insert on the proximal phalanges. These muscles have active control over the height of the longitudinal arch. They lie just beneath the plantar aponeurosis and are innervated by medial or lateral branches of the plantar nerve (Fig. 16).

Abductor hallucis

The abductor hallucis muscle rises from the medial border of the foot and calcaneus forming a portion of the calcaneal canal. The flexor digitorum longus and flexor hallucis longus tendons pass deep to its belly. It passes forward to insert on the medial base of the proximal phalanx with the lateral head of the flexor hallucis brevis. At the metatarsophalangeal joint its tendon blends with the medial capsule of the hallux.

The abductor hallucis functions to stabilize the great toe. In the formation of hallux valgus, this tendon may slip beneath the first metatarsal head, contributing to internal rotational deformity of the great toe and acting as a flexor rather than as an abductor. Treatment of bunion and hallux valgus requires realignment of this tendon to prevent reoccurrence.

Flexor digitorum brevis

The flexor digitorum brevis muscle arises from the calcaneus and the deep aspect of the plantar aponeurosis and an intermuscular septum. It rapidly forms four tendons, which tendons then pass through arches of the vertical septa of the plantar aponeurosis. They penetrate the fibro-osseous tunnel beneath the metatarsals where each tendon then divides to allow the flexor digitorum longus to pass through it. The tendons then insert on the proximal plantar aspect of the middle phalanx.

The function of the flexor digitorum brevis is to flex the toes through flexion of the proximal interphalangeal joints and to actively maintain the longitudinal arch of the foot. In 63% of anatomical specimens there may be an abnormality in this muscle, usually involving the fifth toe and occasionally the fourth toe (Nathan & Gloobe 1974). This muscle is a significant deforming force in hammer toe. Often a spur forms at the origin of this muscle, beneath the calcaneus.

Abductor digiti minimi

The abductor digiti minimi (abductor digiti quinti) arises from the lateral aspect of the calcaneus and plantar aponeurosis and the lateral intermuscular septum distally. It passes through the plantar aponeurosis to insert on the lateral proximal aspect and the plantar plate on the fifth toe.

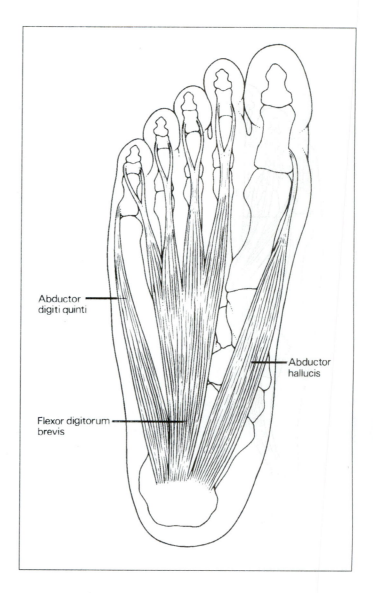

Figure 16

Intrinsic muscles of the foot. First layer

It functions to abduct and flex the small toe and helps maintain the longitudinal arch of the foot. Variations of the abductor digiti minimi, including accessory muscles, are common.

Second layer

The second layer of muscles in the plantar aspect of the foot consists of muscles primarily for controlling toe motion (Fig. 17).

Quadratus plantae

The quadratus plantae has an origin of two heads. The lateral tendinous head arises from the calcaneal tuberosity, the long plantar ligament, and the calcaneal cuboid ligament. The medial fleshy head arises from the medial calcaneus and medial part of the long plantar ligament.

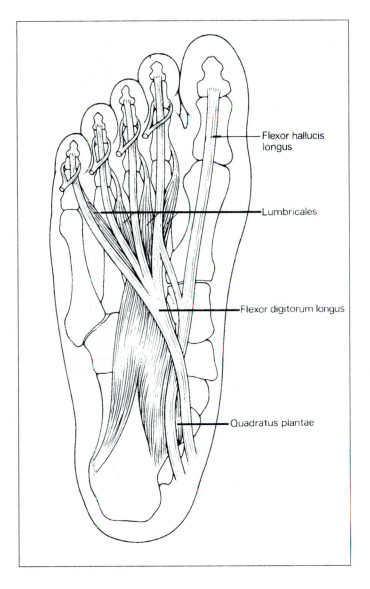

Figure 17

Intrinsic muscles of the foot. Second layer

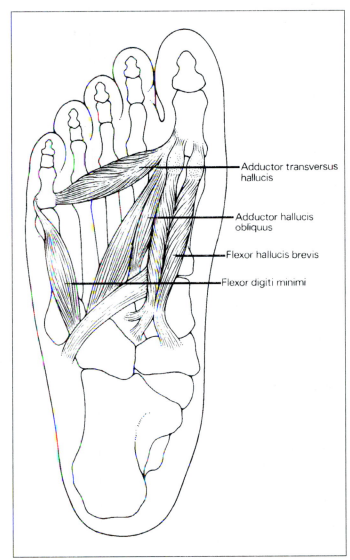

Figure 18

Intrinsic muscles of the foot. Third layer

The medial head forms the lateral border of the calcaneal canal, the two heads uniting at the apex of the canal. The muscle inserts on the deep surface of the common tendon and each of the separate tendons of the flexor digitorum longus. The insertion includes the tendon to the fifth toe and the anastomotic tendon between the flexor digitorum longus and the flexor hallucis longus. The muscle is constant but its course and insertions have unlimited variations. The absence of the muscle is rare.

The quadratus plantae functions to aid flexion of the toes through the flexor digitorum longus tendons.

Lumbricals

There are four lumbricals. These are small fusiform muscles, which arise from the segmented tendons of the flexor digitorum longus shortly after their division from the common tendon. They pass along the medial aspect

of each metatarsal head and are numbered one to four, from medial to lateral. They pass beneath the deep transverse metatarsal ligament to insert on the medial aspect of the extensor hood along with additional fibres from the interossei muscles.

They function to extend the proximal interphalangeal joints. Paralysis or absence contributes to clawfoot deformity.

Third layer

The third layer of muscles is related to the first and fifth toes (Fig. 18).

Flexor hallucis brevis

The flexor hallucis brevis muscle takes its Y-shaped origin medially from the metatarsal portion of the tibialis posterior tendon as that tendon inserts. The lateral head takes its origin from the plantar surface of the cuboid and lateral cuneiform bones as well as from the medial intermuscular septum. The muscle divides into two parts. The smaller lateral head lies in a groove of the first metatarsal. The muscle courses distally. The lateral head joins the plantar plate and encompasses the lateral, fibular sesamoid along with the adductor hallucis muscle beneath the metatarsal head. It then passes distally to insert on the base of the proximal phalanx with the adductor hallucis muscle.

The medial head is larger than the lateral head and passes forward to attach to the medial aspect of the plantar plate and the medial sesamoid. It is joined by the tendon of the abductor hallucis muscle and inserts on the medial plantar part of the proximal phalanx.

This muscle functions to flex and stabilize the metatarsophalangeal joint of the hallux. The sesamoids serve to increase the distance from the centres of rotation of the metatarsophalangeal joint and, therefore, to increase the leverage of this muscle in flexing the great toe and stabilizing the longitudinal arch.

Adductor hallucis

The adductor hallucis has two heads: an oblique head and a transverse head. The oblique head has a long origin from the base of the cuboid, the second, third and fourth metatarsal bases and the sheath of the peroneus longus muscle. It may form an arch for the lateral neurovascular bundle. The transverse head takes its origin from the plantar plates and the transverse metatarsal ligaments of the third, fourth and fifth toes.

The belly of the oblique portion of the muscle is near the flexor hallucis brevis muscle. The transverse and oblique portions pass dorsal to the deep transverse metatarsal ligament. The muscle inserts on the lateral aspect of the lateral sesamoid as well as on the plantar lateral aspect of the base of the proximal phalanx and part of the extensor aponeurosis.

The muscle functions to flex and adduct the hallux, and it is a significant deforming force in the formation of hallux valgus.

Flexor digiti minimi

The flexor digiti minimi muscle arises from the medial plantar aspect of the base of the fifth metatarsal, the sheath of the peroneus longus tendon and the cuboid. It courses slightly laterally along the fifth metatarsal to insert on the plantar plate and the base of the proximal phalanx near the insertion of the abductor digiti minimi and also to the opponens digiti quinti which has been found to be present in 50% of anatomical specimens (LeDouble 1897).

This muscle functions to aid in the control of the fifth toe and adds bulk to the lateral aspect of the foot.

Fourth layer

The fourth layer consists of the interosseus muscles. They are divided into two groups, four dorsal interossei

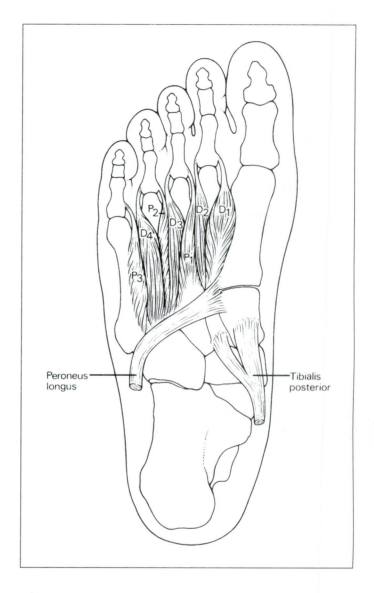

Figure 19

Intrinsic muscles of the foot. Fourth layer

and three plantar interossei. They are named according to their function with respect to the second ray (Fig. 19). Those that move the toes toward the longitudinal axis of the second ray are adductors and those that move the toes away from that axis are abductors. The tendons of two additional muscles are included in the fourth layer. These are the sling muscles of the foot, the tibialis posterior tendon entering from the medial side and the peroneus longus tendon from the lateral side.

The interossei have the least mobility of any muscle in the foot. They are bipenniform in shape and arise from both metatarsals from which they take origin. Each muscle passes distally, dorsal to the transverse metatarsal ligament.

The interossei stabilize the toes, flex the metatarsophalangeal joints and through their attachments to the extensor hood, extend the proximal interphalangeal and,

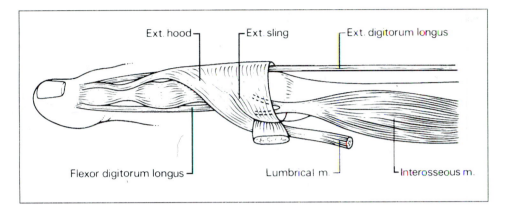

Figure 20

Muscles and tendons of the lesser toes with extensor sling and hood

therefore, the distal interphalangeal joints (Sarrafian & Topouzian 1969).

Dorsal interossei
The dorsal interossei arise from the first, second, third, fourth and fifth metatarsals. They insert on the abductor sides of the second, third and fourth proximal phalanges with respect to the long axis of the second toe. They also insert, in part, into the extensor hood of each toe (Fig. 20). The first dorsal interosseous muscle forms an

arch at its origin. Here the dorsalis pedis passes from the dorsum of the foot between the first and second metatarsals to the deep plantar arterial arch.

Plantar interossei
The three plantar interossei take origin from beneath the dorsal muscles and are smaller in size than their dorsal counterparts. They take origin from the third, fourth, and fifth metatarsals and insert on the adductor sides of the third, fourth and fifth rays and on the extensor hood also.

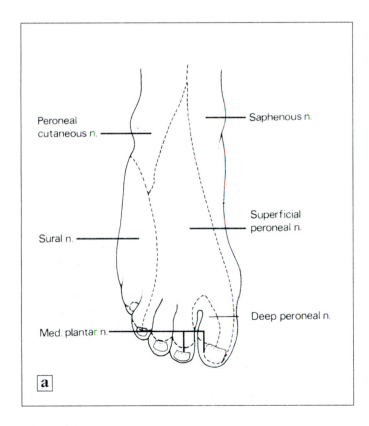

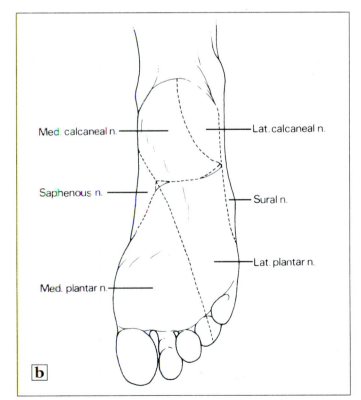

Figure 21

Sensory innervation of the foot by cutaneous nerves. (**a**) Dorsal surface (**b**) Plantar surface. Med. = medial; Lat. = lateral

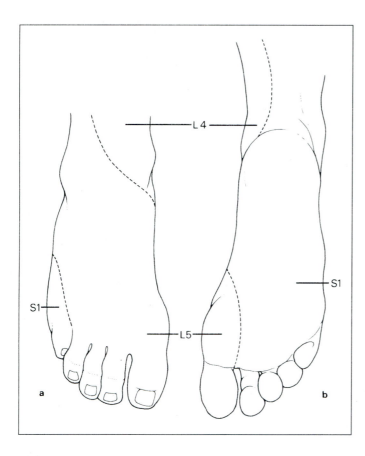

Figure 22

Sensory innervation of the foot by spinal segments. (**a**) Dorsal surface (**b**) Plantar surface. S = Sacral; L = Lumbar

Innervation

Saphenous nerve

The saphenous nerve is a terminal branch of the femoral nerve, which has its origin in the second to fourth lumbar segments of the spinal cord. At the knee, the saphenous nerve lies deep to the sartorius muscle, pierces the fascia lata between the sartorius and the gracilis muscles and then passes medial to the tibia in the leg, just posterior to the greater saphenous vein. There are two branches distally. The smaller one terminates at the ankle, the larger one gives sensation anterior to the medial malleolus and along the medial border of the foot (Fig. 21).

Sciatic nerve

The cutaneous and muscular innervation to the leg, ankle and foot is derived from the sciatic nerve. The origin of its components includes a peroneal portion and a tibial portion. The peroneal portion derives from the posterior divisions of the ventral rami of the lumbosacral plexus and originates from the fourth lumbar to the second sacral segments of the spinal cord (Fig. 22). The tibial portion of the nerve derives from the fourth lumbar to the third sacral nerve roots and forms from the anterior divisions of the ventral rami of the lumbosacral plexus.

Disease entities masquerading as disease of the foot, including diseases of the anterior horn cell and dorsal ganglia, can be caused by injury or irritation to peripheral nerves or lumbosacral nerve roots. Referred symptoms to the foot can include weakness, paralysis, numbness, pain, and paraesthesia. Common lesions affecting the lumbosacral region include entrapment of nerve roots, herniated nucleus pulposus, tumour and fracture.

Sural nerve

The main sensory nerve of the leg is the sural nerve. It is a branch of the tibial nerve arising in the posterior superior popliteal fossa. It passes down the posterior aspect of the calf where it pierces the posterior fascia in the middle of the calf. It communicates with the cutaneous branch of lateral popliteal nerve at the posterolateral border of the lateral malleolus, 1 cm from the malleolar tip. Its distribution then is to the lower and posterior portion of the lateral malleolus and the lateral aspect of the foot.

Common peroneal nerve

The common peroneal nerve is the smaller of the two branches of the sciatic nerve that separate from the sciatic nerve in the popliteal fossa. It courses laterally, passing over the tendon of the biceps femoris and lateral head of the gastrocnemius, and beneath the posterior and lateral aspect of the knee joint. It then curves beneath the head of the fibula where it is quite vulnerable to external pressure. As it passes into the anterior portion of the leg, it divides into a superficial and a deep branch.

Superficial peroneal nerve

The superficial peroneal nerve, also known as the musculocutaneous nerve, is a branch of the common peroneal nerve between the peroneus longus muscle and the neck of the fibula. It descends along the anterior aspect of the leg, innervating the peroneus longus and

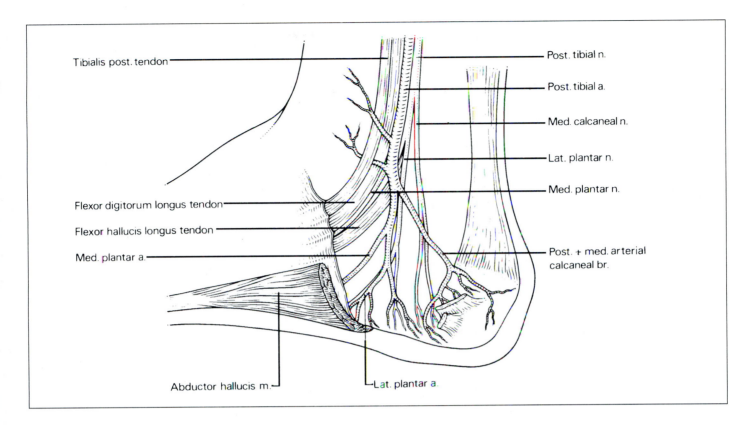

Figure 23

Posteromedial compartment of the ankle showing the relationship of nerves, arteries and tendons. Post. = posterior; n. = nerve; a. = artery, m. = muscle; Med. = medial; Lat. = lateral; br. = branch

peroneus brevis muscle, and it then pierces the fascia 10–15 cm above the lateral malleolus (Kosinski 1926). It continues subcutaneously and at approximately 6 cm above the lateral malleolus splits into a medial dorsal cutaneous branch and an intermediate dorsal cutaneous branch. These branches then give sensory innervation dorsally to the first to fourth, and part of the fifth toes. Occasionally, portions of the nerve are replaced by sural nerve distribution.

Deep peroneal nerve

The deep peroneal nerve is also called the anterior tibial nerve. In the anterior compartment following the branching of the superficial peroneal nerve, motor branches pass to the extensor hallucis longus, tibialis anterior, extensor digitorum longus and the peroneus tertius muscles. The sensory nerve then descends along the lateral side of the anterior tibial artery, passing deep to the superior extensor retinaculum behind the extensor hallucis longus. It passes beneath the inferior extensor retinaculum with the dorsalis pedis artery onto the dorsal aspect of the foot. It lies between the extensor hallucis longus and extensor digitorum longus tendons at 2 and 1.5 cm above the ankle joint. It lies beneath the exten-

sor hallucis longus pulley at the ankle and divides into a medial and lateral branch 1 cm above the ankle joint. These branches innervate the ankle joint anteriorly.

The medial branch then lies lateral to the dorsalis pedis artery between the extensor hallucis brevis and the extensor digitorum longus. It passes to the second toe to give sensory innervation to the first web space.

The lateral branch gives off a motor branch to the extensor digitorum brevis and sensory branches to the tarsometatarsal joints, metatarsophalangeal joints and interphalangeal joints of the lesser toes.

The cutaneous distribution of the deep branch of the peroneal nerve is variable, but most variations include sensation to the first web space (Anatomical Society of Great Britain and Ireland 1891–1892). It is therefore of important diagnostic significance in that when decreased sensation is present in the first web space, a differential diagnosis must include deep peroneal nerve impaired function as with anterior compartment syndrome or impending peroneal nerve palsy.

It is important to recognize the course of such nerves when making surgical incisions on the lateral or anterior aspect of the foot. Inadvertent sectioning of the sural nerve or peroneal sensory nerve can create a pseudoneuroma in addition to creating an asensory portion of the foot.

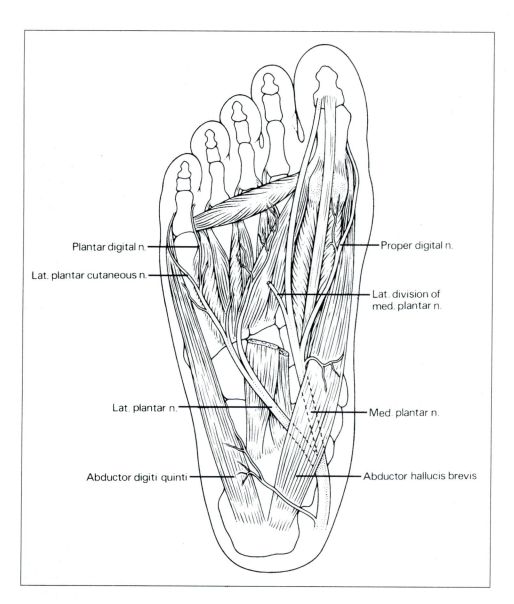

Plantar digital n.

Lat. plantar cutaneous n.

Proper digital n.

Lat. division of
med. plantar n.

Lat. plantar n.

Med. plantar n.

Abductor digiti quinti

Abductor hallucis brevis

Figure 24

Medial and lateral plantar nerves of
the foot

Tibial nerve

The tibial nerve, also known as the posterior tibial or medial popliteal nerve, is the larger portion of the sciatic nerve. It begins in the popliteal fossa following the branching of the common peroneal nerve and passes superficial to the popliteal artery and vein at the popliteus muscle, where it enters the deep posterior compartment of the calf. It then passes beneath the soleus muscle with the posterior tibial artery and vein.

In the lower leg it gives off a branch to the flexor hallucis longus muscle which lies lateral to it. It courses along the medial border of the Achilles tendon (Fig. 23). The tibial nerve branches into the medial and lateral plantar nerves 1 and 1.5 cm above the medial malleolus.

Medial calcaneal nerve

The medial calcaneal cutaneous nerve branches from the tibial nerve in the lower leg. It courses inferiorly and posteriorly to the medial border of the Achilles tendon and to the medial and posterior heel. There is an anterior branch and a plantar branch which innervates the sole and the medial aspect of the foot.

Medial plantar nerve

The medial plantar nerve is larger and more anterior than the lateral plantar nerve. It passes with the tibial artery and vein into the upper chamber of the calcaneal canal and contains motor branches to the abductor hallucis brevis, flexor digitorum brevis, and first lumbrical muscles (Fig. 24).

Proper digital nerve

The proper digital nerve is a branch of the medial plantar nerve. It sends a motor branch to the flexor digitorum brevis and also gives sensation to the medial aspect of the hallux, the sole and the ball of the foot. If this nerve is injured during corrective surgery for bunion or through disease of the sesamoids, then pseudoneuroma or an asensory medial border of the hallux can result.

The motor branches enter the lateral sides of the abductor hallucis and flexor digitorum brevis along the wall of the medial compartment at the base of the first metatarsal.

First common digital nerve

The first common digital nerve lies between the flexor hallucis longus tendon and the flexor digitorum longus. It gives sensation to the lateral side of the hallux and the medial side of the second toe. This nerve lies protected in fat along with the lateral bifurcation of the first plantar metatarsal artery.

A motor branch passes to the first lumbrical. The second and third common digital nerves may have an anastomosis with part of the fourth common digital nerve. Each of the nerves bifurcates in the fatty soft tissue at the level of the metatarsal heads. Each digital branch then passes along the inferior plantar medial and plantar lateral side of the respective toes, plantar to the flexion crease of that toe. These are sensory nerves to the plantar aspects and tufts of the toes.

The most common neuroma of the foot occurs at the bifurcation of the common digital nerve – the so-called Morton's neuroma. The most common position for such a neuroma is at the bifurcation of the third common digital nerve in the web space between the third and fourth toes.

Lateral plantar nerve

The lateral plantar nerve passes into the calcaneal canal posterior to the tibial artery. The first branch passes laterally to the abductor digiti quinti (minimi), arising at the medial border of the flexor digitorum brevis between the quadratus plantae and the flexor digitorum brevis muscles. It penetrates the deep side of the muscle and gives its motor branch to the quadratus plantae muscle. The nerve to abductor digiti quinti passes deep to the origins of abductor hallucis and flexor digitorum brevis, and proceeds laterally to its muscle.

Superficial branch

This branch of the lateral plantar nerve arises between the flexor digitorum brevis and the abductor digiti quinti. It is the sensory branch to the outer sole area, and it also gives a motor branch to the short flexor of the fifth toe and the fifth toe opponens. Occasionally a branch goes to the interossei of the fourth metatarsal space. The fourth and fifth common digital nerves are then formed from this nerve. It ultimately becomes the lateral plantar cutaneous nerve. Occasionally, it provides anastomotic branches to the third common digital nerve.

Deep branch

The deep branch of the lateral plantar nerve follows the lateral plantar artery into the lower calcaneal canal and courses between the adductor hallucis and the interossei muscles. It gives small motor branches to the lateral three lumbricals and to the interossei muscles of the second, third, and fourth spaces. It also innervates the transverse head of the adductor hallucis.

Blood vessels

Arterial system

Anterior tibial artery

The arteries of the leg branch from the popliteal artery at the knee which divides into three smaller arteries in the leg. The anterior tibial artery branches from the popliteal artery at the lower border of the popliteus muscle and passes over the interosseous membrane and the tibialis posterior. Along with the venae comitantes, it lies on the interosseous membrane, between the tibialis anterior and extensor digitorum longus muscles, and then the tibialis anterior and extensor hallucis longus muscles. It passes beneath the superior extensor retinaculum and the inferior extensor retinaculum where it becomes the dorsalis pedis artery. It gives off anterior branches to the medial and lateral malleoli deep to the extensor tendons, and also anastomoses with tarsal arterial branches to form a rich collateral circulation about the ankle.

Dorsalis pedis artery

The dorsalis pedis artery begins at the ankle joint line. It lies medial to the deep branch of the peroneal nerve. Laterally, it sends a branch to the sinus tarsi and the first dorsal metatarsal artery. It also gives off the arcuate artery after which it passes into the plantar aspect of the foot at the proximal end of the first intermetatarsal space (Fig. 25). In the foot, it becomes the first plantar

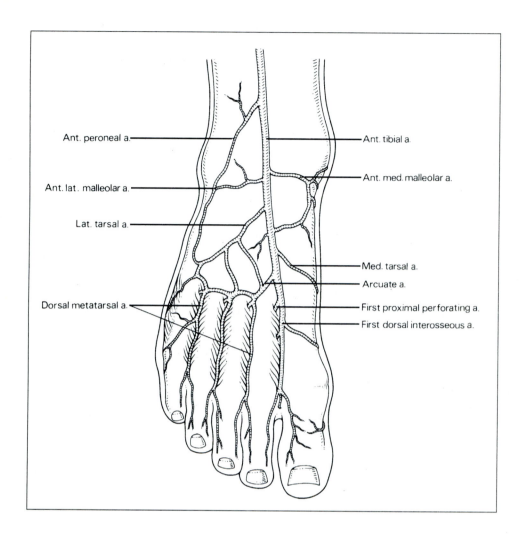

Ant. peroneal a.———————————————— Ant. tibial a.

Ant. lat. malleolar a.———————————— Ant. med. malleolar a.

Lat. tarsal a.————————————————

Med. tarsal a.
Arcuate a.

Dorsal metatarsal a.—————————— First proximal perforating a.
First dorsal interosseous a.

Figure 25

Dorsal arteries of the foot and ankle. Ant. = anterior; lat. = lateral; med. = medial

metatarsal artery and connects with the deep arterial arch. There is great variation of the arterial system in the foot (Edwards 1960, Huber 1944). The artery may be deviated laterally or may be quite thin. These characteristics are of important surgical significance, because the remaining posterior tibial artery may, at times, be the sole arterial blood supply to the foot.

Absence of the dorsalis pedis artery occurs in about12% of specimens studied (Huber 1944).

Posterior tibial artery

As the popliteal artery continues, it becomes the posterior tibial artery at the inferior border of the popliteus muscle. At this point, the artery passes deep to the soleus muscle, and continues along the medial border of the Achilles tendon along with the tibial nerve and its accompanying veins (Fig. 26). It then passes beneath the flexor retinaculum, between the flexor digitorum longus medially and flexor hallucis longus laterally. At this point, the artery lies medial to the nerve. It then divides into medial and lateral plantar arteries divided by the interfascicular transverse septum at the calcaneal canal.

Medial plantar artery

The medial plantar artery courses above the interfascicular septum and the lateral plantar artery passes below, each with its nerve. The medial plantar artery passes deep to the abductor hallucis and flexor digitorum brevis muscles and lies parallel to the flexor hallucis longus tendon. It gives off two branches: a superficial branch and a deep branch. The superficial branch lies on the plantar side of the flexor hallucis brevis muscle and on the tibial side of the flexor hallucis longus tendon. It anastomoses with the first plantar metatarsal artery, and supplies the first three intermetatarsal spaces and the medial four toes. The small deep branch terminates on the deep plantar arch (Fig. 27).

Lateral plantar artery

The lateral plantar artery passes under the interfascicular septum into the lower calcaneal canal and into the middle compartment of the foot. It passes under the quadratus plantae muscle and forms an arch anastomosing with the dorsalis pedis artery which has penetrated from the dorsal to the plantar aspect of the

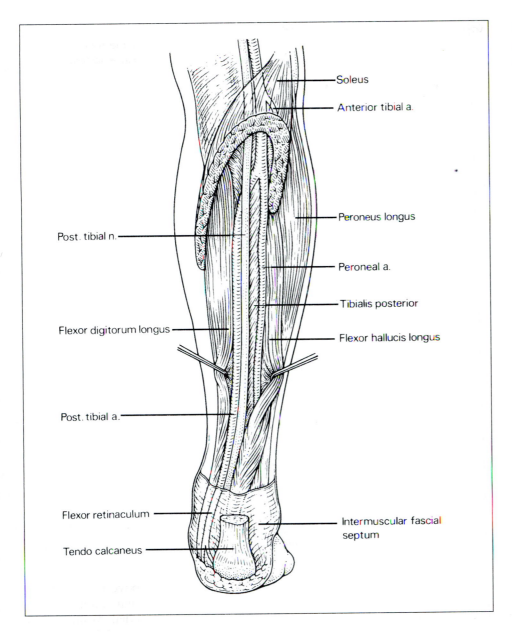

Soleus

Anterior tibial a.

Peroneus longus

Post. tibial n.

Peroneal a.

Tibialis posterior

Flexor digitorum longus

Flexor hallucis longus

Post. tibial a.

Flexor retinaculum

Intermuscular fascial septum

Tendo calcaneus

Figure 26
Arteries of the calf. Post. = posterior;
n. = nerve; a. = artery

foot in the proximal first intermetatarsal space. This forms the plantar vascular arch.

A superficial plantar arterial arch is formed when the common digital arteries anastomose with one another. The digital plantar arteries arise from this arterial arch.

Peroneal artery
The peroneal artery branches from the posterior tibial artery 3 cm beyond the branching of the anterior tibial artery in the deep posterior compartment of the leg. It runs along the posterior aspect of the fibula beneath the flexor hallucis longus muscle. At the lateral malleolus it anastomoses with the lateral malleolar branches of the anterior tibial artery. There is a great variability in the size and position of this artery.

Venous system

The venous system of the ankle and foot is quite variable in its position, as it is in the rest of the body. On the dorsum of the foot, two groups exist, a superficial and a deep system. The superficial venous group lies above the superficial fascia and includes the saphenous veins. This thin, small group of veins drains the dorsal aspect of the toes and then forms the major dorsal venous arcade on the dorsum of the foot. The veins converge at the anterior ankle and also lead into the deep venous system.

Greater saphenous vein
The greater saphenous vein is the largest vein that drains blood from the dorsum of the foot. It lies just anterior

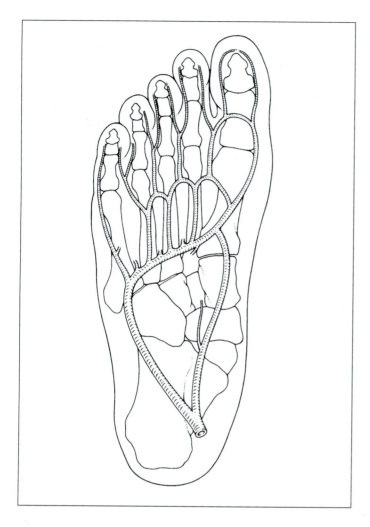

Figure 27

Plantar arteries of the foot

to the medial malleolus at the ankle. Its valves prevent reflux of blood into the foot as well as oedema. It courses along the medial aspect of the calf in the subcutaneous tissue receiving communicating branches from the deep calf to end in the femoral vein.

Lesser saphenous vein

The lesser saphenous vein lies posterior and lateral to the lateral malleolus. Smaller than the greater saphenous vein, it drains blood from the lateral aspect of the foot and the lateral arch.

These veins are easily visualized, fairly constant in their position and are often used as donors in vascular grafts. Incompetent valves can lead to superficial venous varicosities.

Venae comitantes

The deep venous system of the dorsal foot consists of the venae comitantes of the dorsalis pedis artery and its tributaries. Such major arteries often have two veins

accompanying them. The venae comitantes communicate with the greater saphenous vein through the medial malleolar vein. They also communicate with the lesser saphenous vein through the anterior lateral malleolar vein and the metatarsal veins through perforating veins. Valvular incompetence of the deep system of the veins leads to chronic oedema and venous stasis.

Plantar veins

The plantar aspect of the foot also has two systems of veins. The superficial system is intradermal as well as subdermal and consists of a thin mesh of vessels on the sole. It drains to both the medial and lateral margins of the foot. This system of veins is valveless and communicates with the deep plantar venous system. The deep plantar veins accompany the medial and lateral plantar arteries and form a deep plantar venous arch. This in turn drains the metatarsal veins. Valves within the larger veins permit the superficial venous system to drain into the deep system. Surgical stripping of incompetent superficial veins is successful if a competent deep venous system is present. Weight bearing in the stance phase of gait assists in emptying the deep plexus of veins in the foot through a pump-like mechanism of cyclic plantar pressure when walking.

Lymphatic system

The lymphatics of the ankle and foot comprise a superficial and deep system. The superficial system drains the skin of the toes, the sole and the heel. There is a large plexus of minute vessels on the dorsum of the foot. These vessels follow the course of the greater and lesser saphenous veins to terminate at the inguinal lymph nodes and less frequently at the popliteal node.

The deep system drains the deeper tissues. These tiny vessels are aligned with the major arteries of the foot and end proximally in the popliteal node. In performing a lymphangiogram, tiny lymphatic vessels are injected with contrast medium to determine if obstruction is present or if there is spread of carcinoma to nodes through the system. Chronic obstruction of this system with parasites permits large woody oedema to develop as in elephantiasis.

Integument

Skin

Dorsal skin

The skin on the dorsum of the foot is thin and supple. Loose attachments to the underlying subcutaneous tissue permit it to be moved easily over tendons. There are cleavage lines which are oriented obliquely along the lateral border of the foot, but longitudinally along the medial border. Thus, surgical incisions in these respective areas should be planned accordingly.

Plantar skin

The skin of the sole of the foot is thickened and closely adherent to the subcutaneous tissue. The thickness of the epidermis approaches 4–5 mm over the areas of increased weight bearing on the heel and on the ball of the foot. Skin here lacks sebaceous glands and epocrine glands which are present elsewhere in the body. These glands with their oily secretions would compromise the friction of the foot–floor interface if they were present. Eccrine glands, however, are profuse on the sole. These are sensitive to both adrenergic and cholinergic stimuli. Thus, the sole of the foot will become sweaty when one is excited. The sensitivity of the sole is greatly increased compared to that of the dorsum of the foot.

The skin of the sole is closely bound to the plantar aponeurosis through septa. These septa run from the dermis to the aponeurosis in the ball and toes. Between these septa are fat globules, which act as a cushion during walking. In the heel, septa connecting the calcaneus to the skin are arranged in a layered, counterspiralling fashion to act as a shock absorber during heel strike.

In planning a surgical incision on the plantar aspect of the heel, circulation, weight bearing and the formation of postsurgical scars must be considered along with an anatomical approach for adequate surgical exposure. Replacing a tender callous with a painful surgical scar through a poorly planned surgical approach is poor judgement.

Nails

The toenails consist of three layers, they function to protect the distal toes. The medial and lateral borders of the nail lie in a nail groove. The germinal portion of the nail lies 3–4 mm proximal to the cuticle border. Trauma, infection, or surgical incisions into this area can affect the germinal tissue, permanently altering the shape of the nail as it grows. The nail of the great toe grows the slowest of all nails, requiring from nine months to one year to regenerate following removal. The distal border of the great toenail is subject to pressure and trauma.

References

Anatomical Society of Great Britain and Ireland 1891–1892 Report of Commitee of the Collective investigation on the distribution of cutaneous nerve on the dorsum of the foot. J Anat Physiol 26: 89

Charles R H 1893–1894 Morphological peculiarities in the Punjab and their bearing on the question of the transmission of acquired characters. J Anat 28: 1–19, 271–278

Cummins J E, Anson J B, Carr W B, Wright R R, Hauser D W E 1946 The structure of the calcaneal tendon (of Achilles) in relation to orthopedic surgery with additional observations on the plantaris muscle. Surg Gynecol Obstet 83: 107

Dameron T B Jr 1975 Fractures and anatomical variations of the proximal portion of the fifth metatarsal. J Bone Joint Surg 57A: 788

Edwards E A 1960 Anatomy of the small arteries of the foot and toes. Acta Anat 40: 81

Greenfield G B 1969 Radiology of Bone Diseases. J. B. Lippincott Company, Philadelphia

Hecker P 1924 Etude sur le peronier du tarse: Variations des peroniers lateraux. Arch Anat Histol Embryol 3: 327

Huber J F 1944 The arterial network supplying the dorsum of the foot. Anat Rec 80: 373

Kelikian H 1965 Functional Anatomy of the Forefoot in Hallux Valgus, Allied Deformities of the Forefoot and Metatarsaligia. W. B. Saunders Company, Philadelphia, pp 27–42

Kewenter U 1936 Die Sesambeine des I Metatarso-phalangeal-gelenks des Menschen. Acta Orthop Scand (Suppl.) 2: 43

Kosinski C 1926 The course, mutual relations and distribution of the cutaneous nerve of the metazonal region of the leg and foot. J Anat 60: 274

Laidlaw P L 1904 The varieties of the os calcis. J Anat Physiol 38: 138

LeDouble A F 1897 Traite des Variations du Système Musculaire de l'Homme et de leur Signification au Pointe de Vue de l'Anthropologie et Zoologique. Vol. II. Schleicher Frères, Paris. pp 327–360, 402–408, 413–421, 425–427

Mann R A 1984 Rupture of the tibialis posterior tendon. In: Murray J A (ed) Instructional Course Lectures. American Academy of the Orthopedic Surgeons Vol. XXXIII, pp 302–309

Manter J T 1946 Distribution of compression forces in the joints of the human foot. Anat Rec 96: 313

Nathan H, Gloobe H 1974 Flexor digitorum brevis: Anatomical variations. Anat Anz, 135: 295

Pankovich A M, Shivram M S 1979 Anatomical basis of variability in injuries of the medial malleolus and the deltoid ligament: International Anatomica studies. Acta Orthop Scand 50: 217

Pfitzner W 1896 Beitrage zur Kenntniss des Menschlichen Extremitatenskelets: VI. Die Variationen in Aufbau des Fussskelets. In: Schwalbe (ed): Morphologische Arbeiten. Gustav Fischer, Jena, pp 245–527

Sammarco G J 1985 Biomechanics of the foot. In: Frankel V H, Nordin M (eds) Biomechanics of the Skeletal System. Lea and Febiger, Philadelphia, pp 193–220

Sarrafian S K, Topouzian L K 1969 Anatomy and physiology of the extensor apparatus of the toes. J Bone Joint Surg 51A: 669

Spalteholz W 1903 Hand Atlas of Human Anatomy, Volume 1. J. B. Lippincott, Philadelphia, pp 219–223

Swinyard C A 1969 Limb Development and Deformity: Problems of Evaluation and Rehabilitation. Charles C. Thomas, Springfield

Suggested reading

Frankel V H, Nordin M 1985 Basic Biomechanics of the Skeletal System. Lea and Febiger, Philadelphia.

Grant J C B 1956 An Atlas of Anatomy. 4th edn. Williams and Wilkins, Philadelphia.

Sarrafian S K 1983 Anatomy of the Foot and Ankle, Descriptive, Topographic, Functional. J. B. Lippincott Company, Philadelphia.

Woodburne R T 1961 Essentials of Human Anatomy. Oxford University Press, New York.

I.2 Terminology

John Kirkup

For the surgeon, descriptive language demands firstly, consideration of anatomical, functional, pathological and operative concepts and secondly, communication with patients, podiatrists, shoe fitters and other groups who employ their own words. Even if hindfoot, inversion, clubfoot, hallux valgus, triple fusion, instep, and so on cast doubts within and between each group, they have a long history and cannot readily be discarded. Nonetheless, attempts by the Collège International de Médicine et de Chirurgie du Pied (1977, 1978) and others to clarify the surgical terminology are worthwhile, even if agreement is incomplete and recommendations tardily adopted.

Latin remains the basis of anatomical description, as advised by the Basle Nomina Anatomica (His 1895) and its revisions, and it is also the source of many clinical terms. The precision and international acceptance of Latin encourages its retention; to speak a common language clarifies our practice and, above all, benefits our patients.

What is the foot?

Anatomists recognize the ankle joint as the junction of the foot and leg, whereas surgeons perceive it to be a potential site of pathology which influences the attitude and function of the foot. As ankle integrity depends on ligaments connecting the foot to malleoli and also on the interosseous ligament of the inferior tibiofibular joint, the surgical foot includes these structures and the contiguous tibia and fibula, the so-called ankle bones of the layman.

Surgically, the foot is divided into forefoot and hindfoot (not to be confused with the feet attached to the foreleg and hindleg of quadrupeds), at the level of the tarsometatarsal joints (Lisfranc's articulation).

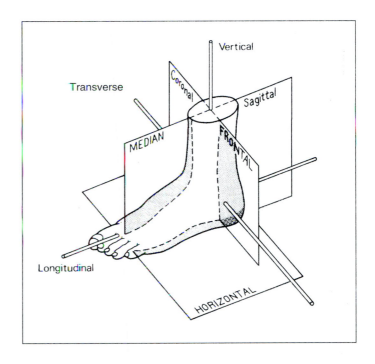

Figure 1

Reference planes and theoretical axes of movement

Planes and axes

The reference planes of the trunk apply to the feet (Fig. 1); median and frontal are recommended as having wider appeal internationally than sagittal and coronal. The axes of potential movement related to these planes

Table 1 Relationship of planes to theoretical and actual axes and movements				
Axis		*Plane*	*Movement*	
Theoretical	*Actual*		*Theoretical*	*Actual*
Transverse	Bimalleolar	Median (Sagittal)	Flexion Extension	Plantarflexion Dorsiflexion
Longitudinal	Peritalar (Henke's)	Frontal (Coronal)	Inversion Eversion	Supination Pronation
Vertical		Horizontal	Adduction Abduction	

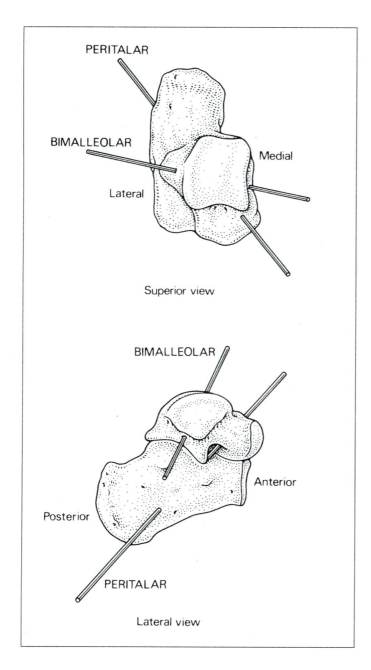

Figure 2

Actual axes of hindfoot movement

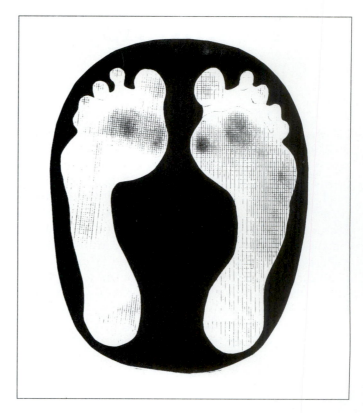

Figure 3

Normal standing footprints illustrating concept of two half pedestals uniting to form a single supporting column

are theoretical only, as it is impossible for the foot to rotate (invert–evert) in the frontal plane about a longitudinal axis or for it to abduct–adduct in the horizontal plane about a vertical axis (Table 1). If flexion–extension (plantarflexion–dorsiflexion) in the median plane suggests a transverse axis, it is actually about an oblique bimalleolar axis (Fig. 2).

Given that one foot cannot function normally on its own, clearly both feet are needed to constitute a single unit of stability and locomotion. Indeed, Ellis (1889) commented that the feet must not be regarded as two pedestals but as two halves of one divided. Studying a pair of normal footprints emphasizes this point (Fig. 3) and supports the clinical convention of naming deformity with reference to the median plane of the body (Fig. 4). This reference line, formerly employed by European anatomists, is ignored in modern anatomical terminology, which is based on median planes passing through the second ray of each foot. We thus have the paradox of hallux valgus being aggravated by adductor hallucis (see Fig. 4), whereas elsewhere in the body, valgus is associated with abductor muscles. As Warwick (personal communication, 1977) asserts, there are two terminologies and clinicians must cope with both!

Shapes and attitudes

Pes cavus (high arch), normalus, planus (flat) and convexus (rocker-bottom) describe the shape of the sole in relation to the horizontal, through the median plane of the first ray (Fig. 5a). Pes varus and valgus describe the attitude of the hindfoot determined by estimating the inclination of the calcaneum to the vertical when the standing heel profile is viewed from behind (Fig. 5b).

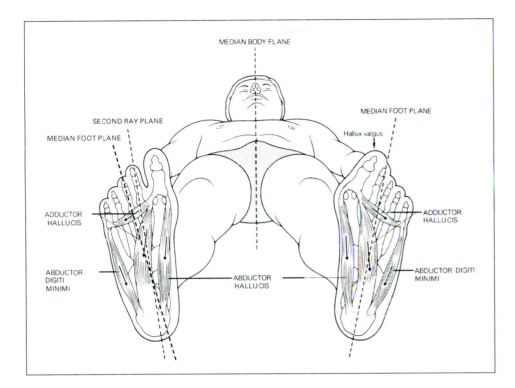

Figure 4

The foot and body planes separate anatomical and surgical terminologies. Hallux valgus is appropriate to the body plane and not to the foot plane; if the latter is the reference plane, then anatomical logic makes this deformity hallux varus (with acknowledgements to Mantegna and Gary M. James)

However, a specific deviation at the tarsometatarsal junction necessitates the qualification metatarsus varus; metatarsus adductus is not correct for it suggests the action of an adductor muscle when this is actually named abductor hallucis (see Fig. 4). Strictly, pes varus and valgus indicate deviation about the vertical axis only whereas, more often than not, the foot is also twisted about its longitudinal axis (see Table 1), in which circumstance, pes supinatus and pronatus are preferred.

In the median plane, pes equinus and calcaneus usually denote fixed attitudes of the foot with reference to its accepted neutral right-angle position with the leg. Mobile equinus may be masked when standing still, and the terms drop-foot or paralytic equinus are more precise.

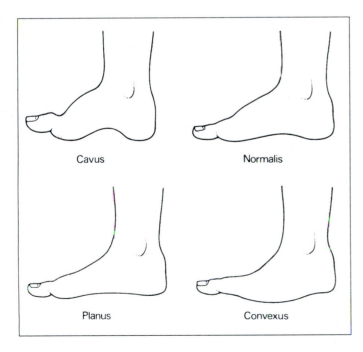

Figure 5(a)

Sole shapes

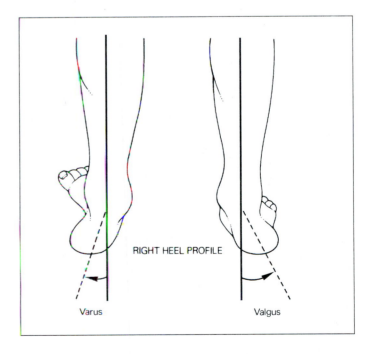

Figure 5(b)

Standing heel profile from behind

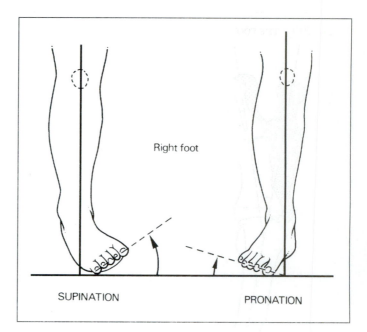

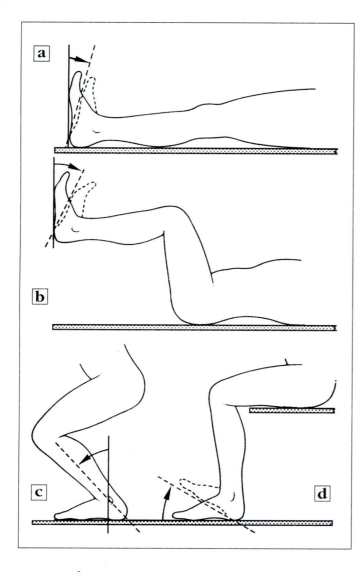

Figure 7

Supination and pronation measured lying or sitting, by estimating the angle of the plane of the sole relative to the horizontal or imagined floor line, with the leg vertical

Figure 6

Foot dorsiflexion: (a) lying, with knee extended; (b) lying, with knee flexed, the range increases; (c) weight bearing, as in climbing stairs, the range increases to the maximum; (d) sitting, an intermediate range similar to (b). It is easiest to measure the plane of the sole relative to its neutral position at 90° to the leg

Combinations of attitude generate compound terms, such as talipes equinovarus, which, if describing the three accepted deformities of clubfoot, is more accurately talipes equinosupinatus. Combinations of shape and attitude include planovalgus and cavovarus. Any tendency to use planus, valgus and pronatus as interchangeable synonyms for flatfoot should be resisted.

Movements

As already observed, active independent movements of inversion, eversion, adduction and abduction are not possible and it is best to describe peritalar joint inversion–adduction as supination and eversion–abduction as pronation (see Table 1 and Fig. 2).

The academic debate as to whether approximation of the foot dorsum towards the shin is flexion or extension can be continued ad infinitum, and for this reason the explicit terms dorsiflexion and its opposite plantar flexion are recommended. In estimating the range of these movements, considerable variation is possible, depending on foot and knee posture, gravity and weight bearing (Fig. 6). Thus, when climbing stairs or crouching down, dorsiflexion may far exceed that possible when supine on a couch with the knee extended; further, an intermediate figure is likely if sitting with knee flexed at 90°. As it is difficult to estimate plantar flexion in a weight bearing subject, the best compromise is to measure both plantar and dorsiflexion passively with the knee flexed with the subject either supine or seated (see Figs. 6b and d). These movements include contributions from the subtaloid and midtarsal joints as well as from ankle joints; these can only be separated by radiography, and hence clinical measurement of plantar and dorsiflexion is never a measure of isolated ankle movement. During walking the significant factor is the position of the sole of the foot relative to the leg; moreover, it is easier to place a goniometer along the lateral margin of the sole than to try to estimate the centre of ankle joint movement and the line of the talar neck (see Fig. 6). Similarly, pronation and supination encompass contributions from joints other than the

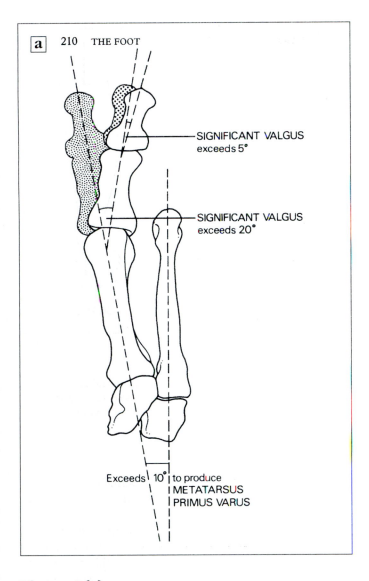

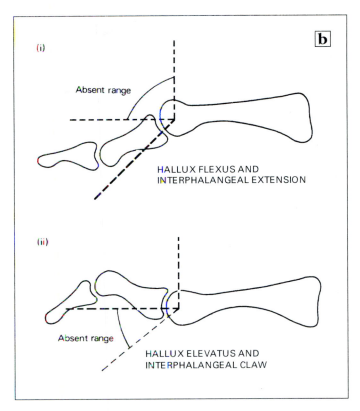

Figure 8(b)

(i) Hallux flexus: no dorsiflexion at the metatarsophalangeal joint. (ii) Hallux elevatus: no plantar flexion at the metatarsophalangeal joint combined with plantar flexion or clawing at the interphalangeal joint

Figure 8(a)

Suggested angles to determine significant metatarsus primus varus, valgus at the metatarsophalangeal and at the interphalangeal joints. Measured on standing radiograph

peritalar complex, and likewise clinical estimates of these movements are most useful when the flat of the sole is the indicator, measured relative to the horizontal plane (Fig. 7). Although individual tarsal joint movements can be calculated, with some difficulty, it is the global range of plantar flexion, dorsiflexion, supination and pronation which determine weight-bearing posture and function.

Further problems of the hallux

Hallux valgus or hallux subluxans?

Hallux valgus describes only one vector of what is usually a three-dimensional deformity associated with

rotational subluxation of the sesamoids and proximal phalanx, which, in extreme cases, leads to dislocation. It would be more accurate to say hallux valgus et tortus, the latter indicating the medial torsion of the hallux; however in some instances fixed flexion or extension is also present. To avoid a lengthy formula based on deformity, a plea is made to describe the actual pathology, and hallux subluxans is suggested. Nevertheless, the valgus component remains a useful indicator, and can be measured accurately on a standing radiograph to determine diagnosis and to monitor progress. Figure 8a suggests relevant angular measurements.

Hallux rigidus or hallux arthriticus?

Rigidus implies fixity whereas, in current practice, hallux rigidus also encompasses mobile joints with diminished dorsiflexion (Kessel & Bonney 1958). Vainio (1956) defines rigidus as 20° or less of passive dorsiflexion at the metatarsophalangeal joint. However, patients with pain and arthritic changes in this joint frequently have a range greater than 20°, and a terminology descriptive of the pathology is more accurate. Thus, in the osteoarthritic case, hallux arthriticus is appropriate, and in rheumatoid arthritis, which generates complex deformities (Kirkup et al 1977), hallux rheumatoideus or rheumatoid hallux is suggested.

Hallux flexus and hallux elevatus

Flexus denotes absence of dorsiflexion and the assumption of a plantar flexed attitude, whereas elevatus denotes absence of plantar flexion and a dorsiflexed attitude (Fig. 8b). Hallux flexus is often associated with interphalangeal hyperextension, and hallux elevatus with interphalangeal clawing, whilst the extremes of these deformities may result in metatarsophalangeal dislocation (Kirkup 1978).

References

Collège International de Médicine et de Chirurgie de Pied 1977 Seminar report. Chirurgia del Piede 1: 589

Collège International de Médicine et de Chirurgie de Pied 1978 Seminar report. Chirurgia del Piede 2: 157

Ellis T S 1889 The human foot. Churchill, London. p 3

His W 1895 Die anatomische Nomenclatur. Veit, Leipzig

Kessel L, Bonney G 1958 Hallux rigidus in the adolescent. J Bone Joint Surg 40B: 668

Kirkup J R, Vidigal E, Jacoby R K 1977 The hallux and rheumatoid arthritis. Acta Orthop Scand 48: 527

Kirkup J R 1978 Dislocation of the hallux in rheumatoid arthritis. Chirurgia del Piede 2: 87–93

Vainio K 1956 The rheumatoid foot. Ann Chir Gynaec Fenn Supplement 1

Wood Jones F 1944 Structure and function as seen in the foot. Baillière, London. p 5

I.3 Biomechanics

David N Condie

Introduction

Mechanics is the study of the effects of forces upon bodies. Biomechanics is therefore the study of the effects of forces on human bodies, or rather the tissues that form the human body. This discussion of the biomechanics of the foot and ankle will consider how the tissues of the ankle joint and the foot respond to the forces that arise as a result of the joint movements associated with activities such as standing and walking.

The ankle joint

Joint structure

The ankle joint is an integral component of the 'kinematic chain' associated with lower limb function. In particular, it is responsible for the manner in which the foot is presented to the ground. Clearly, any impairment of ankle joint function can have a serious effect upon foot function and vice versa. For practical purposes, the ankle joint may be regarded as a 'ginglymus' or hinge-type joint. Movement at the joint takes place between the 'mortise' formed by the bones of the leg and the 'tenon' shaped talar trochlea.

Some authors have analysed the shapes of the corresponding articular surfaces in an attempt to define the precise nature of the permissible joint motion (Barnet & Napier 1952). It will be obvious, however, that a full examination of this subject must take into account the role of the associated collateral ligaments.

The collateral ligaments

The precise anatomy of these important structures has been described elsewhere, however from a biomechanical standpoint, the ligamentous complex on each side of the ankle may be considered as comprising anterior, medial and posterior components. On the medial side of the ankle, these consist of the tibionavicular, tibiocalcaneal and posterior tibiotalar ligaments, which collectively constitute the deltoid ligament; on the lateral side, they consist of the more discrete anterior talofibular, calcaneofibular and posterior talofibular ligaments (Fig. 1).

All of these components take their proximal attachment on the appropriate malleolus and fan out to take their distal attachment on the anterior and posterior

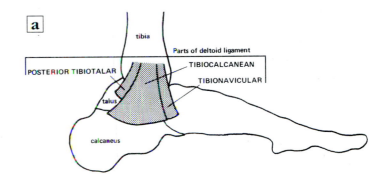

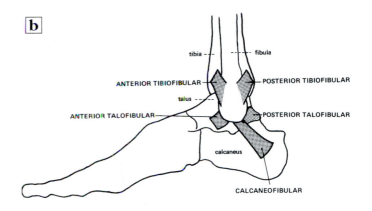

Figure 1

The principal components of: (a) the medial; and (b) the lateral collateral ligaments

surfaces of the talus and the medial and lateral surfaces of the calcaneus. An understanding of the manner in which these ligaments interact with the joint structure to achieve stability and yet permit normal movement at the ankle joint may be obtained by studying the clinical literature relating to ligament injuries to the ankle. In addition, a few investigators have reported the results of tests designed specifically to clarify the role of the individual ligamentous components (Leonard 1949, Anderson 1952, Close 1956, Rasmussen & Tovberg–Jensen 1982, Rasmussen et al 1982, Johnson & Markolf 1983, Rasmussen et al 1983, Rasmussen & Kromann–Andersen 1983).

The composite pattern that emerges from these sources may be summarized by considering each of the types of force (and moment) which the joint will be

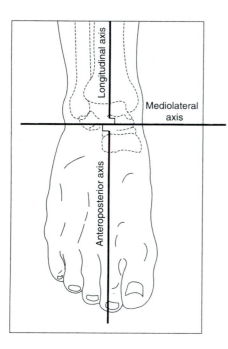

Figure 2

The ankle joint reference axis system

subjected to during normal physical activities. A reference system of orthogonal axes has been defined for this purpose (Fig. 2).

An anterior or posterior force acting on the foot will tend to cause displacement of the talus with respect to the leg. These movements, however, in the normal intact ankle joint will be prevented by tension developed in the two posterior or anterior ligamentous components respectively (Fig. 3a). A longitudinal force acting proximally will of course result in pressure between the talar trochlea and the opposing tibiofibular articular surfaces, while a distally directed force will be resisted by all the ligamentous structures, but most importantly by the medial components (Fig. 3b). A medial or lateral force acting upon the foot will be resisted principally by contact between the sides of the trochlea and the corresponding articular surfaces on the malleoli and the associated ligaments (Fig. 3c).

A moment acting about the anteroposterior axis will be resisted by tension developed in the medial component of the appropriate ligament (Fig. 3d). A moment acting about the longitudinal axis will be resisted by tension developed in the appropriate diagonal pair of

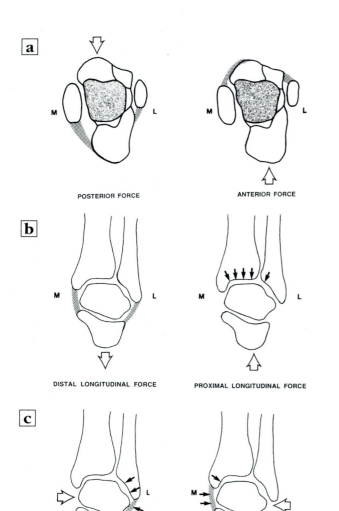

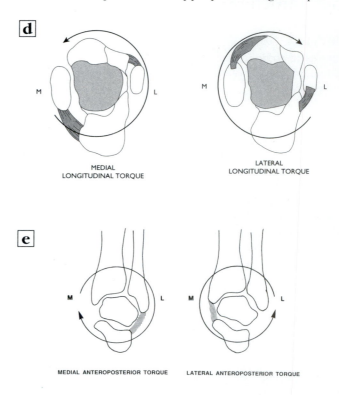

Figure 3

Joint and ligamentous mechanisms responsible for resisting: (a) anteroposterior forces; (b) longitudinal forces; (c) mediolateral forces; (d) moments about an anteroposterior axis; (e) moments about a longitudinal axis

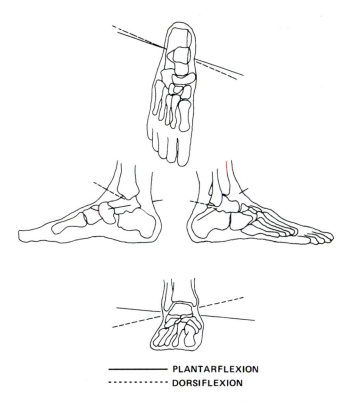

PLANTARFLEXION
DORSIFLEXION

Figure 4

The axis of motion of the ankle joint

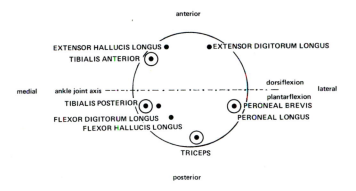

Figure 5

Diagrammatic representation of the positions of the tendons of the ankle joint muscles relative to the ankle joint axis

anterior and posterior components, e.g. a medial torque will result in tension in the anterior lateral component and the posterior medial component (Fig. 3e).

The one remaining type of external force action is a moment about the transverse axis, which it would appear is not resisted, at least within the normal range of motion, by either articular or ligamentous structures. The absence of bony resistance to motion is readily explained by the curved shape of the trochlea when viewed in the sagittal plane. The explanation for the lack

Table 1 The ankle joint plantarflexion and dorsiflexion muscles

Dorsiflexors	
Tibialis anterior	– principal
The long toe extensors	
Extensor digitorum longus	
Extensor hallucis longus	
Peroneals	– secondary
Longus	
Brevis	
Plantarflexors	
Triceps surae	– principal
Gastrocnemius	
Soleus	
The long toe flexors	
Flexor digitorum longus	
Flexor hallucis longus	
Tibialis posterior	– secondary

of collateral ligament resistance lies in their fan shaped distribution, which results in the lines of action of all six components passing through the transverse axis with the consequence that they are not affected by motion about this axis.

Axis of motion

From the preceding discussion, it may be seen that the axis of motion of the normal ankle joint is in fact dictated both by the shapes of the articulating surfaces on the foot and leg and by the positions of the attachments of the collateral ligaments and their restraining effects.

The resulting axis of motion has been successfully determined by several investigators (Hicks 1953, Isman & Inman 1969, Sammarco et al 1973) and found to vary somewhat throughout the range of motion of the joint (Fig. 4). An acceptable approximation, however, would be to consider the axis as passing transversely through the tips of the tibial and fibular malleoli.

The ankle musculature

Control of the forces tending to cause motion about the ankle joint axis is achieved by the action of the ankle joint musculature. Ten muscles have their origin upon the leg, cross the ankle joint and insert upon the foot. The type of control exerted by each muscle may be deduced (as first proposed by Steindler 1935) by considering the line of action of its tendon (as it crosses the joint line) with respect to the joint axis (Fig. 5). In this manner the action of each muscle may be identified as either dorsiflexion or plantarflexion.

The relative importance of each muscle may be judged by considering two factors – its bulk and the length of its lever arm. Using these criteria, the tibialis anterior and the triceps surae may be clearly identified as the principal dorsiflexors and plantarflexors respectively, with the peroneal muscles and the tibialis posterior having important secondary roles as plantarflexors (Table 1).

Ankle joint function during walking

Kinematic and ground reaction force data may be combined to define the motion of the ankle joint and the associated external joint moment throughout the walking cycle (Bresler & Frankel 1948, Brewster et al 1974, Stauffer et al 1977) (Fig. 6). Equilibrium considerations will dictate which group of muscles (plantarflexors or dorsiflexors) must be active to resist the external moment, and electromyographic recordings permit more detailed identification of the precise phasic muscle activity (University of California 1953).

At heel contact the foot is typically plantigrade. Often a momentary dorsiflexion movement is detectable as the heel strikes the ground. Almost immediately, however, the direction of motion reverses and the ankle joint plantarflexes until the sole of the foot makes contact with the ground. During this phase of the gait cycle, the line of action of the ground reaction force is behind the ankle joint and the consequent external joint moment has a plantarflexing action. The observed activity of the dorsiflexor muscles (notably tibialis anterior) is required to ensure that the foot is lowered in a controlled manner until full foot contact with the ground is achieved.

This form of muscular activity is referred to as 'eccentric' activity, in which the muscle is lengthening while in a contractile state and, by doing so, absorbing the mechanical energy associated with the initial phase of stance.

Once foot flat is achieved the direction of joint motion reverses. This requires a contraction of the same muscle group to overcome the external joint moment which still has a plantarflexing action. By mid-stance the ankle joint is once again virtually plantigrade and the line of action of the ground reaction is now in front of the joint axis, resulting in an external dorsiflexion moment. Initially, the ankle joint continues to dorsiflex, requiring eccentric activity on the part of the plantarflexors (notably the triceps surae) to control the rate of dorsiflexion and prevent collapse.

Finally, as the heel leaves the ground, the direction of joint motion reverses once again as active plantarflexion commences, with the plantarflexors contracting to provide the energy necessary to overcome the external dorsiflexion moment.

The ankle joint muscular activity during the stance phase may, therefore, be summarized as comprising, for each group of muscles (plantarflexors and dorsiflexors),

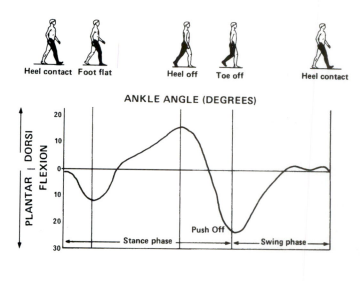

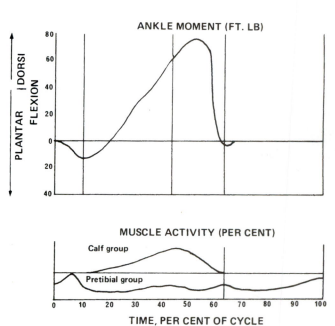

Figure 6

Ankle joint motion, external joint moments and associated muscle activity during normal level walking (from Piezer & Wright 1970, with permission)

a period firstly of 'eccentric' activity, during which mechanical energy is being absorbed, followed by a period of 'concentric' activity, during which the energy necessary to pull and then push the body mass forward is generated.

During the swing phase, the foot is held in a slightly dorsiflexed position with the dorsiflexors acting to resist the external plantarflexion moment resulting from gravitational and inertial effects upon the swinging foot.

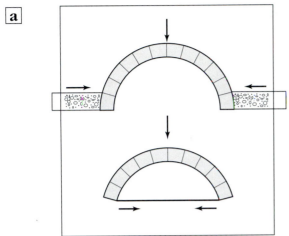

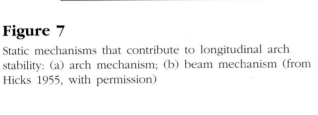

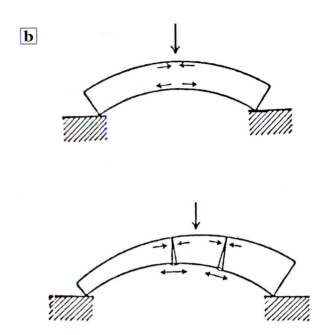

Figure 7

Static mechanisms that contribute to longitudinal arch stability: (a) arch mechanism; (b) beam mechanism (from Hicks 1955, with permission)

Joint and muscle forces

If the positions of muscle lines of action and ligamentous attachments are estimated, it is possible to calculate the magnitude of the forces that will be generated in these tissues to resist the external force and moment actions and the consequent ankle joint forces (Brewster et al 1974, Stauffer et al 1977, University of California 1953). In the most recent published investigations, Proctor and Paul (1982) reported maximal muscle forces occurring during normal level walking of 2.5 times body weight in the triceps surae and approximately body weight in the tibialis anterior, peroneal and tibialis posterior muscles. Joint forces of twice body weight and four times body weight were calculated for the early stance and later stance phases respectively. It should be noted, however, that this study assumed that no tension was developed in any of the components of the collateral ligaments. If this assumption is challenged, it would have the effect of increasing the magnitude of the resultant joint forces.

The foot

The weight-bearing structure

The foot is the site of transmission of the substantial forces, which are developed during physical activities, between the ground and the body. During normal walking on the level, these forces are directed initially onto the heel. The specially adapted fatty tissues of the heel pad are particularly suited to the absorption of the

energy resulting from the large forces occurring at impact and during subsequent loading of the limb. Once the foot is flat and until the heel leaves the ground as push-off is initiated, the supporting forces are shared between the heel and the ball of the foot with only a small contribution from the lateral aspect of the foot.

The ability of the foot to withstand these forces without collapsing is attributed to the so called 'arch structure' of the foot, and its effectiveness is a function of a number of both structural and neuromuscular mechanisms. All the longitudinal arches of the foot have a common posterior pillar, the calcaneus. The medial three arches, which are the most easily recognized, are formed by the calcaneus, the talus, the navicular, a cuneiform, a metatarsal and its associated phalanges. The lateral two arches, which are significantly flatter, are formed by the calcaneus, the cuboid, a metatarsal and its phalanges.

The 'static' integrity of the arches is considered as being achieved by two mechanisms. The arch mechanism likens the foot to the arch of a traditional hump-backed bridge which depends for its security on the inward forces applied by its end buttresses. In the foot these inward forces are created by the tie action of the plantar aponeurosis extending from the heel to the proximal phalanges (Fig. 7a). The beam mechanism (Hicks 1955) proposes that the plantar ligaments extending between each of the elements of the arch, the individual bones, in effect convert it into a single semi-rigid member (Fig. 7b).

The transverse arch of the foot is formed by the metatarsal heads and relies on similar static mechanisms for its integrity. Although less evident than the longitudinal arch, all metatarsal heads make contact with the ground during weight bearing. The importance of its existence is most clearly demonstrated in pathological situations when the normal pressure distribution on the forefoot can become seriously disrupted, with disastrous consequences.

Once the heel leaves the ground the total ground reaction force acts through the forefoot. The resulting very high bending moment acting upon the longitudinal arches would most certainly result in damage to these tissues but for two further 'dynamic' protective mechanisms. Reference has already been made to the tie action of the plantar aponeurosis. Electromyographic studies have revealed the additional important role of the intrinsic muscles of the foot located in this structure, which, it has been experimentally demonstrated, contract just as the heel leaves the ground, thus reinforcing this action (Hicks 1956, Mann & Inman 1964) (Fig. 8).

Furthermore, as the heel rises the toes are forced into hyperextension. Since the distal attachment of these muscles is on the base of the proximal phalanges, this motion, which has been likened to a 'windlass' action (Hicks 1954), will have the effect of further increasing the tension in the aponeurosis (Fig. 9).

The foot joints and their motions

The most important joint within the foot structure is without question the subtalar joint. This joint is formed by the articulations between the articular surfaces on the plantar aspect of the talus and the calcaneus posteriorly and the head of the talus and the navicular anteriorly. These bones are constrained by their ligamentous attachments, such that joint motion takes place about an oblique axis, passing through the neck of the talus downwards and laterally (Hicks 1953, Isman & Inman 1969, Manter 1941) (Fig. 10).

The terms commonly accepted to describe these motions are supination, which may be regarded as a combination of plantarflexion, inversion and internal rotation (or adduction), and pronation, that is, combined dorsiflexion, eversion and external rotation (or abduction).

The second principal joint of the foot is the mid-tarsal joint, which is formed by the articulations between the talus and the navicular and between the calcaneus and the cuboid. The motions occurring at this joint complex have been described as occurring about two distinctly different axes (Manter 1941), one of which – the so called transverse axis — permits a small degree of flexion–extension; the other – referred to as the oblique axis – corresponds closely to the subtalar joint axis (Fig. 11).

As has been noted, the articulation between the head of the talus and the navicular forms part of both the subtalar and the mid-tarsal joints. Perhaps understandably, the type of motion possible at the mid-tarsal joint at any instant appears to be dependent on the position of the subtalar joint (Elftman 1960).

The articulations of the rays of the foot all permit a small degree of independent flexion or extension. More significant, however, is their combined motion, whereby

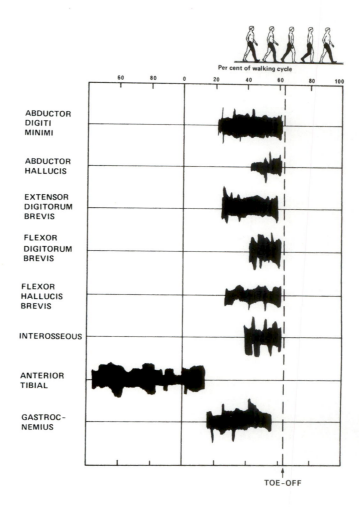

Figure 8

Activity of the intrinsic muscles during level walking in a person with a normal foot (from Mann & Inman 1964, with permission)

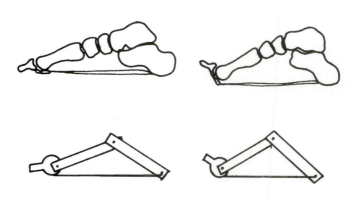

Figure 9

Windlass action of the metatarsophalangeal joints (from Hicks 1954, with permission)

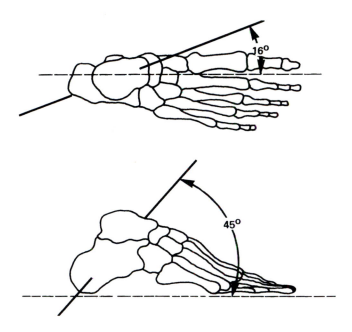

Figure 10

The axis of rotation of the subtalar joint (from Manter 1941, with permission)

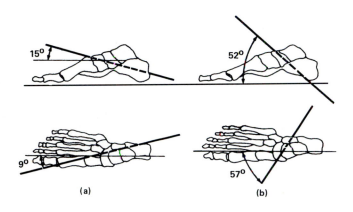

(a)　　　　　　(b)

Figure 11

The axes of rotation of the mid-tarsal joint: (a) the longitudinal axis, (b) the transverse axis (from Manter 1941, with permission)

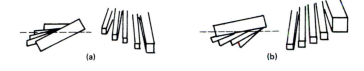

(a)　　　　　　(b)

Figure 12

The combined motion of the forefoot rays: (a) pronatory twist, (b) supinatory twist (from Hicks 1953, with permission)

reciprocal flexion and extension of opposite sides of the forefoot results in an effective inversion–eversion (or supination–pronation) motion of the forefoot relative to the hindfoot (Hicks 1954) (Fig. 12).

The subtalar joint musculature

The muscles that control movement at the subtalar joint are exactly the same as those that control ankle joint motion, and it is possible to deduce the type of control they will exert and their relative importance using the same methodology employed for the ankle joint musculature (Steindler 1935) (Fig. 13). In this manner it is possible to identify the peroneal muscles as the principal pronators and both the triceps surae and the tibialis posterior as major supinators (Table 2).

The function of the foot joints during walking

Investigations of the function of the foot joints during physical activities are comparatively rare, almost certainly because of the practical problems created by their size and complexity. Many authors have drawn attention to the link between inversion–eversion of the foot and internal–external rotation of the leg, sometimes erroneously referred to as a 'torque convertor', which is a result of the oblique alignment of the subtalar joint axis, without attempting to explain its significance.

The action of the subtalar joint was studied intensively at the University of California between 1953 and 1967 (Close & Inman 1953, Wright et al 1964, Close et al 1967). When the conclusions of the most recent of these studies are considered in combination with even earlier investigations of the transverse or longitudinal rotations of the lower extremities during walking conducted at the same institution (Levins et al 1948), it is possible to formulate an explanation of the role of not only the hindfoot joints but also the forefoot rays (Fig. 14).

During the swing phase and approximately the first 15% of the stance phase, the pelvis rotates internally. If the foot is to maintain its alignment relative to the direction of progression it is necessary for the leg to achieve a corresponding degree of external rotation relative to the pelvis.

External rotation of the leg at the hip joint during this phase of the walking cycle was recorded during the previously mentioned early study (Levins et al 1948), and a very small degree of external rotation at the knee joint is also detectable as the leg comes into full extension; however, the sum of these motions is significantly short of that required. The more recent studies (Close & Inman 1953, Wright et al 1964, Close et al 1967), however, clearly demonstrate that during the early stance phase the hindfoot pronates and, by this action, achieves the necessary additional degree of internal rotation (Fig. 15a).

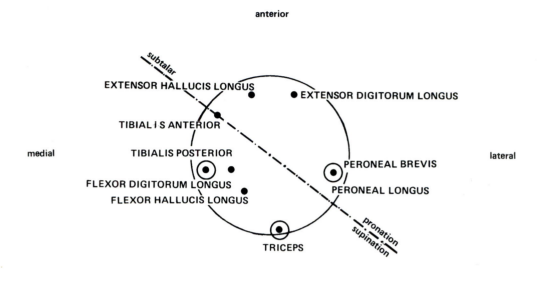

Table 2 The subtalar joint supinator and pronator muscles

Supination	
Triceps surae	– principal
Gastrocnemius	
Soleus	
Tibialis posterior	– principal
The long toe flexors	
Flexor digitorum longus	
Flexor hallucis longus	
Tibialis anterior	
Pronation	
Peroneals	– principal
Longus	
Brevis	
The long toe extensors	
Extensor digitorum longus	
Extensor hallucis longus	
Tibialis anterior	

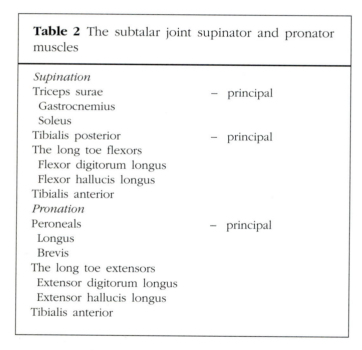

Figure 14

Subtalar joint motion and associated longitudinal rotation of the tibia during normal level walking

During the remainder of the stance phase, the direction of pelvic motion reverses and it becomes necessary for the leg to rotate internally with respect to the pelvis if slippage between the foot and the ground is to be avoided. Once again, the previously measured rotations at the hip and the knee have been demonstrated to be inadequate and it is only by virtue of the coincidental hindfoot supination which occurs during this phase of the cycle that the requisite degree of internal foot rotation is achieved (Fig. 15b).

As has been previously described, supination and pronation of the hindfoot, in addition to producing inter-

nal and external rotation, also result in inversion and eversion of the foot. Clearly this action could seriously disturb the normal distribution of the plantar forces across the forefoot, resulting in excessive pressure and, ultimately, discomfort. Experimental studies of foot pressure demonstrate that under normal circumstances this problem does not arise and one is, therefore, forced to conclude that reciprocal motion of the rays of the forefoot

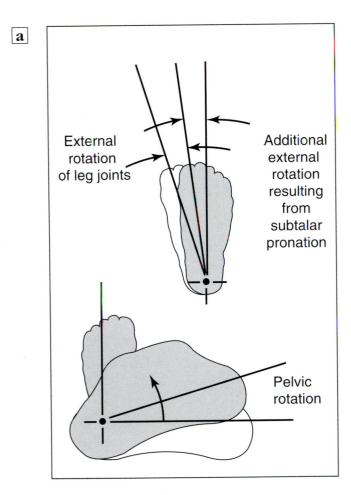

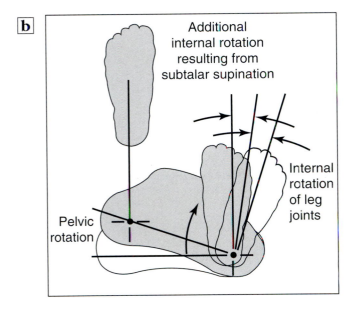

Figure 15

Longitudinal rotation of the lower limbs and pelvis during normal level walking (viewed in the transverse plane)

is occurring, resulting in compensatory forefoot supination during early stance, and pronation during late stance.

Forces and pressure on the foot

Only one study (Proctor & Paul 1982) has experimentally estimated the force occurring in the subtalar joint. They reported mean peak values of 2.43 and 2.84 times body weight in the posterior talocalcaneal facet and a composite anterior talocalcaneal and talonavicular facet. Obviously, since the same muscles are responsible for the control of both the ankle and the subtalar joints, the previously reported calculated values for muscle tension result from the equilibrium requirements for both joints.

Computer models have been developed to permit the estimation of the forces developed both within the individual elements of the arch structure and the soft tissues responsible for its preservation. Simkin (1982) reported that for a 500 newton load applied to the ankle tensile forces of 360 newtons and 100 newtons respectively were experienced by the plantar aponeurosis and the long plantar ligament, and compressive forces of 170 newtons and 150 newtons are generated at the first and third tarsometatarsal joints respectively.

A wealth of experimental data is available relating to magnitude and distribution of the loading on the plantar aspect of the foot which results from the various structural mechanisms described. For example, force plate data have been employed to plot the locus of the centre of pressure of the ground reaction force (Fig. 16). This form of plot illustrates how the centre of pressure is located initially on the heel, moves rapidly along the lateral aspect of the foot towards the metatarsal heads and finally shifts medially to lie between the first and second metatarsal heads during late stance.

Perhaps more clinically significant are the data regarding pressure distribution resulting from the many well established floor-mounted pressure measurement devices and the more recently available in-shoe devices (Duckworth et al 1982, Lord et al 1986). Typical maximum pressures on the sole of a normal foot during level walking of 0.3 megapascal on the heel and metatarsal heads and 0.4 megapascal on the hallux have been measured using these techniques (Fig. 17).

Uneven or sloping surfaces

Virtually all the mechanisms described and the experimental data reported here relate to standing or level walking. In practice, the foot and ankle have to adapt to walking on surfaces of widely varying orientation. It seems reasonable to postulate that the ankle joint, with its transverse axis of rotation, provides an obvious means of accommodating uphill or downhill slopes and that the subtalar joint with its oblique axis of motion offers a means of accommodating side slopes to a limited degree.

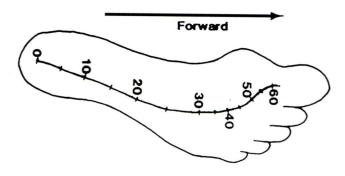

Figure 16

Centre of pressure motion over the sole of the foot during normal level walking (from Nicol and Paul 1988, with permission)

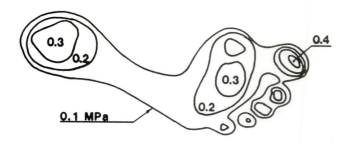

Figure 17

Maximum pressures experienced over the sole of a normal foot during normal level walking (from Nicol and Paul 1988, with permission)

The only published study of such situations (Wright et al 1964) does indeed illustrate the anticipated shifts in the ranges of motion of these joints under the circumstances described.

References

Anderson K J 1952 Recurrent anterior subluxation of the ankle joint. J Bone Joint Surg 34A: 853–860

Barnet C H, Napier J R 1952 The axis of rotation at the ankle joint in man. Its influence on the form of the talus and the mobility of the fibula. J Anat., 86: 1–9

Bresler B, Frankel J P 1948 Forces and moments in the leg during level walking. University of California, Berkeley. Prosthetic Devices Research Project, Series 11, Issue 12

Brewster R C, Chao E Y, Stauffer R N 1974 Force analysis of the ankle joint during the stance phase of gait. 27th ACEMB Alliance for Engineers, Philadelphia

Close J R 1956 Some applications of the functional anatomy of the ankle joint. J Bone Joint Surg 38A: 761–781

Close J R, Inman V T 1953 The action of the subtalar joint. University of California, Berkeley. Prosthetic Devices Research Project, Series 11, Issue 24

Close J R, Inman V T, Poor P M, Todd F N 1967 Function of the subtalar joint. Clin Orthop 50: 159–179

Duckworth T, Betts R P, Frank C I 1982 The measurement of pressure under the foot. Foot Ankle 3: 130–141

Elftman H 1960 The transverse tarsal joint and its control. Clin Orthop 15: 41–46

Hicks J T 1953 The mechanics of the foot. I. The joints. J Anat 87: 345–357

Hicks J T 1954 The mechanics of the foot. II. The plantar aponeurosis and the arch. J Anat 88: 25–30

Hicks J T 1955 The mechanics of the foot. III. The foot as a support. Acta Anat 25: 34–45

Hicks J T 1956 The mechanics of the foot. IV. Action of muscles of the foot in standing. Acta Anat 27: 180–192

Isman R E, Inman V T 1969 Anthropometric studies of the human foot and ankle. Bull Prosthet Res 10–11: 97–129

Johnson E E, Markolf K L 1983 The contribution of the anterior talofibular ligament to ankle laxity. J Bone Joint Surg 65A: 81–88

Leonard M H 1949 Injuries of the lateral ligaments of the ankle. J Bone Joint Surg 31A: 373–377

Levins A S, Inman V T, Blossmer J A 1948 Transverse rotations of the segments of the lower extremity in walking. J Bone Joint Surg 30A: 859–872

Lord M, Reynolds D P, Hughes J K 1986 Foot pressure measurement: a review of clinical findings. J Biomed Eng 8: 283–294

Mann R A, Inman V T 1964 Phasic activity of intrinsic muscles of the foot. J Bone Joint Surg 46A: 469–481

Manter J T 1941 Movements of the subtalar and transverse tarsal joints. Anat Rec 80: 397–410

Nicol A C, Paul J P 1988 Biomechanics. In Helal B, Wilson D (eds) The Foot. Churchill Livingstone, London. pp. 75–86

Piezer C, Wright D W 1970 Human locomotion. In: Murdoch G (ed) Prosthetic and Orthotic Practice. Edward Arnold, London

Proctor P, Paul J P 1982 Ankle joint biomechanics. J Biomech 15: 627–634

Rasmussen O, Kromann-Andersen C 1983 Experimental ankle injuries. Analysis of the traumatology of the ankle ligaments. Acta Orthop Scand 54: 356–362

Rasmussen O, Kromann-Andersen C, Boe S 1982 Deltoid ligament. Functional analysis of the medial collateral ligamentous apparatus of the ankle joint. Acta Orthop Scand 54: 36–44

Rasmussen O, Tovborg-Jensen I 1982 Mobility of the ankle joint. Recording of rotary movements in the talo-crural joint in vitro with and without the lateral collateral ligaments of the ankle. Acta Orthop Scand 53: 155–160

Rasmussen O, Tovborg-Jensen I, Hedeboc J 1983 An analysis of the function of the posterior talofibular ligament. Intern Orthop 7: 41–48

Sammarco C J, Burstein A H, Frankel V H 1973 Biomechanics of the ankle: a kinematic study. Orthop Clin North Am 4: 75–96

Simkin A 1982 Structural analysis of the human foot in standing posture. PhD Thesis, University of Tel Aviv

Stauffer R N, Chao E Y, Brewster R C 1977 Force and motion analysis of the normal, diseased and prosthetic ankle joint. Clin Orthop 127: 189–196

Steindler A 1935 Mechanics of normal and pathological locomotion in man. Chas C Thomas, Springfield, Illinois

University of California, Berkeley 1953 The pattern of muscular activity in the lower extremity during walking. Prosthetic Devices Research Project, Series 11, Issue 25

Wright D G, Desai S M, Henderson L W H 1964 Action of the subtalar and ankle joint complex during the stance phase of walking. J Bone Joint Surg 46A: 361–382

II.1 History and Examination

David L Grace

History

The treatment of a foot disorder cannot proceed until an accurate diagnosis is made. The diagnosis depends on properly conducted history taking and clinical examination, aided where necessary by subsequent special investigations. Good history taking requires experience, patience, and good communication skills. It relies on the brief rapport that is established between the patient and doctor. The history should focus predominantly on the foot problem, but the patient's general health may require further enquiry, as may other general factors such as occupation, hobbies and sport.

Pain

This is usually the chief presenting symptom and can be considered in detail under a number of headings:

Duration

How long the patient has suffered pain is clearly important, and it is surprising how often this information is omitted from the case notes. The pain can be acute or chronic; intermittent or constant; it can be related to particular activities or it may be present at rest.

Mode of onset

This can be sudden, such as a traumatic incident, or gradual.

Rate of progression

Has this been a gradual deterioration, or has the pain been static for a period of time followed by more rapid deterioration? It is often the latter which prompts patients to seek medical attention. Are symptoms episodic? If so, what is the typical duration of a period of pain and the average interval of freedom from pain?

Severity

This is notoriously difficult to evaluate since pain is so subjective and may be greatly dependent upon emotional factors. Visual analogue scales may be helpful. This can be assessed verbally by asking patients to grade their own pain on a scale of 1 to 10, where 1 would be very mild discomfort, 5 would be moderate to severe pain and 10 would be excruciating. Perhaps a more objective way of assessing pain severity is to ask the patient to describe what limitations have been imposed upon his or her physical activities as a result of the pain. Clearly, for example, a patient who voluntarily persists in jogging 5 miles a day is unlikely to be experiencing severe pain. The severity of the pain may determine what type of treatment to offer.

Location

The location of the pain is vital to diagnosis. Patience is required to extract full details of the site or sites of pain in the foot and ankle by getting the patient to map out with the finger exactly where the pain is felt. This might mean asking if pain is present in a certain area and seeking the patient's agreement or denial. Specific questions may have to be formulated for patients who have difficulty in accurately localizing the pain. Perseverance is sometimes necessary, particularly with garrulous or anxious patients. This is particularly so in patients who have had previous failed foot surgery.

When patients describe where they feel pain, they may do so with a sweeping gesture, perhaps with the palm of the hand, which gives a very poor indication of where the pain is actually felt in a relatively small structure like the foot. Asking the patient to indicate with the finger tip is often rewarded by the designation of a much smaller area. Well-localized pain on one or other side of a nail fold, for example, greatly simplifies the diagnosis. Conversely, widespread pain requires more careful analysis, and generalized foot pain occurs in conditions such as reflex sympathetic dystrophy, in some systemic conditions and in dysvascular feet. In patients who have pain in several areas that seem to overlap, it may be helpful to divide the foot up into broad zones by placing a hand across the mid foot and asking, 'Do you feel the pain more towards the toes, or more towards the ankle?' (Fig. 1). Subsequent questioning may further narrow down the exact sites of pain. Similarly, with forefoot pain

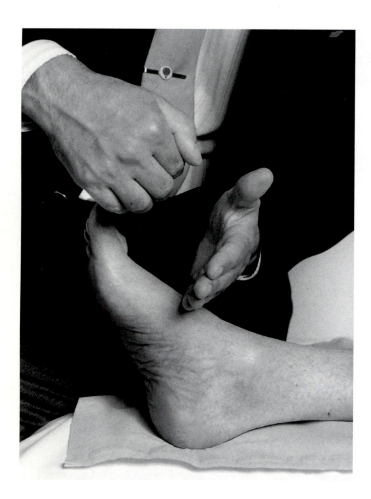

Figure 1

'Which side of this line do you feel most pain?' For vague historians with diffuse or poorly localized pain, division of the foot into 'front' and 'back' may help to assign the pain into broad regions

that is poorly localized, it may be helpful to enquire specifically if pain is felt chiefly in the big toe, or alternatively in the remaining toes. In this respect, it is most important to determine whether first ray pain is more or less severe than lateral metatarsal pain, particularly if surgery to the first ray is being considered.

If symptoms are bilateral, it is important to know whether both feet are as bad as each other, or whether one is considerably worse. A useful question to ask is, 'Would you be seeking treatment today if both of your feet were only as painful as the least painful foot?'

Radiation

Pain confined to a single area without radiation suggests a local pathology such as medial prominence pain in hallux valgus or dorsal first metatarsophalangeal joint (MTPJ) pain in hallux rigidus. Pain due to corns or callosities is highly localized without radiation, but pain from neural structures may radiate proximally or distally in the limb.

Nature and character

Neurogenic pain is suggested by sharp shooting pain or 'electric shocks', 'pins and needles' or numbness. Pain may be throbbing and worse with dependency, suggesting infection or abscess formation.

Timescale

Pain first thing in the morning may suggest an inflammatory aetiology such as ankylosing spondylitis or rheumatoid arthritis. Plantar fasciitis pain is often felt immediately on waking at the start of the day, and may then ease after a few minutes.

Precipitating causes

Specific activities or footwear may provoke some conditions, such as an interdigital neuroma. Pain in osteoarthritis and stress fractures are generally activity related.

Relieving factors

Relief by removing footwear suggests pain due to rubbing or shear forces on a bony prominence, or an interdigital neuroma. Other relieving factors include local measures such as massage or rubbing the foot, warming the foot, or resting the foot with elevation after a period of exercise.

It should not be forgotten that foot pain may be due to more proximal pathology, such as neural irritation from a diseased spine or ischaemia due to arterial occlusion. In these cases, walking provokes pain, reaching a crescendo after a specific period of time or distance and forcing the patient to stop and rest.

Appearance

Patients often seek treatment for deformity. In some instances the cosmetic appearance of the foot may be equally as important, or more important, to them than pain or function. Patients with hallux valgus may be self-conscious about their appearance when walking barefoot or in sandals.

Many patients worry about future deterioration. Is the deformity becoming worse with time? How quickly did it appear? How rapidly is it progressing? Sudden onset of pain followed by a rapidly progressing flat foot in a middle-aged or elderly person suggests tibialis posterior tendon pathology.

Swelling

Patients may present because of a lump in the foot such as a ganglion or plantar fibromatosis. Both of these are generally easy to diagnose. Some swellings may be inter-mittent, such as a ganglion, which may burst and later reappear. Clearly, a steadily enlarging swelling in an unusual location or of an uncertain nature should raise suspicion of a tumour. Soft tissue swelling due to fluid retention may cause generalized oedema of the ankle and foot, especially following injuries and in systemic conditions such as cardiac failure.

Instability

The patient's chief complaint may be of recurrent giving-way of the foot or ankle, such as that commonly experienced with torn lateral ankle ligaments. There may be clicking or snapping, as for example, when the peroneal tendons are unstable. Patients may complain of a grating or crunching sensation in an osteoarthritic joint.

Functional impairment

In this respect it may be necessary to obtain a detailed occupational history to include hobbies and sports. Clearly a patient is significantly disabled if he is genuinely unable to work because of a foot problem. Other disabilities due to generalized disease or other affected joints in the leg require consideration. For example, rheumatoid arthritics with multiple joint involvement in the lower limbs may have considerable functional impairment. The hip and knee may contribute to this more than the foot. This is of great importance when determining priorities and sequence of treatment.

Walking distance

This may be restricted by pain, weakness, or both. It may also be adversely affected by co-existent lower limb disorders. Patients may find it difficult to express how far they can comfortably walk in terms of distance, and may find it helpful to describe their limits in terms of 'blocks' rather than in yards or metres. It is surprising how often patients say things like, 'I can only just reach the shops at the bottom of the avenue', when the questioner is totally ignorant of the geography of the location being described. Patients may also find it easier to describe their walking distance in terms of time, e.g. 5 or 10 minutes before having to stop and rest. Again, recent or gradual deterioration in walking distance may need to be ascertained.

Footwear

This may give the clinician a clue to the cause of some foot problems, such as the typical forefoot deformities of bunion and hammer toes caused by prolonged wearing of ill-fitting shoes. Furthermore, information about footwear may give an indication about the severity of pain. If severe, a woman may find herself having to wear unfashionable styles. Many secretaries are in the habit of kicking off their high-heeled shoes under the desk at work because their feet are uncomfortable. Patients with severe systemic disorders such as diabetes or rheumatoid arthritis may have been forced into wearing slippers for much of the time or have already been advised to wear custom or surgical shoes because of their disease. Patients may complain of their feet distorting newly purchased footwear; this is especially likely if they have large bunions. Ignorance about where to purchase more sensible styles of shoe locally may need to be remedied.

General health status

This requires thorough enquiry, since many systemic diseases may be reflected in the foot and are sometimes the sole cause of the foot disorder. Vascular disorders or back pain may well give a clue to the underlying cause of foot pain.

Family history

A positive family history is common in patients with hallux valgus, and may suggest that the deformity is more likely to progress. Some of the neuromuscular disorders and pes cavus may also be transmitted.

Previous injury

It is important not to overlook this as a possible aetiological factor. Injury may not have been due to a single sudden incident but may be due to repetitive strains such as dance, running or other sporting activity, or may be occupationally related. Is the patient seeking compensation following an injury?

General factors

It may still not be entirely clear at this stage exactly why the patient has sought medical attention. Has this been self-motivated, or was the referral suggested by the family doctor, a physiotherapist, podiatrist, chiropodist, the spouse, a friend, neighbour or shoe shop assistant? Occasionally the question, 'Why have you come to see me today?' is met with the response, 'I went to see my doctor about something else and he suggested I came to see you about my deformed foot, even though it isn't hurting me!' In the case of children, consultation is often at the instigation of the grandmother, who has aroused concern in the child's parents.

Many patients consult a specialist because of worry or concern that the condition will deteriorate. They may want to know if future problems might be potentially preventable by early orthotic or surgical intervention, even if their feet are asymptomatic at the time.

The preceding description of history taking is exhaustive. In a busy clinic, expediency dictates that history taking generally proceeds rather like an algorhythm. Successive questions are determined to some extent by the patient's response to a previous question rather than following a predetermined sequence. Hence, a patient complaining of shooting pain in the third and fourth toes might prompt immediate enquiry into its character, timescale, radiation, and its relationship with footwear, since the clinician will suspect a Morton's interdigital neuroma. It would be unnecessary to extract a detailed history in a patient with a simple ingrowing toenail.

Previous surgery

If symptoms are present following previous surgery, the precise nature of the original symptoms and any immediate benefit after surgery, or any change in symptoms afterwards needs clarification. It is notable that patients with failed previous foot surgery often have more diffuse symptoms resulting from a mild or overt reflex sympathetic dystrophy. These feet can require very careful evaluation. The ability to assess a patient's aspirations, goals of treatment and expectations of surgery needs to be realized at the time of history taking.

Clinical examination

As in other parts of the body, the standard orthopaedic approach of LOOK, FEEL, MOVE is followed.

Look

The foot is inspected during walking, standing, and either lying down or sitting. As with history taking, much of this can reasonably be omitted if the diagnosis appears simple or obvious. The foot may require observation in the following ways:

1. Patient walking wearing a shoe and/or orthosis.
2. Patient walking without the shoe or orthosis.
3. Weight-bearing unshod foot observed from in front, the side and behind.
4. Foot standing on tip toe observed from behind.
5. Foot observed with patient sitting or lying (offloaded).

These will now be considered in turn.

Walking in shoe or orthosis

In the context of orthotic assessment for patients with more major foot problems such as congenital deformities and neurological and post-traumatic disorders, gait analysis by inspection should not be omitted. This should focus not only on the position of the foot during each phase of the gait cycle but also on hip and knee function. The need for walking aids such as crutches is noted. Abnormal patterns of shoe wear should become obvious at this stage, and any unusual loading pattern of the foot will later demand a closer inspection for signs of pressure or keratoses. Does the orthosis properly control foot position during the stance phase? Is the orthosis inappropriate? Is it broken or incorrectly applied? Does the orthosis facilitate easier walking compared with when it is not used?

Patient walking without a shoe or orthosis

Abnormal loading patterns can again be identified and instability with collapse of the forefoot, mid-foot or hindfoot during loading can be observed. Some gait patterns are characteristic, such as the high steppage gait and forefoot strike of a drop foot. Toe heel gait may be present in a patient with fixed equinus, because of cerebral palsy. An antalgic gait, with reduced duration of stance phase, confirms a patient's complaint of pain. Ankle or hindfoot collapse into varus or valgus during the stance phase may indicate severe joint destruction or motor weakness. Do the toes reach the ground during walking and do they have propulsive function?

While gait analysis can provide useful information, it has its limitations when done by simple observation only (Saleh & Murdoch 1985). The complex rotations in the leg, especially in the mid-foot and hindfoot during the various phases of gait, generally occur too quickly to be easily differentiated by the human eye. These can really be assessed only by slow motion video or cine camera or other laboratory methods. Similarly, the motions in the hip and knee cannot easily be related to those in the foot by simple observation. The ability to squat, and the ability to walk on tiptoe and on heels can give a good assessment of joint mobility and motor power.

Standing from in front

Mild muscle wasting may suggest disuse atrophy due to a painful condition. More severe wasting may be present following lower motor neurone lesions such as poliomyelitis, peripheral nerve injuries and hereditary neuropathies. Foot posture is observed and any obvious swellings or lumps are noted. Static deformities can be easily assessed by observing the standing foot from in front, especially forefoot deformities such as the common conditions of hallux valgus and hammer toes. The degree of correctability of hallux valgus can be assessed by trying to push the big toe straight when the foot is loaded (Fig. 2).

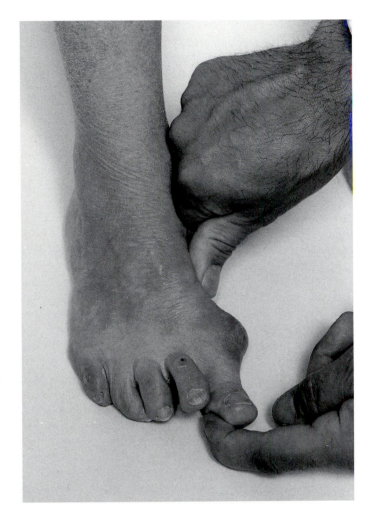

Figure 2

With the foot loaded, an attempt to passively straighten the hallux at the first metatarsophalangeal joint will indicate: (a) the ease of surgical correction, and hence which type of operation to perform; (b) whether or not the second hammer toe will have enough space to sit in if it alone is surgically straightened

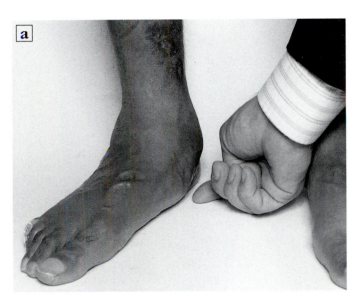

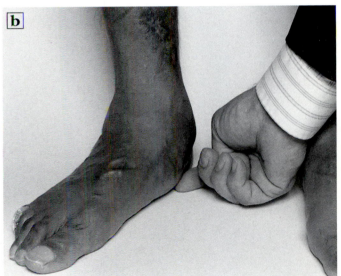

Figure 3

This rather flat-foot fails to accommodate the finger-tip under the head of the talus

Standing from the side

The height of the longitudinal arch is more easily observed when standing viewed from the side. Although extreme shapes, such as gross pes planus or pes cavus, are easily identified, lesser degrees of deformity are more difficult to quantify. A crude test of normality of the height of the medial arch is to see if the tip of a finger can comfortably be placed between the ground and the skin underlying the head of the talus (Fig. 3).

Standing from behind

Muscle wasting in the calf is easily assessed in standing viewed from behind. The margins of the Achilles tendon are usually very clearly defined but may be less distinct in pathologies affecting the tendon or where there is dependent oedema. The width, shape and position of the heel can be observed. A crude test is to imagine a line drawn along the lateral border of the Achilles tendon just above its insertion extended down along the lateral side of the heel, and comparing this with a line in the midline of the calf (Fig. 4). In normality, the angle between the two lines is usually around 10°. Marked variations from this can be readily spotted (Fig. 5a).

An abducted mid-foot will have a positive 'too many toes' sign. The examiner observes from close to the floor directly behind the patient, who is standing with both feet slightly apart and with symmetrical posture. The sign is positive if the examiner can see the third (or second) toe, beyond the heel. Typically, the sign is observed in patients who have a ruptured tibialis posterior tendon, or pes planus due to a variety of causes.

Standing on tiptoe

The patient is then asked to stand on tiptoe whilst the foot is still observed from behind. The patient should first stand on tiptoe on both feet and then one foot at a time, if that is possible. This is an important test, as the normal heel inverts and the medial longitudinal arch rises as the hindfoot supinates. At the same time the tibia externally rotates, owing to the torque convertor function of the subtalar joint. These movements can be observed. They are of particular importance in assessing pes planus in children, since heel inversion and raising of the arch confirms that the deformity is mobile and is therefore unlikely to be due to serious pathology. The same movements (i.e. arch rising and inversion of the heel) can also be tested during relaxed standing by passively dorsiflexing the big toe, thus tightening the plantar fascia by the windlass effect (Hicks 1954). If the subtalar joint is stiff, or if the posterior tibial tendon has stretched or ruptured, heel inversion will not take place. In this respect it is important to test unilateral tiptoe standing, since the patient may 'cheat' by using the normal side to gain elevation without actually loading the abnormal side or the patient may attempt to flex the knee. Comparison can thus be made with the normal side.

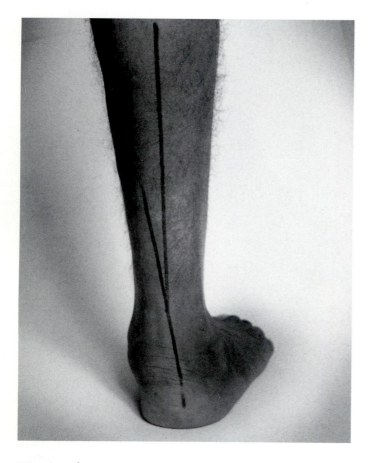

Figure 4

Assessment of heel position. This does not normally exceed 10° of valgus

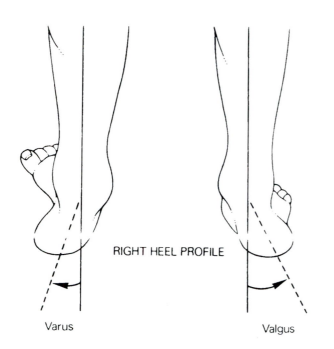

Figure 5a

Standing heel profile from behind (right foot)

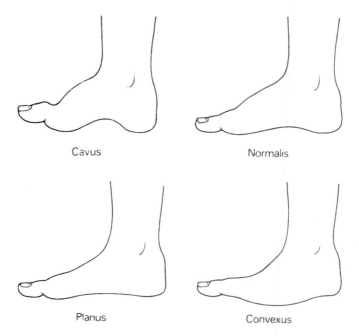

Figure 5b

Sole shapes

If a major hindfoot deformity such as varus or valgus is seen, it is important to determine whether it is fixed or mobile during weight bearing, because it may be suitable for orthotic treatment if it can be passively corrected.

By this stage it is possible to define the basic type of foot shape when viewed from the side (Fig. 5b). The basic foot shape when seen from above can easily be recorded by simply performing an outline drawing of the weight-bearing foot on a piece of paper. If necessary, an outline of the patient's shoe can be superimposed, thus demonstrating to the often surprised patient that the shoe is nowhere near wide enough for the foot; this is especially true of those that have severe metatarsal splaying.

Sitting or lying

The unloaded foot is then inspected, and it is easiest for the examiner to sit down in front of the patient with the foot in his lap. The following are specifically sought:

Colour Areas of pigmentation or depigmentation are sought, together with the state of the cutaneous vessels, including visible veins. The presence of pigmented naevi is noted. A dusky discoloration of the toes may suggest vascular impairment, and areas of black skin will signify necrosis or areas of gangrene following traumatic or vascular insults.

Swellings A closer inspection can now be made of any obvious lumps or bumps that may present in the skin or subcutaneous tissues. Swelling around joints suggests synovitis, effusion or osteophytes. Dependent oedema is easily apparent at this stage of the examination.

Deformity Major foot deformities have already been ascertained in the loaded foot.

Skin This is observed for dryness, skin rashes, scars, localized callosities, corns and hyperkeratotic lesions. These indicate overload or shear forces, and correlate with the patient's pain localization. Sinuses and ulcers may be apparent and are obviously important in diabetics and those with impaired sensation. Dermatoglyphic pattern is identified.

Muscle wasting Small muscle wasting in the foot can be observed at this stage.

Shoes These are observed for abnormal signs of wear under the heel and sole. Collapse of the medial or lateral heel counter occurs respectively in valgus and varus deformities of the hindfoot. Distortion of the toebox may have occurred in patients with fixed severe hallux valgus or hammer toes. A variety of shoe modifications and orthoses may have been applied to the inside or outside of the shoe and these indicate the measures taken by the patient to seek comfort.

Feel

Tenderness

The foot is now systematically prodded with the examining finger to elicit tenderness over bony prominences such as those present in hallux valgus and the common toe deformities. Tenderness is sought along the course of tendons, nerves, ligaments and joint-lines. Point tenderness strongly suggests a very localized pathology and may be confined to a very small area of hyperkeratosis. This might be on the tip of the toe, over a proximal interphalangeal joint or under a metatarsal head or sesamoid bone. Localizing tenderness in this way is very important in some conditions, such as interdigital neuroma, where even the tip of a finger may be too blunt an instrument to define the precise area of maximum tenderness. In this situation, it is sometimes helpful to use the blunt end of a pencil or pen for this purpose.

In eliciting areas of tenderness, the examiner clearly needs to have a thorough knowledge of surface anatomy and of the bony and soft tissue structures below the skin. It might be important to distinguish, for example, tenderness over the anterior talofibular ligament from the calcaneofibular ligament or the subjacent peroneal tendons. It is relatively easy to localize tenderness along a large tendon such as the Achilles tendon, but more difficult with smaller or deeper seated ones such as the tibialis posterior tendon.

Swellings

These should be felt at this stage. The nodules of plantar fibromatosis are easily palpable within the plantar fascia. Synovial swellings, ganglia and other cysts are also easy to feel and should be transilluminated in a darkened room to distinguish them from solid swellings if doubt exists. As with swellings anywhere in the body, a note is made of the dimensions, the surface characteristics, the consistency, the transilluminability, the degree of tenderness, and the degree of tethering both to the skin and to deeper tissues.

Skin

The skin is felt to determine its dryness, mobility, elasticity and texture. Temperature may be reduced in an ischaemic foot or raised in reflex sympathetic dystrophy, inflammation or infections. Skin can be thin and shiny, or like tissue paper in atrophic conditions or in rheumatoid disease. Scars are palpated for tenderness and tethering and can be percussed to indicate painful cutaneous neuromas and Tinel signs.

Vascular status

Dorsalis pedis and posterior tibial pulses are felt and skin temperature, capillary refilling and atrophic changes, such as dryness of skin and loss of hair, are sought. Impaired nutrition due to poor vascular supply, either generally or locally in the foot, will result in trophic changes.

Neurological status

Motor power is tested in patients who may have neuro-muscular disorders by palpating the muscle bellies in the leg and foot during resisted contraction. Power is graded conventionally on a scale of 0 to 5 (Medical Research Council 1943). Ankle reflexes and Babinski responses are tested if a more proximal neurological problem is suspected. Sensation is tested along the usual lines with either light touch or pinprick sensation and vibration sensation. Areas of hypo- or hyperaesthesia can be outlined. Sometimes quite specific individual nerve terri-tories can be identified as abnormal, such as the web space and toe numbness in interdigital neuroma and in severe tarsal tunnel and anterior tibial nerve compres-sion syndromes.

Move

The range of motion is checked both actively and passively in the ankle, subtalar joint complex, mid-foot and forefoot including the hallux and lesser toes. They are tested systematically and can be compared to an expected normal range on the opposite side or to a perceived normal range in the general population. Excessive joint movement (joint laxity or instability) or reduced or absent motion (ankylosis or arthrodesis) can be determined. Pain or crepitus on movements are noted, as these are often present in osteoarthritic joints. Abnormal movements or clicks may occur with peroneal tendon subluxation.

Fig. 6 shows how the passive range of motion in the ankle is tested. The clinical measurement of ankle motion is somewhat unreliable (Backer & Kofoed 1989), and is certainly not as accurate as a lateral radiograph taken at both extremes of position. Nonetheless most normal feet have an average ankle dorsiflexion of around 20° and plantar flexion of 40°. An increase in the range of dorsiflexion when the knee is flexed suggests gastroc-nemius rather than soleus tightness in patients with cerebral palsy.

Assessment of subtalar joint movement is even more difficult, since this occurs about an axis that is oblique to the three main planes of movement. Hence the arc of motion must be assessed three dimensionally, allow-ing the foot to dorsiflex, abduct and evert in one direc-tion and to plantarflex, adduct and invert in the other. Most feet will have an average eversion of 20° and inver-sion of 40°, but there is quite a wide variation amongst normal individuals, especially in those who have gener-alized joint laxity. Accurate measurement of these angles

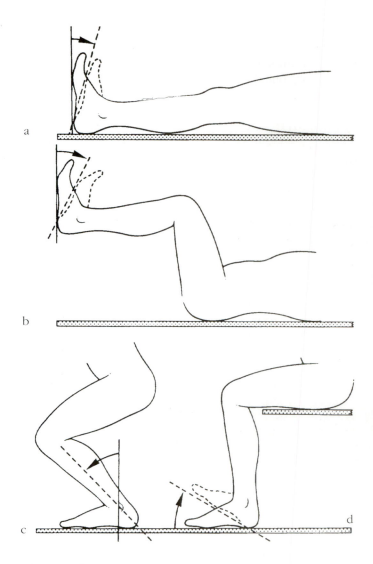

Figure 6

Foot dorsiflexion: (a) lying, with knee extended; (b) lying, with knee flexed, the range increases; (c) weight bearing, as in climbing stairs, the range increases to the maximum; (d) sitting, an intermediate range similar to (b). It is easiest to measure the plane of the sole relative to its neutral position at 90° to the leg

and the estimation of the neutral position can be diffi-cult, and the most accurate way is to examine the patient prone with the knee flexed, with a goniometer applied to the heel in the coronal plane, as shown in Fig. 7. Inevitably when performing this measurement, true subtalar movements will be slightly overestimated because a little ankle motion will come into play. Conversely, if the ankle joint is fixed and subtalar motion is tested with the ankle held rigidly at 90°, true subtalar movements will be under-recorded. The anterior drawer test at the ankle is performed if instability due to torn lateral ligaments is suspected. The amount of forward displacement of the ankle mortice is visually estimated, and can be confirmed by stress radiography (Grace 1984).

A small amount of gliding motion occurs at the mid-tarsal joints but this is not measurable clinically. If the mid-foot is held firm, some idea of the mobility in the tarsometatarsal joints can be ascertained, but this is difficult to quantify.

The hallux is tested for motion both at the metatarsophalangeal joint and at the interphalangeal joint. The foot should be at 90° to the leg, and dorsi- and plantarflexion of the metatarsophalangeal joint should be measured by referring the line of the proximal phalanx to the sole of the foot rather than to the first metatarsal. Average passive dorsiflexion of this joint is 70°; plantarflexion is somewhat less. Excessive dorsiflexion is a good sign of generalized joint laxity whereas reduced motion is expected in a patient with hallux rigidus. Motion at the interphalangeal joint of the hallux is measured by recording the angle between the proximal and distal phalanges. In most people there is very little dorsiflexion, although passive plantarflexion can be 90° or more. Fixed hyperextension deformity can be present if there is osteoarthritis at the first metatarsophalangeal joint. It is rarely necessary to measure joint motion in the lesser toes. However, motion of these joints may produce pain if they are swollen. Also, it may be important to stress the base of the proximal phalanx to test for instability, especially in the second toe. Table 1 outlines the average passive range of movements in the second toe.

Certain pathologies may demand specific manoeuvres; an example of this is transverse forefoot compression producing a Mulder's click in the appropriate web space in feet with interdigital neuroma. This is especially significant if it provokes the characteristic pain. The extent of passive correctability of a hallux valgus deformity can be tested by attempting to straighten the toe, and the concertina test demonstrates how stiff the deformity is and how easy or difficult surgery is likely to be. This may even determine the type of operation selected. In the former test, the examiner attempts to align the hallux with its metatarsal shaft with the patient standing. If it is possible to get them parallel, or even over-corrected to a varus position, the joint is lax and should correct easily at surgery. In a stiff, fixed deformity, the toe will remain in a valgus position however hard it is pushed (see Fig. 2). In the latter test, the weight-bearing hallux is pushed towards the ankle in line with the second metatarsal shaft in order to simulate the forces acting on the first ray during the 'toe-off' phase of gait. With increasing hallux valgus angles, the first metatarsophalangeal joint buckles medially, with shortening and collapse of the first ray due to incompetence and stretching of the medial capsule.

A suspected Achilles tendon rupture will demand a close inspection for signs of a gap in the tendon and the 'squeeze test' may demonstrate discontinuity in it (Thompson & Doherty 1962). Another useful sign of

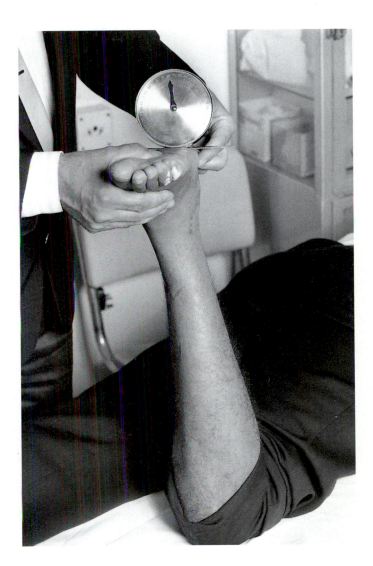

Figure 7

Using a gravity goniometer to accurately measure movements in the subtalar complex

Table 1 Average passive range of movements in the 2nd toe (degrees)

	MTPJ	PIPJ	DIPJ
Dorsiflexion	90	0	10
Plantarflexion	70	80	40

Achilles tendon rupture is to observe the position of both feet from the side with the patient lying prone, relaxed, and with the feet hanging over the end of the couch. On the side of the rupture, the foot drops straight down vertically, whereas on the normal side, the tension within the calf muscles causes the ankle to lie in some equinus.

General examination

Finally, the hips, knees, spine, upper limb and the central nervous system may demand attention, since some conditions affecting the foot may show up elsewhere in the body, e.g. nystagmus in cases of Freidreich's ataxia or small muscle wasting in the hands in hereditary sensorimotor neuropathies. Any neuromuscular disorder will warrant a thorough examination of the lower limb. Proximal muscle power and signs of muscle wasting, fasciculation or spasticity are sought. Vibration sense, proprioception and heel-shin coordination are tested. Straight leg raising should be checked and if this is limited it may suggest a prolapsed intervertebral disc. Inspection of the lower back may reveal cutaneous abnormalities in patients with spina bifida occulta or spinal dysraphism, which again might be the cause of a foot abnormality. Systemic diseases such as diabetes and rheumatoid arthritis may be manifest elsewhere.

References

Backer M, Kofoed H 1989 Passive ankle mobility. Clinical measurement compared with radiography. J Bone Joint Surg 71B: 696–698

Grace D 1984 Lateral ankle ligament injuries. Clin Orthop 183: 153–159

Hicks J 1954 The mechanics of the foot II. The plantar aponeurosis. J Anat 88: 25–30

Medical Research Council 1943 Aids to the investigation of peripheral nerve injuries Revised 2nd Edition. London

Saleh M, Murdoch G 1985 Defence of gait analysis. J Bone Joint Surg 67B: 237–241

Thompson T, Doherty J 1962 Spontaneous rupture of tendo Achilles: a new clinical diagnosis test. J Trauma 2: 126–129

III INVESTIGATIONS

III.1 Radiology

N Ann Barrington

Modalities available

Plain film

The standard plain film anteroposterior (AP) or dorsi-planar (DP) and oblique views of the foot may be supplemented by AP and lateral weight-bearing views which are a more physiological representation of the relationship of the bones of the foot and ankle. Various measurements can be made from these films (Meschan 1970). Steel et al (1980) have drawn up charts of normal measurements.

The anatomy of the hind foot and ankle is best demonstrated on the lateral view (Fig. 1). The calcaneal pitch or angulation is an indicator of the height of the bony framework of the foot. The range given by Steel et al is 11–30°. An angle of 11° or below indicates a low framework, as in pes planus. An angle over 30° indicates abnormally high pitch.

An important angle described by Boehler lies at the bisection of two lines drawn along the superior aspect of the calcaneum: one on the posterosuperior aspect and one extending back from the superior aspect of the anterior part of the calcaneum to the uppermost mid point. The range of normal for the angle is 28–48°. The angle is usually decreased in fractures of the calcaneal body and may be the only obvious sign of trauma on the lateral film.

The midtalar and midcalcaneal lines bisect to form an angle of 25–50° near the anterior margin of the cuboid (Templeton et al 1965). This angle is reduced in club foot and rocker bottom deformity, and increased in flat foot and pes cavus.

An angle formed by the intersection of a line drawn along the inferior margin of the fifth metatarsal and a line drawn along the inferior margin of the calcaneum ranges from 150 to 175° (Templeton et al 1965). The angle is increased in pes planus and rocker bottom deformity.

The talocalcaneal angle on the dorsiplanar weight-bearing view ranges from 30 to 50° in infants and young children but in children over five the angle is less in the range of 15–30° (Templeton et al 1965). A line drawn through the axis of the calcaneum should point to the

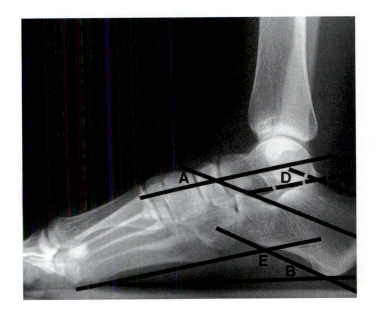

Figure 1

Normal measurements: weight-bearing lateral radiograph. Angle A: lateral talocalcaneal angle (midtalar and midcalcaneal lines); angle B: calcaneal angle of inclination; angle D: Boehler's angle; angle E: fifth-metatarsocalcaneal angle (Templeton)

fourth metatarsal, and a line through the axis of the talus should point to the head of the first metatarsal (Fig. 2). With varus deformity of the heel, the talocalcaneal angle is usually decreased and in valgus heel deformity it is increased. Heel valgus or varus cannot be determined directly in weight-bearing lateral or dorsiplanar views.

Samuelson et al (1981) described a radiographic technique to evaluate and document hindfoot position but this is now more easily evaluated with CT, although this lacks the advantage of weight-bearing. An AP standing view of the ankle may show subluxation at the talonavicular joint not suspected on non-weight-bearing views as a cause of hindfoot valgus. Ono & Hayashi (1974) have described a tomographic method of measuring heel valgus or varus.

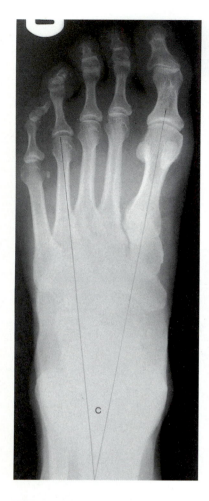

Figure 2

Normal measurements: weight-bearing anteroposterior
radiograph: dorsiplanar view (weight-bearing) showing
talocalcaneal angle (angle C)

The accuracy of measurements in two dimensions
made on three-dimensional structures has been disputed
(Perry et al 1992) and from experience reproducibility of
some of these measurements is in question. However,
some method of comparative measurement is useful,
although many orthopaedic surgeons and radiologists,
having a good knowledge of the normal appearances,
will be satisfied with a subjective impression.

Besides plain film evaluation, there are now many
other techniques available for further radiological assessment of the foot and ankle. Ultrasound, computed
tomographic scanning (CT), isotope bone scanning,
arthrography and magnetic resonance imaging (MRI) can
all be used to investigate specific problems.

MRI, with its multiplanar imaging potential has revolutionized musculoskeletal imaging and is unprecedented
for visualization of soft tissue and bone marrow. Since
it is expensive and availability is limited, it should be
used appropriately and not automatically as a first-line
investigation. Older, established techniques such as
screening and tomography still play an important role
and are too often omitted. Stress and standing views are
of particular importance in assessing integrity of
ligaments and tendons around the foot and ankle. The
relationships of the bones in congenital or acquired
deformity may change considerably on weight-bearing.

Computed tomography

In CT imaging, unlike in conventional radiography and
tomography, the information is processed by a computer
which allows manipulation of the display to visualize
bone and soft tissue (Andre & Resnick 1988). The information can be reformatted into simulated three-dimensional images and other planes (Fishman et al 1987). CT
scanning is of particular value in imaging the small
curved bones of the mid and hindfoot (Heger & Wulff
1985). It is able to demonstrate the three parts of the
subtalar joint, the intertarsal joints and the ankle joint
without the overlapping of bones. It is more sensitive
than linear tomography but does not replace it; the two
techniques are complementary.

A standard CT examination of the foot and ankle
consists of high resolution 4-mm section images in
coronal and axial planes. The coronal plane is the best
to show the tibiotalar and subtalar regions and the axial
plane for the talonavicular, calcaneocuboid and
tarsometatarsal joints. Seltzer et al (1984) described a
range of important normal measurements which can be
made in the hindfoot on coronal CT. They found remarkable symmetry between the two feet in normal volun-
teers. In the posterior part of the subtalar joint the 'heel
valgus angle' can be measured between the long axes
of the tibia and the calcaneum and was found to
measure 5.2° ± 1.6° (Fig. 3). The sustentacular angle
measures the angle of elevation of the sustentaculum tali
from the horizontal plane. This measures about 18.3° ±
1.3° (Fig. 4). Ono & Hayashi (1974) describe a similar
angle but this uses the horizontal of the ankle mortice
for reference; the measurement can be made from simple
anteroposterior tomographic cuts.

In the anterior part of the subtalar joint the medial
displacement of the talar head with respect to the calcaneum – the talar offset angle – was 5.2° ± 1.8° (Seltzer
et al 1984). The plantar talocalcaneal angle can be
measured accurately on the axial or plantar views and
should measure 20.1° ± 2.1°. Evaluation of the forefoot
is easier with plain films than with CT.

Radionuclide scanning

Radionuclide scanning or scintigraphy is a sensitive method
of detecting abnormality at a cellular level (Alazraki 1988).

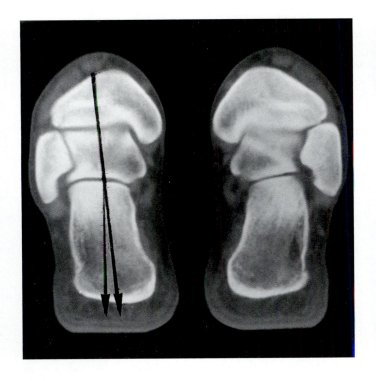

Figure 3

Normal heel valgus angle: coronal CT scan through ankle and subtalar joints

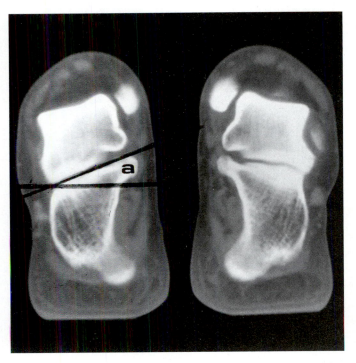

Figure 4

Normal sustentacular angle: coronal CT scan anterior to Fig. 3

99m Technetium diphosphonate (99mTcMDP) provides a unique physiological method of imaging bone and joint disease. It is thought that the 99mTcMDP is adsorbed onto normal bone, especially at sites of osteoblastic activity reflecting bone metabolism and skeletal vascularity (Siegal et al 1976). Any process disturbing the normal balance of bone production and resorption can produce an abnormality on a bone scan. Infection, inflammation, tumour and occult fractures can all be detected before there would be any plain film changes.

Radionuclide bone scanning is used to screen for bone metastases but in the peripheral skeleton, including the foot, its main use is to investigate bone pain (Williams et al 1991). Poor spatial resolution and specificity are the limitations of the technique. A normal scan virtually rules out any underlying bone lesion. An abnormal one will locate the site of pathology for further imaging. Ideally, a three-phase scan provides most information about the lesion, since it assesses vascularity. This is usually reserved for suspected inflammatory and infective lesions since it doubles the gamma camera time. Immediate and blood pool images at 5–10 minutes are followed by the routine images at 3–4 hours which are acquired in several projections (Fig. 5) depending on any abnormal findings and the clinical indications.

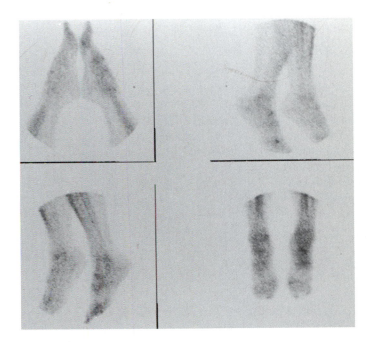

Figure 5

Normal 99mTcMDP scan (bone phase): this patient was asymptomatic. Slight patchy distribution of isotope can be expected, owing to the high sensitivity of this technique

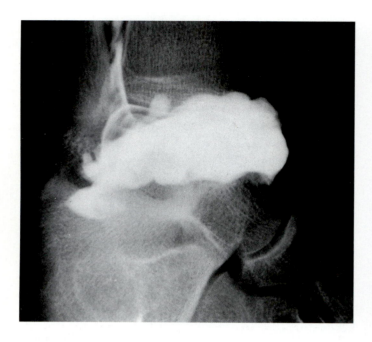

Figure 6

Normal ankle arthrogram: AP oblique view. Slight extension
of contrast between the tibia and fibula is normal

In the event of an equivocal or non-diagnostic
99mTcMDP scan and if chronic or recurrent infection is
suspected, leucocytes labelled with gallium 67, indium
III or 99mTc may also be employed.

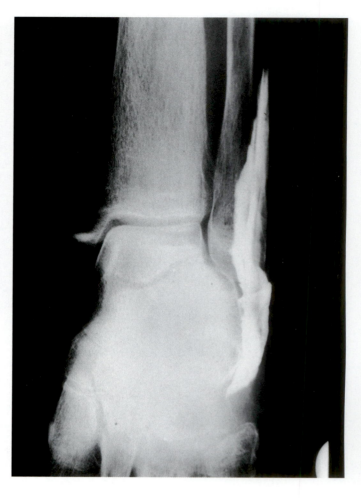

Figure 7

Normal ankle tenogram: contrast injected into the common
peroneal sheath does not communicate with the ankle joint

Contrast studies

The use of contrast in the investigation of the foot and
ankle is limited. Ankle arthrography (Fig. 6) or peroneal
tenography (Fig. 7) can be used in the diagnosis of
ligamentous tears by introducing contrast directly into
either the ankle joint or the common peroneal tendon
sheath (Resnick 1988). In chronic infection contrast can
be introduced into a skin sinus via a small catheter to
define communication with underlying bone and to
delineate sequestra in order to facilitate surgical removal.

main structures, including muscles, tendons, fascia, cartilage, fat and fluids.

Ultrasonography can be used to differentiate between
solid and cystic lesions and to detect joint effusion or
soft tissue fluid collections. It can assess tissue characteristics of tendons and ligaments (Fornage & Rifkin
1988) and help to detect non-opaque foreign bodies in
the sole of the foot (Kaplan et al 1989).

Diagnostic ultrasound

In experienced hands, diagnostic ultrasound is successfully used to solve soft tissue skeletal problems and is
of particular value when MRI is not available. Some
experienced users such as Thermann et al (1992) demonstrate the great potential of ultrasound in understanding
foot and ankle disorders and have studied the
sonographic patterns of the pathological changes of the

Magnetic resonance imaging

This is now a well-established technique for imaging the
skeletal system (Murphy 1988). With recent technical
refinements, the image quality has improved and peripheral joints such as the foot and ankle can be well visualized (Schweitzer & Resnick 1992). Its multiplanar
imaging potential enables muscles, tendons, ligaments
and bone marrow all to be demonstrated without using

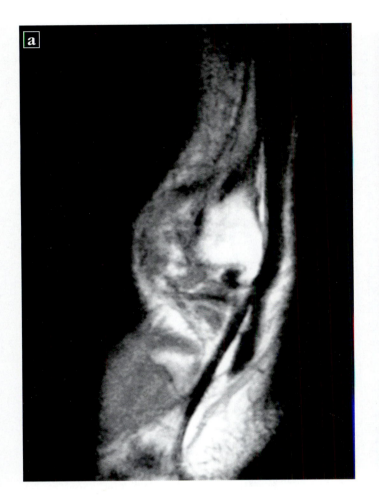

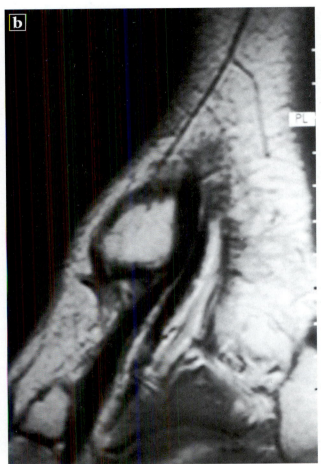

Figure 8

Normal ankle tendons: sagittal MRI (SE T1-weighted). (a) Lateral tendons. Peroneal brevis lies closest to the lateral malleolus; peroneal longus lies behind, diverges and disappears under calcaneum. (b) Medial tendons. Tibialis posterior lies behind the medial malleolus and behind this is the tendon of flexor hallucis longus

ionizing radiation. Calcification and bone does not produce a signal and MRI is therefore unreliable in defining small loose bodies or areas of calcification.

To demonstrate small structures such as tendons and ligaments thin contiguous slices of 3 mm are essential (Fig. 8) to detect subtle abnormality. For larger lesions 5 mm slices can be employed. The tissue contrast is controlled by choice of pulse sequence. The higher resolution of T1-weighted sequences provides good anatomical detail. On this sequence subcutaneous fat and, consequently, bone marrow have the brightest signal. Hyaline cartilage is less bright; muscle, fluid, tendons and ligaments are, in that order, even less bright. The T2-weighted image resolution is not as good, but fluid has a high signal and is bright, thus highlighting most pathological processes. Subcutaneous fat and bone marrow are less bright, followed by tendons and ligaments which are less bright on this sequence also. As well as standard sequences additional ones are now available – for example, to shorten scanning time and to suppress the signal from fat.

Unlike with CT, images can be obtained directly in any plane. Axial, coronal and sagittal planes are the standard ones, but it is neither necessary nor practical to acquire both T1- and T2-weighted images in all three planes. Usually two series are obtained in two orthogonal planes. Further sequences can be reserved for difficult diagnostic cases.

It is important to be familiar with the normal MRI appearances before pathological processes can be appreciated (Ferkel et al 1991, Schweitzer & Resnick 1992, Heron 1993) (Fig. 9).

Ossification and normal variants

A knowledge of the accessory ossicles and normal variants in the foot is particularly important (Fig. 10). They have been well documented (Kohler & Zimmer

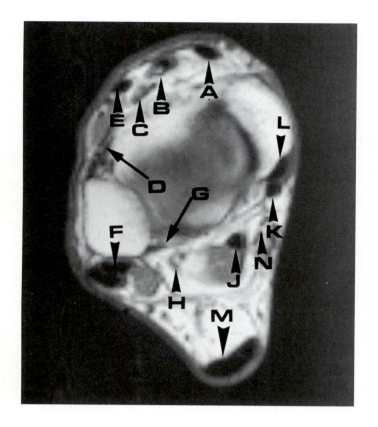

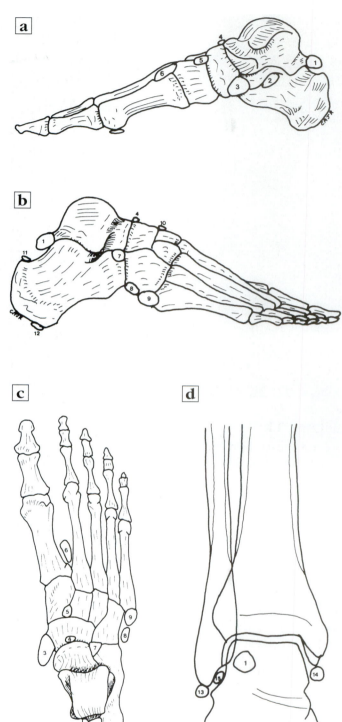

Figure 9

Normal MRI anatomy: T1-weighted SE axial section at level
of ankle joint. A, Tibialis anterior tendon; B, extensor
hallucis longus tendon; C, anterior tibial artery and vein and
sural nerve; D, anterior talo-fibular ligament; E, extensor
digitorum longus tendon; F, peroneus longus and brevis
tendons; G, posterior talo-fibular ligament; H, peroneal
artery; J, flexor hallucis longus tendon; K, flexor digitorum
longus tendon; L, tibialis posterior tendon; M, Achilles
tendon; N, posterior tibial artery, vein and nerve

1968, Lawson 1985, Keats 1988, Romanowski &
Barrington 1991, Silverman & Kuhn 1993) as being
anatomical and physiological curiosities but they often
give rise to symptoms or are misinterpreted as fractures.
Two important, potentially painful, normal variants in the
foot are the os trigonum and the os tibiale externum (see
pp. 76–7). See also Chapter V.5.

The bipartite epiphysis sometimes seen in the proximal phalanx of the hallux (Fig. 11), the extra apophysis
at the base of the fifth metatarsal and the accessory
ossicle in the region of the anterior process of the calcaneum (Fig. 12) can all be misdiagnosed as fractures. An
area of medullary trabecular thinning in the lateral aspect
of the calcaneum is a common incidental radiological
finding not uncommonly misdiagnosed as tumour or cyst
(Fig. 13).

Figure 10

The accessory ossicles of the foot. (a) Medial aspect. (b)
Lateral aspect. (c) Superior aspect. (d) AP view of the ankle.
1, Os trigonum; 2, os sustentaculi; 3, accessory navicular; 4,
os supranaviculare; 5, os intercuneiforme; 6, os
intermetatarseum; 7, os calcaneum secundarium; 8, os
peroneum; 9, os vesalianum; 10, os infranaviculare; 11, os
accessorium supracalcaneum; 12, os subcalcis; 13, os
subfibulare; 14, os subtibiale; 15, intercalary bone (from
Romanowski & Barrington 1991, with permission)

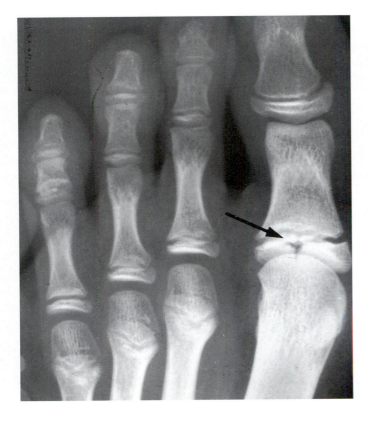

Figure 11

Normal variant: bifid epiphysis of proximal phalanx of hallux (arrow)

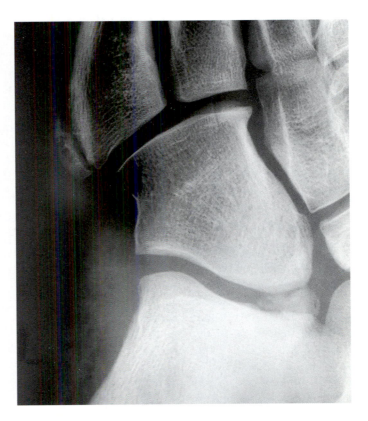

Figure 12

Normal variants: accessory ossification centres base of fifth metatarsal and in anterior process of calcaneum

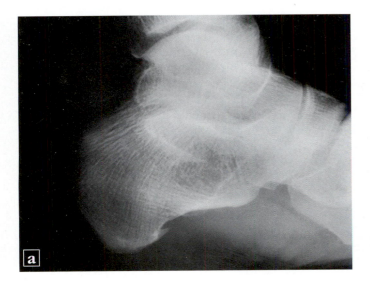

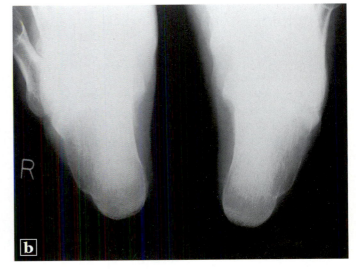

Figure 13

Normal variant: bilateral trabecular thinning in lateral aspect of calcaneal body. (a) Lateral radiograph. (b) Axial CT scan

Common deformities

Many congenital and acquired foot deformities can be diagnosed on plain radiographs.

Hallux valgus

Metatarsus primus varus with hallux valgus, whether idiopathic or acquired, is the commonest foot deformity (Piggot 1960). Corrective procedures can be planned on the plain films (Mitchell et al 1958, Carr & Boyd 1968, Karasick & Wapner 1990). Abduction of the hallux with an angle between the first metatarsal and great toe of 10–20° indicates mild hallux valgus, 20–30° moderate and between 30 and 45° severe. There may be associated subluxation at the first metatarsophalangeal joint. The angle between the first and second metatarsal is normally 9° or less (Mitchell et al 1958, Carr & Boyd 1968). Relative lateral displacement of the sesamoid bones, prominence of the metatarsal head medially with 'cratering' on its medial surface and degenerative changes are common associated radiological features. Eustace et al (1993) have shown that as the intermetatarsal angle increases, so does the degree of first metatarsal pronation; they measured the movement of the inferior tuberosity of the base of the proximal phalanx in 20 cadaveric feet. On pronation, the tuberosity moved lateral to the midline. They showed that pronation and varus deviation of the first metatarsal are both linked in aiding tendon imbalance, which leads to hallux valgus.

Congenital metatarsus adductus and varus

This is a common congenital deformity whereby on the dorsiplanar view a line drawn through the long axis of the talus passes either through the base of the first metatarsal or medial to it. The talocalcaneal angles are normal or slightly increased. The forefoot is adducted and the metatarsals often overlapped. On the lateral view, normal or increased dorsiflexion of the foot is seen. The lateral talocalcaneal angle is normal or slightly increased, and the first metatarsal is noticeably higher than the fifth.

Congenital vertical talus

This is rare and not to be confused with idiopathic flat foot or other foot deformities. On the dorsiplanar view, there is an increase in the talocalcaneal angle. The heel is in severe valgus, and the talar axis line lies a long way medial to the first metatarsal. A 'neutral' lateral, together with one in full plantar flexion, should be taken

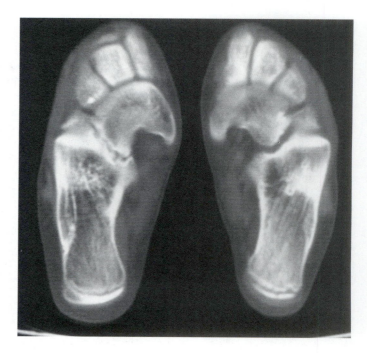

Figure 14

Tarsal coalition: axial CT scan shows bilateral calcaneonavicular coalition. The right one is fibrocartilaginous; the left one is incomplete. Note the increase in size of both navicular bones

(Eyre-Brook 1967). On the neutral lateral view, the calcaneum is in equinus and the anterior end tilted down. The talus tilts towards the vertical and the lateral talocalcaneal angle is much increased. The talus may develop an hour-glass shape. The forefoot dorsiflexes at midtarsal level, with the development of a convex plantar surface or 'rocker bottom' deformity (Freiberger et al 1970). The navicular dislocates dorsally on the talus, and in the infant the position can be inferred from the position of the medial cuneiform and first metatarsal. The lateral view with plantar flexion will demonstrate retention of the dorsal dislocation of the navicular, whereas in severe idiopathic flat foot, any apparent dorsal navicular dislocation will disappear.

Club foot (congenital talipes equinovarus)

On the dorsiplanar view, the talocalcaneal angle approaches 0° or is reversed. Both the midtalar and midcalcaneal lines point well lateral to the normal position. The forefoot is in varus and adducted, with overlapping metatarsal bones. On the lateral view, the midtalar and midcalcaneal lines are more or less parallel. A line drawn through the midtalus and a line drawn through the long

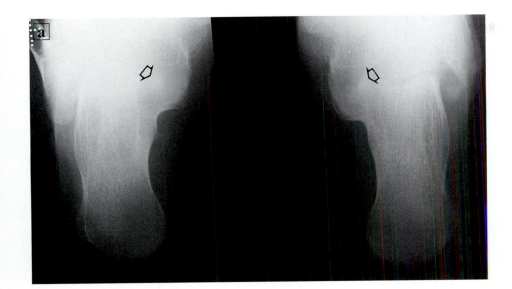

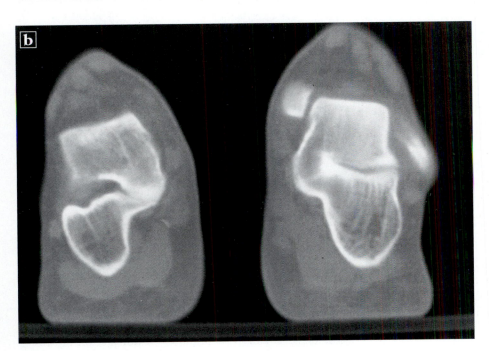

Figure 15

Tarsal coalition: bilateral talocalcaneal coalitions demonstrated. (a) Axial calcaneal view (arrows). (b) Coronal CT

axis of the first metatarsal form an obtuse angle, whereas these two lines normally coincide. A late radiological feature is the development of a flat-topped talus.

Pes cavus

In this condition, often associated with neuromuscular disorders (Brewerton et al 1963), the medial and sometimes the lateral longitudinal arch of the foot is high. The dorsiplanar view looks normal. On a standing lateral view, an increase in the lateral talocalcaneal angle may be seen. An angle is present between a line through the midtalus and a line drawn through the shaft of the first metatarsal. The heel may be in varus or valgus.

Pes planovalgus (flat foot)

This is a diagnosis often made on subjective clinical impression. The main role of radiology in the painful flat foot is to exclude other treatable conditions.

Dorsiplanar and lateral weight-bearing views provide functional assessment and allow for easier reproducibility for follow up. On the dorsiplanar view, the talocalcaneal angle is increased with the heel in valgus. In many cases, the line through the long axis of the talus runs medial to the first metatarsal, while the long axis of the calcaneum normally lies near the fourth metatarsal base. On the lateral view, with an element of plantar flexion of the talus, the lateral talocalcaneal angle is increased. In

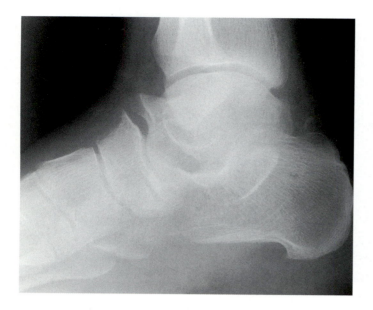

Figure 16

Tarsal coalition: talar beak due to abnormal stresses in relation to a talocalcaneal bar

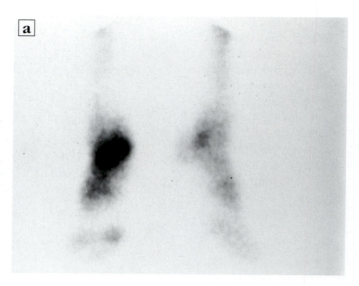

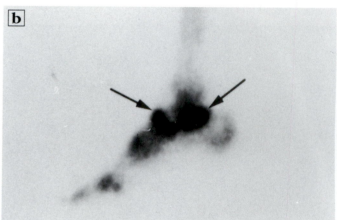

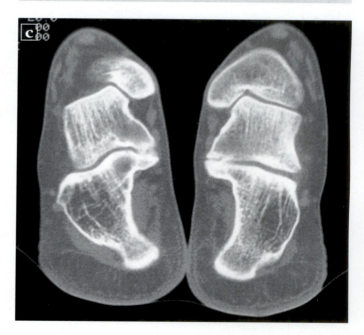

addition, in this condition, a line drawn through the axis of the first metatarsal makes an angle with a line drawn through the axis of the talus, whereas in a normal foot these two lines coincide with no angulation. In unexplained peroneal spastic flat foot, a bone scan will locate or rule out any focal bony cause such as symptomatic tarsal coalition (Deutch et al 1982, Goldman et al 1982).

Tarsal coalition

The talocalcaneal (TC) and calcaneonavicular (CN) are the commonest coalitions. TC coalitions ossify at about 12–16 years and CN at 8–12 years (Jayacumar & Cowell 1977). Talonavicular and calcaneocuboid coalitions are much rarer. Fusion may be bony, cartilaginous, or fibrous and may be between two or more bones. Harris & Beath (1948) showed that most cases of peroneal spastic foot are due to coalitions. A medial talocalcaneal bridge was the most common.

With modern imaging techniques there is less reliance on plain film assessment, although this should still include dorsiplanar and lateral weight-bearing films to measure the talocalcaneal angle and to detect associated abnormalities. The CN coalition is usually well demonstrated on an oblique view of the foot: it may be fibrocartilaginous or bony. A CT scan is a more sophisticated method of showing these (Fig. 14). There may be signs of degenerative change at the site of coalition if the fusion is incomplete or in adjacent joints placed under

Figure 17

Tarsal coalition. (a) Anterior view and (b) medial view of 99mTcMDP scan; (c) CT scan, in patient with bilateral fibrocartilaginous talocalcaneal bars. Only the one on the right was symptomatic with focal increase in isotope uptake in subtalar and talonavicular joints

stress. The axial calcaneal view (Harris & Beath 1948) (Fig. 15a) may show a TC coalition, not suspected on the basic views, which can be confirmed on CT (Fig. 15b). The navicular on the side of the coalition may be larger (Chambers 1950). Because subtalar movement is severely restricted by subtalar fusion, and to a lesser extent with CN fusion, the forces between the talus and navicular are altered, probably to a hinge-type movement, resulting in a dorsal talar beak (Fig. 16) (Jayacumar & Cowell 1977). It has been suggested that patients showing this abnormality do less well surgically (Inglis et al 1986). If the obliquity of the midfacet coalition in relation to the posterior one on the axial radiograph or CT reaches 20° or more a coalition is most probable (Harris & Beath 1948).

Isotope bone scanning provides a physiological assessment of the painful flat foot and increased uptake will be shown in the region of a symptomatic coalition (Deutch et al 1982, Goldman et al 1982) (Fig. 17). CT is now well established in demonstrating coalition (Wechsler et al 1992) which may also be shown in the asymptomatic foot (see Fig. 4). Beckley et al (1975) reported as many as 25% of feet with asymptomatic coalitions. The width of the coalition can be measured and is important to the surgeon: Salomao et al (1992) found the average coalition width was 13 mm, with a range of 9–16.4 mm.

Traumatic conditions of bone and cartilage

Many painful conditions of the foot and ankle are related to trauma which may be recent, due to chronic stress or related to a complication of an old injury. Conversely, pain attributed to trauma may be related to some pre-existing condition. The importance of an accurate history of the mechanism of injury and a thorough examination cannot be overemphasized, since this will influence the choice and sequence of radiological investigation.

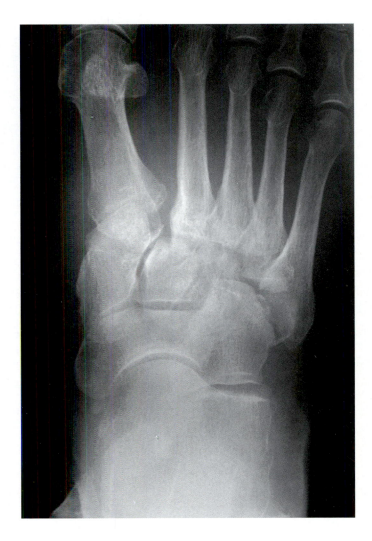

Figure 18

Lisfranc's fracture dislocation: there is a step deformity between the second metatarsal base and the middle cuneiform, with lateral subluxation of the second to fifth metatarsals. There is associated cuboid fracture

Acute injury

For the radiological appearances of most acute traumatic conditions of the foot and ankle the reader should refer to dedicated texts (Rogers 1982, Resnick et al 1988a). The diagnosis of some injuries which may be initially overlooked will be discussed. In tarsometatarsotarsal or Lisfranc subluxations, subtle disruption of continuity of the line joining the medial borders of the second metatarsal base and the intermediate cuneiform is an indicator of significant ligamentous damage (Fig. 18). In midfoot injury the lateral view only may show navicular damage, either complete fracture (Fig. 19) or avulsion reflecting ligamentous damage (Fig, 20). Both talar neck

and navicular fractures may be complicated by avascular necrosis, and early diagnosis is important. In hindfoot injuries, oblique views of the ankle show the subtalar articulation, and an axial view will show fractures in the long axis of the calcaneum. Fractures of the anterior process of the calcaneum are easy to miss (see Fig. 20) (Renfrew & El-Khoury 1985), if not specifically sought. CT is useful in demonstrating injuries of the midfoot (Goiney et al 1984) and hindfoot (Smith & Staple 1984, Heger et al 1985), and in particular calcaneal fracture dislocations (Heger et al 1985), showing subtalar joint involvement and position of fragments which may cause impingement or displacement of the peroneal tendons (Fig. 21). In unilateral injury, by scanning both feet,

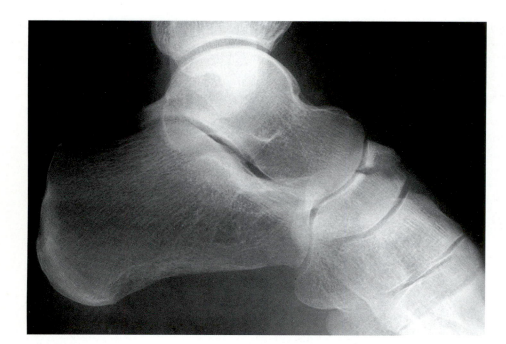

Figure 19

Navicular fracture: this fracture was not visible on the routine AP and oblique projections

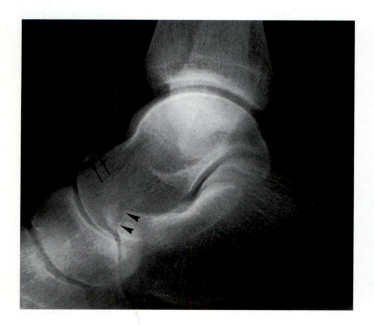

Figure 20

Fracture anterior process of calcaneum: this fracture (arrowheads) is often overlooked. There are also avulsion injuries from the talus (arrows) and adjacent navicular

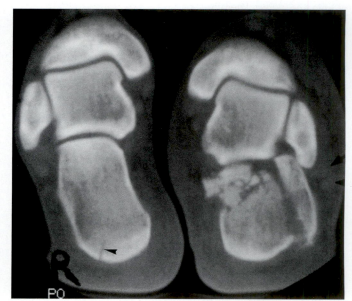

Figure 21

Calcaneal fractures: coronal CT scan shows a left comminuted and a right crack fracture. The left fracture involves the subtalar joint and causes impingement and displacement of the peroneal tendons (arrows). There is also a crack fracture through the right calcaneum (arrowhead)

distortion of the hindfoot and loss of heel contour can be compared with the normal side. MRI in calcaneal fractures has been evaluated (Zeiss et al 1991) but has limited ability to image small bone fragments, which are more easily seen on CT.

When plain films fail a bone scan will usually detect a fracture (Burkus et al 1984). MRI is more specific in demonstrating bone contusion, fracture and articular cartilage damage, but it is not usually available for routine evaluation of acute injuries.

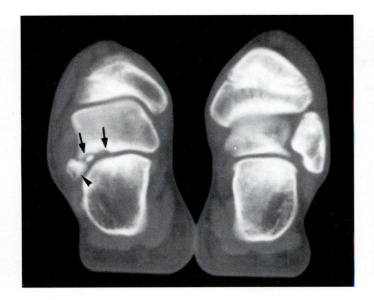

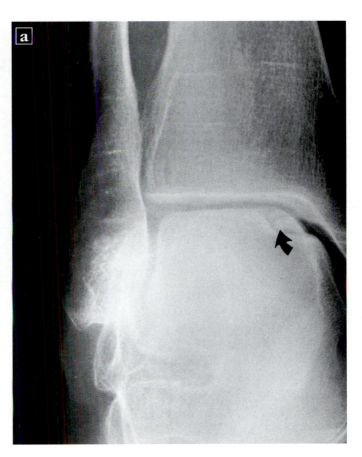

Figure 22

Osteochondral fracture of talus: coronal CT scan in a 14-year old boy shows large talar osteochondral defect in relation to the subtalar joint (arrows). A fragment of bone remains within the defect laterally. Medial to this, fragments have probably been shed into the joint. The fragment of bone lying laterally (arrowhead) was assumed to be an old ununited fracture through the lateral process of the talus

Osteochondral injuries

Transchondral fractures and osteochondritis dessicans are considered traumatic in origin (De Ginder 1955, Berndt & Harty 1959). Although sometimes recognized after acute injury, they may be overlooked until later complication develops. These are often related to the talar dome, although other joints may be involved (Fig. 22). Because of the insensitivity of subchondral bone, it is not always possible to define the exact time and mechanism of injury, nor can the contribution of non-traumatic causes be ruled out (Berndt & Harty 1959, De Ginder 1955). Berndt and Harty (1959) have proposed that the mechanism of medial and lateral talar dome fractures might be due to shearing and rotary forces often associated with ligamentous injury around the ankle. They proposed a classification from an undisplaced fragment with intact articular cartilage to a detached fragment. Loose fragments may present with pain and locking. Radiographs of the ankle with obliques, and screening if necessary, may show the site of injury (Smith et al 1977, Newberg 1979) (Fig. 23a&b). CT will show the site and size of a lesion and the position of loose fragments but not the integrity of the articular cartilage (see Fig. 22). For this, arthrography, arthrotomography, CT arthrography or MRI can all be employed. The degree of late phase uptake on a bone scan has been shown to be directly proportional to the severity of the lesion

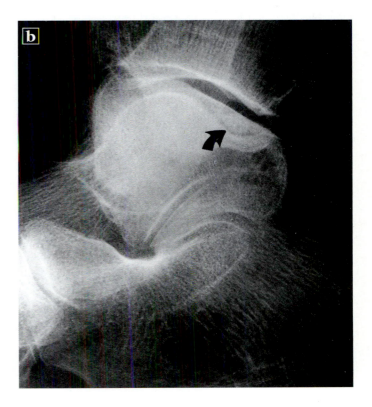

Figure 23

Osteochondral injury of talus: an area of osteochondritis dessicans (arrow) found on the medial talar dome in a patient with recurrent inversion injury of the ankle. (a) Anterior view. (b) Lateral view

(Cahill & Berg 1983): i.e. the greater the uptake the greater the probability of a loose fragment. There may be no increase in uptake in stage 1 lesions where the articular cartilage is intact (Mesgarzadeh et al 1987, Anderson et al 1989), but the sensitivity of MRI may show talar dome cysts in these injuries in the absence of plain film changes (Fig. 24) and following an old apparently healed osteochondral lesion (Fig. 25). Several series have shown its value in staging osteochondral injuries (Mesgarzadeh et al 1987, Anderson et al 1989, De Smet et al 1989), although it may overestimate articular cartilage damage (De Smet et al 1989). High signal on T2-weighted images between the fragment and the rest of the bone can be due to fluid tracking around the lesion through damaged articular cartilage but it can also be due to granulation tissue or persisting signal change in the damaged articular cartilage, which is no longer seen arthroscopically (De Smet et al 1990). Deutch (1992) suggests that when there is no joint effusion this pitfall can be surmounted by injection of intra-articular gadolinium (1 in 200 normal saline). Talar dome lesions are best shown on oblique coronal and sagittal images using T1-weighted, T2-weighted and STIR sequences.

Avascular necrosis

Post-traumatic avascular necrosis of the talar dome is common, particularly with talar neck injuries, where it occurs in 80–90% of displaced fractures (Canale & Kelly 1978). First indication of avascularity is seen on a lateral radiograph between 5 and 8 weeks after injury by the presence or absence of subchondral bone resorption in the talar dome (Hawkins 1970). For this resorption to occur, an intact blood supply is needed. If relying on plain films alone, the diagnosis is usually delayed for 1–3 months until osteoporosis of the surrounding bone highlights the relative sclerosis (Fig. 26a&b) which may be accompanied by collapse of the articular surface.

MRI is the best method of diagnosing and monitoring the healing phase of avascular necrosis (Mitchell & Kressel 1988, Coleman et al 1988, Genez et al 1988). Mitchell & Kressel (1988) have proposed a grading system for staging osteonecrosis based on alteration in signal intensity in relation to the pathological process. In the early stages it may be difficult to differentiate oedema from fracture, and that from osteonecrosis. It is easier to differentiate in the sub-acute and later stages (Fig. 27a&b). A 'double-rim sign' may be seen at the interface of the dead and the viable bone and is a useful diagnostic feature.

Fatigue and stress fractures

Fatigue fractures occur in normal bone with repeated stress as in military recruits, athletes and dancers (Wilson

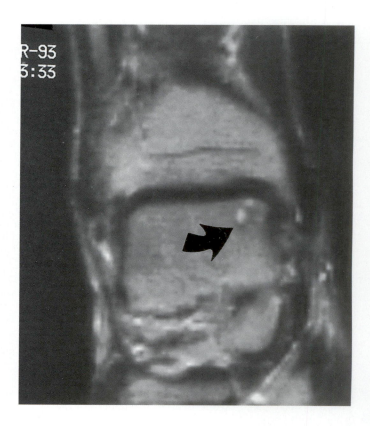

Figure 24
Subchondral injury: professional footballer with ankle pain. Plain films and isotope scan were normal. Oblique coronal T2-weighted SE MRI scan shows subchondral fluid filled cysts in medial talar dome (arrow) likely to be due to recurrent trauma

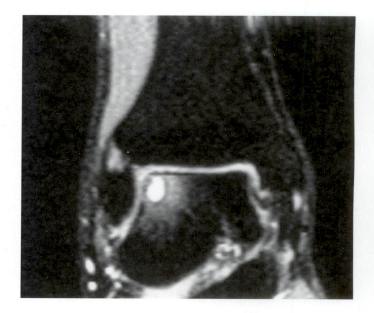

Figure 25
Osteochondral injury: oblique coronal T2-weighted GE MRI scan showing subtalar cyst with surrounding increased signal thought to be due to granulation tissue 3 years after a small osteochondral fracture. Plain films showed no evidence of osteoarthrosis and had been considered normal

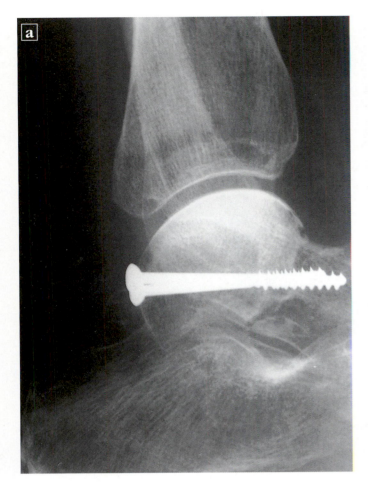

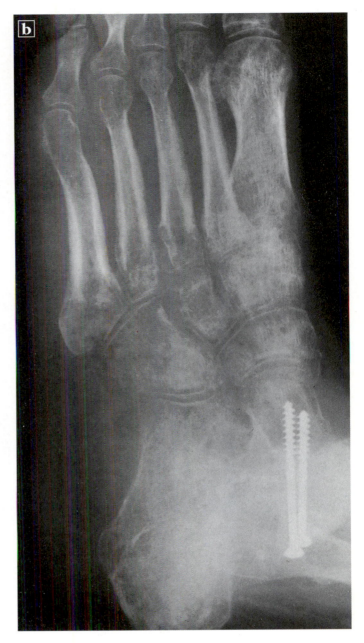

Figure 26

Talar neck fracture. (a) Lateral view at 5 weeks still shows fracture line and sclerosis in proximal talar fragment. There is no subchondral bone resorption, suggesting loss of blood supply. (b) Four weeks later there has been progressive subchondral bone resorption in all bones except the talar dome, which subsequently collapsed. The degree of patchy osteoporosis is consistent with Sudeck's atrophy or 'reflex motor dystrophy', a finding that was supported clinically

& Katz 1969, Schneider et al 1974, Greaney et al 1983). Insufficiency fractures occur in bone weakened by conditions such as osteoporosis (Fig. 28), osteomalacia, rheumatoid arthritis (Miller et al 1967) and neurological disorders.

These fractures are common in the calcaneum (Winfield & Dennis 1959), navicular (Goergen et al 1981, Torg et al 1982, Pavlov et al 1983), metatarsals and distal tibia and fibula. Stress fractures (Fig. 29) of the medial malleolus are associated with running and jumping (Schils et al 1992); although fractures may also result from abnormal stresses after bunion surgery (Ford & Gilula 1977, Frede & Lee 1983). Scintigraphy plays an important role in diagnosing occult stress fractures (Geslien et al 1976, Saunders et al 1979, Rupani et al 1985) (see Fig. 28a&b). Rupani et al (1985) found the three-phase scan provides most information, but this cannot be justified on a routine basis in a busy department.

In a series of 55 navicular stress fractures (Kiss et al 1992) CT was considered suitable for detection and follow up, although it was felt that small fractures could be missed. Stress fractures can also be confirmed by MRI (Lee & Yao 1988) (Fig. 30), which may also demonstrate other traumatic lesions, but at present in most centres MRI is used only where the plain films and scintigram are not diagnostic and when an early diagnosis without radiation exposure is important, as in professional athletes.

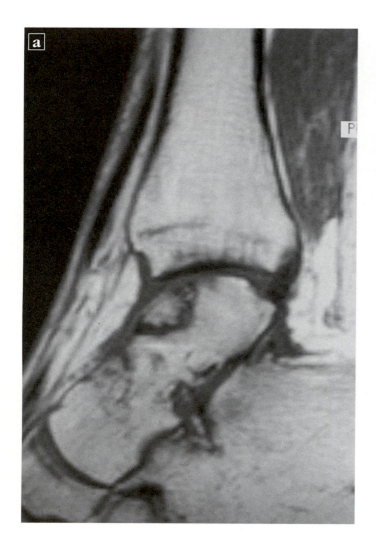

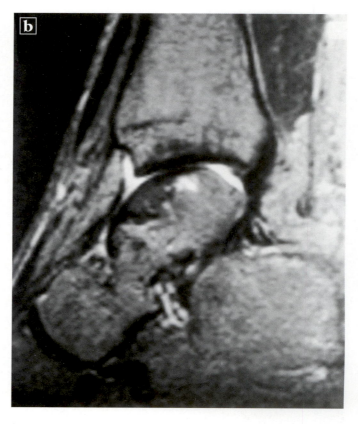

Figure 27

Segmental avascular necrosis of talus. (a) Sagittal T1-weighted and (b) sagittal T2-weighted SE MRI sequences show changed signal in infarcted anterior talar dome. At this stage the articular surface remained intact

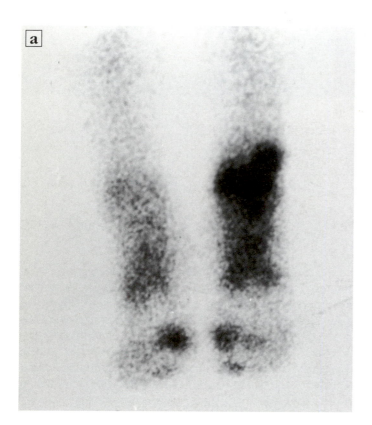

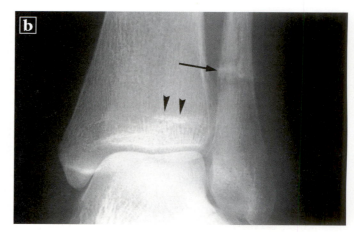

Figure 28

Stress fractures tibia and fibula: osteoporotic stress fractures in 70-year-old woman following increased activity. (a) 99mTcMDP scan shows increased focal uptake at fracture sites and in bilateral osteoarthritic first metatarsophalangeal joints. There is also generalized increase in isotope uptake throughout the left foot and ankle which is a common non-specific finding, reflecting disuse or immobilization of a limb. (b) AP radiograph: arrow shows fibular and arrowheads show tibial fractures

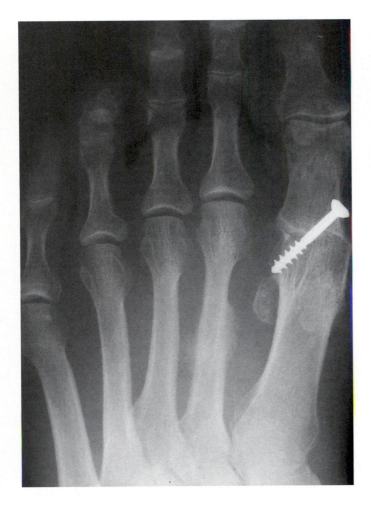

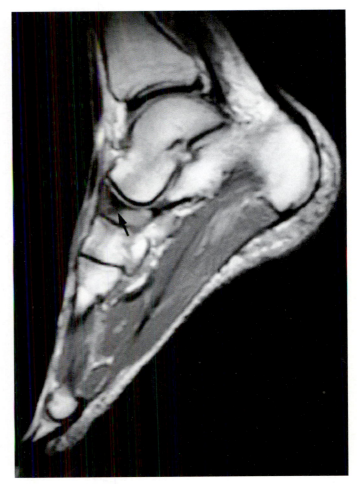

Figure 29

Stress fracture of second metatarsal following first
metatarsophalangeal fusion

Figure 30

Stress fracture navicular: 20-year-old professional footballer
with non-specific foot pain. Sagittal T1-weighted SE MRI scan
shows reduced signal in upper half of navicular due to
fracture (arrow) which subsequently showed on plain films.
An isotope scan would also have suggested the diagnosis

Late traumatic changes

Post-traumatic foot pain may be due to degenerative
disease or fibrous union or nonunion of a fracture.
Osteoarthritis may follow an intra-articular fracture,
especially in weight bearing joints. McMaster (1978)
postulated a traumatic cause for hallux rigidus, relating
it to repeated osteochondral damage. Fracture uptake on
a bone scan should gradually return to normal over
about 9 months. Significant increase in focal uptake
persisting after this time is relevant, especially when
considering prognosis and in medicolegal claims after
injury. In Fig. 31a&b fractures through the third and
fourth metatarsal bases are still visible 18 months after
injury, and the intense but nonspecific isotope uptake
confirms complication such as fibrous or nonunion. The
scan must be interpreted with up-to-date radiographs,
since other conditions including osteoarthrosis may

produce identical uptake (Fig. 32a&b). Sometimes CT or
MRI are needed to confirm the cause for the uptake
when plain films fail to define any abnormality.

Growth plate damage

Growth plate injuries may cause permanent damage and
may not be suspected at the time of injury. The distal
tibial growth plate is particularly vulnerable, and the
younger the child, the greater the potential for the development of deformity. Bony bridging between epiphysis
and metaphysis may result from unrecognized or inadequately treated Salter IV injuries. This can be best
defined by fine tomographic cuts in anteroposterior (Fig.
33) and lateral planes for pre and postoperative assessment. In the older child an isotope scan will confirm
whether there is residual growth potential or whether
the damaged growth plate has fused.

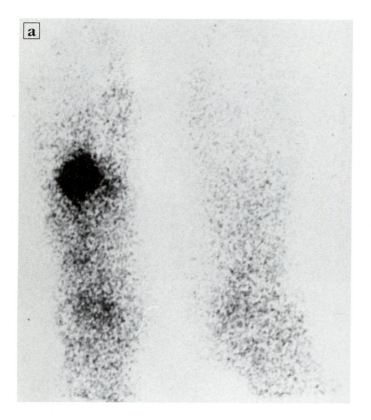

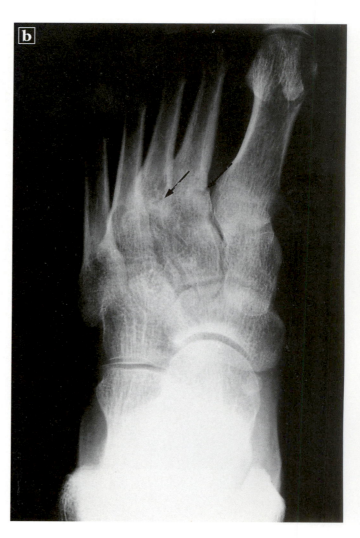

Figure 31

Delayed union metatarsals. (a) 99mTcMDP scan shows
intense uptake in midfoot following crush injury 18 months
previously. (b) AP radiograph shows residual fracture lines in
second and third metatarsal bases (arrows) at site of uptake,
consistent with delayed union

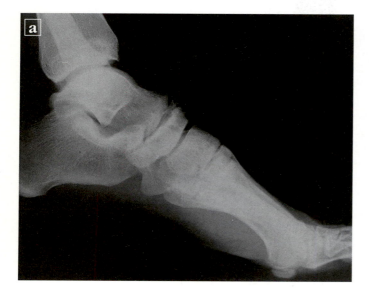

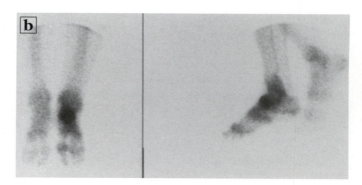

Figure 32

Osteoarthrosis talonavicular joint. (a) A lateral radiograph
shows evidence of degenerative change in this joint
following an old navicular fracture. (b) A 99mTcMDP scan
provides physiological correlation

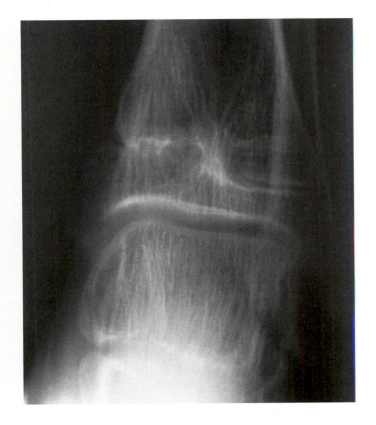

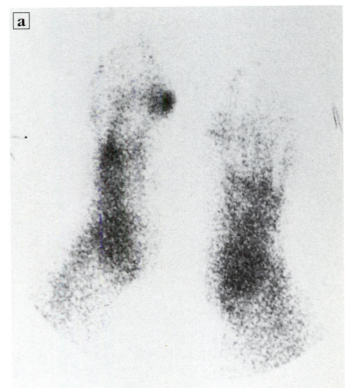

Figure 33
Deformity following Salter IV injury: AP tomograph of ankle shows site of bony tethering causing increasing varus deformity of the foot

The osteochondroses and similar conditions

The osteochondroses are a group of conditions occurring in the immature skeleton. Radiologically they all tend to show fragmentation and sclerosis. Several similar conditions affecting the feet will also be considered, owing to their radiological similarity, although pathologically they are different (Omer 1981, Katz 1981, Resnick et al 1988b). It is probable that trauma plays some part in the pathogenesis of all these disorders (Douglas & Rang 1981). Conditions with similar appearances occur in the adult skeleton affecting the sesamoid bones and normal ossicles. In all these conditions, scintigraphy may be positive long before plain film changes are seen. MRI is more specific, but the simpler diagnostic techniques are usually adequate.

Freiberg's infraction

Described by Freiberg in 1914, this is considered to be due to avascular necrosis. The initial radiographs often

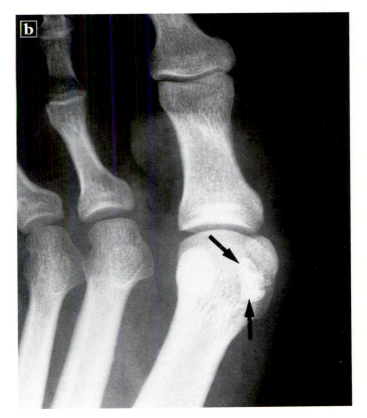

Figure 34
Osteochondritis of sesamoid. (a) 99mTcMDP bone scan shows focal uptake in medial sesamoid bone. Radiographs were normal initially. (b) Six weeks later the medial sesamoid shows sclerosis and fragmentation (arrows) and pain resolved after its excision

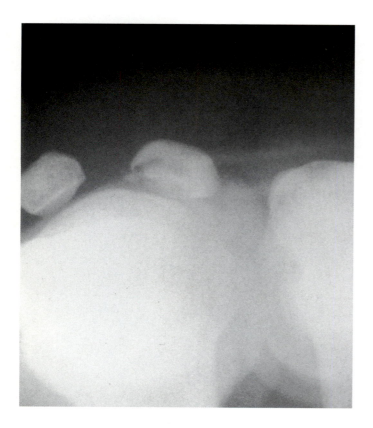

Figure 35

Osteochondritis of sesamoid: tangential view confirmed fragmentation and sclerosis in the lateral sesamoid bone when routine views proved equivocal

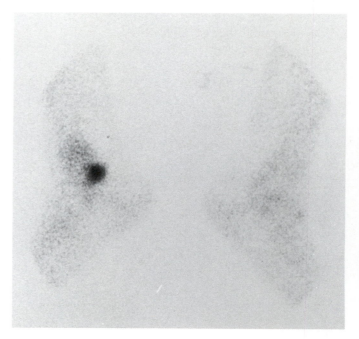

Figure 36

Os trigonum syndrome: positive 99mTcMDP bone scan confirms the suspected diagnosis

show slight flattening and sclerosis of the second, and occasionally third metatarsal head, which may collapse. Periosteal new bone forms around the metatarsal neck in an attempt at healing. Widening of both sides of the joint may result, with premature closure of the growth plate and subsequent development of osteoarthritis.

Kohler's disease

Early radiographs show increase in density, fragmentation and flattening of the navicular but with preservation of the joint space. Because of the variable pattern of navicular ossification the diagnosis should be made with caution. Isotope bone scanning may show a reduction followed by an increase in uptake (McCauley & Kahn, 1977).

Sesamoiditis

Bipartite or tripartite sesamoid bones must not be mistaken for fractures, which are rare in these bones.

Osteochondritis occurs more in females than males and in the mature rather than immature skeleton, between the second and third decades (Ogata et al 1986). Initial radiographs are normal but an isotope scan will show increased uptake in the affected sesamoid bone (Fig. 34a&b). Fragmentation may develop with repeated trauma. A tangential view may confirm the suspected diagnosis if the routine films are equivocal (Fig. 35).

Sever's disease

Although this is historically called an 'osteochondrosis', it is now accepted that the sclerotic appearance of the secondary calcaneal ossification centre is a normal developmental appearance, although this apophysis like any other can suffer avulsion injury.

Os trigonum syndrome

The os trigonum is a common accessory ossicle, which has anatomical continuity with the back of the talus. With repeated forcible plantar flexion, this may become symptomatic, resulting in the 'talar compression' or 'os trigonum' syndrome. It is common in footballers and ballet dancers (Hamilton 1982, Quirk 1982, Brodsky & Khalil

1987, Maffulli et al 1990, Wenig 1990). Wredmark et al (1991) described the condition in 13 Swedish ballet dancers who were diagnosed and treated surgically for this syndrome. The presence of an os trigonum on the plain films with an appropriate history raises the possibility of the diagnosis, which should be confirmed by an isotope bone scan (Johnson et al 1984, Martin 1989). In chronic cases fragmentation of the os trigonum may be seen on serial plain films (Romanowski & Barrington, 1991), but an isotope bone scan is still advocated to confirm that this is the current cause of symptoms (Fig. 36).

The accessory navicular

This is a recognized but less well-known cause of foot pain related to trauma in a normal ossicle (Lawson 1985). Lawson et al (1984) described three types of accessory navicular: type 1 is a completely separate ossicle (os tibiale externum); type 2 ossicle forms a fibrocartilaginous synchondrosis with the rest of the navicular; type 3 is total incorporation of the ossicle into the navicular resulting in a bony prominence medially. In type 2 traction from the tibialis posterior tendon may cause a chronic avulsive strain. Although the diagnosis may be suspected clinically, initially plain films may be normal apart from soft tissue swelling medially, and the diagnosis needs to be confirmed by a bone scan. In a series of 10 patients suffering from this syndrome (Romanowski & Barrington 1992) all related to abnormal stress due to sporting or occupational activity. If the diagnosis is delayed, the ossicle may become fragmented, causing considerable swelling and pain (Fig. 37).

Injuries to tendons and ligaments

When soft tissue injury is suspected in the foot and ankle, stress and weight-bearing views, contrast studies and ultrasound can all contribute to the assessment. Tendon injury can be due to direct trauma or excessive or repeated tension (usually related to sporting activity). Tendons weakened by age or disease are more prone to damage. Predisposing factors include corticosteroid therapy, diabetes, inflammatory or crystal arthropathies and renal failure. Inflammation and myxoid degeneration may lead to partial intrasubstance or complete ligamentous tears.

In experienced hands, ultrasonography is useful in the assessment of tendon injuries (Fornage & Rifkin 1988, Kaplan et al 1989, Thermann et al 1992). It can suggest the presence, type and extent of a lesion, and can monitor change with time (Fornage & Rifkin 1988). CT and MRI have differences in sensitivity and accuracy but both are excellent for imaging tendons (Rosenburg et al 1988a). When MRI is not available, CT is an adequate substitute,

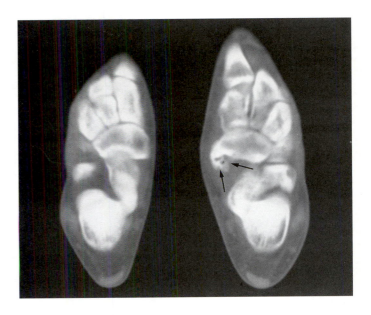

Figure 37

Symptomatic tibiale externum: axial CT scan shows swelling in relation to a fragmented type 2 os tibiale externum (arrows), confirming the isotopic findings (from Romanowski & Barrington 1992, with permission)

and it even has advantages when there are associated bony abnormalities or tendonous calcification (Rosenburg et al 1987a). However, MRI is the method of choice overall because of its higher contrast resolution and its direct multiplanar capabilities (Beltran et al 1987, Rosenburg et al 1988a, Rosenburg et al 1988b, Mink 1992a).

On MRI, intact ligaments show homogeneous low signal on all pulsing sequences, owing to their lack of water content. Thin contiguous slices of 3 mm are necessary to visualize subtle signal changes within them. Tendons are best scanned parallel and perpendicular to the long axis and are best demonstrated longitudinally in the sagittal plane, and cross-sectionally in the axial or oblique axial plane, using at least two pulse sequences.

Tendon injuries

The Achilles tendon may become inflamed with overuse of the calf muscles, and it is the tendon most susceptible to rupture. Achilles tendon injuries can be divided into acute tendinitis and peritendonitis, chronic tendonitis, acute and chronic partial tears and complete ruptures (Mink 1992a). The Achilles tendon has no sheath, and the inflammatory process starts in the paratenon (Brody 1980).

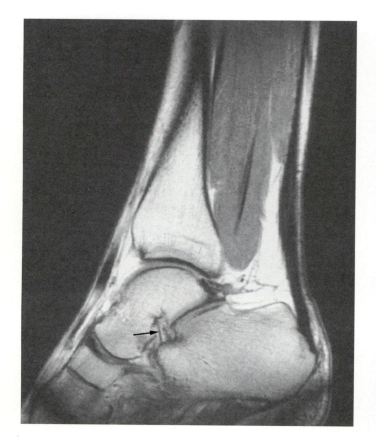

Figure 38

Achilles tendonitis: sagittal T1-weighted SE MRI scan showing fusiform swelling of tendon. This is the earliest sign of abnormality. A normal tendon should have the same diameter throughout its length. A normal interosseous talocalcaneal ligament is shown on this section (arrow)

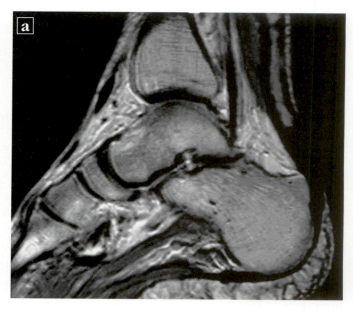

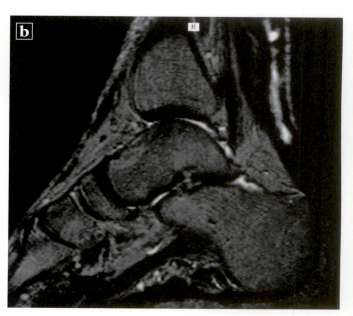

Figure 39

Achilles tendon tear: sagittal SE MRI scans showing thickened irregular tendon containing abnormal signal within it. (a) Intermediate on T1-weighted and (b) high on T2-weighted due to extensive intrasubstance tear

Ultrasonography is useful in imaging the Achilles tendon (Blei et al 1986, Fornage 1986) and in differentiating between tendon damage that requires surgery and damage that can be treated conservatively (Mathieson et al 1988). On CT and MRI, the normal tendon has a flat, slightly concave, anterior margin, appearing slightly cresent-shaped, except close to its insertion into the calcaneum, where it is ovoid. Fusiform thickening and widening of the tendon confirm chronic tendinitis (Quinn et al 1987, Weistabl et al 1991). Initially, there may be no signal change within the tendon on MRI, and alteration in shape may be the only sign (Fig. 38). The anteroposterior dimension of the tendon should not exceed 8 mm (Mink 1992a), and its anterior border should be flat or concave. Peritendinitis is shown as oedema around the tendon, which appears as high signal on T2-weighted sequences.

In chronic inflammation, small foci of intratendinous mucoid degeneration develop (Brody 1980, Quinn et al 1987), which progress to longitudinal intrasubstance splits (Fig. 39a&b). This is shown by linear and globular foci of low signal on T1-weighted, and high signal on T2-weighted, sagittal images. Many studies have found MRI useful in predicting the extent of tendinitis, the degree of rupture and the state of the edges of torn tendons (Reinig et al 1985, Daffner et al 1986, Marcus et al 1989, Keene et al 1989, Weinstabl et al 1991). Although sensitive, it is not specific in differentiating

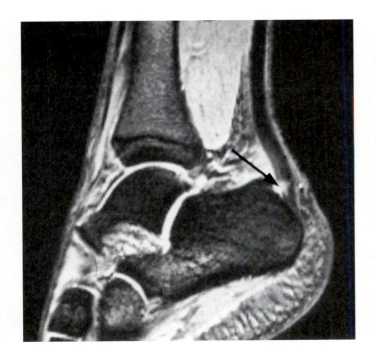

Figure 40

Achilles tendon tear: sagittal T2-weighted GE MRI scan
showing partial thickness horizontal tear (arrow) near its
calcaneal attachment

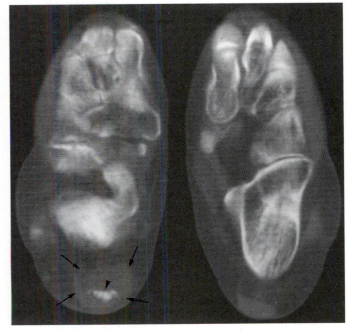

Figure 41

Achilles calcific tendonitis: axial CT scan showing normal left
tendon, and swollen right tendon (arrows) with
intrasubstance calcification (arrowhead)

between chronic inflammation and myxoid degeneration
with partial or early intrasubstance rupture, unless an
area of discontinuity is seen. This usually occurs several
centimetres above the calcaneum, although avulsion
injuries can occur at its calcaneal attachment. Fig. 40
shows a partial thickness tear on the anterior border
proximal to its attachment to the calcaneum. With
complete disruption, fat signal may be interposed
between the torn ends. Fraying of the tendon edges may
be associated with retraction of the proximal end. Keene
et al (1989) found good correlation between the images
and the surgical findings. Axial sequences may reveal
fluid or inflammation not only within the Achilles tendon
but also in other tendons and ligaments around the
ankle, which may or may not be pathological. Axial CT
images will show the size and shape of both tendons
and any areas of attenuation or thickening. It has the
advantage of visualizing intratendinous calcification not
visible on plain films or even MRI (Fig. 41).

Rupture of the tibialis posterior tendon (PTT) occurs
classically in middle-aged females. The tendon is one of
the main stabilizers of the hindfoot, and with chronic
tears attenuation results in an insidious, unilateral flat
foot deformity with associated talar plantar flexion,
valgus heel and forefoot abduction (Fig. 42a) (Funk et
al 1986). Intrinsic degeneration of the tendon fibres tends
to occur near the tendon insertion into the navicular,

owing to mechanical wear as it passes under the medial
malleolus. Weight-bearing lateral views may confirm the
loss of the convex arch and show subluxation of the
talonavicular and the naviculocuneiform joints (see Fig.
42b&c).

High-resolution CT and MRI now suggest the diagnosis of PTT injuries prior to exploration (Rosenburg et al
1988a, 1988b) (Fig. 43a&b). MRI will demonstrate the
nature of partial or complete tears better than CT does
and will demonstrate an associated synovial effusion.
Partial (or Grade 1) tears are hypertrophied regions
containing heterogeneous signal. Grade 2 tears are due
to longitudinal splitting in attenuated sections in tendons.
The tendon may thin to half or a third of its usual size.
Sometimes the splits are long and divide the tendon into
two. Complete tears (type 3) show a gap. The retracted
tendon appears wider than usual and can be mistaken
for the swollen tendon seen in type 1 injury, if the tendon
is not fully visualized in continuity (Rosenburg et al
1988b).

The peroneal tendons pass behind the lateral malleolus
in a common synovial sheath and are held in position by
thick retinacula. The superior peroneal retinaculum may
rupture secondarily to trauma to the lateral side of the
ankle, resulting in partial or complete dislocation or in
entrapment of the peroneal tendons (Rosenburg et al
1986). This is particularly associated with calcaneal

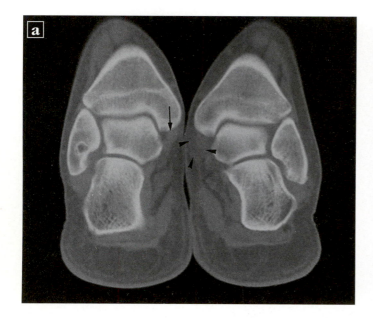

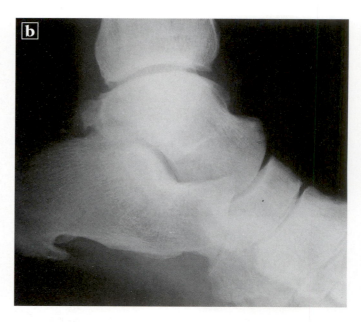

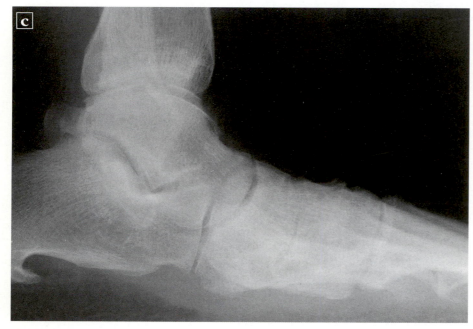

Figure 42

Tibialis posterior tendon degeneration in a 60-year-old woman with left-sided progressive flat foot deformity. (a) Coronal CT scan showing swollen tendon (arrowheads) and valgus heel. On the right a normal tibialis posterior tendon is shown just below the medial malleolus (arrow). (b) Non-weight-bearing lateral radiograph. (c) Weight-bearing radiograph. Note the change of position of the medial cuneiform in relation to the navicular between the two films. A thin attenuated degenerate tendon was found at operation

fractures (Rosenburg et al 1987b). CT or MRI will show the relationship of the tendons to the bony fragments (Fig. 44).

The flexor hallucis longus (FHL) passes posterolaterally to the PTT and flexor digitorum longus, over the back of the talus between the medial and lateral tubercles under the sustentaculum and along the plantar surface of the foot to insert into the great toe. The FHL becomes inflamed in ballet dancers and footballers (Fig. 45), but synovial fluid may be seen in all tendon sheaths on the plantar aspect of the foot in active asymptomatic patients (Fig. 46a&b).

The tendon of the anterior tibialis tendon starts just above the ankle joint. It has its own synovial sheath, which may become inflamed in relation to traumatic or inflammatory disease. Unlike the plantar tendons, fluid in its sheath is always significant. The tendon attaches to the first metatarsal base and medial cuneiform.

Fusiform swelling, splitting and synovitis may be seen in all tendon injuries.

Ligamentous injuries of the ankle

Most ligamentous injuries around the ankle are adequately seen on plain radiographic studies (Sclafani 1985, Clanton 1989) in conjunction with the clinical assessment. Stress views of the ankle mortice, preferably under general or local anaesthetic may detect instability

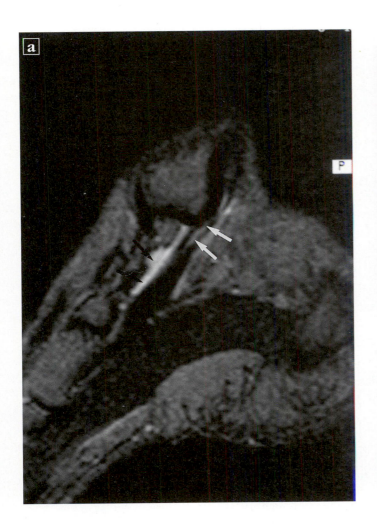

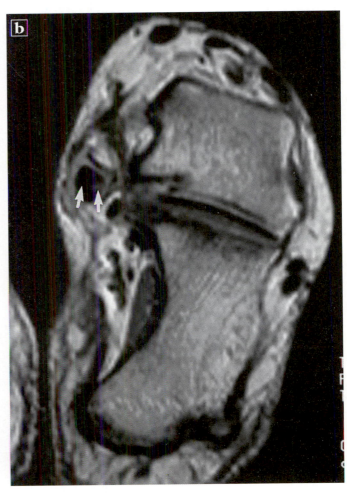

Figure 43

Tibialis posterior tendon tear: MRI scan. (a) Sagittal T2 SE-weighted sequence showing high signal along tendon due to an intrasubstance longitudinal tear (white arrows) as it passes beneath the medial malleolus. There is peritendinous oedema distal to this shown by high signal (black arrows). (b) Oblique axial proton density sequence confirms high signal across the tendon (white arrows)

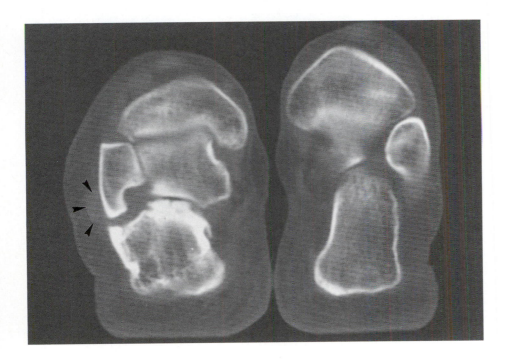

Figure 44

Peroneal tendon subluxation: coronal CT of ankles showing old right calcaneal fracture resulting in impingement of the fibula and displacement of the peroneal tendons (arrowheads). Note the normal left peroneal tendons

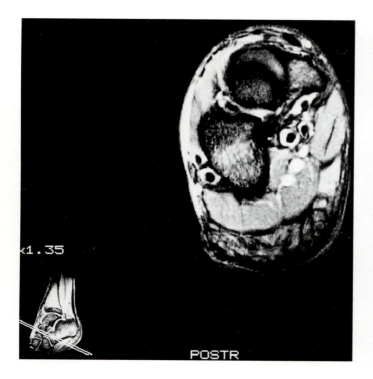

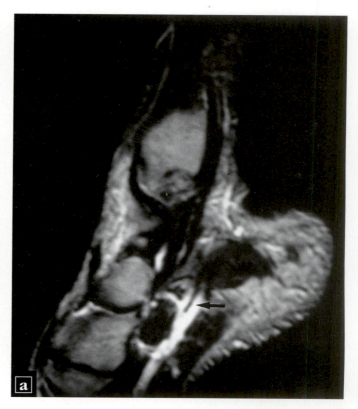

Figure 45

Normal fluid filled flexor tendon sheaths: T2-weighted GE oblique axial MRI scan of the right hind foot in a professional footballer scanned after inversion injury. The high signal in the soft tissue laterally is due to soft tissue swelling. The high signal around all the plantar flexor tendons is due to synovial sheath effusions, a normal finding with repeated activity

and demonstrate talar tilt or subluxation but are limited in acute injuries, owing to splinting from pain and spasm. Ankle arthrography or peroneal tenography has been shown to be more reliable in demonstrating the integrity of the calcaneofibular (CF) ligament, if it is carried out soon after injury (Sauser et al 1983). Peroneal tenography is considered by some to be more accurate than ankle arthrography (Blanchard et al 1986). Intercommunication between the common peroneal tendon sheath and the ankle joint with either technique confirms damage to the CF ligament (Fig. 47), since the CF and the posterior talofibular ligaments are closely applied to the medial aspect of the peroneal tendon sheath.

Although the normal ligamentous anatomy can be defined on MRI (Erickson et al 1990b, Ferkel et al 1991, Schneck et al 1992), it is seldom used as a first-line investigation for acute ligamentous injuries. Its value is still being evaluated (Schneck et al 1992, Mink 1992b). Most ligamentous complexes cannot be shown on one image but their integrity needs to be assessed in more than one plane and on contiguous images. It may be difficult to differentiate between a poorly visualized and a torn

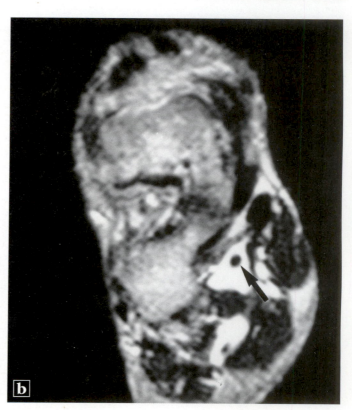

Figure 46

Tenosynovitis flexor hallucis longus tendon: T2-weighted SE MRI scan shows high signal around tendon (arrows) in (a) sagittal and (b) oblique axial planes. This excess fluid was considered to be relevant in this case, correlating with a clinical diagnosis of tenosynovitis following excessive unaccustomed footballing activity

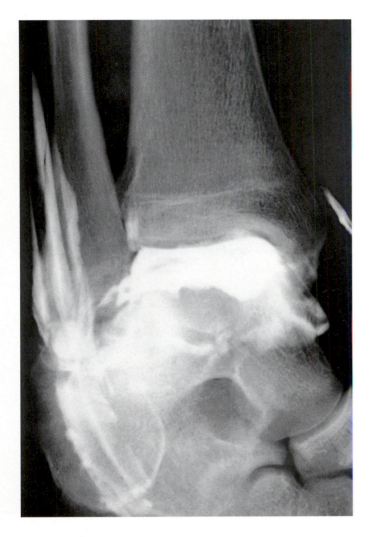

ligament, especially when the injury is not recent. An examination showing a normal ligament is more conclusive than one where a ligament is not shown, since this could mean injury to it or simply that it has not been imaged in the correct plain. Figs. 48a&b show normal CF and posterior talofibular ligaments respectively. Detection of associated abnormalities, such as chondral damage to the talar dome, may imply an underlying ligamentous injury (Berndt & Harty 1959). Similarly, inflammation and oedema are often shown in association with partial, rather than complete, ligamentous disruptions.

The cervical and talocalcaneal intraosseous ligaments (IOL) (see Fig. 38) help to stabilize the hindfoot and, if torn, cause pain, weakness and instability known as the 'sinus tarsi syndrome' (Clanton 1989). In 70% of cases, associated damage to the lateral ligament (Meyer et al 1988, Beltran et al 1990) was found. Rupture of the IOL is best seen on sagittal MRI sequences. Residual oedema and disorganized soft tissue will be shown in the tarsal tunnel on T2-weighted images in acute subtalar ligamentous strains (Klein & Spreitzer 1993).

The inflammatory arthropathies

The radiological features of rheumatoid arthritis and the seronegative spondyloarthropathies have certain similarities. They all involve synovial and cartilaginous joints (Mason et al 1959, Weissberg et al 1978). Bursae, tendons, ligaments and synovium may all be affected as well as

Figure 47

Ankle arthrogram showing calcaneofibular ligament tear: communication between the ankle joint and peroneal tendon sheath confirms damage to this ligament

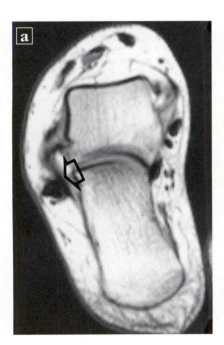
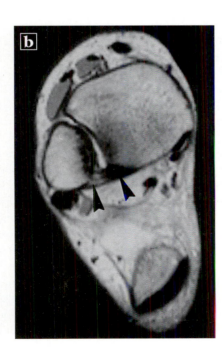

Figure 48

Normal ankle ligaments: T1-weighted SE MRI scans. (a) Oblique axial through subtalar joint showing calacaneofibular ligament (open arrow). Note its close proximity to the peroneal tendons. (b) Axial above ankle joint showing posterior tibiofibular ligament (arrow heads). Note fan-shaped fibular attachment

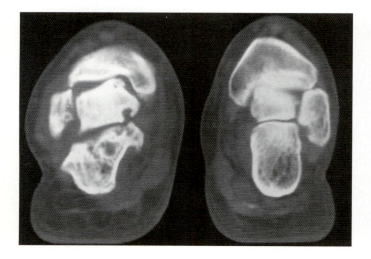 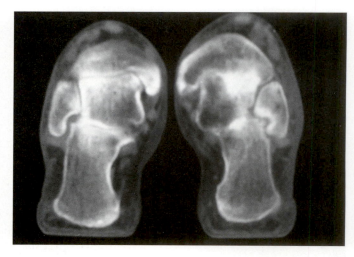

Figure 49

Rheumatoid arthritis: coronal CT scan of both ankles and subtalar joints. On the right severe erosion has caused collapse of calcaneal articular surface

Figure 50

Rheumatoid arthritis: severe articular cartilage destruction in subtalar and ankle joints. On the left there is calcaneal impingement of the fibula and sclerosis either side of the ankle joint owing to secondary osteoarthritis

bone. The distribution and extent of the abnormalities differ between the diseases (Resnick & Niwayama 1988c). By understanding the pathological processes, differentiation can be made between them, and the early radiological signs are more likely to be recognized (Resnick & Niwayama 1988a). The diagnosis depends largely on the clinical assessment and on good quality radiographs, although more modern imaging techniques may help in diagnosing some of the soft tissue complications.

In the foot and ankle weight-bearing views are important in assessing subluxations and deformities. CT scanning is useful in showing the joints of the hindfoot (Seltzer et al 1984) in order to plan arthrodesis and other surgical procedures. Increased heel valgus angles and flattened sustentacular angles can be measured (Seltzer et al 1984), and impingement on tendons, erosions and secondary degenerative change may be detected. Scintigraphy using 99mTcMDP will show the extent of the disease earlier than will clinical assessment and radiographic changes, and it can monitor the response of inflammation to treatment (Gerster et al 1977, Weissberg et al 1978, Mottonen et al 1986). MRI is extremely sensitive in demonstrating synovitis, synovial hypertrophy and joint effusion, as well as other complications of the disease (Bjorkengren et al 1989).

Rheumatoid arthritis

The radiological changes of rheumatoid arthritis have been extensively described (Bywaters 1954, Kirkup et al 1974, Calabro 1975, Resnick 1975, Videgal et al 1975, Resnick 1976, Kirkup et al 1977). The disease tends to involve synovial joints, bursae and tendon sheaths. In the foot there is a predilection for metatarsophalangeal joints and proximal interphalangeal joints as well as the tarsus and calcaneum.

Soft tissue swelling and juxta-articular osteoporosis are the earliest changes seen radiologically. Erosions commence at the joint margins, developing between the articular cartilage and the attachment of the joint capsule and spreading to involve the articular surface. This means larger erosions are seen on the metatarsal heads than in the adjacent phalanges (Martel et al 1980). The first erosions are often seen in the lateral aspects of the fifth metatarsal heads followed by the medial aspects of the heads of the other metatarsals (Fletcher & Rowly 1952, Thould & Simon 1966). Enlarging bony defects with destruction accompany the progressive loss of joint space. In the great toe, erosions of the sesamoids (Resnick et al 1977) are best shown on tangential views. Alignment abnormalities are common. Hallux valgus is commonest, occurring in 70% of cases reviewed by Videgal et al (1975). Calabro (1975) found the incidence was commoner in women and increased with the duration of the disease. Hallux rigidus, chisel toes and hallux elevatus are also seen (Kirkup et al 1977). Resnick (1975) found abnormalities in the first metatarsophalangeal articulation related to the rheumatoid process in up to 50% of foot radiographs.

Lateral sesamoid dislocation is associated with lateral drift of the flexor hallucis longus tendon, resulting in widening of the intermetatarsal spaces between the first and second toes and between the fourth and fifth toes, thus broadening the forefoot. Fibular deviation of the toes may occur with subluxation and dislocation due to

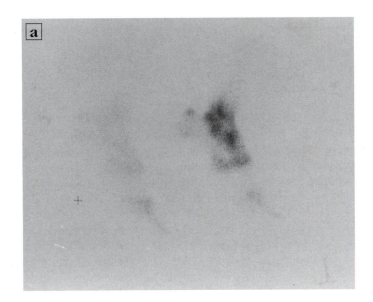

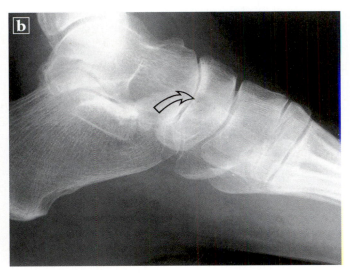

Figure 51

Rheumatoid arthritis. (a) A 99mTcMDP bone scan locates site of disease in this 20-year-old woman. (b) Plain films show corresponding loss of articular cartilage in the talonavicular joint with a subarticular erosion in the navicular (arrow). The subtalar joint was also narrowed

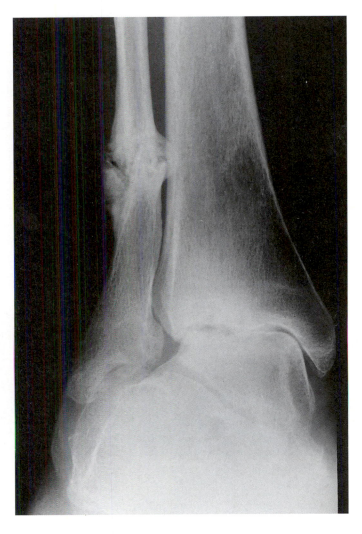

Figure 52

Rheumatoid arthritis: a standing AP view of the ankle shows a healing fibular stress fracture. There is ankle joint disease, a valgus hindfoot and fibular impingement

hyperextension at the metatarsophalangeal joints and flexion at the proximal interphalangeal joints. The fifth toe is usually spared.

Deformities in the midfoot and hindfoot, particularly pes planus and pes planovalgus, may be seen late in the disease. Subtalar views or CT may be needed to demonstrate fully hindfoot joint disease. Subtalar joint erosion may cause collapse of the weight-bearing surfaces (Fig. 49). Calcaneal subluxation may result in a valgus heel deformity and fibular impingement (Fig. 50). A valgus hindfoot deformity was found in 53 of 100 feet (50 adults) by Kirkup et al (1974). Tarsal fusion was found

in 25 tarsal bones after an average of 19 years' disease. Scintigraphy may indicate occult disease overlooked on initial films (Fig. 51a&b). Stress fractures are common in patients with rheumatoid arthritis (Fig. 52) (Miller et al 1967). Synovitis, synovial hypertrophy and joint effusion are common complications, as are the deformities due to bone destruction and ligamentous damage.

MRI is superior to plain films in detecting early cysts and erosions (Poleksic et al 1993). Gubler et al (1993) found that the subarticular cysts in the 'cystic' form of rheumatoid arthritis did not enhance with intravenous gadolinium, which suggests that they are truly

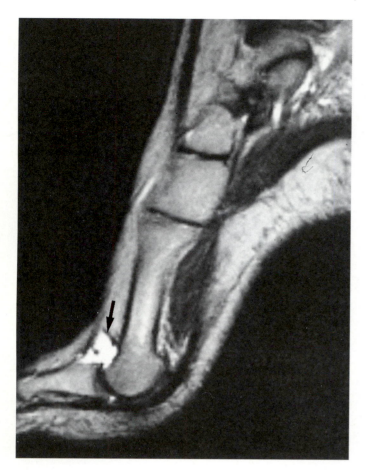

Figure 53

Rheumatoid arthritis: T2-weighted SE sagittal MRI showing high signal in relation to the first metatarsophalangeal joint due to synovitis and fluid (arrow) not suspected on plain films or scintigraphy. High signal was also shown in relation to the other metatarsophalangeal joints on more lateral sections

intraosseous and do not contain synovium. MRI may detect inflammatory change earlier than does scintigraphy (Fig. 53). T2-weighted sequences will show, but not differentiate between, swollen synovium and joint effusion. A recent study suggests that intravenous gadolinium enhancement may help with this differentiation (Bjorkengren et al 1989).

MRI will also detect synovial proliferation and cysts in the sinus tarsal bones (Klein et al 1993, Erickson et al 1990a) in patients presenting with sinus tarsi syndrome, which may not be shown by other techniques.

The seronegative arthropathies

Changes in peripheral joints in the seronegative arthropathies tend to be poorly recognized, which often leads to late diagnosis (Hammerschlag et al 1991).

The seronegative arthropathies have certain basic similarities (Resnick 1979) involving cartilaginous articulations in the axial skeleton with occasional involvement of synovial joints of the peripheral skeleton. The synovial inflammatory changes are less florid than in rheumatoid arthritis. Classic radiological features in the peripheral skeleton include asymmetrical joint involvement, absence of osteoporosis, presence of soft tissue swelling and joint space narrowing, which may lead to osseous erosion and bony fusion. Bony proliferation is characteristic and may be intra- or extra-articular involving sites of tendon and ligamentous attachments (Resnick & Niwayama 1977). In the foot, common sites are the plantar and posterior aspects of the calcaneum in relation to the plantar fascia and Achilles tendon attachments (Gerster et al 1977). Radiographs may be normal or may show irregularity and sclerosis at the site of the increased 99mTcMDP uptake due to the enthesiopathy (Fig. 54ab&c). Fluffy periosteal new bone may also develop along shafts of the phalanges and metatarsals and around the ankle joint. Destruction in relation to the distal interphalangeal joints resulting in the 'cup and pencil' appearance and resorption of the phalangeal tufts are classic features of psoriatic arthropathy (Martel et al 1980). The disease may progress to arthritis mutilans. Mason et al (1959) made a comparative radiological study of Reiter's disease, rheumatoid arthritis and ankylosing spondylitis, and found Reiter's disease has a predilection for the feet, involving them twice as often as the hands. Chand and Johnson (1980) found in a review of 91 feet in 61 patients with Reiter's disease that the radiological changes matched the clinical findings and that the type and location of the foot pain should alert the clinician and the radiologist to suspect the diagnosis. In a series of 25 patients with long-standing ankylosing spondylitis 15% had involvement of the feet (Resnick 1974). Changes were seen in the metatarsophalangeal joints with erosion and bony proliferation, especially on the medial sides of the metatarsal heads. In all the seronegative conditions, periostitis of the phalanges and metatarsals occasionally proceeds to bony ankylosis.

The crystal arthropathies

The commonest crystal induced arthropathies are calcium pyrophosphate deposition (CPPD) and gout. Less commonly, periarticular aggregates of hydroxyapatite crystals (HA) may be a cause for severe local pain and inflammation in the foot and ankle.

Calcium pyrophosphate deposition arthropathy

In the foot, CPPD arthropathy tends to affect the talocalcaneonavicular complex (Reginato et al 1970). Both the acute symptoms and the late radiographic changes may

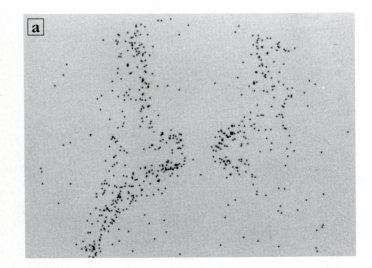

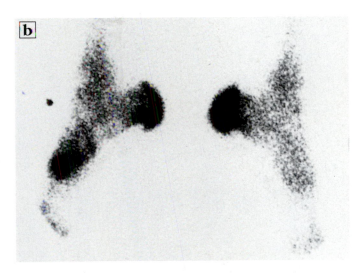

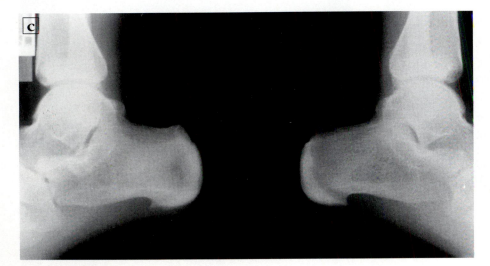

Figure 54

Reiter's disease: 20-year-old man with painful heels. (a) Perfusion and (b) delayed phase 99mTcMDP scans show increased perfusion in both heels and in the region of the right metatarsals matched by superficial bony uptake on delayed bone phase. (c) Radiographs show erosions and bony proliferation on plantar surfaces of both calcanei due to enthesiopathy

be mistaken for other conditions such as gout, infection, rheumatoid arthritis and other inflammatory arthropathies. The diagnosis in the foot is more likely to be considered if there are characteristic changes in other joints.

Gout

The radiology of gout (Watt & Middlemiss 1975) reflects the clinical and pathological features (Resnick & Niwayama 1988b). During an acute attack there is soft tissue swelling around the affected joint, and the swelling disappears when the attack subsides. As the disease progresses, eccentric nodular soft tissue prominence or tophi develop. When calcification occurs within these tophi, it tends to form peripherally as a faint cloud-like radio-opacity. An overhanging bony rim develops as these enlarge. Distinctive radiological features of gout occur late compared with other arthropathies with initial preservation of joint space and relative lack of

osteoporosis. The plain films may be normal even after recurrent attacks. Erosions eventually occur due to tophaceous deposits and many be intra-articular, para-articular or some distance from the joint (Fig. 55). The erosions often develop a sclerotic rim resulting in a well defined 'punched-out' appearance.

The commonest site of involvement in the foot is the first metatarsophalangeal joint, followed by the fifth. Erosions tend to occur medially and dorsally in the first metatarsal head. Rarely, a severely destructive arthropathy can occur. Biochemical and clinical confirmation is usual, but plain films can monitor the rate of progression of the bony and cartilaginous changes.

Calcium hydroxyapatite deposition

HA deposition can occur in the foot (Weston 1959, Gruneberg 1963): patients present with periarticular pain and soft tissue swelling mimicking other conditions such

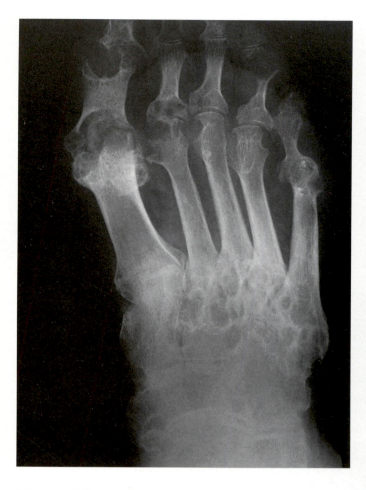

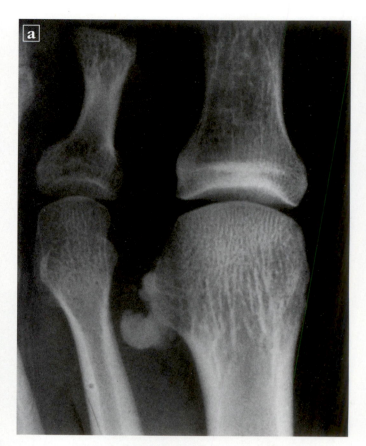

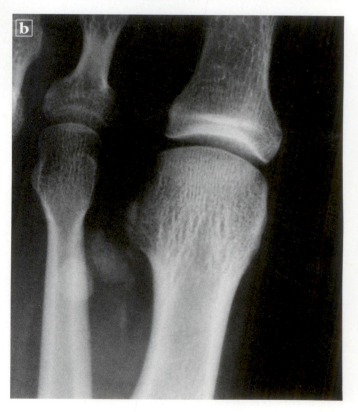

Figure 55

Gout: multiple well defined 'punched out' erosions with a sclerotic edge are typical of gouty arthritis. These may be away from the joint undercutting it as in the second and fifth metatarsal heads. Bone density is preserved

as infection and gout. In the foot and ankle, deposits may be seen in relation to the Achilles tendon, the peroneus longus tendon and the flexor tendons of the forefoot (Holt & Keats 1993). Initially, the HA crystal deposits are thin, cloud-like and poorly defined, and they gradually become much denser and better defined. Although often as dense as bone, close observation shows the homogeneous nature of the deposit is quite different and distinctive. The aggregate of crystals may disperse slowly, as it developed (Fig. 56a&b), or may suddenly shed into adjacent soft tissues, joint or bursa.

Tumours and tumour-like lesions

Soft tissue tumours and tumour-like lesions are common in the foot and ankle and are mainly benign, whereas bone lesions, especially malignant ones, are rare (Dahlin & Unni 1986, Mirra 1989, Huvos 1991). Many lesions, not

Figure 56

Hydroxyapatite deposition: unexplained pain in the forefoot. (a) There are dense areas of calcification between the first and second metatarsal head. Two weeks later the calcification is fading (b) and eventually it disappeared

strictly tumours, are clinically indistinguishable. Kirby et al (1989) studied 83 patients presenting with suspected foot tumours: they found that 87% were benign and that of the malignant ones nearly half were synovial sarcomas. Ganglion cysts were the commonest benign lesions, followed by plantar fibromatosis.

Bone destruction or erosion may occur in lesions within or adjacent to bone. Soft tissue components are not reliably shown on plain films unless they contain some distinguishing feature such as calcium, bone or air. In the small curved bones of the mid and hindfoot, CT may define abnormalities not seen on plain films, such as the intramedullary and extraosseous soft tissue component and its relationship to vessels and joints. It also defines the margins of the bony component, which may be thinned, expanded or breached. It can help to differentiate between benign and malignant soft tissue lesions (Sunderman & McQuire 1988, Moskovic et al 1992), but MRI is now considered the best overall method of imaging and staging these (Petasnick et al 1986, Berquist et al 1989, Keigley et al 1989, Wetzel & Levine 1990, Kerr 1992, Greenfield et al 1993). Although indicators such as the signal characteristics (Wetzel & Levine 1990) or lesion size (Armstrong et al 1992) may help in the diagnosis, in most cases it is not possible to differentiate between benign and malignant (Kransdorph et al 1989, Crim et al 1992). Calcification and gas in the soft tissues may be overlooked by MRI (Totty et al 1986). CT using two- and three-dimensional reformations contributes greatly to the planning of therapeutic irradiation (Magid 1993) and is more readily available than MRI. In both CT and MRI, a skin marker makes it easier to define the suspected lesion and to plan the imaging planes.

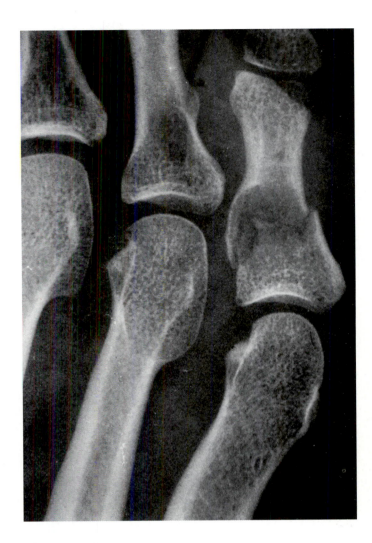

Figure 57

Enchondroma: expansile bony lesion containing speckled calcification and presenting with pathological fracture

Benign bone tumours

Osteoid osteomas and enchondromas are the most commonly encountered benign bone tumours in the foot (Dahlin & Unni 1986). Enchondromas are well-defined, expansile lesions common in metatarsals and phalanges and can be diagnosed on plain films. They may contain calcification and often present as a pathological fracture (Fig. 57).

Up to 10% of osteoid osteomas occur in the foot, especially in the talus (Shereff et al 1983), and their diagnosis depends on clinical suspicion, since the plain films are often normal. An isotope bone scan with vascular phase is needed to locate the lesion (Helms et al 1984) (Fig. 58ab&c). Classically, uptake is increased in all phases, although subperiosteal (Lander et al 1986) and intra-articular lesions may show atypical radiological appearances (Helms et al 1984, Caesar-Pullicino et al 1992) (Fig. 59). Tomography or high resolution fine section CT (Aisen & Glazer 1984, Lander et al 1986) are required to demonstrate the confirmatory central lucency

and sclerotic nidus (Fig. 58c). This can be ablated by introducing a percutaneous needle under CT control (Doyle & King 1989).

Different densities measured by Hounsfield units will help distinguish synovial fluid, blood, fat and fibrous tissue on CT. Fluid levels may be shown on CT and MRI in some lesions, especially aneurysmal bone cysts, but this appearance is nonspecific and can be seen in cysts, tumours and even fibrous dysplasia (Tsai et al 1990).

Malignant bone tumours

Malignant bone tumours are rare in the foot. Ewing's sarcoma is commonest and has a 3–4% incidence (Reinus et al 1985). The plain films show periosteal layering and bone destruction, which may be indistinguishable from

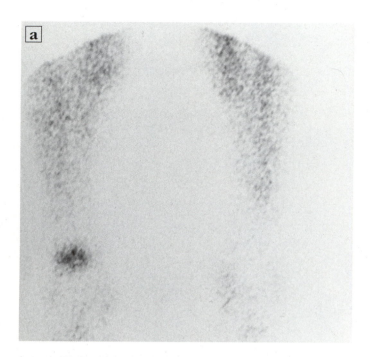

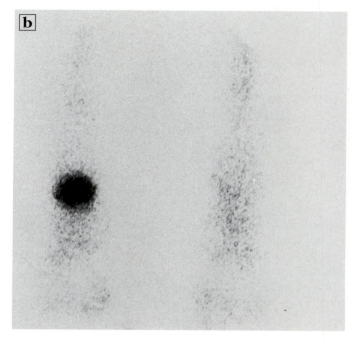

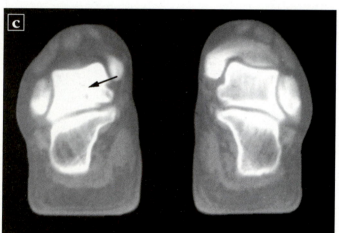

Figure 58

Osteoid osteoma of talus. (a) Increased perfusion and (b) increased delayed phase uptake by 99mTcMDP is typical of this tumour. (c) Coronal CT scan shows small lucent area with sclerotic centre confirming the diagnosis

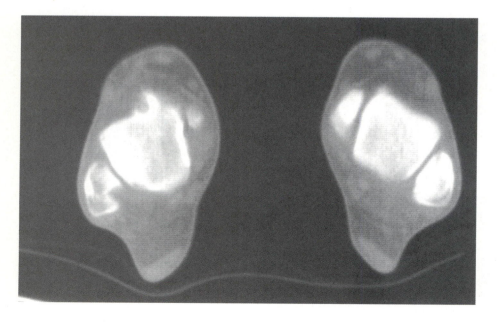

Figure 59

Sub-periosteal osteoid osteoma talus: axial CT scan locates lesion localized by a positive isotope scan

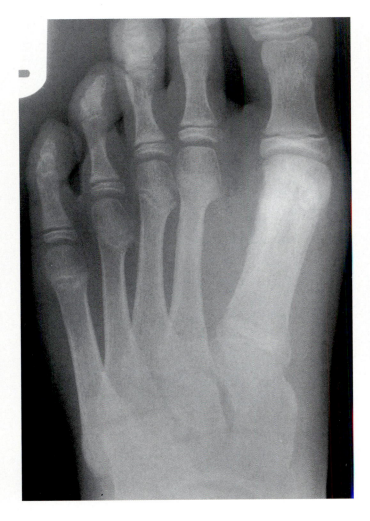

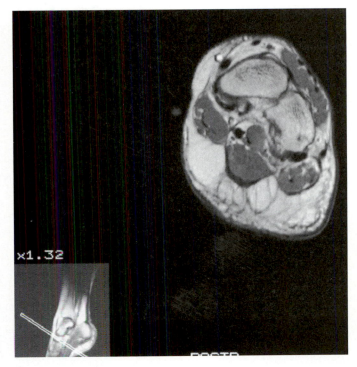

Figure 61

Lipoma: T1-weighted SE oblique coronal MRI sequence shows a well defined high signal lesion in the medial aspect of foot due to a lipoma

Figure 60

Ewing's tumour of first metatarsal: layers of periosteal new bone formation have similar appearance to chronic osteomyelitis

chronic osteomyelitis (Fig. 60). Scintigraphy, CT and even MRI, although highly sensitive, may be no more specific. CT will demonstrate the interface between normal and abnormal bone and will detect periosteal reaction, which may be the first indicator of tumour recurrence or progression (Magid 1993). It can demonstrate the soft tissue component and its relationship to important structures.

Metastases occasionally arise in the feet, most commonly in tarsals and metatarsals (Zindick et al 1982), and may mimic primary malignancies.

Benign soft tissue tumours and tumour-like lesions

Soft tissue masses in the foot are commonly due to benign conditions such as lipomas, haemangiomas, neuromas, plantar fibromatosis and ganglion (Kirby et al 1989). On MRI, some of these benign conditions show a specific signal pattern, which may – if taken in context with the site and clinical picture – suggest a particular tissue diagnosis (Kransdorph et al 1991).

Lipomas can be distinguished from other lesions by their low attenuation on CT and by the fat signal on MRI (Fig. 61). They are well-marginated, lobulated mass lesions, which may be traversed by strands of fibrous tissue and may contain fine calcification. However, there are variants of lipoma that contain other tissue components and therefore have different characteristics on MRI (Kransdorph et al 1991) and tend to mimic liposarcoma.

Hemangiomata are uncommon in the foot and tend to occur medially in the plantar aspect (Tubiolo et al 1986). Angiography or MRI angiography will identify feeding vessels (Fig. 62), and these can then be removed surgically or embolized.

Pigmented villonodular synovitis is a synovial proliferative disorder of unknown aetiology (Granowitz et al 1976), that can affect joint, tendon sheath or bursa. Plain films may be unhelpful unless the lesion causes pressure erosion on bone or a soft tissue mass is shown. The knee and hip are most commonly affected, followed by the ankle and small joints of the feet and hands (Dorwart et al 1984). Synovial pigmentation due to haemosiderin from recurrent haemorrhage produces paramagnetic

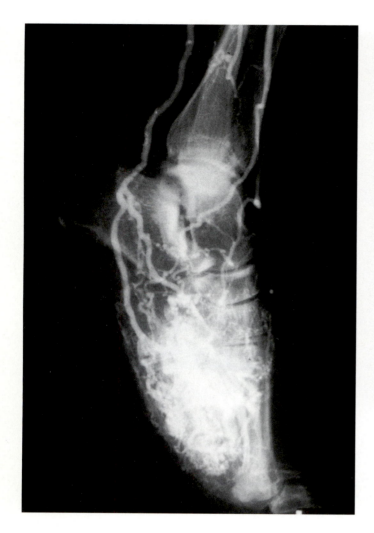

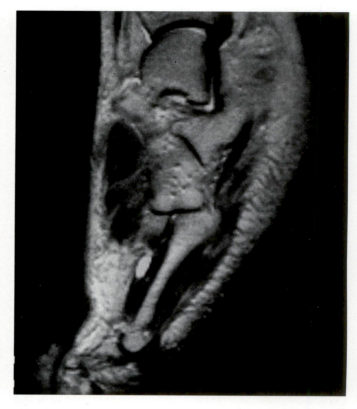

Figure 63

Ganglion: sagittal T2-weighted SE MRI sequence showing high signal area between metatarsals. The appearances are non-specific but were in keeping with the clinical diagnosis of a ganglion cyst

Figure 62

Hemangioma: angiogram showing feeding vessels with view to embolization

effects on MRI. Characteristic areas of low signal on T1- and T2-weighted sequences are classic, interspersed with signal change related to fresh blood from more recent haemorrhage. Interdigital or Morton's neuromas are not tumours but considered to be fibrosing degenerative or traumatic lesions around a digital nerve (Reed & Bliss 1973). The clinical diagnosis is usually apparent. They can be shown on ultrasound as a hypoechoic mass parallel to the long axis of the metatarsals (Redd et al 1987) which can also be detected by MRI (Fieldman et al 1989).

Ganglia present as fluctuant swellings, which can be detected by ultrasound and particularly well on MRI (Fig. 63). T2-weighted sequences are best to show the relationship of the ganglion to the joint capsule (Fieldman et al 1989). They tend to be lobulated and often partitioned by fibrous septae. Pseudopodia extend along fascial planes, and small capsulated cysts may extend into adjacent joints or tendon sheaths (McEvedy

1962). Other lesions, including tumours, can have similar signal characteristics.

The fibromatoses are another group of benign lesions that are infiltrative and liable to recurrence (Aviles et al 1971). In the foot, these tend to be superficial in the form of plantar fibromatosis and present as a firm nodule on the sole of the foot. The extent of the condition is best assessed by MRI (Quinn et al 1991) (Fig. 64a&b). The lesions are well defined by subcutaneous soft tissue, being low signal on T1-weighted images and low to intermediate on T2-weighted images.

Neurofibromata show relatively high signal on T2-weighted MRI images, reflecting the high fluid content in the endoneural matrix, although focal low signal areas may also be present on this sequence. They are not encapsulated and may infiltrate the soft tissues.

Malignant soft tissue tumours

MRI, with its multiplanar imaging potential, has revolutionized the investigation and management of malignant

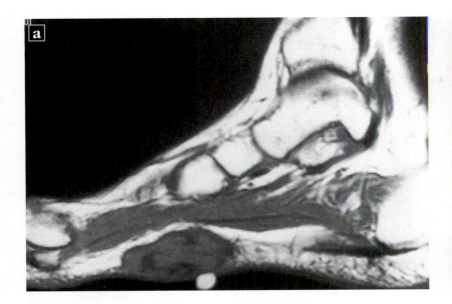
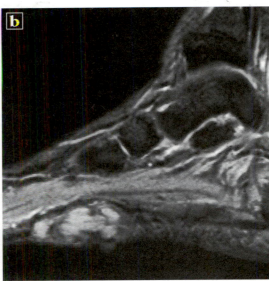

Figure 64

Plantar fibromatosis. (a) Sagittal T1-weighted and (b) sagittal T2-weighted SE sequences show extent of a plantar soft tissue swelling. Mixed signal characteristics were shown and appearances, although compatible with, are not specific for this lesion

soft tissue lesions, although CT is also useful when MRI is not available. Classically, tumour appearance on MRI is intermediate signal on T1-weighted (grey) and high signal on T2-weighted images (white), although in most tumours or mass lesions there is a degree of heterogenicity. The signal pattern may be modified by haemorrhage, calcium, fat or necrosis. High signal intensity on T1-weighted images suggests fat or blood; low signal on T2-weighted images suggests high cellularity due to fibrous tissue, bone, calcium or haemosiderin. Involvement of bone and spread to bone marrow can be demonstrated by the relatively low signal of the tumour compared to the higher signal of the marrow fat on the T1-weighted or proton density sequence (Fig. 65ab&c). Although MRI is unreliable for differentiating between benign and malignant lesions, it can define the extent of the lesion. It is useful in assessing recurrent disease after surgery (Reuther & Mutschler 1990, Huvos 1991), although after radiation therapy the inflammatory response may be indistinguishable from tumour (Vanel et al 1987). The effect of chemotherapy on bone and soft tissue tumours and their imaging characteristics is still being evaluated (Erlemann et al 1990).

Bone and soft tissue infection

The diagnosis of bone and soft tissue infection, particularly in the foot, remains a major diagnostic problem. The plantar surface is prone to puncture wounds, foreign bodies and skin ulceration. The risk is much greater in patients with neuropathic conditions, such as diabetes and rheumatoid arthritis, where pressure points, such as the calcaneum and metatarsal heads, are particularly vulnerable to skin infection (Zlatkin et al 1987), which may spread to osteomyelitis and septic arthritis if diagnosis is delayed. Open fractures and surgical procedures may be complicated by osteomyelitis. Clinicopathologicoradiological correlation of all types of skeletal sepsis are covered comprehensively by Resnick and Niwayama (1988d).

Acute osteomyelitis

Plain radiographs are normal for days to weeks after onset of symptoms (Resnick & Niwayama 1988e). The first radiological sign is osteoporosis, followed by periostitis. With modern imaging allowing early diagnosis, plain film changes are seldom seen in acute infection but may indicate a foreign body. Ultrasound can also locate non-opaque foreign material (Kaplan et al 1989). Because of the insensitivity of radiographs, it is usual to proceed to a 99mTcMDP bone scan. The specificity can be increased by employing the three-phase technique (Gilday et al 1975, Gold et al 1991), which in most cases differentiate between cellulitis and osteomyelitis (Fig. 66ab&c). The sensitivity of the three-phase technique decreases in neonates (Gilday et al 1975, Handmaker 1980, Sullivan et al 1980), where a negative or equivocal scan should be followed by a 67-gallium scan (Lisbona & Rosental 1977, Alazraki et al 1985a, Schauwecker 1992). Sensitivity is also reduced when there is bone remodelling as in acute

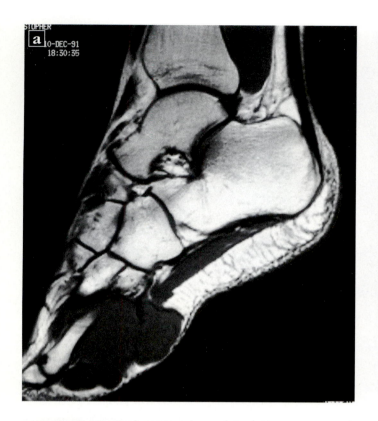

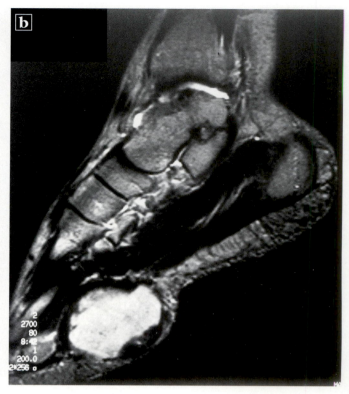

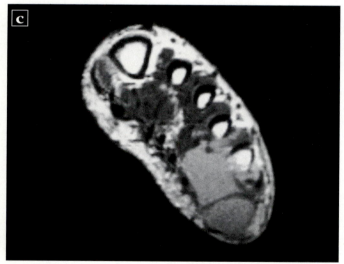

Figure 65

Rhabdomysarcoma. (a) and (b) Sagittal T1- and T2-weighted sequences show a large mass lesion destroying the fourth metatarsal and infiltrating the marrow. (c) Proton density oblique coronal sequence

complicating osteomyelitis (Schauwecker et al 1984) (discussed below).

CT is more sensitive than plain films in detecting early infective changes (Kuhn & Berger 1979) and can be used to evaluate an area of focal uptake on a bone scan. MRI has higher sensitivity than CT in diagnosing early changes of acute skeletal infection (Chandnani et al 1990), and, when available, has the advantages of no irradiation, of multiplanar imaging potential and of high tissue contrast. It provides excellent appreciation of bone marrow, joint and soft tissue abnormality in skeletal inflammatory and infective processes (Tang et al 1988, Unger et al 1988, Yuh et al 1989). Although it is consid-

ered to provide the most accurate picture in skeletal infection with distinct advantages over CT and isotope studies (Beltran et al 1988), the routine plain films and three-phase 99mTcMDP scan are usually adequate in the diagnosis of acute skeletal infection. MRI is more justified in complicated and chronic situations.

Sub-acute and chronic osteomyelitis

Sub-acute osteomyelitis may present as a Brodie's abscess in children and young adults, affecting the distal tibial metaphysis and tarsals, particularly the calcaneum.

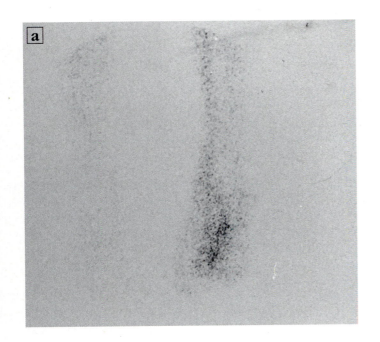

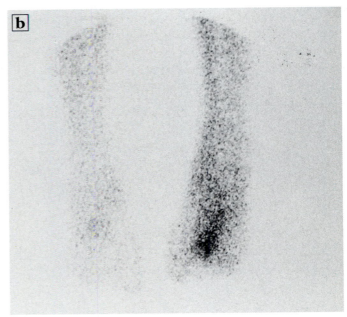

Figure 66

Septic arthritis after penetrating injury. (a) Perfusion, (b) blood pool, and (c) delayed phases of 99mTcMDP bone scan show isotope accumulation around the third metatarsophalangeal joint. Plain film changes did not develop because of early diagnosis and treatment

Plain films are usually diagnostic and show a multiloculated lucency with a sclerotic rim. Although often indolent, these may reactivate with spread of infection across the growth plate to the epiphysis and joint, resulting in synovitis and septic arthritis. Articular cartilage and subchondral bone destruction may lead to arthrodesis, and growth plate damage to premature epiphyseal closure or valgus/varus deformity. Tomography may provide useful information if surgery is considered. A 99mTcMDP scan will show absence of growth plate uptake, if this has closed prematurely.

Chronic osteomyelitis may result from an inadequately treated acute haematogenous infection or may occur after an open fracture or surgical procedure. Thickening and sclerosis of cortical bone forms an involucrum, with cavitation and sequestration inside it. There may be soft tissue collections of pus and debris, and joints may be primarily or secondarily involved. Radiographic features (Fig. 67) may also persist after treatment, and a 99mTcMDP bone scan may remain positive after antibiotic treatment, owing to bone remodelling rather than persisting infection (Alazraki et al 1985a). It is claimed (Alazraki et al 1985b, Israel et al 1987) that by following a three-phase 99mTcMDP bone scan by 24-hour images, accuracy is improved since the ratio of the lesion uptake to normal bone should continue to increase

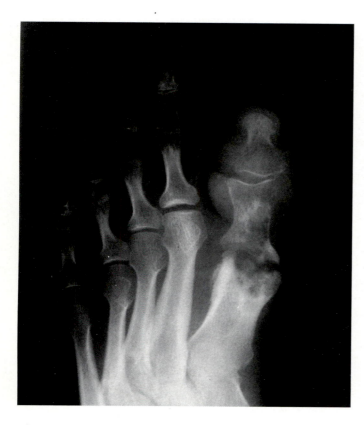

Figure 67

Osteomyelitis and septic arthritis: late diagnosis of an infected first metatarsophalangeal joint in this immunosuppressed patient resulted in destruction of the joint and spread of the infection proximally to destroy the metatarsal shaft. Distally there is early involvement of the interphalangeal joint which is subluxed due to pus formation

during the fourth phase in infection. This is claimed to be useful in evaluating ischaemic feet.

For detecting recurrent infection in chronic osteomyelitis, white cells labelled with 111 indium can be employed (Schauwecker et al 1984, Merkel et al 1985, Schauwecker 1989, Seabold et al 1990, Jacobson et al 1991). More recently, 99mTcHMPAO-labelled white cells have been used. This technique provides better image quality owing to the far greater radioactivity and can be prepared in the laboratory from a kit (Schauwecker 1989, Hovi et al 1993). However, all white cell labelling techniques are tedius and time-consuming.

In chronic osteomyelitis CT can show medullary cavity and cortical involvement; in conjunction with conventional tomograms it can enable planning for the surgical approach to remove sequestra (Fig. 68) (Seltzer 1984).

MRI can distinguish between soft tissue and bony infection and between cellulitis and abscess formation (Unger et al 1988, Yuh et al 1989), both important factors in surgical management. Ultrasound can also define fluid collections. Differentiation of areas of 'healed' from active infection may be difficult (Erdman et al 1991) even with MRI. Sinus tracts show as areas of linear increased signal, extending through the bony cortex to the skin on T2-weighted images. The high signal helps to differentiate a sinus from an old retracted scar. Sequestra are not as well shown with MRI as on CT, and small ones may be missed, especially when thicker-image slices are taken. Detection of articular cartilage destruction may be seen more easily on T2-weighted and STIR sequences in the presence of joint fluid. Erdman et al (1991) found the differentiation between reactive oedema and extension of the infective process difficult in the early phases, since in 60% of cases in their series of septic arthritis marrow oedema was subsequently shown to be reactive and not infective.

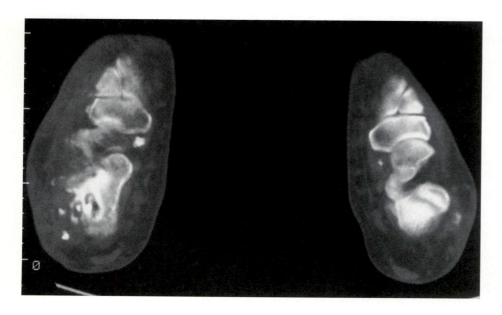

Figure 68

Chronic osteomyelitis: axial CT scan of feet shows cavitation in the right calcaneum. Sequestra are present both within and extruded out of the bone

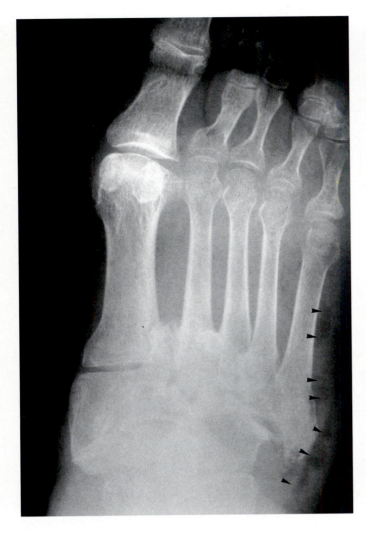

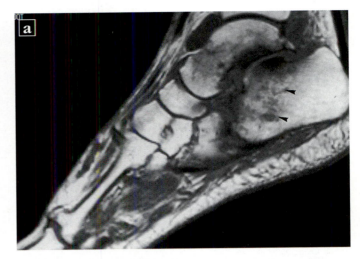

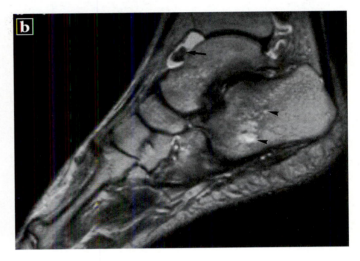

Figure 69

Diabetic foot: Neuropathic and infective changes are present. There is disorganization of the midfoot and evidence of a gas forming infection in the soft tissues (arrow heads)

Figure 70

Diabetic foot: MRI scans. (a) Sagittal T1-weighted and (b) sagittal T2-weighted SE sequences show reduced and increased signal respectively across the calcaneum (arrow heads) but no cortical bone destruction was shown. Appearances represented a stress fracture. Joint effusion and intra-articular loose body are features of the neuropathic joint damage

A review article (Schauwecker 1992) concludes that, although MRI has the best resolution of bone against soft tissue, the results are no better than the three-phase 99mTcMDP scan, which is adequate in most clinical situations.

Many chronic foot infections involving bone are found in neuropathic conditions, especially diabetes, and the associated diagnostic problems are discussed separately.

The neuropathic foot

Diabetes is the commonest cause of neuropathic bone and joint disease in the foot and presents a particular diagnostic problem, since neuropathic and infective changes may coexist. Lack of pain appreciation and of awareness of skeletal damage results in joint effusions and micro- (or frank) fractures, followed by subluxation and eventually complete disorganization of the joint. The midtarsal region is particularly susceptible, but the ankle may also be affected. Radiological features include disorganization with formation of varying amounts of loose fragments and debris (Newman 1981, Cofield et al 1983, Zlatkin et al 1987) with preservation or even increase in bone density. Damage can progress rapidly and one author (Goldman 1982) suggested this developed over a range of 1–15 months. The rate of destruction may be so severe that it mimics an infective cause. Other factors may contribute to the demise of the joints, such as ataxia, steroid injection and osteoporosis. Fig. 69 shows neuropathic midfoot changes of disorganization

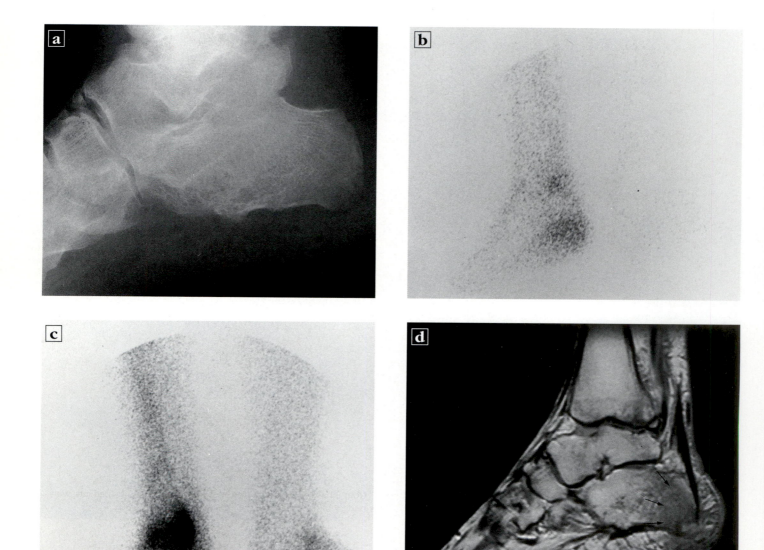

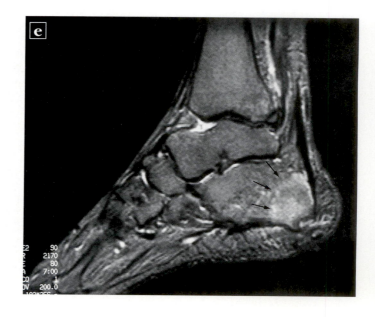

Figure 71

Neuropathic foot: 24-year-old woman with spina bifida and
skin ulceration. (a) Cortical destruction and gas in soft
tissues at the back of the heel are shown on radiograph,
with (b) increase in perfusion, and (c) delayed phase isotope
uptake in calcaneum and in medial malleolus. (d) T1-
weighted and (e) T2-weighted SE MRI sequences show
alteration in marrow signal, which is low on T1 and high on
T2 (arrows), radiating from the area of cortical destruction.
Osteomyelitis was confirmed in both calcaneum and medial
malleolus on exploration

associated with a gas-containing soft tissue abscess due to anaerobic infection. A neuropathic feature, also seen in leprosy and rheumatoid arthritis, is circumferential resorption of the metatarsal shafts such that they become spindled and pointed. Felson (1970) relates this to neurovascular abnormality.

Pre-existing neuropathic changes, particularly fractures and ischaemia, result in over-diagnosis of infection on plain films and 99mTcMDP radionuclide studies in diabetics (Maurer et al 1986, Unger et al 1988). It is suggested (Seabold et al 1990) that a combined TcMDP/111-indium scanning sequence may help to differentiate between neuropathic and infective change. Schauwecker (1989) found better results with this technique in neuropathic feet than in osteomyelitis at other sites, owing to less background artefact and lack of 111-indium leucocyte uptake in the normal bone marrow; Larcos et al (1991) also found it useful in the diabetic foot.

Yuh et al (1989) compared MRI favourably with scintigraphy in the diabetic foot. Other studies (e.g. Berquist et al 1985) found MRI more accurate than CT and plain films; 111-indium leucocyte scans were the method of choice after surgery. Unger et al (1988) found that the absence of abnormal marrow signal in a diabetic patient with cellulitis and skin lesions rules out osteomyelitis. Further studies support the role of MRI in the diabetic foot (Beltran et al 1988, Erdman et al 1991, Durham et al 1991). The main problem with MRI is differentiating between marrow oedema from microfractures and from osseous infection (Moore et al 1991).

Fig. 70a&b shows sagittal MRI images in an 18-year-old diabetic girl with progressive foot pain and deformity. There is intra-osseous oedema (high signal on T2-weighted scans) within the calcaneum, owing to a fracture, and bony debris within the anterior part of the ankle joint. No articular cartilage or subchondral bone erosion was shown to suggest infection, despite the large joint effusion. Fig. 71abcd&e shows cortical bone destruction over the back of the calcaneum in a 24-year-old patient with spina bifida. A 99mTcMDP scan shows increased perfusion and delayed uptake in this site and also in the medial malleolus. MRI sequences confirm osteomyelitis due to spreading infection from skin ulceration.

Infection of a tendon sheath may result from direct spread from adjacent tissues. A small amount of fluid is commonly seen in tendon sheaths of the foot and ankle, particularly in the active, but a larger amount suggests pathology. However, MRI will not reliably distinguish between infective and sterile tenosynovitis.

In conclusion, MRI can help to differentiate between infective and traumatic changes in the diabetic foot, provided the images are interpreted with other investigations and with the pitfalls in mind (Erdman et al 1991). In a few cases, in the event of recent neuropathic fractures, it will not be possible to rule out infection by any imaging technique. Conversely, a normal MRI scan is reassuring, since it tends to rule out infection.

Other foot infections

In vascular insufficiency and neurological deficit, there is a higher incidence of clostridial and non-clostridial gas-forming infections (see Fig. 69).

Tuberculous dactylitis involves the small tubular bones of the hand and foot (Eideken et al 1963). It commonly occurs before the age of five. Soft tissue swelling is followed by expansion of bone, which appears cystic (spina ventosa). Spread along the bone to involve joints with sequestration and sinus tract formation is common in childhood.

For bone changes in tropical diseases, such as maduromycosis, leprosy yaws and ainhum, the reader is referred to dedicated texts on tropical disease of bone (Reeder 1970) and to Chapter VIII.1.

References

Aisen A M, Glazer G M 1984 Diagnosis of osteoid osteoma using computed tomography. J Comput Assist Tomogr 8: 175–178

Alazraki N 1988 Radionuclide techniques. In: Resnick D and Niwayama G (eds) Diagnosis of Bone and Joint Disorders 2nd edn. W B Saunders: Philadelphia. 1: 460–505

Alazraki N P, Fierer J, Resnick D 1985a Chronic osteomyelitis. Monitoring by 99mTc phosphate and 67Ga-citrate imaging. Am J Roentgenol 145: 767–771

Alazraki N, Dries D, Datz F et al 1985b Value of a 24 hour image (four phase bone scan) in assessing osteomyelitis in patients with peripheral vascular disease. J Nucl Med 26: 711–717

Anderson I F, Chichton K J, Gratton-Smith T et al 1989 Osteochondral fractures of the dome of the talus. J Bone Joint Surg [Am] 71: 1143–1152

Andre M, Resnick D 1988 Computed tomography. In: Resnick D and Niwayama G (eds) Diagnosis of Bone and Joint Disorders 2nd edn. W B Saunders: Philadelphia. 1: 143–202

Armstrong S J, Wakely C J, Goddard P R et al 1992 Review of the use of MRI in soft tissue lesions. Clin Radiol 46: 311–317

Aviles E, Arlen M and Miller T 1971 Plantar fibromatosis. Surgery 69: 117–120

Beckley D E, Anderson P W, Pedegana L R 1975 The radiology of the subtalar joint with special reference to talocalcaneal coalition. Clin Radiol 26: 333–341

Beltran J, McGhee R B, Shaffer P B et al 1988 Experimental infections of the musculoskeletal system: Evaluation with MR imaging and Tc-99m MDP and Ga67 scintigraphy. Radiology 167: 167–172

Beltran J, Munchow A M, Khabiri H et al 1990 Ligaments of the lateral aspect of the ankle and sinus tarsi: MR imaging. Radiology 177: 455–458

Beltran J, Noto A, Herman L J et al 1987 Tendons: High field strength surface coil MR imaging. Radiology 162: 735–740

Berndt A L, Harty M 1959 Transchondral fracture (osteochondritis dissecans) of the talus. J Bone Joint Surg [Am] 41: 988–1020

Berquist T H, Brown M L, Fitzgerald R H et al 1985 Magnetic resonance imaging: Application in musculoskeletal infection. Magn Reson Imaging 3: 219–230

Berquist T H, Ehman R I, King B F et al 1989 Value of MR imaging in differentiating benign from malignant soft tissue masses. Study of 95 lesions. Am J Roentgenol 155: 1251–1255

Bjorkengren A G, Geborek P, Rydholm F et al 1989 MR imaging of the knee in acute rheumatoid arthritis: synovial uptake of gadolinium DTPA. Am J Roentgenol 155: 329–332

Blanchard K S, Finlay B D L, Scott D J A et al 1986 A radiological analysis of lateral ligament injuries of the ankle. Clinical Radiol 37: 247–251

Blei C L, Nirschl R P, Grant E G 1986 Achilles tendon: US diagnosis of pathologic conditions. Radiology 159: 765–767

Brewerton D A, Sandifer P H, Sweetman D R 1963 The aetiology of pes cavus. Br Med J 2: 659–661

Brodsky A E, Khalil M A 1987 Talar compression syndrome. Foot Ankle 7: 338–344

Brody N 1980 Running injuries. CIBA Clin Symp 32: 1–64

Burkus J K, Sella E J, Southwick W O 1984 Occult injuries of the talus diagnosed by bone scan and tomography. Foot Ankle 4: 316–324

Bywaters E G L 1954 Heel lesions of rheumatoid arthritis. Ann Rheum Dis 13: 42–51

Caesar-Pullicino V N, McCall I W, Wan S 1992 Intra-articular osteoid osteoma. Clin Radiol 45: 153–160

Cahill R B, Berg C B 1983 99mTc phosphate compound joint scintigraphy in the management of juvenile osteochondritis dissicans of the femoral condyles. Am J Sports Med 11: 329–335

Calabro J J 1975 A critical evaluation of the feet in rheumatoid arthritis. Arthrit Rheum 5: 19–29

Canale S T, Kelly F B Jn 1978 Fractures of the neck of the talus. Long term evaluation of 71 cases. J Bone Joint Surg [Am] 60: 143–156

Carr C R, Boyd B M 1968 Correctional osteotomy for hallux valgus and matatarsus primus varus. J Bone Joint Surg [Am] 50: 1353–1367

Chambers C H 1950 Congenital anomalies of the tarsal navicular with particular reference to the calcaneo-navicular coalition. Br J Radiol 23: 580–586

Chand Y, Johnson K 1980 Foot and ankle manifestations of Reiter's syndrome. Foot Ankle 1: 167–172

Chandnani V P, Beltran J, Morris C S et al 1990 Acute experimental osteomyelitis and abscesses. Detection with MR imaging versus CT. Radiology 174: 233–236

Clanton T 1989 Instability of the subtalar joint. Orthop Clin North Am 20: 583–591

Cofield R H, Morrison M J, Beabout J W 1983 Diabetic neuropathy in the foot: Patient characteristics and pattern of radiographic change. Foot Ankle 4: 15–22

Coleman B G, Kressel H Y, Dalinka M K et al 1988 Radiographically negative avascular necrosis: detection with MR imaging. Radiology 168: 525–528

Crim J R, Seeger L L, Yao L et al 1992 Diagnosis of soft tissue masses with MR imaging: Can benign masses be differentiated from malignant ones? Radiology 185: 581–586

Daffner R, Reimer B L, Lupetin A R et al 1986 Magnetic resonance imaging of Achilles tendon ruptures. Skeletal Radiol 15: 619–621

Dahlin D C, Unni K K 1986 Bone Tumours. General Aspects and Data on 8,542 Cases 4th edn. Charles C Thomas: Springfield

De Ginder W L 1955 Osteochondritis dissicans of the talus. Radiology 65: 590–598

De Smet A A, Fisher D R, Bernstein M I et al 1989 Value in MR imaging in staging osteochondral lesions of the talus (osteochondritis dissicans): results in 14 patients. Am J Roentgenol 154: 555–558

De Smet A A, Fisher D R, Graf B K et al 1990 Osteochondritis dissicans of the knee: Value of MR imaging in determining lesion stability and the presence of articular cartilage defects. Am J Roentgenol 155: 549–553

Deutch A L 1992 Osteochondral injuries of the talar dome. In: Deutch A L, Mink J H, Kerr R (eds) MRI of the foot and ankle. Raven Press: New York. pp. 111–134

Deutch A L, Resnick D, Campbell G 1982 Computed tomography and bone scintigraphy in the evaluation of tarsal coalition. Radiology 144: 137–139

Dorwart R H, Genant H K, Johnson W H et al 1984 Pigmented villonodular synovitis of synovial joints: Clinical, pathologic, and radiologic features. Am J Roentgenol 143: 877–885

Douglas G, Rang M 1981 The role of trauma in the pathogenesis of the osteochondroses. Clin Orthop Rel Res 158: 28–32

Doyle T, King K 1989 Percutaneous removal of osteoid osteoma using CT control. Clin Radiol 40: 514–517

Durham J R, Lukens M L, Campanini D S et al 1991 Impact of magnetic resonance on the management of diabetic foot infections. Am J Surg 162: 150–154

Eideken J, De Palma A F, Moskowitz H et al 1963 'Cystic' tuberculosis of bone. Clin Orthop Rel Res 28: 163–168

Erdman W A, Tamburro F, Jayson H et al 1991 Osteomyelitis: Characteristics and Pitfalls of diagnosis with MR imaging. Radiology 180: 533–539

Erickson S J, Quinn S F, Kneeland J B et al 1990a MR imaging of the tarsal tunnel and related spaces; normal and abnormal findings with anatomical correlation. Am J Roentgenol 155: 323–328

Erickson S J, Smith J W, Ruiz M E et al 1990b MR imaging of lateral collateral ligament of the ankle. Am J Roentgenol 156: 131–136

Erlemann R, Sciuk J, Bosse A et al 1990 Response of osteosarcoma and Ewings sarcoma to preoperative chemotherapy: assessment with dynamic and static MR imaging and skeletal scintigraphy. Radiology 175: 791–796

Eustace S, O'Byrne J, Stack J et al 1993 Radiographic features that enable assessment of first metatarsal rotation: the role of pronation in hallux valgus. Skelet Radiol 22: 153–156

Eyre-Brook A L 1967 Congenital vertical talus. J Bone Joint Surg [Br] 49: 618–627

Felson B 1970 Letter from the editor. Semin Roentgenol 5: 325–326

Ferkel R D, Flannigan B D, Elkins B S 1991 Magnetic resonance imaging of the foot and ankle: Correlation of normal anatomy and pathologic conditions. Foot Ankle 11: 289–305

Fieldman F, Singson R D and Staron R B 1989 Magnetic resonance imaging of para-articular and ectopic ganglia. Skeletal Radiol 18: 353–358

Fishman E K, Magid D, Robertson D D et al 1987 Advances in CT Imgaing of Musculoskeletal Pathology. In: Scott W W, Magid D, Fishman E K (eds) Computed Tomography of the Musculoskeletal System. Churchill Livingstone: Edinburgh. pp. 213–239

Fletcher D E, Rowly K A 1952 The radiological features of rheumatoid arthritis. Br J Radiol 25: 282–295

Ford L T, Gilula L A 1977 Stress fractures of the middle metatarsals following the Keller operation. J Bone Joint Surg 59: 117–118

Fornage B D 1986 Achilles tendon: US examination. Radiology 159: 759–764

Fornage B D, Rifkin M D 1988 Ultrasound examination of tendons. Radiol Clin N Amer 26: 87–107

Frede T E, Lee J K 1983 Compensatory hypertrophy of bone following surgery on the foot. Radiology 146: 347–348

Freiberger R H, Hersch A, Harrison M O 1970 Roentgen examination of the deformed foot. Sem Roentgenol 5: 341–353

Funk D A, Cass J R, Johnson K A et al 1986 Acquired adult flat foot deformity secondary to posterior tibial tendon pathology. J Bone Joint Surg [Am] 68: 95–102

Genez B M, Wilson M R, Houk R W et al 1988 Early osteonecrosis of the femoral head: detection in high-risk patients with MR imaging. Radiology 168: 521–524

Gerster J C, Vischer T L, Bennani A et al 1977 The painful heel. Comparative study in rheumatoid arthritis, ankylosing spondylitis, Reiter's syndrome and generalised osteoarthrosis. Ann Rheum Dis 36: 343–348

Geslien G E, Thrall J H, Espinona J L et al 1976 Early detection of stress fractures using 99mTc-polyphosphate. Radiology 121: 683–687

Gilday D L, Paul D J, Paterson J 1975 Diagnosis of osteomyelitis in children by combined blood pool and bone imaging. Radiology 117: 331–335

Goergen T G, Venn-Watson E A, Rossman D J et al 1981 Tarsal navicular stress fractures in runners. Am J Roentgenol 136: 201–203

Goiney R C, Connell D G, Nichols D M 1984 CT evaluation of tarsometatarsal fracture-dislocation injuries. Am J Roentgenol 144: 985–990

Gold R H, Hawkins R A, Katz R D 1991 Bacterial osteomyelitis: Findings on plain radiography, CT, MR and scintigraphy. Am J Roentgenol 157: 365–370

Goldman A B 1982 Some miscellaneous joint diseases. Semin Roentgenol 17: 69–80

Goldman A B, Pavlov H, Schneider R 1982 Radionuclide bone scanning in subtalar coalitions: Differential considerations. Am J Roentgenol 138: 427–432

Granowitz S P, D'Antonio J, Mankin H L 1976 The pathogenesis and longterm end results of pigmented villonodular synovitis. Clin Orthop 114: 335–351

Greaney R B, Gerber F H, Laughlin R L et al 1983 Distribution and natural history of stress fractures in U.S. marine recruits. Radiology 146: 339–346

Greenfield G B, Arrington J A, Kudryk B T 1993 MRI of soft tissue tumours. Skeletal Radiol 22: 77–84

Gruneberg R 1963 Calcifying tendinitis in the forefoot. Br J Radiol 36: 378–379

Gubler F M, Algra P R, Maas M et al 1993 Gadolinium-DTPA enhanced magnetic resonance imaging in bone cysts in patients with rheumatoid arthritis. Annals Rheum Dis 52: 716–719

Hamilton W G 1982 Stenosing tenosynovitis of the flexor hallucis longus tendon and posterior impingement upon the os trigonum in ballet dancers. Foot Ankle 3: 74–80

Hammerschlag M D, Rice J R, Caldwell M D et al 1991 Psoriatic arthritis of the foot and ankle: Analysis of joint involvement and diagnostic errors. Foot Ankle 12: 35–39

Handmaker H 1980 Acute haematogenous osteomyelitis: Has the bone scan betrayed us? Radiology 135: 787–789

Harris R I, Beath T 1948 Aetiology of peroneal spastic flat foot. J Bone Joint Surg [Br] 30: 624–634

Hawkins L G 1970 Fractures of the neck of the talus. J Bone Joint Surg [Am] 52: 991–1002

Heger L, Wulff K 1985 Computed tomography of the calcaneus: Normal anatomy. Am J Roentgenol 145: 123–129

Heger L, Wulff K and Seddiqui M S A 1985 Computed tomography of calcaneal fractures. Am J Roentgenol 145: 131–137

Helms C A, Hattner R S, Volger J B I 1984 Osteoid osteoma: Radionuclide diagnosis. Radiology 151: 779–784

Heron C 1993 Magnetic resonance of the foot and ankle. The Foot 3: 1–10

Holt P D, Keats T E 1993 Calcific tendinitis: a review of the usual and unusual. Skeletal Radiol 22: 1–9

Hovi I, Taavitsainen M, Lantto T et al 1993 Technetium-99m-HMPAO labelled leucocytes and Technetium-99m-labelled human polyclonal immunoglobulin G in diagnosis of focal purulent disease. J Nucl Med 9: 1428–1434

Huvos A G 1991 Bone tumours: diagnosis, treatment and prognosis 2nd edn. W B Saunders: Philadelphia

Inglis G, Buxton R A, McNicol M F 1986 Symptomatic calcaneonavicular bars. The results 20 years after surgical excision. J Bone Joint Surg [Br] 68: 128–131

Israel O, Gips S, Jerushalmi J et al 1987 Osteomyelitis and soft tissue infection: Differential diagnosis with 24 hour/4 hour ratio of Tc99m MDP uptake. Radiology 163: 725–726

Jacobson A F, Harley J D, Lipskey B A et al 1991 Diagnosis of osteomyelitis in the presence of soft tissue infection and radiological evidence of osseous abnormalities: Value of leucocyte scintigraphy. Am J Roentgenol 157: 807–813

Jayakumar S, Cowell H R 1977 Rigid flatfoot. Clin Orthop Rel Res 122: 77–84

Johnson R P, Collier B D, Carrera G 1984 The os trigonum syndrome: use of bone scan in the diagnosis. J Trauma 24: 761–764

Kaplan P A, Anderson J C, Norris M A et al 1989 Ultrasonography of post-traumatic soft-tissue lesions. Radiol Clin N Amer 27: 973–982

Karasick J, Wapner K L 1990 Hallux valgus deformity: preoperative assessment. Am J Roentgenol 155: 119–123

Katz J F 1981 Non articular osteochondroses. Clin Orthop Rel Res 158: 70–76

Keats T E 1988 Atlas of Normal Roentgen Variants that may Simulate Disease 4th edn. Chicago: Year Book. pp. 670–746

Keene J S, Lash E G, Fisher D R et al 1989 Magnetic resonance imaging of Achilles tendon ruptures. Am J Sports Med 17: 333–337

Keigley B A, Haggar A M, Gaba A et al 1989 Primary tumours of the foot: MR imaging. Radiology 171: 755–759

Kerr R 1992 Tumours and tumourlike lesions of soft tissue and bone. In: Deutch A L, Mink J H, Kerr R (eds) MRI of the Foot and Ankle. Raven Press: New York. pp. 223–279

Kirby E J, Shereff M J, Lewis M M 1989 Soft-tissue tumours and tumour-like lesions of the foot. J Bone Joint Surg [Am] 71: 621–626

Kirkup J R, Videgal E, Jacoby R K 1974 Ankle and tarsal joints in rheumatoid arthritis. Acta Orthop Scand 3: 50–52

Kirkup J R, Videgal E, Jacoby R K 1977 The hallux and rheumatoid arthritis. Acta Orthop Scand 48: 527–544

Kiss Z S, Khan K M, Fuller P J 1992 Stress fractures of the tarsal navicular bone: CT findings in 55 cases. Am J Roentgenol 160: 111–115

Klein M A, Spreitzer A M 1993 MR imaging of the tarsal sinus and canal: Normal anatomy, pathologic findings, and features of the sinus tarsi syndrome. Radiology 186: 233–240

Kohler A, Zimmer E A 1968 Borderlands of the Normal and Early Pathologic in Skeletal Roentgenology. New York: Grune & Stratton. pp. 459–530

Kransdorph M J, Jelinek J S, Moser R P Jr et al 1989 Soft tissue masses: diagnosis using MR imaging. Am J Roentgenol 153: 541–547

Kransdorph M J, Moser R P J, Meis J M et al 1991 Fat containing soft tissue masses of the extremities. Radiographics 11: 81–106

Kuhn J P, Berger P E 1979 Computed tomographic diagnosis of osteomyelitis. Radiology 130: 503–506

Lander P H, Azouz E M, Marton D 1986 Subperiosteal osteoid osteoma of the talus. Clin Radiol 37: 491–493

Larcos G, Brown M, Sutton R 1991 Diagnosis of osteomyelitis of the foot in diabetic patients: Value of 111In-leukocyte scintigraphy. Am J Roentgenol 157: 527–531

Lawson J P 1985 Symptomatic radiographic variants in extremities. Radiology 157: 625–631

Lawson J P, Ogden J A, Sella E et al 1984 The painful accessory navicular. Skeletal Radiol 12: 250–262

Lee J K, Yao L 1988 Stress fractures: MR imaging. Radiology 169: 217–220

Lisbona R, Rosenthal L 1977 Observations on the sequential use of 99m-Tc-phosphate complex and 67-Ga imaging in osteomyelitis, cellulitis, and septic arthritis. Radiology 123: 123–129

Maffulli N, Lepore L, Francobandiera C 1990 Traumatic lesions of some accessory bones of the foot in sports activity. J Am Podiatr Med Assoc 89: 86–90

Magid D 1993 Two-dimensional and three-dimensional computed tomographic imaging in msculoskeletal tumours. Radiol Clin N Am 425–447

Marcus D S, Reicher M A, Kellerhouse L E 1989 Achilles tendon injuries: The role of MR imaging. J Comput Assist Tomogr 13(3): 480–486

Martel W, Stuck K W, Dworin A M et al 1980 Erosive osteoarthrosis and psoriatic arthritis. Am J Roentgenol 134: 125–135

Martin B F 1989 Posterior triangle pain: the os trigonum. J Foot Surg 28: 312–318

Mason R M, Murray R S, Oates J R et al 1959 A comparative radiological study of Reiter's disease, rheumatoid arthritis and ankylosing spondylitis. J Bone Joint Surg [Br] 41: 137–148

Mathieson J R, Connell D G, Coopersberg P L et al 1988 Sonography of the Achilles tendon and adjacent bursae. Am J Roentgenol 151: 127–131

Maurer A H, Millmond S H, Knight L C et al 1986 Infection in diabetic osteoarthropathy: Use of indium labelled leucocytes for diagnosis. Radiology 161: 221–225

McCauley R G K, Kahn P C 1977 Osteochondritis of the tarsal navicular. Radioisotopic appearances. Radiology 123: 705–706

McEvedy B V 1962 Simple ganglia. Br J Surg 49: 585–594

McMaster M J 1978 The pathogenesis of hallux rigidus. J Bone Joint Surg [Br] 60: 82–87

Merkel K D, Brown M L, Dewarjee M K 1985 Comparison of indium labelled leucocyte imaging with sequential technetium/gallium scanning in the diagnosis of low-grade musculoskeletal sepsis. J Bone Joint Surg [Am] 67: 465–476

Meschan I 1970 Radiology of the normal foot. Seminars Roentgen 5: 327–340

Mesgarzadeh M, Sapega A A, Bonakdarpour A et al 1987 Osteochondritis dissicans: analysis of mechanical stability with radiography, scintigraphy, and MR imaging. Radiology 165: 775–780

Meyer J, Garcia J, Hoffmeyer P et al 1988 The subtalar sprain: A roentgenographic study. Clin Orthop 226: 169–173

Miller B, Markheim H R, Towbin M N 1967 Multiple stress fractures in rheumatoid arthritis. J Bone Joint Surg [Am] 49: 1408–1414

Mink J H 1992a Tendons. In: Deutch A L, Mink J H, Kerr R (eds) MRI of the Foot and Ankle. Raven Press: New York. pp. 135–172

Mink J H 1992b Ligaments of the ankle. In: Deutch A L, Mink J H, Kerr R (eds) MRI of the Foot and Ankle. Raven Press: New York. pp. 173–197

Mirra J M 1989 Bone Tumours. Clinical, Radiologic and Pathologic Correlation. Lea & Febiger: Philadelphia.

Mitchell C L, Fleming J L, Allen R et al 1958 Osteomybunionectomy for hallux valgus. J Bone Joint Surg [Am] 40: 41–59

Mitchell D G, Kressel H Y 1988 MR imaging of early avascular necrosis. Radiology 169: 281–282

Moore T E, Yuh W T C, Kathol M H et al 1991 Abnormalities in the foot in patients with diabetes mellitus: Findings on MR imaging. Am J Roentgenol 157: 813–816

Moskovic E, Serpell J W, Parsons C et al 1992 Benign mimics of soft tissue sarcomas. Clin Radiol 46: 248–252

Mottonen T, Hannonen P, Rekonen A et al 1986 Joint scintigraphy and erosions. Annals Rheum Dis 45: 966–967

Murphy W A 1988 Magnetic resonance imaging. In: Resnick D and Niwayama G (eds) Diagnosis of Bone and Joint Disorders 2nd edn. W B Saunders: Philadelphia. pp. 1: 203–244

Newberg A H 1979 Osteochondral fractures of the dome of the talus. Br J Radiol 52: 105–109

Newman J H 1981 Non-infective disease in the diabetic foot. J Bone Joint Surg [Br] 63: 593–596

Ogata K, Sugioka Y, Urano Y et al 1986 Idiopathic osteonecrosis of the first metatarsal sesamoid. Skel Radiol 15: 141–145

Omer G E Jn 1981 Primary articular osteochondroses. Clin Orthop Rel Res 158: 33–40

Ono K, Hayashi H 1974 Residual deformity of treated congenital club foot. J Bone Joint Surg [Am] 56: 1577–1585

Pavlov H, Torg J S, Freiberger R 1983 Tarsal navicular stress fractures: Radiographic evaluation. Radiology 148: 641–645

Perry M D, Mont M A, Einhorn T A et al 1992 The validity of measurements made on standard foot orthoroentgenograms. Foot Ankle 13: 502–507

Petasnick J P, Turner D A, Charters J R et al 1986 Soft-tissue masses of the locomotor system: Comparison of MR imaging with CT. Radiology 160: 125–133

Piggott H 1960 The natural history of hallux valgus in adolescence and early adult life. J Bone Joint Surg [Am] 42: 749–760

Poleksic L, Zdravkovic I, Jablanovic B et al 1993 Magnetic resonance imaging of bone destruction in rheumatoid arthritis: comparison with radiography. Skeletal Radiol 22: 577–580

Quinn S F, Murray W T, Clark R A 1987 Achilles tendon: MR imaging at 1.5 T. Radiology 164: 767–770

Quinn S F, Erickson S J, Dee P M et al 1991 MR imaging in fibromatosis: Results in 26 patients with pathologic correlation. Am J Roentgenol 156: 539–542

Quirk R 1982 Talar compression syndrome in dancers. Foot Ankle 3: 65–68

Redd R A, Peters V J, Emery S F et al 1987 Morton Neuroma: Sonographic evaluation. Radiology 171: 415–417

Reed R J, Bliss B O 1973 Morton's neuroma. Arch Pathol 95: 123–129

Reeder M M 1970 Tropical diseases of the foot. Semin Roentgenol 5: 378–406

Reginato A M, Valenzuela F R, Martinez V C et al 1970 Polyarticular and familial chrondro-calcinosis. Arthritis Rheum 13: 197–212

Reinig J W, Dorwart R H, Roden W C 1985 MR imaging of a ruptured Achilles tendon. J Comput Assist Tomogr 9: 1131–1134

Reinus W R, Gilula L A, Seigal G P et al 1985 Radiographic appearance of Ewing sarcoma of the hands and feet: Report from the Intergroup Ewing Sarcoma Study. Am J Roentgenol 144: 331–336

Renfrew D L, El-Khoury G Y 1985 Anterior process fractures of the calcaneus. Skel Radiol 14: 121–125

Resnick D 1974 Patterns of peripheral joint disease in ankylosing spondylitis. Radiology 110: 523–532

Resnick D 1975 The interphalangeal joint of the great toe in rheumatoid arthritis. J Can Assoc Radiol 26: 255–262

Resnick D 1976 Roentgen features of the rheumatoid mid and hind foot. J Can Assoc Radiol 27: 99–107

Resnick D 1979 Radiology of seronegative spondyloarthropathies. Clin Orthop Rel Res 148: 38–45

Resnick D 1988 Arthrography, tenography and bursography. In: Resnick D and Niwayama G (eds) Diagnosis of Bone and Joint Disorders 2nd edn. W B Saunders: Philadelphia. pp. 1: 412–427

Resnick D, Niwayama G 1977 On the nature and significance of bony proliferation in 'rheumatoid variant' disorders. Am J Roentgenol 129: 275–278

Resnick D, Niwayama G 1988a Rheumatoid arthritis and the seronegative arthropathies. In: Resnick D, Niwayama G (eds) Diagnosis of Bone and Joint Disorders 2nd edn. W B Saunders: Philadelphia. pp. 3: 894–953

Resnick D, Niwayama G 1988b Gouty arthritis. In: Resnick D, Niwayama G (eds) Diagnosis of Bone and Joint Disorders 2nd edn. W B Saunders: Philadelphia. pp. 3: 1618–1671

Resnick D, Niwayama G 1988c A target area approach to articular disorders: A synopsis. In: Resnick D, Niwayama G (eds) Diagnosis of Bone and Joint Disorders 2nd edn. W B Saunders: Philadelphia. pp. 3: 1912–1938

Resnick D, Niwayama G 1988d Osteomyelitis, septic arthritis, and soft tissue infection: the mechanism and situations. In: Resnick D, Niwayama G (eds) Diagnosis of Bone and Joint Disorders 2nd edn. W B Saunders: Philadelphia. pp. 4: 2525–2618

Resnick D, Niwayama G 1988e Osteomyelitis, septic arthritis, and soft tissue infection: the organisms. In: Resnick D, Niwayama G (eds) Diagnosis of Bone and Joint Disorders 2nd edn. W B Saunders: Philadelphia. pp. 4: 2647–2754

Resnick D, Goergen T G, Niwayama G 1988a Physical injury. In: Resnick D, Niwayama G (eds) Diagnosis of Bone and Joint Disorders 2nd edn. W B Saunders: Philadelphia. pp. 5: 2757–3008

Resnick D, Goergen T G, Niwayama G 1988b The osteochondroses. In: Resnick D, Niwayama G (eds) Diagnosis of Bone and Joint Disorders 2nd edn. W B Saunders: Philadelphia. pp. 5: 3288–3334

Resnick D, Niwayama G, Feingold M L 1977 The sesamoid bones of the hands and feet. Participators in arthritis. Radiol 123: 57–62

Reuther G, Mutschler W 1990 Detection of local recurrent disease in musculo-skeletal tumours. Magnetic resonance imaging versus computed tomography. Skeletal Radiol 19: 85–90

Rogers L F 1982 Radiology of Skeletal Trauma. Churchill Livingstone: New York

Romanowski C A J, Barrington N A 1991 The accessory ossicles of the foot. The Foot 2: 61–70

Romanowski C A J, Barrington N A 1992 The accessory navicular – an important cause for medial foot pain. Clin Radiol 46: 261–264

Rosenburg Z S, Cheung Y, Jahss M H 1988a Computed tomography scan and magnetic resonance imaging of ankle tendons: an overview. Foot Ankle 8: 297–307

Rosenburg Z S, Cheung Y, Jahss M H 1988b Rupture of posterior tibial tendon: CT and MR imaging with surgical correlation. Radiology 169: 229–235

Rosenburg Z S, Feldman F, Singson R D 1986 Peroneal tendon injuries: CT analysis. Radiology 161: 743–748

Rosenburg Z S, Feldman F, Singson R D et al 1987a Computed tomography of ankle tendons. Radiology 166: 221–226

Rosenburg Z S, Feldman F, Singson R D et al 1987b Peroneal tendon injury associated calcaneal fractures: CT findings. Am J Roentgenol 149: 125–129

Rupani H D, Holder L E, Espinola D A et al 1985 Three phase radionuclide bone imaging in sports medicine. Radiology 156: 187–196

Salamao O, Napoli M M M, Egydio de Carvalho A Jr et al 1992 Talocalcaneal coalition. Diagnosis and surgical management. Foot Ankle 13: 251–256

Samuelson K M, Harrison R, Freeman M A R 1981 A roentgenographic technique to evaluate and document hindfoot position. Foot Ankle 1: 286–289

Saunders A J L, Sayad T F, Hilson A J W et al 1979 Stress fractures of the lower leg and foot. Clin Radiol 30: 649–651

Sauser D D, Nelson R C, Lavine M H et al 1983 Acute injuries of the lateral ligament of the ankle: comparison of stress radiography and arthrography. Radiology 148: 653–657

Schauwecker D S 1989 Osteomyelitis diagnosed with In-111-labelled leucocytes. Radiology 171: 141–146

Schauwecker D S 1992 The scintigraphic diagnosis of osteomyelitis. Am J Roentgenol 158: 9–18

Schauwecker D C, Park H M, Mock B H et al 1984 Evaluation of complicating osteomyelitis using 99mTcMDP, Indium 111 granulocytes, and Ga 67 citrate. J Nucl Med 25: 849–853

Schils J P, Andrish J T, Piraino D W et al 1992 Medial malleolar stress fractures: Review of the clinical and imaging features. Radiology 185: 219–221

Schneck C D, Mesgarzadeh M, Bonakbarpour A et al 1992 MR imaging cf the most commonly injured ankle ligaments. Part 1. Normal anatomy. Radiology 184: 499–506

Schneider H J, King A Y, Bronson J L et al 1974 Stress injuries and developmental changes in lower extremities in ballet dancers. Radiology 113: 627–632

Schweitzer M E, Resnick D 1992 Normal anatomy of the foot and ankle. In: Deutch A L, Mink J H, Kerr R (eds) MRI of the Foot and Ankle. Raven Press: New York. pp. 33–65

Sclafani S J A 1985 Ligamentous injury to the lower tibiofibular syndesmosis: Radiographic evidence. Radiology 156: 21–27

Seabold J E, Flickinger F W, Kao S C S et al 1990 Indium-111 leukocyte/technesium-99m MDP bone and magnetic resonance imaging: Difficulty in diagnosing osteomyelitis in patients with neuropathic osteoarthropathy. J Nucl Med 31: 549–556

Seltzer S E 1984 Value of computed tomography in planning medical and surgical treatment of chronic osteomyelitis. J Comput Assist Tomogr 8: 482–487

Seltzer S E, Weissman B N, Braunstein E M et al 1984 Computed tomography of the hindfoot. J Comput Assist Tomog 8: 488–497

Shereff M J, Cullivan W J, Johnson K A 1983 Osteoid osteoma of the foot. J Bone Joint Surg [Am] 65: 638–641

Siegal B A, Donovan R L, Alderson P O et al 1976 Skeletal uptake of 99mTc diphosphonate in relation to local bone blood flow. Radiology 120: 121

Silverman F N, Kuhn J P 1993 The bones: normal and variants. In: Caffey's Paediatric X-Ray Diagnosis 9th edn. Mosby: St Louis. pp. 1510–1518

Smith G R, Winquist R A, Allan T N K, Northrop C H 1977 Subtle transchondral fractures of the talar dome: A radiological perspective. Radiology 124: 667–673

Smith R V, Staple T W 1984 Computed tomography scanning techniques of the hindfoot. Clin Orthop Rel Res 177: 34–38

Steel M W, Johnson K A, Dewitz M A et al 1980 Radiographic measurements of the normal adult foot. Foot Ankle 1: 151–158

Sullivan D C, Rosenfield N S, Ogden J et al 1980 Problems with the scintigraphic detection of osteomyelitis in children. Radiology 135(3): 731–736

Sunderman M, McQuire M H 1988 Computed tomography or magnetic resonance for evaluating the solitary tumour or tumour-like lesion of bone? Skeletal Radiol 17: 393–401

Tang J S, Gold R H, Bassett L W et al 1988 Musculoskeletal infection of the extremities: Evaluation with MR imaging. Radiology 166: 205–209

Templeton A W, McAllister W H, Irwin D Z 1965 Standardisation of terminology and evaluation of osseous relationships in congenitally abnormal feet. Am J Roentgenol 93: 374–381

Thermann H, Hoffman R, Zwipp H et al 1992 The use of ultrasonography in the foot and ankle. Foot Ankle 13: 386–390

Thould A K, Simon G 1966 Assessment of the radiological changes in the hands and feet in rheumatoid arthritis. Annals Rheum Dis 25: 220–228

Torg J S, Pavlov H, Cooley L 1982 Stress fractures of the tarsal navicular: a retrospective review of 21 cases. J Bone Joint Surg [Am] 64: 700–712

Totty W G, Murphy W A, Lee J K T 1986 Soft tissue tumours: MR imaging. Radiology 160: 135–141

Tsai J C, Dalinka M K, Fallon M D et al 1990 Fluid-fluid level: A non specific finding of tumours of bone and soft tissue. Radiology 175: 779–782

Tubiolo A J, Jones R H, Chalker D K 1986 Cavernous haemangioma of the plantar forefoot. A literature review and case report. J Am Podriatr Med Assoc 76: 164–167

Unger E C, Moldofsky P J, Gatenby R et al 1988 Diagnosis of osteomyelitis by MR imaging. Am J Roentgenol 150a: 605–610

Vanel D, Lacombe M J, Covanet D et al 1987 Musculoskeletal tumours: Follow-up with MR imaging after treatment with surgery and radiation therapy. Radiology 164: 243–245

Videgal E, Jacoby R K, Dixon A et al 1975 The foot in chronic rheumatoid arthritis. Ann Rheum Dis 34: 292–297

Watt I, Middlemiss H 1975 The radiology of gout. Clin Radiol 26: 27–36

Wechsler R J, Karasick D, Schweitzer M E 1992 Computed tomography of talocalcaneal coalition: imaging techniques. Skeletal Radiol 21: 353–358

Weissberg D, Resnick D, Taylor A et al 1978 Rheumatoid arthritis and its variants: Analysis of scintiphotographic, radiographic and clinical examination. Am J Roentgenol 131: 665–673

Weistabl R, Stiskal M, Neuhold A et al 1991 Classifying calcaneal tendon injury according to MRI findings. J Bone Joint Surg [Br] 73: 683–685

Wenig J A 1990 Os trigonum syndrome. J Am Podiatr Med Assoc 80: 278–282

Weston W J 1959 Tendinitis calcaria on the dorsum of the foot. Br J Radiol 32: 495

Wetzel L H, Levine E 1990 Soft tissue tumours of the foot. Value of MR imaging for specific diagnosis. Am J Roentgenol 155: 125–130

Williams P H, Monaghan D, Barrington N A 1991 Undiagnosed foot pain: the role of the isotope bone scan. The Foot 1: 145–149

Wilson E S Jn, Katz F N 1969 Stress fractures. An analysis of 250 consecutive cases. Radiology 92: 481–486

Winfield A C, Dennis J M 1959 Stress fractures of the calcaneus. Radiology 72: 415–418

Wredmark T, Carlstedt C A, Bauer H et al 1991 Os trigonum syndrome: a clinical entity in ballet dancers. Foot Ankle 11: 404–406

Yuh W T C, Corson J D, Baraniewski H M et al 1989 Osteomyelitis of the foot in diabetic patients: Evaluation with plain film, 99m Tc-MDP bone scintigraphy, and MR imaging. Am J Roentgenol 152: 795–800

Zeiss J, Ebrahim N, Rusin J et al 1991 Magnetic resonance imaging of the calcaneus: Normal anatomy and application in calcaneal fractures. Foot Ankle 11: 264–273

Zindick M R, Young M P, Daley R J et al 1982 Metastatic tumours of the foot. Clin Orthop Rel Res 170: 219–225

Zlatkin M B, Pathria M, Sartoris D J et al 1987 The diabetic foot. Radiol Clin North Am 25: 1095–1105

Acknowledgments

I would like to thank my radiological colleagues at the Northern General and Royal Hallamshire Hospitals, Sheffield, for their help in preparing this chapter.

III.2 Radiography

Andrew Milne

Plain radiographs of the foot and ankle are amongst the most commonly performed radiographic examinations. CT scans and MRI images are gradually replacing some of the more specialized plain views. This chapter looks at the standard films that are useful in investigating foot and ankle disorders, as well as some of the specialized views that have been found to be useful in clinical practice. The chapter also discusses some of the general considerations that are important in imaging, and the techniques involved in the more specialized areas.

Plain radiographs

The foot

Anteroposterior or dorsiplantar view
The patient sits on the X-ray table with the knee flexed and the sole of the foot positioned on the X-ray cassette so that two views can be taken, one on each side of the film (Fig. 1a). The knee is slightly internally rotated to bring the foot flat onto the film. The beam is centred to

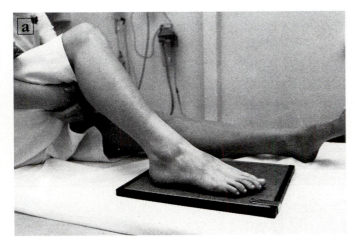

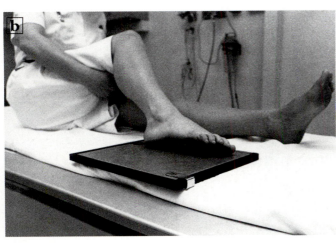

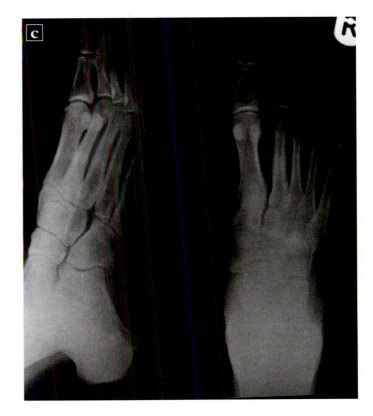

Figure 1

(a) Basic position for dorsiplantar view. (b) Oblique view of the foot. (c) Radiograph showing alignment and appearance of bones in the normal foot

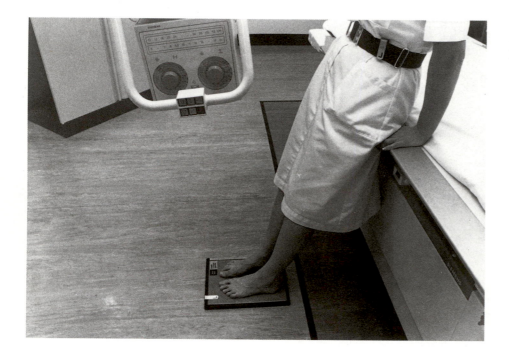

Figure 2
Position for a weight-bearing view of both feet

the film and collimated appropriately. A lead marker is applied to indicate orientation and the film is exposed.

Oblique view

The patient sits as described above and moves the foot onto the other side of the film. The knee is internally rotated further so that the sole of the foot is at approximately 45° to the film (Fig. 1b). An exposure is made as before.

Both these views can be taken with the patient in the chair, on a trolley, or supine in bed if necessary, without any reduction in image quality.

Lateral view

For this view, a separate film is required. The patient sits on the X-ray table and the limb concerned is externally rotated so that the knee is close to the surface of the table. The beam is centred to the middle of the foot and collimated.

Weight-bearing views

Anteroposterior weight-bearing view

The film is placed on a non-slip surface, and the patient stands on the cassette and leans back to rest with the body at 10° to the vertical against a suitable support, usually the X-ray table (Fig. 2). The feet are positioned slightly apart. The beam is centred to the midline of the film so that it is equidistant between the two feet and collimated to the film, the tube being angled 10° towards

the ankle joint. The film is exposed to include both feet on the single image.

Lateral weight-bearing view

The patient stands on a suitable step so that the film can be positioned medial to the foot, and the beam can be centred to the lateral border of the foot using a horizontal ray. A step with a recess to allow the film to fall below the level of the sole of the foot is ideal. For safety and to allow this image to be produced, a specially designed step system with a safety handle is desirable. X-ray tube supports have a restricted lower limit of travel, which will make this view impossible when the patient is standing on the floor. The film must be allowed to fall below the edge of the foot by whatever method can be devised, or information will be lost from the image.

Sesamoid views

The patient sits on the X-ray table with the leg fully extended and the foot dorsiflexed to 90° and placed on the film. The beam is directed vertically downwards with the toes fully dorsiflexed, if necessary by means of traction with a bandage. The beam is centred to the mid-point of the foot just behind the toes, and collimated.

The ankle

Anteroposterior view

The patient sits on the X-ray table with the lower limb fully extended and the ankle placed on an X-ray cassette.

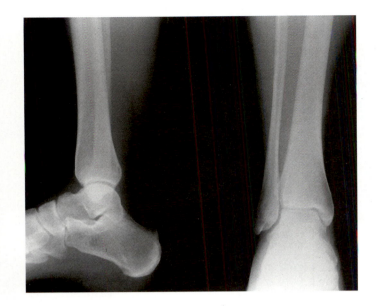

Figure 3

Lateral and anteroposterior radiographs, showing alignment of bones and their appearance in the normal ankle

The film is divided into two halves (Fig. 3) and the ankle is placed so that the axis of the foot is internally rotated approximately 8° in order to show the ankle mortise. The beam is centred to the midline of the ankle joint and collimated to the cassette. The exposure is made. It is important that the foot is dorsiflexed so that the calcaneum is not rotated upwards, which would obscure the fibula. If the ankle view does not show the mortise well, then a so-called mortise view can be obtained with similar positioning but with up to 12° internal rotation. A good view of the mortise is essential in trauma investigations.

Lateral views

The patient lies supine on the X-ray couch, the limb is rotated externally and the knee is flexed and slightly raised off the surface of the table. The beam is collimated and centred to the medial malleolus; the foot should be dorsiflexed to 90°.

Oblique view

The patient extends the lower limb fully and the limb is internally rotated 45°. The foot must be dorsiflexed or

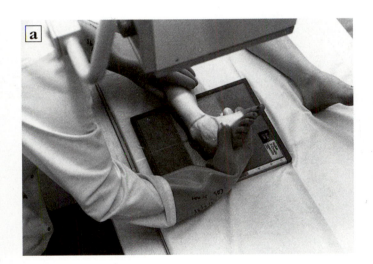

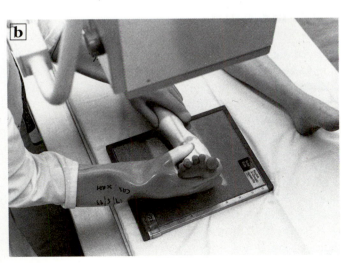

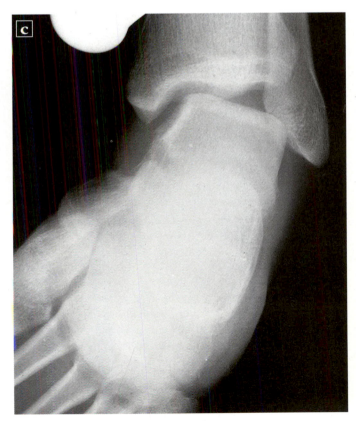

Figure 4

(a) Medial stress view showing technique for applying stress while maintaining the anteroposterior position. (b) Lateral stress view. (c) Resulting radiograph showing marked rotation of the talus

Figure 5

Radiographs showing the resulting talar shift following stress applied to the foot, anteriorly to the right foot and posteriorly to the left foot

the tip of the fibula will be hidden by the calcaneum. The beam is centred to the ankle joint and collimated to the cassette.

Stress views

Forced eversion–inversion views

These views are taken to demonstrate ligament damage or laxity, and they must be performed with the aid of the referring clinician or radiologist. The patient is supine with the feet near the end of the X-ray table, and the limb fully extended. Wearing a pair of lead gloves, the clinician grips the calcaneum and exerts a force medially (Fig. 4a) and then laterally (Fig. 4b) while the ankle is X-rayed in the AP position. Any laxity will be shown by a widening of the joint line at the lateral side for medial stress (Fig. 4c) and at the medial side for lateral stress.

Forced anterior and posterior subluxation views

The clinician must be involved. The limb is lifted from the table surface by means of a small block placed under the heel, and a force is applied in the downward direction on the lower tibia. The film is placed lateral to the limb and the tube is directed horizontally and centred on the malleolus.

Similarly, the block is moved to a position below the distal tibia, and the foot is gripped firmly and pulled in a downward direction, with the film again placed in the lateral position. Any laxity or damage to the ligaments will be demonstrated by the opening of the joint surfaces (Fig. 5). These images can also be produced with the limb externally rotated into the lateral position, using firm manual traction.

The calcaneum

Lateral views

The position for this view is similar to that for the lateral view of the ankle joint, except that the beam is centred to the mid-point of the calcaneum and collimated.

Axial views

The limb is fully extended and dorsiflexed in the antero-posterior position. Dorsiflexion can be aided by traction applied by means of a bandage wrapped around the sole of the foot and held in the patient's hands. The beam is centred to the mid-axis of the calcaneum using a tube angle of 60° cephalad, and collimated.

This can be a difficult view to take, especially in trauma cases, where this position is sometimes impossible to achieve. Oblique views can be taken with 45° internal and external rotation, but CT scanning is often the investigation of choice in cases of fractured calcaneum.

Axial weight-bearing views

The patient stands on a large X-ray plate with the knees slightly flexed, the tibia being approximately 10° to the vertical (Fig. 6a). The beam is angled 30° towards the toes and centred to the midline between the heels, and collimated so that a good length of the tibia is included on the film. This view will demonstrate the tibiocalcaneal angle (Fig. 6b). The beam is incident to the limb from exactly the opposite direction to the supine technique (Harris & Beath, 1948).

Subtalar joints

The patient sits on the X-ray couch with the limb fully extended. The foot is dorsiflexed and two views are taken with 50° internal and external rotation respectively. The beam is centred to the midline of the joint in each case and the tube is angled 15° towards the head (Fig. 7). The beam is collimated and the exposure made.

Views of hindfoot position

This technique will allow the visualization of the weight-bearing hindfoot position. However, it requires a specialized stand to support the patient and the film. The patient stands on a perspex shelf, which allows two

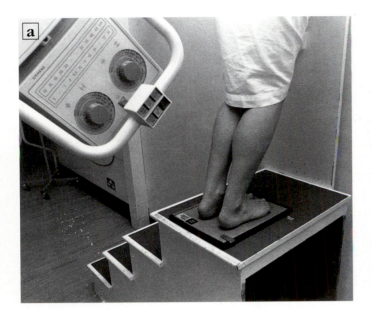

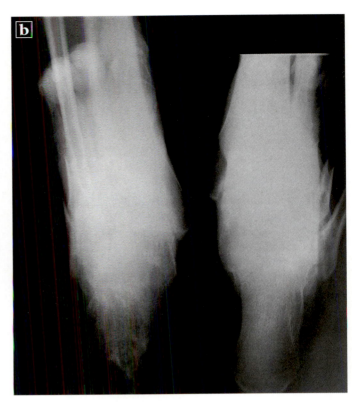

Figure 6
(a) Position for the weight-bearing view of the tibiocalcaneal angle. (b) Radiograph showing a marked valgus calcaneum following trauma

Figure 7
Radiograph showing subtalar joints

exposures to be made on the same film. The first one is very similar to the anteroposterior ankle view, with the malleoli equidistant from the film. Without the patient moving, the beam is angled 20° towards the head, and re-centred relative to the malleoli. A second exposure is made, and a composite image is formed, which shows the body of the calcaneum and the ankle joint. This can be used to document the position of the calcaneum relative to the ankle, using the method of Samuelson et al (1981).

Tomography

This well-established method of imaging can be useful in many instances where plain films are found not to provide sufficient information. The technique involves the use of a moving tube–film system, which rotates around a fulcrum. If the tube and the film are moving at the same speed, but in opposite directions, then those structures within the body that are at the same level as the fulcrum will be sharply in focus on the film. Thus

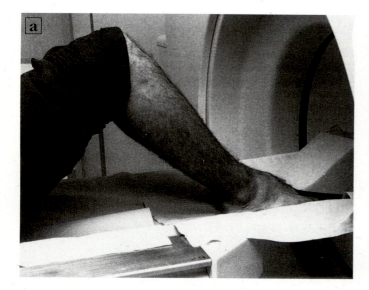

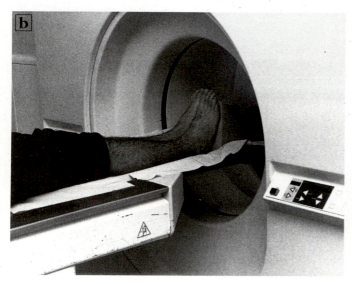

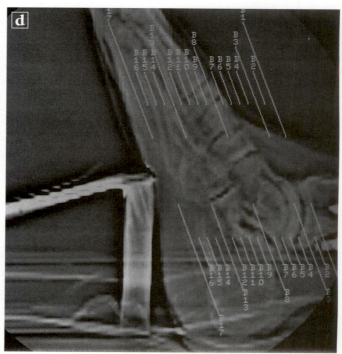

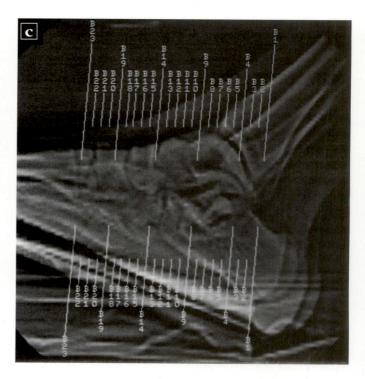

Figure 8

(a) Patient positioning of hindfoot CT scans. (b) Patient positioning for calcaneal scans of both feet. (c), (d) Scanograms showing the position of the cuts for each type of CT scan

an image is formed which can be defined at any chosen level within the body. Simple tomography is available in most imaging departments.

Computed tomography

CT scanning is fast becoming the method of choice for many of the more complex questions that can be answered radiologically. Patients undergoing CT scanning are often very intimidated by the technology and fearful of going into the enclosed space within the scanner.

Positioning may be quite difficult, particularly when only one limb is to be included in the scan field. In cases of multiple trauma or when the patient is being intensively nursed it is sometimes wise to delay scan requests until the patient is in a more stable condition. For scans of the foot and ankle, the patient is positioned supine with the affected limb immobilized (Fig. 8a,b). If both limbs are to be included they must be positioned so that they are in a comparable position from side to side. The limb may be dorsiflexed or plantar-flexed as necessary, and a scanogram is usually produced to indicate the starting position and the cut levels required (Fig. 8c,d). The clinician must remember that absolute cooperation is required from the patient; if this is not possible, anaesthesia must be considered.

CT scanning is a technique that delivers a high effective radiation dose to the patient.

Magnetic resonance image scanning

MRI scanning is the latest imaging modality to gain wide acceptance. It is noninvasive and ideal for imaging the soft tissues. The problems for the patient are similar to those encountered with CT scanning.

There is also a problem related to metallic implants in the body, such as paramagnetic surgical clips, the displacement of which can be disastrous (Carter et al, 1994). Claustrophobia is a problem with some patients.

Patients with hip replacements and other such implants may be excluded from MRI scanning, owing to the effect of metal on the magnetic fields induced. There can be problems with induced currents causing metal components to heat up to very high temperatures. Patients undergoing limb reconstruction using external fixators and other such devices are excluded from this imaging option where the area of interest may be poorly seen owing to artefacts caused by the metalwork. Pacemakers and devices with magnetically or electronically operated switches, such as cochlear implants, are contraindications for MRI scanning.

Positioning problems are similar to those encountered in CT scanning.

General technical considerations

Plaster of Paris
A limb in plaster is difficult to X-ray. The plaster obscures detail and prevents correct positioning of the limb. Plaster must be removed before imaging if a high-definition view is required. Films for position in plaster are commonly taken to monitor the healing process after fracture manipulation or fixation, but they are rarely able to provide the clinician with all the information required.

The new types of resin-based casts degrade image quality to a lesser extent and also require less X-ray exposure; they should be used whenever possible.

Film–screen combination
A high-resolution film and screen combination is required for examinations of the foot and ankle. This 'slower' type of system provides a good range of contrast while keeping radiation dose at a reasonable level. Standard systems, such as would be used for abdomen or chest, should not be used. The possibilities of using digital radiography, with its very broad contrast range, is being explored in centres where this technology is available.

Radiation protection and radiation dose
Gonad shields are required for patient protection when carrying out plain films of the foot and ankle. Their importance is even greater in CT scanning because of the higher doses required. In plain radiography of the foot, as a general principle the beam should not be directed at the gonads. A record is kept of effective doses given to a patient, and X-ray examinations are kept to the minimum required to provide adequate information for clinical management.

CT scanning increases patient dose by the order of several magnitudes.

MRI scanning is noninvasive and the use of this technique should be encouraged whenever clinically appropriate.

References

Carter P H, Paterson A M Thornton M L, Hyatt A P, Milne A, Pirrie J R 1994 Chesney's Equipment for Student Radiographers, 4th edition. Blackwell Scientific Publications, Oxford. p. 308

Harris R I, Beath T 1948 Aetiology of peroneal spastic flat foot. J Bone Joint Surg 30B: 624–634

Samuelson K M, Harrison R, Freeman M A R 1981 A roentgenographic technique to evaluate and document hindfoot position. Foot Ankle 1: 286–289

Acknowledgements

I would like to express my thanks to my models, radiographers Ms D McGarty and Ms D Parrott, and also to Mr P Heath and Mr M Buckley for their kind assistance. Thanks also to Dr N A Barrington for her support and encouragement.

III.3 Ankle Arthroscopy

Mark S Myerson

Introduction

Over the past decade, our understanding of the pathophysiology of disorders of the ankle has expanded. Intra-articular anatomy and soft-tissue, chondral, and bony defects of the tibia and talus have been clarified. Substantial advances in ankle arthroscopy have evolved through improved instrumentation and the use of mechanical distraction, without which the field of vision is limited to the anterior third of the joint. Distraction has enabled us to perform a global evaluation of the joint, including the anterior and posterior compartments, without causing scuffing and damage to the articular surfaces. Our understanding of soft-tissue pathology and its application to functional instability of the ankle is increasing. Newer innovative techniques, such as arthroscopic ankle arthrodesis, combine the advantages inherent in arthroscopy with current methodologies of fracture fixation. Arthroscopic evaluation of the ankle joint allows us to directly examine the articular cartilage and soft tissues, all of which are discussed below.

Arthroscopic anatomy

Integral to the success of ankle arthroscopy is a thorough understanding of the surface and intraarticular anatomy. The surface landmarks of the ankle are demarcated by the malleoli. The tip of the fibula is approximately 2 cm distal and posterior to the medial malleolus. The joint line is 2.5 cm proximal to the tip of the fibula and approximately 1 cm proximal to the medial edge of the medial malleolus. The surface structures from medial to lateral are the thick anterior tibial tendon medially and the extensor hallucis and extensor digitorum communis tendons lying centrally over the joint. More laterally, the peroneus tertius tendon runs obliquely across the ankle to its insertion on the base of the fifth metatarsal. These tendons should be identified and marked before commencing the procedure.

There is minimal subcutaneous tissue separating the joint cavity from the skin. Neurovascular structures are therefore at particular risk, but they are easily palpable and must be identified preoperatively. The deep peroneal nerve and dorsalis pedis artery lie in the sulcus between the extensor digitorum and extensor hallucis tendons and deep to the extensor retinaculum. This deeper location is vulnerable when performing a synovectomy, as little separates the neurovascular bundle from the capsule. The superficial peroneal nerve bifurcates 6 cm proximal to the level of the fibula into the dorsal medial and the dorsal intermediate cutaneous nerves (Adkison et al 1991). The dorsal intermediate cutaneous nerve is more lateral, lying immediately lateral to the peroneus tertius tendon, and is in a more vulnerable location. The dorsal intermediate cutaneous nerve can be easily identified preoperatively, particularly in thin patients, by plantarflexing the fourth toe. The nerve becomes prominent, and its location should be marked.

The posterolateral aspect of the ankle is contained by the fibula and the peroneal tendon immediately posterior and adjacent to it. The sural nerve lies almost midway between the peroneal and Achilles tendons and should be avoided with the posterolateral portal.

The anterior articular surface of the joint is not horizontal, and undulations along its surface provide the basis for the anterior portals. Just lateral to the medial malleolus, the articular surface is recessed by approximately 4 mm, creating a notch that forms the anteromedial portal between the medial malleolus and the anterior tibial tendon. There is a slightly rounded distal projection from the tibia centrally, where it juts out to correspond to a similar concavity on the dorsal surface of the talus. It is not easy, therefore, to sweep the arthroscope under the tibia across the joint from side to side, and this has to be performed anterior to the tibia or across the talar neck. The fibula is situated between 1.5 and 2 cm posterior to the anterior articular edge of the tibia. When viewing the lateral aspect of the joint from the anteromedial portal, the fibula is therefore not visible. To see the anterior aspect of the fibula, the arthroscope is gently introduced through the anteromedial portal and then carefully swept across the tibiotalar surface.

The posterior articular surface of the tibia lies more distally than its anterior edge. This distal projection is increased by the condensation of soft-tissue structures posteriorly, including the transverse ligament, which is adherent to the inferior tibiofibular ligament and easily visible with mechanical distraction. The ligament is covered with synovium; with dorsiflexion of the ankle, it remains attached to the tibia and, as the talus moves distally, a synovial-lined recess is exposed. This recess should also be carefully examined, particularly for loose bodies. An additional posterior structure that is occasionally seen from an anterior portal is the tibial slip, which extends from the edge of the posterior talofibular ligament obliquely to the medial edge of the transverse ligament.

The anterior talofibular ligament (ATFL) should be routinely inspected to differentiate it from pathological conditions, as this is a common site for soft-tissue lesions. The ATFL is partly intracapsular and is intra-articular. When torn, the hemorrhagic cellular exudate occasionally does not resolve. During the healing process, the inflammatory tissue hypertrophies and forms a variable fibrous mass over the anterior talofibular recess. When debriding this hypertrophic tissue, care must be taken not to resect too deeply, as the remnant of the ligament is likely to be debrided. Similarly, on the medial aspect of the joint, the deep portion of the deltoid ligament is easily visible and may also be involved in a pathologic inflammatory process. The tibiofibular joint is synovial lined, and proliferative synovitis, which occurs in inflammatory, degenerative, and post-traumatic conditions, commonly affects this joint. The transverse tibiofibular ligament and posterior talofibular ligament are extra-articular and not normally seen arthroscopically. However, the posterior talofibular ligament may become hypertrophied as a result of trauma, in which case it becomes visible as a posterior bulge. Patients with this condition present with posterior ankle pain; the pathologic tissue is amenable to resection.

Almost the entire visible surface of the talus is covered by articular cartilage. Most of the dome of the talus is visible through either of the anterior portals. Approximately 50% of the dome is visible without distraction; the amount visualized can be increased to about 80% with distraction. If further visualization posteriorly is required from an anterior portal, then the 70° arthroscope can be used. Anteriorly, the neck of the talus is visible from either the anteromedial or anterolateral portals. The talar neck is not often involved in a pathologic process; however, it is commonly covered with loose or adherent osteophytes in post-traumatic degenerative conditions. Arthroscopic management of these degenerative arthritides may be difficult, as many of these osteophytes are intracapsular and not intra-articular.

Arthroscopic technique and positioning

Anesthesia

Although general anesthesia is preferred, local anesthesia may be used occasionally for arthroscopic examination of the joint, provided one is certain that only anterior joint pathology is present. However, general anesthesia is preferred for a thorough evaluation of a joint that may require mechanical distraction. If local anesthesia is used, 10 to 15 cm³ of a mixture of 1% xylocaine and 0.5% bupivicaine with admixed epinephrine is instilled into the joint and 2 cm³ are instilled into each portal 30 minutes before commencing the procedure.

Patient positioning

The patient is placed in a supine position with the hip and knee flexed and the ankle supported with a sterile holder, depending on the method of distraction used. With the patient in the supine position and the ankle free, the anterior portals are easily accessible. If the posterolateral portal is used, the limb must be internally rotated or a sterile ankle holder used. A tourniquet is always applied to the thigh, although it is not always inflated.

Initial procedures

The joint is inflated first with 10–15 cm³ of saline or the local anesthetic mixture. I use small incisions for the portals with a No 11 blade to puncture the skin only, and a hemostat is then used to spread the subcutaneous tissue longitudinally. This moves the subcutaneous structures, such as tendons and nerves, out of the way and also minimizes the portal size, which prevents fluid extravasation. A blunt obturator is then used to enter the joint; this is twisted around in a circular motion to free up the tissues. The arthroscope is then inserted.

It is important in ankle arthroscopy to maintain high fluid inflow and outflow, which I accomplish with gravity, using continuous overhead saline inflow. An arthroscopy pump may be used to maintain high volume and pressure, but it can be quite dangerous in the ankle because of fluid extravasation, and I do not recommend its use.

Portals

Before induction of anesthesia, all of the anterior and posterior soft tissue structures are carefully marked out. The anteromedial portal is located in the sulcus in between the medial malleolus and the anterior tibial tendon and is confirmed by insertion of a No 22 needle. The anterolateral portal is located immediately lateral to the tendon of the peroneus tertius and medial to the dorsal intermediate cutaneous branch of the superficial peroneal nerve at the level of the joint. Although this may be located before insertion of the arthroscope, it is easier to find by turning the arthroscope toward the skin so that the light source highlights the subcutaneous soft tissues.

I use the anteromedial portal for insertion of the arthroscope, preferably directly over the joint line. If it is more than 1 cm inferior or below the joint line, difficulty will be experienced in visualizing the lateral aspect of the joint, particularly more posteriorly. If this portal is made directly over the joint line, there is enough room

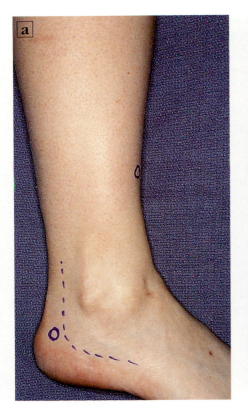
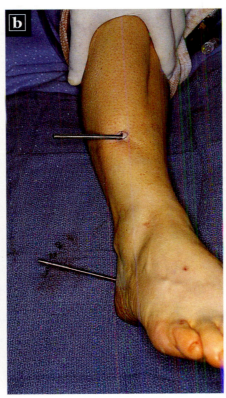
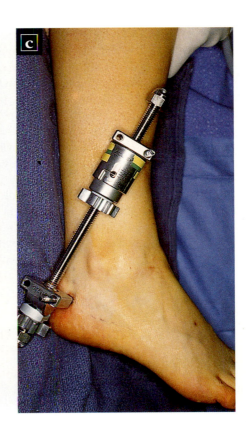

Figure 1

(a) Placement of the pins for the external fixator/distractor is demonstrated. (b) Note the slight convergence of the pins which facilitates exposure and prevents eccentric distraction of the ankle joint. (c) The position of the sural nerve and portal for placement of the lateral pin for the distractor is demonstrated; the distractor is applied as shown

inferiorly for an accessory anteromedial portal. The joint is quickly inspected anteriorly and the anterolateral portal is selected as described above.

The anterocentral and posteromedial portals are fraught with potential complications, and are not recommended under any circumstances. The posterolateral portal is particularly useful for fluid inflow and is also used to evaluate posteromedial lesions of the talar dome. With the arthroscope anteromedially, the portal is located with a No 22 needle, 5 mm medial to the peroneal tendon and 1 cm proximal to the tip of the fibula. The posterior articular margin of the tibia is 5 mm lower than the anterior margin, and this overhang must be taken into consideration with this portal.

Distraction

If improved visualization is required, then some form of distraction of the joint is necessary. This may be accomplished through invasive or non-invasive means. The simplest form of non-invasive distraction is through the use of a sterile stocking bandage wrapped around the midfoot and then hitched onto the surgeon's foot to apply distraction. A commercially available non-invasive soft-tissue distractor is available and may be the preferred method for distraction.

Mechanical distraction may be performed invasively using calcaneal and tibial pins (Fig. 1). The pins for the latter system are threaded and are inserted after predrilling with a 3.2 or 3.5 mm drill bit. Alternatively, a threaded trochar tipped Steinmann pin may be used. The tibial pin is inserted 6 cm proximal to the joint line from lateral to medial, slightly posterior to the anterior tibial crest. The anterior tibial muscle is pushed posteriorly with a clamp or trochar and the pin is inserted using a power tool. Although it has been recommended that only one cortex be used, I have inserted the pin across both cortices as this method inhibits the angulation tendency of the pins. A No 22 needle is used to locate the inferior surface of the calcaneus, and then the inferior pin is inserted 1–2 cm proximal to its inferior edge, engaging both the lateral and medial cortices of the calcaneus. It is important to angulate the distal pin approximately 20–30° caudally (toward the tibial pin) in order to prevent varus angulation of the ankle joint during distraction. The distraction should be initiated slowly and should never exceed 50 pounds of force (as read on the distractor). During the course of the arthroscopic distraction, some relaxation of the ligaments occurs due to inherent elastic deformation; in this case, more distraction can be applied. The gradual application of distraction is particularly important in patients with arthrofibrosis.

Most authors recommend insertion of these pins laterally in the tibia and calcaneus. However, there is a tendency when using this unilaterally applied distractor for the ankle to tilt into varus, which may decrease visualization medially. If this occurs, the fixator pins may be inserted medially in the tibia and talus directly inferior to the medial malleolus. This is particularly relevant when attempting to visualize the medial and posterior surfaces of the talus.

Osteochondral lesions of the talus

Etiology and diagnosis

The terminology for osteochondral defects of the talus can be quite confusing, and whether this represents a traumatic or idiopathic etiology, the generic term of transcondylar talar dome lesions is applicable (Baker et al 1986, Berndt & Harty 1959, Flick & Gould 1985, Guhl et al 1993, O'Farrell & Costello 1982, Ferkel & Scranton 1993). Whether these lesions are idiopathic in nature and represent a pathologic fracture of necrotic bone as a result of ischemia or whether they are traumatic in etiology, it is my preference to use the term osteochondral lesions of the talus (OLT) to describe these lesions. The etiology of the transchondral lesion is certainly controversial, yet most authors currently recognize the predominant effect of trauma in producing these lesions. The medial OLT is typically produced by an inversion and plantarflexion injury with external rotation of the tibia on the talus. Lateral lesions are caused by inversion with simultaneous dorsiflexion of the ankle.

Berndt & Harty (1959) classified these fractures into four stages based upon the radiographic appearance:

stage 1,   a small subchondral compression fracture;
stage 2,   a partially detached osteochondral fragment;
stage 3,   a completely detached osteochondral fracture without displacement; and
stage 4,   a displaced osteochondral fracture.

Although this classification scheme is still used today, it is outdated. Plain radiographs may underestimate the extent of the defect and, particularly in stage 1 and stage 2 defects, they do not adequately demonstrate discontinuity. Most surgeons currently use a classification system based on a computed tomography (CT) scan or the arthroscopic appearance of the lesion. With an arthroscopic staging system, irregularities and subtle defects of the chondral surface are clearly identified and can be appropriately treated.

Surgical treatment

Any patient with a symptomatic OLT should be treated surgically, regardless of the stage. However, since stage 1 lesions are rarely symptomatic and are theoretically quiescent, they should probably be treated initially with physical therapy and rehabilitative modalities.

One may be able to treat a stage 2 lesion with restriction of activity and physical therapy, but these patients rarely obtain permanent relief. If these patients are prepared to modify their activities, it is possible that, with time, the chondral surface may stabilize. Most patients, however, will experience repetitive bouts of discomfort with exercise over a period of years until the lesion is treated surgically. Given the propensity for further softening and fibrillation of the chondral surface with potential for loose body formation, these symptomatic lesions should be treated surgically.

These patients will describe a variety of symptoms (including aching, a sensation of clicking or snapping, or pain and swelling of the ankle after exercise), none of which seem to be specific. A common presentation is an ankle sprain that does not get better with time or therapy. Some athletes can manage their regular day-to-day activities but become symptomatic after exercise.

The defect is usually visible on routine radiographs. The medial lesions are typically posterior and the lateral lesions are anterior; these locations appear to be consistent with the proposed pathogenesis. In addition to these radiographs, I further clarify the position of the OLT with lateral radiographs in maximum plantarflexion and dorsiflexion. The OLT is then further defined with CT. CT (but not magnetic resonance imaging) is useful to plan the extent of surgery, since it defines precisely the exact size and depth of the lesion as well as the location of any loose bodies.

The lateral lesions are usually anterior on the talus and are accessible through an arthrotomy. However, the medial lesion is typically more posterior and can seldom be reached through an anteromedial arthrotomy (Fig. 2). Some clinicians have therefore advocated an osteotomy of the medial malleolus, whereas others have described grooving of the anterior surface of the tibia over the lesion in order to expose the talus satisfactorily. These approaches involve substantial soft-tissue and bony trauma, with the added risk of malunion or nonunion of the medial malleolus. Arthroscopy is currently the surgical method of choice for approaching OLT.

The arthroscopic procedure is performed under general anesthesia. Mechanical distraction is used to improve visualization, although anterolateral lesions of the

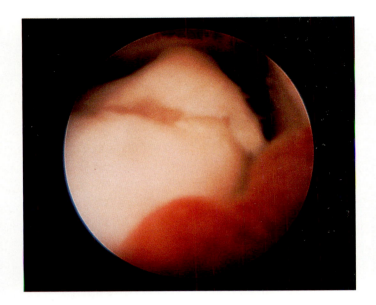

Figure 2

This acute medial osteochondral lesion of the talus was more anterior than most medial lesions. Demonstrated is a markedly unstable lesion and associated anteromedial synovitis

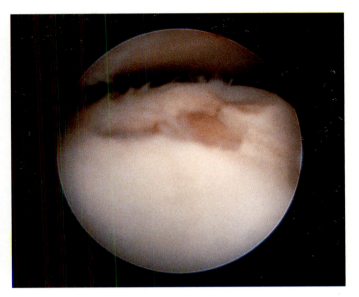

Figure 3

The appearance of an anterolateral osteochondral lesion of the talus following debridement and prior to drilling of the talus

talus are more readily accessible and distraction may not always be required. I am able to determine the need for distraction preoperatively with accurate localization of the lesion and, in particular, the accessibility of the talus with the foot in maximum plantar flexion.

After a synovectomy, the arthroscope is reintroduced into the anterolateral portal for access to the medial lesion. A thorough inspection of the joint has to be made, particularly for evidence of loose bodies. The cartilage is carefully probed to determine softening and to accurately stage the lesion. The posterior compartment is best inspected through a posterolateral portal. The OLT is debrided with an angled curette, a ring curette, a grasper, and a banana knife. The OLT often fragments and cannot be excised in one piece; therefore, care must be taken to avoid leaving small fragments behind. All degenerated cartilage and necrotic subchondral bone has to be removed (Fig. 3). The final steps in the procedure are to prepare the bed of the defect by a combination of drilling and curettage. Before drilling the crater, the hard necrotic subchondral bone must be removed. This is best achieved with a straight and angled curette, depending on the size and location of the lesion.

For the anterolateral lesions, I use a No 20 spinal needle to ensure that the pin enters the talus perpendicular to the OLT. The needle is inserted along the anterior edge of the tibia with the foot in maximum plantarflexion. The needle is removed and exchanged for a 0.062-inch diameter Kirschner wire, which is then used to drill four to six holes, depending on the size of the OLT.

It is more difficult to reach the medial lesions. The posteromedial lesions are best visualized through a posterolateral portal, and the instruments are inserted anteriorly with drilling through the medial malleolus. The transmalleolar approach is particularly useful in posteromedial OLT. Although the talar defect can be visualized from the anteromedial or posterolateral portals, there is no room for passage of the operating instruments from either of the anterior portals. With distraction, the anterolateral or posterolateral portal for visualization and the anteromedial portal for the operating instruments are occasionally sufficient. The initial debridement and removal of the defect may be accomplished with an angled curette introduced from the anteromedial portal but, if the lesion is in the anterior third of the talus, the final preparation of the crater with drilling can be satisfactorily accomplished only from the medial portal. This approach is contraindicated in a child with open epiphyses. I use a 0.062-inch diameter Kirschner wire introduced from the anteromedial cortex of the distal tibia. Although blind triangulation with the transmalleolar pin is difficult, this has been my preferred method. More recently, a mini-drill guide (Micro Vector) has been developed with a retractable tip and offset guide that precisely positions the drill pin over the talar lesion.

Without the drill guide, once in position with the pin, movement of the ankle will allow the insertion of three or four holes in one plane. If the lesion is large, the drill has to be repositioned for another set of holes.

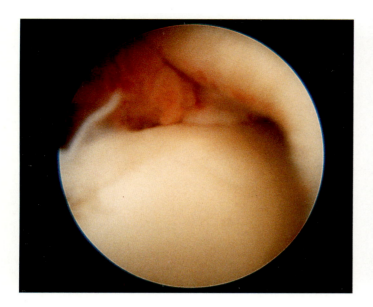

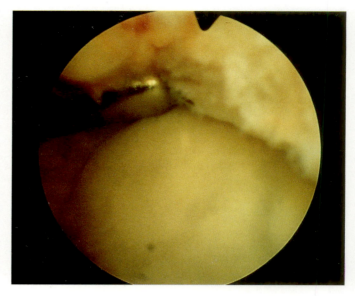

Figure 4

This patient experienced chronic pain in the anterior ankle. Arthroscopic evaluation demonstrated anteromedial synovitis, which was subsequently identified as pigmented villonodular synovitis

Figure 5

Hypertrophy and inflammation of the anterior inferior tibiofibular ligament is demonstrated with the arthroscope introduced anteromedially and the shaver anterolateral

Anterior soft tissue pathology

Soft-tissue pathology in the ankle is generally synovial in origin and includes various inflammatory synovitides and the more common forms of post-traumatic synovitis (Bassett et al 1990, Drez et al 1982, Ferkel et al 1991, Guhl 1986, Martin et al 1989, Wolin et al 1950). Although rheumatoid arthritis frequently involves the ankle, it has been my experience that arthroscopic synovectomy of the ankle in these patients has a limited role. Ideally, a synovectomy should be performed before the development of radiographic changes of joint space narrowing. However, by the time the patients are symptomatic, these changes have already occurred, and the beneficial effect of the synovectomy is minimal. As with other joints, it is almost impossible to perform a complete synovectomy of the ankle, even using distraction. Nevertheless, patients who present early enough in the course of the disease may benefit from a synovectomy.

Synovial chondromatosis and pigmented villonodular synovitis are two other conditions that are amenable to arthroscopic debridement (Fig. 4). Synovial osteochondromatosis has a variable presentation. The condition evolves slowly over a period of years, and the diagnosis and treatment differ for each phase of its development. During stage 1, there is involvement only of synovium, and the exact diagnosis can only be made arthroscopically.

Pigmented villonodular synovitis is non-specific and should be treated by as total a synovectomy as possible. If synovial thickening is identified posteriorly, then the distractor should be used to obtain adequate exposure for a more extensive debridement. The diagnosis is confirmed if chondral elements are found among areas of acute and chronic synovitis. During the second stage of activity, multiple chondral bodies form within the synovium, may break off into the joint, and may be diagnosed on arthrography or magnetic resonance imaging. The inflammatory synovitis becomes quiescent during the third stage, but many (even hundreds of) osteochondral fragments remain in both intra-articular and intrasynovial locations. Since a complete synovectomy cannot be performed, the recurrence rate is high. During stage 2, there are literally hundreds of these small and relatively soft fragments in the joint that are difficult to retrieve. During stage 3, the small intra-articular osteochondral fragments are easily removed; however, there are many intracapsular fragments, and some form an osseous union with the adjacent talus, usually necessitating an arthrotomy to complete the debridement.

Localized forms of synovitis occur more commonly. These are usually located anterolaterally and follow an episode of trauma, typically an ankle sprain (Fig. 5). After an ankle sprain or even a minimally displaced fracture, a hemarthrosis develops and is followed by a cellular reaction around the ATFL. Instead of this resolving, a proliferative fibrosis and finally synovitis and adhesion formation occur. These lesions are usually anterolateral and correspond to tears of the ATFL. Although less common, chronic post-traumatic antero-medial synovitis from a tear of the deep portion of the deltoid ligament may also occur.

The symptoms are all non-specific. However, patients will describe aching discomfort, a sensation of fullness, a build-up of pressure, and swelling. Occasionally, patients report a clicking, particularly with twisting motions. Athletes are unable to perform cutting motions. Marked local tenderness and focal synovitis are present. Pain is exacerbated by plantarflexion inversion movements for lateral lesions and dorsiflexion eversion for the medial lesions. Localized tenderness is present anterior to the lateral malleolus directly over the joint line and is associated with palpable synovitis. There is no ankle instability, but the term 'functional ankle instability', anterior capsular impingement syndrome, or, more commonly, anterolateral impingement syndrome of the ankle is used to describe the condition. Wolin et al (1950) were the first to describe a thickened band of tissue between the fibula and the talus that occurred after trauma, calling it 'meniscoid'. Although the tissue differs pathologically from a true meniscus, the hyalinized connective tissue from the talofibular joint capsule is probably a more advanced histologic form of the more common post-traumatic anterolateral synovitis. If symptomatic, I treat this post-traumatic focal synovitis with renewed physical therapy, emphasizing isokinetic exercise, diathermy ultrasound, and non-steroidal anti-inflammatory medication. If these fail, I use a local cortisone injection, which is effective in approximately half of these patients. Arthroscopy is used for those who remain symptomatic.

If one is certain of the extent of the anterior pathology, the arthroscopy may be performed under local anesthesia. This is followed by instillation of 10 cm³ of a local anesthetic. An initial evaluation is performed with the arthroscope anteromedial and the operating instruments anterolateral. The pathologic tissue is consistently found in the talofibular recess in the region of the ATFL. Debridement is performed with a motorized 3.5 mm full-radius resector shaver, followed by use of a basket punch forceps to abrade the lesion. Care should be taken to avoid debriding any remaining functional ATFL.

There appears to be histologic gradation of pathologic tissue, particularly in the anterolateral ankle, from flimsy adhesions to tougher fibrous tissue, and finally to the so-called meniscoid lesion, which by all accounts appears to be fibrocartilaginous tissue similar to the meniscus of the knee joint. These focal lesions are generally anterior. Occasionally, the entire anterior and anterolateral joint is filled with dense adhesions and not much can be seen. Typically, I commence the debridement with a motorized shaver and, as debridement progresses, more of the joint surfaces can be seen. I have found the 3.5 mm full-radius resector shaver to be useful for the initial debridement. A basket forceps and rongeur are then used to complete the debridement.

Posterior soft-tissue lesions

The incidence of posterior soft-tissue impingement is not as high as that of anterolateral impingement. Focal synovitis and adhesions occur, but additional pathology may be associated with hypertrophy of the transverse tibiofibular ligament or a posterior meniscus of the ankle. The transverse tibiofibular ligament extends from its origin on the distal fibula adjacent to the posterior talofibular ligament. It extends around the posterior margin of the joint to the edge of the medial malleolus. It lies directly below the posterior tibiofibular ligament. Before the use of mechanical distraction, lesions of the transverse tibiofibular ligament were not commonly recognized. However, over the past few years since I have been using distraction more frequently, it has been easy to recognize the normal and pathologic forms of this ligament. Hypertrophy of the ligament with or without fibrillation and synovitis may occur. A true posterior meniscus is rare and has been previously documented only in marsupials.

Posterolateral impingement is common in dancers, particularly during *pointe* maneuvers. In these cases, the presentation is similar to other forms of posterior impingement, but it is not associated with a bony block to plantarflexion, such as an os trigonum. Ankle pain is diffuse and, although vague, it is limited to the posterior aspect of the joint. This is worsened with exercise and using stairs, during which descent is particularly difficult. Dorsiflexion of the foot is painless. Clinically, it is difficult to differentiate the lesion from other posterior ankle pathology, but it is anterior to the more common retrocalcaneal bursitis. Tenderness is located slightly internally, which differentiates it from the lesion of the os trigonum that occurs on the medial aspect of the talus. These patients are best treated by conservative modalities, much as those described for the anterior lesions. Achilles tendon stretching is particularly useful. If symptoms persist after physical therapy treatments, the posterior ankle is injected with cortisone and the patient is placed in a short leg walking cast with the foot positioned in 5° of dorsiflexion. Magnetic resonance imaging is particularly useful in differentiating posterior ankle pathology and, in rare circumstances, has demonstrated a meniscus.

Arthroscopic ankle arthrodesis

As an alternative to more traditional techniques of ankle fusion, arthroscopic arthrodesis is an innovative approach that combines current technologies of arthroscopy with compression fixation of the joint. It is likely that, with improvements in instrumentation and technique, the arthroscopic procedure will become more appealing. The indications for arthroscopic arthrodesis

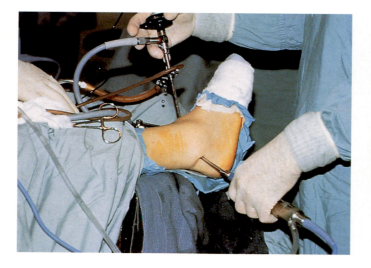

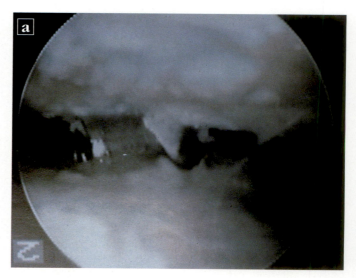

Figure 6

Arthroscopic ankle arthrodesis performed with the arthroscope anteromedial and the shaver posterolateral. The distractor is applied medially so as not to interfere with the posterolateral portal

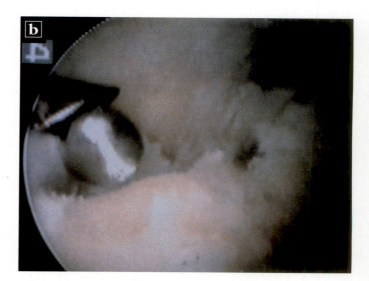

are the same as for conventional fusion, and include debilitating arthritis of the joint refractory to conservative treatment modalities. The arthroscopic technique can be used in most patients, provided both sagittal and horizontal plane alignment of the tibiotalar joint is normal and no substantial bone loss has occurred.

I have previously reported on the arthroscopic approach to ankle arthrodesis with a significantly more rapid rate of arthrodesis when compared to a traditional open method (Myerson & Allon 1989, Myerson & Quill 1991). I attributed this to decreased periosteal stripping and devascularization compared to open arthrodesis. The rapid and high rate of fusion makes this approach an appealing alternative, particularly where the need for early ambulation is imperative. Patients with vascular disease, dermatologic disorders, and those with other general medical contraindications to a major surgical procedure can also benefit from the arthroscopic arthrodesis.

The arthroscopic procedure is tedious. Despite an improving learning curve, it still takes almost twice as long to perform as an open arthrodesis. Adequate visualization of the joint is sometimes difficult. Because of the narrow field of operative exposure, arthritis visualization in the setting of severe post-traumatic conditions may be difficult. I routinely use distraction and recommend intermittent fluoroscopic imaging throughout the procedure. Anterolateral and anteromedial portals are used (Fig. 6).

Distraction should be performed cautiously due to severe scarring, contracture, and arthrofibrosis, and the distraction pins should not be allowed to bend. During the course of the debridement, some soft-tissue laxity occurs, and more distraction can be applied. Once

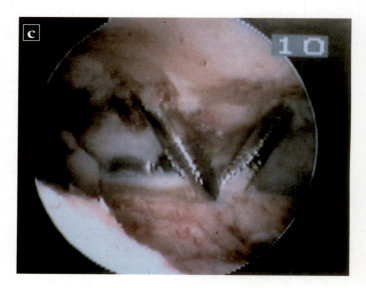

Figure 7

(a) Severe degenerative ankle arthritis, treated with debridement (b), and arthroscopic arthrodesis.
(c) Arthroscopic view of cannulated guide pins introduced from the tibia into the talus

debridement commences, the available space increases, further facilitating full posterior access and visualization. The initial debridement and synovectomy is performed with a 4.5 mm shaver, carefully debriding the talofibular and medial malleolar recess (Fig. 7). Curettage and burring are alternately used to denude the articular surfaces, followed by a high-speed cannulated burr, which results in smooth bleeding bone surfaces (Fig. 7b). The contour of the ankle should be preserved, and squaring off of the joint should be avoided. A chisel is not generally necessary. Optimally, the talus should fit snugly into the rounded off mortise.

The foot is then positioned in neutral dorsiflexion, 5° of valgus and 5° of external rotation, and guide pins from a cannulated large screw system are inserted fluoroscopically (Fig. 7c). The distractor is then dismantled, and the screws are inserted. The first screw is inserted through the posterior tibial cortex into the talus anteromedially, and the second screw is inserted from the medial malleolus into the lateral talus, just anterior to the posterior facet. More recently, I have used a third screw introduced from the fibula directed medially into the talus. Although this screw does not provide compression, it controls rotation.

Postoperative care

I routinely suture the portal punctures to prevent egress of any remaining inflow fluid, which may result in a synovial fistula. A compression bandage is applied; it may be removed and reapplied after three days. Swelling is a serious problem if the foot is left in a dependent position, and limb elevation and non-weight-bearing on crutches should be enforced until asymptomatic. During this period of time, patients are encouraged to elevate the extremity and perform range of motion exercises as soon as comfort permits. Generally, patients are non-weight-bearing for approximately 10–14 days. After the more extensive debridements for OLT, patients are kept non-weight-bearing for approximately 4 weeks. I am not certain that this makes a difference, but the prolonged period of non-weight-bearing may enhance the fibrocartilage 'filling in' of the defect. This depends on the size of the lesion, and smaller shallow defects probably do just as well with earlier weight bearing. Occasionally, a postoperative hemarthrosis may occur that is extremely painful; this can be aspirated.

Complications of ankle arthroscopy

Complications of ankle arthroscopy are relatively rare and are generally minor problems that resolve in time (Barber et al 1990, Drez et al 1982, Ferkel et al 1993).

True infection is also rare; when it occurs, it is superficial and limited to the portals. I have encountered mild skin problems on occasion, but these all appeared superficial and resolved with local wound care with peroxide or Betadine dressing changes and five days of oral antibiotic therapy. Sinus formation has been reported by Guhl (1986), with four cases in his first series of 69 patients. This was related to problems with triangulation when he used accessory portals that were too close to each other. One of the problems peculiar to the ankle is that there is minimal subcutaneous tissue and, with repeated passage of instruments through the portals, the tissues are prone to break down. This has occurred when switching frequently from medial to lateral portals and should be minimized by using small plastic cannulas for the arthroscope and instruments. I have experienced this problem on occasion when performing arthroscopic ankle arthrodesis or other procedures that involve extensive manipulation of instruments. It is probably caused by the size of the instruments, as I use the large (4.8 mm and 5.5 mm) motorized shavers. None of these patients developed chronic drainage or infection of these sinuses, although this has been described by Guhl (1986). In my experience, attention to wound care with frequent dressing changes resolved this problem within a few days.

Neurovascular complications have been described. These should be avoided with careful placement of portals. Before the procedure, the structures over the anterior ankle are carefully marked out. Particular attention should be paid to palpation of the deep peroneal nerve, dorsalis pedis artery, saphenous vein and nerve, and the branches of the superficial peroneal nerve. Although this works well medially and anteriorly, it is sometimes difficult to palpate the superficial peroneal nerve. In thin ankles, this nerve is easily palpated and can be rolled under the fingers. However, in obese patients or those with swollen ankles, this nerve has to be identified indirectly by the superficial skin and bone markings, or by its presumed course adjacent to the extensor digitorum and peroneus tertius tendons.

When introducing the arthroscope or instruments, a very small skin incision is made with a No 11 blade. The tissues are spread longitudinally with a small hemostat, and a blunt probe is then used to enter the joint. Under no circumstances should the knife blade be introduced too deeply. Not only can this cause inadvertent laceration of nerves, but the portal created by this technique is too large, and fluid egress may become a problem.

The arthroscope is introduced initially anteromedially and then turned anteriorly to visualize the soft-tissue structures and skin anterolaterally before creating the anterolateral portal. This avoids puncturing the lesser saphenous vein and possibly the superficial peroneal nerve. Neuromas of the deep and superficial peroneal nerve may be permanent. I have seen two unfortunate patients who now have permanent disability from injury to the deep peroneal nerve as a result of imprecise portal placement. One patient has a severe neuritis of the deep peroneal nerve that triggered a reflex sympathetic dystrophy, which has not resolved with treatment. From the other patient's description, it would appear that a motorized shaver was used to perform an anterior synovectomy that was carried too superficially, debriding the entire deep peroneal nerve in the process. There is a tendency to continue debridement with the shaver at times knowing that you are in a 'safe' area. I make it a rule to always keep the tips of the shavers and operating instruments in full view while performing the debridement. Doing so will not only avoid inadvertent damage to soft-tissue structures, it will also prevent articular cartilage scuffing. The latter problem is difficult to quantify, but is a very real problem. This is a complication that should no longer occur now that satisfactory modes of distraction are available.

Occasional massive swelling intraoperatively causes problems with visualization. Although this may not be construed as a complication, I had to abandon a procedure midway because of excessive fluid extravasation during the procedure. This used to be a common problem years ago, but no longer seems so since I have been using mechanical distraction more frequently. Furthermore, the size of the portals should be kept as small as possible, minimizing potential extravasation between the arthrotomy portal and the instrument. Some clinicians maintain that the use of an arthroscopy pump will also minimize extravasation. If a tourniquet is being used, this should be deflated to avoid further extravasation of fluid into the anterior compartment of the leg.

References

Adkison D P, Bosse M J, Gaccione D R, et al 1991 Anatomical variations in the course of the superficial peroneal nerve. J Bone Joint Surg 73A: 112–114

Baker C L, Andrews J R, Ryan J B, 1986 Anthroscopic treatment of transchondral talar dome fractures. Arthroscopy 2: 82–87

Barber F A, Click J, Britt B T 1990 Complications of ankle arthroscopy. Foot Ankle 10: 263–266

Bassett F H, Gates H S, Billys J B, et al 1990 Talar impingement by the anteroinferior tibiofibular ligament. A cause of chronic pain in the ankle after inversion sprain. J Bone Joint Surg 72A: 55–59

Berndt A L, Harty M 1959 Transchondral fractures (osteochondritis dissecans) of the talus. J Bone Joint Surg 41A: 988–1020

Drez D Jr, Guhl J F, Gollehon D L 1982 Ankle arthroscopy. Technique and indications. Clin Sports Med 1: 35–45

Ferkel R D, Scranton P E Jr 1993 Arthroscopy of the ankle and foot. J Bone Joint Surg 75A: 1233–1242

Ferkel R D, Guhl J F, Van Buecken K, et al 1993 Complications in ankle arthroscopy: analysis of the first 518 cases [abstr]. Orthop Trans 16: 726–727

Ferkel R D, Karzel R P, Del Pizzo W, et al 1991 Arthroscopic treatment of anterolateral impingement of the ankle. Am J Sports Med 19: 440–446

Flick A B, Gould N 1985 Osteochondritis dissecans of the talus (transchondral fractures of the talus): review of the literature and new surgical approach for medial dome lesions. Foot Ankle 5: 165–185

Guhl J F 1986 New techniques for arthroscopic surgery of the ankle: preliminary report. Orthopedics 9: 261–269

Guhl J F, Ferkel R D, Stone J W 1993 Other osteochondral pathology – fractures and fracture defects. In: Guhl J F (ed) Foot and Ankle Arthroscopy. Slack Inc, Thorofare (NJ). pp 131–139

Martin D F, Curl W W, Baker C L 1989 Arthroscopic treatment of chronic synovitis of the ankle. Arthroscopy 5: 110–114.

Myerson M S, Allon S M 1989 Arthroscopic ankle arthrodesis. Contemp Orthop 19: 21–27

Myerson M S, Quill G 1991 Ankle arthrodesis. A comparison of an arthroscopic and an open method of treatment. Clin Orthop 268: 84–95

O'Farrell T A, Costello B G 1982 Osteochondritis dissecans of the talus. The late results of surgical treatment. J Bone Joint Surg 64B: 494–497

Wolin I, Glassman F, Sideman S, et al 1950 Internal derangement of the talofibular component of the ankle. Surg Gynecol Obstet 91: 193–200

III.4 Foot Pressure Measurement

History and development

Rami J Abboud and David I Rowley

Introduction

The human foot is a complex multi-articular structure consisting of bones, joints and soft tissues, and it plays an extremely important role in the biomechanical function of the lower extremity. It is controlled both by intrinsic and extrinsic muscles and is the only part of the body acting on the ground. The foot provides support and balance during standing, and it affects stabilization of the body during both the weight bearing and propulsion phases of gait. During the stance phase – between heel strike and toe off – the foot has to adapt to a constantly changing pattern of loading consequent to the shifting location of the centre of mass of the body. The foot must also be relatively compliant in order to cope with uneven ground, yet be simultaneously capable of maintaining its functional integrity.

When the foot contacts the ground, an equal and opposite force to body impact, the ground reaction force (GRF), develops. The GRF changes in both direction and magnitude as the body propels itself forward or backward. This force is proportional to an infinite discrete area on the plantar surface of the foot when in contact with the ground and is defined as 'foot pressure'. This pressure encompasses both vertical and horizontal pressure, i.e. plantar vertical pressure and shear pressure.

Foot pressure measurement has long been an area of interest for many different professional groups, including orthopaedic surgeons, prosthetists and orthotists, footwear manufacturers, rehabilitation engineers, clinicians, and those involved in biomedical or biomechanical research. These professions need a clinical system of measuring foot pressure that is reliable, easy to calibrate and user-friendly, and preferably suitable for the investigation of foot and its related problems on a daily basis.

During the past century, many attempts have been made to develop a suitable technique for the measurement of the distribution of pressure underneath the plantar surface of the foot. The methods that have been proposed have been extensive and have ranged from simple devices to extremely complex ones. The existing systems can be classified in four different groups.

1. Instruments that measure the vertical pressure between the plantar surface of the foot and the ground, known as barefoot pressure devices, e.g. the dynamic pedobarograph (DPBG) (Betts & Duckworth 1978, 1985, Betts et al 1980).

2. Instruments that measure the vertical pressure between the plantar surface of the foot and the shoe, and measure the in-shoe pressure, e.g. GaitScan (Nevill 1991, Abboud 1989, McLauchlan et al 1994, Akhlaghi 1995, Nevill et al 1995).

3. Instruments that measure the vertical pressure between the sole of the shoe and the ground (Miyazaki & Iwakura 1978).

4. Instruments that measure either shear pressure (Lord et al 1992) or both vertical and horizontal pressures, such as the Parotec system.

Barefoot pressure systems

The earliest attempts at measuring pressure gave only qualitative information, this being highlighted in a paper by Beely (1882). Beely described a method of obtaining load patterns under the plantar surface of the foot by standing subjects barefoot on a thin, lined bag filled with freshly mixed plaster of Paris. He postulated that the rapidly setting plaster would capture the impression of the parts of the foot carrying load, the highest load causing the deepest impression. Despite the fact his method has failed to measure pressure pattern, it has laid down the principle of orthotic casting which was developed over the years to include both weight bearing and non-weight-bearing casting. His technique is still used by researchers investigating the gait cycle by studying footprints of someone walking on sand, clay or mud. Variations of this technique were reported by Muskat (1900), Seitz (1901), Momburg (1908), and Elftman (1934). Frostell (1925) and Abramson (1927) added to this technique a contact medium between the foot and the measuring device to prevent deformation of the foot during testing.

The earliest technique to measure plantar foot pressure distribution can be attributed to Morton in 1935, who provided one of the first semiquantitative methods for recording plantar loading. This kinetograph employed the ability of rubber to deform under loads. The deformation is seen to be proportional to the load applied, a principle which has been used by later researchers (Betts & Duckworth 1978). Harris & Beath (1947) adopted Morton's technique to facilitate easier calibration. Their design was later developed into three levels of ridges on a rubber mat (Fig. 1). These differing levels of ridges produce the effect of an increased density of ink in areas

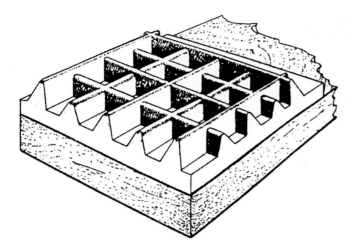

Figure 1

Harris–Beath three-dimensional ridges mat

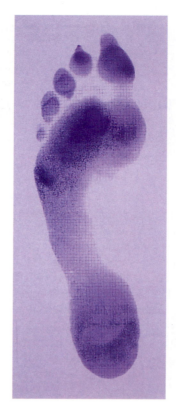

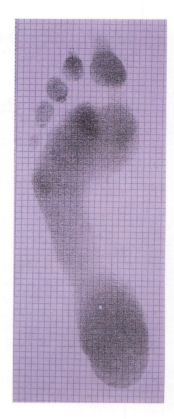

Figure 2

Harris–Beath printout

Figure 3

Podotrack printout of the same subject in Fig. 2

of high pressure when the subject stands on the mat. The pressure 'intensity' obtained from this system is somewhat dependent upon the amount of ink placed on the rubber mat and cannot be controlled or standardized. However, Silvino et al (1980) devised a way to calibrate the Harris–Beath mat by using a contact area of known size and weight, thus enabling qualitative and semi-quantitative information. A typical Harris–Beath printout is presented in Fig. 2.

Many other researchers have adopted the technique: Henry & Waugh (1975) used the system to study the effects of foot surgery on foot function and loading. Rose et al (1985) investigated flat feet in children with this system; Welton (1992) used it to develop a clinical tool for normal children and skeletally mature individuals. In his 30-year study, Welton subdivided his subjects into different groups, following age, sex, weight and pathology, and he subjectively analysed the footprints obtained and correlated these with clinical findings.

Most recently, in 1993, a new barefoot pressure system known as the 'Podotrack' (PDT) has been developed by Medical Gait Technology (Netherlands). This system is based on the principle of the Harris–Beath mat, and it makes use of a chemical reaction with a carbon paper. No special mat is required (Fig. 3). This system has several advantages over the Harris–Beath mat: it has a standard ink layer (designated by the carbon paper); it is calibrated – a plastic card provided with the system shows different grey scales proportional to pressure (Fig. 4); it is portable, strong and flexible; it can be fixed to the floor by means of two sticky strips and is antistatic and anti-allergic. It provides repeatable results of 61% of foot presure values when compared with those obtained from the DPBG (Barnes 1994). In his project, Barnes carried out a comparative study between the PDT and DPBG by placing the PDT paper on top of the DPBG

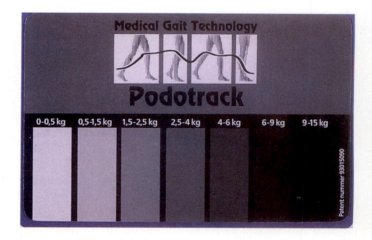

Figure 4

Podotrack pressure card

plastic sheet. The subjects then walked over both systems and data were recorded simultaneously in real time. This system has been described by van Ijzer (1993) as 'The new generation Harris mat'. The PDT system can be very useful as a first-stage assessment in any foot clinic before referral to a specialized laboratory.

Grieve et al (1980) used a sheet of aluminium foil (450 × 250 mm²) sandwiched between a 5 mm sheet of high density foam and a rubber undermat. This equipment was able to detect and measure peak pressures. The upper surface of the rubber mat was embossed with a pyramidal lattice, with a 3.54 mm interval. When pressure was applied to the foam, the aluminium foil beneath it deformed, the depth of penetration being proportional to the load applied.

Elftman (1934) described a device that used a light source and a cine-camera to show a series of dots and squares on a glass plate, the size and density of the dots indicated the pressure applied. This device proved to be of an immense value in the development of electronic optical scanners and video cameras to produce both qualitative and quantitative information (Tsuchiya 1972, Miura et al 1974, Beyerlein 1977).

Another entirely new concept was used by Barnett (1954) when designing his 'Plastic Pedobarograph'. His system was able to provide a record of the force distribution under the feet, and consisted of 640 rods of transparent perspex, each 10 mm² and 15 mm high, packed into a matrix 40 × 16, surrounded by a perspex jacket, giving an area of 37 × 15 cm². Position of foot contact and change in position of the horizontal lines due to force applied were filmed from the side at a speed of 30 frames/second. The data obtained included a two-dimensional graph representing foot pressure when viewed horizontally from the lateral side of the rods, and this was photographed and quantified.

Devices similar to Elftman's but using different optical principles have been described by Hertzberg (1955) and Chodera (1957). Chodera's 'Pedobarograph' consisted of a polyvinylidene chloride (PVC) sheet with near random roughness in contact with a smooth glass plate into which light was shone from the edges. Patterns produced from the scattered light were recorded by a monochrome camera and processed electronically to give pressure contours. Microcomputers have recently been used to generate high-quality colour images, the Pedobarograph platform has been embedded in a walkway (Fig. 5) and in turn linked to a computer to provide quantitative data.

Much of this work has been carried out by Betts & Duckworth (1978, 1980, 1985); this has led to the DPBG (Fig. 6). The DPBG consists of a pressure platform, 600 × 600 mm², and an adjustable measurement area of 380 × 280 mm², big enough for any foot size. The DPBG system has greater measurement resolution (6 mm²) and greater pressure resolution (0.04 kg/cm²) than any other system. The DPBG is at least four times more precise than any other pressure measurement technique which optimizes the interpretation of the data for clinical diagnosis. The sampling rate is adjustable with a maximum rate of 30 Hz. A disadvantage of the DPBG is that it is not portable.

The results from the DPBG for any given subject have been found to be consistent and repeatable to within

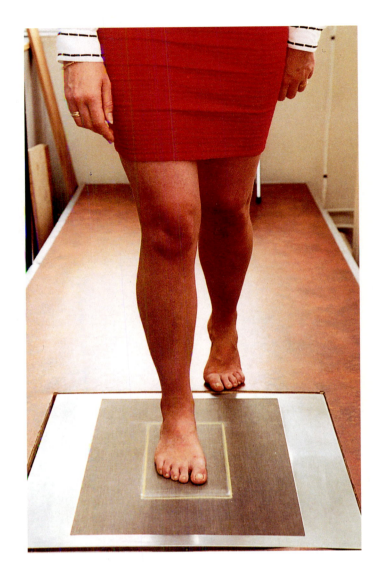

Figure 5

Pedobarograph platform embedded in a walkway

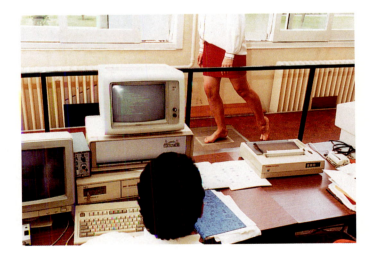

Figure 6

The Dynamic Pedobarograph

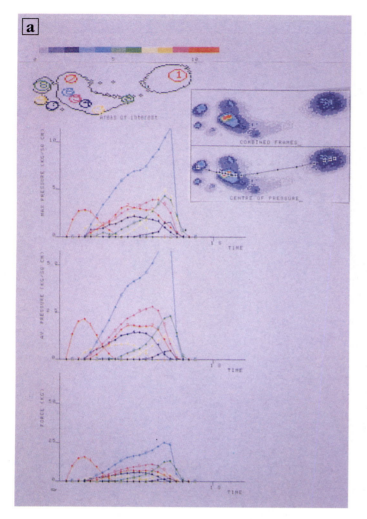

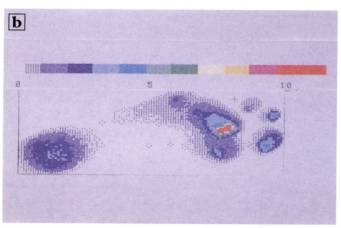

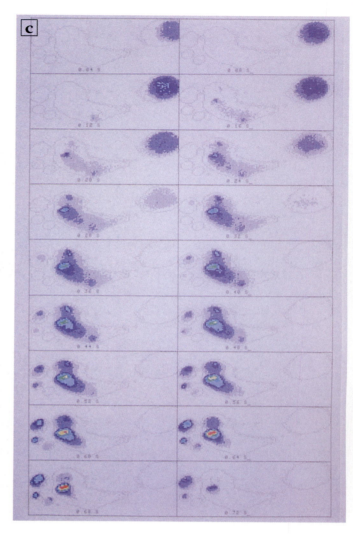

Figure 7

Dynamic Pedobarograph printout (same foot on H&B, PDT, DPBG) showing (a) maximum pressure, average pressure and vertical tone over time; (b) an overall loading of the foot on a contour map; and (c) specific load:time graphs to areas of specific interest

5–10%, this error being due to the main factor of foot step to step variation caused by the swinging of the pelvis. The information obtained from the DPBG can be shown graphically (Fig. 7).

The basic system (Fig. 8) consists of glass plate illuminated at its edges by strip lights. The top surface of the glass plate is covered with a thin sheet of opaque reflective plastic on which the subject walks. At the points of contact, the light is refracted out of the glass sandwich and reflected via a mirror positioned at 45° to the

horizontal underneath the DPBG platform to a video camera. The camera is in turn connected to a microcomputer where the data are stored, analysed and displayed. The amount of light scattered is proportional to pressure. Early systems suffered from an error of 10–15% in calibration because of viscoelasticity and temperature effects of the PVC used. This has been overcome with computer-based systems by dynamically relating the integrated light output to the total force measured by force transducers (Kistler) under the glass

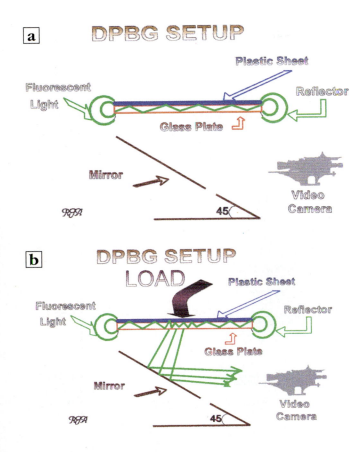

Figure 8

(a) The set up of the Dynamic Pedobarograph. (b) Under load

plate (Franks et al 1983) with detailed information obtained by Betts & Duckworth (1978, 1980, 1985). Since its development, the DPBG has been used extensively in clinical application as well as research.

Arcan & Brull (1976) described an optical principle that allows for collection of quantitative data on pressure distribution and measurement of load pressures simultaneously over the entire contact area. This device was used clinically by Aharanson et al (1980), and a similar principle was used by Leduc et al (1979) to investigate forefoot loading using a photoelastopodometry technique. Simkin & Stokes (1982) constructed an apparatus that was located in the floor, thus enabling subjects to walk across it. It consisted of 500 plungers inserted vertically into a metal frame and resting, at their lower hemispherical ends, on a sheet of glass coated with a photoelastic material. A plate size of 350 × 350 mm enabled one foot to be studied at a time, subjects walking barefoot along a walkway at their normal walking speed. Dhanendran (1979) suggested that the device used by Amar (1923), consisting of rubber balls and spring displacement to measure the two horizontal components of force, was the first force plate. Lord (1981), in her review, suggests that the harp-

like instrument of Basler (1927) is one of the earliest. His plate was divided into ten beams, each of which was balanced and stabilized by a metal wire. This device, when subjected to force, would place tension on the wire, thereby changing the frequency emitted by the wire. The first modern force plate was probably that constructed by Cunningham & Brown (1952). This was able to measure directly all four components of force and the coordinates of the instantaneous centre of pressure by using strain gauges mounted on each of four tubular aluminium columns. This original force plate of Cunningham & Brown was used as a basis by Harper et al (1961), who used all the characteristics of the earlier force plate and added cinematographic principles to capture the contact area of the foot during the stance phase of the gait cycle.

Sakorecki & Charnley (1966) described their system for measuring vertical components of force using both mechanical and optical methods, originally to study the effect of hip replacements on the gait cycle. In a study by Grundy et al (1975) the Skorechi–Charnley plate was ussed to investigate the centre of pressure under the foot during walking.

In 1972, Hutton & Drabble designed a force plate using twelve beams, each 9.5 mm wide and separated by a 2 mm gap, giving a 406 × 140 mm load-sensitive insert located in a 7 metre walkway. This insert could be rotated through 90°, and a strain gauge was used to record the vertical component of load on each beam during the stance phase of the gait cycle. By alignment of the beams parallel to or at right angles to the direction of progression of gait, either the mediolateral or the anteroposterior distribution of the foot pressure could be studied. A twelve-channel UV recorder produced twelve simultaneous curves of force against a base of time. This device was further developed by Stokes et al (1974).

Dhanendran et al (1978) described a variation on the beam principle that involved a full matrix force plate consisting of 128 cells arranged 16 by eight, each cell being 14 mm square and supported by a strain gauge ring. A minicomputer was used for on-line recording of data and for immediate processing. Manley (1979) also used the beam technique, but he used 16 transparent parallel beams mounted in a walkway transverse to the direction of walking. In order to calculate the total load and centre of pressure, force transducers were placed at the end of each beam, a camera was placed to show the contact load of the foot during recordings, and another camera was placed to obtain information from the lateral aspect showing the leg and foot. Using this same technique, Hutton & Dhanendran (1981) investigated the mechanics of the hallux. In 1985, Beverly et al investigated silastic arthroplasty of the hallux.

A strain gauge load cell within two force plates was used by Pelisse & Mazas (1975) in their study of the effectiveness of prosthetic knee and ankle joints. They measured the vertical and two horizontal components of force and the point of application..

An alternative design of load cell was used by Nicol & Henning (1978), who described a force transducer consisting of a 48×24 cm rubber mat, each side of which was covered by 16 conducting strips in orthogonal directions, which produced a framework of 256 capacitors. Arvikar & Seireg (1980) constructed a platform to measure the vertical loads under each of five metatarsal heads and the heel, and Draganich et al (1980) reported a different approach – the combination of a piezoelectric force plate measuring the three components of force and a matrix of switches. The matrix was capable of measuring foot contact area digitally as a sequence of switch closures. West (1987) questioned the usefulness of this innovation as a clinical tool.

Kistler Instruments Ltd (Switzerland) have produced a multicomponent measuring platform–load cell that is widely used in medical engineering applications. It can be used with a force platform as well as with a pressure platform such as the DPBG. The Kistler transducer is capable of measuring forces and moments in three orthogonal directions by using four load cells, one at each corner. The accuracy, reliability, and calibration have resulted in the piezoelectric being used at research as well as clinical centres investigating gait and foot pressure analysis (Kirtley et al 1985).

Scranton & McMaster (1976) developed a completely original method for measuring the momentary distribution of force under the foot, using a liquid crystal sheet of cholesteric crystals to determine the dynamics of pressure distribution under the weight bearing foot. Increases in pressure caused by foot contact on the sheet resulted in a proportional colour change from light to dark shades of blue; these colour changes were recorded by camera..

In 1983, Hirokawa & Ezaki described the development of an automatic gait measurement system capable of collecting successive footsteps both barefoot and shod. This system has been used by Hirokawa in 1987 and 1989 for the study of normal gait characteristics.

As modern technology has advanced, many researchers have turned their attention to the development of high-resolution pressure mats, thus providing a powerful tool for a full objective foot investigation. In addition to the DPBG, a commercially available system, known as the 'Musgrave Footprint', was developed at the Musgrave Park Hospital, Belfast, UK. The first commercially available system (in 1985) was based upon a matrix of 32×16 conductive foam rubber transducers. The system suffered from calibration problems and the data obtained were only qualitative. In 1987, a major change in the system was carried out by replacing the foam with Force Sensing Resistor material (FSR), which led to the first specially developed matrix of 2048 sensors of 5×5 mm^2 each. The properties of the material allowed calibration of the system and the software was upgraded to run on any compatible computer. The system was still limited in its ability to provide quantitative data by poor transducer performance. Since then, the system has gone through many changes and

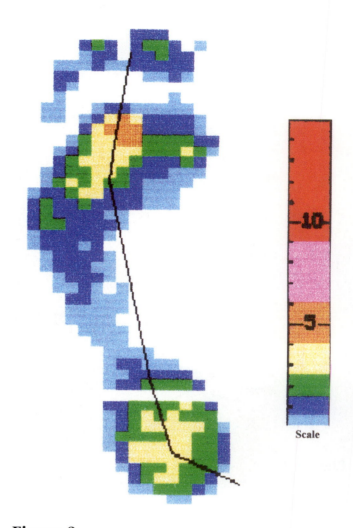

Figure 9

Musgrave printout (same foot on H&B, PDT, DPBG)

improvements, and the existing system consists of two footplates of $642 \times 297 \times 38$ mm^3 with an active area of the plate of 394×194 mm^2. Each plate contains 2048 sensors (5×5 mm^2), which have an electronically maximum scanning speed of 113 777 sensors per second with a sensitivity from 0.1–17 kg/cm^2. The system is calibrated statically and dynamically using a hydraulic probe. This system is the fifth generation Musgrave Footprint Mark 3; it can run on any computer and is supported by publications (Borton & Stephens 1994, Bennett & Duplock 1993, Roggero 1993, Corrigan 1993) (Fig. 9).

A system, known as the EMED system has been developed in Germany by Novel GmbH. It has been on the market since 1986. A large variety of EMED systems exist, and each comes with a modified software package depending on the system specification ·and capability. Novel GmbH has produced a diversity of systems that can be used in different areas, from clinical to industrial. The systems differ in size, weight, number of sensors, resolution, sampling frequency, and hence also in price (Table 1).

Table 1. EMED systems

EMED	Sensor Area	Record/Frequency	Sensor resolution
EMED-SF-1	500×300 mm²	max 100 Hz	1 sensor per cm²
EMED-SF-2	645×341 mm²	max 70 Hz	2 sensors per cm²
EMED-SF-4	570×322 mm²	max 50 Hz	4 sensors per cm²
EMED-SF-Tires	420×417 mm²	max 40 Hz	4 sensors per cm²
EMED-SL	360×190 mm²	max 50 Hz	2 sensors per cm²
MINI-EMED	350×160 mm²	max 16 Hz	3 sensors per cm²
MICRO-EMED	85, 170, 256 sensors	100, 50, 20 Hz respectively	9 sensors per cm²
Pedar	256 sensors	50–100 Hz	?

Table 2 Podinamic systems

Platform	PS1	PS2	PS3
Dimension (mm)	$475 \times 430 \times 0.7$	$950 \times 430 \times 0.7$	$1425 \times 430 \times 0.7$
Number of sensors	2544	5088	7632
Matrix elements	53×48	53×96	53×144
Thickness (mm)	72	72	72

The EMED software package is divided into four parts: data calibration, data collection, analysis and display/printout. The system has been used extensively by researchers and is supported by a considerable number of publications (Hennig 1991, Phillipson 1994, Chen et al 1994, Becker et al 1994). It is thought to be as reliable clinically as the other existing systems, though manufacturers do not recommend pressure systems for the automated production of insoles.

In 1990, Zeno Buratto SpA an Italian company began to develop a pressure measurement system, Podinamic Sensor, ACP (Computerized Pressure Analysis). It consists of a platform equipped with pressoceptors, protected by a layer of rubber, of FSR type, which makes use of the semi-conductive property of special materials inserted between two layers of polymer colaminates with interlaced electrodes. When pressure is exerted, the contact area between the semi-conductive material and the electrodes increases, causing a resistance decrease as a result. The sensor is 0.8×0.8 mm² in size, and has a sensitivity range between 250 g/cm² and 10 kg/cm², with nominal pressure of 10–20 kg/cm². The company developed three kinds of pressure platform, PS1, PS2 and PS3 (Table 2).

The first platform is capable of capturing one footstep whereas the other two are capable of collecting multiple barefoot steps up to a maximum of three steps. This makes the Podinamic pressure platform the first barefoot pressure system capable of measuring multiple footsteps. Data collection is done by using new scanning technology and a 32-bit analogue-to-digital converter. The sampling rate used at the moment is 250 Hz with a possibility, in the near future, to upgrade it to 500 Hz. The system comes with a powerful two-dimensional and three-dimensional software package to display pressure data in a variety of formats as well as calculating the angle of walking of both feet, which can be useful to measure postural sway. As the sensor is stable (company information), it needs to be calibrated only once. Despite the fact that the company proclaims an installation of over 200 systems in Europe, throughout my search I could not find a single publication using the system or any clinical validity.

The Belgian company Clinical Interactive Research market two systems based around their multiple sensor mat: the Electropostugraph (ELP), and the electropodograph (EPG). The mat consists of 1024 sensors and is again based on the Nicol capacitive pressure mat. The software is capable of presenting only relative percentage values. The system is not widely used.

In-shoe pressure measurement

An instrumented insole presents an attractive method of registering foot loading during normal and sport activities of a shoe-wearing subject. Providing that the insole is sufficiently thin, it can be slipped into any footwear and gives an assessment of the interaction of the foot with a particular shoe. Over the last two decades with the fast increase of electronic and computer technology, there has been a growing tendency towards the measurement of the foot–shoe interface and hence an increase in the development of in-shoe pressure systems. This is widely believed to reveal more information about foot pressure behaviour than the traditional barefoot pressure and force platforms. Furthermore, insole systems can record successive steps in walking. As the majority of people in the West wear shoes, in-shoe information would be of tremendous value for clinical assessment and shoe and orthotic design, as well as for pre- and postoperative rehabilitation.

Another method of recording continuous pressure information is by the attachment of pressure pads, either directly to the sole, or to the footwear from the inside or on the sole of the shoe. The available in-shoe pressure transducers can be summarized as follows: capacitive, strain gauge, force sensitive resistive film (FSR), piezoelectric, microcapsules, projection devices, hall effect and magnetoresistive, conductive polymers, and shear pressure. Although frequently referred to as 'pressure' transducers, most of these transducers measure load, which is related to 'average pressure' by the parameter of transducer area (Pressure = Force/Area). It is then obvious that different results are obtained at the same site by similar transducers of different sizes. Cavanagh et al (1992) in their review attempted to detail the existing in-shoe systems as well as identifying some of the existing systems with their advantages and disadvantages.

As early as 1947, Schwartz and Heath developed a system using small capacitive disc transducers; however, many calibration and performance difficulties were encountered. In 1964, Schwartz et al reported a different system of twelve 12.5 mm diameter piezometric discs which were attached to the plantar surface of the foot under the great toe and the first, third and fifth metatarsal heads, and under the medial and lateral aspects of the heel on both sides. A flexible cable connected each disc to a galvanometer, and a record of all twelve channels against a time base was achieved. Although a static calibration curve demonstrates the reproducibility of the transducers over the pressure range 0–2 kg/cm² (0 to 200 kPa) within a 5% limit, the curve is nonlinear over about 0.5 kg/cm². No dynamic calibration is given or discussed, despite the fact that the system had been used in gait studies.

Bauman & Brand (1963) taped capacitive pressure pads 100 mm² in area and 1 mm thick to the sole of the foot, with transducers located beneath the five metatarsal heads, the great toe, and the heel. Each transducer was attached by flying leads to an amplifier and pin recorder where peak pressures were recorded. Only static calibrations were carried out; these showed a nonlinearity which was compensated by special amplifiers. Furthermore, these transducers suffered from thermal drift, and thermal effects should always be taken into consideration when dealing with in-shoe measurement. This system was later redesigned by Hennacy & Gunther (1975). They used piezoelectric crystal elements as an alternative transducer material. Dynamic calibration was accomplished using a pressure varying relative to each other at frequencies between 20 and 70 per minute, which is considered to be very low to calibrate for a normal dynamic walking pattern where pressure variations can reach up to 50 Hz.

Miyazaki et al (1986) used a capacitive technique to monitor foot loading. An insole was designed from a 2 mm sponge rubber sheet sandwiched between two 50 μm copper foils, the whole constituting a capacitor. A sound is generated when the desired load is obtained during physiotherapy applications.

A commercially available system, the Computer Dyno Graphy (CDG) which uses special slippers with 8 pre-positioned transducer sites is marketed by a Dutch company, Infotronic. The transducers are capacitive and are of relatively large dimensions (30 × 30 × 1.5 mm³).

Novel GmbH include a thin flexible insole as part of their EMED systems (see page 129) for dynamic pressure measurement. Trials using the insole have been undertaken at several places, though there were difficulties because of internal breakages. The insole consisted of a matrix of around only 70 transducer elements, resulting in a relatively coarse spatial resolution. However, the 'Pedar' system, which consists of 256 sensors, is claimed by the company to overcome all the troubles that occurred in the past. The system is accompanied by powerful two-dimensional and three-dimensional software and a reliable hydraulic calibration system (personal communication).

A complex flexible system with a matrix of hundreds of elements (Tekscan) has been initially developed for the shoe manufacturer Scholl. The insole is composed of two polymer layers, each deposited with 4 mm strips of FSR material, one longitudinally and the other transversely. The main aim of the development of this system was for it to be used in Scholl's own high-street shoe stores and hence the main system features were to present powerful graphics to show to the public. This system has been modified to a microthin capacitive pressure sensor, FSCAN (Tekscan Inc, Boston, Massachusetts). The pressure sensor retains 960 individual sensor cells, at an interval of 5 mm, which can be trimmed to each individual's foot size. The sensing range of each individual cell is 56 to 868 kPa (0.56 to 8.68 kg/cm²). Data are collected at a sampling rate of 100 Hz. This system comes with a powerful software in two-dimensional and three-dimensional visual and graphical presentations of pressure and force. Ironically, the FSCAN system suffers from its own advantage, being thin. It wrinkles while being inserted inside the shoe and while the wearer is walking; hence it is prone to track failure and faulty data are more likely to be collected. Rose et al (1992) assessed the system thoroughly and found that two insole sensors would give different results when used on the same subject; consequently the system can be said to suffer from calibration problems. In addition, they found that there was a decline in sensitivity of 20.5% when used 12 times. Removing the insole pad and subsequently replacing it into the shoe also affected the pressure measurements. Despite these variations, the authors studied the 'effect of heel wedges on plantar pressure distribution and centre of force'. This was followed by other studies: Hayda et al (1994) utilized the FSCAN to investigate the 'effect of metatarsal pads and their positioning', and Lord & Hosein (1994) used it to study the effect of pressure redistribution by moulded inserts in diabetic footwear.

In 1973, Lerreim & Serek-Haussen produced a different type of transducer made of silicon beam strain gauge, which was 12 mm in diameter and 2.5 mm thick. This was embedded in a polyvinylidene chloride insole. These transducers were placed by referring to an X-ray film positioned under the metatarsal heads and connected by a lead to a multichannel recorder. Soames et al (1982) developed 16 transducers with a beryllium copper body and a centrally situated cantilever. A semiconductive strain gauge was attached to the cantilever to indicate bending upon application of forces. Unfortunately, this could only be used on an unshod foot and on a firm floor due to the need of a film surface underneath the transducers.

Frost & Cass (1981) described strain gauge load cells mounted individually into 10 mm cut out holes of a rubber insole with a thickness of 1.6 mm. Transducers were mounted within the holes of the insole and held in place by the lead-out wires. There was a high risk of wire breakage during use. This system suffered from bending artifacts, and hence the insole had to be worn barefoot and used on a flat ground, which made it useless as an in-shoe tool.

An ultra-thin (0.9 mm) Entran silicon strain gauge transducer to measure forefoot pressure at pre-determined sites on the plantar surface of the foot was described by Bransby-Zachary et al (1990). They use their transducers for the assessment of footwear as well as orthosis by measuring relevant foot pressure variables: pressure peak height, pressure time integral and step duration.

An unusual study of the pressures of ballet *pointe* shoes was carried out by Teitz et al (1985) by using small strain gauge pressure transducers with a sensitive area of 2.7 mm² at the tips of the first and second toes to investigate ballet shoe design.

Conductive and resistive films (FSR) have featured prominently in recent developments. Two most attractive characteristics of FSR transducers are that they are very thin and flexible. Early versions tended to act like on–off switches and suffered from poor resolution and huge temperature drift as well as bending effect problems, especially when used inside shoes. Langer Biomechanics group introduced their first FSR pressure in-shoe system, the Electrodynogram (EDG), as early as 1982. The system consisted of 14 flexible force transducers that can be positioned underneath discrete locations of the plantar surface of the foot. This system was followed by another EDG device consisting of seven disposable FSR transducers for each individual foot. These are placed at chosen points of interest. The transducers are connected to a data logger than can be worn around the waist. It has been used in several clinical applications (Feehery 1986). However, these FSR transducers still suffer from calibration problems, temperature drift and most of all breakage.

Peruchon et al (1989) have used a matrix insole made of conductive elastomeric sheet laid upon a flexible Kapton layer with 2×127 printed electrodes. Electromechanical properties of the conductive rubber were the main difficulties encountered, making transducer life limited to around 100 uses. More systems using FSR technology have been designed since FSR has become readily available. Hence, the development of the Lega system by a Belgian biomedical company, Clinical Interactive Research (CIR). The system consists of two flexible printed insoles with eight fixed transducer sites; the insoles are available in six sizes. Bending artifacts were one of many problems experienced by the system. In 1988, Maalej et al used a conductive polymer pressure sensor array to investigate in-shoe pressure distribution beneath the second metatarsal head for one subject. A four-by-four array was constructed, each element measuring 5×5 mm² The study found that the sensor should be at least 7 mm in diameter in order to cover the peak pressure under the MHs. The sensor system has been altered and used recently by Chang et al (1994) to investigate 'plantar pressure alterations using metatarsal pads'. Eight discrete interlink conductive polymer pressure transducers of 1.5 cm diameter and 0.25 mm thickness were located under the calcaneus, the medial longitudinal arch, the metatarsal shaft region, the metatarsal heads, and the hallux. The system allowed long-term continuous recording of up to 2 hours at 40 Hz. The transducers under the metatarsal heads are prone to bending, which can cause excessive hysteresis in data collection and hence unpredictable errors.

In 1990, the Italian company, Zeno Buratto, produced their Podinamic Soles system based on the same technology as their platforms. They produced three different kinds of soles with 48, 64, 96 and 144 sensors per insole. This system can work at a selectable frequency from 50–250 Hz.

In general, FSR has the drawback of being an active transducer material and therefore requiring an energizing signal. It has been found to be difficult to calibrate, owing to its ageing and wear characteristics and its high temperature coefficient and sensitivity especially around body temperature.

A number of research groups have used piezoelectric materials, such as the flexible polyvinyledine fluoride (PVDF), to develop their transducers. The attractive characteristic of the piezo films is that it requires no external voltage source, unlike other transducers. The piezoelectric effect results in the generation of charge when the material is deformed. After the charge has been collected on electrodes, it is converted into a voltage proportional to applied pressure. Pedotti et al (1984) used 200 μm PVDF film to produce a very thin insole with 16 aluminium deposited electrode sites, each 6 mm in diameter. The insole suffered from serious calibration problems, owing to bending. A very detailed system was reported by Hennig et al (1982), who developed a flexible silicon rubber insole embedded with 499 lead zirconate titanate piezoelectric elements. The system was very complicated, since 499 charge amplifiers were used. The transducers were tested and calibrated separately using a mechanical loading frame and a Kistler type 9322A quartz reference transducer. In 1988, Gross et al developed a system of eight discrete PZT piezoelectric transducers, $4.84 \times 4.83 \times 1.3$ mm^3 in dimension. A new generation of the PVDF film, known as Kynar film, produced by Penwalt Corporation, was used by Bhat et al (1989). They published various papers on transducer development using the new PVDF with a thickness of only 52 μm. The film was sandwiched between two insulating mylar film layers and the whole taped to a metal backing plate with a total dimension of $42 \times 19 \times 2$ mm^3.

The latest in the development of transducers using Kynar PVDF films was carried out by Nevill (1991). He tackled most problems other systems suffered from. He paid great attention to transducer cross-talk, bending and edge effect of piezo film, thermal drift, relative fragility, poor fatigue resistance, wiring, and – most of all – calibration, using a quasidynamic jig. The PVDF film, which is a long chain semi-crystalline polymer CH2-CF2, has several advantages compared to other transducers: high level of piezoactivity, wide frequency range of $10^{-8}–10^6$ psi (pounds/in^2), low acoustic impedance which matches human tissue impedance, faithful reproduction of input forces, its ease of cutting and its high stability coefficient, providing resistance to moisture and most chemicals (0.01% water absorption). This GaitScan system consists of eight piezoelectric discrete transducers per individual insole of $10 \times 10 \times 2.8$ mm^3 in dimensions. The copolymer film used (0.5 mm), was sandwiched between a sheet of printed circuit board (1.3 mm) and a brass sheet (1 mm), and embedded in a customized insole (Abboud 1989) of 1.8 mm of rubberized cork and 1 mm of regenerated leather, providing flexibility and rigidity in the vertical direction. The insole material compound was developed by Abboud (1989) during a study to find the best material to be used with these piezoelectric transducers.

The transducers are connected to a pre-amplifier box located above the ankle, which is then connected to a conditioning console. The system has a frequency response between 0.01 Hz and 200 Hz and an adjustable sampling rate from 50–200 Hz. It can capture up to 20 seconds of data with a transducer sensitivity range from 0–2000 kPa. This system has been used extensively for research as well as clinical applications.

An early system by Bauman & Brand (1963) used small dye-filled capsules sandwiched between two layers of foam. The capsules fractured under a certain load releasing dye onto a sock inside the shoe. This system was used to measure the pressure of the foot–shoe interface. Silvino et al (1980) adapted Harris mat for in-shoe use and made some attempts to provide quantitative results. Grieve & Rashdi (1984) used a more sophisticated method – an aluminium foil sheet was placed on top of an insole with pyramidal projections. The sheet deformed under pressure and an optical scanner was used to measure the deformations.

An important variable of in-shoe measurement – shear pressure – is still a big mystery, and until now there is not a single reliable system available on the market. This area has been tackled by Tappin et al (1980), who designed an integral magnetoresistive transducer, 15.69 mm in diameter and 2.3 mm thick. The transducer was attached to particular areas of the plantar surface of the foot using double sided tape. Pollard et al (1983) carried out similar work in an attempt to investigate footwear. In 1991, Tappin & Robertson continued Pollard's work using their own magnetoresistive transducers. They showed that shear forces occur for around 73–80% of the stance phase under the forefoot. Lord et al (1992) described a methodology for use of a shear transducer, 16 mm in diameter and 4 mm in thickness, based on the magnetoresistive principle. In her study, she located the shear transducer in the metatarsal head region. The exact placement of the transducer was determined by direct pressure distribution obtained by the FSCAN system, as she found that palpation is inaccurate by an average of 2 cm in the anteroposterior direction. This is highly unlikely to happen as the skin movement under the metatarsal heads will never be more than a couple of millimeters. This error can easily be obtained either by mispalpating the area of metatarsal head or by wrinkling and breakage of FSCAN tracks.

The author has used palpation for the last 6 years when locating GaitScan transducers, and during our latest study we proved a reliability of 95% in locating the metatarsal (McLauchlan et al 1994; Fig. 10). Further development on the GaitScan technique was carried out by Akhlaghi (1995) to measure shear pressure in two horizontal planes. Unfortunately, there is not enough information or clinical application of the system as yet. Laing et al (1992) described the development of a low profiled shear transducer that can be stuck to the plantar surface of the foot. The system is not fully developed.

A system, known as Parotec and marketed by a company called Kraemer, consists of pre-fixed transducers of up to 24 sensors using hydrocell technology. The company claims that this system is capable of collecting both shear and vertical pressure simultaneously. However, this system suffers from calibration problems and pressure insensitivity. Maximum pressure recorded can be up to 5 kg/cm² which is considered to be very low.

Sole-shoe transducer

In 1978, Miyazaki & Iwakura provided a portable device with the intention of recording total ground contact rather than to investigate load distribution. Their strain gauge transducers, 6 mm in thickness, were embedded and flushed to the sole of the shoes avoiding any interference with subjects' gait. They were located under the heel and metatarsal heads areas and were 65 × 35 mm² and 85 × 35 mm² respectively. Results obtained from these transducers, when compared with a force plate, showed that the errors were well within 10% of full scale for cadences under 110 steps per minute. The cut-off frequency of the system was 30 Hz, adequate for most purposes (Lord 1981). Nevertheless, the transducers demonstrated independency, which enabled individual heel and sole force to be calculated. This method proved to be of great help and can reveal considerable information for shoe designers and manufacturers, especially of sports shoes. The load pattern obtained can be related to the wearing of shoes, and hence a modular sole which can correct or accommodate any abnormality can be produced. Ranu (1987, 1989) described a shoe upon the sole of which five triaxial load cells measuring 19 × 19 × 8 mm³ were attached.

These types of transducer or systems have not appealed to researchers or clinicians. However, most barefoot systems can be used to record the interface between the shoe and the ground.

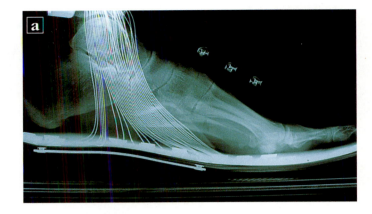

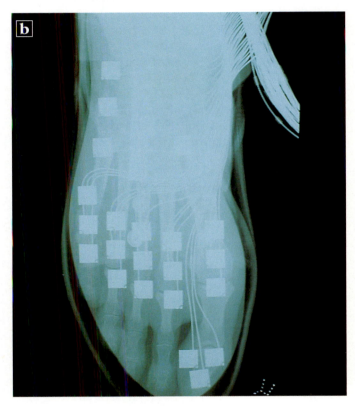

Figure 10

(a) Lateral and (b) anteroposterior radiographs taken during development of the GaitScan matrix with 32-transducer per insole show accurate location of the metatarsal heads and transducers by palpation

The dynamic system in clinical practice

Thomas Duckworth and Roderic P Betts

The patient whose postoperative record is shown in Fig. 11 was a 50-year-old female who suffered from hallux valgus affecting her left foot and who had been treated by a Keller operation. This procedure often renders the great toe functionless and tends to cause a greater load to fall on the metatarsal heads. This effect is well illustrated in the pressure record, in which the second, and particularly the first, metatarsal heads show very high peak pressures, the curve for the first going off-scale completely and the first metatarsal being loaded throughout a high proportion of the footstep time. In this case a preoperative print was not obtained, but this might well have shown a high loading under the first metatarsal head, a finding that would probably contraindicate the use of a Keller operation.

The second example (Fig. 12) illustrates a true pre- and postoperative comparison, the patient being a 53-year-old male suffering from bilateral hallux rigidus, with pain in the first metatarsophalangeal joints. There was no metatarsalgia, but he was having difficulty in finding suitable shoes, as he had an abnormally broad fitting. The tracing taken immediately prior to operation shows a noticeable concentration of pressure under the hallux. This falls just outside the normal range in absolute terms, but when seen in conjunction with the pressure distribution under the foot as a whole, the loading on the big toe is abnormally high. This is a common feature of hallux rigidus where dorsiflexion of the metatarsophalangeal joint is restricted. In some patients with severe pain from the hallux rigidus, this characteristic pattern is not seen, probably because the gait is adjusted to avoid high loads on the great toe and the weight is borne preferentially on the lateral side of the foot. In these circumstances, if the patient is asked to try to ignore the pain and walk normally, the high pressure under the hallux at the toe-off becomes apparent. This patient was treated by metatarsophalangeal arthroplasty using a Swanson-type implant. The procedure was satisfactory in relieving symptoms, the patient was able to go on an Alpine walking holiday less

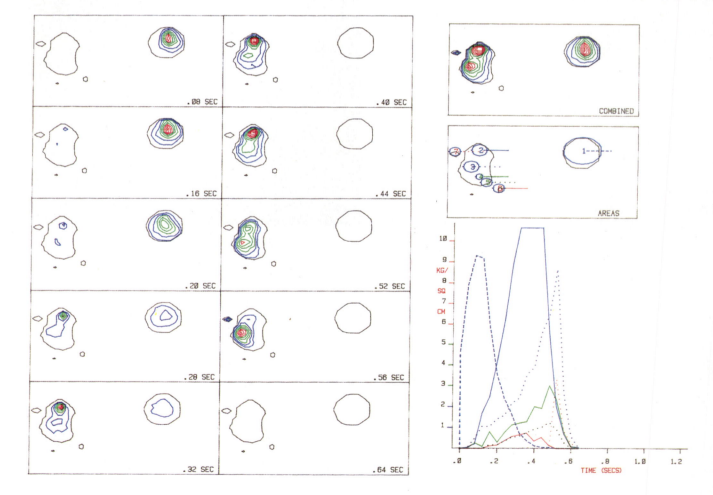

Figure 11

The colour plotter output for the left foot of a 50-year-old female treated by a Keller operation for hallux valgus. Postoperative result

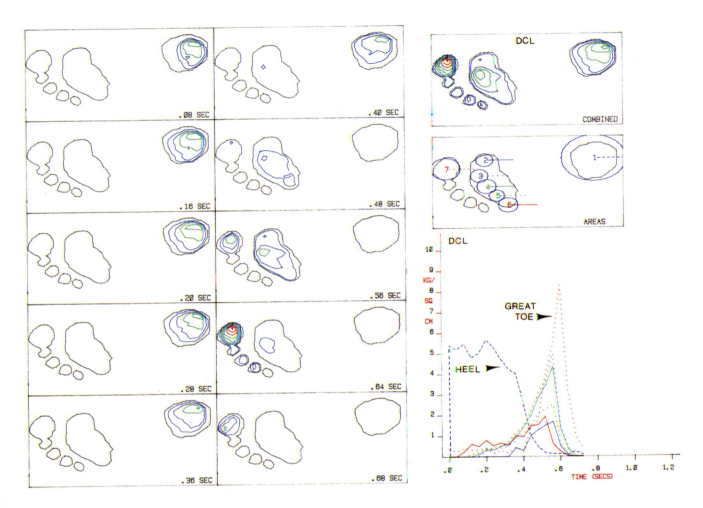

Figure 12

The colour plotter output for the left foot of a 53-year-old male treated by bilateral metatarsophalangeal joint replacements for hallux rigidus. Preoperative result

than three months after surgery, and he was able to wear normal shoes. The postoperative recordings (Fig. 13) show a change in distribution of pressure with an increase under the second metatarsal head, but still with some function retained under the big toe. It is this preservation of big toe function that is claimed to be the advantage of this particular operative procedure, and the value of this method of assessment is obvious.

These two examples could be amplified to show the characteristic patterns found in a wide range of common conditions and following surgical and orthotic procedures. As described, the foot pressure measurement system can be used to design insoles and other shoe modifications and is, to some extent, useful in checking whether the desired effect has been achieved. It is possible to use the device with the patient wearing shoes, provided the sole is not too thick and rigid and the pattern on the sole is not too pronounced. The pressure recording is somewhat diminished in definition, but the general pattern is easily distinguishable.

The second aspect of pressure management with the dynamic system which is currently proving to be of clinical value is that of the detection of points of high loading that might have significance in the development of pressure problems. This aspect was touched upon in discussion of the static system and experience has shown that both techniques are of value in this respect. This can be illustrated by reference to results obtained in diabetic patients (Boulton et al 1983, Betts & Duckworth 1985).

The factors responsible for the development of ulceration are undoubtedly complex and have been considered by a number of authors (Brand 1979, Bauman et al 1963, Kosiak 1961, Price 1964). Saboto et al (1982) demonstrated a highly significant association between the presence of an ulcer and the ground pressure beneath the foot. Their pressure measurements were made using a static system and they found that, in some patients, pressure sores occurred at sites where the pressure did not appear to be high and, not surprisingly, sores did not inevitably develop at all high pressure sites. They felt it was likely that areas other than those developing high pressures during standing probably occurred during walking. Their patients suffered from leprosy and presented very similar problems to those seen in diabetics.

Boulton et al (1983), showed that it is feasible to define a group of diabetic patients who are particularly

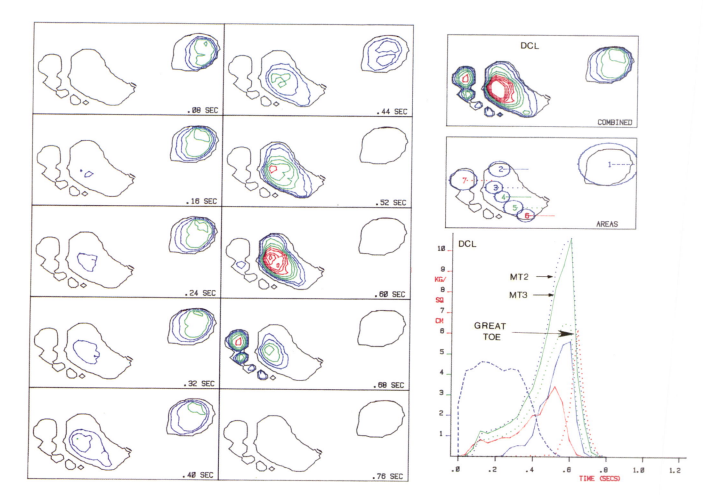

Figure 13

The same patient as illustrated in Fig. 12. Postoperative result

at risk of developing pressure sores and that these patients can be screened by using a series of simple clinical tests, of which the most useful proved to be the vibration perception threshold (VPT). These patients at risk can then be subjected to foot pressure analysis with a view to detecting those areas of the foot that are at particular risk because of the high pressures occurring. In a comparison of static and dynamic measurements used for this purpose, Betts & Duckworth (1985) found that, in order to detect all areas at risk, both techniques were required. In a series of 82 diabetic patients and 41 nondiabetic controls, it was found that all patients with neuropathy and a history of foot ulceration had abnormally high plantar pressures. This was also the case in 31% of diabetic patients with neuropathy but no history of ulceration. However, high pressures occurred in only 17% of patients with diabetes but no neuropathy, and in only 7% of nondiabetic subjects. In every group, there were a number of feet that were abnormal on both the static and the dynamic measurements, but also some feet that were detected as abnormal by only one of the two techniques of measurement. It was concluded that, for the most effective screening, a combination of both techniques was required.

For the purpose of this screening, threshold values of $1.75 \, \text{kg/cm}^2$ for the static measurements and $10 \, \text{kg/cm}^2$ for the dynamic measurements were taken as being those above which the foot could be considered to be at risk of developing pressure ulceration. These figures are based on normal values given above, but, clearly, it is likely that the time during which the pressure remains above this value is also likely to be important, and this factor was considered in the same study. If the information obtained from this kind of screening is to be of value, it must presumably lie in the design of protective footwear and perhaps of corrective operations, and the importance of making a complete assessment cannot be overemphasized. If, for example, only a static measurement is made, a high-spot may be detected and a suitable modification to the shoe may be made to off-load this area. There may, however, be another area or a different area of high loading when measured during walking, and this means that, unwittingly, the modification may be so designed that additional pressure is applied to such an area, thereby increasing the risk of ulceration.

Similar screening of feet at risk of pressure ulceration is now carried out by the authors in a range of other neurological conditions, particularly in children with spinal dysraphism, where the combination of deformity and sensory loss, together with a lack of insight by the patients into their condition, makes this a very vulnerable group. Dynamic measurements have proved to be a valuable addition to the static measurements which were originally planned for these children. It is in this group also that pre- and postoperative analysis has shown that some of the surgical procedures which have been widely used for correcting the deformities have had a surprisingly poor success rate.

References

Abboud R 1989 Evaluation of an inshoe pressure measuring system. MSc thesis, Dundee University

Abramson E 1927 Zur Kenntnis der Mechanik des Mittelfusses. Skand Archiv Physiol 51: 175–234

Aharanson Z, Voloshin A, Steinbach T V, Brull M A, Fanne I 1980 Normal foot–ground pressure pattern in children. Clin Orthop Rel Res 150: 220–223

Akhlaghi F 1995 An In-shoe Biaxial Shear Force Transducer Utilising Piezoelectric Copolymer Film and the Clinical Assessment of In-shoe Forces. University of Kent, Canterbury

Akhlaghi F, Daw J, Pepper M, Potter M J 1994 In-shoe step-to-step pressure variations. Foot 4: 62–68

Arcan M, Brull M A 1976 A fundamental characteristic of the human body and foot. The foot–ground pressure pattern. J Biomech 9: 453–457

Arvikar R, Seireg A 1980 Pressure distribution under the foot during static activity. Engineering Med 9: 99–103

Barnes D 1994 A comparative study between two barefoot pressure measuring systems. BMSc thesis, University of Dundee

Barnett C H 1954 A plastic pedograph. Lancet ii: 273

Basler A 1927 Bestimmung des auf die einzehen Sohlen bezirke wirkenden Teilgwitches des menschlichen Körpers. Abderhaldens Hamduch 5: 559–574

Bauman J H, Brand P W 1963 Measurement of pressure between the foot and the shoe. Lancet i: 629–632

Becker H P, Rosenbaum D, Zeithammel G, Gerngross H, Claes L 1994 Gait pattern analysis after ankle ligament reconstruction. Foot Ankle 15: 477–482

Beely F 1882 Zur Mechanik des Stehens über die Bedentung des Fussgewolbes beim Stehen. Langenbecks Archiv für klinische Chirurgie 27: 457

Bennett P J, Duplock L R 1993 Pressure distribution beneath the human foot. J Am Podiatr Med Assoc 83: 674–678

Betts R P, Duckworth T J 1978 A device for measuring plantar pressures under the sole of the foot. Engineering Med 7: 223–228

Betts R P, Franks C I, Duckworth T J, Burke J 1980 Static and dynamic foot pressure measurement in clinical orthopaedics. Med Biol Eng Comput 18: 674–684

Betts R P, Duckworth T J 1985 Plantar pressure measurements and prevention of ulceration in the diabetic foot. J Bone Joint Surg 67: 79–85

Beverly M C, Horan F T, Hutton W C 1985 Load cell analysis following silastic arthroplasty of the hallux. Int Orthop 9: 101–104

Beyerlein H R 1977 Apparatus for the synchronous measurement of pressure distribution and components of the resulting force under the human sole. Z Orthop 115: 778–782

Bhat S, Webster J G, Tompkins W J, Wertsch J J 1989 Piezoelectric sensor for foot pressure measurement. IEEE Engineering in Medicine and Biol Sci 11th Annual International Conference – Instrumentation Rehabilitation and Biomechanical Measurements. pp. 1435–1436

Borton D C, Stephens M M 1994 Basal metatarsal osteotomy for hallux valgus. J Bone Joint Surg 76B: 204–209

Boulton J M, Hardisty C A, Betts R P et al 1983 Dynamic foot pressure and other studies as diagnostic and management aids in diabetic neuropathy. Diabetes Care 6: 26–33

Brand P W 1979 Management of the insensitive limb. Phys Ther 59: 8–12

Bransby-Zachary M A P, Stother I G, Wilkinson R W 1990 Peak pressures in the forefoot. J Bone Joint Surg 72B: 718–721

Cavanagh P, Hewitt Jr F G, Perry J E 1992 Inshoe plantar pressure measurement: a review. Foot 2: 185–194

Chang A H, Abufaraj J U, Harris G F, Ney J, Shereff M J 1994 Multistep measurement of plantar pressure alterations using metatarsal pads. Foot Ankle 15: 654–660

Chen H, Nigg B, Koning J 1994 Relationship between plantar pressure distribution under the foot and insole comfort. Clin Biomech 9: 335–341

Chodera J 1957 Examination methods of standing in man. Czeckoslovak Academy of Sciences, Prague, vol. 1–3

Corrigan J P, Moore D P, Stephens M M 1993 Effect of heel height on forefoot loading. Foot Ankle 14: 148–151

Cunningham D M, Brown G W 1952 Two devices for measuring the forces acting on the human body during walking. Proc Soc Exp Stress Analysis 9: 75–90

Dhanendran M 1979 A Minicomputer Instrumentation System for Measuring the Force Distribution under the Feet, PhD thesis, PCL

Dhanendran M, Hutton W C, Parker Y 1978 The distribution of force under the human foot – an on line measuring system. Measurement Control 11: 261–264

Draganich L F, Andriacchi T P, Strongwater A M, Galante J O 1980 Electronic measurement of instantaneous foot-floor contact patterns during gait. J Biomechanics 13: 875–880

Elftman H O 1934 A cinematic study of the distribution of pressure in the human foot. Anat Record 59: 481–491

Feehery R V Jr 1986 Clinical applications of the Electrodynogram. Clin Podiatr Med Surg 3: 609–612

Franks C I, Betts R P, Duckworth T 1983 Microprocessor-based image processing system for dynamic foot pressure studies. Med Biol Eng Comput 21: 566–572

Frost R B, Cass C A 1981 A load cell and assembly for dynamic pointwise vertical force measurement in walking. Engineering Med 10: 45–50

Frostell G 1925 Beitrag zur Kenntnis der vorderen Stützpunkte des Fusses, sowie des Fusswinkels beim Stehen und Gehen. Z Orthop Chir 47: 3–54

Grieve D W 1980 Monitoring gait. Br J Hosp Med 24: 198–204

Grieve D W, Rashdi T 1984 Pressures under normal feet in standing and walking as measured by foil pedobarography. Annals Rheum Dis 43: 816–818

Gross T S, Bunch R P 1988 Measurement of discrete vertical in-shoe stress with piezoelectric transducers. J Biomed Eng 10: 261–265

Grundy M, Blackburn P A, Tosh R D, McLeish R D, Smidt L 1975 An investigation of the centres of pressure under the foot while walking. J Bone Joint Surg 57B: 98–103

Harper F C et al 1961 The forces applied to the floor by the foot in walking. National Building Studies Research, paper No 32. HMSO, London

Harris R I, Beath T 1947 Army Foot Survey. Report of National Research Council of Canada, Ohawa

Hayda R, Tremaine M D, Tremaine K et al 1994 Effect of metatarsal pads and their positioning: a quantitative assessment. Foot Ankle 15: 561–566

Hennacy R A, Gunther R 1975 A piezoelectric crystal method for measuring static and dynamic pressure distributions in the feet. J Am Podiatr Ass 65: 444–449

Hennig E M, Cavanagh P R, Albert H T, Macmillan N H 1982 A piezoelectric method of measuring the vertical contact stress beneath the human foot. J Biomed Eng 4: 213–221

Hennig E, Rosenbaum D 1991 Pressure distribution patterns under the feet of children in comparison with adults. Foot Ankle 11: 306–311

Henry A P J, Waugh W 1975 The use of footprints in assessing in results of operations for hallux valgus. J Bone Joint Surg 57B: 478–481

Hertzberg H T E 1955 Some contributions of applied physical anthropology to human engineering. Ann N Y Acad Sci 63: 616–629

Hirokawa S 1989 Normal gait characteristics under temporal and distance constraints. J Biomed Eng 11: 449–456

Hirokawa S, Ezaki T 1983 Development of walkway system to measure distance and temporal factors of gait, and to undertake gait-analytical study through the system. Jpn J Med Electron Biol Eng 21: 9–16 (paper in Japanese)

Hirokawa S, Matsumara K 1987 Gait analysis using a measuring walkway for temporal and distance factors. Med Biol Eng Comput 25: 577–582

Hutton W C, Dhanendran M 1981 The mechanics of normal and hallux valgus feet – a quantitative study. Clin Orthop Rel Res 157: 7–13

Hutton W C, Drabble G E 1972 An apparatus to give the distribution of vertical load under the foot. Rheum Phys Med 11: 313–317

Hutton W C, Parker Y 1979 Quantitative assessment of normal and pathological foot function. Engineering Med 8: 69–74

Kirtley C, Whittle M W, Jefferson R J 1985 Influence of walking speed on gait parameters. J Biomed Eng 7: 282–286

Kosiak M 1961 Etiology of decubitus ulcers. Arch Phys Med Rehabil 42: 19

Laing P, Deogan H, Cogley D, Crerand S et al 1992 The development of the low profile Liverpool shear transducer. Clin Physiol Meas 13: 115–124

Leduc A, Reyns I, Liegois E, Levray P H, Lievens P 1979 Load sharing within the forefoot. In: Kenedi R M, Paul J P, Hughes J (eds) Disability: proceedings of a seminar on rehabilitation of the disabled. Macmillan Press, Baltimore. pp. 182–184

Lerreim P, Serek-Haussen F 1973 A method of recording plantar pressure distribution under the sole of the foot. Bull Prosthet Res 118–125

Lord M 1981 Foot pressure measurements: a review of methodology. J Biomed Eng 3: 91–99

Lord M, Hosein R 1994 Pressure redistribution by molded inserts in diabetic footwear: a pilot study. J Rehab Res Dev 31: 214–221

Lord M, Hosein R, Williams R B 1992 Method for in-shoe shear stress measurement. J Biomed Eng 14: 181–186

Maalej N, Webster J G, Tompkins W J, Wertsch J J 1988 A conductive polymer pressure sensor array. IEEE Eng in Medicine & Biol Sci 11th Annual International Conference. pp 1116–1117

Manley M, 1979 Discussion contribution plus figure. In: Kennedy et al (eds) Disability. MacMillan, Basingstoke. pp 185–190

McLauchlan P T, Abboud R J, Randall G C, Rowley D I 1994 Use of an in-shoe pressure system to investigate the effect of two clinical treatment methods for metatarsalgia. Foot 4: 204–208

Miura et al 1974 Photographic method of analysis of the pressure distribution of the foot against the ground. In: Nelson R C, Morehouse C A (eds). Biomechanics IV. University Park Press, Baltimore. pp. 482–487

Miyazaki S, Iwakura H 1978 Foot-force measuring devices for clinical assessment of pathological gait. Med Biol Eng Comput 16: 429–436

Miyazaki S, Ishida A, Iwakura H, Takino K et al 1986 Portable limb-load monitor utilizing a thin capacitive transducer. J Biomed Eng 8: 67–71

Momburg 1908 Der Gang des Menschen und die Fussgeschwulst. Bibliothek von Color 25: 34

Morton D J 1935 The Human Foot. Columbia University Press, New York

Muskat G 1900 Beitrag zur Lehre vom menschlichen Stehen. Archiv Anat Physiol, Physiologische Abteilung 24: 285–291

Nevill A J 1991 A Foot Pressure Measurement System Utilising PvdF and Copolymer Peizoelectric Transducers. PhD Thesis, University of Kent, Canterbury

Nevill A J, Pepper M G, Whiting M 1995 In-shoe foot pressure measurement system utilising piezoelectric film transducers. Med Biol Eng Comput 33: 76–81

Nicol K, Henning E M 1978 Measurement of pressure distribution by means of a flexible, large surface mat. Biomechanics VI-A. University Park Press, Baltimore. pp 374–380

Pedotti A, Assente R, Fusi G, DeRossi D, Dano P, Domenici C 1984

Multisensor piezoelectric polymer insole for pedobarography. Ferroelectrics 60: 163–174

Pelisse F, Mazas Y 1975 A computer-directed measuring device to analyse pathological gait [in French]. C R Acad Sci Hebd Seances Acad Sci D 280: 2613–2616

Peruchon E, Julian J M, Rabischong P 1989 Wearable unrestraining footprint analysis system. Applications to human gait study. Med Biol Eng Comput 27: 557–565

Phillipson A, Dhar S, Linge K, McCabe C, Klenerman L 1994 Forefoot arthroplasty and changes in plantar foot pressures. Foot Ankle 15: 595–598

Pollard J P, LeQuesne L P, Tappin J W 1983 Forces under the foot. J Biomed Eng 5: 37–40

Price E W 1964 The etiology and natural history of plantar ulcer. Lepr Rev 35: 259

Ranu H S 1987 Normal and pathological human gait analysis using miniature triaxial shoe-borne load cells. Am J Phys Med 66: 1–11

Ranu H S 1989 A quantitative method of measuring the distribution of forces under the different regions of the human foot: during normal and abnormal gait. IEEE Engineering in Medicine and Biology Society 11th Annual International Conference – Biomechanics of the Upper and Lower Extremities. 824–825

Roggero P, Blanc Y, Krupp S 1993 Foot reconstruction in weight bearing area. Eur J Plast Surg 16: 186–192

Rose G K, Wetton E A, Marshall T 1985 The diagnosis of flat foot in the child. J Bone Joint Surg 67B: 71–78

Rose N, Feiwell L A, Cracchiolo A C 1992 A method for measuring foot pressure using a high resolution, computerized insole sensor: the effect of heel wedges on plantar pressure distribution and centre of force. Foot Ankle 13: 263–270

Saboto S, Yosipovitch Z, Simkin A, Sheskin J 1982 Plantar trophic ulcers in patients with leprosy. Int Orthop (SICOT) 6: 203–208

Sakorecki, Charnley 1966 The design and construction of a new apparatus for measuring the vertical forces executed in walking: a gait machine. J Strain Analysis 1: 429

Schwartz R F, Heath A L 1947 The definition of human locomotion on the basis of measurement with description of oscillographic method. J Bone Joint Surg 29: 203–213

Schwartz R P, Heath A L, Morgan D W, Towns R C 1964 A quantitative analysis of recorded variables in the walking pattern of normal adults. J Bone Joint Surg 46A: 324–334

Scranton P E, McMaster J H 1976 Momentary distribution of forces under the foot. J Biomech 9: 45–48

Seitz L 1901 Die vorderen Stutzpünkte des Fusses unter normalen und pathologischen Verhaltnissen. Z Orthop Chir 8: 37–78

Silvino N, Evanski P M, Waugh T R 1980 The Harris and Beath footprinting mat: diagnostic validity and clinical use. Clin Orthop Rel Res 151: 265–269

Simkin A, Stokes I A F 1982 Characterization of the dynamic vertical force distribution under the foot. Med Biol Eng Comput 20: 12–18

Soames R W, Blake C D, Stoll J R R, Goodbody A, Brewerton D A 1982 Measurement of pressure under the foot during function. Med Biol Eng Comput 20: 489–495

Stokes I A, Stott J R, Hutton W C 1974 Force distributions under the foot. A dynamic measuring system. Biomed Eng 9: 140–143

Tappin J W, Pollard J, Beckett E A 1980 Method of measuring 'shearing' forces on the sole of the foot. Clin Phys Physiol Meas 1: 83–85

Tappin J W, Robertson K P 1991 Study of the relative timing of shear forces on the sole of the forefoot during walking. J Biomed Eng 13: 39

Teitz C C, Harrington R M, Wiley H 1985 Pressures on the foot in pointe shoes. Foot Ankle 5: 216–221

Tsuchiya K 1972 Labour Welfare Projects Corporation, Prosthetics Centre Bioengineering Lab. Keisokn to Seigyo 11: 56–57

van Ijzer M 1993 The Podotrack, a new Generation Harris Mat. Podopost 39–41

Welton E A 1992 The Harris and Beath footprint: interpretation and clinical value. Foot Ankle 13: 462–468

West P M 1987 The clinical use of the Harris and Beath footprinting mat in assessing plantar pressures. Chiropodist 337–348

III.5 Electrodiagnosis

Colin G Barnes

Introduction

Electrodiagnosis is the study of nerve and muscle function and, therefore, is an investigation to be undertaken only after careful clinical assessment. It is rarely the only investigation required; usually it must be considered alongside radiographic techniques, haematological and biochemical studies, and biopsies.

Electrodiagnosis is never confined to the foot alone, but almost all electrodiagnostic investigations of the leg extend to the foot. Consideration of electrodiagnosis in a textbook devoted to the foot therefore demands discussion of investigation of the entire leg.

Clinical symptoms and signs that may indicate the need for electrodiagnostic investigation include:

1. Pain – sharp or shooting, as in typical nerve root lesions (e.g. sciatica) or nerve entrapment (e.g. tarsal tunnel syndrome).

2. Muscle weakness and wasting – typically including foot drop and deformity that can be confirmed objectively, indicating either nerve root, anterior horn cell or peripheral nerve lesions; or involving proximal muscles as in primary muscle disease.

3. Paraesthesiae and numbness – following dermatomes, as in root lesions, or following peripheral nerve distribution, as in nerve entrapment syndromes.

4. Tinel's sign – the production of pain and paraesthesiae in a nerve's distal distribution by tapping over the nerve at the site of a lesion (e.g. typically over the posterior tibial nerve behind the medial malleolus in a tarsal tunnel syndrome).

Classification of neuromuscular diseases has been well summarized by Swash & Schwartz (1981) and may be outlined as follows:

1. Neurogenic
   a. disorders of anterior horn cells
      (i)   spinal muscular atrophies
      (ii) motor neurone disease
      (iii) poliomyelitis and viral disorders   .
   b. disorders of motor nerve roots
   c. peripheral neuropathies
      (i)   genetically determined
            (a) peroneal muscular atrophy
            (b) hypertrophic
            (c) acute intermittent porphyria
            (c) amyloid
      (ii) acquired
            (a) mononeuropathies
                traumatic

entrapment
neuralgic amyotrophy
vasculitis
   (b) polyneuropathies
       inflammatory, e.g. Guillain–Barré
       metabolic, e.g. diabetes mellitus
       toxic and drug induced
       in malignant disease
       infective e.g. diphtheria
       connective tissue disorders
   d. disorders of neuromuscular transmission
      (i)   myasthenia gravis
      (ii) myasthenic syndrome (Eaton–Lambert)
      (iii) botulism
2. Myopathic
   a. genetically determined
      (i)   muscular dystrophies
      (ii) benign myopathies of childhood
      (iii) metabolic myopathies
      (iv) myotonic syndromes
   b. endocrine
      (i)   thyroid
      (ii) parathyroid and osteomalacia
      (iii) pituitary (acromegaly)
      (iv) steroid
   c. inflammatory
      (i)   idiopathic
            (a) polymyositis
            (b) dermatomyositis
            (c) in malignant disease
            (d) sarcoidosis
      (ii) infectious
            (a) viral
            (b) bacterial
   d. drug induced

Electrodiagnosis aims at distinguishing between neurogenic and myopathic conditions and, within these two main groups, between root and peripheral nerve lesions; peripheral polyneuropathies and isolated nerve lesions; anterior horn cell disease and disorders of neuromuscular transmission; and inflammatory and other forms of myopathy.

Reference to specialized works is necessary for a detailed account of electrodiagnostic techniques, for example Swash & Schwartz (1981), Kimura (1983), Licht (1971), and Marinacci (1968a). Electrodiagnostic investigation of the foot and leg, as in other parts of the body, involves electromyography and nerve conduction studies, the latter including assessment of late responses which in turn includes reflex latencies.

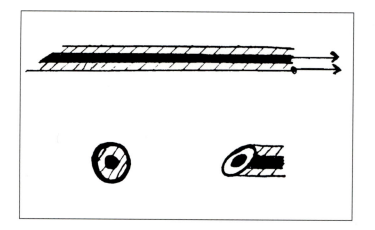

Figure 1

Diagram of concentric needle electrode – the central core is a wire (solid shading) threaded through a hollow hypodermic needle from which it is insulated (cross hatching). The tip of the needle is therefore a concentric bipolar electrode

Electromyography

Concentric needle electrodes (Fig. 1) are now used for routine electromyography, which involves the detailed study of four aspects of the electrical action potentials of individual muscles (Table 1). Surface electrodes may be used in studies of the patterns of contraction of different muscles in composite movements (e.g. walking or running) but do not permit sufficiently detailed investigation of neuromuscular pathology. Conversely, unipolar needles are used for specialized investigation of single muscle fibres.

Insertional activity

The insertion of a needle into a resting muscle produces a very brief spontaneous burst of muscle action potentials representing the underlying physiological state of the muscle. Thus a short run of normal motor units lasting for only just longer than the movement of the needle during insertion may be seen in normal muscle, fibrillation or positive potentials (see below) in denervated muscle, and short duration polyphasic units in myopathy. Long trains of high frequency discharges with decreasing frequency, likened to a 'dive-bomber', occur in myotonia.

All insertional activity is more easily provoked in denervated, myopathic, and polymyositic muscle.

Table 1 Outline of major electrographic findings in normals and in neuromuscular disease

	Insertional activity	Spontaneous activity	Volitional activity	Evoked potential
Normal	Transient – normal units	None	Biphasic or triphasic units up to 2 mV amplitude – complete interference pattern	Biphasic or triphasic 8–10 ms
Denervation	Transient or increased – normal units, fibrillation	Fibrillation Positive potentials	Reduced interference pattern, or no activity, incomplete denervation – normal units – giant polyphasics in long-standing disease	Complete – no evoked potential Partial – dispersed, polyphasic and prolonged (20–40 ms)
Myopathy	Increased – small polyphasics	None or fibrillation in polymyositis	Small, short duration polyphasic potentials	
Spinal muscular atrophy	Transient	Fibrillation	Denervation pattern (as above)	Denervation pattern (as above)
Motor neurone disease	Increased	Fibrillation Positive potentials Fasciculation	Reduced interference pattern Giant polyphasics	

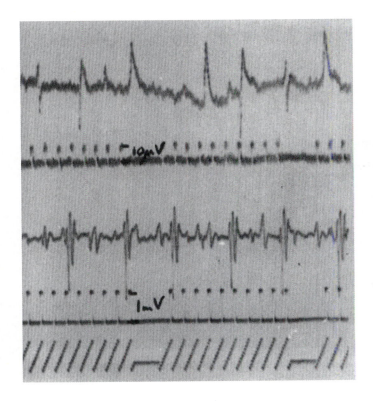

Figure 2

Fibrillation and positive potentials (upper tracing); incomplete interference pattern during maximal volitional contraction (lower tracing) indicating partial denervation

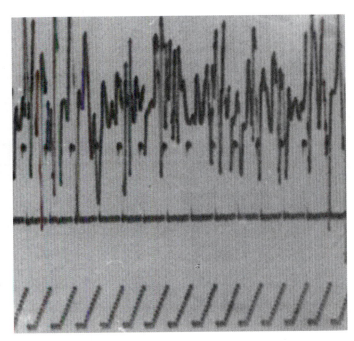

Figure 3

Extensor digitorum brevis muscle – normal EMG with complete interference pattern (calibration 1 mV)

Spontaneous resting activity of muscle

Normal relaxed muscle is electrically silent when the burst of insertional activity provoked by insertion or movement of the needle has ceased. Spontaneous activity is sought by sampling multiple areas of muscle and may be found in lower motor neurone denervation (fibrillation and positive potentials) and anterior horn cell disease (fasciculation).

Fibrillation and positive potentials

Fibrillation (Fig. 2) represents the spontaneous repetitive contraction of isolated muscle fibres producing electromyographically a short duration (1–5 ms), low amplitude (10–300 µV) spike potential with a repetition rate of 2–30 per second (Buchtal & Rosenfalck 1966). Positive potentials occur irregularly, having an initial fast positive deflection and slower decay with a negative phase, of longer duration (up to 20 ms) and larger amplitude (up to 120 µV) than fibrillation (Buchtal & Rosenfalck 1966).

Both these spontaneous potentials are indicative of lower motor neurone denervation of muscle, and develop within 10–21 days of the onset of denervation.

They are considered to be diagnostic if they persist for at least 1 minute and are detected in at least three sites in the muscle being studied (Leyshon et al 1981).

Fasciculation

Fasciculation is the irregular spontaneous firing of a motor unit; it represents, electromyographically, the motor action potential of a group of muscle fibres. The shape, size, duration, and repetition rate vary greatly. Fasciculations are polyphasic, with a larger amplitude and longer duration than fibrillation (up to 25 ms) and with positive potentials (up to 1000 µV). The repetition rate is very variable, from one per second to as little as one per minute (Hjorth et al 1973).

Although fasciculation may be benign, it occurs in anterior horn disease, when many muscles are affected, in radiculopathies, and occasionally in peripheral nerve lesions when muscles supplied by those roots or nerves only are affected.

Active motor units

Voluntary contraction of normal muscle produces biphasic or triphasic action potentials, which summate as the strength of contraction is increased. Thus minimal contraction will produce individual action potentials while maximal contraction will produce a pattern that

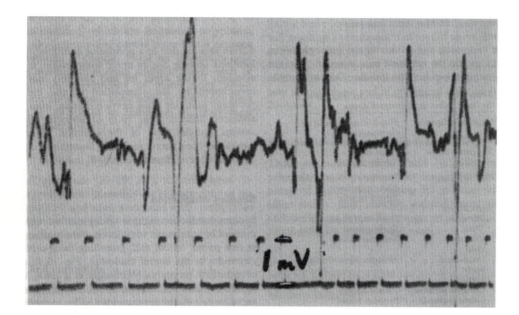

Figure 4

Giant polyphasic units

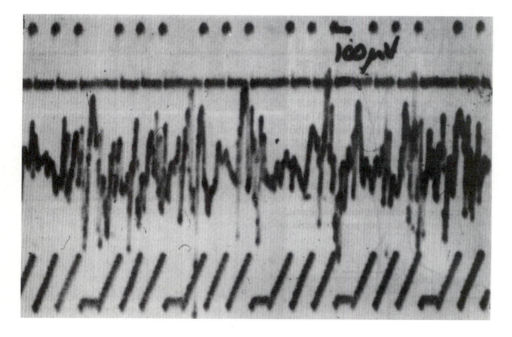

Figure 5

Short duration small amplitude polyphasic units in myopathy

completely obliterates the base line of the tracing (complete interference pattern). Polyphasic units may be seen in normal muscle and are accepted as normal if they occupy up to 5% of the tracing. A normal action potential duration is from 2–10 ms with an amplitude of 100 µV to 2 mV (Fig. 3). Partial denervation of a muscle leads to an incomplete interference pattern during the maximum voluntary contraction that can be achieved (see Fig. 2).

Giant polyphasic units

Giant units (Fig. 4) of up to 25 mV amplitude and up to 30 ms duration, which are frequently polyphasic, occur in long-standing partial lower motor neurone denervation of muscle. These are thought to arise from reinnervation from adjacent motor units or even from hypertrophy of motor units whose innervation is intact. Some authorities accept a giant unit of over 8 mV as an indication of denervation (Leyshon et al 1981).

Small amplitude polyphasic units

Small amplitude (25–150 µV), short duration (1–2 ms) polyphasic potentials are characteristic of the myopathies, and when associated with spontaneous fibrillation potentials indicate an inflammatory polymyositis (Fig. 5).

Evoked potentials

The muscle action potential evoked in a muscle by stimulation of its motor nerve is normally biphasic or triphasic 8–12 ms duration, and up to 5 mV amplitude. In the presence of complete denervation, as in nerve section, stimulation of the nerve above the lesion will not result in any muscle contraction. Partial nerve lesions, and hence partial denervation, will result in a combination of loss of nerve fibres, decreased excitability of some neurones, and changes in conduction velocity in others. This results in a dispersed evoked action potential which may be polyphasic and of prolonged duration (e.g. 20–40 ms).

Muscles investigated in the foot and leg

These are summarized in Table 2. The basic principles are that myopathies are predominantly proximal, neuropathies causing diffuse denervation affect mainly distal muscles, and individual nerve and root lesions demand investigation of the muscles supplied by those nerves and roots.

Table 2 Representative muscles investigated in the major pathological groups of disease

Suspected diagnosis	Muscle(s) investigated by electromyography
Myopathy/polymyositis	Quadricepts
	Tibialis anterior
Polyneuropathy	Extensor digitorum brevis
	Abductor hallucis
	Tibialis anterior
Nerve lesions	
Femoral	Quadriceps femoris
Tibial	Gastrocnemius and soleus
Posterior tibial	Abductor hallucis
(medial and lateral plantar)	Abductor digiti minimi
Common peroneal	Tibialis anterior
(lateral popliteal)	Peroneus longus
Deep peroneal	Extensor digitorum brevis
Nerve root lesions	See Table 3

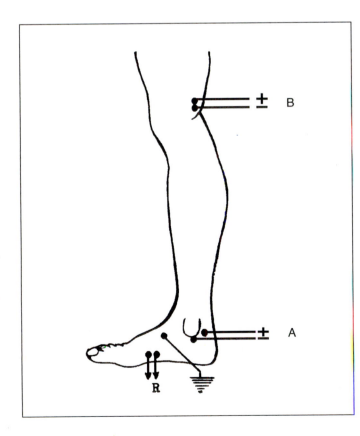

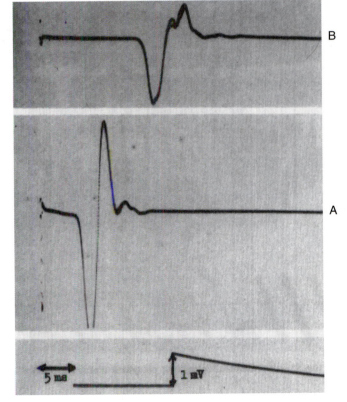

Figure 6

Diagram of motor conduction study of the medial popliteal/posterior tibial nerve with resultant tracings (R = surface or needle electrodes recording from the abductor hallucis muscle; A = stimulation behind the medial malleolus; B = stimulation in the popliteal fossa)

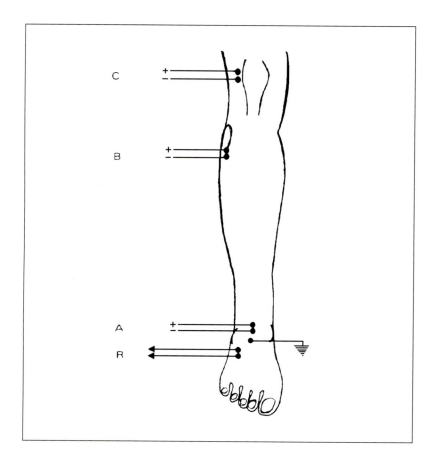
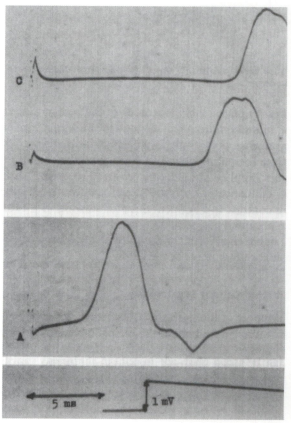

Figure 7

Diagram of motor conduction study of the common peroneal (lateral popliteal nerve) with resultant tracings. (R = surface or needle electrodes recording from extensor digitorum brevis muscle; A = stimulation at anterior surface of ankle; B = stimulation at neck of fibula; C = stimulation in popliteal fossa)

Nerve conduction

Motor conduction

The principle of measuring motor conduction velocity depends on the stimulation of a nerve at at least two points and measuring the latency between stimulus and the resultant muscle action potential (M-response) in a distal muscle. This will allow assessment of diffuse slowing due to a peripheral neuropathy, or localized slowing due to nerve compression. In the lower leg and foot this may be investigated by the stimulation of the medial popliteal/posterior tibial nerve recording from the abductor hallucis (Fig. 6) or abductor digiti minimi muscles, and of the common peroneal (lateral popliteal) nerve recording from the extensor digitorum brevis muscle (Fig. 7).

Sensory conduction

Sensory conduction in the lower leg and foot may be assessed by antidromic stimulation of the sural nerve at

two points on the calf, recording from surface electrodes at the lateral malleolus (Fig. 8) and over the fifth metatarsal (McGuigan et al 1983), and by orthodromic stimulation of the medial plantar nerve by ring electrodes round the hallux, recording from surface electrodes at the ankle inferomedial to the medial malleolus (McGuigan et al 1983). This enables slowing or loss of sensory nerve conduction to be assessed in the diagnosis of peripheral neuropathy, and localized abnormalities to be assessed as in the tarsal tunnel syndrome.

Late responses

F-response

The F-response (F-wave) is a late muscle potential resulting from stimulation of the nerve to that muscle which conducts antidromically and electrically activates the anterior horn cell, which then transmits an impulse down the motor nerve past the original point of stimulation to activate the muscle. As the configuration of the F-wave may vary with repeated stimuli the fastest of 10

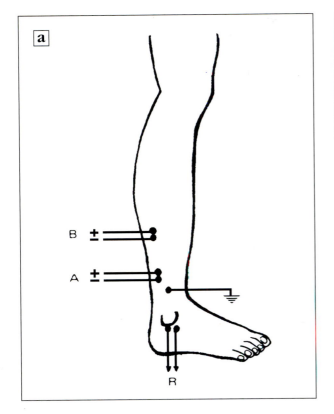

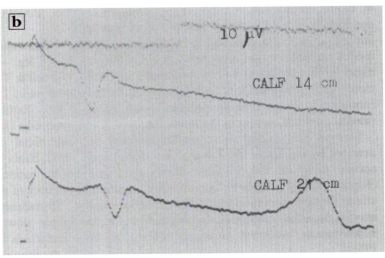

Figure 8

Sural nerve (antidromic) sensory conduction (a) diagram of points of recording (R) and stimulation (A and B) (b) resultant tracing

responses is taken as the latency. The latency thus represents the conduction from the point of stimulation to the anterior horn cell and back down the length of the nerve to the muscle (Swash & Schwartz 1981).

The F-wave therefore follows the M-response (Fig. 9) and as the point of nerve stimulation is moved proximally the latency of the M-response increases and the latency between the M and F responses decreases (Magladery & McDougal 1950, Kimura 1983).

The F-wave or proximal nerve conduction velocity may be calculated by measuring the distance from the point of stimulation to the spinous process of L2 vertebra, thereby estimating the distance to the anterior horn cell and using the following formula (Kimura 1978):

F–velocity (m/s) =

distance stimulating electrode to spine L2 (cm)

$$\overline{}$$

½ (F-wave latency – M latency – 1 ms)

(1 ms is allowed for central delay.)

This may be used to investigate proximal nerve function and is abnormal in Charcot–Marie–Tooth disease, polyneuropathy, e.g. Guillain–Barré syndrome (Kimura 1978), proximal entrapment neuropathies, and radiculopathies.

H-reflex

The H-reflex is a monosynaptic reflex derived from stimulating the medial popliteal nerve and recording

from the soleus muscle. This is mediated by the S1 nerve root, and a difference of over 1.5 ms between the two legs is considered to be abnormal on the side with the longer reflex time (Braddom & Johnson 1974).

T-reflex

The T-reflex, or tendon jerk, is analogous to the H-reflex. The Achilles tendon is tapped with a reflex hammer, this triggers the electromyograph time base while recording from surface electrodes placed over the calf muscles. A difference of over 2 ms indicates a slowing in the S1 nerve root (Malcolm 1951) (Fig. 10).

Peripheral neuropathy

Peripheral neuropathy implies symmetrical involvement of multiple peripheral nerves with a centripetal progression. The symptoms are paraesthesiae, which may be painful, numbness or disturbance of sensation in a glove-and-stocking distribution, and weakness of peripheral muscle groups.

Electromyography

In advanced and severe cases of polyneuropathy, electromyography of peripheral muscles will reveal partial denervation, the severity and extent of which depends on the rapidity of onset, severity and duration of the neuropathy.

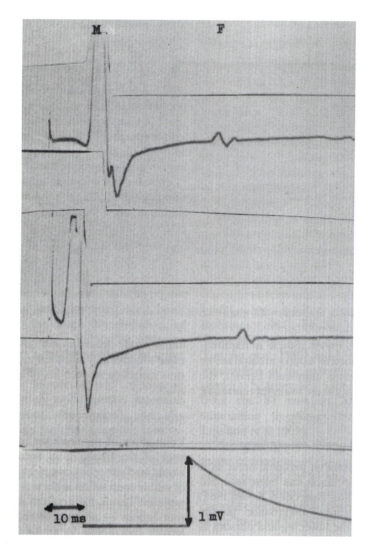

Figure 9

F-wave produced by stimulation of the common peroneal nerve at the ankle (lower tracing) and neck of fibula (upper tracing) recording from the extensor digitorum brevis muscle. (M = muscle contraction; F = F-wave)

Nerve conduction

Slowing of sensory nerve conduction, or loss of sensory nerve potentials, occurs early in peripheral neuropathy and is followed or accompanied by a slowing of motor conduction velocity. Thus, sural nerve conduction will be slow or absent, distal motor latency (ankle to extensor digitorum brevis muscle; medial malleolus to abductor hallucis and abductor digiti minimi muscles) will be prolonged, and the motor conduction velocity will be slowed in the common peroneal (lateral popliteal) and tibial (medial popliteal) nerves in the lower leg.

Slowing of proximal nerve conduction may be detected by studies of the F-wave. This occurs early in the Guillain-Barré syndrome (Kimura 1978). Diabetic neuropathy typically affects sensory more than motor nerve function, and may be detected in newly diagnosed diabetics with improvement following treatment (Ward et al 1971).

Entrapment neuropathy

Four entrapment neuropathies occur in the foot and lower leg – the medial tarsal tunnel syndrome (Kopell & Thompson 1960, Johnson & Ortiz 1966, Marinacci 1968b, Fu et al 1980, McGuigan et al 1983, Radin 1983), the anterior tarsal tunnel syndrome (Marinacci 1968b), entrapment of the superficial peroneal nerve (Kopell & Thompson 1963, Banerjee & Koons 1981), and entrapment of the common peroneal (lateral popliteal) nerve at the neck of the fibula. Entrapment of a nerve results in a segmental motor slowing, and slowing or loss of sensory conduction with a reduction or loss of the amplitude of the sensory action potential.

Peripherally placed entrapment, as in the case of the tarsal tunnel syndrome analogous to the carpal tunnel

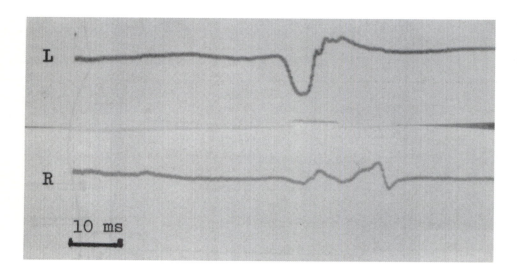

Figure 10

Ankle jerk – recording of ankle jerks showing a delay of 2.5 ms on the right (R) compared to the left (L)

syndrome, thus results in a delay of the distal latency from the point of stimulation at the ankle to the muscles supplied in the foot. This is in contrast to a segmental motor slowing in the more proximal course of a nerve as in common peroneal nerve entrapment at the neck of the fibula.

(Medial) Tarsal tunnel syndrome

The entrapment of the posterior tibial nerve under the retinaculum behind the medial malleolus is usually known as the tarsal tunnel syndrome. Marinacci (1968b) however distinguishes this from the less common anterior tarsal tunnel syndrome (see below).

Electromyography
Muscles supplied by branches of the posterior tibial nerve are sampled for evidence of denervation; thus the abductor hallucis (medial plantar nerve) is usually chosen. Since the symptoms may be similar to those produced by lesions of nerve roots or nerves proximal to the ankle it may be necessary, in difficult cases, to sample muscles above the ankle which would not show evidence of denervation in a tarsal tunnel syndrome.

Motor nerve conduction
The tibial (medial popliteal) nerve is stimulated behind the medial malleolus just proximal to the retinaculum and in the popliteal fossa, the resultant muscle action potential being recorded with needle or surface electrodes from the abductor hallucis or abductor digiti minimi muscles.

The distal latency (medial malleolus to abductor hallucis/abductor digiti minimi) will be delayed, while motor conduction velocity in the lower leg remains normal in contrast to a peripheral neuropathy (Johnson & Ortiz 1966, Marinacci 1968b, Fu et al 1980, McGuigan et al 1983). A delay in the distal latency of more than 2SD from the mean for the laboratory is considered abnormal.

Sensory nerve conduction
Sensory conduction in the medial plantar nerve may be studied by stimulating the hallux with ring electrodes and recording from surface electrodes placed over the posterior tibial nerve behind the medial malleolus. However potentials are small, McGuigan et al (1983) reporting a mean of 1.3 µV, and abnormalities may therefore be taken to support the diagnosis in conjunction with motor and electromyographic abnormalities.

Anterior tarsal tunnel syndrome

Marinacci (1968b) describes the entrapment of the terminal branch of the deep peroneal nerve at the ankle. This is rare, and electrodiagnostic study is analogous to that of the (medial) tarsal tunnel syndrome. Electromyography of the extensor digitorum brevis muscle and motor nerve conduction study of the common peroneal (lateral popliteal) by stimulation over the dorsum of the ankle, at the neck of the fibula, and in the popliteal fossa recording from the extensor digitorum brevis muscle is required. The diagnosis is confirmed by a delay in distal motor latency (ankle to extensor digitorum brevis), the motor conduction velocity in the lower leg remaining normal.

Superficial peroneal nerve entrapment

Entrapment of the superficial peroneal nerve as it emerges from the deep fascia has been recorded (Kopell & Thompson 1963, Banerjee & Koons 1981) causing pain and sensory disturbance in the anterolateral aspect of the lower leg and dorsum of the foot sparing the fifth toe. As the nerve has an entirely cutaneous sensory function electrodiagnostic confirmation of the lesion is not possible. However because of the similarity of symptoms with an L5 nerve root lesion, investigation to exclude such a root lesion (see below) may be necessary.

Common peroneal (lateral popliteal) nerve entrapment

Common peroneal nerve entrapment at the neck of the fibula is common; it causes footdrop and sensory disturbance. This must be distinguished from an L4 or L5 root lesion. Thus electromyography would demonstrate denervation in all anterior and lateral tibial muscles and in the extensor digitorum brevis, thus including muscles supplied by roots L4, L5, and S1.

Motor nerve conduction
Stimulation of the common peroneal nerve at the neck of the fibula in an entrapment neuropathy leads either to a complete absence, or equality, of visible contraction in the anterior and lateral tibial muscles. This is distinct from an inequality in nerve root lesions – absence or reduction of peroneus longus contraction

in an L5 root lesion, and of tibialis anterior contraction in an L4 root lesion.

Stimulation of the common peroneal nerve in the popliteal fossa, below the neck of the fibula and at the ankle, recording from the extensor digitorum brevis, will reveal a normal distal latency (ankle to extensor digitorum brevis) and motor conduction velocity in the lower leg (between neck of fibula and ankle) but a segment of slowed conduction around the neck of the fibula (popliteal fossa to neck of fibula).

Anterior horn cell diseases

Anterior horn cell diseases are characterized by those of viral origin, classically poliomyelitis, and those of progressive and chronic type, classically motor neurone disease.

Poliomyelitis

Acute poliomyelitis is now virtually never seen. It is characterized by the early onset of the denervation changes of fibrillation and positive potentials at rest, and reduction of action potentials on volition which, in the most severely affected muscles, may be completely absent. These changes develop within the first month of the onset of clinical weakness.

Reinnervation occurs to a variable extent and may be complete. Chronic denervation is characterized by the presence of giant polyphasic units. Motor and sensory nerve conduction studies are normal.

Motor neurone disease

Progressive wasting and weakness of muscles is most obvious in the upper limbs but may affect lower limbs, particularly the feet. Degeneration of neurones in the spinal cord and motor neurones themselves thus gives a combined pattern of upper and lower motor neurone lesions.

Electromyographic features at rest are those of spontaneous fibrillation and positive potentials (lower motor neurone denervation) and also fasciculation potentials (anterior horn cell involvement). On volition a reduced pattern with reduced recruitment of activity on progressive voluntary exertion and the presence of giant polyphasic units is typical.

Motor and sensory nerve conduction studies remain normal.

Nerve root compression

Electromyography

Electromyography is a useful and accurate method of investigating nerve root compression, complementing routine radiological and scanning techniques. It has, however, been largely superseded by more recent imaging techniques, particularly MRI. Its value is based on the detection of lower motor neurone denervation in both limb and paraspinal muscles supplied by the affected root, delay in the F-response to the appropriate muscle; and a delayed latency of the H-reflex and ankle jerk in S1 root lesions or of the knee jerk in L4 root lesions.

The techniques for detecting individual nerve root lesions by investigating the lower limbs are summarized in Table 3. Paraspinal muscles may also need to be investigated and may be the only site of abnormal EMG findings (Johnson & Melvin 1971).

The accuracy of electrodiagnostic detection of nerve root lesions has been compared with clinical assessment, myelography (radiculography), and computed tomography (CT). In 1950, Shea et al recorded that preoperative electromyography correctly indicated the nerve root involved as confirmed at operation in 90% of 60 patients. Subsequent studies indicated an accuracy of between 62 and 100% in electromyographic diagnosis both of the existence of a nerve root lesion and of the specific root involved (Marinacci 1955, Shea & Woods 1955, Crue et

Table 3 Electrodiagnostic abnormalities of nerve root lesions (Leyshon et al 1981, Tonzola et al 1981)

Nerve root	EMG abnormalities in limb muscles	Late responses
L 4	Quadriceps femoris Tibialis anterior	Delayed knee jerk
L 5	Tibialis anterior Extensor hallucis longus Extensor digitorum longus Peroneus longus Gastrocnemius – lateral head Extensor digitorum brevis	Prolonged or absent F-reflex in extensor digitorum brevis
S 1	Gastrocnemius – medial head Soleus Abductor hallucis	Prolonged or absent F-reflex and H-reflex in soleus Prolonged or absent ankle jerk

al 1957, Knutsson 1959, 1961, Kambin et al 1962, Flax et al 1964, Leyshon et al 1981, Tonzola et al 1981, Khatri et al 1984). In all reports electromyography was shown to correlate well with operative findings, and better than clinical assessment, myelography, radiculography, or CT scanning alone, although no single technique was entirely accurate.

It has been shown that electromyographic evidence of partial denervation may persist after previous spinal surgery, thus making assessment of such patients with persistent symptoms notoriously difficult (Johnson & Melvin 1971, Leyshon et al 1981).

Denervation of muscles supplied by several nerve roots in both legs may be present in lumbar spinal stenosis and the cauda equina syndrome. Thus electromyographic assessment of both legs is necessary when symptoms are those of caudal claudication, and it has been shown that nerve roots involved may be at, below or even above the level of the stenosis (Young et al 1981, Seppalainen et al 1981, Bartleson et al 1983).

Nerve conduction studies

Standard motor and sensory conduction studies do not assist in the diagnosis of radiculopathy as such studies are normal (Eisen et al 1977, Leyshon et al 1981). If there is any suspicion that the clinical manifestations may arise from a peripheral neuropathy then sural nerve (sensory) conduction should be measured as an initial assessment of peripheral nerve function.

F-response
Delay in the F-response (see above) is indicative of a proximal nerve lesion including those of the roots. Thus, by investigation of this response in the common peroneal nerve recording from the extensor digitorum brevis muscle, or in the tibial nerve recording from the abductor hallucis muscle, one may detect proximal lesions in the L5 and S1–2 nerve roots respectively (see Table 3) (Tonzola et al 1981).

H-response and T-reflex
These techniques (see above) are only useful in detecting S1 nerve root lesions by study of the H-reflex to the soleus and the ankle jerk T-reflex, and possibly by studying the knee jerk in L4 root lesions.

References

Banerjee T, Koons D D 1981 Superficial peroneal nerve entrapment. J Neurosurg 55: 991–992

Bartleson J D, Cohen M D, Harrington T M, Goldstein N P,

Ginsburg W W 1983 Cauda equina syndrome secondary to long-standing ankylosing spondylitis. Ann Neurol 14: 662–669

Braddom R I, Johnson E W 1974 Standardisation of H reflex and diagnostic use in S1 radiculopathy. Arch Phys Med Rehab 55: 161–166

Buchtal F, Rosenfalck P 1966 Spontaneous electrical activity of human muscle. Electroencephalogr Clin Electromyogr 20: 321–326

Crue B L, Pudenz R H, Shelden C H 1957 Observations on the value of clinical electromyography. J Bone Jt Surg 39A: 492–500

Eisen A, Schomer D, Melmed C 1977 An electrophysiological method for examining lumbosacral root compression. Can J Neurol Sci 4: 117–123

Flax H J, Berrios R, Rivera D 1964 Electromyography in the diagnosis of herniated lumbar disc. Arch Phys Med Rehab 45: 520–524

Fu R, DeLisa J A, Kraft G H 1980 Motor nerve latencies through the tarsal tunnel in normal adult subjects: standard determinations corrected for temperature and distance. Arch Phys Med Rehab 61: 243–248

Hjorth R J, Walsh J C, Willison R C 1973 The distribution and frequency of spontaneous fasciculations in motor neurone disease. J Neurol Sci 18: 469–474

Johnson E W, Melvin J L 1971 Value of electromyography in lumbar radiculopathy. Arch Phys Med Rehab 52: 239–243

Johnson E W, Ortiz P R 1966 Electrodiagnosis of tarsal tunnel syndrome. Arch Phys Med Rehab 47: 776–780

Kambin P, Smith J M, Hoerner E F 1962 Myelography and myography in diagnosis of herniated intervertebral disc. J Am Med Ass 181: 472–475

Khatri B O, Barvah J, McQuillen M P 1984 Correlation of electromyography and tomography in evaluation of lower back pain. Arch Neurol 41: 594–597

Kimura J 1978 Proximal versus distal slowing of motor nerve conduction velocity in the Guillain-Barré syndrome. Ann Neurol 3: 344–350

Kimura J 1983 Electrodiagnosis in disease of nerve and muscle: principles and practice. F A Davis, Philadelphia

Knutsson B 1959 Electromyographic studies in the diagnosis of lumbar disc herniation. Acta Orthop Scand 28: 290–299

Knutsson B 1961 Comparative value of electromyographic, myelographic and clinical neurological examinations in diagnosis of lumbar root compression syndrome. Acta Orthop Scand (suppl) 49: 1–35

Kopell H P, Thompson W A L 1960 Peripheral entrapment neuropathies of the lower extremity. New Engl J Med 262: 56–60

Kopell H P, Thompson W A L 1963 Superficial peroneal nerve. In: Peripheral Entrapment Neuropathies, The Williams & Wilkins Co., Baltimore. Ch 7, p 39

Leyshon A, Kirwan E O'G, Wynn Parry C B 1981 Electrical Studies in the diagnosis of compression of the lumbar root. J Bone Jt Surg 63B: 71–75

Licht S (ed) 1971 Electrodiagnosis and electromyography. 3rd edn. Waverly Press Inc., Baltimore

McGuigan L, Burke D, Fleming A 1983 Tarsal tunnel syndrome and peripheral neuropathy in rheumatoid disease. Ann Rheum Dis 42: 128–131

Magladery J W, McDougal D B Jr 1950 Electrophysiological studies of nerve and reflex activity in normal man. 1. Identification of certain reflexes in the electromyogram and the conduction velocity of peripheral nerve fibres. Bull Johns Hopkins Hosp 86: 265–290

Malcolm D S 1951 A method of measuring reflex times applied in sciatica and other conditions due to nerve root compression. J Neurol Neurosurg Psychiatry 14: 15–24

Marinacci A A 1955 Clinical Electromyography. San Lucas Press, Los Angeles

Marinacci A A 1968a Applied Electromyography. Lea and Febiger, Philadelphia

Marinacci A A 1968b Neurological syndromes of the tarsal tunnels. Bull LA Neurol Soc 33: 90–100

Marinacci A A 1968c Evaluation of lumbar herniated disc. In:

Applied Electromyography. Lea and Febiger, Philadelphia. Ch 22, p 218

Radin E L 1983 Tarsal tunnel syndrome. Clin Orthop 181: 167–170

Seppalainen A M, Alaranta H, Soini J 1981 Electromyography in the diagnosis of lumbar spinal stenosis. Electromyogr Clin Neurophysiol 21: 55–66

Shea P A, Woods W W 1955 Electromyography as an aid in clinical diagnosis. Arch Intern Med 96: 787–793

Shea P A, Woods W W, Werden D H 1950 Electromyography in diagnosis of nerve root compression syndrome. Arch Neurol Psychiatry 64: 93–104

Swash M, Schwartz M S 1981 Neuromuscular disease: a practical approach to diagnosis and management. Springer Verlag, Berlin

Tonzola R F, Ackil A A, Shahani B T, Young R R 1981 Usefulness of electrophysiological studies in the diagnosis of lumbosacral root disease. Ann Neurol 9: 305–308

Ward J D, Barnes C G, Fisher D J, Jessop J D, Baker R W R 1971 Improvement in nerve conduction following treatment in newly diagnosed diabetics. Lancet i: 428–430

Young A, Dixon A K, Getty J, Renton P, Vacher H 1981 Cauda equina syndrome complicating ankylosing spondylitis: use of electromyography and computerised tomography in diagnosis. Ann Rheum Dis 40: 317–322

III.6 Vascular Assessment

Amar S Jain

There is increased morbidity following foot surgery in general as a result of delayed wound healing and delayed restoration of function. This may be due to multiple factors. Meticulous surgery, and a well-structured and controlled postoperative management programme is essential for a successful outcome, but the foot has the inherent problem of being a distal organ of locomotion and being vulnerable to dependent oedema. There is also a comparative lack of soft tissue padding between the bones and the dorsal skin.

All operations must aim at the best possible result but in some instances a poor result cannot be avoided. The risk of failure must be taken into account when deciding on the indications for surgery and in planning the operation. Examination of the foot follows the lines adopted for any other part of the body; i.e. observation, palpation, test for sensation, and then radiography and special investigations. The vascular assessment should include assessment tissue perfusion and nutrition.

Inspection

The first important point to be noted is the colour of the skin as this is an indication of the condition of the circulation. This should be noted with the leg both dependent and in the elevated position since postural changes are important in some conditions such as thromboangitis obliterans. In vascular deficiency thickening of the nails, loss of hair and occasional peripheral cyanosis are observed.

Condition of the skin

The skin condition should be observed next. Excessive sweating and a clammy, sodden surface is common in many nervous disorders, both functional and organic, whereas in other conditions, such as diabetic neuropathy, there is reduced sweating, which leads to dry plantar skin and a tendency to scale and crack. An imprint on the dorsal skin caused by stockings or the strap of a shoe should be noted. It is an indication of oedema not sufficient to produce the characteristic pitting seen in severe degrees.

Palpation

The dorsalis pedis artery can be palpated on the dorsal surface of the foot. It lies between the extensor hallucis

longus tendon and the common extensor tendon. The posterior tibial artery can be palpated behind the medial malleolus about one-third of the way between it and the heel. One pulse at least should be palpable, preferably tibialis posterior. Diabetic neuropathy also alters the normal regulation of the microcirculation, leading to thickening of the capillaries and arterial venous shunting. This causes a warm, dry foot with a pounding pulse and distended veins.

Temperature

The dorsum of the hand is a very sensitive structure and it is used to feel the skin temperature. With experience, up to 1°C difference can be appreciated. Atherosclerosis and diabetes mellitus are the commonest conditions that lead to vascular insufficiency.

Atherosclerosis

It is estimated that 5% of men over the age of 50 years suffer from peripheral vascular disease (PVD). The disease itself never presents in isolation. PVD may occur as a consequence of atherosclerosis. The most important factor in the development of PVD is atherosclerosis of major vessels.

A review of the literature shows that the following factors play an important part in the development of atherosclerosis. One must, therefore, look for these risk factors in the vascular assessment of the foot.

1. Smoking
2. Hypertension
3. Diabetes
4. Hyperlipidaemia
5. Ageing
6. Male sex
7. Family history

Diabetes mellitus

The prevalence of known diabetes mellitus in the UK is approximately 1% of the population (Neil et al 1986). This may be a conservative estimate, as American literature has shown as high a rate as 5% (Levin 1987). Since diabetes is more common in people over the age of 50, the prevalence is expected to rise further as the population becomes progressively older. Between 12 and 15% of the diabetic population present with foot problems, including neuropathy and PVD, which will ultimately

Table 1 Features of ischaemic and diabetic ulcers	
Ischaemic Ulcer	*Diabetic Ulcer*
Foot cool	Foot warm
Painful	Painless
Veins not dilated	Veins dilated
Ulcer not surrounded by thick skin (hyperkeratosis)	Ulcer surrounded by thick hyperkerotic skin
Pulses absent	Ulcer commonly occurs on the plantar surface under the metatarsal heads
	Ulcer has a pink punched out base

affect the skeletal structure, sensation and circulation. Some patients present with ulcers. Certain features help in differentiating between ischaemic and diabetic ulcers (Table 1, Figs 1, 2).

Special investigations

Vascular assessment of the foot is rather difficult as most available investigations do not accurately predict wound healing after surgery. Clinical experience has shown that a warm foot does not necessarily mean increased vascularity. In the same way a cool foot may heal satisfactorily. However, clinical examination is the main part of the assessment, but a number of special investigations can help further in assessing the foot.

Haematological and blood chemistry investigations

Haematological and blood chemistry estimations, such as haemoglobin estimation, blood viscosity, plasma protein and white cell count can give some indication of likely wound healing. Serum albumin level above 3.5 gm/dl (Dickhaut et al 1984) and a total leucocyte count over 1500 per mm^3 seen to predict satisfactory wound healing.

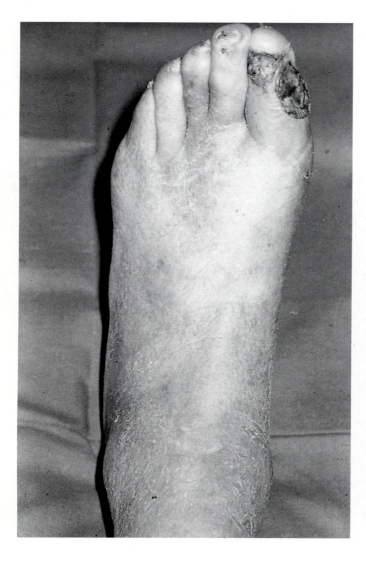

Figure 1

Ischaemic ulcer

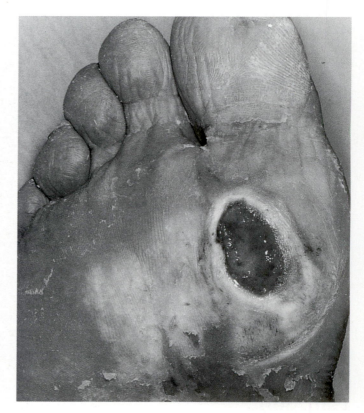

Figure 2

Diabetic ulcer

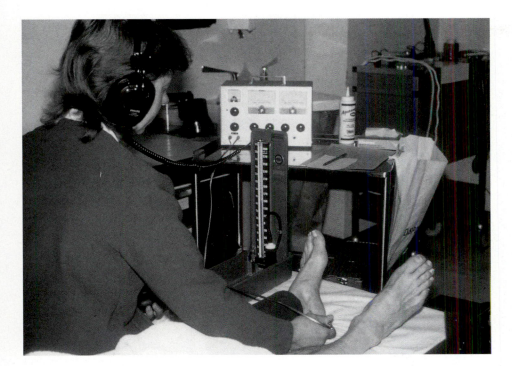

Figure 3

Pressure measurement by Doppler ultrasound

Measurement of pressure index (Doppler probe)

Doppler ultrasound enables blood flow to be monitored in impalpable arteries. It has become widely accepted as a standard method for noninvasive vascular assessment (Fig. 3). It is a less than precise method but is undoubtedly useful if taken within the context of sound clinical assessment. (See further p. 156.)

Exercise testing

If the level of Doppler ankle pressure is equivocal then exercise testing should be carried out. The increased muscle blood flow required for exercise should result in a fall in the ankle pressure in the presence of arterial disease. Arterial disease leads to a significant fall in ankle pressure. Conversely, if there is no fall it suggests that there is no major arterial problem.

The test is usually carried out with the patient on a treadmill. If for any medical reason the patient is unable to use the treadmill, then ankle pressure can be measured after hyperaemia induced by ankle flexion and extension or after release of an occlusive thigh tourniquet.

Transcutaneous oxygen tension measurement

Transcutaneous oxygen tension measurement enables the measurement of oxygen tension in the skin (TcPO$_2$). This measurement depends on the notion that, at equilibrium, the partial pressure of oxygen which diffuses through to the surface of the skin will reflect the oxygen tension of the underlying tissue (Fig. 4). The

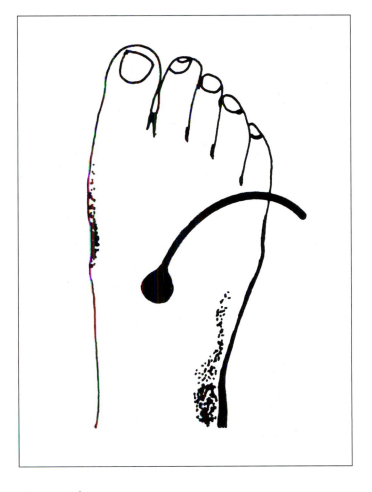

Figure 4

Measurement of the transcutaneous oxygen tension by oximetry

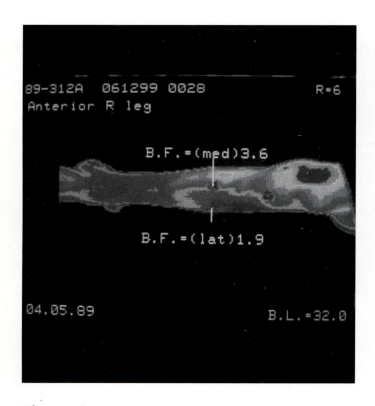

Figure 5
Thermography showing skin blood flow measurement carried out by radioactive isotope

measurement is carried out using an oxygen electrode probe together with a heating element and a temperature sensor. The electrode, which is clipped on to a ring, is placed at the site of measurement. The resting TcPO$_2$ measurement is of little value by itself, but in combination with the exercise test it can help in the assessment of the vascular insufficiency. (See further pp. 155–6.)

Local blood flow measurement

A quantitative measurement of skin blood flow at the precise level of surgery is an added help in predicting wound healing. Radioactive isotope has been used for this purpose, and it has proved to be a good indicator of tissue viability, especially below the level of the knee (Malone et al 1981, Spence et al 1988). However, its clinical use in the foot has not been proved.

Thermography

Infrared thermography has been used in vascular assessment for the last 20 years. Recently, high-resolution digital systems have become available, and when linked to a microcomputer, the output from these systems can be quantified (Fig. 5). It is now possible to obtain an accurately calibrated thermal map of the limb, which provides a highly acceptable assessment.

Andrea Cracchiolo III

Clinical methods used to assess peripheral circulation in the foot and ankle area have mostly been performed to select a proper amputation level. However, a vascular evaluation is also critical in some patients who are to have elective surgical procedures on their foot or ankle, and occasionally in patients who have sustained trauma and require treatment.

Doppler flow measurement

Of all the laboratory studies, ankle brachial indices performed with ultrasound Doppler have been the 'gold standard' for measuring blood supply and predicting wound healing. However, in patients with calcified noncompressible vessels, ankle–brachial indices may lead to falsely elevated measures of blood flow. Continuous wave Doppler ultrasound velocimetry can provide useful qualitative information in assessing the peripheral arterial circulation (Johnston et al 1981). In addition, it can yield quantitative results that may detect and localize peripheral arterial occlusive disease. Most commercial instruments provide an audio output that allows the examiner to listen to blood flow in the peripheral arteries, and an output that can make recordings of the Doppler flow velocity wave form. The audio signal allows the examiner to assess the blood flow in the peripheral arteries qualitatively and also to measure the systolic blood pressure at the ankle. The Doppler blood flow velocity waveform can provide quantitative information used in assessing and localizing peripheral occlusive disease (Figs 6, 7).

Wagner (1981) evaluated transcutaneous Doppler ultrasound using a stethoscope to measure systolic blood pressure in the lower extremity. He used systolic pressures at the ankle to establish an ischemic index by dividing the ankle pressure by the brachial artery

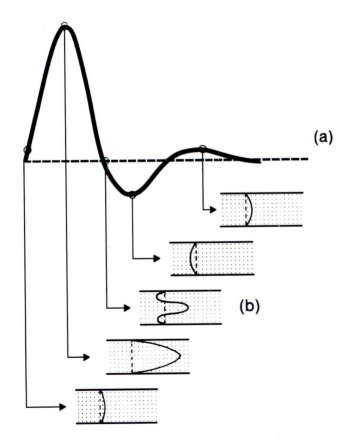

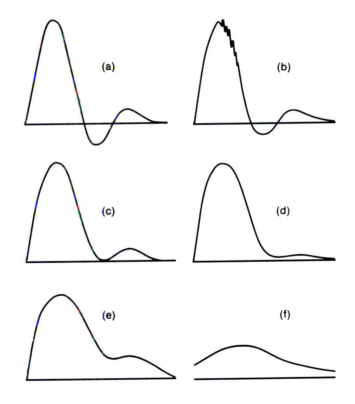

Figure 6

(a) The mean instantaneous blood flow velocity wave from a normal femoral artery. The vertical axis is velocity with forward flow above the dotted line and reverse flow below. The horizontal axis is time. (b) Velocity profiles at specific instants of time

Figure 7

(a–f) Progressive arterial stenosis alters the shape of the distal velocity wave form. With increasing arterial stenosis, the blood flow velocity wave form becomes progressively dampened. (Adapted from Johnston et al 1981)

pressure. It was established that an index of 0.45 in a diabetic patient and 0.35 in a nondiabetic was sufficient to ensure healing of the wound following a surgical procedure. He realized that patients with calcific vessels would have systolic pressures that were abnormally high. However, even when the index was over 1.0 he felt that an operation could be performed in such patients if there was pulsatile flow, suitable skin and no infection.

Brodsky (1994) recommended obtaining a vascular consultation if the ratio of ankle pressure to arm pressure was below 0.45, or if there was no pulsatile flow and in cases of artificially elevated pressures (ratio over 1.0).

Transcutaneous oxygen tension

Transcutaneous oxygen tension ($TcPO_2$) measured by superficial skin sensors is an effective method of measuring oxygen delivery to the skin. $TcPO_2$ measurements are noninvasive, do not require radioactive isotopes, can be performed at any location on the limb, and can be performed in the absence of pulses that are palpable or able to be assessed by Doppler. In a study of 37 patients undergoing below-knee amputation, Burgess et al (1982) measured a mean below-knee $TcPO_2$ of 16 ± 15 mmHg in the group who did not heal their amputations, compared to 42 ± 11 mmHg in the group who healed ($p < 0.01$). In all patients who had $TcPO_2$ over 40 mmHg, the below-knee amputations healed primarily. Six of seven patients with failed below-knee amputations were also smokers.

Wyss et al (1988) studied 162 patients undergoing 206 amputations. They found a significantly increasing risk of failure of healing with decreasing $TcPO_2$ ($p < 0.01$). In those patients with $TcPO_2$ under 20 mmHg, the probability of healing was 4%, whereas with $TcPO_2$ over 20 mmHg, the probability of failure was 4%. The authors cautioned, however, that $TcPO_2$ does not represent an absolute threshold measurement for healing, because in four out of 11 sites with $TcPO_2$ values of zero, the wounds still healed. Furthermore, $TcPTcPO_2$ O_2 values measured proximal to the knee had little predictive value for healing above-knee amputations. Interestingly, the values for $TcPO_2$ did not relate to the diagnosis and were not affected by whether the patient was a diabetic or a nondiabetic.

Finally, Pinzur et al (1992) performed 38 amputations in the foot and ankle and measured $TcPO_2$ preoperatively. When $TcPO_2$ was over 30 mmHg, 92.3% (24/26) healed; for $TcPO_2$ values of 20–29 mmHg, six out of eight healed; and for $TcPO_2$ under 20 mmHg, two out of four healed. The authors concluded that $TcPO_2$ values of 30 mmHg were highly predictive of wound healing.

The consensus seems to be that transcutaneous oxygen tension measurement is a useful study in addition to the standard ankle brachial Doppler indices, particularly when the patient has calcified vessels and the Doppler indices may be falsely elevated. Values for $TcPO_2$ under 20 mmHg indicated severe ischemia, while values over 30 mmHg are more predictive of successful wound healing. However this test cannot give an absolute assurance of wound healing. Many of the patients in the above studies also had prior revascularization operations. The surgeon's clinical judgement and assessment of all the clinical findings is critical. To this is added the quantitative ischemic risk provided by the tests.

References

Brodsky J W 1994 Surgical treatment and reconstruction of the diabetic foot. In: Gould J S (ed) Operative Foot Surgery. W B Saunders, Philadelphia, pp 209–224

Burgess E M, Matsen F A, Wyss C R, Simmons C W 1982 Segmental transcutaneous measurement of PO_2 in patients requiring below-the-knee amputation for peripheral vascular insufficiency. J Bone Joint Surg 64A: 378–382

Dickhaut S C, DeLee J C, Page C P 1984 Nutritional status: importance in predicting wound-healing after amputation. J Bone Joint Surg 66A: 71–75

Dormandy J, Mahir M, Ascady G 1989 Fate of the patient with chronic leg ischaemia. J Cardiovasc Surg 30: 50–57

Johnston K W, Maruzzo B C, Kassam M, Cobbold R S C 1981 Methods for obtaining processing and quantifying Doppler blood velocity waveforms. In: Nicolaides A N, Yao J S T (eds) Investigation of Vascular Disorders. Churchill Livingstone, New York, London, pp 532–558

Levin M E 1987 Understanding your diabetic patient. Clin Paediatr Med Surg 4: 315–330

Malone J M, Leal J M, Moore W S et al 1981 The 'gold standard' for amputation level selection: xenon-133 clearance. J Surg Res 30: 449–455

Neil H A W, Gatling G, Mather A M 1986 A reassessment of the prevalence of non-diabetes in England and Wales. Diabetic Med 3: 360a

Pinzur M S, Sage R, Stuck R, Ketner L, Osterman H 1992 Transcutaneous oxygen as a predictor of wound healing in amputations of the foot and ankle. Foot Ankle 13: 271–272

Spence V A, McCollum P T, Walker W F 1988 Recommendations for the objective determination of the level of limb viability. In: Murdoch G, Donovan R G (eds) Amputation Surgery and Lower Limb Prosthetics. Blackwell, Oxford

Wagner F W 1981 The dysvascular foot: a system for diagnosis and treatment. Foot Ankle 2: 64–122

Wyss C R, Harrington R M, Burgess E M, Matsen F A 1988 Transcutaneous oxygen tension as a predictor of success after an amputation. J Bone Joint Surg 70A: 203–207

IV PAEDIATRIC AND CONGENITAL CONDITIONS

IV.1 Congenital Talipes Equinovarus (Club Foot)

Malcolm F Macnicol

Congenital talipes equinovarus (club foot) is encountered as an orthopaedic problem in approximately two live births per 1000. Inconsequential positional deformities including calcaneovalgus, often incorrectly labelled 'talipes', are at least three times as common. Nevertheless, now that neonatal hip instability (developmental dysplasia of the hip) is recognized and splinted effectively in maternity units with a careful screening programme (Macnicol 1990), the structural club foot is the most frequent congenital limb anomaly that requires surgical treatment. Between one third and one half of the affected infants will present with bilateral club feet and boys present twice or three times as often as girls.

The confusion surrounding the details of treatment of this condition arises from:

1. uncertainties about the aetiology of the deformity, and hence its prognosis;
2. a related inadequacy in grading the severity of the deformity prior to conservative or operative management; and
3. a lack of convincing long-term reviews of treatment based upon prospective assessment and unbiased comparisons of technique.

Aetiology

The natural position of the embryonic foot resembles talipes equinovarus between the eighth and 10th intrauterine weeks (Kawashima & Uhthoff 1990), but it is unclear whether the persistence of this deformity results from exogenous factors, such as fetal moulding, or from endogenous or intrinsic factors, such as blastemal (cartilaginous) defects, idiopathic fibrosis or abnormal tendon attachments. Handelsman & Badalamente (1981) investigated the appealing theory

that a large proportion of children with club foot suffer from a neuromuscular imbalance affecting the lower leg particularly. An increased proportion of Type I (slow twitch) muscle fibres was demonstrated in comparison with normal controls, and the peronei were more obviously involved than the other calf muscles. There was a general decrease in the size rather than the number of myofibrils, and fibrosis within the muscle reduced its excursion. An infiltration of myofibroblasts within the medial ligamentous tissue of club feet, similar to that seen in Dupuytren's contracture, suggests that muscle and ligament blend pathologically to produce the rigidity of the foot.

It is important to examine the child completely. Talipes equinovarus may present in hypermobile infants, particularly those with myelodysplasia or Down's syndrome, or the 'stiff syndrome', seen in arthrogryposis (Fig. 1), the fetal alcohol syndrome or the Freedman Sheldon syndrome. These atypical cases behave differently from the classical club foot in an overtly normal child, and disappointing results may attend the standard operation, whether from overcorrection or relapse. Conditions associated with equinovarus of the foot are shown in Table 1. In rare cases, severe and progressive

Table 1 Conditions associated with equinovarus of the foot

Myelodysplasia (spina bifida)
Down's syndrome
Diastrophic dwarfism and other skeletal dysplasias
Constriction band syndrome
Freedman–Sheldon syndrome
Arthrogryposis
Congenital myopathy
Fetal alcohol syndrome

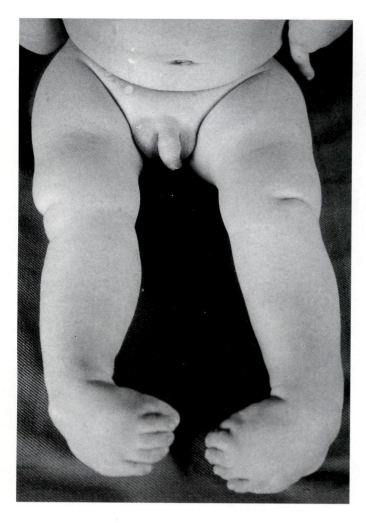

Figure 1

Atypical club foot presents as a regular problem in the child with arthrogryposis. A standard soft-tissue release may lead to disappointing results, although even talectomy may fail to correct the later problem of forefoot deformity

deformities are later shown to be the first manifestation of a central nervous system neoplasm.

Pathological anatomy

Not only is club foot multifactorial but the resulting deformities illustrate a spectrum of abnormality, both in terms of anatomical extent and severity (rigidity). Crudely, most clinicians grade the foot as follows:

1. postural ('resolving')
2. moderate ('tendons tight')
3. severe ('joint contracture')

The deformity is therefore part of a continuum, with varying degrees of talonavicular subluxation, as

described by Scarpa in 1802. Harrold & Walker (1983), in one of the few papers that has attempted to report results in relation to the severity of the deformity, found that 90% of grade I feet did well after treatment, whereas only 10% of grade III were successfully dealt with. The severe deformity certainly continues to bewilder and disappoint the surgeon, and there is some value in dividing grade III into typical and atypical cases, where the latter is the very rigid, small foot, often encountered in other syndromes. Delayed, more extensive surgery for these atypical cases should be followed by a prolonged period of plaster splintage.

Two other grades of club foot are recognized as separate entities. Firstly, the false correction produced by strapping or plasters, with residual equinus, persisting bunching of the foot, and a mildly incompetent and supinated first ray should be recognized and usually merits surgical release later in the first year of life. Radiography is often helpful in making this decision. Secondly, the relapsed and often very stiff foot after unsuccessful initial surgery merits a different grading since a variety of soft tissue and skeletal abnormalities are present (Fig. 2).

Clinical appearances

The clinical appearances of the club foot include a small inverted heel with a deep posterior crease above it. The loss of the normal, bulbous contour of the calcaneum is usually obvious. The lateral malleolus is shifted posteriorly to a varying degree, and the skin anterior to this appears loose (the 'devil's thumbprint'). Supination and adduction of the midfoot and forefoot produce a deep, vertical, medial crease where the talonavicular joint is subluxed. The medial border of the foot is therefore concave in contrast to the convex lateral border.

The hindfoot equinus masks a midfoot varus which becomes apparent if only a posterior release is carried out. The ankle is externally rotated, a product of the posteriorly positioned lateral malleolus, but the tibia often develops internal torsion. The navicular is closely applied to the medial malleolus, and in the more rigid foot the head and neck of the talus are also deviated medially, away from the axis of the body of the talus (Carroll et al 1978). The talus prolapses anteriorly from the ankle mortise while the plantarflexed calcaneum moves posteriorly as it is drawn up. Proximally, calf wasting is increasingly obvious as the baby's fat is lost; however, careful serial measurements of volume will always disclose that the calf and foot were also smaller at birth, so that the muscle loss is not progressive. In the older child genu recurvatum and knock knee are promoted by the fixed equinus, and intoeing will persist due to 'medial spin' of the uncorrected hindfoot (Tarraf & Carroll 1992).

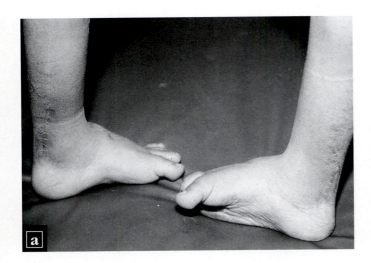

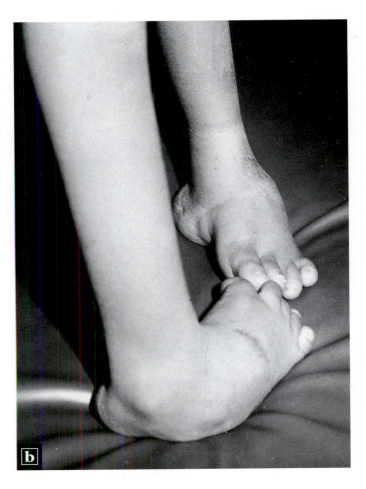

Figure 2

Relapsed club feet after several surgical procedures using longitudinal posteromedial incisions. (a) Note the supination and medial rotation. (b) Note the pipestem calf and heel inversion

Radiography

Simons (1977) described the use of radiographs to define the severity of the hindfoot distortion. The angles subtended by the long axes of the talus and calcaneum, viewed from both lateral and anteroposterior projections, offer an indirect means of assessing the club foot (Fig. 3). Adding the two talocalcaneal angles should produce an 'index' of 50° or more if the foot has been satisfactorily corrected.

Unfortunately, it is notoriously difficult to position the foot acceptably for these composite but essentially uniplanar radiographs. Even if a board is placed firmly under the sole of the dorsiflexed foot, as recommended, some degree of artefact is introduced as the projections attempt to define a complex, three-dimensional, rotational deformity. Similarly, attempts at viewing the 'flat top' talus characteristic of severe deformity (Hutchins et al 1985) are open to misinterpretation.

The fallacies inherent in assessing the talocalcaneal angle radiographically before the respective bones are fully ossified were demonstrated by Herzenberg et al (1991) who used a three-dimensional computer model of the relevant bones. In particular, the ossification centre of the talus was shown to be eccentric in club foot, and is placed anterior to the main mass of the body. Hence, attempts at defining the alignment of the talus and calcaneum from the apparent long axis of the ossified nucleus inevitably introduce an erroneous depiction of the true anatomy. Yet, if this artefact is accepted as proportional to the severity of the deformity, a good case can still be made for the retention of radiographs as a useful discriminant in deciding whether to operate on the occasional, borderline (grade I–II) foot. Postoperatively, the x-ray appearances of the older foot are also helpful in determing the success of correction and the relationship of the talus and navicular.

Surgical management

This is based upon Syme's operative principles. He recommended in the 1860s an early release and splintage to maintain the position, and later contended that a rebalancing of tendon pull produced better correction in the long term.

Aims

Surgical release should yield a plantigrade foot with good ankle movement. It should not produce further stiffness, and sensation must be preserved. These simple aims are actually quite difficult to achieve, and it is still

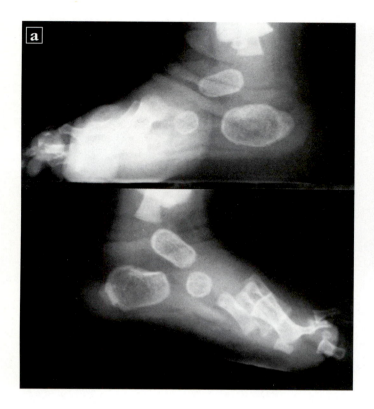

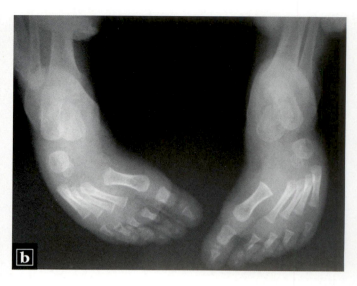

Figure 3

Lateral (a) and anteroposterior (b) radiographic projections of the right foot deformities and reduction in the talocalcaneal angles

common to encounter both undercorrected, deformed feet and overcorrected, stiff feet.

The Edinburgh approach relies upon neonatal assessment of the club foot followed by a period of strapping twice weekly. This not only reduces the initial deformity but also separates the grade I foot from the true, structural deformities. It is not acceptable to persist with strapping for much longer than three months, as skin reddening, abrasions and even superficial pressure sores may develop. Therefore it is advisable to change to weekly long leg casts or mobile bracing until a decision has been made about recommending surgery. In all but the most obviously postural deformities the parents of the child are warned that surgical intervention may be required. The decision to operate is only confirmed after a trial period with strapping applied by a physiotherapist with a special interest in club feet.

Conservative management is inappropriate for the complete care of most grade II feet and all grade III feet. Using serial plasters, Laaveg and Ponseti (1980) achieved an overall success rate of only 12.5%, while Ghali et al (1983) achieved a 48% established correction rate after regular manipulation and splintage.

Timing

Although neonatal surgical correction has been described (Pous and Dimeglio 1978, Ryöppy & Sairanen 1983) the general view prevails that this is unnecessarily early. The surgery is difficult and the margin for error small. Some grade I feet may be operated upon unnecessarily and the tiny, very stiff grade III foot is a formidable proposition even under magnification. In some centres, too, there is inadequate provision for safe anaesthesia at this

Table 2 Disappointing results after the conservative management of club foot

	Technique	Success Rate
Laaveg & Ponseti (1980)	Serial plasters	12.5%
Ghali et al (1983)	Manipulation and splintage	48%
Seringe & Atia (1990)	Stretch & Strap	30%

Figure 4

The age at operation of 152 clubfeet
(1982–1991)

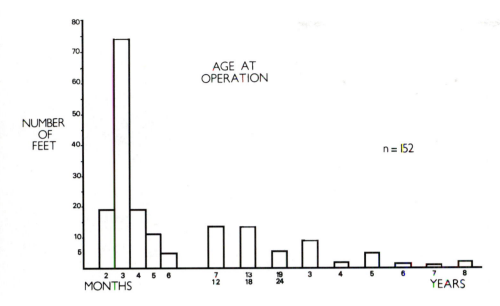

age. Ryöppy states that plaster splintage is then required until the child is walking, and this demands a prolonged period of regular, out-patient attendance.

Turco (1979) recommended that surgical release should not be attempted until 1 year of age, when the child is beginning to stand and walk. This is advantageous, since weight bearing is corrective in its own right, and the dissection is easier to accomplish in the larger foot. Hence, for the very tight and 'clenched' foot, later surgery is appealing. A prolonged period of plaster cast splintage, and further deformity of the tarsal bones must inevitably be accepted if surgery is recommended as late as this.

Therefore, for the majority of grade II and III feet operation is usually scheduled at 3–6 months of age (Fig. 4). Many surgeons prefer to offer surgery at this stage (Attenborough 1966, Green and Lloyd-Roberts 1985, Porter 1987a,b). The foot is large enough to allow a careful identification and release of pathological tethers (Ghali et al 1983) but does not usually require fixed splintage for more than a few months. If the balance of muscle forces around the hindfoot is restored, and the talonavicular joint is stabilized, light splints or stretching alone will suffice to hold the correction until the child is walking.

When the grade III foot is very small and stiff, prolonged stretching and casting are advised since surgical release may be difficult to achieve fully. There is no convincing evidence that delay in operation adversely affects the result, and it is imperative that a full and careful dissection is achieved. Therefore surgery is recommended later in the first year of life, as it is with arthrogryposis and other syndromes (see Table I) where the result may be unpredictable.

Extent

It is now generally accepted that surgical release should involve the majority of the peritalar tissues. Release of

the Achilles tendon alone is completely inadequate, and the posterior release of Attenborough (1966) is felt to be insufficient. While a certain variety of surgical judgement is appropriate, depending upon the severity of the deformity and the operative effects of progressive release, a minimum surgical procedure should include:

1. Achilles tendon lengthening
2. extensive ankle capsular release
3. peripheral subtalar capsular release
4. full talonavicular capsular release
5. release of fibrotic bands (tethers) below the medial malleolus and behind the lateral malleolus.

The tendon of tibialis posterior, often much enlarged, is considered to be a major deforming force and should therefore be 'Z' lengthened, but the long toe flexors, the plantar fascia and abductor hallucis muscle, and the calcaneocuboid joint are not universally released. Turco (1979) popularized the posteromedial dissection, which was then extended to a lateral–posteromedial release (McKay 1983a,b). The extensive 'hanging foot' operation of Simons (1985) has few adherents as there is an unease that a stiff, overcorrected foot may result. For instance, a complete subtalar release which includes the interosseous ligaments may produce lateral calcaneal shift and fixed valgus of the hindfoot. However, the presence of medial subluxation of the cuboid should be recognized, in association with the talonavicular malalignment, and it warrants correction in the severe structural deformity (Thometz and Simons 1993).

The exposure of the peritalar pathoanatomy is much facilitated by the transverse skin crease incision known as the 'Cincinnati approach' (Crawford et al 1982; Brougham & Nicol 1988). A combined posterolateral longitudinal and a medial transverse approach is also

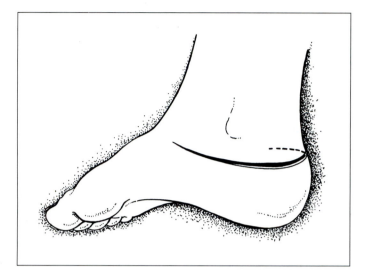

Figure 5

The Cincinnati incision allows a full exposure of the posteromedial structures and can be extended readily to the talonavicular and calcaneocuboid joints

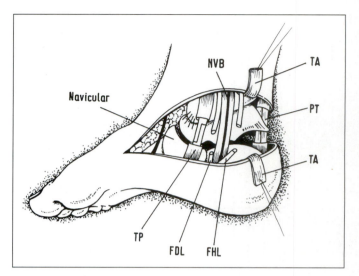

Figure 7

A full release of the ankle and subtalar joints is ensured, preserving only the anterior tibiotalar fibres in front of the tibialis posterior tendon (TP) sheath. Flexor hallucis longus (FHL) and flexor digitorum longus (FDL) are sectioned only in the very tight foot, and the peroneus longus and brevis tendons (PT) are carefully retracted while their sheaths are sectioned fully.

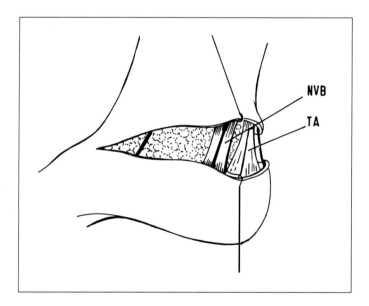

Figure 6

The neurovascular bundle (NVB) is carefully exposed and the Achilles tendon (TA) Z lengthened 1–1.5 cm, retracting the proximal skin flap and undermining it by blunt dissection

effective (Carroll et al 1978) but the cosmetic advantages of the Cincinnati incision make it particularly appealing.

A 'middle ground' surgical release is effective in all but the most severe grade III feet. It is recognized that stretching of unreleased tethers is possible, so that tissues are not severed unnecessarily. The lateral–posteromedial release of the ankle and subtalar joints does not include

the calcaneocuboid joint unless 'first ray competence' (Ghali et al 1983) fails to result from talonavicular and plantar release. The navicular must be freed to the extent that it can be placed over the anterolateral aspect of the talar head, and it is rarely necessary to transfix the foot with K wires as recommended by Turco (1979), Carroll et al (1978) and McKay (1983a,b).

The stages in the operation are illustrated in Figs 5, 6, and 7. It should be noted that the medial lamina of the Achilles tendon is released distally since this helps to lessen the deforming, varus pull of the tendon. Sharp dissection with a scalpel should be very cautious since the articular cartilage is easily damaged. When the Achilles tendon is released by the Z cut, which is preferred to an oblique transection of the tendon 'on the flat', excellent exposure of the ankle and subtalar joints is achieved, once the neurovascular bundle has been isolated and gently retracted with a moistened tape.

The invertor–evertor imbalance is partially corrected by lengthening the Achilles and tibialis posterior tendons, the shortening of the flexor hallucis and digitorum longus being corrected by progressive stretching in plaster. Conversely, the overstretched peroneal muscles will adaptively contract, so that surgical shortening of the tendons by reefing (Porter 1987b) is unnecessary. The tibiotalar portion of the deltoid ligament, contiguous with the deep portion of the tibialis posterior tendon sheath, is left intact and ensures that the hindfoot will not hyperpronate. The Z lengthened Achilles and posterior tibial

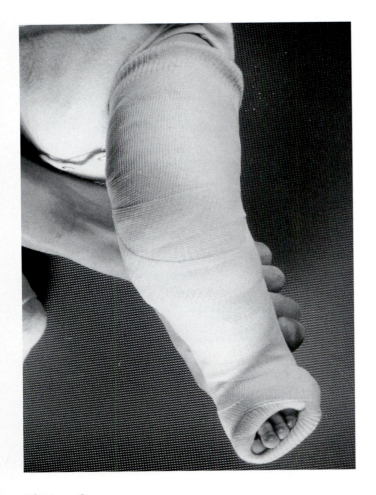

Figure 8

A long leg cast with the foot dorsiflexed and everted. Later in the first year further casting may be required occasionally in order to stretch up the foot, and a 1–2 month period of splintage is also required in 20% of feet during the 1–2 year old stage when the foot is growing rapidly

Table 3 Criteria used by Macnicol (1994) in reporting the early results of the Cincinnati approach. The scores were subtracted from 130 to grade the results

Objective Findings

1.	Ankle dorsiflexion	>10°	0
		6–10°	−5
		0–5°	−10
		0°	−20
2.	Heel position	0–5° of valgus	0
		>5° of valgus	−5
		varus	−10
3.	Forefoot alignment	neutral or corrects passively	0
		0–5° of angulation	−5
		5° of angulation	−10
4.	Bimalleolar angle (McKay 1983a,b)	>80°	0
		70–80°	−5
		<70°	−10
5.	Anteroposterior talocalcaneal angle (Simons 1977)	>25°	0
		20–25°	−5
		<20°	−10
6.	Lateral talocalcaneal angle: (Simons 1977)	>35°	0
		20–25°	−5
		<25°	−10
7.	Triceps surae strength	stands on tiptoes (affected foot)	0
		stands on tiptoes (both feet)	−5
		unable to stand on tiptoes	−10
8.	Flexor hallucis longus	functioning	0
		non-functioning	−10
9.	Scar	narrow and insensitive	0
		widened or sensitive	−5
10.	Subtalar pain	none	0
		occasional ache	−5
		with activity	−10
		disabling	−20
11.	Shoe wear	comparable to other side	0
		increased laterally	−5
12.	Games	no difficulty	0
		slight limitation	−5
		unwilling to participate	−10

tendons are carefully repaired with a horizontal mattress and further circumferential 'tacking' sutures, using an absorbable material such as 3–0 or 2–0 vicryl. Skin closure is achieved loosely with interrupted or subcuticular stitches of the same material, remembering that considerable gapping may occur if the foot is to be held initially in the neutral position. The rapid epithelialization across the wound at this age means that skin healing is well advanced at two weeks, when the long leg cast is changed to one with the foot in the fully corrected (dorsiflexed and everted) position.

The long leg neutral cast can be applied before releasing the tourniquet, but it should be well padded and must be split if circulatory return is not rapid. Sometimes the position of the ankle and knee will have to be adjusted if the toes do not pink up quickly. A second, long leg cast in the fully corrected position is applied at 2 weeks postoperatively (Fig. 8), and this is exchanged for a short leg cast after a further 4 weeks. If the foot is slightly tight or oedematous after 10 weeks, a further complete plaster or a night splint is advised. The foot must be kept in its fully corrected posture and failure to maintain this at such a critical stage in healing may lead to later problems with inadequate correction.

Results

Macnicol (1994) has reported the early results of the Cincinnati approach, avoiding the use of pins. The grading system of Laaveg & Ponseti (1980) and McKay (1983b) was modified to provide a scoring of the feet in terms of symptoms, function and the clinical appearances, including radiography. The feet were rated by subtracting the score derived from the criteria in Table 3 from 130 points, grading the outcome as follows:

Excellent	115–130 points
Good	100–114 points
Fair	85–99 points

Standing radiographs are taken using anteroposterior and lateral projections (Simons 1977) and the bimalleolar angle (McKay 1983a,b) is measured from a tracing of the foot (Fig. 9).

The transverse, posterior (Cincinnati) incision should not be stretched up too rapidly. Superficial skin necrosis may be produced by suture tension and the skin should either be closed loosely with absorbable sutures or not at all. There is a 5% incidence of initial wound healing with granulation tissue (Fig. 10), controlled effectively with silver nitrate local application, and four scars have remained hypertrophic in the last 150 cases (2.7%). Slight widening is apparent in approximately 20% of cases, but the cosmetic effect, compared to longitudinal incisions, is invariably good.

Overall excellent and good results were achieved in over 80% of feet, comparing well with the success rate

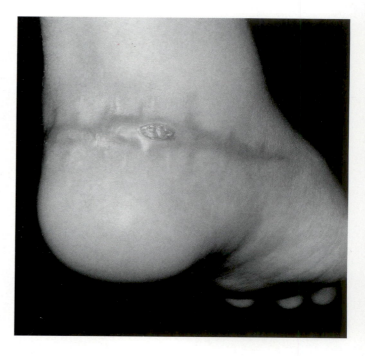

Figure 10

Superficial wound breakdown occurs if excessive correction of the position of the foot in the early postoperative stage leads to skin tension. The use of sutures in the skin may be unnecessary

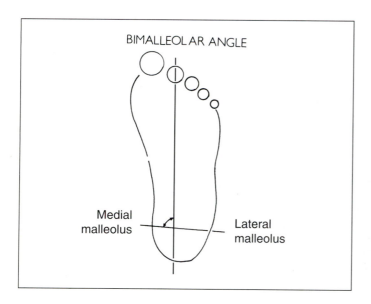

Figure 9

The bimalleolar angle (McKay 1983a,b) describes the degree to which the medial and lateral columns of the foot have been realigned

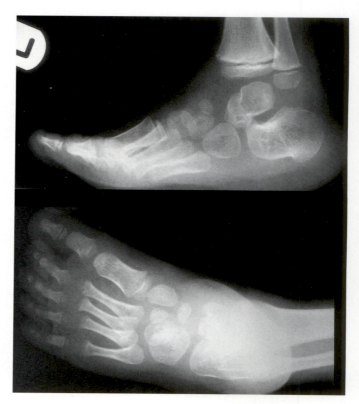

Figure 11

Irregular ossification of the head of the talus and persisting malreduction despite the use of transfixion K wires in a foot referred for further treatment

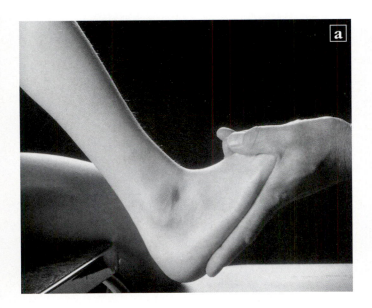
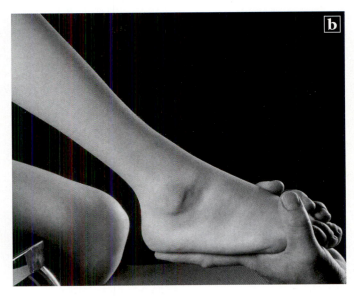

Figure 12

Assessment of dorsiflexion (a) and plantarflexion (b) should ensure that the hindfoot is held centrally below the tibia

from conservative management (see Table 2) and improving upon the operative results reported by Hutchins et al (1985), Porter (1987b) and Brougham & Nicol (1988) who achieved 75% satisfactory results using K wire fixation. Pin tract infections have been reported as a result of the transfixion technique, while cartilage may be readily damaged (Fig. 11).

Ankle (hindfoot) dorsiflexion and the total residual range of ankle movement are useful indicators of the degree to which hindfoot function has been restored. It is rare, for instance, to find that residual heel varus correlates with a flexible hindfoot. The normal range of hindfoot motion (plantar flexion and dorsiflexion) is between 60° and 70° (Giannestras 1967). Simons (1985) reports a total range of approximately 30° after extensive dissection. McKay (1983a,b), utilizing a hinged cast to maintain movement, reported an average of 58° when lateral–posteromedial release was combined with sheath recession of the flexor sheath to prevent scarring of the flexor hallucis longus tendon; these modifications apparently improved his earlier result of just under 40°. The current series produced an average dorsiflexion of 14° (0–20°) and plantarflexion of 35° (20–73°), giving a mean range of 49° (Figs. 12,13).

The total range of ankle motion correlates in linear fashion with the talocalcaneal index of Simons (1977), although the r value is low. A closer correlation (r = 0.38, p = 0.02) is seen between the bimalleolar angle and the talocalcaneal index (Fig. 14) with satisfactory and permanent correction achieved when the bimalleolar angle is 70° or more and the talocalcaneal index above 50° (combined AP and lateral angles).

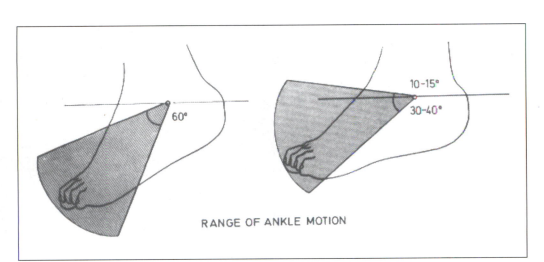

RANGE OF ANKLE MOTION

Figure 13

The average preoperative and postoperative ranges of ankle movement. The total arc of movement is altered dorsally but rarely increases

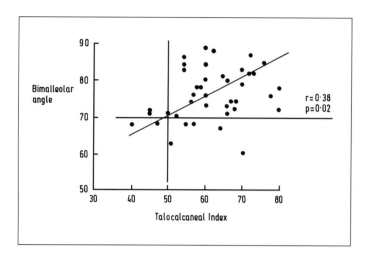

Figure 14

The correlation between the bimalleolar angle and the talocalcaneal index

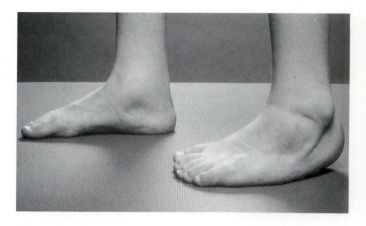

Figure 15

Inadequate correction has resulted in residual equinus of the left hindfoot and an early midfoot breach

An AP talocalcaneal angle of 25 ± 8 degrees was achieved, and the comparable lateral angle was 35 ± 9 degrees, giving a mean index of 60°. Reliance upon radiography is unwise, but poor results are invariably found when the index is less than 50° with concomitant absence of dorsiflexion, hindfoot varus and 'medial spin' (bimalleolar angle of less than 60°). The horizontal bean-shaped foot that is described by the term medial spin is a relatively common finding after clubfoot surgery. The deformity arises as a result of incomplete release, not only of the talonavicular joint but also of the inferior lamina of the tibialis posterior tendon, the bifurcate ('Y') calcaneocuboid ligament and the posterolateral tethers in varying degrees.

Push-off power is weakened in all children with structural club feet, but both the range and strength of ankle plantarflexion must be preserved as fully as possible. Restitution of gastrocnemius and soleus pull-through is obviously important, and the Achilles tendon after Z or oblique cut lengthening usually heals in a narrowed but functioning way. Adhesion to scars will be limiting, however, and is seen in a significant portion of children when a longitudinal scar is explored. The flexor hallucis longus and flexor digitorum longus tendons should be left intact, or their tendon sheaths recessed, in order to preserve toe flexion. Most children will then be able to walk on tiptoe, albeit with some heel 'dip'. In addition to the inevitable long-term weakness of plantarflexion and dorsiflexion, there will be the characteristic difference in calf bulk and foot size. Split shoe sizes will be required only in some of the severely affected feet, since an insole and orthopaedic felt below the tongue or strap of the shoe will ensure adequate hindfoot and midfoot hold. A shoe filler should not be inserted in the toe cap or box, although heel inserts are occasionally helpful. Heel wear and the alignment of the shoe upper is rarely

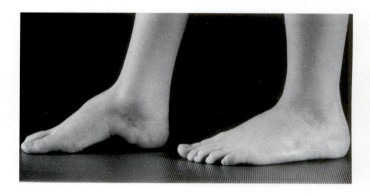

Figure 16

Calcaneocavus after a lateral–posteromedial release of the right foot through a Cincinnati incision

asymmetrical in the late postoperative case, but a slight increase in lateral sole wear is often noted.

When the foot is undercorrected the following secondary deformities develop:

1. genu recurvatum, sometimes with increased valgus
2. external tibial torsion
3. external rotation of the ankle mortise
4. hindfoot equinus.

These mask the presence of fixed midfoot varus and forefoot supination.

Complications

Surgical treatment faces three principal problems which will lead to the familiar complications of the clubfoot operation:

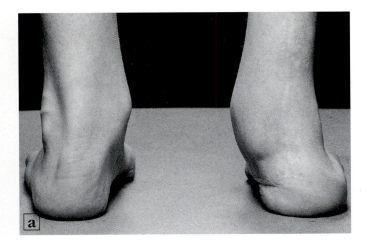

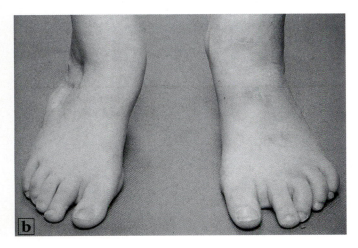

Figure 17
Overcorrection has produced fixed hindfoot valgus (a) and pronation of the foot (b). In this referred case the tendon of tibialis posterior had not been repaired

Table 4 Complications of surgery for club foot	
Lack of correction	Inadequate release
	Inadequate splintage
Overcorrection	Excessive release
	Diagnostic error
Technical error	Injury to joint surfaces (stiffness, pain)
	Injury to arterial supply (causalgia, gangrene)
	Injury to posterior tibial or sural nerves
	Wound edge tension (ischaemia, infection)
	Transfixion pin damage

1. lack of correction, either due to inadequate release or inadequate later splintage (Figs 15,16);
2. overcorrection, which is usually impossible to reverse fully (Fig. 17); and
3. technical errors at the time of surgery.

Surgical precision is dependent upon a thorough knowledge of the anatomy, which is often aberrant, and experience in the proper use of instruments. Sharp dissection is vital in some of the soft tissue dissection, for instance, but may be very damaging to the cartilaginous tarsal structures. Gentle spreading of tissues and potential spaces, pivotal manipulations of the foot and the preservation of tendon function are all learnt by experience, within the narrow confines of the surgical field. Magnification loupes are worthwhile in the smallest feet, but it may equally be appropriate to delay surgical release until the child is older. Delayed surgery, until the time of the first birthday, does not appear to affect results adversely (Pous and Dimeglio 1978, McKay 1983a,b).

It is important to realize that the clubfoot deformity results from a considerable number of conditions, and these may adversely affect the surgical result. One should beware of the hypermobile child, and unpredictable results may also follow surgical release in the child with neurological deficit, skeletal dysplasia and a variety of dysmorphic conditions. Bilateral clubfoot deformities are usually more resistant, and later developmental or cerebral abnormalities may appear.

The complications of surgery (Table 4) include incomplete release with medial spin, dorsal subluxation of the navicular, fixed heel valgus or calcaneus from excessive dissection, talar avascular necrosis, loss of sensation in the foot, scar hypersensitivity and skin sloughing or gangrene. Significant damage to the posterior tibial neurovascular bundle always imperils the foot as the anterior tibial (dorsalis pedis) arterial supply is deficient to a varying degree. The peroneal artery is readily damaged if the posterolateral release is careless, and hence vascular insufficiency is produced. Correcting the foot too rapidly will also extinguish much of the arterial supply, and will exacerbate oedema secondary to venous stasis. Preservation of the tendons of the flexor hallucis longus and flexor digitorum longus goes some way towards preventing this danger.

Long-term outcome

Most papers report relatively short-term results and the value of recent surgical modifications is impossible to assess fully. The radical releases that entail major separation of the talus from the calcaneum by transecting the interosseous subtalar ligaments run a considerable risk of irreversible overcorrection. There is also the concern

Table 5 Secondary surgical procedures for recurrent equinovarus deformity

1.	Repeated release	posteromedial talonavicular calcaneocuboid plantar
2.	Tendon transfer	tibialis anterior (TATT) (sometimes transferred back medially at a later date) tibialis posterior (useful in a proportion of neurologically abnormal feet)
3.	Conservative skeletal procedures	shortening of lateral column combined with medial release (calcaneocuboid fusion, excision of anterior calcaneal process, cuboid enucleation) realignment of calcaneum (lateral closing wedge easier to accomplish than medial opening wedge) midfoot osteotomies supramalleolar osteotomy
4.	Distraction with or without excisional osteotomies (Ilizarov and other external fixation devices)	
5.	Radical skeletal procedures	triple arthrodesis and other hindfoot and midfoot fusions

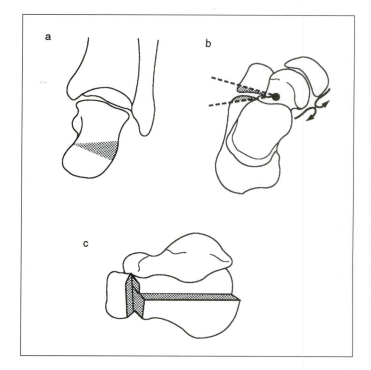

Figure 18

(a) Closing wedge (lateral excisional) calcaneal osteotomy.
(b) The Evans procedure, consisting of the calcaneocuboid laterally based excision wedge osteotomy and a talonavicular release.
(c) Calcaneal T osteotomy

that the relationship between the midfoot joints will be adversely affected, particularly if they are pinned out of position.

Inadequate dissection and inefficient postoperative splintage will also present the problem of recurrent deformity, although regular 3–6-month monitoring and a recourse to later plaster splintage lessens this risk during the first 3 years of life when the skeleton is growing most rapidly. Night splints and parental manipulation of the feet help to maintain the corrected position, so that recurrence is relatively rare, especially after the age of three. Later osteotomies, external fixation and distraction or arthrodeses have been unnecessary over the last 10 years of the Edinburgh series.

The procedures that may be necessary in later childhood are shown according to their different categories in Table 5. As a general rule soft tissue release is applicable as a repeat procedure until the age of 3 years, and as late as 6–8 years (see Fig. 4) if a mildly uncorrected foot is presented, with no antecedent surgery or where only the Achilles tendon has been released. Tendon transfers are only appropriate if the foot is mobile and reasonably well corrected; in other words, when the deformity is largely dynamic.

Correction of the incompletely released or untreated foot becomes more and more difficult as the tarsal bones mature and ossify. Soft tissue release will not achieve the same success since skeletal deformity is increasingly predominant.

Osteotomies of the calcaneum (Dwyer 1959; Mitchell 1977) offer limited scope in terms of realigning the heel, and may leave the basic joint incongruity unaltered (Fig. 18a). The Evans procedure (Evans 1961; Graham & Dent 1992) combines a calcaneocuboid excisional wedge arthrodesis with a further medial (principally talonavicular) release (Fig. 18b). While it straightens the bean-shaped (horizontally breached) foot it makes no impact upon residual supination, and of course it leaves residual hindfoot malalignment untouched. As a rule, it is best to preserve joint motion, and skeletal procedures tend to stiffen the foot. Triple arthrodesis inevitably makes a small foot smaller, and must not be considered until skeletal growth is near to completion, preferably after the age of 12 years.

For the cavovarus foot, in which the heel is inverted, Dwyer (1959) introduced a closing wedge osteotomy. This is based laterally but leaves a heel that is small and high. Dwyer later described an opening wedge calcaneal osteotomy (1963) but the soft tissue tension and post-surgical scar make this a difficult procedure as the heel is effectively being lengthened.

Torok (1980) discussed the use of wedge osteotomies for the neglected club foot, but large tarsometarsal wedge arthrodeses (Jahss 1980) inevitably result in stiffening and do not address the primary deformity. Calcaneal displacement osteotomies, which found a place in the management of neurological deformity, have been modified by Pandey et al (1980) who described a calcaneal T-osteotomy, combining lateral displacement of the posterior calcaneum with an open wedge, its fulcrum at the neck of the calcaneum (Fig. 18c). The procedure was used with reasonable success for 72 feet in 60 children (aged 3–12 years). The heel is broadened and the cavovarus is partially corrected. However, additional metatarsal osteotomy or lateral wedge midfoot osteotomy was required to correct the adduction in some cases, and persistent cavus required further dorsal wedge tarsectomy. In four feet skin sloughing was a significant complication.

Stretching of the soft tissues and skin remains a guiding principle in the management of club foot, and hence it is not surprising that distraction devices have been described by both Joshi (1994, personal communication) and Ilizarov (1991). Grill & Franke (1987) described the use of the Ilizarov distractor for relapsed and neglected club foot. Proximally, two wires are passed horizontally through the upper third of the tibia and fixed under tension to a ring. Transverse wires are inserted distally through the posterior calcaneum and the necks of the metatarsals (Fig. 19a), each fixed to a semicircular ring. The tibial and heel rings are attached by three bars, and the heel and metatarsal semicircular rings by links that allow ankle dorsiflexion. A hinged bar also connects the anterior portion of the tibial ring to the metatarsal ring.

Correction of the components of the deformity can proceed simultaneously and takes 1–3 months, followed by a further 1–3 months in the device, and then 3–4 months in a plaster cast. The method avoids bone resection and shortening of the foot, although compression of articular cartilage is likely to cause long-term stiffness in its own right. Application of the Ilizarov principle of tissue histogenesis has gained enthusiastic support (Grant et al 1992, Paley et al 1992, O'Doherty et al 1992). The technique was used by de la Huerta (1994) for seven adults (aged 19–24) with 12 neglected club feet. The fixation time varied from 5–8 months and complete correction was obtained in all patients. The adductus deformity recurred in three feet and stiffening of the forefoot was significant, but no worse than before the procedure.

Distraction alone may not suffice, and hence the Ilizarov technique may have to be combined with U or V osteotomies (Fig. 19b). The child or adult must be prepared for the lengthy treatment time, and in some children this form of management may cause behavioural upset. Nevertheless, correction by distraction of this sort

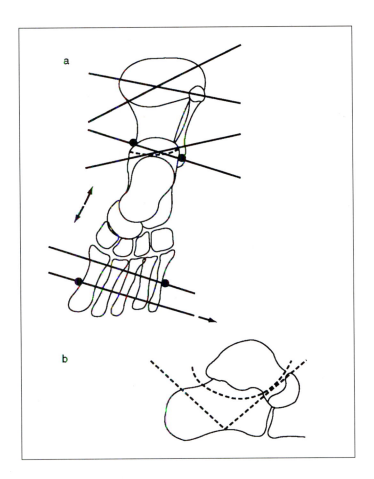

Figure 19

(a) Transfixion pins are inserted in the tibia, hindfoot and forefoot. (b) Correction is enhanced by U or V osteotomies through the hindfoot. The posterior limb of the V osteotomy is preferred to the complete V cut, which is rarely required

represents a considerable advance, and offers a further solution to the difficult problem of severe, late club foot deformity. Talectomy and supramalleolar osteotomy are best avoided in all but the most severely deformed cases.

Clinical experience with external fixation and distraction is limited, and long-term results are still unavailable. Problems with pin tract infection and psychological disturbance in the child treated by this method should not be underestimated, although severe, late deformity with poor skin cover may make the Ilizarov technique the only solution. Tibial osteotomies are largely inappropriate, although heavily scarred feet may make further hindfoot procedures impossible, so that a more proximal osteotomy is a tempting solution to the persistently internally rotated foot. While the fibula and the ankle mortise are externally rotated, the tibia itself is medially deviated. Any decision to commit the child to radical osteotomies should therefore, in view of the complexity of the pathological anatomy, be preceded by CT scanning and three-dimensional imaging if available.

In conclusion, a proper concern for the appropriate diagnosis and early treatment of the club foot deformity should make late surgery unnecessary. Irrespective of the surgical approach used, the preoperative and postoperative management remains vital to the success in correcting this most common of the childhood deformities.

References

Attenborough C G 1966 Severe congenital talipes equinovarus. J Bone Joint Surg 48B: 31–39

Brougham D I, Nicol R O 1988 Use of the Cincinnati incision in congenital talipes equinovarus. J Pediatr Orthop 8: 696–698

Carroll N C, McMurtry R, Leete S F 1978 The patho-anatomy of congenital clubfoot. Orthop Clin North Am 9: 225–232

Crawford A H, Marxen J L, Osterfeldt D L 1982 The Cincinnati incision: a comprehensive approach for surgical procedures of the foot and ankle in children. J Bone Joint Surg 64A: 1355–1358

de la Huerta F 1994 Correction of the neglected club foot by the Ilizarov method. Clin Orth Rel Res 301: 89–93

Dwyer F C 1959 Osteotomy of the calcaneum for pes cavus. J Bone Joint Surg 41B: 80–86

Dywer F C 1963 The treatment of relapsed club foot by insertion of a wedge into the calcaneum. J Bone Joint Surg 45B: 67–75

Evans D 1961 Relapsed club foot. J Bone Joint Surg 43B: 722–733

Ghali N N, Smith R B, Clayden A D, Silk F F 1983 Results of pantalar reduction in the management of congenital talipes equinovarus. J Bone Joint Surg 65B: 1–7

Giannestras N J 1967 Foot Disorders. Medical and Surgical Management. Lea & Febiger, Philadelphia

Graham G P, Dent C M 1992 The Dillwyn–Evans operation for relapsed club foot: long-term results. J Bone Joint Surg 74B: 445–448

Grant A D, Atar D, Lehman W B 1992 The Ilizarov technique in the correction of complex foot deformities. Clin Orth Rel Res 280: 94–103

Green A D L, Lloyd-Roberts G C 1985 The results of early posterior release in resistant club foot: a long-term review. J Bone Joint Surg 67B: 588–593

Grill F, Franke J 1987 The Ilizarov distractor for the correction of relapsed or neglected club foot. J Bone Joint Surg 69B: 593–597

Handelsman J E, Badalamente M A 1981 Neuromuscular studies in club foot. J Pediatr Orthop 1: 23–32

Harrold A J, Walker C J 1983 Treatment and prognosis in congenital club foot. J Bone Joint Surg 65B: 8

Herzenberg J E, Carroll N C, Christofersen M R, Lee E H, White S, Munroe R 1991 Club foot analysis with three-dimensional computer modelling. J Pediatr Orthop 8: 257–262

Hutchins P M, Foster B K, Paterson D C, Cole E A 1985 Long-term results of early surgical release in club foot. J Bone Joint Surg 67B: 791–799

Ilizarov G A 1991 Transosseous Osteosynthesis: Theoretical and Clinical Aspects of the Regeneration and Growth of Tissue. Springer-Verlag, Berlin

Jahss M H 1980 Tarsometatarsal truncated-wedge arthrodesis for pes cavus and equinovarus deformity of the fore part of the foot. J Bone Joint Surg 62A: 713–722

Kawashima T, Uhthoff H K 1990 Development of the foot in prenatal life in relation to idiopathic club foot. J Pediatr Orthop 10: 232–237

Laaveg S J, Ponseti I V 1980 Long-term results of treatment of congenital club foot. J Bone Joint Surg 62A: 23–81

Lichtblau S 1973 A medial and lateral release operation for club foot. A preliminary report. J Bone Joint Surg 55A: 1377–1384

Lloyd-Roberts G C, Swann M, Catterall A 1974 Medial rotation osteotomy for severe residual deformity in club foot. J Bone Joint Surg 56B: 37–43

Macnicol M F 1990 Results of a 25-year screening programme for neonatal hip instability. J Bone Joint Surg 72B: 1057–1060

Macnicol M F 1994 The surgical management of congenital talipes equinovarus (club foot) Current Orthop 8: 72–82

McKay D W 1983a New concept of and approach to club foot treatment: Section II – correction of the club foot. J Pediatr Orthop 3: 10–21

McKay D W 1983b New concept of and approach to club foot treatment: Section III – evaluation and results. J Pediatr Orthop 3: 141–148

Mitchell G P 1977 Posterior displacement osteotomy of the calcaneus. J Bone Joint Surg 59B: 233–235

O'Doherty D P, Street R, Saleh M 1992 The use of circular external fixators in the management of complex disorders of the foot and ankle. The Foot 2: 135–142

Paley D, Catagni M, Argnani F, Prevot J, Bell D, Armstrong P 1992 Treatment of congenital pseudarthrosis of the tibia using the Ilizarov technique. Clin Orth Rel Res 280: 81–93

Pandey S, Jahss M H, Pandey A K 1980 'T'-osteotomy of the calcaneum. Int Orthop 4: 219–224

Porter R W 1987a Congenital talipes equinovarus: I – resolving and resistant deformities. J Bone Joint Surg 69B: 822–825

Porter R W 1987b Congenital talipes equinovarus: II – a staged method of surgical management. J Bone Joint Surg 69B: 826–831

Pous J G, Dimeglio A 1978 Neonatal surgery in club foot. Orthop Clin North Am 9: 233–240

Ryöppy S, Sairanen H 1983 Neonatal operative treatment of club foot. A preliminary report. J Bone Joint Surg 65B: 320–325

Seringe R, Atia R 1990 Idiopathic congenital club foot: results of functional treatment (269 feet). Rev Chir Orthop 76: 490–501

Simons G W 1977 Analytical radiography of club feet. J Bone Joint Surg 59B: 485–489

Simons G W 1985 Complete subtalar release in club feet: part II – comparison with less extensive procedures. J Bone Joint Surg 67A: 1056–1065

Tarraf Y N, Carroll N C 1992 Analysis of the components of a residual deformity in club feet presenting for operation. J Pediatr Orthop 12: 207–216

Thometz J G, Simons G W 1993 Deformity of the calcaneocuboid joint in patients who have talipes equinovarus. J Bone Joint Surg 75A: 190–195

Torok G 1980 Surgical treatment of the neglected clubfoot. In: Lehman WB (ed) The Clubfoot. JB Lippincott, Philadelphia pp 87–96

Turco V J 1979 Resistant congenital club foot. One-stage posteromedial release with internal fixation. J Bone Joint Surg 61A: 805–814

IV.2 Local Congenital Disorders

Antonio Viladot

In 15% of the 841 congenital systemic disorders reviewed in the *National Foundation Birth Defects Compendium*, there were partial abnormalities of the foot (Bergsma 1973). From an aetiological point of view, most of the syndromes can be classified according to the following groups (Zimbler & Craig 1976): (a) local manifestations of generalized genetic disturbances of the skeleton (e.g. osseous dysplasia); (b) isolated defects of the extremities in the embryo (e.g. polydactyly); and (c) anomalies associated with disorders of other parts of the body (hand–foot–uterus syndrome). This last group is much less common.

We shall consider congenital disorders of the foot in two groups: foot disorders in systemic diseases, and isolated malformations of the foot and ankle.

Alterations of the foot in systemic diseases

Alterations of the dermatoglyphics of the foot

Between the 11th and 12th week of fetal development, a shrinking of the inner surface of the epidermis can be seen, which is followed by the appearance of ridges. In the palms and soles these are accentuated, giving place to crests in which the canals of the sudorific glands are found, the mouths of which open on the surface of the skin. Among these crests there are small wrinkles that run in the same direction. As the fetus grows, this pattern also becomes more marked and it then remains unchanged throughout life. It will even regenerate after severe trauma if the deep layer of the epidermis is not destroyed.

An impression of the footprint can be made by painting the sole of the foot with ink, as for fingerprints (Viladot 1954). If this is done carefully, one can evaluate the dermatoglyphic prints. Photopodograms are produced by brushing the plantar aspect of the foot with photographic developer and pressing the foot onto photographic paper that has previously been exposed to the light (Fig. 1).

Awareness of footprints has existed for a long time, and they were classified in 1892 by Francis Galton. The fingers then acquired greater importance in legal medicine, for identification. Only more recently has attention been recalled to the dermatoglyphics of the sole, especially by Cummins & Midlow (1961) and

Penrose & Loesch (1969); they have evaluated the relation of these prints to chromosomic alterations. These can also show the action of teratogenic agents which have acted in early phases of fetal development, such as rubella or thalidomide.

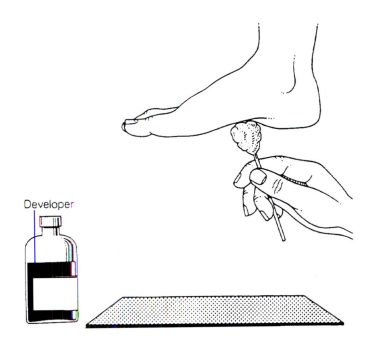

Developer

Figure 1

Technique for obtaining the photopodogram

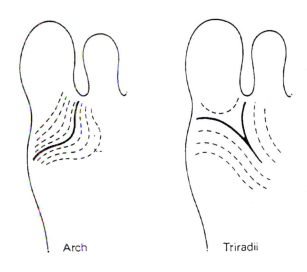

Arch   Triradii

Figure 2

Identification of plantar prints

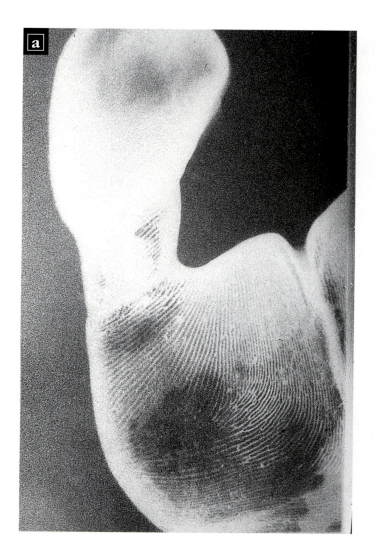
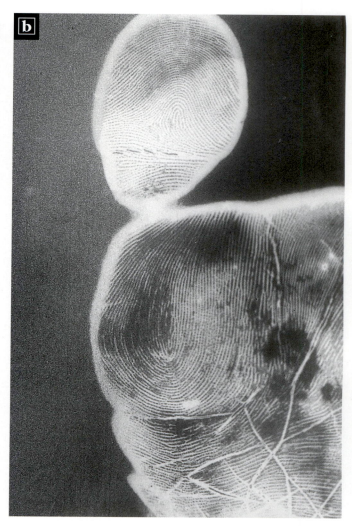

Figure 3

(a) Photopodogram of the halluceal area in a child with Down's syndrome; (b) Same area in a normal foot

For identification of the plantar prints the following elements are taken into account (Fig. 2):

1. The presence of arches or loops when the print lines turn at an angle of 180°. Two arches closely united give rise to double or twin arches. When two arches are fused, forming a concentric pattern, they give origin to a whorl.
2. Triradii occur at the point of fusion of three areas of parallel lines. At the centre they form a delta composed by three points; their fusion forms an angle of approximately 120°.
3. It is also of interest to count the number of ridges from the nucleus of an arch to the delta that forms the centre of the triradii.

The alterations that appear in Down's syndrome are typical: in the halluceal area (skin that is under the head of the first metatarsal), there is a reduction of the print,
which is limited by a line of ridges in the form of an arch or by ridges that go from the first commisure toward the medial part of the foot. The distal loops of the fourth interdigital area occur three times more frequently than in the normal population. Another characteristic is a marked tendency for the proximal triradii to displace toward the fibular border (Fig. 3).

The toes present more arches and fewer whorls than the fingers. A diminished number is found in Down's syndrome.

More recently, Lewis (1983) has studied the types of dermatoglyphics in various feet with metatarsus varus. She reaches the following conclusions: (a) there is no great difference between one foot and the other; (b) there is a great difference in dermatoglyphic patterns between the sexes; (c) even though she believes that the dermatoglyphics can be altered in early genetic changes, she did not find important differences in those cases with metatarsus varus.

The foot in Ehlers–Danlos syndrome

This disease, which is characterized by great laxity of the skin, was described in 1901 by Ehlers and in 1908 by Danlos. The fundamental components of the syndrome are: (a) great decrease in the elasticity and increase in the fragility of the skin, with tendency to erosions and wounds, resulting in hypertrophic scars; (b) calcified spherical nodules; (c) haemorrhagic diathesis of vascular origin, which tends to produce haematomas; (d) joint laxity.

Less frequently are found molluscum pseudotumours under the skin, ocular deviations (strabismus, blue sclerotics) and internal manifestations such as diaphragmatic hernia or aneurysm of the aorta.

Rozman et al (1967) described a case in which, besides the common symptoms of the disease, there was a lymphoedema that affected the mother and her daughter and which was evident at the level of the ankle and the tarsus, where the skin formed many creases.

McKusick (1966) thought the basic defect of the Ehlers–Danlos syndrome was an anomaly of the collagen, with a relative increase of elastic fibres in relation to the collagen. On the other hand, there could have been a loss of adherence and of decussation, which would facilitate greater stretching.

This ligamentous laxity accounts for the presence of flatfoot in most of the patients affected by this disease. It has even been said that the child's flat foot might be a minimal form of the same condition.

A case of this disease was published by Viladot & Rochera (1972), in which there was luxation of the hips and, what is rare, a club foot, which was reducible. Curiously the skin could be freely moved around the deformed skeleton of the foot (Fig. 4).

The foot in arthrogryposis

The term 'arthrogryposis' comes from Greek and means a curved joint. It is a clinical syndrome that appears at birth and affects the limbs, producing multiple joint rigidities with deformities. There is a limitation in the elasticity of the muscles, with muscle fibres decreased in diameter and in number and partly replaced by fibrous tissue and fat. Together with this deviation of the muscular tissue, there are disturbances of the central nervous system in the limbs, with a decrease in number and size of the cells of the anterior horn. Degeneration of the posterior horn has also been described.

Friedlander et al (1968) reviewed 45 patients affected with this disease, and found that the foot was affected in the great majority of cases. It is characteristic that no matter how good the intervention, the deformity relapses very frequently and further interventions are usually necessary.

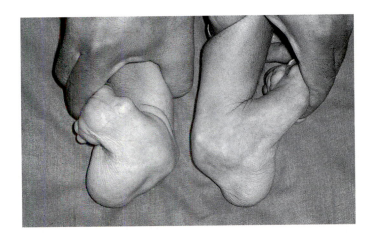

Figure 4
Great laxity of the feet in a patient affected with Ehler–Danlos disease

Dubosset (1982) described three types of malformations that appear in the foot: club foot, direct equinus and vertical talus.

1. Club foot is very resistant to any treatment. It has been said that all severe club feet may be localized forms of arthrogryposis. There are feet in which conservative treatment is ineffective. Soft tissue surgery not only fails, but often the secondary scarring makes the deformity worse. It is for these reasons that the author agrees with Menelaus (1971) and other authors that astragalectomy in these patients is the chosen operation. Despite the apparent biomechanical disaster that this intervention might seem to be, the clinical result is very good. In very small children, a convex prominence in the distal epiphysis of the tibia appears, and this tends to form a new astragalus (Viladot et al 1978).
2. Direct equinus is also frequently a relapsing one. Because of this a transfer of a portion of the Achillis tendon to the forefoot has been suggested.
3. Vertical talus is discussed in Chapter V.1.

The foot in Marfan's syndrome

Arachnodactyly or dolichostenomelia is a congenital dystrophy of the skeleton characterized by notable lengthening and thinning of the bones of the four extremities. It was described by Marfan in 1896.

Besides the fingers and the toes being very long and thin, which gives rise to the name of the disease (arachnodactyly: 'in the form of a spider'), the patients are usually tall and thin, sometimes with a kyphoscoliosis, and exhibit a great ligamentous laxity. In 50% of cases, ectopic calcification and heart lesions are found.

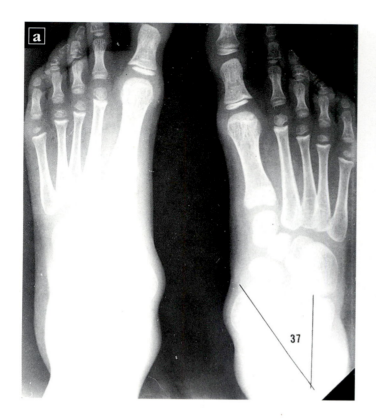 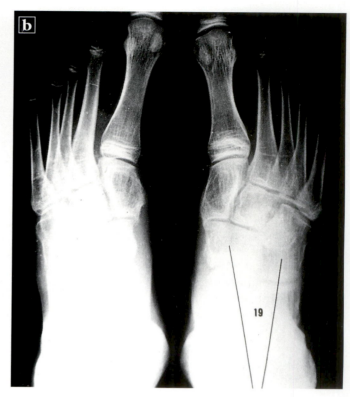

Figure 5

(a) Dorsoplantar radiograph of flat foot secondary to Marfan's syndrome; (b) Same case, 5 years after the operation to correct the sinking of the arch

The feet of these patients are extremely long and thin (Fig 5); the great length of the toes makes it difficult to wear shoes; generally the big toe is much longer than the other toes, and this results in varus or valgus deformities. The great laxity of these ligaments produces a flat foot resistant to conservative treatment. In some cases, the marked deformity has obliged us to operate, with rewarding results.

The foot in dysplasia epiphysealis multiplex

According to Jaffe (1972), dysplasia epiphysealis multiplex is a relatively rare hereditary familial disease that affects skeletal development. It is characterized by anomalies in the evolution of the ossification centres of the epiphysis and apophysis of the bones. The inheritance is transmitted by dominant Mendelian characters. As the abnormality is not lethal, the literature abounds with cases that refer to generations of the same family. At first, the disease affects only the extremities and this differentiates it from Morquio's disease in which the vertebral lesion is characteristic.

The hands and feet show the typical irregularities of the epiphyses of the long bones, which tend to be delayed in their appearance. The ossification centres are underdeveloped and irregular in outline and density. Generally the feet are fat and flattened. The proximal epiphyses to the toe have a conical form (Fig. 6).

The osseous lesions are combined with ligamentous laxity, resulting in a flat foot. Rarely is surgical treatment indicated in these patients. Orthoses should be used to prevent, if possible, the deformities of the feet.

The foot in Duchenne type muscular dystrophy

Progressive muscular dystrophy is a degenerative disease primarily of skeletal muscles and is of genetic origin. It is given the name myopathy because it is a disease of the muscle, characterized by biochemical, pathological and electrical changes in the muscle fibres.

One of the commonest forms is Duchenne dystrophy. The disease appears in infancy, and is transmitted by a recessive sex-related gene. It predominantly affects the male.

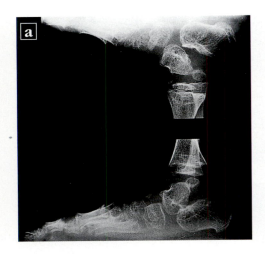

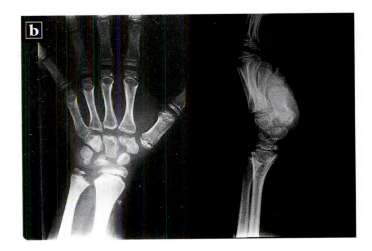

Figure 6

(a) Radiograph of the foot in dysplasia epiphysealis multiplex; (b) the hands of the same patient

Even if the lesion affects the proximal muscular system of the limbs, pelvis and shoulder, it is characteristic that in the beginning there is a false appearance of pseudo-hypertrophy of the calf. If one adds to this the fact that sometimes these children have a flat foot, one can easily fall into the error of attributing the cause of the instability and frequent falls with which the child presents to this condition, missing the diagnosis of a severe muscular lesion.

In doubtful cases, when the child is checked for apparent flatfoot, it is necessary to look for Gower's sign. Sitting the child on the floor, one can observe how he gets up with great difficulty placing his hands over the legs as if climbing up himself. A positive Gower's sign makes electromyography, a study of the muscular enzymes and, if necessary, a muscular biopsy, mandatory to confirm the diagnosis.

The foot in neurofibromatosis

This is a hereditary condition characterized by a malformation of the connective tissue of the central and peripheral nervous system. There are variable anomalies of the skeleton, the skin and the soft tissues (Tachdjian 1976).

The first to relate this disease to the nervous system was von Recklinghausen in 1882, and because of this the disease carries his name.

From the clinical point of view the lesion is characterized by the appearance of 'café au lait' spots on the skin and subcutaneous swellings that grow along the peripheral nerves and the nerve trunks. The tumours of neurofibromatosis can invade osseous tissue, inducing characteristic lesions such as scoliosis or congenital pseudoarthrosis of the tibia.

Another of the disturbances that this disease gives rise to is gigantism. Enlargement of either the whole foot or of one toe can occur. Together with the idiopathic form and arteriovenous fistula, this constitutes the most frequent cause of total or partial gigantism of the foot.

Isolated malformations of the foot and ankle

Many classifications of skeletal malformations have been proposed. In an attempt to systematize them, it is useful to adopt the classification proposed by Werthemann (1966) as quoted by Hans Grebe in *Human Genetics*. The following groups are modified and adapted to congenital malformations of the foot:

1. Numerical alterations of segmentation
    Syndactyly and polydactyly
    Synostosis
    Tarsal bridges
    Ball and socket ankle joint
2. Abnormalities of epiphyseal development
    Aplasia distal epiphysis of tibia
    Aplasia distal epiphysis of fibula
    Aplasia of other bones of the foot
    Supernumerary bones
    The problem of the distal epiphysis of the first metatarsal
3. Hereditary contractures
    Congenital talipes equinovarus
    Calcaneo vertical talus valgus
    Hallux varus
    Other malformations of the toes

4. Joint aplasias
5. Malformations related to alterations of the original
    ectoderm
        Lobster foot
        Syndactyly
6. Constitutional hypertrophy and hypotrophy
        Hypertrophy of the foot
        Megadactyly
        Brachydactyly
7. Lesions caused by amniotic disease

The foot in diastrophic dwarfism

This syndrome is manifest at birth, and the clinical
findings include small stature, soft cystic masses in the
auricle, cleft palate, progressive kyphoscoliosis and
marked shortening of the first metacarpals with proximally set hypermobile thumbs.

In the legs it is characterized by flexion contractures
and varying degrees of webbing of the hips and knees.
In the foot it produces important deformities similar to
arthrogryposis. The most frequent are club foot and
metatarsus varus.

Polydactyly and oligodactyly

Polydactyly and oligodactyly, together with syndactyly,
which often accompanies them, is a malformation known
from ancient times. The Bible (2 Samuel 21: 20) mentions
a family with six fingers and six toes. The surname
Seisdedos (Six fingers, or Six digits) can be found repeatedly in the telephone book of the city of Barcelona.

It is considered that, apart from clubfoot and congenital luxation of the hip, these are the most frequent
congenital malformations of the limbs. Von Verschuer
(1959), in a large study, found 45 cases of polydactyly
per 100 000, 33.9 cases of syndactyly per 100 000 and
1.9 cases of oligodactyly per 100 000.

Polydactyly is an increase in the number of digits,
often associated with a similar deformity of the hand
(Fig. 7). The most frequent reduplications are the ones
that take place at the level of the fifth toe; these do not
always have bones, since many are composed of soft
tissue which forms atrophic lateral toes. Duplications of
the big toe and of the central toes of the foot also occur.

The absence of digits, oligodactyly, occurs less
frequently than polydactyly. It is not caused by embry-
ologic regression but is a primary absence of organo-
genesis. A form of oligodactyly is described as
perodactyly, in which the affected ray adopts the form
of a stump.

As with polydactyly, oligodactyly is often combined
with syndactyly, which will be described later. There are
also disturbances of normal segmentation, alterations of

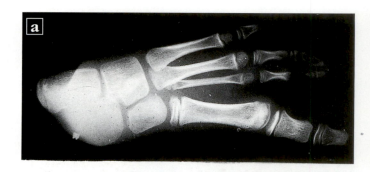
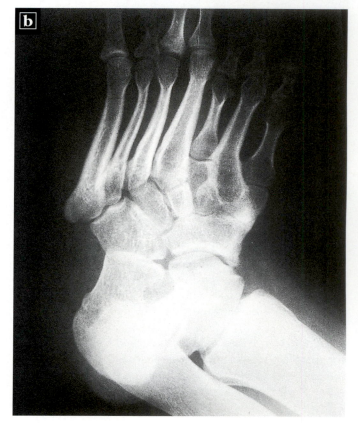

Figure 7

(a) Radiograph of oligodactyly; (b) polydactyly

the metatarsals, which can show either a diminution of
their number or intermetatarsal synostoses and which
may or may not be accompanied by the lack of a toe.

Treatment

Oligodactyly rarely produces discomfort. Because of this
surgical treatment is indicated in very few cases of oligodactyly of the foot.

In the case of polydactyly, besides the aesthetic
consideration, the patient usually has problems fitting
into shoes. In such cases, it is necessary to resort to
surgical treatment. Before doing so, it is essential to

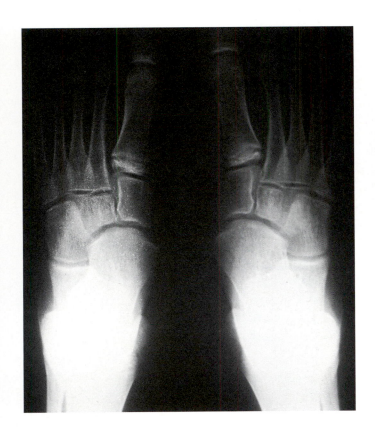

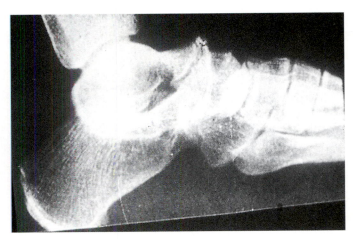

Figure 9

Radiograph of calcaneonavicular bridge

Figure 8

Radiograph of astragalonavicular synostoses

make a careful radiographic study of each case, observing which toe continues the axis of the metatarsal and must be preserved. It is common to find a supernumerary metatarsal, which is best removed.

Osseous synostoses

These affect the bones of the metatarsals and of the tarsus in which there is a congenital absence of the normal division of the bones of the extremities. Often syndactylies are combined with fusion of the metatarsals. At a more posterior level, many sorts of osseous fusions have also been found (Fig. 8).

From a clinical point of view, the importance is in the alteration of the shape of the foot, especially with regard to difficulty with shoes. Functional limitation is generally minimal and these lesions are well tolerated. Therefore, surgical treatment is seldom necessary.

Osseous bridges

In contrast to the osseous synostoses, which generally coexist with great deformity of the foot, osseous bridges or tarsal unions are formed by bars of osseous tissue (synostosis), cartilage (synchrondrosis) or fibrocartilage (syndesmosis) that join one bone to another without significant deformity.

Interest in these arose from the studies of Harris & Hon (1955), who called attention to the possible relation between such bridges and contracted or spastic flatfoot.

Although the tarsal bridges have been known for many years, it was not until 1921 that Slomann showed calcaneonavicular coalition with radiographic oblique views. Besides the studies of the school of Harris (1948, 1965) and Jack (1954), there are those of the Uruguayans, Bado & Garcia-Novales (1951) and especially Ruiz (1976). The Argentinian, Natiello (1966), also wrote on the subject. Even though there are several studies made by Europeans Roger & Meary (1969) and Marqui & Gambier (1953), we have the impression, from personal experience and personal communications with North and South American orthopaedists, that the malformation is much commoner in the New World than in Europe.

Pathological anatomy

Although osseous bridges can occur between the majority of the bones of the foot, the most frequent are the calcaneonavicular and the calcaneotalar. The

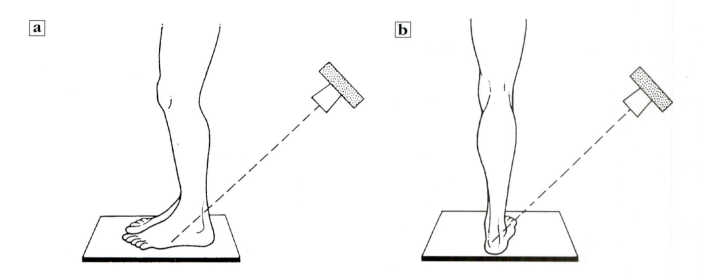

Figure 10
Radiological projections for viewing the osseous bridges: (a) Harris; (b) Slomann

talonavicular and navicular–cuneiform bridges are rarer. Sometimes calcaneonavicular and calcaneotalar bridges coexist (four cases in the statistics of Ruiz 1976). The calcaneonavicular bridge would join the anterointernal portion of the calcaneum with the posteroexternal border of the navicular (Fig. 9).

Often the deformity is asymptomatic. Occasionally it provokes pain at the level of the subastragalar joint and results in a spasm of the peroneus.

Astragalocalcanean bridge (Fig. 10)
The Harris studies (1955) evaluated this union as a cause of contracted flatfoot. We must remember that the subtalar joint is divided into two independent zones, the posterior or 'thalamus', and the anterior or 'sustentaculum tali'. It is at the latter site that unions are usually found. This anterior subastragalar joint can present in three forms: (a) a more or less elliptic form (found in 42% of cases of our studies); (b) in the form of a bean, with a narrowing waist (22% of cases); and (c) divided into two small subjoints (36%).

When there is a bridge, it is at the level of this anterior portion. In these cases, the sustentaculum tali appears irregular and, instead of maintaining a horizontal level, it is found deviated downwards and inwards. Unions of the posterior portion are much rarer. Harris (1955) presents one, and Ruiz (1976) presents two.

Secondary alterations
Osseous bridges alter the biomechanics of the posterior tarsus. Inversion and eversion are complex movements formed by other, smaller ones: pronation and supination, flexion and extension, abduction and adduction, and

anterior sliding 'listhesis' of the astragalus over the calcaneum. These movements occur not only through the subtalar joint, but always together with Chopart's joint. The rigidity of one of these joints alters the biomechanics of the other and produces pain and spasm.

In the astragalocalcaneal bridge, the limitation of movement of the anterior subtalar joint obliges the navicular to course over the astragalar head to compensate for the loss of talocalcaneal movement. In dorsiflexion it produces elevation of the astragalocalcanean ligament, which is submitted to stretching and so provokes the formation of one beak of the talus.

These alterations of the biomechanics provoke inflammatory reactions, with spasm of the peroneus that gives origin to contracted or spastic flatfoot. Rather than being a clinical entity, this is an 'episode' that any flat foot can go through. Shortening of the peronei will occur only if the pain and spasm crisis recurs repeatedly; in these cases, the deformity becomes fixed.

Another, more exceptional, secondary change of an astragalocalcanean synostosis would be the formation of a ball and socket ankle joint, which will be discussed later.

Radiographic diagnosis
Besides the standard radiographic projections that can display tarsal coalitions, there are two other projections which are useful (see Fig. 10).

Harris projection
The patient stands on a radiographic plate and the tube is placed behind and above so that it forms a 45° angle. In this projection, the two subtalar joints can be seen

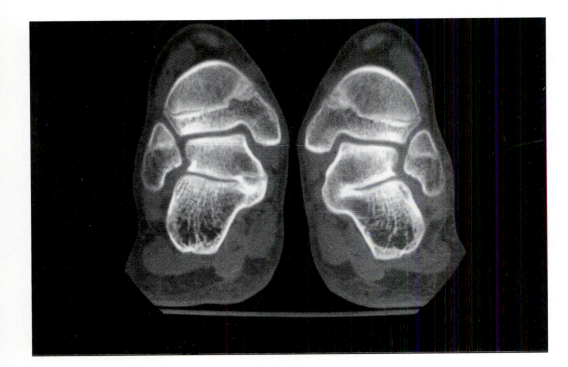

Figure 11
CT scan of
astragalocalcaneal bridge

clearly, separated by the tarsal canal. The posterior is seen on a more inferior plane, the anterior slightly above. Both, in normal feet, are horizontal. In the abnormal osseous bridge, irregularities of the sustentaculum tali joint can be seen; it is oblique posteriorly and medially. Sometimes an osseous island is seen.

Slomann projection
The foot is placed so it is resting over a cassette at 45°. The beam is placed laterally and above the foot. In this way all the types of union are apparent – syndesmosis, synchondrosis and synostosis.

Nowadays the diagnosis is easier with magnetic resonance imaging (MRI) or CT (Fig. 11).

Treatment
Management, given the irregular results of surgical treatment, is initially conservative. The use of plantar supports in the cases of calcaneonavicular unions, especially if this is partial, can give relief. In the forms of contracted foot, infiltration of the tarsal sinus with novocaine has given good results. This is preferred to injecting corticosteroids, as they sometimes provoke discomfort for a few days, and, what is worse, may cause fat atrophy that leaves small patches of depigmentation of the skin. In cases where conservative treatment fails, resort is made to surgical treatment. The proposed surgical interventions are:

Resection of the calcaneonavicular bridge
This was proposed by Bentzon in 1928. It is done through a lateral incision, similar, though smaller, to that for triple arthrodesis; extensor digitorum brevis is disinserted and then the bridge is seen very clearly. A complete resection must be performed; if not ankylosis will recur very easily. It can be useful to place a fragment of muscle between the calcaneum and the navicular. Postoperatively, compression bandages for 10 days suffice.

Resection of the astragalocalcanean bridge
This has been proposed by Jayakumar & Cowell (1977), who resect the small crest that joins the anterior subtalar area. The results are usually very uncertain, either because the resection is insufficient or because it affects a great part of the articular surface in which case overloading of the posterior joint is provoked.

Lengthening the peronei
Even if we have affirmed that the contracted foot is an isolated episode of spasm of the peronei, within the history of the disease, if this repeats frequently then a retraction of the peroneal tendons occurs. The confirmation of this is that infiltration of the tarsal sinus does not relax the tension. In this case, elongation of the tendons of one or both peronei by Z-plasty is successful. It is generally done as a complement to the previously mentioned procedures. In cases where this produces discomfort, resection of the beak of the talus can be performed.

If all the previously mentioned procedures fail, and if the condition is very painful, there is no other alternative but to carry out a triple arthrodesis.

Ball and socket ankle joint

This deformity is characterized by the astragalar trochlea, which instead of having a semicylindrical form, has a

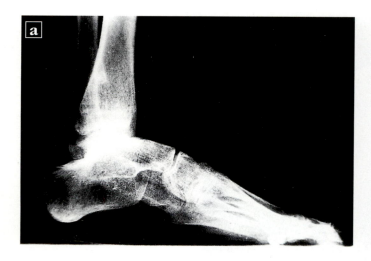

Figure 12

Radiographs of ball and socket ankle joint

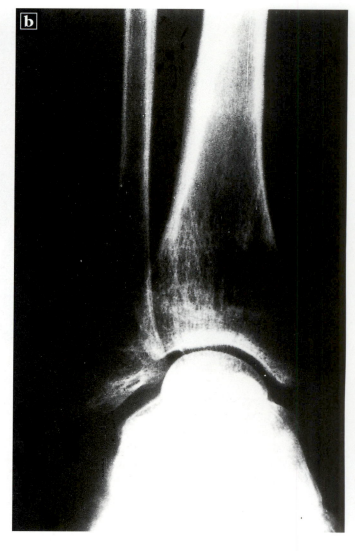

spherical structure (Fig. 12). The tibiofibular mortice also adjusts to this same form.

The deformity was first described by Lamb in 1958. Since then, many articles have been published on this subject (Imhauser 1970, Penrose 1974, Channon & Brotherton 1979). The Spanish authors, Peinado & Cañadell (1977), added two personal observations to 45 cases published in the world literature up until 1977.

Aetiopathology

The deformity is produced in an attempt to compensate for the movement of inversion–eversion of the subtalar joint, blocked by some osseous malformation. It confirms what has been said previously: in 75% of these cases, tarsal synostosis is found. This explanation is also supported by the fact that in those cases in which it has been practised in very small children, a Grice's style arthrodesis of the subtalar joint secondarily has provoked this deformity (Schreiber 1963).

There is also a frequent association of this disease with multiple congenital anomalies, as in the case of

Murakami (1975), who associated it with Nievergelt–Pearlman syndrome. Mendes & Lima (1978) presented five cases in the same family. Two of them exhibited anomalies in the sacroiliac joint.

Treatment

Being a compensatory anomaly, treatment is not necessary.

Aplasia of the distal epiphysis of the tibia

The absence of the tibia can be total or partial; the latter can affect the proximal extremity or the distal extremity.

We are especially interested in this latter type. It can be associated with other more proximal anomalies of the limb, but aplasia of the inner portion of the foot is almost constant. Curiously the lack of rays of the foot is usually less in aplasias of the tibia than in those of the

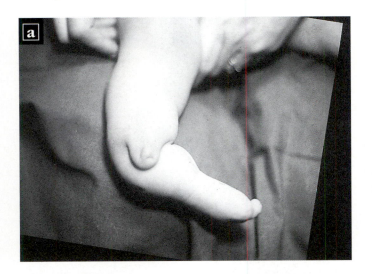

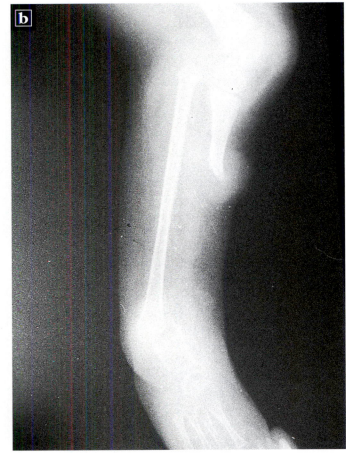

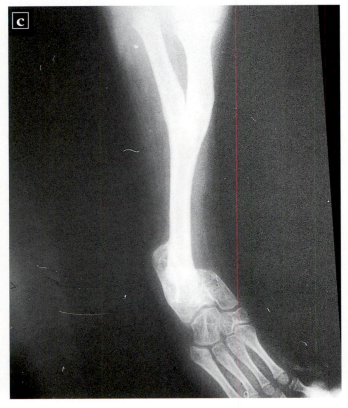

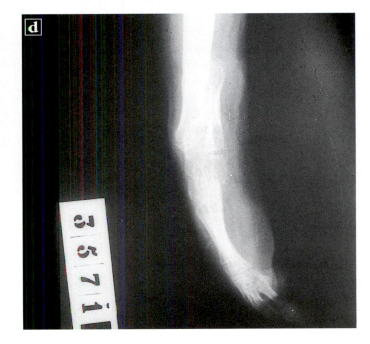

Figure 13

Aplasia of the tibia: (a) clinical aspect; (b) radiology; (c) and
(d) the same case, 3 years after a tibia–fibula synostosis,
which placed the foot in full equinus to compensate for the
shortening

fibula. Generally the fibula is of normal length or at least
more so than the tibia. This places the foot in a marked
varus in relation to the leg. This varus is often seen to
be increased by an aplasia of the first ray that makes
the whole forefoot deviate inwards.

Many types of tibial aplasia can be distinguished radiologically: in type I the tibia is not seen. In type II the
tibia is seen in its proximal portion, but not the distal
portion. In type III the distal portion is seen, but not the
proximal portion. Finally, in type IV all the tibial

diaphysis is seen, but it is shortened and the foot is in an equinovarus position.

In aplasia of the tibia, the fibula is not much altered, contrary to what happens when there are anomalies in the fibula, where the tibia curves.

Treatment

According to Tachdjian (1985), there are various problems produced by tibial hemimelia: (a) severe dysmetria of the lower limbs; (b) absence or instability of the knee and ankle; (c) rotary alterations of the axis of the leg; (d) varus deformity of the foot; (e) deficit of the muscles that control the mobility of the foot and ankle.

Surgical treatment varies depending on the problem and who is treating it. Putti (1929) suggests a transplant of the fibula alongside the tibia and a lengthening fusion of the foot. With support, the fibula hypertrophies. Salo (1978) and the author obtained a good result by fusing the astragalus to the tibia, leaving the foot in complete equinus, which compensated for the shortening (Fig. 13). The foot was put into its new position as if it were the lower extremity of a horse. The prosthesis with a solid ankle cushion heel (SACH) foot could be done more easily and aesthetically in this position than with the foot in a normal position and looking for a lengthening of some 14 or 15 cm. Many authors incline towards Syme's amputation, which they complement, in case of instability of the knee, with a joint fusion. It is always much easier to lengthen an amputated limb by prosthesis than to correct a very deformed foot and a shortened leg.

A much more recent method is that of the Russian Ilizarov (1983), which is based on the placing of a round external fixator that maintains tension with some Kirschner wires through the bone. An osteotomy is done at the level of the zone to be modified or of the bone that is to be enlarged. With distraction, the limb length is augmented; at the same time the desired form is given. The method can radically modify the functional prognosis of these limbs by obtaining not only spectacular lengthening of the extremity, but the correction of the deformities.

Aplasia of the distal epiphysis of the fibula

The fibula fails more frequently than the tibia. Generally, aplasia of the fibula accompanies the complete lack of a large part of the foot.

Coventry & Johnson (1952) divide these malformations into three types: (a) only one extremity is affected, the leg is short but there are no deformities in the tibia or in the foot. There are no functional disturbances. (b) Again in this case the affection is unilateral, but there is

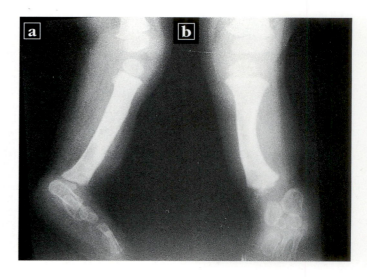

Figure 14

Aplasia of the fibula and outer metatarsals: (a) radiograph of frontal view; (b) profile view

substantial shortening and the tibia is bowed forward. The foot is deformed into equinovalgus and the tarsal bones are hypoplasic or absent (Fig. 14). (c) This type is the most severe, can be bilateral and accompanies other skeletal anomalies.

In the severe cases, the most clinically evident malformation is the shortening of the extremities together with the deviation into valgus of the foot. This is found to be maintained by a strong band of fibrocartilaginous tissue that substitutes for the fibula and maintains the foot in equinovalgus, together with an anterior bowing of the tibia. It is curious that, even when this band does not exist, causes of total aplasia of the distal portion of the peronei are found, but this does not alter the position of the ankle.

Treatment

In those cases where the band exists, surgical treatment must be early. Its removal allows restoration of the ankle to a good position, which an orthosis or an adequate orthopaedic shoe helps to maintain. In those cases where the valgus tends to relapse, an ankle fusion is necessary, giving the foot the necessary equinus to correct for the shortening.

Aplasia of other bones of the foot

Included in this group are malformations ranging from complete aplasia of the foot to the lack of some bones. These cases of osseous aplasia must not be confused with the osseous synostoses previously described. Most notable in this group are the multiple variations that are found in the rays of the foot, often in conjunction with similar deformities in the hands. The date in the development of the embryo at which the pathological gene responsible for anomalies in the digitalization of the hands and feet is induced is between the 6th and 8th week. Cases have been found in connection with thalidomide administration.

Brachyphalangia
This is frequent in the foot, especially at the level of the terminal phalanges; the toes have only one phalanx instead of three. In perodactylia, the terminal phalanx is absent, the form taken being that of a stump.

Schinz et al (1953) have described an extraordinarily frequent specific brachimesophalangeal aplasia of the fifth toe of the foot, which is often associated with the disappearance of those interphalangeal joints which even in normal adults have very limited movement. According to Venning (1966), who has gathered the works of different authors, the proportion of the diminution of the phalanx in these lesser toes would be:

1. Fifth toe with two phalanges: 40% of Europeans and 75% of Japanese
2. Fourth and fifth toes with two phalanges: 2% of Europeans
3. Third, fourth and fifth toes with two phalanges: 1% of Europeans
4. Three phalanges on the four last toes: 55% of Europeans and 25% of Japanese

The triphalangeal big toe is extremely rare.

This phenomenon was interpreted by Pfitzner (1890) (who found it in 36% of cases) as an adaptation of the osseous pieces to the erect attitude – a phenomenon of evolution that will increase with each new generation. According to this theory, fusion of the last three toes of the foot would follow and finally they would tend to disappear, leaving the forefoot formed only by a principal toe, the big toe, and another accessory toe.

Brachiphalangia is also associated with the trichorhinophalangeal syndrome. This is formed by a triad which, besides the alteration of the phalanges of the hands and feet, shows a diminution of growth, weak hair with precocious baldness, and a flat nose, well separated from the upper lips (Beals 1973).

The changes in the phalanges are associated with a conical epiphysis in the proximal extremity of the first phalanx (Fig. 15). According to Venning (1966) there are two types of proximal epiphysis in the phalanx: one has the regular form of a fringe placed dorsal to the corresponding metaphysis, the other presents a conical form with the point facing into the diaphysis. This anomaly is accompanied by a disappearance of the proximal epiphysis of the second and third phalanx and of a diminution in length of the tarsus and metatarsus.

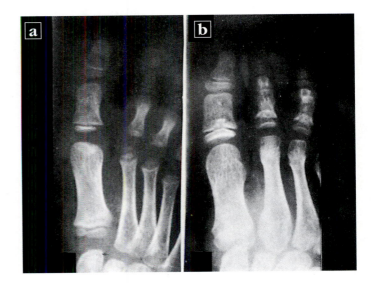

Figure 15
Radiographs of (a) normal foot; (b) conical epiphysis

Giedion (1967) classifies the conical epiphysis into 38 types. Some are found in children with normal feet but the great majority appear in children with congenital malformations, both systemic and localized.

Brachimetapody
This means diminution in the length of the metatarsals. It is less common than brachiphalangia, but it has more clinical importance. It can affect all the metatarsals and has the following characteristics:

1. Shortening of the first metatarsal. This has been masterfully described by Dudley Morton (1952), and it constitutes one of the special characteristics of the atavistic foot. It is recalled that in the feet of primates, with a shortened first ray, the metatarsal deviates into valgus and the sesamoid is retracted or deviated medially. A ligamentous laxity facilitates the separation between the first and second cuneiform, which further increases the varus of the first ray. Together with hallux valgus that generally accompanies this disease, it constitutes one of the most frequent deformities of the forefoot.
2. Aplasia of the fourth metatarsal. Curiously, this fourth metatarsal is frequently found to be affected by an early fusion of its distal extremity. It is seen frequently together with alterations of the poliomyelitic foot, or in clubfoot, but it can appear as an isolated deformity of the forefoot.

The problem of this deviation is that whilst the foot carries on growing, the ray gets shorter so on reaching

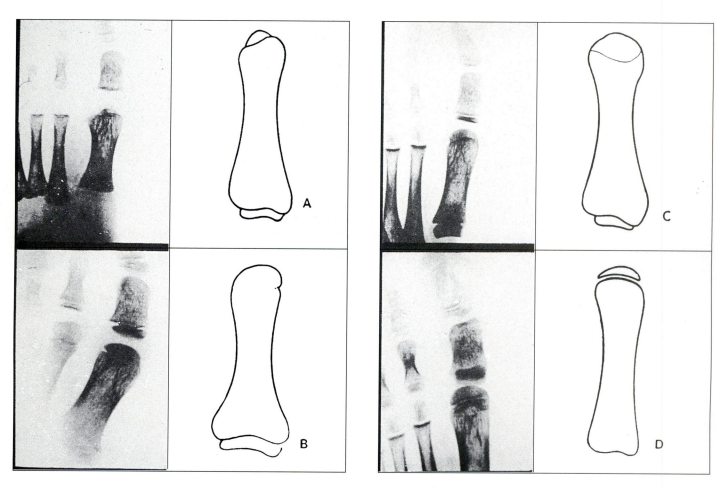

Figure 16

Variations of the distal epiphysis of the first metatarsal, as shown on radiograph: (A) small epiphyseal shadow; (B) partial fissure; (C) complete epiphysis; (D) real epiphysis separated from the rest of the bone

skeletal maturity, there is a kind of aberrant toe located on the dorsal surface of the metatarsal, which represents a serious problem when fitting shoes.

Although various operations have been proposed for trying to restore the length of the metatarsal, the amputation of the whole of the affected ray is recommended. If the precaution is taken to amputate the distal two-thirds of the metatarsal, the cosmetic and functional result is excellent. The adjacent metatarsals are approximated and these substitute for the affected ray.

Supernumerary epiphysis

It is relatively common to encounter a supernumerary epiphysis in the distal portion of the first metatarsal or metacarpal. It is well known that the first metatarsal differs from the rest, and has the epiphysis at its proximal end. This led Meckel (1932) to consider long ago that the metatarsal was the proximal phalanx of the big

toe. The big toe would thus correspond to the triphalangeal type that characterizes all the rest. The bone that would correspond to the first metatarsal would be the medial cuneiform bone. This could be the reason why triphalangeal thumb is less frequent.

The author studied this for the first time with Gonzalez Casanova in 1973 (Viladot & González Casanova 1973), and a study was published by Rochera & Rabat in 1980, dealing with an independent nucleus of ossification that appears in the distal epiphysis of the first metatarsal. In an examination of 400 X-rays of children aged between 2 and 8 years, we found this bilaterally in 53 cases (13%) and with a greater proportion appearing in the male (77% of the cases).

The form is variable; the following groups were differentiated (Fig. 16):

1. Small epiphyseal shadow separated from the rest of the bone by a thin line
2. Appearance of a partial fissure between epiphysis and metaphysis

3. A complete fissure
4. In older children there is a real epiphysis, totally separated from the rest of the bone.

It is interesting that in the majority of cases (83%) this alteration appears in individuals with a longer big toe (Egyptian foot) and a metatarsal 'index plus' type. This observation, together with the fact that it appears rather more in males would give credit to the idea that this malformation is a sign of evolution and would tend to represent in the foot, the triphalanx that sometimes appears in the thumb. This would be the converse anomaly to the atavistic Morton's metatarsal.

The pathological influence that this epiphysis could have is as follows. (a) By increasing the length of the metatarsal, it gives an 'index plus' metatarsal formula, which favours the development of hallux rigidus. (b) The alteration in the ossification that occasionally has been observed in this distal epiphysis may produce an osteonecrosis similar to Freiberg–Köhler II disease, which can appear in the other metatarsals. (c) The localized vascular alterations of the epiphyseal nucleus would explain some cases found with osteochondritis dissecans.

Hereditary contractures

Vertical talus

This was described for the first time in 1914 by Henken and by Nove-Josserand in 1923, as congenital valgus convex foot. Since then, it has received a varied nomenclature. Rocher (1913) calls it foot in 'piole', and Mau (1930), foot in 'balance', both describing the clinical aspects of the foot. Giannestras (1967) calls this type of foot 'congenital rigidus flat foot'. Tachdjian (1985), concentrating on the principal anatomopathologic characteristic of this condition, proposed calling it 'teratologic luxation of the astragalonavicular joint'.

The pathogenic cause of this congenital malformation is unknown. Lamy & Weisselman (1939) attributed it to a delay in development occurring during the first quarter of intrauterine life, Rocher & Pouyanne (1934) to a muscular imbalance (Fig. 17).

Some histories of hereditary and familial forms have been described. The lesion can be unique or associated with other systemic malformations, such as arthrogryposis, Hurler's syndrome, Marfan's syndrome, Down's syndrome, etc. It is also frequently associated with spina bifida and cerebral palsy. Isolated forms are rare; in a review by Viladot et al (1980) of over 20 flat feet, there were only five cases. They are more frequent when accompanying other malformations. Sharrard & Grosfield (1968) found that in spina bifida it appeared in 20% of cases.

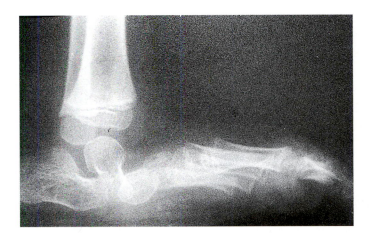

Figure 17
Radiograph of vertical talus valgus foot

Pathological anatomy
The vertical talus (astragalus) flat foot presents differently from other types of flat feet and can be summarized as: (a) valgus of the heel with a displacement of the astragalus downward, forward and medially on the hindfoot; (b) abduction and (c) supination of the forefoot; (d) the heel is in equinus.

It also presents characteristics such that some osteoarticular, vascular, ligamentous, muscular and cellular tissue alterations can be distinguished (Patterson et al 1966, Drennan & Sharrard 1971).

Osteoarticular alterations
The astragalus is longer than normal, but has a shorter neck. The navicular is found luxated superiorly and fixed in this position. The astragalonavicular luxation is the key to this malformation (Fig. 18). When there is no astragalonavicular luxation, we can speak of a flat foot with a vertical talus, more or less severe, but this is a different disease to the one we are referring to here.

The calcaneum is found in equinus and in valgus. There are alterations at the level of the subtalar joint with a hypoplasia of the anterior facet, and with a change in the sustentaculum tali.

Vascular alterations
In a study (Ben Mechamen & Butler 1974) made of feet with congenital malformations, the authors noticed that the major blood supply came from arteries on the dorsum of the foot, contrary to the normal foot, as if there was a greater need of blood supply to the dorsum than to the sole.

Musculoligamentous alterations
There is retraction of the anterior tibial muscles, extensor longus, common extensor to the toes, short lateral peroneus and triceps. The posterior tibial and the

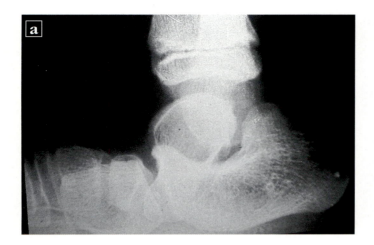

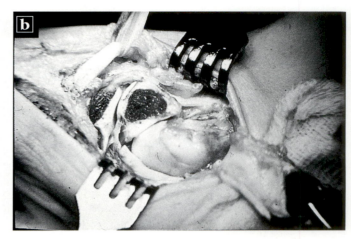

Figure 18

The commonest deformity of the vertical astragalus foot is the astragalonavicular luxation. (a) Radiograph; (b) peroperative findings

peroneus muscle tendons are found displaced forward, acting as dorsiflexors instead of acting as plantar flexors. Sometimes, in more severe cases, the tendons form bow strings at the level of the dorsum of the ankle. The triceps surae has an insertion wider than normal into the valgus calcaneum.

There are also important ligamentous retractions that help maintain the deformity. The calcaneonavicular ligament, or 'spring ligament', is found elongated and thinner, because of the pressure of the head of the astragalus.

Subcutaneous cellular tissue
This tissue that normally covers the plantar aspect of the heel, is found displaced laterally leaving the longitudinal arch, which has disappeared or is reversed, unprotected.

Diagnosis
Diagnosis can be made at birth by the rocker bottom that the foot presents, the head of the astragalus being palpable in the sole. Medially it is sometimes possible to palpate the navicular on the dorsum. The rigidity that presents from birth characterizes this deformity and permits one to differentiate it clinically from the talus valgus foot and other malformations.

Walking is not usually delayed. The foot is already so deformed that it does not worsen the gait, but progressively becomes more painful with the passage of time. The disease has bad prognosis and it eventually incapacitates the patient.

Radiological examination
The astragalus lies in the axis of the tibia, and this does not change with dorsiflexion and plantar flexion, which

leads to a differential diagnosis to other types of abnormalities of the foot.

The calcaneum is in equinus and its inferior surface is convex; the astragalocalcanean angle is increased and reaches the right angle. At 3 years of age, the navicular is ossified and a complete luxation of the navicular over the neck of the talus can be shown radiographically. This astragalonavicular luxation, as we have noted, is pathognomonic of the vertical astragalus flat foot. The forefoot is supinated, the first metatarsal being in dorsiflexion.

Treatment
Although some authors (Becker et al 1974) propose conservative treatment in the first weeks of life, based on manipulation and a plaster bandage, in most cases this is not sufficient and surgical treatment is necessary, since it is very difficult to reduce the astragalonavicular luxation.

Surgical treatment
There are various aspects to be considered in discussing the surgical treatment of the disease:

1. It is necessary to remember the musculotendinous contracture that maintains the deformity, namely the shortening of the extensors and the anterior peroneus and the Achilles tendon. It is for this reason that the tendons must be elongated to achieve complete peritalar relaxation in all of these cases (Fitton & Nevelos 1979).
2. While trying to correct the astragalonavicular luxation, the surgeon can be presented with a problem that arises because of the elongated astragalus and the dorsal luxation of the navicular: there

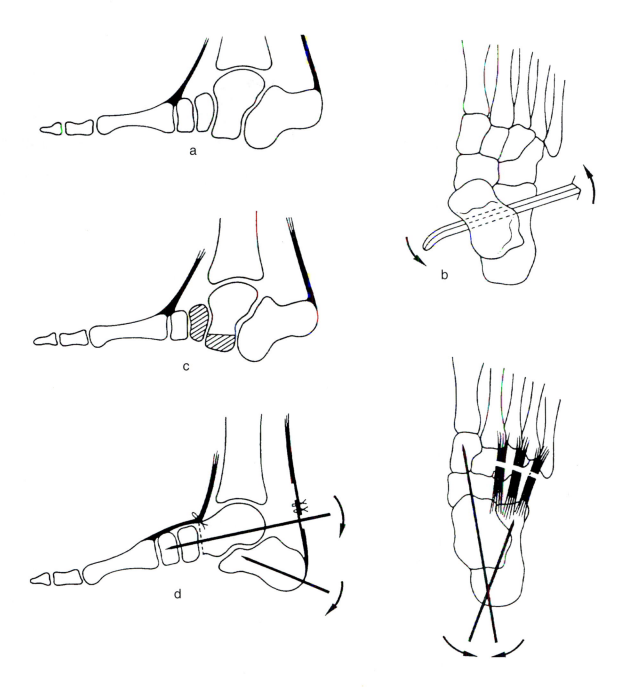

Figure 19

Surgical techniques. (a) Preoperative aspect; (b) placing the astragalus over the calcaneum; (c) correction of the astragalonavicular luxation; it is often necessary to remove either the navicular or the head of the astragalus; (d) elongating the Achilles tendon, sectioning of the extensors, fixing the anterior tibial to the head of the astragalus. The correction is maintained with Kirschner wires

can be difficulty in reducing the astragalus to the horizontal and replacing the navicular in front of the talus head, since the length of these bones is then too great to model a normal arch. In these cases, there is no other remedy but to excise bone. For this, the total or partial removal of the navicular or resection of the head of the astragalus has been recommended (Eyre-Brook 1967, Colton 1973, Robbins 1982).

3. Maintenance of the correction can be achieved by using Kirschner wires to stabilize the foot long enough to allow the smooth parts to accommodate themselves. In a more definitive way, stabilization can be obtained by suturing the anterior tibial tendon to the neck of the astragalus, to elevate the level (Tachdjian 1985). Grice (1959) proposes the Malvarez–Grice arthrodesis of the subtalar joint (Malvarez 1966).

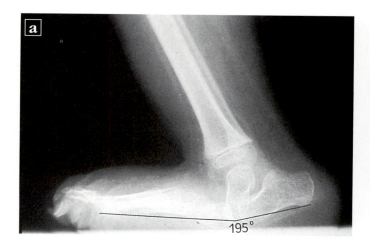

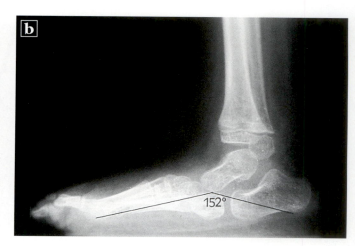

Figure 20

Radiographs of vertical talus: (a) preoperative condition; (b) postoperative condition

In view of all these facts, we choose to adopt a bilateral approach when operating on the vertical talus, according to the following technique (Fig. 19):

1. A medial incision is made extending from the anterior quarter of the foot to the level of the malleolus. An osteoperiosteal flap, based posteriorly, is lifted, containing the tibialis posterior, and reaches the insertion of the anterior tibialis. In this way the astragalonavicular joint and the cuneiform can be seen, exposing the astragalonavicular luxation.
2. A lateral incision is made beneath the lateral malleolus and ascending to the external aspect of the ankle. Through it the Achilles tendon is lengthened, the common extensor to the toes and the abundant fibrous bands of the dorsum are sectioned, and with them the tendon of the anterior peroneus.
3. Entry is made with a blunt instrument from the outside of the sinus tarsi, passing below the neck of the astragalus, which is elevated and placed over the calcaneum. At the same time, the inner part must be checked to see if correction is possible.
4. In case this correction is not possible, the head of the astragalus is resected and modelled. Rarely is the navicular removed.
5. The tibialis anterior tendon is fixed to the neck of the astragalus through a point that crosses the astragalar neck.
6. The best position of the bones is secured with Kirschner wires. Viladot et al (1980) have proposed a useful method using two relatively rigid needles, one of which crosses the talus, navicular and cuneiform, while the other crosses the calcaneus longitudinally. With this they can correct the astragalocalcanean sagittal angle and the horizontal line of the same bones, which is generally too open.
7. The wound is closed.

A compression bandage fixes the bones of the tarsus in position, and 15 days later the bandage is removed. The Kirschner wires must remain in place for a minimum period of one month (Fig. 20).

Talus foot

This is generally a postural moulding defect, present at birth. In the most exaggerated cases (Fig. 21) it might be necessary to use a corrective splint.

Hallux varus

This deformity, which is relatively rare, is characterized by a deviation medially of the big toe (Fig. 22). It is generally unilateral and can coexist with other anomalies, such as metatarsus varus, oligodactyly or syndactyly.

The toe is found deviated medially, forming an angle of between 60° and 90° with the medial side of the foot; sometimes the deformity is increased at the level of the interphalangeal joint, which is angled inward. The pulp and the nail have a normal aspect, but are flat and widened.

Aetiopathology
This condition presents in two circumstances:

1. As a secondary deformity to metatarsovarus or even to clubfoot. In these cases, the big toe follows the deformity of the metatarsal, and exaggerates it. Sometimes it appears compensating a flat foot.

2. In the primary cases, the deformity of the big toe is found at the level of the metatarsophalangeal joint. Radiologically it was observed that, in its congenital form, the proximal epiphysis appears implanted on the medial face of the head of the metatarsal.

According to McElvenny (1941), together with the deviation of the toe, one or more of the following anomalies may appear:

1. The first metatarsal is generally thicker and shorter than normal.
2. There are usually accessory bones and toes associated with the deformity.
3. There can be a metatarsus varus.
4. A band of firm fibrous tissue extends from the internal side of the big toe to the base of the first metatarsal.

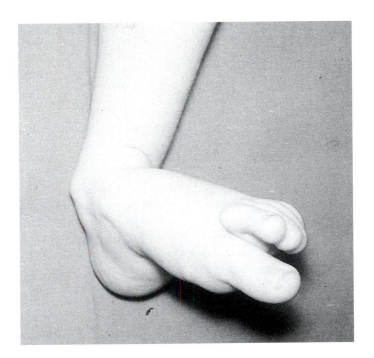

Figure 21

Talus foot

Treatment

In congenital cases, conservative treatment almost never gives good results. Surgical treatment is difficult, because the deformity has a great tendency to relapse, and because of this it should be done as early as possible.

Surgical technique

As is usual, we perform the operation under haemostasis and general anaesthesia.

1. A medial longitudinal incision is made and dissection of the abductor tendon, generally thickened, is carried out. Sometimes, from the body of the muscle a strong fibrous band inserts itself at the level of the terminal phalanx.
2. All the elements that maintain the deviation of the toe and medial arthrotomy of the joint are removed.
3. A cuneiform incision is made in the interdigital commisure between the first and second toes, removing the small spindle of skin with the object of creating a syndactyly proximally, between these toes and in the suture.
4. External arthrotomy of the metatarsophalangeal joint is carried out next. Sometimes it is necessary to remove a small aberrant bone and to remove a supernumerary phalanx that is usually found in this area. It is sometimes necessary to remove the lateral sesamoid to obtain correction.
5. These steps are taken to correct the deviation of the toe. If this is not possible (frequently after infancy), a resection of the proximal portion of the phalanx, as in Brandes–Keller intervention, is performed.
6. Both wounds are sutured. On the medial side, the tendon of the abductor remains plantar. To maintain the correction it is useful to place a suture connecting the pulps of the first and second toes for 10 days. Some authors practise syndactyly between the first and second toes (McElvenny 1941, Montero 1967).

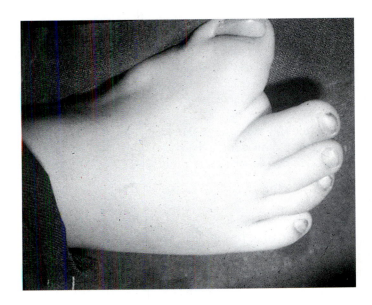

Figure 22

Hallux varus

The forefoot is supported by an elastic bandage and antivarus shoes worn for at least a year.

McElvenny (1941) contributes a technical modification in sectioning the tendon of the extensor digitorum brevis to the big toe from its muscle and passing it through a canal drilled in the diaphysis of the metatarsal, so that it pulls the phalanx laterally. The same tendon is passed through a loop that enfolds the tendon of the long extensor and keeps this in position.

Joint aplasia

Aplasias of the interphalangeal joints of the outer toes are frequent, especially at the level of the fifth toe, fusing to form short phalanges. They receive different names, such as 'hereditary phalangic synostosis', and 'congenital digital rigidity'.

According to Capecchi et al (1968), the diminution of the number of phalanges occurs in two phases: first is found a progressive reduction of the length of the corresponding phalanx, followed later by a diminution of the joint line between the phalanx fated to disappear and the distal phalanx.

To some authors (Testut & Latajet 1932), these ankyloses are due to the wearing during many generations of narrow shoes that immobilize these last joints, which, having no function, tend to disappear. These joint rigidities, according to their frequency, can go through different phases:

1. Joint hypoplasias of the first degree: minimal joint rigidity
2. Joint hypoplasia of the second degree: fibrous ablation of the joint cavity
3. Joint hypoplasia of third degree; osseous fusion across the joint cavity (synostosis of the phalanges)
4. Complete joint aplasia.

Even though the interphalangeal fusion almost always involves the fifth toe, it can coexist in various finger joints of the hand or of the other toes. The deformity is hereditary.

Lobster clawfoot

Also called ectrodactyly, this is so described because in its anterior portion the foot has a large cleft that reaches the midfoot. Laterally, two divergent pillars are formed, the appearance being reminiscent of a lobster claw (Fig. 23).

In its typical form, the deformity is bilateral and is inherited as an autosomal dominant characteristic. Even if it presents as an isolated deformity, it usually occurs together with a similar deformity in the hand.

Radiologically there is an aplasia of the central metatarsals, sometimes total, and in others forming small stumps. In a personal case it was evident that the central metatarsals, without the corresponding toes, were going to articulate with the first and fifth metatarsals. Radiologically the impression was that the development

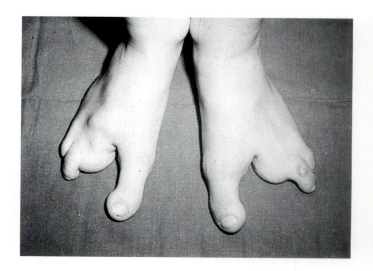

Figure 23

Lobster foot

of these central metatarsals increased the divergence of each of the lateral segments of the foot.

There are cases in which this anomaly is found to be well tolerated. In others it provokes different types of disturbance: (a) of aesthetic character, especially if associated with anomalies of the hand, which can cause psychological problems for the patient; (b) because of the uneven development of the different rays, some of them are excessively prominent, which leads to an alteration in the pressure points of the sole of the foot; and (c) the excessive divergence of the rays creates a width of the forefoot that impedes the wearing of normal shoes.

Treatment

Closure of the fissure of the forefoot by means of cutaneous suture is of no value in isolation. The skeleton must be very carefully studied in each case. Consideration of the aesthetics should not cloud judgement of the functional aspects. In a case in which there was great divergence of the first and fifth metatarsals, the problem was solved by resecting the divergent central metatarsal; having done this, a simple arthrotomy of the cuneometatarsal joint permitted the metatarsals to be placed in correct alignment, obtaining an excellent result, both aesthetic and functional. In another case, the metatarsals had to be aligned by shortening and resecting a portion of the diaphysis.

Syndactyly

Syndactyly is characterized by the union of two or more toes in only one cutaneous cover (Fig. 24). The condition is frequently associated with polydactyly.

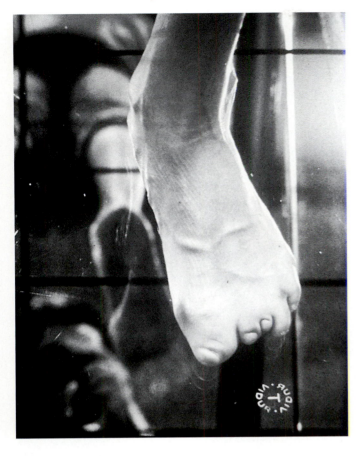

Figure 24

Polysyndactyly

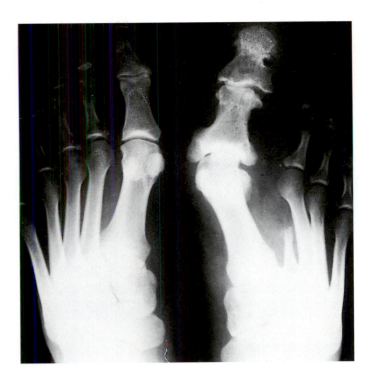

Figure 25

Radiograph of gigantism of the big toe. The second ray had been amputated

Among the syndactylies, different degrees can be found, with regard to the extent of the connection (depending on how much of the length of the toe is involved) or to the number of rays affected.

In the foot, the most frequent is cutaneous partial syndactyly, that appears commonly between the second and third toes. Polysyndactyly usually affects the big toe or the fifth toe. Being tolerable, syndactylies of the foot do not necessarily require treatment.

Constitutional hypertrophies

It is necessary to differentiate the hypertrophies of the toe that are due to tumorous or vascular disorders from those that are related to a congenital aetiology. Among the first type are lipomas, the haemangiomas and lymphangiectasis. All of these can cause considerable hypertrophy of the whole foot or leg.

Congenital hypertrophies can affect all the foot or a part of it. Isolated hypertrophy of a toe is not uncommon

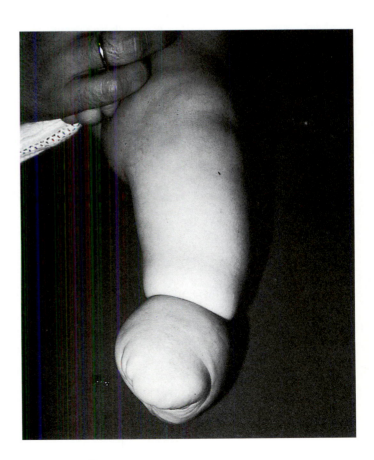

Figure 26

An intermediate form of amniotic rings producing distal atrophy

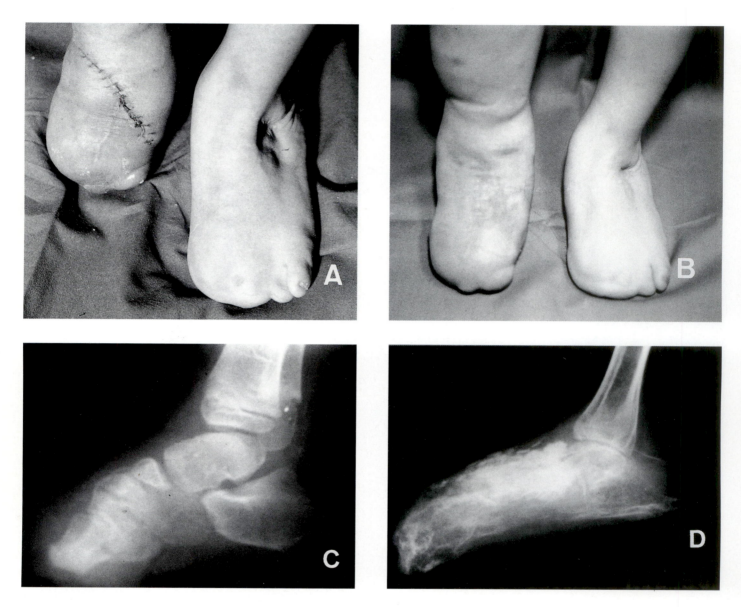

Figure 27

Enlargement of the forefoot by Ilizarov's technique: (A) before and (B) after operation; (C) radiograph before operation; (D) radiograph after operation.

(Fig. 25). Different to false tumorous hypertrophy, we are concerned here with a major overgrowth of all the tissue elements. Congenital hypertrophy can present in three forms:

1. Without histological alteration. There is a total hypertrophy of the foot or of a part of it, but without any anatomopathological alterations beside the greater growth.
2. In relation to von Recklinghausen's disease. It occurs frequently here, together with tumours of the peripheral nerves. The same alteration that causes changes in ectodermal and dermal development that characterize the disease is responsible for the gigantism.

3. In relation to arterovenous fistulas. These can produce a global alteration of the leg, foot or toe. They are not always found by arteriographic examination. Sometimes, similar to the occurrence in von Recklinghausen's disease, the condition begins with pigmentation of the skin. From this comes the name of phakomatosis used by some authors to label the hypertrophy. This also happens with Klippel–Trennaney disease.

Treatment
The problem of gigantism is in fitting shoes. In some cases, attempts to control growing by binding children's feet has been tried. The results are always very poor.

Surgical therapy is indicated only in those cases in which there is an excessive growth of a toe. If this is not the big toe, it is better to practise complete amputation of the ray. When there is a great quantity of soft tissue, Tachdjian (1985) recommends doing the operation in two stages: first the proximal phalanx and the spare adipose tissue of a toe is resected, and then syndactylized with previous removal of the soft tissue of the adjacent toe.

Lesions caused by amniotic disease

Amniotic rings

The constriction band is a rare malformation that appears in one in 10 000 births. Most authors are unanimous in affirming that the condition is not caused by endogenous or genetic factors, but by amniotic bands, which can appear in an isolated form that include only one foot or both extremities. One toe alone is seldom affected.

The alterations provoked in the foot range from the simple ring without alteration of the vital part, to the complete amputation of the affected part. Intermediate forms produce distal atrophy (Fig. 26).

Treatment

With a Z-plasty done in the ring, a good correction can be obtained.

Until recently, the treatment was merely orthesic. Nowadays, using Ilizarov's technique (1983), it is possible to obtain lengthening of the absent digit. Figure 27 shows a case operated on by our colleague, Dr R Mascaro. After a medial tarsal osteotomy, a distraction was applied until the length of the foot was the same as the contralateral foot. To maintain the lengthening bone grafts were necessary.

References

Bado J L, Garcia-Novales J 1951 Pié valgo espástico: consideraciones clínicas y fisiopatológicas. An Ortop Traumatol 4: 191

Beals R 1973 Richo-rhino phalangeal dysplasia. J Bone Joint Surg 55A: 821

Becker P E, Andersen H, Reimann I 1974 Congenital vertical talus – reevaluation of early manipulative treatment. Acta Orthop Scand 45: 130

Ben Mechamen Y, Butler J 1974 Arteriography of the foot in congenital deformities. J Bone Joint Surg 56A: 1625

Bentzon P C K 1928 Coalitio calcaneo naviculars mit besonderer Bezungnahme auf die operative Behandlung des durch diese Anomalie bedingten Plattfusses. Verh Dtsch Orthop 23: 269

Bergsma D 1973 Birth Defects. Williams & Wilkins Co., Baltimore

Capecchi V, Cicala G, Grisafulli A 1968 Le ossa sopranumerari del piede. Acta Orthop Ital X 1

Channon G M, Brotherton B J 1979 The ball and socket ankle joint. J. Bone Joint Surg 61B: 85

Colton C L 1973 The surgical management of congenital vertical talus. J Bone Joint Surg 55B: 566

Coventry M B, Johnson E W 1952 Congenital absence of fibula. J Bone Joint Surg 34A: 941

Cummins H, Midlo C 1929 The topographic history of the volar pads (walking pads: tast ballen) in the human embryo. Embryology 20: 103

Cummins H, Midlo C 1961 Fingerprints, palms and soles. Dover Publications Inc., New York

Danlos M 1908 Un cas de cutis laxa avec tumeurs par contusion chronique des coudes et des genous (xanthome juvenile pseudo-diabétique de M M Hallopeau et Mace de Lépinay). Bull Soc Franc Derm Syph 19: 70

Drennan J C, Sharrard W J W 1971 The pathological anatomy of congenital convex pes valgus. J Bone Joint Surg 53B: 455

Dubosset J 1982 Arthrogrypose. Encyc Med Chir 15201 A 10: 4.7.09

Ehlers E 1901 Cutis laxa, Neilgung zu Haemmorrhagien in der hautlockerung mehrerer Artilationen. Derm Z T: 173

Eyre-Brook A L 1967 Congenital vertical talus. J Bone Joint Surg 49B: 618

Fitton J M, Nevelos A B 1979 The treatment of congenital vertical talus. J Bone Joint Surg 61B: 481

Friedlander H L, Westin W, Wood W L 1968 Arthrogryposis multiplex congenita. A review of forty-five cases. J Bone Joint Surg 50A: 89

Galton F 1892 Fingerprints. Macmillan, London

Giannestras N J 1967 Foot Disorders. Medical and Surgical Management. Lea & Febiger, Philadelphia

Giedion A 1967 Cone-shaped epiphyses of the hands and their diagnostic value: The tricho-rhino-phalangeal syndrome. Ann Radiol 10: 322

Grice D S 1959 The role of subtalar fusion in the treatment of valgus deformities of the feet. Instr Course Lect 16:

Harris R I 1948 Aetiology of peroneal spastic flat foot. J Bone Joint Surg 30B: 624

Harris R I 1965 Retrospect personal spastistic flat foot (rigid valgus foot). J Bone Joint Surg 47A: 1657

Harris R I, Hon F R C 1955 Rigid valgus foot due to talocalcaneal bridge. J Bone Joint Surg 37A: 169

Henken R 1914 Contribution a l'étude des formes osseuses du pied plat valgus congénital. Thesis, Lyon

Ilizarov G A 1983 Abstracts of the 1st International Symposium on experimental theoretical and clinical aspects of transosseous osteosynthesis in the method developed in Kurgan Scientific Research Institute, Kurgan

Imhauser G 1970 Kubelformige Knöchelgelenke bei angeborchen Fuss und zel Synostesen. Z Orthop 108: 247

Jack E A 1954 Bone anomalies of the tarsus in relation to peroneal spastic flatfoot. J Bone Joint Surg 26B: 530

Jaffe H L 1972 Metabolic, Degenerative, and Inflammatory Diseases of Bones and Joints. Lea & Febiger, Philadelphia

Jayakumar S, Cowell H R 1977 Rigid flatfoot. Clin Orthop 122: 77–84

Lamb D 1958 The ball and socket ankle joint. A congenital abnormality. J Bone Joint Surg 40B: 240

Lamy L, Weisselman L 1939 Congenital convex pes valgus. J Bone Joint Surg 21: 79

Lewis J 1983 A study of metatarsus varus. PhD Thesis, University of East Anglia, Norwich

McElvenny R T 1941 Hallux varus. Q Bull North West Med Sch 19: 277

McKusick V A 1966 Heritable disorders of connective tissue. C V Mosby, St Louis

Malvarez O 1966 Artrodésis calcáneo astragalina extra-articular en el pié pronado paralítico. Estudio sobre 400 casos. Bol Trabajos Soc Arg Ortop Traumat 33: 246

Marfan A B 1896 Un cas de déformation congénitale des quatre membres, plus prononcée aux extremites caracterisée par l'allongement des os avec un certain degré d'amincissement. Bull Mem Soc Med Hop 13: 22

Marqui E de, Gambier R 1953 Le sinozifosi del tarso nel piede piatio valgo conttrato. Chir Org Mov 38: 350

Mau K 1930 Muskelbefunde und ihre Bodentung beim angelborerer Klumpfussleiden. Arch Orthop Unfallchir 28: 202

Meckel 1932 In: Testut L, Latarjet A (eds) Tratado de Anatomía Humana. Salvat Editores, Barcelona

Mendes A, Lima C 1978 Tornozelo concavo-convexo. Rev Ortop Traumat 4: 109

Menelaus M B 1971 Talectomy for equinovarus deformity in arthrogryposis and spina bifida. J Bone Joint Surg 53B: 468

Montero M 1967 Técnicas para el hallux valgus congénito. Rev Ortop Traumat 11: 509

Morton D 1952 The Human Foot. Columbia University Press, New York

Murakami Y 1975 Nievergelt–Pearlman syndrome with impairment of hearing. J Bone Joint Surg 57B: 367

Natiello O 1966 Pie plano y anomalías del tarso. Bol Trabajos Soc Arg Ortop Traumat 31: 136

Nove-Josserand 1923 Formes anatomiques du pied plat. Rev Orthop 10: 117

Patterson W R, Fitz D A, Smith W S 1966 The pathologic anatomy of congenital convex pes valgus. J Bone Joint Surg 50A: 458

Peinado A, Cañadell J M 1977 Articulación del tobillo concavo-convexo. Rev Ortop Traumat 21: 79

Penrose J H 1974 Tarsal synostosis and the ball and socket ankle joint. J Bone Joint Surg 56B: 202

Penrose L S, Loesch D 1969 Dermatoglyphic sole patterns: a new attempt at classification. Hum Biol 41: 427

Pfitzner I 1932 (quoted by Testut L, Latarjet A). Tratado de Anatomía Humana. Salvat Editores, Barcelona

Pfitzner W 1890 Beiträge zur Kenntnis der Misbildungen des menschlichen Extremitätenskeletts. Schwalbes Morph Arch Anat 8: 332

Putti V 1929 The treatment of congenital absence of the tibia or fibula. Chir Organi Mov 7: 513

Recklinghausen F von 1882 Über die multiplen Fibrome der Haut und ihre Beziehung zu den multiple Neuromen. Verlag V A Hirschwald, Berlin

Robbins H 1982 Disorders of the Foot Vol. I. W B Saunders Co., Philadelphia

Rocher H L 1913 Les raideurs articulaires congénitales multiples. J Med Bordeaux 84: 722

Rocher H L, Pouyanne L 1934 Pied plat congénital par subluxation sous astragalienne congénitale et orientation verticale d'astragale. Bordeaux Chir 5: 249

Rochera R, Rabat E 1980 The growth of the first metatarsal bone. Foot Ankle 1: 117

Roger A, Meary R 1969 Les synostoses congénitales des os du tarse. Rev Chir Orthop 55: 721, Paris

Rozman C, Jurado-Grau J, Elizalde C 1967 Síndrome de Ehlers–Danlos con linfedema. Presentación Familiar Med Clin 44: 237

Ruiz S 1976 El pié contracturado por malformaciones tarsales congénitas. Rev Soc Ortop Traumat Uruguay 11: 52

Salo Orfila J 1978 Conducta terapéutica en les aplàsies esquelètiques de la cama. Ann Med 64: 120

Schinz H R, Baensch W R, Friedl E, Vehlinger E 1953 Rongendiagnóstico. Salvat Editores, Barcelona

Schreiber R R 1963 Congenital and acquired ball and socket of the ankle joint. Radiology 84: 940

Sharrard W G W, Grosfield J 1968 The management of deformity and paralysis of the foot in myelomeningocele. J Bone Joint Surg 50B: 456

Slomann 1921 On coalition calcaneo-navicularis. J Orthop Surg 3: 586

Tachdjian M 1985 The Child's Foot. W B Saunders Co., Philadelphia

Testut L, Latarjet A 1932 Tratado de Anatomía Humana. Salvat Editores, Barcelona

Venning P 1966 Variation of the digital skeleton of the foot. Clin Orthop 16: 26

Verschuer O von 1959 Genetik des Menschen. Urban & Schwarzenberg, Munich

Viladot A 1954 Nuevo método de exploración estática del pie: El fotopodograma. Clin Lab LVII, 335: 144

Viladot A 1984 Patología del Antepié, 3rd edition. Ediciones Toray, Barcelona

Viladot A, González Casanova J C 1973 Malformaciones congénitas del antepié. Actualités Med Chir Pied 7: 97

Viladot R, Rochera R 1972 La enfermedad de Ehler–Danlos. Annals Medicina 58: 227

Viladot R, Valenti J, Palazón N 1978 La astragalectomía del piede torso infantil. Chir piede 2: 17

Viladot R, Valenti J, Ubierta M T 1980 El peu plas 'vertical talus'. Communication to the Sociedad Catalana de Cir Ortop y Traumato, Barcelona

Werthemann 1966 Die Entwicklungsstörungen der Extremitäten. Quoted by Hans Grebe in: Becker P E (ed) Hum Genet Vol. II. Editores Toray, Barcelona

Zimbler S, Craig C 1976 Symposium on birth defects and the orthopedic surgeon. W B Saunders Co., Philadelphia

IV.3 Myelomeningocele

Nigel S Broughton and Malcolm B Menelaus

Myelomeningocele is a congenital abnormality caused by failure of the neural tube to close. It results in abnormal innervation to the segments involved and in deficiencies of the posterior part of the vertebral bodies. There is involvement of multiple organs, including bladder, bowel, vascular, and the musculoskeletal system, and there are abnormalities of sensibility.

The incidence of myelomeningocele has decreased in recent years, owing to improved maternal screening and selection programs, but there are still a significant number of children with myelomeningocele born in our hospital, who are managed to maturity (Broughton et al 1993).

The orthopaedic management of myelomeningocele is aimed at fulfilling the child's maximum physical and social potential within the limits imposed by the congenital anomaly. We aim to perform the minimum number of operations and immobilize the child as little as possible, and so we advocate multiple procedures under the one anaesthetic and procedures that keep postoperative immobilization to a minimum (Menelaus 1980).

Accurate assessment of the neurosegmental level of the child is important, as it allows a reasonable prediction of the expected functional ability of the child. This should be repeated regularly so that any significant deterioration can be appreciated and the child investigated for a tethered cord or cord syrinx.

Expectations of outcome for different spinal levels

In general terms, children with strong quadriceps muscles and hip abductors can be expected to be good walkers. Of those with good quadriceps and poor abductors, most can walk with aids. Most children with no quadriceps or abductor power prefer a wheelchair as they approach skeletal maturity, although there may be a period between the ages of 3 and 10 years when the child may walk with reciprocating gait orthoses or the parawalker.

Our aim is to keep children mobile. In children with lesions at the thoracic level, we are increasingly finding that this is best achieved and is most energy efficient in a wheelchair.

Young children enjoy being upright and we use braces plus aids to encourage this; however, when the child finds he can be more mobile, expend less energy and cover longer distances in a wheelchair, this is not discouraged. In thoracic L1 and L2 level children, our early treatment is directed towards good orthotic fitting to allow an upright posture, but we are aware that our surgery should also be compatible with a wheelchair existence in the future. We discuss this likely outcome with the parents at an early stage, so when the child does decide to opt for a wheelchair for improved mobility there is no sense of guilt or disappointment within the family.

The foot

The problems of the foot in myelomeningocele

The foot in children with myelomeningocele can give rise to significant problems. This is due to a combination of fixed deformity, reduced sensation, reduced proprioception and poor or inappropriate muscle action.

Fixed deformity may be due to muscle imbalance. This can be due to normally innervated muscles with paralysed antagonists, or it may occur where spasticity of muscles produces imbalance against normally innervated or paralysed antagonists (Fig. 1). Deformity may arise from intrauterine posture or from habitually assumed posture after birth. Some children with equinovarus deformities at birth resemble cases of arthrogryposis multiplex congenita with rigidity of joints and absence of normal creases (Fig. 2).

The main complications of the foot in myelomeningocele children are the development of neuropathic ulcers and joints in an insensate, stiff, deformed foot (Lindseth 1982).

The goals of treatment

The main goal of treatment is to produce a plantigrade foot which is not stiff or deformed and to prevent the complications of neuropathic ulcers and joints (Tachdjian 1990). In the non-walker, prevention of ulcers is important but it is also important to the child's self esteem that the foot be plantigrade so it can be placed in a shoe and appear to be normal resting on the foot plate of a wheelchair. In the walker treatment should be aimed at allowing normal walking without the development of deformity and where necessary the comfortable fitting of an ankle-foot orthosis (AFO).

The principles of treatment

The principles of treatment in the myelomeningocele foot are:

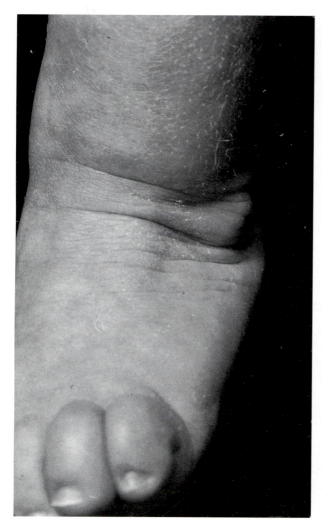

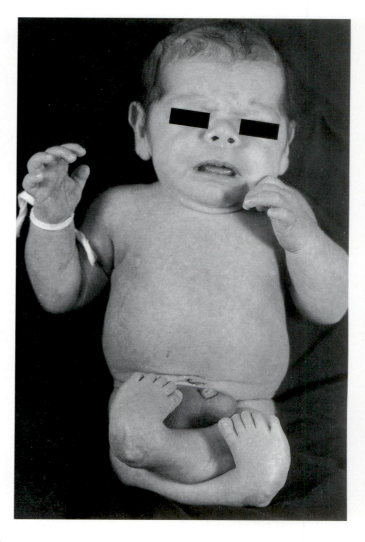

Figure 1

Spasticity of the peroneus tertius leading to calcaneovalgus posture of the foot

Figure 2

Child with myelomeningocele plus gross arthrogrypotic type talipes equinovarus deformity. In addition the knees are fixed in extension and there is gross fixed flexion deformity of the hips

1. Correct the muscle imbalance causing the deformity. This is generally done by release but occasionally by lengthening. Muscle transfer commonly fails by producing over-correction and we now do few tendon transfers other than tibialis anterior to the heel in the calcaneus foot. A flail foot after tendon release which can easily be braced is better functionally than a foot with persisting muscle imbalance and recurrent deformity or overcorrection.
2. Correct the deformity by operative means. Splintage cannot correct deformity in these circumstances and our aim is to perform operative correction to reduce the length of time orthoses are used. Under 10 years of age we generally use soft tissue release or lengthening and, over 10 years of age, bony correction.
3. Treatment should not be delayed unnecessarily. It can be started in the first year of life when convenient,

the child is thriving and coordinated with treatment of other systems.
4. A fixed varus deformity will inevitably create problems. A complete correction by surgery is necessary as a partial correction will always require further surgery in the future. A valgus deformity is better tolerated and surgery can be delayed until appropriate.

Types of deformity

Foot deformity is common in myelomeningocele. In our patients with high level myelomeningocele (thoracic, L1, L2 and L3) we found significant foot deformity in 220 (89%) of 248 feet, and in those with foot deformity, 78%

Table 1 Foot deformities in 248 feet of children with high level myelomeningocele

No deformity	28
Equinus	70
Equinovarus	47
Equinovalgus	9
Calcaneovalgus	46
Calcaneus	18
Calcaneovarus	6
Valgus	16
Varus	3
Paralytic convex pes valgus	5

required surgery to correct the deformity (Table 1). Spasticity of muscles controlling the foot was detected in 36 (51%) of the 70 calcaneus feet and in 22 (17%) of the 126 equinus feet.

The deformities were symmetrical in 94 children. In six children asymmetrical spasticity of muscles accounted for the asymmetry, but in 24 children there was no obvious explanation to account for the asymmetry (Broughton et al 1994).

Even in patients who have no voluntary muscle activity below the knee, there is a high incidence of foot deformity. Spasticity accounts for some of these deformities and, although habitually assumed posture may account for others, there are a significant number of children with asymmetrical foot deformities which do not appear to be due to muscle imbalance or habitually assumed posture. In fact, in many of these children we were unable to identify an aetiological cause for the deformity.

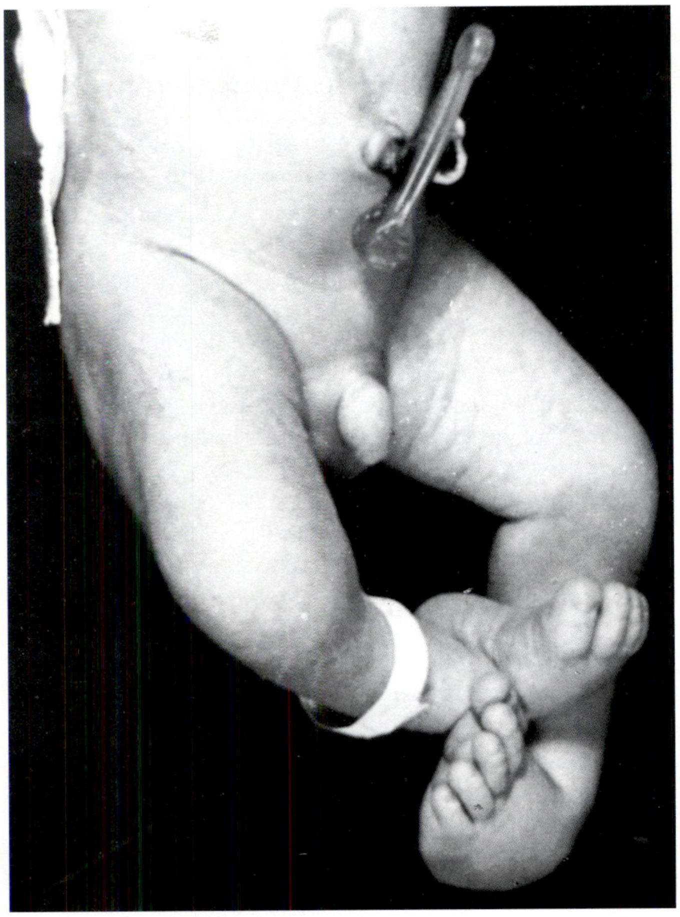

Figure 3

Child with myelomeningocele and bilateral talipes equinovarus deformity; these feet have a similar degree of deformity to that seen in uncomplicated club feet and lack the extreme rigidity of the arthrogrypotic type deformities (illustrated in Fig. 2)

Equinovarus

Equinovarus deformity usually presents at birth. It can often be a severe stiff deformity similar to that seen in arthrogryposis (see Fig. 2). It should always be treated, as a fixed varus deformity is the most troublesome deformity of the foot giving rise to a small area of weight-bearing and eventual ulceration over the base of the fifth metatarsal (Fig. 3). Conservative treatment is ineffective, and surgery is necessary in virtually all patients. Surgery should be extensive as recurrence is common and overcorrection is unlikely.

In the neonatal period, treatment is started with the application of well-padded above-knee plaster casts to correct deformity. These are changed frequently while the baby is still hospitalized, and later at 2–4 weekly intervals as circumstances allow. The rationale for cast treatment is to stretch the skin over the defect so that later surgery is easier; the deformity is unlikely to resolve without surgery.

The Achilles tendon is always short although it may not be obvious at birth, and a closed tenotomy should be performed when convenient between 3 and 6 months. This can usually be done without anaesthetic as the overlying skin is insensate. Between the age of 6 months and a year when the child is thriving, a postero-medial release is performed. Both sides are done at one operation if the deformity is bilateral.

We use a Cincinnati incision for good exposure of all posterior and medial structures (Crawford et al 1982). Because the rate of recurrence is high, excision of a section of the Achilles tendon, tibialis posterior, flexor hallucis longus and flexor digitorum longus is performed rather than lengthening. A posterior ankle release and a full subtalar release, including division of the interosseous ligaments, is performed. Overcorrection is rare, so division of both layers of the medial (deltoid) ligament is performed. By following down tibialis posterior, the navicular is identified and a full talonavicular release is performed. If necessary a calcaneocuboid release is performed from the medial side.

When a full reduction can be achieved, a K wire is passed through the talus to hold the talonavicular joint in the reduced position. The wire is left prominent between the 1st and 2nd metatarsals. The wound is then closed and a firm backslab applied to hold the foot in a corrected position without putting undue tension on the wound. If the skin seems stretched, then a less than perfect position is accepted at this point.

After two weeks, under anaesthetic the backslab is removed, the wound inspected and the K wire removed. At this point, a full correction can usually be obtained without any danger to the skin edges. An above-knee plaster cast is maintained until 12 weeks after the operation. An AFO can be fitted at this stage but we try to avoid the use of resting splints to maintain correction. Although the risk of recurrence is high, the use of AFOs does not seem to influence this.

Using the technique as outlined above, we have always been able to obtain adequate correction with the Cincinnati approach but we recognize its limitations in posterior exposure and necrosis of the skin edges if too much tension is applied to the skin repair. For gross equinus, we would consider the use of a posterolateral and medial two-incision approach as described by Carroll (1988). Walker (1971) has described an interesting flap technique to bring some of the redundant skin on the lateral side of the foot across the dorsum of the foot in order to offload the medial skin repair, but we have not had to use this.

If the deformity recurs, repeat posteromedial releases are performed and these can be combined with lateral column shortening if there is significant adduction. The lateral column shortening can be altered according to where the maximum deformity seems to be, using a calcaneocuboid joint excision and fusion or decancellation of the cuboid or distal calcaneum.

If the deformity recurs despite these measures and the demands on the foot are such that trophic ulceration is likely, then further surgery may be necessary. In the past, we have used talectomy but now find that, although this corrects the deformity well, it leaves the malleoli close to the weight bearing area and there are problems with orthotic fitting (Menelaus 1971). We now use variations on the Verebelyi–Ogston procedure with decancellation of the talus and cuboid to allow collapse of these bones and correction of the deformity.

There is no place for tendon transfers in the equinovarus foot. We have tried transferring tibialis anterior laterally in nine feet, but the results were unsatisfactory as they tended to overcorrect to calcaneocavus feet. Five tibialis posterior transfers to the dorsum of the foot have been performed in this institution in these circumstances, but the transfers were all weak or non-functioning and the results were unsatisfactory (Williams 1976).

We have also tried supramalleolar osteotomies for varus deformities but find the deformity invariably recurs,

so we no longer use this technique in these circumstances.

If deformity is still present at maturity, we have found triple arthrodesis to be a useful operation (Olney & Menelaus 1988). This is performed as an excisional wedge procedure from the lateral side and as long as the excision has been accurate and there is good bony apposition we use a plaster cast to maintain the correction. When the swelling has reduced, a firm well fitting plaster is applied and weightbearing allowed after six weeks. We prefer not to use staples in these circumstances.

In nine triple arthrodeses for varus deformity, followed for an average of 10 years, three had developed painful pseudarthroses of the talonavicular joint, two of which responded well to revision. In general, these adolescents had no deterioration of walking ability, less trouble with trophic ulcers and shoe fitting and less use of AFOs and calipers. Although others have reported rapid degeneration with Charcot-like changes at the ankle after triple arthrodesis (Duncan & Lovell 1978), this has not been our experience.

In some children with recurrent deformity who are too young or in whom a triple arthrodesis seems inappropriate, a calcaneal osteotomy could be used for a varus foot with or without cavus. This is done in the style of Dwyer, but we use a lateral approach and a combination of excisional wedge and a lateral slide to obtain a correction, then a temporary K wire to maintain the correction. This has reduced our incidence of problems of wound healing when the medial approach was used.

For pure adductus deformity, a medial release and lateral column shortening in the style of Dillwyn Evans or basal metatarsal osteotomies can be used. However, we have not had to use the calcaneal osteotomy, the Dillwyn Evans or the basal metatarsal osteotomies often in these circumstances.

Equinus

This abnormality is less troublesome than an equinovarus deformity and its treatment can be less vigorous. Although some authors recommend splinting from birth with regular changes, we recognize that surgery is usually necessary and successful and recommend a closed tenotomy of the Achilles tendon at about 3 months. If the deformity develops at a later stage, an open division may have to be combined with a posterior ankle release. The plaster is maintained for 6 weeks, then walking is allowed.

Calcaneus

This is a common deformity in myelomeningocele. It is generally seen in patients with L5 neurosegmental lesions, but also in children with high-level lesions and spasticity of the tibialis anterior (Fig. 4). It is due to unbalanced activity in the ankle extensors. Tibialis anterior overactivity generally produces the deformity, but this is usually accompanied by unbalanced activity in peroneus tertius and sometimes in extensor digitorum communis; rarely there is displacement of the peronei in front of the lateral malleolus as an added factor in the production of calcaneus deformity. Commonly, a foot that is deformed into calcaneus will later, whether or not it is treated, develop associated valgus deformity.

The deformity is invariably progressive and the heel becomes increasingly large and the forefoot narrow and undeveloped. The child has a gait characterized by a calcaneus 'hitch'. If the deformity is ignored it becomes fixed and shoe fitting becomes difficult. By teenage years recurrent trophic ulceration occurs commonly over the prominent heel.

Because the deformity is invariably progressive it demands treatment and only surgical treatment is effective. We find this is best carried out at the age of 4–5 years, but we would operate sooner if there is progressive calcaneus deformity producing symptoms.

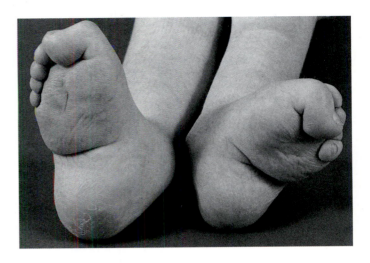

Figure 4

Bilteral calcaneocavus deformity in a patient with myelomeningocele with paralysis below L4

Transfer of tibialis anterior to heel

If the function of tibialis anterior is strong and normal, we perform a transfer of tibialis anterior to the heel. The tendon is divided at its insertion, drawn out through an incision four fingers' breadth above the ankle joint, passed through a window in the interosseous membrane and brought down lateral to the Achilles tendon. It is then passed through a drill hole in the tuberosity of the os calcis and sutured over a button in the sole. The tension is such that the ankle is in 20–30° equinus. Subsidiary fixation is obtained by suturing the tendon to the Achilles tendon. A below knee cast is worn for 6 weeks, then walking is encouraged, usually in an AFO initially (Bliss & Menelaus 1986).

Rarely this operation is followed by progressive equinus deformity such that the tendon transfer requires lengthening. A more common complication is progressive depression of the first metatarsal head owing to unbalanced activity of the peroneus longus. This may require later dorsal wedge excision at the base of the first metatarsal.

If the calcaneus deformity is fixed, the transfer of tibialis anterior is combined with an anterior ankle release. This is performed through a 'lazy S' incision. Extensor tendons and tibialis anterior are divided, and then anterior capsulotomy is performed until the ankle can be placed in a position of 20° of equinus.

Tenodesis of Achilles tendon to fibula

If the function of tibialis anterior is weak or spastic, we perform tenodesis of the Achilles tendon to the fibula with release of tibialis anterior and overactive extensors and an anterior ankle release if the calcaneus deformity is fixed. The Achilles tendon is divided at the musculotendinous junction. A hole is drilled in the fibular metaphysis and

the Achilles tendon passed through this and sutured to itself with the ankle in 20° of equinus. Sometimes the stimulation of growth, brought about by the drilling of the fibular metaphysis, tends to correct valgus at the ankle mortice which may accompany calcaneus deformity.

The foot is immobilized in a cast in 20° of equinus for 6 weeks. In some patients the tenodesis stretches and the patient has to use AFOs and in some the tenodesis contracts with growth and requires lengthening.

If the patient is unlikely to walk we may sometimes do a simple tibialis anterior release with or without an anterior ankle release for fixed calcaneus. However, for those who are likely to be ambulators, even for a short period, we feel they are better served by tenodesis of the Achilles tendon to the fibula, where tibialis anterior is weak or spastic.

If the presentation is late, at the age of 10–14 years, we would not perform a tibialis anterior transfer nor an Achilles tenodesis, but perform an anterior ankle release and tibialis anterior release.

In feet that have a combination of calcaneus and cavus, a calcaneal osteotomy should be considered (see below).

Valgus feet

In general, valgus feet give rise to less trouble than varus feet and can be controlled more easily by orthoses. They give rise to problems because of ulceration over the prominent medial malleolus in adolescence, and are frequently associated with an external rotation deformity of the tibia.

The deformity may be present at the ankle or subtalar joint or a combination of the two. Clinical examination and weight-bearing radiographs can help to differentiate where the deformity is; sometimes a CT scan through the hind foot is useful.

Ankle valgus

Clinically this can be recognized by palpation of the distal tip of the lateral malleolus at a level above the medial malleolus. Dias (1978) has described a relative shortening of the fibula of 1.3 mm per year where the soleus is paralysed. In the normal child up to the age of 5, the distal fibular growth plate is above the talar dome, level with it at the age of 5, after which it becomes progressively lower than the talar dome to be 3 mm lower at maturity. In the child with myelomeningocele, the distal fibular growth plate is commonly seen above the talar dome with an associated wedge-shaped distal tibial epiphysis.

The valgus ankle can be improved by tenodesis of the Achilles tendon to the fibula, which helps prevent the progressive shortening of the distal fibula. This is particularly useful in the calcaneovalgus foot, when a tibialis anterior to heel transfer is performed.

The wedge shaped distal tibial epiphysis can be improved by a medial arrest of the distal tibial epiphysis. To be effective this has to be performed before the child is 6 years. We generally use a small fragment screw through the tip of the medial malleolus passing across the growth plate; this is less bulky than the staple previously employed.

A supramalleolar osteotomy is performed to correct this deformity over the age of 6 years, and preferably not before 10 years (Fig. 5). We perform this 1 cm above the growth plate by excision of a medial-based wedge together with an oblique distal fibular osteotomy. Any rotational deformity can be corrected at the same time and fixation is by staples or two crossed K-wires. We have experienced delayed union and wound breakdown following this procedure. There are also more complex wedge excision techniques described that allow distal medial displacement in an attempt to give the ankle and foot a better shape and weight-bearing axis, but we have not found these to be necessary (Wiltse, 1972).

Subtalar valgus

This can present in the first years of life owing to spastic peroneal muscles (see Fig. 1). Spastic peroneals should be released and the deformity held with an AFO. If the deformity is more severe a subtalar release and tenodesis of the Achilles tendon may be required.

If an orthosis is unable to control the deformity we would perform a bony correction between the ages of 5 and 10. In the past we have performed a Grice extra-articular subtalar fusion using tibial graft to avoid shortening of the fibula. We have also used bank bone in these circumstances to avoid graft site problems. Where

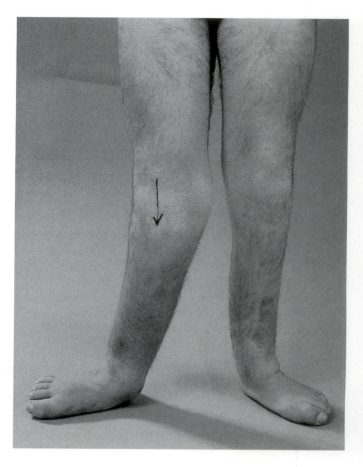

Figure 5

Gross external tibial torsion of the right tibia in a boy with an L5 lesion. Note the associated planoabductovalgus deformity of the right foot. The left foot had previously been similarly deformed and has been subjected to supramalleolar osteotomy

appropriate, we would now use a calcaneal osteotomy in a manner similar to Dwyer. By using a medial approach and excising a medial based wedge, the heel can be shifted medially and held by a Steinmann pin which is removed at 8 weeks. When close to skeletal maturity, we use a lateral inlay triple arthrodesis (Figs. 6, 7 and 8).

A precisely measured rectangle of bone from the borders of the talus, navicular, cuboid and calcaneum is removed. A matching rectangle of bone is harvested from the upper tibia and countersunk into position. The subtalar joint is also roughened with an osteotome and some cancellous bone from the tibia pushed into the joint. The foot is more stable after this procedure than after an excisional triple, and the foot is not shortened (Williams & Menelaus, 1977).

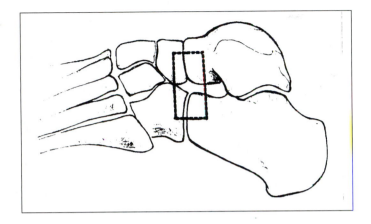

Figure 6

The site of the removal of a rectangle of bone from the junction of the subtalar and mid tarsal joints

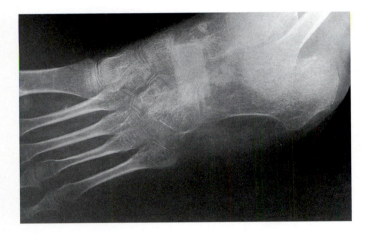

Figure 7

The postoperative radiographic appearance of lateral inlay triple arthrodesis at the time of removal of the cast at 3 months. The rectangle can be clearly seen

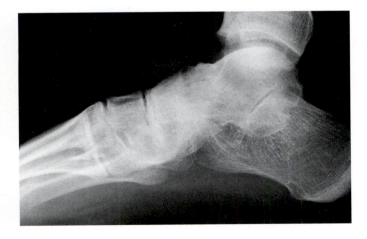

Figure 8

The appearance of the foot at the age of 19 years. Sound arthrodesis is evident

We have found this to be a successful operation with few recurrences and usually there is an improvement in orthotic use and shoewear difficulties. Although Charcot changes in the ankle have been described following this procedure, this has not been our experience. Failure of fusion of the triple arthrodesis has been unusual (Olney & Menelaus, 1988).

Ankle plus subtalar valgus

Each deformity should be addressed separately, as outlined in the above sections. Correction near to maturity would usually consist of a lateral inlay triple arthrodesis with a supramalleolar osteotomy which would normally have a rotational correction for the associated external rotation abnormality of the tibia (Figs. 9, 10, 11 and 12).

An ankle fusion is rarely indicated as failure is common resulting in a Charcot type joint (Fig. 13).

Cavus deformity

Cavus deformity is usually accompanied by heel varus. It is seldom seen under the age of 4 years. A cavus element may appear in feet that were previously equinovarus despite treatment, or it may appear in previously normal feet. Initially the deformity is mobile but it becomes increasingly rigid and fixed with age.

A soft-tissue plantar release is appropriate in the first 5 years of life for those feet without significant bony deformity. After the age of 5 it is usually necessary to combine this with bony procedures.

Osteotomy of the base of one or several of the metatarsals is performed when the plantaris element of the forefoot is significant and fixed. The procedure is performed with a plantar release. Longitudinal K-wire fixation is used to prevent the need for pressure from a plaster cast, which carries the risk of trophic ulceration. In late cases, often with calcaneus, a pistol grip deformity of the calcaneus can result in ulceration over the tip of the heel. A calcaneal osteotomy is performed in order to horizontalize the tuberosity. If the osteotomy is curved it may be possible to rotate the tuberosity into a horizontal position. However, more commonly we find it necessary to excise a dorsally based wedge from the tuberosity and any varus or valgus deformity can be corrected at the same time. Again the position is best maintained by the use of a horizontal K-wire. This procedure would generally be combined with plantar release and sometimes with osteotomy of the bases of the metatarsals.

Triple arthrodesis is appropriate in the child close to skeletal maturity who has a degree of deformity that is producing pressure effects.

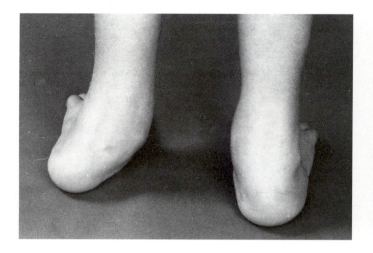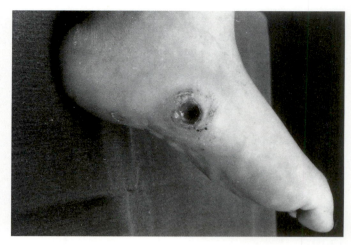

Figures 9 and 10

Gross valgus deformity of the left foot of a 13-year-old girl with an L5 lesion. Note the pressure sore on the medial aspect of the foot

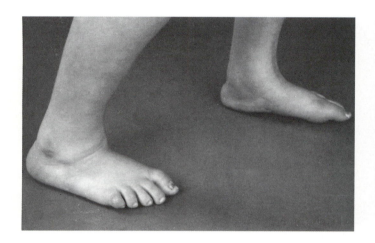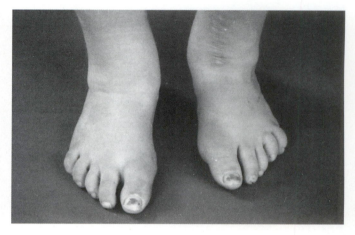

Figures 11 and 12

The postoperative appearance of the feet of the child illustrated in Fig. 5, following lateral inlay triple arthrodesis of the right foot plus supramalleolar osteotomy of the lower tibia to correct external tibial torsion plus ankle valgus

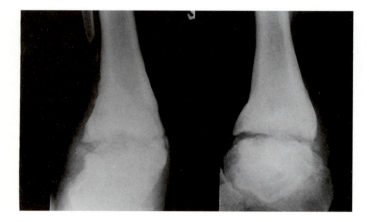

Figure 13

Failure of attempted arthrodesis of the ankle in spina bifida. There has been successful subtalar fusion

Paralytic convex pes valgus

Although much has been written about paralytic convex pes valgus, it is an unusual deformity with an incidence of about 2%. It is commonly but not always bilateral and it can occur with any neurosegmental level. If it presents at birth, it is similar to the congenital vertical talus, but a less rigid form that develops slowly over the first years of life is also seen.

The talus is plantarflexed and the calcaneum is dorsiflexed and rotated laterally. The navicular with the rest of the foot sits adjacent to the neck of the talus rather than on the distal articular surface of the talus, which is plantarflexed and can be felt at the apex of the convexity of the medial aspect of the foot (Figs. 14 and 15).

If the foot is completely paralysed with no voluntary motor activity, the procedure consists of tenotomy

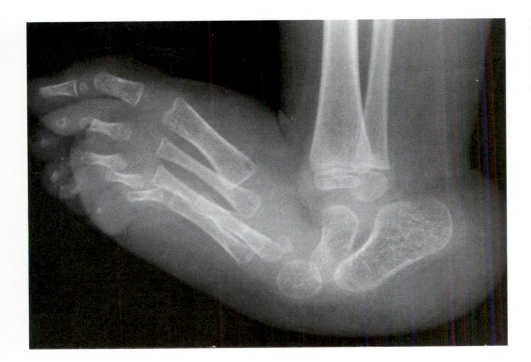

Figure 14

Radiographic appearances in paralytic convex pes valgus (vertical talus) in patient with spina bifida

of all foot motors, a complete subtalar and talonavicular release and temporary fixation with K-wires. This is usually performed in the first year of life. It is achieved by a Cincinnati approach with a lateral extension beyond the calcaneocuboid joint. All the tendons on the dorsum of the foot and the peroneals are released. The Achilles tendon, flexor hallucis longus, flexor digitorum longus and tibialis posterior are all released and a posterior ankle release performed. The subtalar joint is released from the lateral side and completed on the medial side and a talonavicular release is performed so the talus can be reduced on to the navicular. A K-wire is run from the posterior talus to hold the reduced talonavicular joint, and the calcaneum is held reduced under the talus by a further wire run in from the plantar aspect of the calcaneum into the talus.

If the correction is difficult to hold or if the operation is performed late, then a Grice–Green lateral inlay subtalar arthrodesis is added to the above procedure. The wires are removed at 6 weeks and plaster immobilization is used for 3 months postoperatively. A carefully moulded AFO is then used to control planus, heel valgus and the flail ankle.

If there is voluntary activity in the foot, one of two transfers may be performed in addition to the above procedures. The peroneus brevis can be transferred across the back of the ankle into the sheath of tibialis posterior and the navicular directly or onto the tendon of tibialis posterior, together with a transfer of tibialis anterior to the neck of the talus (Duckworth & Smith 1974). Alternatively the single transfer of tibialis anterior to the neck of the talus has been described (Walker & Cheong-Leen 1973).

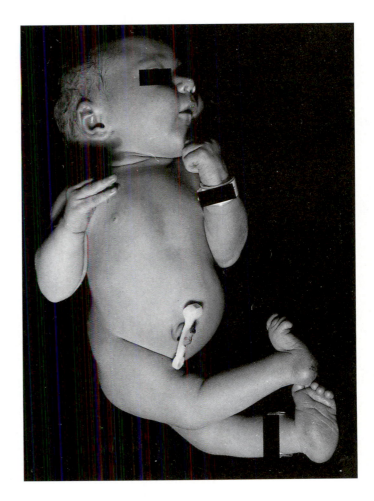

Figure 15

The clinical appearances of the feet of the child in Fig. 14. Note recurvatum deformities of the knees and fixed flexion deformities of both hips

Toe deformity in spina bifida patients

Historically, the toe deformity that has been long associated with myelomeningocele is syndactylism (Fuchs 1909, quoted by De Vries 1928). It was Fuchs who coined the word myelodysplasia, and he mentions syndactylism of the second and third toes as one of the features of the condition. In fact, we have only twice noted syndactylism of the toes in 359 feet of children with spina bifida.

The commonest toe deformities are:

1. hallux malleus with or without a pronation deformity of the hallux;
2. claw hallux; and
3. clawing of the lesser toes.

Combinations of the above deformities are commonly seen in patients with all levels of lesions. Parents are generally concerned at the appearance of the toes and fear that problems will arise because of these obvious deformities. In fact it is seldom that the toe deformities (with the exception of hallux malleus with pronation deformity) lead to pressure problems. Toes that are flail may tend to curl up inside the sock when the child is being dressed and the parent may have to straighten out the toes, but this does not lead to pressure problems or other difficulties.

Chilblains are common in the lesser toes whether they are deformed or not.

Hallux malleus with or without a pronation deformity

There is a fixed flexion deformity of the IP joint of the hallux. Frequently the entire hallux is pronated from the MP joint distally such that the medial border of the hallux, the medial border of the IP joint and the pulp adjacent to the medial border of the toe nail become the weight-bearing areas for the toe (Fig. 16). This is particularly liable to happen in patients who have planovalgus feet in association with external tibial torsion. Recurrent trophic ulceration is seen most in L4 and L5 patients who are good walkers but who have anaesthetic toes and the deformity as described.

Trophic ulceration may occur along the medial border of the hallux. There may be ingrowing of the medial aspect of the toe-nail in these circumstances. If there are no specific problems then the deformity is best ignored. If recurrent ingrowing toe-nails occur, this is best treated by wedge resection as for ingrowing toe-nails in other circumstances.

For hallux malleus plus pronation deformity with recurrent trophic ulceration, interphalangeal fusion is appropriate. In addition to correcting the flexion deformity of the IP joint, the surgeon should rotate the IP joint as much as possible in a supination direction and then transfix the opposed bony surfaces with two heavy

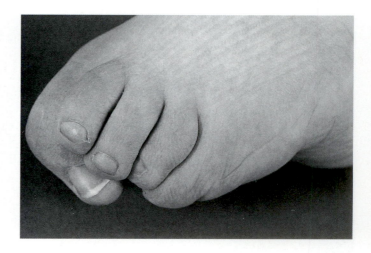

Figure 16

Hallux malleus with pronation of the hallux

K-wires. In general, fusion will occur, but we have had failure of fusion in the spina bifida patient. If the deformity of the IP joint is not gross, but there is gross pronation deformity, then we have performed flexor tenotomy of the long flexor tendon and osteotomy through the proximal phalanx. The osteotomy together with the IP joint are held in the corrected position (e.g. one of supination of the osteotomy and extension of the IP joint) by two longitudinal K-wires.

Claw hallux

Clawing of the hallux (hyperextension of the MP joint with flexion of the IP joint) is less common than hallux malleus, in spina bifida patients. Minor degrees of this deformity do not produce pressure effects and can be ignored. It may be necessary to suggest shoes or boots with a high toe cap. Paralytic clawing of the hallux, if mobile, can sometimes be treated by tenodesis of the flexor hallucis longus (Sharrard & Smith 1976). This procedure is appropriate for children up to the age of about 11 years; over this age interphalangeal joint fusion is appropriate (under this age it is likely to fail).

If flexion of the MP joint allows the IP joint to be fully extended, then tenotomy of the flexor hallucis longus tendon is appropriate. Whilst this would be unacceptable for the nonparalysed patient, this procedure does not lead to significant disability in patients with paralysis below L4 and L5. If flexion of the MP joint has no effect on the IP joint and the problems from pressure warrant surgical management, than interphalangeal fusion is performed in a routine fashion. The Robert Jones tendon transfer has been performed in the past but with the passing years the tendon transfer becomes weaker, and we now merely perform interphalangeal fusion with tenotomy of extensor hallucis longus.

Clawing of the hallux may be associated with the same pronation deformity that is seen with hallux malleus and it requires some supination at the IP joint, together with extension at the IP joint, as the optimum position for fusion.

Clawing of the lesser toes

Again, this deformity is commonly seen and, unless problems are recurring as a result of pressure effects, it is best ignored. In fact it is seldom that there are pressure effects.

If there are problems and if passive correction of the MP joint allows the IP joint to be extended, then open flexor tenotomy of long and short flexor tendons is the procedure of choice. This is done through a plantar incision between the proximal and distal flexor creases of the toes. If there is mild flexion deformity of the PIP joint, the capsule of this joint can be tenotomized through the same incision.

If there is fixed deformity, filleting of the distal half of the proximal phalanx is generally appropriate. Patients with fixed deformity are generally adults. We prefer filleting to IP fusion as it removes the problem of 6 weeks with Kirschner wires in the toe (which may lead to ulceration of the pulp or low-grade infection of the toe in the spina bifida patient).

Under-riding toes may be treated by flexor tenotomy if the deformity is mobile or by filleting of the distal half of the proximal phalanx if the deformity is fixed.

References

Bliss D G, Menelaus M B 1986 The results of transfer of the tibialis anterior to the heel in patients who have a myelomeningocele. J Bone Joint Surg 68B: 1258

Broughton N S, Menelaus M B, Cole W G, Shurtleff D B 1993 The natural history of hip deformity in myelomeningocele. J Bone Joint Surg 75B: 760

Broughton N S, Graham G P, Menelaus M B 1994 The high incidence of foot deformity in high-level spina bifida patients. J Bone Joint Surg 76B: 548

Carroll N 1988 Pathoanatomy and surgical treatment of the resistant club foot. AAOS Instructional Course Lectures 37: 93

Crawford A H, Marxsen J L, Osterfeld D L 1982 The Cincinnati incision: A comprehensive approach for surgical procedures for the foot and ankle in childhood. J Bone Joint Surg 64A: 1355

De Vries E 1928 Spina bifida occulta and myelo-dysplasia with unilateral clubfoot beginning in adult life. Am J Med Sci 175: 365

Dias L S 1978 Ankle valgus in children with myelomeningocele. Dev Med Child Neurol 20: 627

Duckworth T, Smith T W 1974 The treatment of paralytic convex pes valgus. J Bone Joint Surg 56B: 305

Duncan J W, Lovell W W 1978 Hoke triple arthrodesis. J Bone Joint Surg 60A: 795

Fuchs A 1909 Über den klinischen Nachweis kongenitaler Defektbildungen in den unteren Rückenmarksabschnitten ('Myelodysplasie'). Wien Med Wochensch 59: 2141

Lindseth R E 1982 Myelomeningocele. In: Drennan J C (ed) The Child's Foot and Ankle. Raven Press, New York, p. 267

Menelaus M B 1971 Talectomy for equinovarus deformity in arthrogryposis and spina bifida. J Bone Joint Surg 53B: 468

Menelaus M B 1980 The Orthopaedic Management of Spina Bifida Cystica, 2nd edn. Churchill–Livingstone, Edinburgh

Olney B W, Menelaus M B 1988 Triple arthrodesis of the foot in spina bifida patients. J Bone Joint Surg 70B: 234

Schafer M F, Dias L S 1983 Myelomeningocele: orthopaedic treatment. In: Dias L S (ed) The Foot. Williams & Wilkins: Baltimore. p. 179

Sharrard W J W, Smith T W 1976 Tenodesis of flexor hallucis longus for paralytic clawing of the hallux in childhood. J Bone Joint Surg 58B: 224

Tachdjian M O 1990 The neuromuscular system. In: Pediatric Orthopedics 2nd edn. W B Saunders Co., Philadelphia. p. 1795

Walker G 1971 The early management of varus feet in myelomeningocele. J Bone Joint Surg 53B: 462

Walker G, Cheong-Leen P 1973 Surgical management of paralytic vertical talus in myelomeningocoele. Dev Med Child Neurol Supp. 29, 15: 112

Williams P F 1976 Restoration of muscle balance of the foot by transfer of the tibialis posterior. J Bone Joint Surg 58B: 217

Williams P F, Menelaus M B 1977 Triple arthrodesis by inlay grafting: a method suitable for the undeformed or valgus foot. J Bone Joint Surg 59B: 333

Wiltse L L 1972 Valgus deformity of the ankle. J Bone Joint Surg 54A: 595

IV.4 Cerebral Palsy

Kit Song, Charles E Johnston II and John A Herring

Introduction

Definitions

Cerebral palsy is not a specific disease entity, but a descriptive term that encompasses a broad range of clinical symptoms. A recent consensus definition stated that cerebral palsy is an 'umbrella term covering a group of nonprogressive, but often changing, motor impairment syndromes secondary to lesions or anomalies of the brain arising in the early stages of its development' (Mutch 1992). Another commonly used term, static encephalopathy, emphasizes the nonprogressive nature of such disorders. The insult to the brain usually occurs in the neonatal period. Cerebral palsy acquired after the age of 2 years from meningoencephalitis, trauma, or cerebral vascular accident accounts for approximately 10% of all cases (Blasco 1992). The prevalence of cerebral palsy has been estimated at between 1 and 2.5 per 1000 live births. This number has not decreased despite marked improvements in obstetric care and the virtual elimination of kernicterus from Rhesus incompatibility. Increasing survival of low-birth-weight and premature infants has led to increasing numbers of children with diplegia and it is thought that this may account for the consistent number of affected individuals (Kuban 1994). In the USA, the total annual cost to society has been estimated at 5 billion, making cerebral palsy a relatively common and important health problem (Kuban 1994).

It is 150 years since Little described the clinical signs and symptoms of cerebral palsy and attributed it to difficult births. Sir William Osler in 1888 is credited with popularizing the use of the term 'cerebral palsy' and formulating the first classification system based on etiology (Blasco 1992).

The most widely used classification system for cerebral palsy was developed by the American Academy of Cerebral Palsy in the 1950s (Minear 1956). This system is based on physiologic and anatomic descriptions of motor dysfunction. The physiologic classification is dependent on the location of the lesion in the brain. Pyramidal system lesions are generally located in the cerebral cortex or near major motor pathways and result in spasticity. Extra-pyramidal system lesions are often in the brain stem or basal ganglia and lead to dyskinetic (choreoathetoid, dystonic, ballismic) movement disorders. Cerebellar lesions produce an ataxic form of cerebral palsy. Mixed patterns will often occur. The anatomic classification defines what extremities are involved (hemiplegia, diplegia, triplegia, quadriplegia) and may be useful in prognosticating walking ability. Bleck (1987) found that 100% of patients with hemiplegia would ambulate and that 90% of patients with diplegia would eventually become community ambulators.

Although helpful, classification has significant limitations and is difficult to apply with consistency. Blair and Stanley (1985) demonstrated that agreement among trained clinicians was only 55%. This classification also does not address the etiology of the cerebral palsy nor does it provide information about the functional capacity of the individual. Both of these are important considerations in evaluating a patient with motor abnormalities. Cognitive deficits, visual or auditory disturbances, and seizure activity, may accompany cerebral palsy and will have a great impact on the rehabilitative potential of the individual following treatment.

Etiology and pathophysiology

To date, we have a poor understanding of the pathophysiology of cerebral palsy. In the vast majority of cases of cerebral palsy, the cause is unknown (Nelson 1986). Brain asphyxia appears to be the final common pathway resulting in injury, but the antecedent factors leading to the injury remain elusive. Traumatic brain injury, prematurity, and neonatal asphyxia were implicated by Little in his original article as being causative of cerebral palsy. With the increased use of Cesarean section and abandonment of high and mid-forceps deliveries, physical trauma to the brain has become very rare. Although prematurity and low birth weight are risk factors for cerebral palsy, almost 65% of involved children are born at term (Nelson 1986). Experimental neonatal hypoxia models have shown that it is very difficult to create brain injury by hypoxia alone, which suggests that other as yet unknown factors must be present to allow ischemia to produce permanent neuronal injury (Brann 1975). The list of possible factors is very long. Prenatally, viruses, drugs, and other teratogens may make the immature brain susceptible to hypoxia. Genetic syndromes such as familial spastic paraparesis may also be present. Postnatally, prematurity, trauma, infections, kernicterus, and other genetic syndromes may produce cerebral palsy. It is important to be aware of rare progressive neurologic lesions that may masquerade as cerebral palsy so that proper evaluation and treatment may be instituted. For example, tumors, indolent abscesses, hydromyelia, cervical spine instability, Rett's syndrome, and demyelinating disorders must be considered when evaluating a child with motor abnormalities.

The extent and location of neuronal death produces characteristic changes in central nervous system function. Neuronal groups that are most sensitive to hypoxia are in the watershed areas of the cerebral and cerebellar cortex or in the deep nuclei of the brainstem, thalamus, and basal ganglia. Extra-pyramidal and cerebellar lesions will produce dyskinetic or ataxic forms of cerebral palsy in which spasticity will not be a major feature. Experience has shown that surgical intervention in these patients will not give predictable results and should be approached very cautiously. The majority of patients will have pyramidal lesions caused by neuronal death in the cerebral cortex or near the path of the pyramidal tracts. Cortical inhibition to lower, more primitive reflex arcs is lost. This results in an increased sensitivity of muscle spindle units which in turn produces spasticity.

Foot deformities in cerebral palsy are acquired. Tonic reflexes of the foot and ankle normally disappear within the first year of life (Duncan 1960), but in the presence of cerebral palsy they may persist. As muscles repeatedly overact in a spastic manner, they shorten and the joint upon which they act will assume a fixed posture toward the deforming force. Rearrangement of these forces early will result in a return of joints to a more normal position. If deformities remain for many years, especially in the growing child, secondary changes occur in the joint capsules and in the shape of articular surfaces that interfere with realignment. Alterations in skeletal anatomy will then be required to reposition the foot. Even osteotomies or arthrodesis may not prevent progressive deformity in a growing child, however, if the deforming muscle forces are not resolved.

The foot may also become deformed because of stresses from above. An example of this is when hip and knee flexion contractures obligate increased pressure on the metatarsal heads with a resultant dorsiflexion moment on the foot and ankle (Fig. 1). If the triceps sura is spastic, this will cause increased stimulation and equinus contracture. If the muscle is not spastic, it will stretch out and allow excessive dorsiflexion. This posture also forces the foot into external rotation. A valgus stress results at the great toe and may cause a hallux valgus deformity even though no muscle imbalance may exist. Lastly, apparent deformities of the foot may be caused by dynamic or fixed contractures of other joints. An internal foot progression angle due to excessive internal femoral or tibial torsion may mimic varus deformity of the foot and lead to incorrectly applied surgery.

Clinical examination

The evaluation of dynamic and static deformities of the limbs in the patient with cerebral palsy is a process that

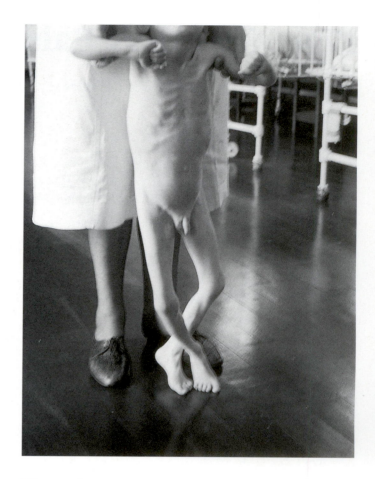

Figure 1a

Crouch gait in which hip and knee flexion cause toe walking. Note that the ankles are plantar flexed, only to the extent necessary to keep the centre of gravity balanced over them. Tendo Achillis lengthening will increase this patient's knee flexion further

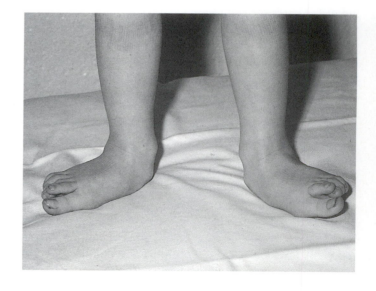

Figure 1b

Pronated, valgus position of feet during quiet standing. The lack of plantar flexion at the ankles is obvious

challenges the clinical interpretative skills of even the most experienced orthopedist. Fear, pain, or excitement can cause mass limb withdrawal responses that will confound an evaluation. Repeated examinations under circumstances where the patient is relaxed, distracted, and unaware of the examiner's scrutiny are essential. Basing a therapeutic decision on a single rapid examination of an irritable child is an invitation to disaster. An uncomfortable child will have excessive tone that will lead to misinterpretation of dynamic imbalances and an overestimation of the magnitude of static contracture.

Motor involvement in cerebral palsy may change over time. It is notable that almost half of all children with cerebral palsy at 1 year of age 'outgrew' or lost motor signs of cerebral palsy by the seventh year (Nelson 1982). On the other hand, one needs to be sure that the patient does have a 'static encephalopathy'. Progressive deterioration of function or spasticity without identifiable risk factors for cerebral palsy should trigger an evaluation by a neurologist and radiographic evaluation of the spine to rule out other causes of the neurological dysfunction.

Initial observation of the patient should be from a distance. In ambulatory patients, posture and gait can be assessed while the child moves freely about the examination room. Inspection should be performed from in front of, behind, and to the side of the patient. Enough room must be present to allow a typical gait pattern for the patient to develop. Lateral trunk posture and an estimation of where ground reaction forces fall in relation to the hip, knee, and ankle axes, will aid in the detection of deformity at those joints (Skinner et al 1985, Wasylenko et al 1983). Position of the forefoot and hind foot during early stance, mid-stance, and swing phase should be noted. Shoe wear and plantar callosities will provide additional information. Finally, balance and the patient's protective reflexes (Bleck 1987), especially posterior and lateral, should be evaluated.

An evaluation of static deformities of the hips, knees, ankle, and feet should be done next. It must be remembered that rapid muscle stretch may trigger mass reflexes. Patience is needed to perform each joint range of motion quickly and slowly to determine if limitation is from muscle spasticity or from fixed contractures. Co-spasticity of the iliopsoas and quadriceps and of the gastrocnemius and soleus has been demonstrated by electromyography (Perry et al 1974, Perry et al 1976). Differentiation of spasticity of these muscles by the Duncan–Ely or Silverskiold test has been shown to be erroneous because of this. Specific tests for muscle strength in the foot are likewise inaccurate, owing to mass firing of agonist and antagonist muscles. Estimations of the degree of voluntary muscle control over specific muscles should be made. Spurious motion in one joint may occur because of compensatory mobility in another. An example of this is the ankle, where dorsiflexion may seem increased because of subtalar eversion if the hindfoot is not held in varus. The rotational profile of the lower extremities should be noted. The combination of femoral anteversion and external tibial torsion may produce a valgus foot. In older patients in whom corrective bony surgery is being considered, these rotational abnormalities may trap the surgeon into misaligning the corrected foot according to the deformity above the ankle (Patterson et al 1950).

Normal gait

Walking is a very complex process. Intricate regulatory mechanisms exist to accomplish the smooth, coordinated movements of normal gait. Interruption of the smooth cascade of motor activity that coordinates muscle activity for gait will result in poor positioning of limb segments with an increase in energy requirements for the individual (Gage 1991).

By convention, gait is described in terms of a gait cycle. A gait cycle begins at the time of foot contact and continues until the same foot strikes the ground again. The gait cycle is divided into stance and swing phases. Stance phase occupies 60% and swing phase 40% of the gait cycle in normal walking. There are two periods of double limb stance when both feet are on the ground at the same time (Fig. 2).

The major functions of the foot and ankle during gait are shock absorption at initial foot contact, providing a stable platform for stance phase, and preserving momentum. Complex motion at the subtalar, midtarsal, and tarsometatarsal joints facilitates these functions. Much of the function of the rest of the lower extremity involves positioning the foot and ankle complex to optimally perform its function. Perry's rocker analysis of the foot and ankle complex in stance is very helpful in understanding the mechanism of these relationships (Perry 1992) (Fig. 3). First rocker begins at the point of heel contact. The initial action of the ankle is to plantarflex with eccentric contraction of the pretibial muscles. Knee flexion increases as increasing load is applied to the foot. These actions dampen the shock of foot contact. Knee flexion contractures, fixed equinus of the ankle, excessive varus or valgus of the foot, or any other process that interferes with pre-positioning of the foot will interfere with these actions.

The second rocker spans the time when the foot is flat on the floor. Advancement of the tibia over the stationary foot occurs here. Eccentric contraction of the triceps sura controls this movement. Knee extension is a passive motion coupled to the ankle by the gastrocnemius. Excessive ankle dorsiflexion or equinus will impede smooth tibial advancement and cause persistent knee flexion or hyperextension.

Third rocker begins at heel rise and ends at toe off. This is the power generation portion of stance. Concentric contraction of the gastrocnemius and soleus lock the ankle in neutral position and provide a stable

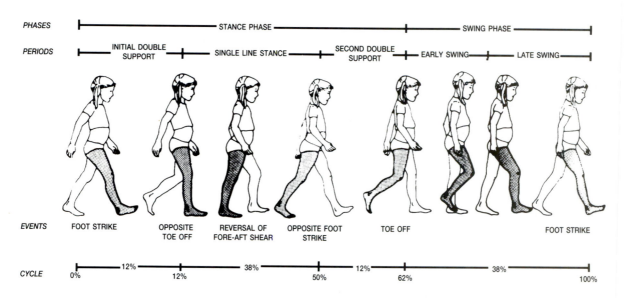

Figure 2

Conventional gait cycle

platform for toe off. Knee flexion is accelerated by the coupling effect of the gastrocnemius. The resultant 'push off' strength may be greatly compromised by an unbalanced foot position or a weak calf.

Normal muscle activity during gait has been studied through dynamic electromyography studies. Fig. 4 lists muscle groups of the calf and foot with their activity during the gait cycle in normal people.

The role of gait analysis

The role of gait analysis in the management of cerebral palsy remains controversial. Observational gait analysis

is known to be much more consistent if done by a single viewer and especially if aided by slow motion videotape (Krebs et al 1985). Expensive modern gait analysis systems now tie together observation by sophisticated infra-red cameras and tracking by elaborate computer software packages. Is the management of the patient with cerebral palsy improved by the addition of this technology? Much has been learned about normal and pathologic gait using these systems (Fig. 5), but to date no prospective outcome study has demonstrated superior clinical results using information generated from gait analysis. A typical modern gait study involves three-dimensional kinematic (joint motion) evaluation,

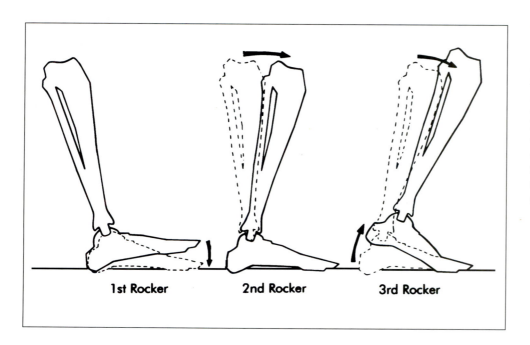

Figure 3

Rocker model of ankle foot motion. In first rocker, contact is made with the heel. The foot plantarflexes with eccentric contraction of the pretibial muscles. In secon rocker, the tibia advances over the foot with eccentric contraction of the triceps surae. In third rocker, the triceps surae concentrically contracts locking the ankle and allowing push-off

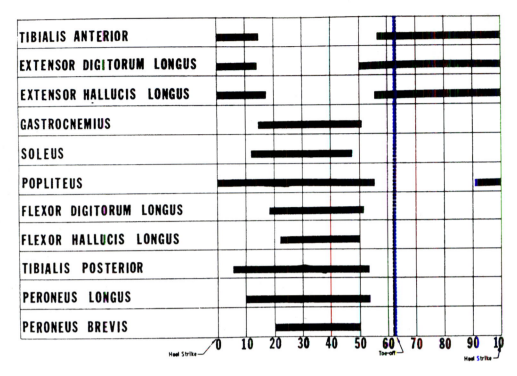

Figure 4

Normative data on muscle activity in the calf and foot during gait

electromyographic (EMG) analysis, and kinetic (joint and ground reaction force) evaluation. Oxygen consumption studies are now also underway in many centers to quantify the metabolic cost of walking and how it is altered by treatment.

The major limitation of gait analysis for the foot and ankle is the inability to accurately model these segments with the computer. Disagreement exists as to the true axis of rotation of the ankle and the many joints of the foot create multiple planes of motion that cannot be accurately traced using the limited number of markers applied to the foot for gait analysis. The equinus ankle with planovalgus foot deformity and apparent dorsiflexion is not well differentiated from true ankle dorsiflexion with some external tibial torsion in gait analysis laboratories. Similarly, hindfoot varus or valgus and forefoot pronation or supination may be difficult to appreciate. On the other hand, gait analysis can provide

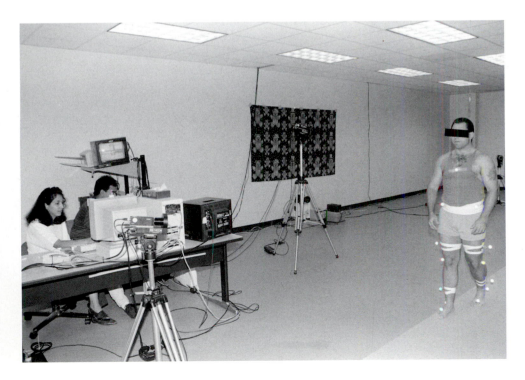

Figure 5

Patient with reflective markers used in modern gait analysis. Note how few markers are used to define the foot

quite a bit of information about deformities of the knee and hip which may affect the ankle and knee. It can also allow observation of multiple planes of motion and of multiple events occurring simultaneously that may escape the unaided eye.

Electromyography information in most labs is generated from surface electrodes which monitor mass activity of a muscle group. For the most part, this information is qualitative and not quantitative. Muscle strength cannot be reliably estimated from the data. Careful selection of lead sites is needed to avoid confusion from simultaneous firing of adjacent muscle groups. Needle EMG benefits from more exact localization of a muscle, but in routine testing has not proven to be more accurate or reliable than surface EMG except for deep muscles such as the posterior tibialis, iliopsoas, and gluteus medius (Kadaba et al 1984, Perry 1992). Electromyographic (EMG) analysis of foot deformities may be useful in cerebral palsy. Much literature has been published about EMG gait analysis of the equinovarus foot to identify muscles that are phasic, spastic, dysphasic, or nonfunctional. This information may be helpful in presurgical planning of tendon transfers or lengthenings.

Joint kinetics as calculated from force plate and kinematic data are becoming increasingly utilized. Distinguishing compensatory mechanisms from true pathologic gait can be done by relating the timing of muscle activity to the ground reaction forces driving limb segments (Gage 1991). Sagittal and coronal planes are best suited for study due to the magnitude of the forces produced by gravity. Transverse plane forces are not yet utilized clinically.

In summary, many limitations still exist for the application of gait analysis to foot deformities in patients with cerebral palsy. It must be remembered that gait analysis is still only a single observation of the patient. Children can have day to day and step to step variability in their walking that may not be realized by study of a single gait cycle. Problems with modeling of the foot and ankle and the relatively small size of these limb segments makes kinematic data suspect at its best. EMG and force plate information have been reported as being useful in preoperative planning. Gait analysis is useful for quantifying deformity preoperatively and changes postoperatively. Newer software systems have begun to explore the possibilities of predicting the effects of tendon lengthenings or osteotomies based on individual patient data and show some promise for the future.

Treatment

Patients with cerebral palsy fall into two large groups, dyskinetic and spastic. Dyskinetic patients will have patterns of involuntary movement and variable tone, which make the results of surgical intervention unpredictable and ill-advised. The majority of patients with cerebral palsy will manifest with spasticity. It is the management of these patients which will be discussed.

Nonoperative therapy

The options for nonoperative treatment of patients with spasticity have grown in number in recent years. In addition to more conventional treatments with physical therapy, casting, and orthotics, medical therapy with botulinum toxin and baclofen have received recent attention. None of these modalities have been shown to have permanent effects or to alter the effects of fixed contractures or deformity.

Physical therapy
The role of physical therapy in cerebral palsy has been hotly debated for years and will undoubtedly remain controversial. A recent consensus conference sponsored by the American Physical Therapy Association concluded that there was not evidence to show the efficacy of physical therapy in the management of cerebral palsy (Campbell 1990). There is only one controlled trial in the literature looking at the effect of physical therapy and it concluded that physical therapy was not effective in advancing motor milestone development in children with spastic diplegia (Palmer et al 1988). In spite of this, physical therapy remains an integral part of many early childhood intervention programs. Although there is no consensus of opinion regarding any aspect of physiotherapy, there is some general agreement that a functional approach tied to realistic goal setting is productive. There is only anecdotal evidence that muscle stretching programs have any benefit. Some authors have advocated a strong role for sports and other recreational activities such as swimming and horseback riding in place of traditional correctional physiotherapy modalities (Bleck 1987). Scrutton & Gilbertson (1975) have summarized their philosophy by recommending exercise to inhibit pathological postural activity and substitute more normal activity. They believe that this intervention should be started by 6–9 months of age in order to be effective.

In our institution, physical therapists play an important role in the screening and motor assessment of involved children. They provide important caregiver education and guidance to environmental adaptations. We believe that programs should be goal-oriented and that goal setting must be realistic. The therapist is frequently in the best position to recommend orthotics or surgery, or a change in direction and goals. Mobility, intellectual development, and self-care often take precedence over prolonged attempts at ambulation.

Casting
Casting has been widely used in the management of cerebral palsy. The two major reasons given for casting

have been to stretch rigid equinus deformities serially in growing children and to suppress the overly sensitive tonic reflexes present in the foot. Duncan (1960) mapped areas of the foot that would elicit specific postural reflexes if cutaneous stimulation were applied. Neurodevelopmental therapists popularized the concept of 'inhibitive' or 'tone reducing' casts during the 1960s and 1970s. Their premise was that inhibition of abnormal patterns of motor activity would facilitate more appropriate patterns of motor function (Bobath 1967). The technique described by Sussman and Cusick (1979) is the one most often utilized. Careful molding of the cast is required. Special attention is paid to providing good heel alignment, correcting any deformity, extending the foot plate beyond the toes, extension of the metatarsophalangeal joints, and reducing contact in the reflexogenic areas of the foot. Casts are changed weekly and weightbearing is encouraged. In the setting of spasticity, flexible deformity, and persistent tonic foot reflexes, it has been felt by several authors (Sussman & Cusick 1979, Mott & Yates 1981, Duncan & Mott 1983, Westin & Dye 1983, Bleck 1987, Donovan & Aronson 1989, Rick & Eilerts 1993) that properly applied short leg casts may decrease the need for surgery, decrease lower and upper extremity tone, and improve function. The period of casting varies from 3–6 weeks with orthotic use for 3–12 months following casting.

Exactly how casting might promote accelerated motor development is not explained by existing studies. Control groups of untreated patients are lacking in these studies and improvements in functional ambulation due simply to neurologic maturation cannot be excluded. Decreases in plantar flexor spasticity have been measured after casting, leading to speculation that elongation of intrafusal muscle sarcomeres reduces the dynamic sensitivity of the stretch reflex (Otis et al 1985).

Serial casting can be useful for the treatment of ankle equinus in the growing child. Dynamic equinus may lead to knee recurvatum and the combination of deformities can impede early standing and walking. Control of the equinus by casting or with an AFO can improve the knee recurvatum (Fig. 6). Increases in ankle dorsiflexion are documented in several studies (Westin & Dye 1983, Watt 1986, Donovan & Aronson 1989), but treatment effects are short lived and may be lost by 5 months (Watt 1986). Casts are applied in the prone position. Two to six casts may be required to achieve the recommended 10° minimum dorsiflexion (Donovan & Aronson 1989). The use of both short and long leg casts has been reported, but we have not found any advantage of long leg casts.

In our institution, we have moved away from the use of casts for 'tone reduction' and have largely replaced them with well molded aquaplast or polypropylene splints. As suggested by Sussman (1983), we believe these are best applied to children who have gained enough truncal balance to attempt standing and who have a significant amount of extensor thrust. Casting may be used while awaiting brace fabrication. We utilize serial casting in ambulatory diplegic and quadriplegic children under the age of 4 with pure equinus to achieve a plantigrade, braceable foot and to delay surgery.

Orthotic management

There is tremendous variability among treatment centers as to the use of orthotics in patients with cerebral palsy. Some centers brace patients quite heavily, while others do not use braces at all. A great deal has been written about the virtues of orthoses, but much of the literature is in the form of case reports and single-subject studies which cannot be generalized to other patients. Very few studies offer any objective information to suggest that orthotics improve walking in cerebral palsied patients. Some improvements in walking velocity, increases in stride length, and decreases in heart rate have been demonstrated (Mossberg et al 1990). Subjective improvements in standing balance and trunk control have also been observed (Rosenthal 1984, Harris & Riffle 1986, Butler et al 1992). Some decreases in the rate of contracture formation have been observed (Bleck 1987), but delays in surgery have only been a year and the deformity at surgery appears to be as severe as in an unbraced extremity. The means by which orthoses may improve gait, posture, or balance is uncertain. Conventional polypropylene orthoses as described by Hoffer (Hoffer et al 1974) work primarily by stabilizing the foot and ankle in good functional positions. 'Tone-reducing' ankle foot orthoses are fabricated using the principles of inhibitive casting with similar effects on balance and trunk control being reported (Rosenthal 1984, Harris & Riffle 1986, Knutson & Clark 1991).

Orthotics do have some disadvantages. They may be expensive, uncomfortable, cosmetically unattractive, or heavy, and therefore should be used only for specific indications. Orthoses may be useful in dealing with flexible, dynamic deformities, but add little to the management of fixed deformity since they do not alter bony alignment during weight bearing (Ricks & Eilert 1993). In fact, the application of orthotics to an extremity with fixed deformity can lead to pressure sores and should be avoided. No evidence exists that orthoses will hasten motor development and it must be remembered that the major impediment to walking will be the problems with motor control and balance that are characteristic of cerebral palsy.

A wide variety of orthoses exist for foot and ankle deformities in cerebral palsy. Metal braces have largely been supplanted by molded polypropylene designs (Fig. 7). Flexible forefoot and hindfoot abnormalities may be addressed by arch supports, heel cups, University of California Biomechanics Laboratory (UCBL) orthosis, or modifications of the above in which posting and wedging may be added. Hindfoot, ankle, and knee deformities can be managed with supramalleolar ankle foot orthoses (SMO), ankle–foot orthoses (AFO), floor reaction ankle–foot orthoses, or knee–ankle–foot

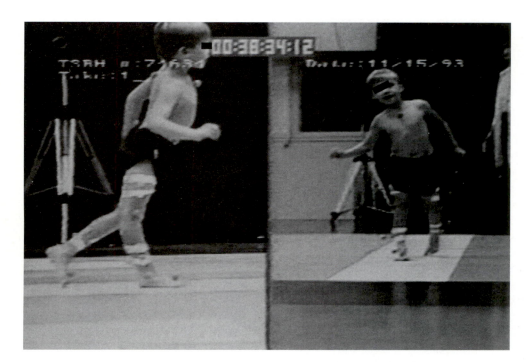

Figure 6a
Diplegic patient with gastrocsoleus spasticity, equinus, and recurvatum at the knee

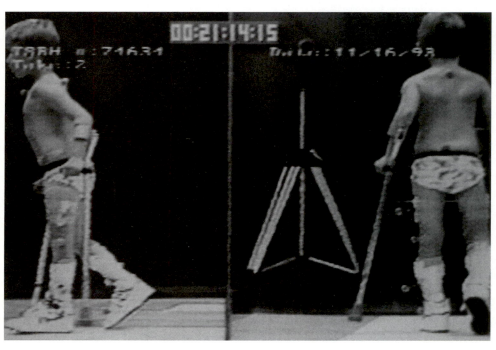

Figure 6b
Improvement in the recurvatum with an AFO

orthoses (KAFO). Higher level bracing was mostly abandoned in the 1960s with the shift to a neurodevelopmental philosophy, but lightweight modern designs may be reviving their use in select situations (Bleck 1987, Knutson & Clark 1991). Many variations are described for each of the basic orthotic designs listed above. A discussion of the relative merits of the various designs and materials is beyond the scope of this text, but the reader should realize that very little evidence exists to favor the use of one orthotic modification over another.

In general, the critical factors for successful application of orthotics to individuals with cerebral palsy are the rationale used in prescribing the orthosis and the skill of the orthotist in the fitting and fabrication of the orthosis. The factors governing selection of a particular orthosis will be highly individualized to the patient. Our own philosophy as to the use of orthotic devices includes the following principles:

1. The prescription of an orthotic should be aimed at accomplishing a specific anatomic goal.
2. The patient should not be hindered.
3. The orthotic should be prescribed for a specific time period at which point the goal should be reassessed.

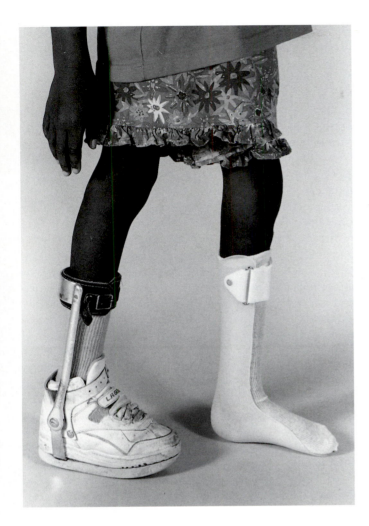

Figure 7

Traditional double metal upright orthosis and polypropylene AFO

In our institution, we use 'tone reducing' AFOs in children with extensor tone who are demonstrating enough truncal balance and control to allow standing. We have seen improvement in dynamic deformities that may facilitate early standing, but we do not believe that an orthosis can make a child without trunk or head control ambulatory. Conventional, molded polypropylene AFOs are utilized in ambulatory children who may have dynamic equinus of the ankle or flexible hindfoot varus or valgus that places the foot in a poor position for weight acceptance and advancement. In heavier children or children with moderate hamstring spasticity and a mild flexion contracture at the knee, we will occasionally use floor reaction AFOs. It is rare that we will use KAFOs in patients with cerebral palsy. Higher level bracing has been reserved for children who are in a postoperative rehabilitation program to provide extra support during the early mobilization phase. Patients are rapidly weaned to lower level bracing.

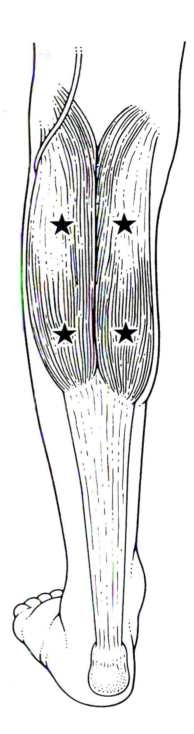

Figure 8

Injection sites for gastrocnemius myoneural blocks

Medical management

Several injectable chemical agents have been reported for the management of spasticity in cerebral palsy. Intramuscular alcohol injections have been utilized by Carpenter (& Mikhail 1972 & Seitz 1980) to aid in the pre-operative assessment of patients with dynamic deformities. He injects a volume of 4 cm³ of 50% ethanol into spastic muscles under local anesthesia and light sedation to reduce muscle spasticity (Fig. 8). The effects last from 5–6 days to 6 weeks and are not known to produce any permanent changes. Carpenter used selective injections of muscles to determine which ones were causing deformity. He also used them to decide whether deformity was from spasticity or fixed contracture in selective cases. Carpenter reported the test to be of no value if there were obvious fixed contractures, athetosis, ataxia, or rigidity and also recommended that it should not be used in patients until they had been under treatment for at least a year. No follow-up detailing exactly how this technique alters treatment has been reported and we presently do not use this technique in our practice. Bleck (1987) has recommended a combination of myoneural blocks and orthosis use for the occasional resistant dynamic equinus.

Botulinum toxin (Botox) has been used in ophthalmology for blepharospasm with good success. Recently, results of its use in cerebral palsy have been reported (Koman 1993). Spasticity is reduced in 12–72 hours after injection and effects last 3–6 months. Few side effects have been noted. This has been proposed as a method by which to delay surgical intervention and to decrease the number of operations needed. At this time, Botox must still be considered investigational in the management of cerebral palsy. We have no personal experience with this drug.

Oral muscle relaxants such as dantrolene, diazepam, and baclofen have been tested in children with cerebral palsy. Side effects such as mental sluggishness have prevented the widespread use of such medications. Furthermore, there has not been any objective evidence to suggest that diazepam truly decreases spasticity. Baclofen has been somewhat effective in spasticity caused by spinal cord injury, but does not seem to be as useful in cerebral spasticity (Bleck 1987, Blackman et al 1992). Intrathecal use of baclofen was first reported in 1985 (Penn 1985) with the reported advantages being higher drug concentrations in the cerebrospinal fluid and more rapid onset of action. Fewer side effects are reported than with oral use (Blackman et al 1992), but meningitis, overdose leading to respiratory depression, and catheter displacement have been reported (Penn 1989). Continuous infusion with implantable pumps is now being attempted (Penn 1992). Improvements in functional outcome have not been demonstrated with any of these agents.

Although many of these agents hold some promise for the future, none can be considered to be a method to be used in the routine management of cerebral palsy at this time. Even commonly used medications such as diazepam have no proven efficacy and should be used cautiously owing to their sedating effects.

Operative management of foot deformities in cerebral palsy

Surgery in patients with cerebral palsy needs to have well-defined goals. A patient can be easily made to look and walk differently, but the critical goal is to improve function. Functional improvements in gait can be made by performing procedures to improve the position of the foot for weight acceptance, allow smooth progression of the tibia over a stable plantigrade foot, stabilize the hindfoot for 'push-off', and facilitate foot clearance during the swing phase of gait. To achieve this, the surgeon must achieve adequate muscle balance about the foot, and correct fixed deformities. The primary modalities available are tendon lengthenings, tendon transfers, osteotomy, and arthrodesis.

Successful surgical intervention in patients with cerebral palsy is dependent on much more than the technical expertise of the surgeon. Patient motivation and intelligence, the degree of spasticity, the presence of dyskinetic (i.e. athetosis, ballismus, dystonic) motor abnormalities, and the presence of deformity at the knee and hip will influence surgical outcomes tremendously and need to be carefully considered in the preoperative evaluation of patients with cerebral palsy. In an effort to avoid what Mercer Rang (1990) called the 'birthday syndrome' of repeated small operations, many centers have adopted an approach of operating on deformity at multiple levels simultaneously. Much of this has come about because of better characterization of the gait abnormalities in cerebral palsy by gait analysis laboratories. This approach has, however, made it crucial that the observer consider the entire patient in the preoperative evaluation. The foot, especially, should never be considered separately from the remainder of the limb.

Selective dorsal rhizotomy

Selective dorsal rhizotomy has been used in the management of spasticity since the late 1800s, but has only recently been enjoying a resurgence. Peacock's series of reports beginning in 1982 (Peacock & Arens 1982) detailed improved gait in children with spastic diplegia and led to increased use of this procedure in the USA. There are few data to describe the specific indications for this procedure and no outcome studies comparing it to traditional soft tissue releases. Stimulation of 50–70 dorsal nerve rootlets is done by EMG from L2–S2, and 25–50% of these are sectioned during the procedure. Weakness is a significant feature for the first 6 months postoperatively and extensive rehabilitation may be necessary. Gait improvements are felt to be secondary to the decreased spasticity and consist primarily of increases in stride length and walking velocity. Casting in the postoperative period has been successful in improving range of motion, but surgery to release contractures may still be necessary in up to 50% of the patients (Dias & Marty 1992, Oppenheim et al 1992). An experienced multidisciplinary team is mandatory to ensure proper patient selection. The procedure is not selective enough to be useful in the treatment of specific lower extremity abnormalities, but it appears to be a useful adjunct in the management of select patients. Reversible chemical rhizotomy through the use of intrathecal baclofen has been undergoing clinical trials for the last 8 years with significant reductions in tone being reported in cerebral palsied patients (Penn & Kroin 1985, Penn et al 1989, Penn 1992, Coffrey et al 1993). Baclofen acts as a gamma-aminobutyric acid agonist and may be administered by either single injection or by continuous infusion from an implantable pump. As with selective dorsal rhizotomy, only generalized changes in tone are produced, and this limits its usefulness in the management of foot and ankle deformities.

Equinus

Etiology and evaluation

The most common problem in the ambulatory child with cerebral palsy is the toe-to-toe gait. Toe walking can cause a significant disruption of the normal mechanisms of gait. There is loss of the heel rocker (1st rocker) which results in a loss of energy absorption as weight is transferred onto the stance leg. The foot rocker (2nd rocker) is also lost, inhibiting progression of the tibia over the stable foot. This may lead to hyperextension of the knee owing to the knee-extension–ankle-planterflexion couple (Simon et al 1978) (Fig. 9). Patients may complain of painful callosities over the metatarsal heads, difficulty with ankle sprains, excessive shoe wear, or calf fatigue and soreness. Persistent equinus of the hindfoot has been postulated as a reason for progressive midfoot valgus deformity and bunion formation (Bleck 1987), but these deformities may also occur in patients who do not have ankle equinus. There has been no conclusive evidence that toe walking is detrimental if limited to childhood.

An equinus foot position alone does not prevent ambulation. The surgeon must resist the temptation to release contractures in an effort to hasten motor development. Children who do not have trunk control or who retain primitive reflexes are unlikely to benefit from a plantigrade foot. Developmental progress instead of chronological age should guide treatment so that the operation will help the child to the next milestone rather than delay it.

Toe walking may be secondary to knee and hip flexion deformities with limited ankle dorsiflexion that forces the child to walk on his toes to keep his center of gravity anterior to the ankles and over the feet (Fig. 10). Toe walking due to hip and knee flexion deformities is best treated by appropriate lengthening of the hamstrings and hip flexors. Use of an ankle foot orthosis alone will not alter the foot position and may, in fact, make walking more difficult by limiting mid and forefoot mobility. Lengthening of the Achilles tendon in this situation will worsen the crouched gait by producing a calcaneus deformity. This pattern will be most common in patients with spastic diplegia, but up to 28% of hemiplegic patients may also have proximal involvement (Winters et al 1987).

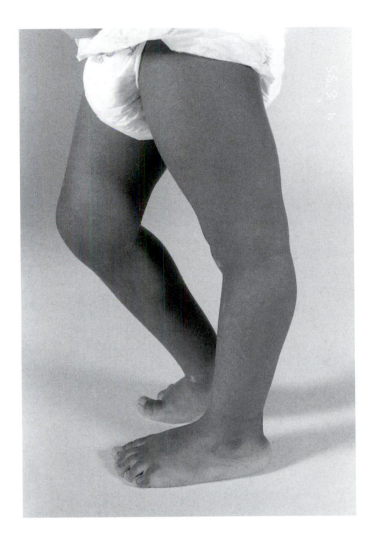

Figure 9

Extensor gait pattern. The ankles are in equinus and the knees hyperextended. Tendo Achillis lengthening is appropriate in this situation

Fixed ankle equinus may also cause toe to toe gait. Ankle equinus is defined as the inability to dorsiflex the ankle above the neutral position. Normal walking requires 10° of ankle dorsiflexion to facilitate foot clearance in swing and tibial advancement over the foot in stance. Dorsiflexion must be measured with the hindfoot locked in varus. Allowing the foot to fall into valgus and pronation may give a false impression of adequate ankle dorsiflexion. It is only in mild cases that surgery is likely to be avoided for equinus deformities. Ziv et al (1984) postulated that the inability of spastic muscles to stretch to their full length led to a failure of growth and contractures. Rang (1990) noted that limb length doubled in the first 4 years of life and doubled again from then until skeletal maturity. These observations may explain the inability of orthoses to prevent contractures and the high rate of recurrence of deformity in children who have surgery at a young age when there is still a large growth potential.

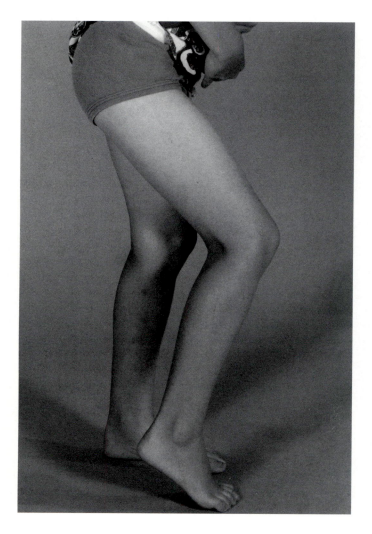

Figure 10

Toe walking secondary to hip and knee flexion deformity. The ankle equinus is modest, but is accentuated by deformity above the ankle

The ability to differentiate the etiology of toe to toe gait is of obvious importance. In the majority of patients, a careful physical examination including observation of gait will allow accurate identification of the problem. Injection of the triceps sura by alcohol has been advocated by both Carpenter & Seitz (1980) and Bleck (1987) as a means of assessing children who have inconsistent walking patterns or where opinions of the treating team may differ. Similarly, botulinum toxin is being used to temporarily induce muscle weakness and reduce spasticity. The duration of effect has been for as long as 6 months (Koman et al 1993). Correlation of the findings after injection to clinical outcome after surgical intervention has not been reported. Equinus may be dynamic, caused by severe spasticity of the gastrocnemius soleus complex (triceps sura), or it may be rigid, caused by true contracture of one or both of these muscles. Studies by

Perry et al (1974) have shown that the triceps sura usually behaves as a unit muscle in spastic conditions. The Silfverskiold test (Silfverskiold 1924) is unable to distinguish between gastrocnemius and soleus activity because there is so much reflex synergy between the two muscles that the contribution of each muscle cannot be isolated. The action of the two muscle units can be distinguished with needle EMGs, but excessive gastrocnemius activity has only been demonstrated in 8% of patients with cerebral palsy, making routine use of EMGs unnecessary (Hoffer & Perry 1983).

Surgical treatment

Many procedures have been used in the treatment of ankle equinus. In general, they fall into one of three categories: recession of the muscle origins, lengthening of the triceps sura, or advancement of the muscle insertion. Silfverskiold (1924) performed an advancement of the gastrocnemius origins that was popular for many years. Recurrence rates of 2.5–16% have been reported if this procedure is used in combination with a partial neurectomy of the nerve to the gastrocnemius (Silver & Simon 1959, Bassett & Baker 1966). Concerns about possible calcaneus deformity, knee recurvatum, and the extensive dissection needed to perform this procedure have limited its use, but Craig & van Vuren (1976) reported excellent results if the procedure was used in combination with an Achilles tendon lengthening. They noted a recurrence rate of only 9% with a 5% rate of calcaneus deformity.

Distal lengthenings of the triceps sura have largely replaced proximal releases, owing to their simplicity. Both open and percutaneous lengthenings using 'Z' lengthenings or sliding techniques have been reported. The simplest Achilles tendon lengthening for the patient is the percutaneous type. Originally reported by White (1943), this may be performed by either a two-cut or a three-cut method. With the two-cut method, a small knife blade is inserted into the center of the tendon just proximal to its insertion onto the calcaneus (Fig. 11). The knife is then rotated to the medial side and pressed against the index finger. With tension on the tendon provided by forced dorsiflexion in the medial half of the tendon, the tendon can be cut without cutting the skin. The knife is removed and inserted again in the center of the tendon just below the insertion of the gastrocnemius muscle belly into the tendon. The knife is turned laterally while maintaining forced dorsiflexion cutting the lateral half of the tendon.

The knee is then extended and the ankle dorsiflexed by a slow, firm pressure. If enough fibers have been cut, the tendon can be felt to give as it lengthens. If the first cut is insufficient, a few more fibers will need to be cut both proximal and distal. These tight strands can be palpated through the skin. The dorsiflexion force should not be excessively applied or the tendon will rupture suddenly, producing too much lengthening.

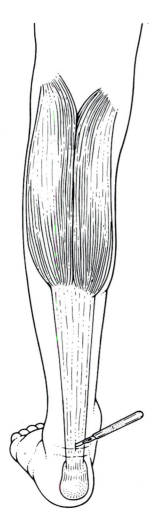

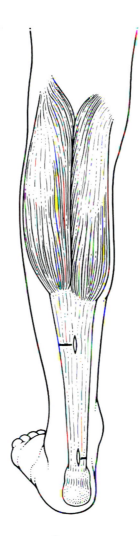

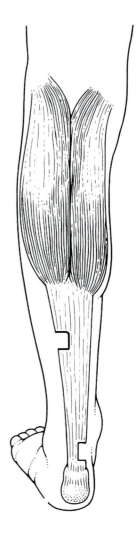

Figure 11a

Technique for percutaneous tendo Achillis lengthening. The surgeon grips the heel between his thumb and index finger and inserts the knife vertically

Figure 11b

The Achilles tendon is hemisected at proximal and distal levels, 2.5 cm apart

Figure 11c

After dorsiflexion of the foot, the tendon elongates through the hemitenotomies. The technique for open two-cut lengthening is identical, except for the skin incision

After the tendon is lengthened, the surgeon should squeeze the calf while offering resistance to dorsiflexion. If the tendon is in continuity, the ankle will plantarflex. If the tendon has ruptured completely at either end, the ankle will not plantarflex and an open repair will be necessary. It may be advisable for the surgeon who is gaining familiarity with the procedure to first perform it open so as to be able to see the anatomy of the tendon better (Fig. 11c).

A three-cut lengthening may also be performed (Fig. 12). The medial half of the tendon is cut just proximal to its insertion and a second medial cut is made at the junction between the gastrocnemius muscle and the tendon. Midway between these two incisions, a lateral hemisection is made. As in the two-step cut, the knee is extended and the ankle dorsiflexed. With the three-step cut, the tendon gives or lengthens more gradually and a distinct slide is often not palpable.

When an open Achilles tendon lengthening is indicated, we prefer sliding lengthenings to a 'Z' type (Fig. 13) because there is less scarring within the tendon. The incisions should be well medial to the tendon in order to leave a buffer of subcutaneous tissue between the incision and the tendon. Using the Hoke method, three cuts are made in the tendon. First, the medial half of the tendon is cut just proximal to the insertion of the tendon. A second medial cut is made just distal to the insertion of the gastrocnemius muscle into the tendon. A third cut is made through the lateral half of the tendon, midway between the first two cuts (see Fig. 12). The knee is then extended and the ankle dorsiflexed until the tendon slides into a lengthened position.

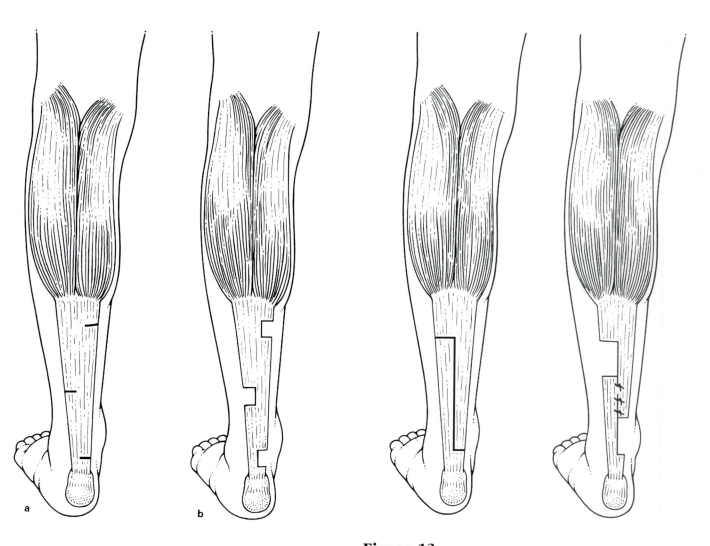

Figure 12a

Three-cut percutaneous (or
open) lengthening

Figure 12b

The tenotomy sites gap open
after dorsiflexion of the ankle

Figure 13

Technique for open 'Z' lengthening of Achilles tendon

The tendon may also be lengthened by a two-cut
method (see Fig. 13). With this technique, the medial
half of the tendon is cut distally as in the Hoke lengthening. The proximal cut is made distal to the myotendinous junction and the posterolateral half of the tendon
is cut. This oblique cut is necessary to allow for the
rotation of the tendon fibers. Again the knee is extended
and the ankle dorsiflexed to neutral. The tendon fibers
will separate as the tendon lengthens. It is not necessary
to suture the tendon. Postoperatively a short-leg plaster
is applied and the patient allowed full weight bearing.
A knee immobilizer is usually necessary for the next few
days to prevent a flexed knee posture, but it may be
discarded after that. The child is allowed regular
footwear after 6 weeks.

The 'Z' lengthening is useful when an exactly
controlled lengthening is desirable, or when the tendon
has been previously lengthened. A 'Z' cut is made in the
tendon such that after lengthening there will be at least

a 3 cm overlap of the tendon. The tendon is repaired
with nonabsorbable sutures (see Fig. 13). The amount of
tension after this type of lengthening is critical to avoid
a calcaneus gait. We usually make this judgment by
pulling the proximal stump distalward with moderate
tension and simultaneously placing the ankle at neutral
dorsiflexion. The tendon is sutured with the amount of
overlap present in this position. If there is severe spasticity and clonus, the ankle is dorsiflexed 5° before suturing the tendon.

There are a number of procedures that have in
common a selective lengthening of the gastrocnemius as
it inserts into the Achilles complex. Strayer (1958)
described a transverse cut in the gastrocnemius fascia
leaving the soleus intact. In the Baker type of lengthening (Baker 1956), an inverted U incision is made through
the gastrocnemius aponeuroses so that the lateral and
medial portions of the muscle remain intact (Fig. 14).
The central tongue is dissected free from the soleus. This

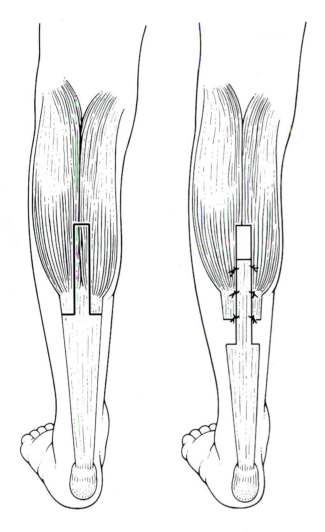

Figure 14

A Baker-type lengthening through the gastrocnemius fascia

tongue should be completely freed from the underlying muscle fibers. The knee is then extended and the ankle dorsiflexed beyond neutral, causing the two segments of the muscle complex to slide apart. A suture is placed at each of the four corners created and the incision is closed. For more dorsiflexion, the surgeon can section the median raphe of the soleus.

Recurrence of equinus has been reported in 9–17% (Sharrard & Bernstein 1972, Lee & Bleck 1980, Graham & Fixsen 1988) and calcaneus deformities in 1–30% (Sharrard & Bernstein 1972, Segal et al 1989) of patients undergoing slide lengthenings of the Achilles tendon. Recurrence rates have been noted to be higher in children who were less than 6 years old at the time of surgery (Lee & Bleck 1980) and in children who did not have preoperative voluntary ankle dorsiflexion (Grant et al 1985). Authors reporting on gastrocnemius lengthenings have noted recurrence rates of 4–48% (Bassett & Baker 1966, Lee & Bleck 1980, Banks 1983, Olney et al 1988), but no calca-

neus deformity in long term follow-up. Patients less than 5 years old and patients with hemiplegia were at highest risk of recurrence of equinus. Because only 8% of patients with cerebral palsy will demonstrate more gastrocnemius than soleus activity, we believe that clinicians without access to dynamic EMGs should probably perform a Z-plasty type lengthening in the majority of these deformities. Perry et al (1974) and Hoffer & Perry (1983) have recommended that gastrocnemius lengthenings should be performed in those patients who have onset of only gastrocnemius activity before midstance.

Recently, attention has been focused on the potential loss of push-off strength resulting from Achilles tendon lengthening. Decreases in functional 'push off' power have been noted in 70% of patients undergoing conventional Z-plasty lengthening versus 50% of patients undergoing Baker type lengthenings (DeLuca et al 1988). Garbarino & Clancy (1985) reported excellent results with Z-plasty lengthenings using a geometric method preoperatively to calculate the amount of lengthening needed. While mathematically simple, this method has been clinically difficult to apply and has not offered a significant advantage to us. Rose et al (1993) demonstrated maintenance of push-off strength, more appropriate timing of energy generation, and improved dynamic range of motion following modified Baker type lengthenings in combination with other lower extremity procedures. Their patients had an average of 4° of ankle dorsiflexion with an extended knee and 10° of dorsiflexion with a flexed knee preoperatively. To our knowledge, no direct comparison of Z-plasty lengthenings to gastrocnemius lengthenings has ever been performed. Future gait laboratory studies will probably help to define more precisely which patient populations may benefit from gastrocnemius lengthening versus more conventional triceps sura lengthenings.

Another method which has been advocated is heel cord advancement. First described by Pierrot & Murphy (1974), good clinical results with no calcaneus deformity were reported by Throop et al (1975) and by Strecker et al (1990). We have no practical experience with this method.

Pes valgus

Etiology and evaluation

A valgus deformity is seen in 20–25% of all cerebral palsy patients and occurs most commonly in spastic diplegia and quadriplegia (Ruda & Frost 1971, Bennett et al 1982). The deformity probably results from several pathological mechanisms working together. Considerable controversy exists in the literature as to which are more important.

The deformity consists of eversion and equinus of the calcaneus with forefoot abduction and pronation (Fig. 15). The talus is plantar flexed owing to loss of support for the head of the talus by the sustentaculum tali and

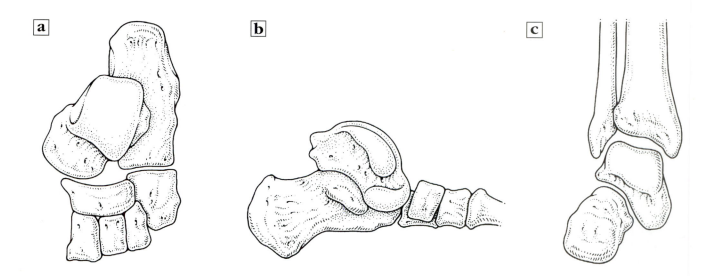

Figure 15

Components of the equinovalgus deformity. The head of the talus is uncovered medially (a,c), and the talus is rotated into a more vertical position due to loss of support of the neck of the talus by sustentaculum tali (b,c). The characteristic 'sag' through the midfoot produces prominence of the talar head in the sole of the foot medially (c), and loss of ankle height

plantar calcaneonavicular ligament, both of which move laterally with the eversion of the anterior end of the calcaneus and the abduction of the navicular. As the forefoot pronates and abducts, the navicular moves laterally. This uncovers the head of the talus, which is then prominent on the medial side of the foot. The deformity is flexible initially, with normal relationships restored by inverting the hindfoot and adducting the forefoot. The degree of concomitant contracture contributing to the deformity is assessed by attempting dorsiflexion with the foot inverted. The examiner will note that unless the forefoot is 'locked' in varus as the hindfoot is dorsiflexed, the entire foot will evert through the subtalar joint, taking the path of least resistance when encountering equinus contracture. The examiner must also beware of a variation on the usual valgus deformity, described by Duckworth (1983), where the forefoot is fixed in relative supination to the hindfoot and does not demonstrate normal flexibility in the midtarsal joints. Passive correction of hindfoot valgus leaves the forefoot fixed in supination. This rare variation, thought to be due to a transverse ('horizontal') deformity of the talus, must be recognized before hindfoot correction is performed or else the forefoot will remain supinated, almost appearing to stand on its lateral rays (Duckworth 1983).

The majority of patients with pes valgus will have a tight Achilles tendon, which makes it attractive to assign to this the role of primary etiologic deformity. Unfortunately, the tight Achilles tendon is not the sole factor, because pes valgus can persist or recur after an adequate Achilles tendon lengthening (Bleck 1987). Furthermore, the 'bow string' theory (Tachdjian 1972,

Bennett et al 1982), where the hindfoot is forced into valgus (the path of least resistance) as the shortest distance to get the heel on the floor after toe-strike in the presence of Achillis tendon contracture, does not account for the observation that patients who have never borne weight (e.g. with severe total body involvement) may have severe equinovalgus feet (Bennett et al 1982).

Lastly, varus deformity associated with equinus contracture is commonly observed in patients with hemiparesis, who are almost invariably good ambulators (Bennett et al 1982, Bleck 1987). Hence, while definitely contributory, Achilles tendon contracture cannot be the sole or primary deformity leading to pes valgus, and the 'bowstring' theory which relies on weight bearing to produce the deformity does not account for the foot deformities associated with equinus in nonambulators and hemiparetics.

Some investigators have implicated peroneal spasticity as contributing to the problem (Tachdjian 1972, Skinner & Lesater 1985, Bleck 1987). Certainly forefoot abduction could be explained by its existence. In addition, Bleck (1987) has analyzed the action of spastic peroneal muscles on the subtalar joint, reasoning that they change the axis of rotation to a more horizontal alignment than the usual obliquity in the sagittal plane. This horizontal alignment would then allow greater eversion of the calcaneus, and block inversion to some extent. It would therefore seem logical, if peroneal spasticity is present, that early lengthening might eliminate or delay the development of a horizontally aligned subtalar joint and forefoot abduction that is induced by a lateral subluxation of the talonavicular joint.

Electromyographic studies of cerebral palsied valgus feet have not shed much light on the etiology of the deformity. Perry & Hoffer (1977) found two patterns of peroneal activity – one in which both peroneus longus and brevis were essentially phasic, and the second where one or both muscles were active continuously (spastic) throughout the gait cycle. Bennett et al (1982) discovered a nonfunctioning tibialis posterior in five of six diplegic patients with pes equinovalgus; conversely, all six hemiplegic patients with pes equinovarus had continuous (spastic) activity of the tibialis posterior muscle. Peroneal function was variable, being both phasic or continuous in both deformities. Barto et al (1984) also found peroneal overactivity in patients with spastic equinovarus, with its significance being uncertain. Skinner & Lester (1985) described three patterns of activity in hindfoot valgus deformities. Hyperactive peroneals with a strong posterior tibial muscle; hyperactive peroneals with a weak posterior tibial; and hyperactive extensor digitorum longus muscles. Thus, the determining factor producing valgus may be a relatively diminished function of the tibialis posterior. Valgus deformity after tibialis posterior tenotomy has been noted previously in cerebral palsy (Bleck 1987) and in normal feet (Tachdjian 1972, D Evans 1975) and in polio where the tibialis posterior was weak. Hence it is not surprising that a nonfunctioning tibialis posterior has been uncovered in equinovalgus feet. Similarly, peroneus brevis transfer to the tibialis posterior has been recommended as a possible solution, especially if the peroneal is phasic (Perry & Hoffer 1977, Bennett et al 1982).

Two other factors producing pes valgus or equinovalgus should be mentioned. Bleck (1987) has drawn attention to persistent fetal medial rotation of the talar neck as the source of the occasional intoeing seen after subtalar arthrodesis, where the heel appears to be satisfactorily aligned. When this deformity is present, alignment of the forefoot to the hindfoot by talonavicular reduction produces a medially rotated foot. Standing radiographs of the ankle for determination of the talar neck angle (in addition to any obliquity of the talar dome itself) are the most assured method of uncovering this deformity preoperatively.

Finally, the rotational and angular alignment of the remainder of the extremity above the ankle must be considered in the etiology of pes valgus. The patient with an adducted, internally rotated thigh and knee flexion contracture during stance phase must apply a valgus, pronating force to the forefoot and midfoot (see Fig. 1b). Very often, there is a compensatory external tibial torsion. The high incidence of pes valgus in diplegic patients may be partly due to the fact that they more frequently demonstrate these thigh, knee, and tibial deformities. The foot deforms in part because of the position dictated by the deformities in the limb above it. Of course, correction of the hip and knee deformities above does not assure a normal plantigrade foot, any more than Achillis tendon lengthening alone does.

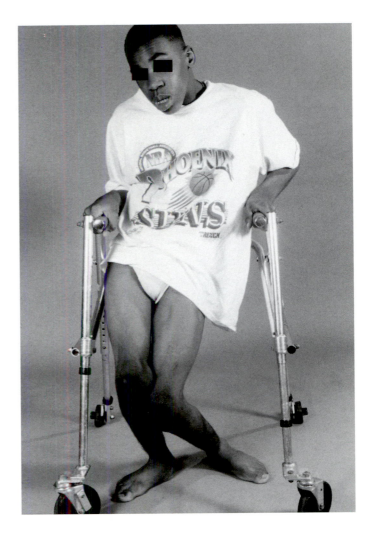

Figure 16

Increasing crouch in a child after isolated Achilles tendon lengthening. Note adducted internally rotated thigh, knee flexion deformity, and external tibial torsion leading to planovalgus foot deformity

However, correction of pes equinovalgus in isolation will frequently lead to a deterioration in gait due to loss of whatever compensation for hip and particularly knee deformities the equinus was providing (Perry et al 1974, 1975, Bleck 1987). The result – increasing crouch gait and the appearance of calcaneovalgus feet (so-called 'over-lengthened' Achilles tendon) – is frequently more debilitating and energy consuming than the original untreated deformities (Fig. 16). Calcaneus deformity induces mandatory knee flexion during stance and increased energy demand on a quadriceps mechanism already compromised by chronic antagonism from spastic hamstrings (Perry et al 1975). Hence isolated treatment of pes equinovalgus without regard to the hip, and especially the knee above, is unwise.

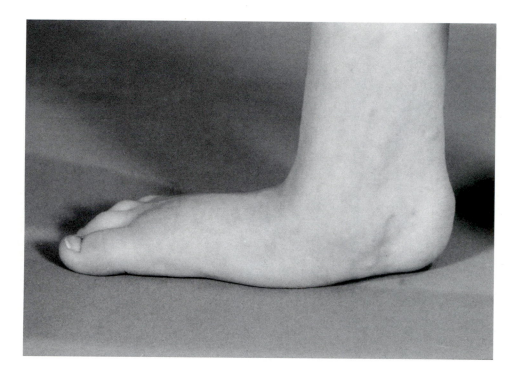

Figure 17

Pes valgus with prominence of the talar head, loss of ankle height, and prominence of the medial malleolus

Treatment

The child under 4 years of age with pes valgus can be managed without surgery in many cases. The deformity at this time is generally flexible and is often associated with an equinus ankle due to contracture of the gastrocnemius and soleus. Attention to the equinus component is usually more important in the younger child. Initially, short leg walking casts, applied with the foot inverted to stretch the Achilles tendon to neutral dorsiflexion, will control the valgus deformity. To maintain control of the foot, a rigid plastic ankle–foot orthosis (AFO) with a high lateral edge to control heel valgus and forefoot abduction may be used. The AFO coupled with a judicious Achilles tendon lengthening as necessary to allow the heel to be contained deeply within orthosis is frequently the only treatment required for pes valgus. A supple foot without a contracture of the Achilles tendon may not require any treatment. Orthotics, special shoes, inserts, and manipulation or stretching programs have not been shown to prevent pes valgus. They have also not been effective in the correction of rigid deformities. Surgical correction is reserved for progressive deformity that is not controlled by orthoses or for a foot that cannot be braced because of severity of deformity. The former rarely occurs before age 6 or 7, while the latter should only be seen in a neglected case in an older child or adolescent. While exact surgical indications are not well defined, surgical correction is appropriate for feet with a painful prominent talar head (Fig. 17), a painful bursa over a medial bunion associated with hallux valgus (Holstein 1980), or a marked loss of height of the ankle

caused by severe heel eversion that exposes a prominent medial malleolus which will not tolerate an orthosis (Bleck 1987).

Soft tissue procedures

Although interest in peroneal tendon transfer or lengthening in valgus deformity has been generated by the use of gait EMG studies (Perry & Hoffer 1977, Barto et al 1984), past use of these procedures has been for the most part unsuccessful, or even contraindicated, owing to the development of reverse deformity. Intramuscular lengthening may be useful in mild valgus deformities (Nather et al 1984), but these deformities generally occur in younger patients with flexible deformities that are best managed by observation or orthoses. Calcaneus deformity can occur when both the peroneal tendons are rerouted anterior to the malleolus (Keats 1974, Samilson & Hoffer 1975, Smith et al 1976, Goldner 1982). Isolated transfer of the peroneus longus without tenodesis of the longus stump to the brevis has been associated with the development of dorsal bunion and varus deformity. In these situations, there is usually a strong tibialis anterior present (Goldner 1981, 1982). Surgery directed towards the peroneal tendons may have an adjunctive role when combined with a subtalar fusion, calcaneal osteotomy, or an Achilles tendon lengthening (Fig. 18), but some authors feel there is no need for muscle balancing after subtalar fusion, and it was rarely needed after calcaneal osteotomy in Silver's series (Silver et al 1974). An electromyographic study demonstrating marked prolongation of peroneal activity would be additional evidence

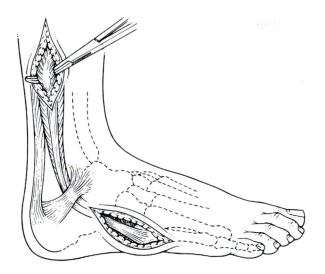

Figure 18

Incisions for peroneal exposure. These two incisions can be combined with lateral subtalar or calcaneal exposure (see Fig. 35). The peroneus brevis exposure for transfer medially is demonstrated

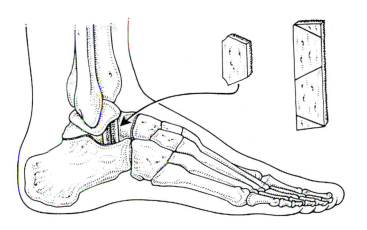

Figure 19

Grice procedure, original technique. The cortical bone grafts prop open the subtalar joint (after Grice 1952)

of the need for peroneal surgery, especially if physical examination documented sufficient strength of the peroneals. Peroneal transfer to aid dorsiflexion must be done with extreme caution, documenting inactivity of other dorsiflexors prior to surgery (Hill et al 1970, Goldner 1981), and never transferring both tendons. Peroneal transfer to the medial side is indicated only when the tibialis posterior is documented to be absent (Perry & Hoffer 1977).

Grice operation and variants
This procedure, initially suggested by William T Green in 1945, and presented in 1950 by Grice to the American Orthopedic Association (Grice 1952), has been widely used as a standard stabilizing operation for paralytic valgus deformity. Initially utilized for polio deformities, its use has been expanded to include valgus deformities in cerebral palsy, myelodysplasia, pes planovalgus, congenital vertical talus, and tarsal coalition (Grice 1959). The basic objective is to correct and stabilize the hindfoot valgus deformity by an extra-articular subtalar arthrodesis, utilizing cortical bone grafts of a sufficient size and strength which, when the sinus tarsi is blocked open by these grafts during manipulative correction of the deformity, will prevent the deformity from recurring by the arthrodesis achieved. As the sinus tarsi is opened, the calcaneal eversion is corrected and the sustentaculum pushed medially to its normal position supporting the talar head and neck (Fig. 19). Subsequent growth of the foot is not impaired because no bone or joint surfaces are excised. Although Grice initially described

the procedure as a temporizing one and assumed a formal triple arthrodesis at skeletal maturity would frequently be necessary, his follow-up report in 1959 indicated that the procedure was often a definitive one.

This procedure has been popular with many authors. A literature review of the major reported series of Grice procedures yields satisfactory results in at least 75% of patients (Baker & Hill 1964, Keats & Kouten 1968, Lahdenranta & Pylkkanen 1972, Banks 1975, Bratberg & Scheer 1977, Nakano & Schmitt 1983, Rosenthal & Candage 1983, Dravaric et al 1989). While criteria for a satisfactory outcome are not always described and frequently vary, Grice's own series (5 to 13 year follow-up) had 79% satisfactory results after the initial procedure, 85% satisfactory results when dislodged grafts and muscle imbalance (secondary to poliomyelitis) were dealt with, and a 94% fusion rate (Grice 1959). In the largest series of cases (286), Tohen et al (1969) reported 77% satisfactory results and 100% fusion rate. The satisfactory rating indicated a foot without varus or persistent excessive valgus, solid fusion and/or no pain, and maintenance of correction over time (Keats & Kouten 1968, Horstmann & Eilert 1977, Goldner 1982). In series consisting mainly or exclusively of patients with cerebral palsy, results have been reported to be satisfactory in 80–90% of patients in several large series (Baker & Hill 1964, Banks 1975, Bratberg & Scheer 1977, Keats & Kouten 1968, Nakano & Schmitt 1983, Dravaric et al 1989).

Unfortunately, problems with the Grice procedure have also been noted with some regularity. As early as 1964, Pollack & Carrell noted a tendency for 'late' varus (later than 6 months postoperatively) when both peroneal tendons had been transferred at the time of subtalar arthrodesis in valgus deformities secondary to

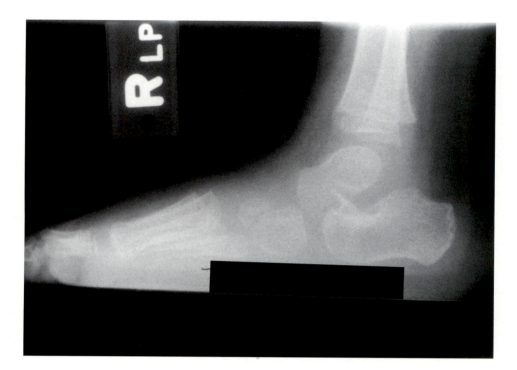

Figure 20

Grice procedure with graft
dislodgement and resorption, with
suspected nonunion of subtalar
arthrodesis

poliomyelitis. They reported an 84% fusion rate, but only 62.5% had satisfactory results, with 27.5% failing because of varus deformity. They reasoned that the transfer of both peroneals was responsible though almost half of those having failures also had pseudarthrosis. Ross and Lyne (1980) have reported the worst results with a 64% failure rate and 28% complication rate. They cite problems with unacceptable ankle valgus, nonunion, and loss of position of the bone graft (Fig. 20). In their critical analysis, half of the feet were uncorrected or made worse by the procedure. Progression of ankle valgus was frequent, and was interpreted as transmitting the hindfoot instability to the ankle. Talar exostoses were noted in 60 of 71 radiographs obtained 10 or more years postoperatively, suggesting that this iatrogenic tarsal coalition produces degenerative changes. They also mentioned degenerative changes in the midtarsal joints and rounding of the edges of the talus ('ball-and-socket' ankle joint). Similar problems have been reported by other authors with nonunion and failure rates of up to 50% (Engstrom et al 1974, Moreland & Westin 1986, Bleck 1987). Smith & Westin (1968) reported only 59% satisfactory results with 8-year follow-up in their series of patients with polio. Twenty-nine per cent failed owing to varus deformity of the forefoot. In this series, there was failure to recognize ankle valgus at the time of surgery, with relative overcorrection of the calcaneus required to place it in line with the axis of the tibia. This positioning meant varus of the calcaneus in relation to the valgus tilt of the talus, a common finding in patients with weak plantar flexion and proximal migration of the fibula (now seen most commonly in myelodysplasia). By

placing the calcaneus in a varus position with respect to the talus, the forefoot was felt to be overcorrected into a relatively fixed supinated position. The overcorrected forefoot was unaffected by tendon transfers. This misalignment may also occur in the valgus-variant foot where the forefoot is supinated relative to the hindfoot preoperatively, and is hence oversupinated when the hindfoot is corrected. Duckworth (1983) observes this deformity, termed the 'horizontal talus', primarily in cerebral palsy and myelodysplasia feet.

Valgus deformity is also a well-documented complication of the Grice operation where a fibular pseudarthrosis develops after graft harvesting (Paluska & Blount 1968, Hsu et al 1972, Wiltse 1972) (Fig. 21). Wedging of the distal tibial epiphysis is frequently observed, suggesting inhibition of the lateral half of the distal tibial physis. This may represent pressure inhibition of the outer half of the physis caused by the shift of the weight bearing axis laterally, according to the Heuter–Volkmann principle. Stabilizing the ankle mortise once the fibular malleolus has drifted cephalad can be very difficult (Johnston & Schutte 1984). A number of operative approaches to this deformity have been described, including the creation of a distal tibiofibular synostosis (Langenskiold 1967), a supramalleolar chevron-type osteotomy (Wiltse 1972), distal tibial medial epiphyseal stapling (Paluska & Blount 1968), and iliac bone grafting of the pseudarthrosis to reestablish fibular continuity (Hsu et al 1972). While any of these methods may succeed in stabilizing a progressive ankle valgus, Bleck's recommendation (1987) to avoid the problem altogether by using another graft site seems the most logical approach.

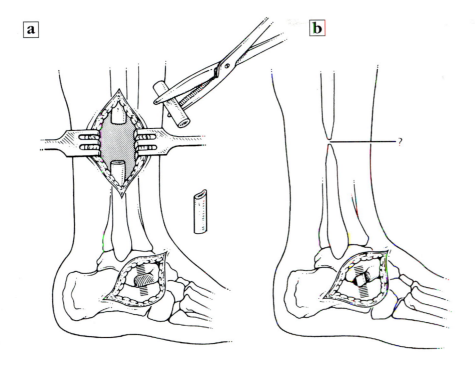

Figure 21

Grice procedure, using distal fibula as the graft site. Pseudarthrosis of the fibula, producing ankle valgus, is an avoidable complication

Brown and Seymour & Evans simultaneously reported in 1968 the use of a fibular graft drilled blindly across the subtalar joint from an anterior fenestration in the talar neck. They attributed the procedure to J S Batchelor of Guy's Hospital, London, and it was intended to provide subtalar stability during growth, just as the Grice operation proposed. Its advantage was technical simplicity in that the sinus tarsi was not exposed, and the technical problems of proper graft placement and graft stability in the subtalar joint were circumvented. The subtalar joint was simply corrected by manipulation, and a fibular strut drilled from the talar neck into the calcaneus provided stability immediately – the fibular acted as internal fixation with eventual arthrodesis. Displacement of the graft, and hence loss of correction, were claimed to be impossible unless the graft fractured, which occurred in two out of 23 of Brown's patients, both of whom were older than usual (over 15 years) and heavy. The procedure was not advocated for such patients. No problems with graft-site pseudarthrosis were mentioned.

However, in 1972 Hsu et al reported fibular pseudarthrosis as a major complication of the Batchelor technique, especially when the graft was harvested from the lower third of the fibula (see Fig. 21). Seventy-one per cent of the grafts taken from the distal third failed to regenerate, with 57% developing significant ankle valgus and cephalad migration of the lateral malleolus. By harvesting the graft from the middle third, the incidence of fibular pseudarthrosis fell to 11%. Subsequently, the same group reported a larger series of patients, all with polio deformities, where only 67% satisfactory results were obtained (Hsu et al 1976). This latter group's unsatisfactory results did not include any ankle

valgus cases from fibular pseudarthrosis; but, instead, failures were due to persistent deformity caused by inadequate manipulative reduction (16%), nonunion of the subtalar arthrodesis with recurrent valgus (14%), and varus overcorrection (3%).

The high incidence of nonunion (graft fracture or resorption) was attributed to the older age (10 years) of the patients in the Hong Kong series. However, further experience with Batchelor's technique has shown pseudarthrosis is to be common – 41% in Gross's series (Gross 1976) – owing to the cortical nature of the graft and its placement in the axis of the subtalar joint rather than parallel to the weight bearing axis as in the original Grice technique. The technical simplicity of the fibular strut placement was offset by the poor biomechanical outcome of such placement. It should not be surprising that cortical grafts placed without a compression deforming force would fracture or resorb. Gross observed late loss of position more than one year postoperatively after the graft had been incorporated by radiographic appearance in 10% of the cases. Gross suggested the procedure was too unreliable to warrant continued usage, since overall results showed only 53% satisfactory.

The Princess Margaret Rose procedure, reported by Dennyson & Fulford (1976), combines internal fixation with a large threaded screw through the talar neck, and sinus tarsi evacuation and extra-articular arthrodesis with cancellous graft from the ilium (Fig. 22). Loss of subtalar correction is prevented by the rigid screw fixation. Rapid arthrodesis (7.5 weeks in Dennyson & Fulford's series) is achieved by using cancellous graft, since cortical graft as a corrective strut is no longer required. Immediate

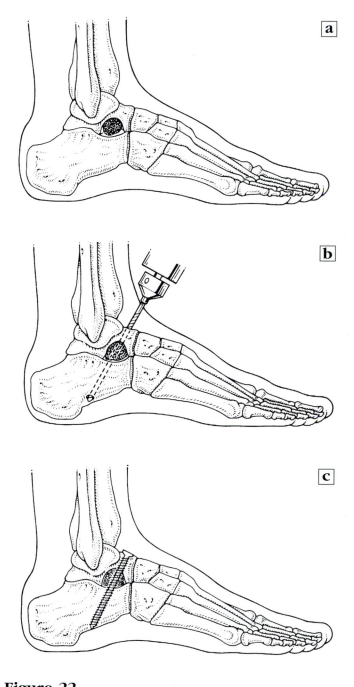

Figure 22

Princess Margaret Rose modification of subtalar arthrodesis.
The subtalar joint is fused with cancellous bone in the sinus
tarsi, and correction maintained with internal fixation

weight bearing is feasible with this technique –
something not allowed for up to 2 months in the previously mentioned procedures. Ninety per cent satisfactory
results and 94% fusion rate were reported. Subsequent
experience (Boss et al 1983, Rosenthal & Candage 1983,
Barasso et al 1984) has confirmed 85–95% satisfactory
results in 131 patients, all but nine of whom had cerebral
palsy. The fusion rate varied from 88–100%. Though
follow-up periods were only 2–3 years, the high fusion

rate, the security of internal fixation to hold the correction of the deformity, and the ability to mobilize the
patients quickly seemed to justify the larger surgical
intervention, including the iliac graft site. At this time,
the Princess Margaret Rose procedure appears to incorporate the best of both Grice and Batchelor techniques
and has the most predictable outcome of the extra-
articular subtalar arthrodesis procedures. A disadvantage
of this method is the possible need to remove the screw
implant in a later procedure.

Calcaneal osteotomy

The advantage of correcting hindfoot deformity by
calcaneal osteotomy is that it retains subtalar motion
while realigning the axis of weight bearing. The preservation of subtalar joint function is important in maintaining normal gait mechanics. The eversion of the foot
which occurs through this joint in early stance phase,
allows for gradual loading of the foot. This provides an
important 'shock absorption' function as weight is
distributed evenly onto the maximum available plantar
surface. Silver et al (1967, 1974) performed a lateral
opening wedge calcaneal osteotomy, and estimated
retention of 50% of subtalar motion, thereby providing
some flexibility to the hindfoot and forefoot to compensate for less than perfect weight bearing alignment – a
margin for error not enjoyed by subtalar arthrodesis.
Maintaining subtalar motion was also mentioned by
Baker & Hill (1964), who found that a smaller opening
wedge under the posterior facet of the subtalar joint
restored normal talocalcaneal alignment, placed the
sustentaculum under the talar neck, and thus solved the
hindfoot deformity without subtalar fusion. Interestingly,
they combined this procedure with the Grice operation
in 10 cases and performed it alone in 31, but did not
indicate specific reasons why the two procedures should
be performed separately or in combination. Dwyer
(1960) indicated that the opening wedge should bring
the heel into the line of weight bearing and thus change
the line of action of the Achilles tendon from an evert-
ing, deforming force to a neutral or inverting one.
Achilles tendon lengthening was performed simultaneously (Fig. 23).

The results of these few series have been comparable
to the best subtalar arthrodesis results. Satisfactory results
have been found in up to 93% of patients. Severe deformity (plantar flexion of the talus of up to 80°) may not
be correctable by calcaneal osteotomy (Bleck 1987).
Silver et al (1974), while providing no guidelines as to
the amount of deformity that can be corrected, do admit
that only flexible valgus feet can be corrected by
osteotomy (fixed or rigid pronated feet require triple
arthrodesis), and that supplemental tendon transfers or
soft tissue procedures were required in 23% of the valgus
deformities. The most common supplemental procedure
was some form of weakening of the triceps sura.

Two other calcaneal osteotomy procedures are useful.
The simplest calcaneal osteotomy for valgus hindfoot

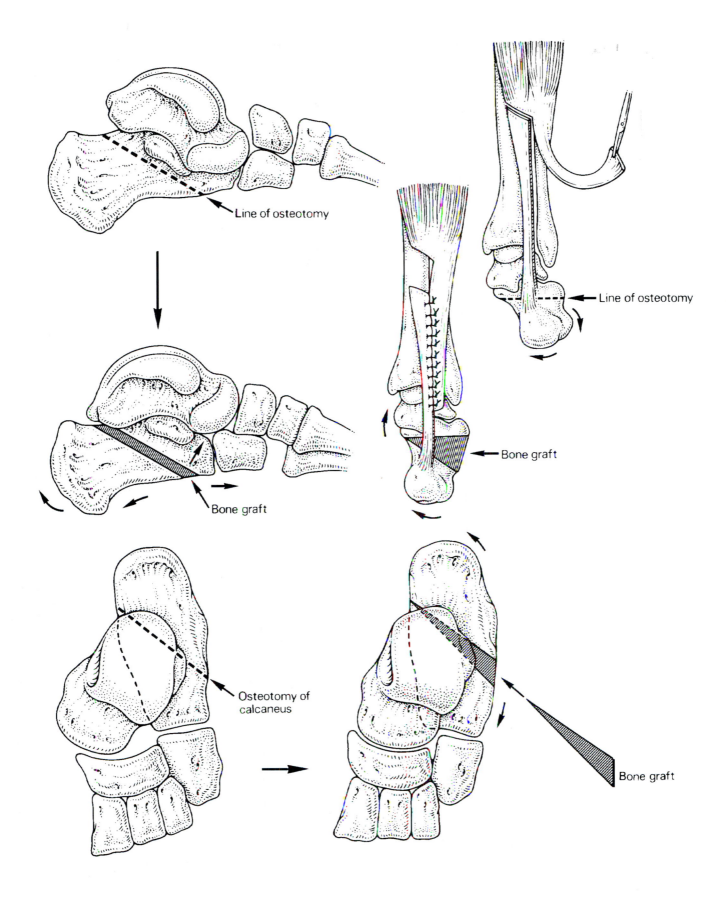

Figure 23

Opening wedge calcaneal osteotomy. The osteotomy elongates the calcaneus in all planes, correcting the varus of the heel by increasing the height of the os calcis laterally. Forefoot abduction is corrected by lengthening the lateral aspect of the foot, pushing the anterior portion of the os calcis distally and medially. Support for the talar neck is produced (after Dwyer 1960)

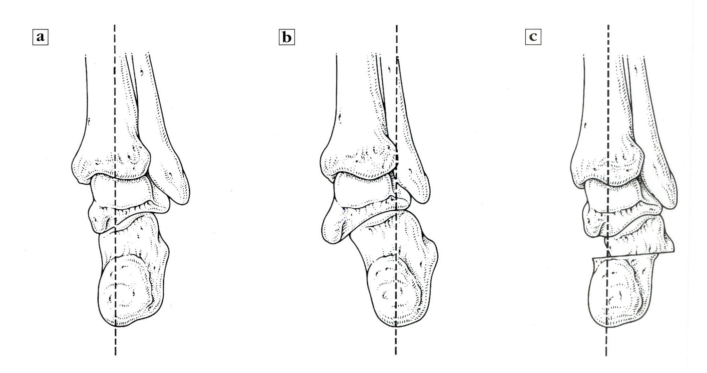

Figure 24

Sliding osteotomy of the calcaneus for correction of valgus deformity. (b) Normal weight bearing alignment (a) is obtained by medial displacement of the distal fragment (c)

was originally described by Koutsogiannis (1971). A transverse, oblique osteotomy from the lateral side is performed, and the posterior fragment simply displaced medially to place the heel beneath the proper weight bearing axis of the tibia (Fig. 24). Excellent results have been reported in 95–100% of treated feet (Koutsogiannis 1971, Trieshmann et al 1980). Rapid union, avoidance of bone grafting, early ambulation, maintenance of subtalar motion, and avoidance of technical complications such as those experienced in the Grice operation – especially in younger children – were reported. The simplicity of the procedure appears to be its major advantage.

D Evans (1975) described an opening wedge osteotomy of the anterior process of the calcaneus to elongate the lateral column of the foot (Fig. 25). This procedure was the reverse of his solution for the relapsed clubfoot where the elongated lateral column of the foot was shortened. Evans noted during correction of paralytic valgus deformity that, as the anterior portion of the calcaneus was pushed distally, the valgus of the hindfoot was noted to improve and the forefoot valgus disappeared. The appropriate new length of the lateral column was reestablished using a tibial cortical bone graft wedged into the vertically oriented osteotomy. In 56 procedures, the results were successful enough to avoid triple arthrodesis. This report showed this method to be successful even in rigid feet. However, D Evans specifically warned against its use in cerebral palsy because of a tendency to overcorrect into equinovarus.

No explanation for this 'tendency' or how to avoid it was specifically offered. Subsequent series reporting results of this procedure in cerebral palsy have not identified overcorrection as a problem (Phillips 1983, Mosca 1995). Many patients require lengthening of the heel cord to prevent equinus resulting from lengthening of the lateral column. Mosca (1995) has successfully used allograft bone graft and also suggests lengthening of the peroneal tendons coupled with medial soft tissue plication and any additional procedures needed to balance the foot dynamically.

Triple arthrodesis

In the symptomatic valgus foot with late, fixed deformity, triple arthrodesis may be appropriate. The established indications are poorly defined except that patients should be at least 12 years of age (Bleck 1984). Surgery prior to 8 years of age produces excessive shortening of the foot and carries with it as much as a 47% failure rate due to paucity of bone apposition in these young feet (Hill et al 1970, Patterson et al 1950).

The need for triple arthrodesis in cerebral palsy has been infrequent. Horstmann & Eilert (1977) reported that only 5% of nearly 900 patients with cerebral palsy underwent triple arthrodesis. Baker & Hill (1964) reported only three out of 72 cerebral palsy patients undergoing surgical procedures for foot deformities needed triple arthrodesis. Valgus deformities account for 30–40% of triple arthrodesis done for all etiologies (Patterson et al

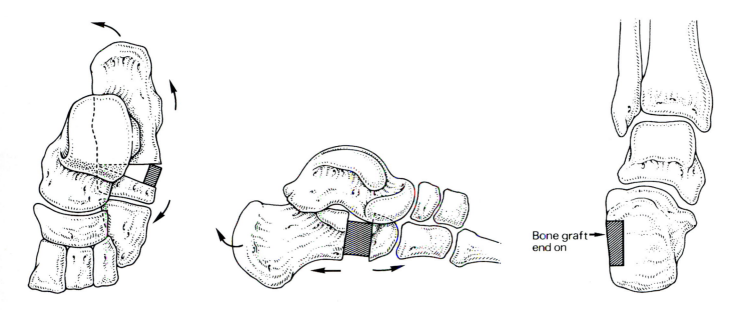

Figure 25

Elongation osteotomy of the calcaneus. The mechanism for correction of the valgus foot by elongation of the lateral column
(after D Evans 1975)

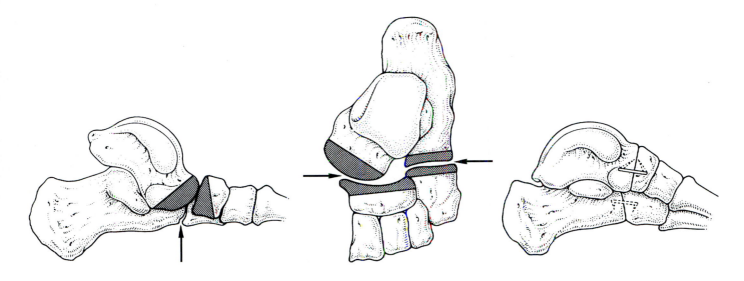

Figure 26

Triple arthrodesis for valgus deformity. Two incisions are necessary to ensure correction, especially the appropriate wedge
removal of the talonavicular joint. Internal fixation is optional (after Coleman 1983)

1950, Wilson et al 1965 Seitz & Carpenter 1974), but in cerebral palsy, valgus deformities predominate, making up 75 out of 112 cases from three different series of triple arthrodesis in patients with spasticity (Horstmann & Eilert 1977, Malekafzali & Rosenthal 1981, Ireland & Hoffer 1985).

As many as 88% of the valgus deformities operated upon continue to have residual deformity (Seitz & Carpenter 1974), and other series show a high incidence of incomplete correction for valgus feet, often in a much greater percentage than for other deformities (Horstmann & Eilert 1977, Coleman 1983). The source of this recurrence or persistence does not seem to be more frequent pseudarthrosis – the incidence in cerebral palsy seems not significantly higher than in other etiologies (Wilson et al 1965, Seitz & Carpenter 1974, Goldner 1981). Rather, it appears to be incomplete correction at the time of surgery, or recurrence after surgery due to persistent neuromuscular imbalance (Patterson et al 1950, Seitz & Carpenter 1974). This may be due to the fact that the procedure is being performed on a long-established, stiff deformity, and that complete correction would require excessively large bone wedges, which would significantly shorten the height and length of the foot (Bleck 1987) (Fig. 26). It may also be due to inadequate surgical exposure through one incision, as outlined by Coleman (1983).

In spite of lack of correction, the clinical results do not seem to suffer. Horstmann & Eilert (1977) found improved stability in walking endurance in 89% of their patients (all deformities), while Malekafzali & Rosenthal (1981) found 100% of their patients improved by increasing activity and decreasing need for crutches or orthoses. Aiona (1990) found that these results were maintained in an average follow-up of 24 years. Other series, while not commenting specifically on changes in functional level, report 79–100% satisfactory results in their cerebral palsy patients (Adelaar et al 1976, Patterson et al 1950). This finding of generally good clinical outcomes in spite of incomplete correction of valgus deformity may be due to residual forefoot pronation, which has been shown by force plate gait analysis to be generally not deleterious (Southwell & Sherman 1981). While all patients with triple arthrodesis demonstrated increased force concentration on the midfoot and metatarsal heads, those with pronated forefeet preferentially loaded the medial two metatarsals with little clinical difficulty. Patients with forefoot supination had increased loading of the lateral three metatarsals with a high incidence of painful callosities.

Nonunion can occur when triple arthrodesis is performed in children. The talonavicular joint is the joint most often affected by pseudarthrosis, and pain can occur (Wilson et al 1965, Ireland & Hoffer 1985, Aiona 1990), but the need for additional surgery for relief of pain has been uncommon in the cerebral palsy population (Seitz & Carpenter 1974, Goldner 1981, Ireland & Hoffer 1985, Aiona 1990). Radiographic degenerative changes in the ankle joint following triple arthrodesis have been observed in 25–58% of patients (Drew 1951, Adelaar et al 1976, Southwell & Sherman 1981, Tenuta et al 1993), but no correlation of these changes with clinical symptoms has been demonstrated. Unfortunately, follow-up of more than 25 years has not been reported and the biomechanical effects of fusing the midtarsal and subtalar joint (Mann 1980) may produce significant problems with time.

In summary, a flexible valgus foot can be a satisfactory weight bearing platform. The mere presence of valgus does not warrant surgery, though a progressive valgus deformity should lead the surgeon to consider maintenance of flexibility by soft tissue release or lengthening before arthrodesis. Triple arthrodesis to correct deformity will generally not lead to complete correction and can result in a stiff foot that will often exhibit radiographic signs of degenerative arthritis in long-term follow-up. The operating surgeon must have a clear surgical indication such as pain, skin breakdown, or intolerance of orthoses or footwear before embarking on this procedure.

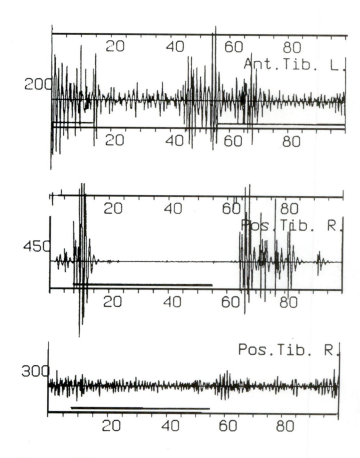

Figure 27

EMG of tibialis anterior and posterior in cerebral palsy. Normal activity represented by the solid line at the bottom of each graph. Top: Out-of-phase activity of the tibialis anterior during mid- to late-stance phase. Middle: Out-of-phase activity of the tibialis posterior with swing phase activity. Bottom: Continuous activity of the tibialis posterior throughout swing and stance phase

Pes varus

Equinovarus foot deformity is seen in about 20–25% of the entire cerebral palsy population and is found most often in patients with hemiparesis (Ruda & Frost 1971, Bennett et al 1982, Drew 1951, Bleck 1987). Observation alone is sufficient for the young child with a mild flexible varus. The use of an orthotic such as an AFO or UCBL orthosis may be helpful in the passively correctable foot. Surgical management is indicated in the child older than 4 years if foot position can no longer be controlled by orthoses. Varus of the hindfoot will result in a supination of the forefoot. Weight bearing will thus be on the lateral border of the foot. Painful callous may develop over the fifth metatarsal base and recurrent ankle sprains may occur (Mann 1980, Bleck 1987). Soft tissue surgery alone will often not be successful over age 10, owing to the development of structural changes in the bony skeleton (Ruda & Frost 1971).

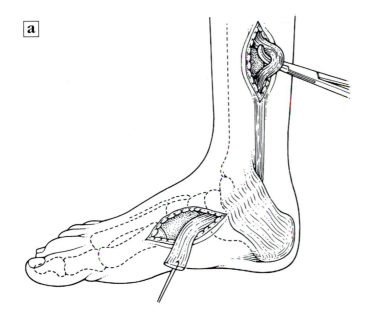

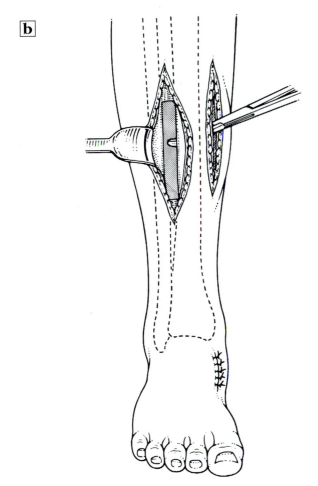

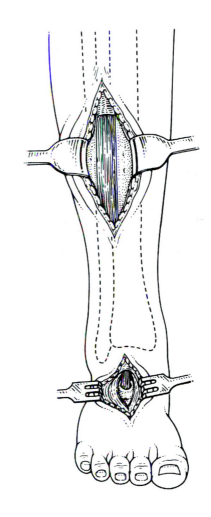

Figure 28

(a) Exposure medially for transfer of the tibialis posterior to the dorsum of the foot through the interosseous membrane. (b) Through an anterior exposure just lateral to the tibia, the contents of the anterior compartment are retracted carefully, and a large window removed from the interosseous membrane. A tunnel is then created bluntly to pass the tibialis posterior from the posterior compartment to the anterior compartment. (c) The transferred tibialis posterior is then tunnelled subcutaneously to the dorsum of the foot, and affixed in the midline through a drill hole in the bone

The etiology of dynamic pes varus has traditionally been felt to be spasticity of the tibialis posterior, with lesser roles assigned to tibialis anterior spasticity, peroneal weakness, and gastrocnemius–soleus spasticity and contracture (Bleck 1987). Electromyographic studies have been extensively used to clarify the etiology of this deformity and indicate the surgical solution in an objective manner. Perry & Hoffer (1977) studied children with varus foot deformity and found that the posterior tibialis had abnormal and continuous stance and swing phase activity

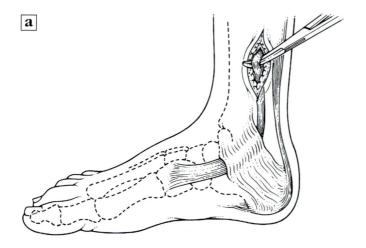

Figure 29a

Exposure of the tibialis posterior proximal to the medial malleolus

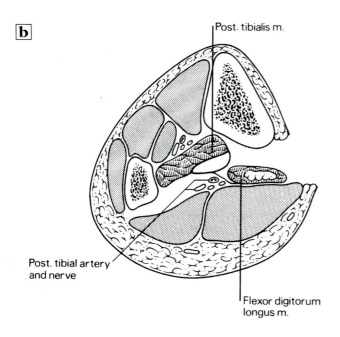

Post. tibialis m.

Post. tibial artery and nerve

Flexor digitorum longus m.

Figure 29b

Location of the tibialis posterior at the level of the myotendinous junction. The tendon is delivered up into the wound after retracting the flexor digitorum longus posteriorly

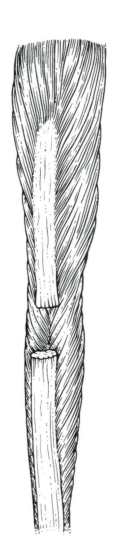

Figure 29c

Lengthening of the tibialis posterior at the myotendinous junction by releasing only the tendinous portion of the muscle. The foot is then everted and dorsiflexed maximally to lengthen the tendinous portion (after Majestro et al 1971)

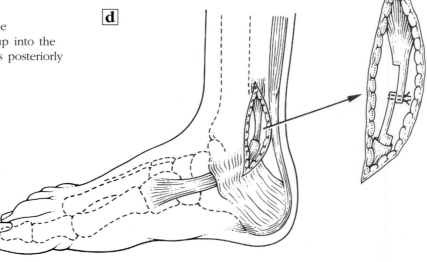
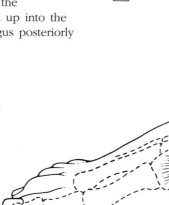

Figure 29d

'Z'lengthening of the tibialis posterior behind the medial malleolus

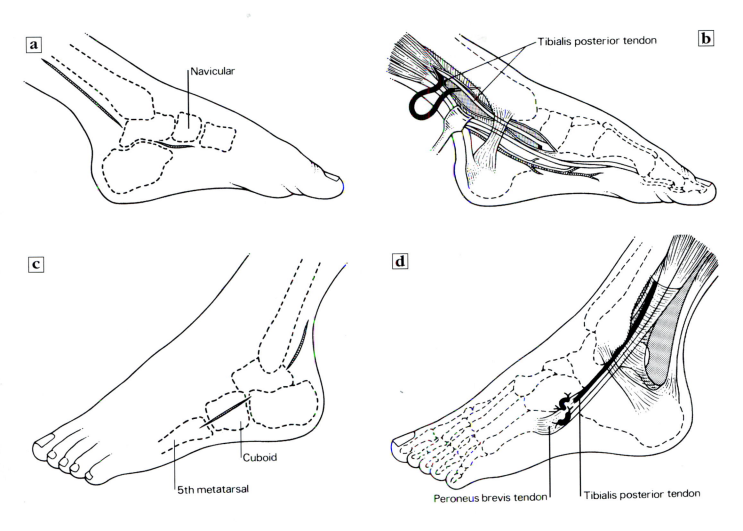

Figure 30

Split transfer of the tibialis posterior. Half of the tendon is detached from its distal insertion, and passed posterior to the tibia and fibula to be woven into the peroneus brevis tendon. Tension on the transferred half should be sufficient to maintain the forefoot in neutral position to slight eversion (after Green et al 1983)

in 73% of their patients, abnormal swing phase activity in 13% of patients, and that the anterior tibialis was overactive in 14% of patients (Fig. 27). Subsequent studies have found a higher percentage of patients with anterior tibialis abnormalities, but have confirmed that the posterior tibialis is the likely cause of varus deformity in the majority of patients (Barto et al 1984, Willis et al 1988).

For each of these three patterns, an operative solution to the deformity has been proposed. With the continuously firing tibialis posterior, the tendon is lengthened with an appropriate lengthening of the Achilles tendon. If the tibialis posterior phase is reversed and the muscle is active during swing phase, the tendon is transferred through the interosseous membrane to the dorsum of the foot. If the tibialis anterior is firing continuously, split transfer of half of its tendon to the cuboid with Achilles tendon lengthening is indicated (Perry & Hoffer 1977, Barto et al 1984).

Surgical treatment

In spite of seemingly clear electromyographic gait analysis evidence of the etiology of this deformity and strong recommendations regarding treatment, there is considerable controversy about the optimal surgical treatment for this disorder. Transfer of the tibialis posterior to the dorsum of the foot has had mixed results (Fig. 28). Several series have reported moderate success with this transfer (Gritzka et al 1972, Banks 1975, Bisla et al 1976, Miller 1982). Bisla had good results in 14 out of 20 patients and noted that the majority of these patients had phase reversal of the tibialis posterior. Failure rates of up to 70% have also been reported. Overcorrection leading to the reverse deformity, a spastic calcaneovalgus deformity, has been a common finding in poor results from anterior transfer (Turner & Cooper 1972, Williams 1976, Schneider & Balon 1977, Miller et al 1982, Root & Kirz 1982). These findings have led to the recom-

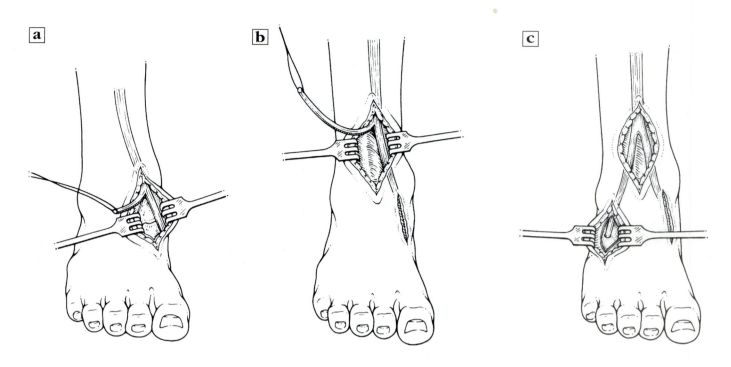

Figure 31

Split transfer of the tibialis anterior. The lateral half of the tendinous insertion is detached and mobilized proximally (a,b), and then transferred subcutaneously to the cuboid, where it is anchored into a drill hole in the bone (c). Tension on the transferred half should be sufficient to maintain the foot in neutral position

mendation that the tibialis posterior be transferred only if confirmation of its swing-phase activity is found on gait electromyography (Miller et al 1982, Bleck 1987). Transfer of the tendon too laterally, and overlengthening of the Achilles tendon combined with the anterior transfer have also been implicated in poor outcomes (Watkins et al 1954, Bisla et al 1976, Bleck 1987).

Good results with subcutaneous transfer of the posterior tibial tendon were reported by Baker & Hill (1964). Bisla et al (1976), however, had patients improve with this procedure in only 25% of cases. A subsequent report by Johnson (1989) reported good correction of the varus in 85% of patients treated with this procedure. We have no personal experience of this procedure.

Concerns about overcorrection with anterior transfer of the tibialis posterior tendon have led several authors to recommend lengthening, especially if gait analysis is not available. Either 'Z' lengthening behind the medial malleolus, or an intramuscular lengthening in the distal leg (Fig 29) is recommended. Both of these procedures can be combined with Achilles tendon lengthening, and good results have been reported in 90% of patients so treated (Banks & Panagakos 1966, Majestro et al 1971, Perry & Hoffer 1977, Bleck 1987). Poor results have also been reported in as many as 50% of patients. Over and under correction occur with the 'Z' lengthening procedure having more poor outcomes than intramuscular lengthening (Ruda & Frost 1971, Root & Kirz 1982). The

best results were in children less than 6 years old. Little improvement was seen in children older than 10 years.

Because of the risk of overlengthening the tibialis posterior, with resultant valgus deformity, the concept of split transfer of the tibialis posterior was introduced by Kaufer (1977), presumably following the example of the split tibialis anterior transfer of Hoffer et al (1974). In this procedure (Fig. 30), the posterior half of the tendon is split longitudinally, detached distally, and transferred to the lateral side of the ankle anterior to the neurovascular bundle but posterior to the tibia and fibula, where it is then woven into the peroneus brevis tendon (Green et al 1983). In this fashion, the posterior half of the transfer, which is attached under tension so that the hindfoot is in neutral to slight eversion, corrects the dynamic varus deformity, but overcorrection is prevented since the anterior half of the tendon remains undisturbed. Some authors also advocate intramuscular tenotomy because of the tension placed on the split transfer (DeLuca 1992). Results of this procedure appear to document its apparent soundness – no valgus deformities have been reported, and because the plantarflexion function of the nontransferred half is retained, no calcaneus deformities were produced, even when the procedure was combined with Achilles tendon lengthening (Green et al 1983, Kling & Hensinger 1983, Medina et al 1989, Snyder et al 1993). Only the series by Green et al (1983) employed preoperative EMG gait analysis.

EMG gait analysis did show either diphasic (stance and swing activity with a period of silence intervening) or continuous activity of the tibialis posterior. The implication is that this procedure is successful by balancing the spasticity of the two arms of the transferred tendon, thereby aligning the hindfoot. Details of the EMG activity of the tibialis anterior were not clarified, but he considered the muscle to be weak and therefore not the offending muscle.

For patients who have out-of-phase activity of the tibialis anterior and a varus forefoot deformity, a split transfer of the lateral half of the tibialis anterior can be performed, as recommended by Hoffer et al (1974) (Fig. 31). The lateral half of the tendon is taken subcutaneously to the lateral cuneiform or to the cuboid and anchored into a drill hole with absorbable suture. The suture is passed to the sole of the foot and tied over a button. Redundancy of the medial limb is almost always present. This can be left redundant or tightened based on the surgeon's discretion. Alternatively, the entire tibialis anterior can be moved to the midline (Goldner 1982). Proponents of split tibialis anterior transfer (Mital & McCarthy 1982, Coleman 1983, Rush 1983, Hoffer et al 1985) state that this muscle is sufficiently strong in cerebral palsy to warrant transferring its lateral half to the cuboid to balance the deforming forces of varus and supination. Lengthening of the Achilles tendon for a fixed equinus deformity is often necessary, and in patients who have continuous activity of the posterior tibialis, an intramuscular lengthening of that muscle is also added (Hoffer et al 1985). Good results have also been reported without using preoperative EMG gait analysis (Barnes & Herring 1992). These authors also recommend intramuscular lengthening of the posterior tibialis tendon and a judicious lengthening of the Achilles tendon.

Many inconsistencies in the management of the equinovarus foot deformity in cerebral palsy remain unresolved. Although there has been much attention paid to the use of EMG in the preoperative assessment of the equinovarus foot (Perry & Hoffer 1977, Bleck 1987), the fact that several series not employing preoperative EMG gait analysis have reported excellent results using either a split anterior tibialis or a split posterior tibialis tendon transfer (Kling & Hensinger 1983, Medina et al 1989, Barnes & Herring 1992, Snyder et al 1993) raises significant questions about the need for this information. EMG activity has never been correlated with strength in cerebral palsy patients. Estimates of voluntary muscle control, degree of spasticity, and the status of agonist and antagonistic muscle groups is not detailed in any of the published series. This is partly due to the difficulty in assessing these signs in a patient with cerebral palsy. Recently, Vaughn et al (1992) has raised questions regarding what constitutes a normal EMG activity pattern of the posterior tibialis. He found that some normal adults had peak posterior tibialis activity in early swing phase and that there was not a standard pattern of activity in his 10 subjects. His review of the literature found that 'normal' activity patterns for the posterior tibialis during gait were based on few patients and that considerable variability was in fact present in those series. Similarly, Davids et al (1993) have questioned the reliability of the 'confusion test' and the EMG activity patterns of the tibialis anterior in determining the contribution of this muscle to dynamic varus deformities. He found that virtually all patients with poor selective control of the tibialis anterior had a positive 'confusion test' and that this did not correlate well with ankle swing phase function.

What, then, is a clinician to do when faced with an equinovarus deformity that is causing significant problems and is not controllable with bracing? EMG gait analysis may be helpful in determining which muscles are behaving abnormally, but is probably not mandatory in the preoperative evaluation. The exception to this is if the surgeon is contemplating anterior transfer of the tibialis posterior through the interosseous membrane. This transfer should not be done unless the EMG gait analysis shows the phase of activity is reversed. Lengthening of the posterior tibialis tendon with appropriate lengthening of the Achilles tendon can provide excellent clinical outcomes. Intramuscular lengthening appears to be more predictable than 'Z' lengthening of the tendon. This procedure has not been as predictable as split tendon transfers in providing a balanced foot. Both the split posterior tibialis transfer and split anterior tibialis tendon transfer with intramuscular lengthening of the posterior tibialis are likely to produce a good clinical result with improvement of the varus foot position. These procedures will generally need to be augmented with a lengthening of the Achilles tendon.

Our preferred method of management of the equinovarus foot is to control it with an orthosis in the child less than 4 when the deformity is generally quite flexible. We will usually perform EMG gait analysis in the older child. If there is clear out-of-phase activity of the tibialis posterior with no abnormality in the tibialis anterior, an anterior transfer of the tibialis posterior to the dorsum of the foot may be performed. There are few children in our practice who fit these criteria. In children with mild dynamic varus and significant equinus deformity, a lengthening of the Achilles tendon with an intramuscular lengthening of the tibialis posterior will be performed. For children with more significant varus deformity, a split transfer of the tibialis anterior to the lateral cuneiform with an intramuscular lengthening of the tibialis posterior and an appropriate lengthening of the Achilles tendon is our procedure of choice. In the occasional patient who has a weak or nonexistent tibialis anterior and strong posterior tibialis activity, a split transfer of the posterior tibialis will be performed. This may also be combined with proximal transfer of the toe extensors if the child appears to be actively recruiting these muscles for ankle dorsiflexion (Tohen et al 1966).

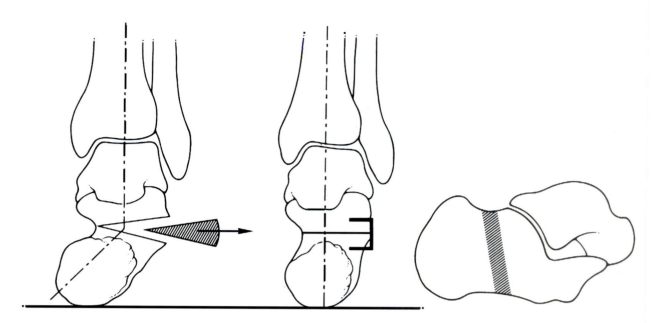

Figure 32
Correction of heel varus by lateral closing wedge osteotomy of the calcaneus. Internal fixation is optional

Fixed (late) deformity

In the older child or the neglected case, a varus deformity of the hindfoot that is not passively correctable will require calcaneal osteotomy to treat the fixed aspect of the deformity. This is a situation in which a spastic tibialis posterior has not been weakened or balanced adequately, and dynamic deformity has persisted long enough to produce skeletal changes (Bleck 1987, Ruda & Frost 1971). The patient with fixed varus will usually have more difficulty with brace tolerance and callosities over the lateral aspect of the foot (Mann 1980).

Provided the midfoot has some flexibility and the supination is not fixed, osteotomy of the calcaneus, accompanied by the appropriate muscle-balancing procedures, is a simple and generally effective means of producing a neutral or slightly valgus hindfoot, while maintaining subtalar motion. Either the lateral closing wedge technique (Fig. 32) (Silver et al 1967, 1974), originally popularized by Dwyer (1959, 1960), or sliding osteotomy (Trieshmann et al 1980) can be utilized to correct fixed heel varus. The muscle-balancing aspect of the procedure cannot be overemphasized, as recurrence of deformity is a result if the deforming forces are not balanced. Fisher & Shaffer (1970) confirmed Dwyer's experience that recurrent deformity was the most likely complication of an otherwise simple and effective procedure. Silver et al (1974) noted that in 213 of their calcaneal osteotomies, other soft tissue procedures were necessary. Bleck (1987) has simply stated that lengthening of the tibialis posterior and Achilles tendon are necessary.

Persistence of deformity into late childhood and adolescence can produce a foot with both hindfoot and midfoot fixed varus. While correction of the two deformities with separate procedures (calcaneal osteotomy and tarsometatarsal capsulotomies or metatarsal osteotomies) has been proposed (Fisher & Shaffer 1970), the deformity is usually found in the midtarsal joints, and is best corrected by triple arthrodesis (Banks 1975, Bleck 1987). Since a foot fixed in varus and supination is usually inadequate as a weight bearing platform (Mann 1980) and produces symptoms of both pain and instability, it is much easier to recommend triple arthrodesis as the surgical solution to a varus foot than, for example, to a valgus deformity. As discussed earlier, valgus feet tend to be flexible, owing to relaxation of the midtarsal joints during hindfoot eversion, allowing broad plantar distribution of weight bearing stress (Mann 1980). Even in the presence of a valgus foot that is rigid from years of spasticity and uncorrected deformity, the midfoot and forefoot may be remarkably plantigrade and there will usually be an acceptable, broad weight bearing surface. Varus feet tend to be rigid, making the even distribution of weight bearing forces impossible, since they are concentrated on the lateral rays of the foot and place rotational stress on the lateral ankle ligaments (Mann 1980, Southwell & Sherman 1981). Triple arthrodesis to correct and stabilize the deformity should be considered in a teenager with pressure sores or gait difficulties from ankle instability and limited weight bearing surface.

The technique for triple arthrodesis for varus deformity has been an orthopaedic standard since Hoke (1921) and Ryerson (1923) described them in the early 1920s. Removal of appropriate wedges based laterally corrects the deformity (Fig. 33). Hoke's method of exposure of the talonavicular joint – removal and

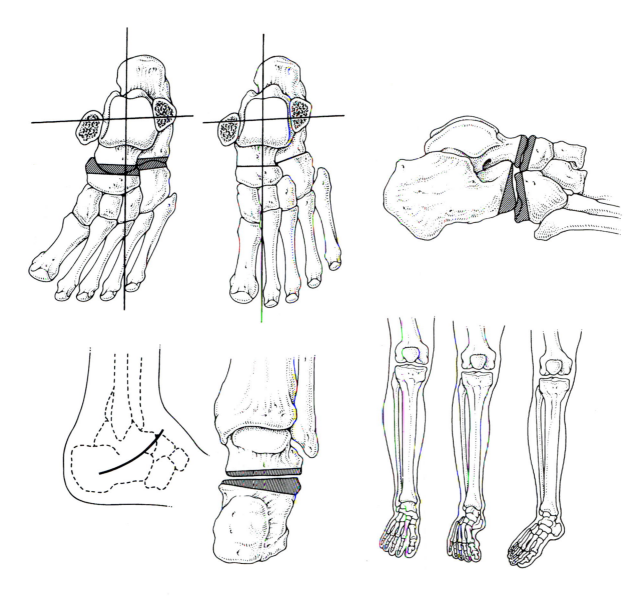

Figure 33

Correction of pes equinovarus by triple arthrodesis. The wedges to be removed can usually be safely excised through a lateral sinus tarsi approach. Note that the foot position must be aligned with the ankle mortise, and *not* aligned with the knee. The foot will be supinated if aligned with the knee in the presence of external tibial torsion (after Coleman 1983 and Patterson 1950)

subsequent replacement of the head of the talus – affords the best exposure of this area (Duncan & Lovell 1978), important for obtaining full talonavicular correction and arthodesis. The principle source of failure of triple arthrodesis is residual deformity, most commonly under-correction of varus deformity because of insufficient bone removal at surgery (Patterson et al 1950, Southwell & Sherman 1981). The other major source of failure – pseudarthrosis, reported in 8.5–23% of cases (Friedenburg 1948, Adelaar et al 1976), which can lead to either pain or recurrence of deformity – occurs at the talonavicular joint in 65–89% of the total pseudarthroses diagnosed (Patterson et al 1950, Coleman 1983, Wilson et al 1965). Hence, adequate talonavicular exposure is a

critical method for gaining adequate exposure. Pseudarthrosis in varus feet is not considered any more likely to be symptomatic than pseudarthrosis after valgus surgery (Patterson et al 1950, Wilson et al 1965, Horstmann & Eilert 1977). Reviews of Hoke procedures agree with near unanimity that pseudarthrosis and under-correction of deformity occur infrequently (Patterson et al 1950, Wilson et al 1965, Duncan & Lovell 1978). The rare occurrence of avascular necrosis of the talus, secondary to damage to the vascular supply of the talus during removal of the talar head in the Hoke procedure has, for the most part, been eliminated as a complica-tion of this procedure by increased awareness of the vascular anatomy of the talus (Duncan & Lovell 1978,

Coleman 1983). The role of internal fixation in decreasing the pseudarthrosis rate is debatable, but many authors recommend it as an important adjunct to obtain solid triple fusion (Bleck 1987). Wilson et al (1965) found only one of 35 talonavicular joints failed to fuse when a staple was used to stabilize it. On the other hand, some of the lowest pseudarthrosis rates (8.5–9%) have been reported in series using no internal fixation.

The overall results of triple arthrodesis for varus deformity give two seemingly contradictory impressions: the deformity is more improved than with valgus triples, but the failures are not uncommon, owing to incomplete correction which is symptomatic (Patterson et al 1950, Horstmann & Eilert 1977, Southwell & Sherman 1981).

Seitz & Carpenter (1974) had 35% incidence of residual deformity (due to undercorrection) in equinovarus feet, compared to 88% valgus feet with residual deformity, yet revised 62.5% residual varus deformities, while none of the valgus feet required revision in spite of their deformity. Similar results have been reported by other authors who emphasize the need for correction of muscle imbalance at the time of arthrodesis (Patterson et al 1950, Drew 1951, Southwell & Sherman 1981). Specifically, a spastic tibialis posterior should be lengthened (Bleck 1987), released (Patterson et al 1950), or transferred to the dorsum if it is the only functioning muscle (Coleman 1983). If the tibialis anterior is present and spastic, it should be split or transferred entirely to the midline (Bleck 1987), released (Patterson et al 1950), or transferred to the dorsum if it is the only functioning muscle (Coleman 1983). If the tibialis anterior is present and spastic, it should be split or transferred entirely to the midline (Goldner 1982, Bleck 1987) especially if peroneals are weak. Achilles tendon lengthening and posterior ankle release must be considered, especially since most feet demonstrate decreased passive dorsiflexion after triple arthrodesis (Adelaar et al 1976, Southwell & Sherman 1981). A role for EMG gait analysis prior to triple arthrodesis might be implied by these recommendations, but to date there have been no reports of this being done.

As it is in triple arthrodesis done for valgus feet, radiographic changes of osteoarthritis are found in the ankles of fused varus feet in longer term follow-up (Drew 1951, Adelaar et al 1976, Duncan & Lovell 1978, Southwell & Sherman 1981, Aiona 1990, Tenuta 1993). There has generally been a lack of symptoms associated with these changes, but the potential for future problems cannot be ignored as the longest average reported follow-up is only 24 years. It has been suggested that patients with cerebral palsy are 'low demand' patients and that this accounts for the low degree of symptoms (Aiona 1990), but most of these asymptomatic patients are only in their fourth decade of life and longer follow-up may reveal significant clinical problems as has been seen in so many other pediatric conditions.

There is little doubt that triple arthrodesis for an equinovarus deformity that is significantly symptomatic

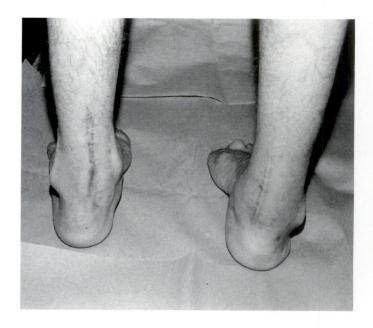

Figure 34a

Residual varus following triple arthrodesis in spastic diplegia

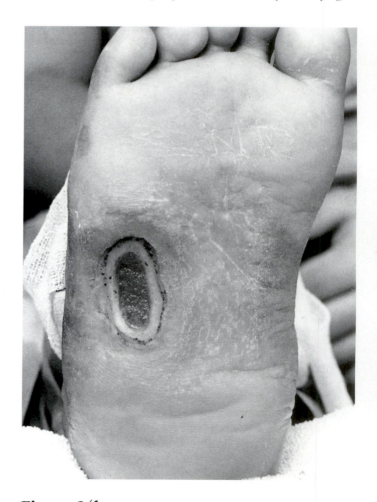

Figure 34b

Plantar surface of the right foot of patient in Fig. 32a. Decubitus over the fifth metatarsal base is due to weight bearing on an inadequate surface in a foot made stiff by arthrodesis

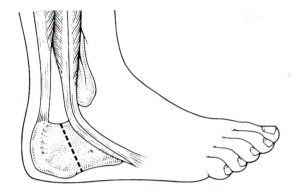

Figure 35a

Superior displacement osteotomy for calcaneus deformity. An oblique osteotomy is made through the body of the calcaneus

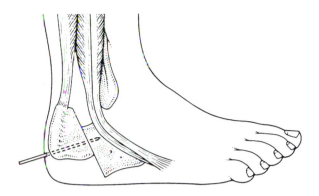

Figure 35b

The posterior segment of the calcaneus is displaced proximally and internally fixed (after Samilson 1976)

or severe is a valuable procedure to improve function in the cerebral palsy patient. There is also little doubt that it is an exacting procedure to perform, for undercorrection of the hindfoot and residual supination of the forefoot, either due to a rotatory malalignment of the forefoot or to failure to align the foot to the ankle mortise, will produce painful symptoms leading to decreased function failure of the procedure (Fig 34). The force plate analysis of Southwell & Sherman (1981) demonstrates the deleterious effects of weight bearing on the lateral three metatarsals, and the apparent lack of problems with increased weight bearing on the medial two metatarsals. Since the margin for error is small, slight valgus and pronation is the desired position in which to stabilize the equinovarus foot. Even with this position, the observance of degenerative changes in the ankle is an ominous development that must be kept in perspective – even though follow-up studies to date have found it to be clinically asymptomatic. Perhaps the most appropriate conclusion should be to avoid the necessity of triple arthrodesis by appropriate and timely surgical management of the muscle imbalance producing pes equinovarus at an early stage of the deformity. In this way, fixed deformity may be avoided and the requirement for triple arthrodesis eliminated altogether.

Calcaneus deformity

The calcaneus deformity may be one of the most difficult management problems encountered in cerebral palsy. The most common cause of calcaneus deformity is the well-intentioned surgeon. Excessive dorsiflexion of the ankle may be either a result or a cause of a crouched gait pattern. At times, a patient who walks with marked knee and hip flexion will gradually overstretch his gastrocsoleus complex. The child will initially walk on

his toes and with time 'sink down' so that the feet are plantigrade. More frequently, a child with a crouching gait pattern undergoes a tendo Achillis lengthening without appropriate attention to the tight hip flexor and hamstring muscles (Rang 1990). In this situation, the gastrocsoleus is functioning as a counter balancing force against the tibia to hold the body up. When the tendon is lengthened, the inevitable result is a marked increase in the knee and hip flexion posture in gait. With the foot now flat, the tibia is free to move forward over the ankle. To make matters worse, this unpleasant situation is often progressive. Decreases in stride length and walking velocity are common in calcaneus gait (Segal et al 1989) and the increased knee flexion requires enormous increases in energy expenditure (Perry & Hoffer 1977). The end result may be a loss of the ability to walk effectively. Anterior subluxation of the peroneal tendons in severe valgus deformity has also been postulated to be a cause of this deformity (Dillin & Samilson 1983). Once subluxated, the peroneal muscles act as dorsiflexors and overpower the ankle plantarflexors.

The best solution to this problem is to avoid it. Overlengthening of the Achilles tendon is most often inappropriate lengthening of the tendon. In most instances, the problem is one of failure to appreciate that the patient walks on his toes because of spasticity of the hip flexors and hamstrings. The incidence of this appears to be decreasing as a heightened awareness of the contribution of the hip and knee flexion contractures becomes more widespread. Gait analysis laboratories have been helpful in documenting adequate ankle dorsiflexion in toe-to-toe gait patterns where contractures above the ankle lead to an apparent equinus position. When an Achilles tendon lengthening is necessary, care must be taken to avoid overlengthening. This is especially true of a percutaneous lengthening, where one should always test the integrity of the muscle–tendon complex by squeezing the calf while observing the ankle

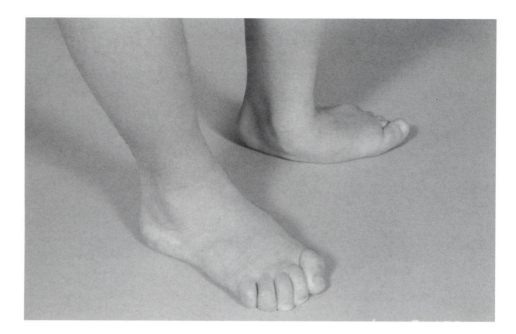

Figure 36a

Pes valgus. Note the tendency for the great toe to be pushed into valgus

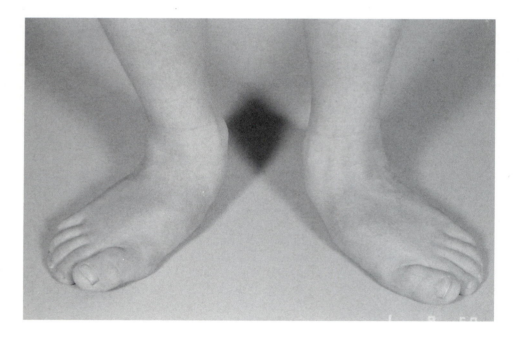

Figure 36b

Pes valgus. Valgus position of all toes

to determine if the foot plantar flexes. When there is any doubt the tendon should be exposed and repaired if necessary. When the calcaneus deformity is established, the first line of treatment is to evaluate again the posture of the extremity. If there is significant residual hip and knee flexor tightness, those muscles should be lengthened. An ankle–foot orthosis or even a knee–ankle–foot orthosis with an anterior shell over the foot and ankle may be helpful, though this rarely solves the problem. Metal braces, even when used with a locked ankle and long metal shoe plate, usually deform rapidly and are mechanically unable to block excessive dorsiflexion.

Tendon transfers for correction of this deformity in cerebral palsy have not been nearly as predictable as in pure paralytic disorders such as polio (Dillin & Samilson 1983). Shortening of the Achilles tendon may be attempted, but we are unaware of any reported series documenting good results with this procedure. The best that can be said for such procedures in this condition is that they occasionally work. As a last resort, a calcaneal osteotomy, calcaneal tenodesis, or even a triple arthrodesis may be performed. The latter procedures will improve the foot configuration, but they are often not adequate in restoring upright posture.

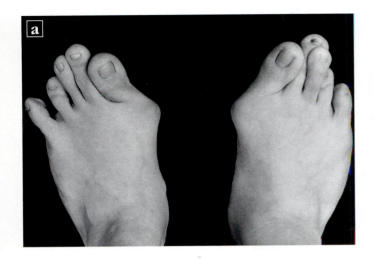

Figure 37a

Hallux valgus in a diplegic patient with equinovalgus feet. The patient has had no previous orthopaedic surgery

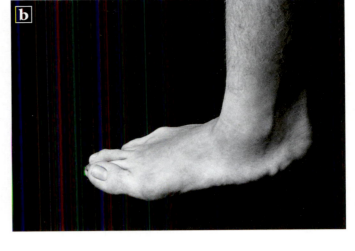

Figure 37b

Lateral view of hallux valgus with equinovalgus foot

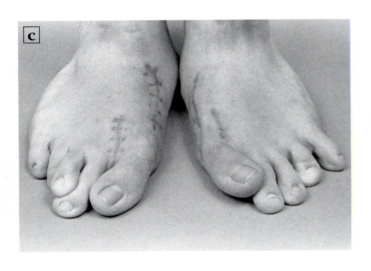

Figure 37c

Early recurrence of hallux valgus (mild) following soft tissue correction and first metatarsal osteotomy. The pronated forefoot position can be appreciated

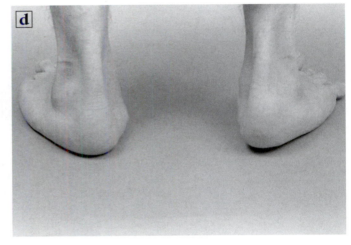

Figure 37d

Persistent equinovalgus postoperatively. No treatment for this part of the foot deformity was undertaken. The forefoot remains in the abducted, pronated position, mechanically encouraging recurrence of hallux valgus

When a calcaneus deformity has progressed to the point where the foot position is inflexible, it may be necessary to perform a calcaneal osteotomy in addition to an Achilles tendon shortening procedure. The first step of the procedure is to perform a plantar release – either percutaneously, or through a short, medial incision. An osteotomy is then made through the calcaneus parallel to the peroneal tendons. When the osteotomy is completed, the posterior fragment of the calcaneus is then displaced backwards and upwards (Samilson 1976, Mitchell 1977) (Fig. 35). If free displacement does not occur, more complete stripping of the plantar fascia and muscle origins from the calcaneus may be necessary. The osteotomy may be fixed in place with a threaded Steinman pin passed upward through the heel. After 3–4 weeks, the pin may be removed and a walking cast applied.

Hallux valgus

Hallux valgus in cerebral palsy appears to be a deformity produced secondarily by several mechanisms. Pes

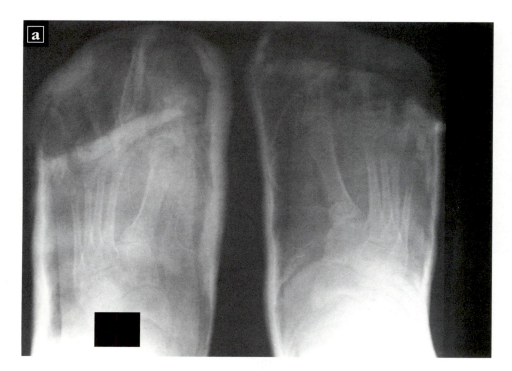

Figure 38a

This 10-year-old diplegic patient underwent bilateral Achilles tendon lengthening and soft tissue correction for hallux valgus combined with proximal first metatarsal osteotomy without internal fixation. The postoperative position of each great toe was thought to be satisfactory. The forefoot appears to be supinated, and the metatarsophalangeal joints both aligned well. The only criticism might be that the casts are not well moulded to the medial side of the foot as noted by the clear space visible

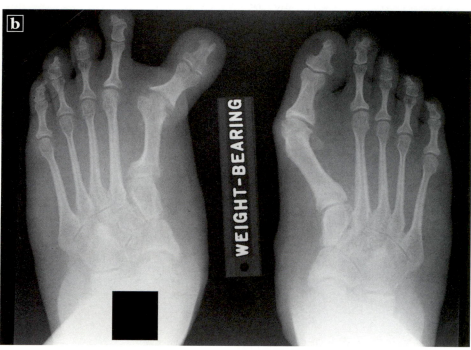

Figure 38b

Six years postoperatively, there is significant recurrence of hallux valgus on the right, and significant hallux varus on the left, in spite of the identical positions in plaster immediately postoperatively. In retrospect, internal fixation of the first metatarsal osteotomies might have prevented the recurrence of the first metatarsal varus on the right, and the settling and resultant shortening of the first metatarsal on the left. Muscle imbalance, and over-plication of the medial capsule, combined with the metatarsal shortening, probably produced the hallux varus complication

equinovalgus with forefoot eversion in an ambulatory patient is probably the most commonly cited cause of hallux valgus; it occurs because the great toe is pushed into valgus during forefoot strike while the foot is everted and externally rotated (Holstein 1980, Goldner 1981, 1982) (Fig. 36). In support of this theory, some authors have noted that an equinovarus foot treated with tibialis posterior lengthening and incomplete equinus correction, thereby producing heel valgus, can develop a hallux valgus where none existed preoperatively (Samilson & Hoffer 1975, Holstein 1980). On the other hand, despite many patients with cerebral palsy having planovalgus foot deformities, the incidence of hallux valgus in cerebral palsy patients is only slightly higher than in the general population. Renshaw (1979) noted 'significant disability' in ambulatory patients in only 14 feet over a 15-year period at Newington, Connecticut, Goldner (1981) treated 26 feet in a 20-year period, and Seaquist et al (1977) similarly had only 26 feet in their review from Rancho Los Amigos, Los Angeles, California. The number of patients with cerebral palsy and significant hallux valgus thus seems rather small.

Spastic muscle imbalance has also been implicated as a causal factor. In the setting of fixed metatarsal adduction, spasticity of the abductor hallucis may lead to a secondary hallux valgus (Bleck 1984). Similarly, a laterally displaced spastic extensor hallucis longus or persisting muscle imbalance in a planovalgus foot from a weak or transferred tibialis posterior may lead to this deformity (Drew 1951, Duckworth 1983, Bleck 1987).

Indications for treatment include pain, gait impairment, and shoe fitting difficulties related to prominent bunion and to toe overlapping (Bleck 1984, Renshaw et al 1979). Patients should be mature before surgery is contemplated so that their neurologic imbalances are static, and lasting correction can be achieved by a combination of bony realignment, arthrodesis, and soft tissue balancing. As noted above, correction of hindfoot deformity is recommended either before or at the same time as the bunion surgery, or the hallux valgus may recur from mechanical forces during stance phase, pushing the great toe back into valgus (Samilson & Hoffer 1975, Renshaw et al 1979) (Fig. 37). If hallux valgus is developing secondary to dynamic spastic metatarsus adductus, abductor hallucis release is preventative (Bleck 1984).

Surgical correction of hallux valgus in cerebral palsy is different from surgical correction of hallux valgus in normal individuals. As previously mentioned, pes equinovalgus deformity needs to be dealt with. Soft tissue releases alone are not recommended (Renshaw et al 1979, Bleck 1984). Most authors favor full soft tissue release and bony realignment. A useful combined procedure is adductor hallucis release, lateral metatarsophalangeal capsulotomy and medial capsular plication, centralization of the extensor hallucis longus, and proximal first metatarsal osteotomy combined with proximal phalangeal osteotomy for bony realignment (Goldner 1981, Bleck 1984, 1987). Since hallux rigidus is a sequela of this deformity, either developing spontaneously or postoperatively, controversy arises over transarticular pinning of the metatarsophalangeal joint. Seaquist et al (1977) and Goldner (1981, 1982) recommend it, while Bleck (1987) reports less stiffness without pinning the joint.

While usually relegated to a salvage procedure, first metatarsophalangeal arthrodesis (McKeever 1952) gave good results in Renshaw's series (Renshaw et al 1979). Its advantages include lasting correction and stability, and an efficacious effect on gait by enabling the great toe to function in the toe-off phase. Force analysis of hallux valgus gait demonstrates marked diminution of pressure and contact time for the great toe, with transfer of these normal weight bearing functions to the lateral metatarsal heads (Hutton & Dhanendran 1981). Although a gait disturbance might be implied by fusion of the great toe metatarsophalangeal joint from lack of dorsiflexion during toe-off (Goldner 1981, Mann 1980), Renshaw actually found the opposite, noting improved loading and contact of the first ray and great toe (Renshaw et al 1979). A properly positioned first

metatarsophalangeal arthrodesis (15–25° of dorsiflexion, slight valgus) has minimal effect on gait in an otherwise normal foot (McKeever 1952, Renshaw et al 1979, Hutton & Dhanendran 1981). We have also found first metatarsophalangeal arthrodesis to be a useful procedure for bunions in neuromuscular feet (Mowery et al 1988). In our patients, it has been used primarily in the management of recurrent deformity after correction of associated hindfoot and rotational abnormalities of the long bones.

Various complications of hallux valgus surgery in spastic patients have been reported (Renshaw et al 1979, Bleck 1987), depending upon the procedures chosen (Fig. 38). They are similar to the common bunion surgery complications familiar to most orthopaedic surgeons and will not be repeated here.

Many patients at risk of developing hallux valgus secondary to an equinovalgus foot deformity will be treated for the latter prior to a significant toe deformity. This may explain the low incidence of problem hallux valgus in the cerebral palsy population. Goldner (1981) and Bleck (1984) feel that early surgery for both problems – correction of hindfoot deformity by calcaneal osteotomy, release of the abductor hallucis and first metatarsal osteotomy – may be preventive. Certainly, the treatment of equinovalgus should proceed at the time when it develops, but it has been our experience that hallux valgus is rarely symptomatic, especially if the alignment of the limb above (thigh internal rotation, knee flexion) has been treated and equinovalgus managed successfully, so that the patient's great toe is not mechanically forced into valgus with each step. Hence, the prophylactic soft tissue release and metatarsal osteotomy are probably not indicated.

Hallux flexus and dorsal bunion

This rather unusual deformity in cerebral palsy is most likely to be a result of imbalance between the extensor hallucis longus (weak) and tibialis anterior (overactive) (Goldner 1981, 1982). The latter elevates the first metatarsal, and in the absence of the former, the toe passively flexes (drops) at the metatarsophalangeal joint, and the metatarsal head is not pushed plantar by the windlass mechanism, as in a clawtoe. In the presence of flexor hallucis longus and brevis spasticity – especially if the triceps sura has been over weakened by, for example, injudicious Achilles tendon lengthening and the toe flexors are overactive to compensate for triceps weakness – the great toe flexes actively and continuously, leading to a marked deformity (Goldner 1981, 1982) (Fig. 39). Usually, lateral deviation of the phalanges accompanies the flexion caused by the spastic flexor hallucis so that hallux valgus with the great toe underlying the second toe is combined with the flexion deformity. The role of the peroneus longus is controversial. McKay (1983) noted weakness or absence (by

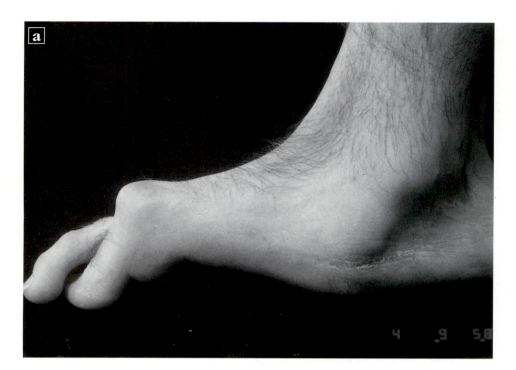

Figure 39a

Dorsal bunion, in a previously operated foot with residual equinovalgus. First metatarsal elevation by the tibialis anterior is obvious

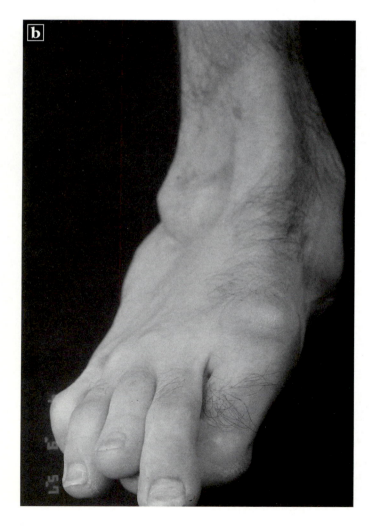

Figure 39b

Dorsal bunion, with significant underlapping great toe (combined hallux valgus and flexus)

transfer) of the peroneus longus in three-fourths of his cases (Fig. 40). Samilson & Hoffer (1975) also implicated weakness of the peroneus longus while, on the other hand, Goldner denies absence of the peroneus longus *per se* as a major cause of the deformity.

The most common situation for hallux flexus to develop in cerebral palsy would probably be where the extensor hallux longus was transferred proximally to aid in dorsiflexion. In a patient with calcaneus deformity due to an over lengthened Achilles tendon and gradual overpull of the toe flexors, clawing and cavus would probably ensue if the extensor hallucis longus is intact. The clinical problem is one of pain on the end of the great toe, footwear difficulty caused by the underlying toe, and possibly toe clearance problems during swing phase if the hallux is markedly flexed (Samilson & Hoffer 1975).

Balancing the muscle pull and removing the deforming force – the flexor hallucis brevis, primarily (McKay 1983) – may be all that is required if the deformity is supple. To this end, McKay transfers the flexor hallucis back from the proximal phalanx to the dorsal neck of the first metatarsal, so that these foot intrinsics become depressors of the first metatarsal head (Fig. 41). The extrinsic toe muscles are left undisturbed. If a varus or valgus deformity exists with the hallux flexus, the appropriate antagonist intrinsic (the adductor for varus deformity; the abductor for valgus) is left undisturbed. Although McKay's patients were predominantly affected by poliomyelitis or had postoperative clubfoot sequela, this procedure failed in only one of 17 patients. Goldner (1981) recommends balancing in cerebral palsy by transferring the flexor hallucis longus to the extensor hallucis longus, proximal to the metatarsophalangeal joint to restore the long extensor function. The tibialis anterior is transferred to the second metatarsal to remove the

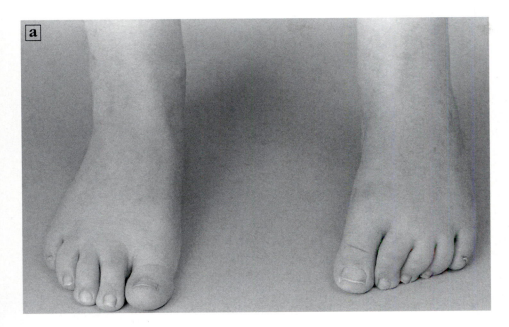

Figure 40a

Residual dorsal bunion following correction of an equinovarus foot in a hemiplegic patient. Peroneal function was weak preoperatively. The patient underwent Achilles tendon lengthening, tibialis posterior lengthening and split anterior tibialis transfer. The lateral half of the tibialis anterior transfer was not felt to be functioning, leaving some residual forefoot varus and first metatarsal elevation

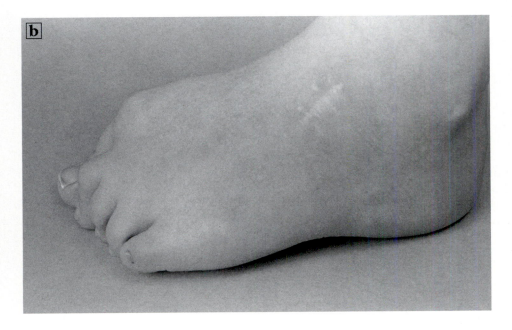

Figure 40b

Lateral view of dorsal bunion. The surgical scar for the lateral transfer of half of the tibialis anterior is visible. The muscle imbalance producing the dorsal bunion is not easily explained, but overpull of the great toe flexors following plantar flexor lengthening combined with persistent supination and dorsiflexion by the functioning medial half of the tibialis anterior, producing first metatarsal elevation, is reasonable

elevating force on the first. Release of hallux valgus as necessary is performed simultaneously. If the dorsal bunion is fixed, the correction of the metatarsal elevation by either metatarsal osteotomy or metatarsal–cuneiform fusion (Lapidus procedure) is required, with metatarsophalangeal capsulotomy to mobilize the flexed toe (Lapidus 1940, Tachdjian 1972). Bleck (1987) also adds cuneiform–navicular fusion, 'Z'-lengthening of the flexor hallucis longus tendon, and sometimes a tenotomy of the insertions of the flexor hallucis brevis muscle.

Toe deformities

Flexion deformities of the toes – claw toes and hammer toes – represent hyperflexion of the proximal inter-phalangeal joints of the toes with hyperextension of the metatarsophalangeal joints in the former, and relative neutral position of the metatarsophalangeal joints in the latter. Neither deformity is common in cerebral palsy and both are almost always due to a muscle imbalance following treatment of a deformity more proximal in the foot. Toe deformities are usually seen in adolescents and adults (Bleck 1987), where previous procedures elsewhere have led to an imbalance which, over time, develops into a toe deformity.

As described under the hallux flexus discussion, an imbalance between the toe extensors (weak) and spastic toe flexors may produce a flexed, hammer toe deformity. Such an imbalance may develop as a result of proximal transfer of the extensor digitorum longus to aid in dorsiflexion of the foot in the presence of spastic flexor

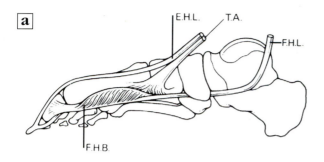

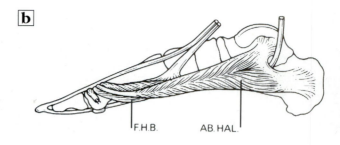

Figure 41

Soft tissue correction of hallux flexus (dorsal bunion). The flexor hallucis brevis (FHB), abductor hallucis (AB.HAL.) and adductor hallucis are transferred from the proximal phalanx to the dorsum of the first metatarsal neck, to produce active depression of the first metatarsal (after McKay 1983)

digitorum longus or intrinsics. Two solutions are recommended. In a nonfixed, dynamic deformity, tenotomy of the toe flexors distally is usually sufficient (Bleck 1987). In a fixed deformity, a standard Jones-type resection of the proximal interphalangeal joint with intramedullary pin fixation will yield stable correction (Jones 1916a).

Clawing of the toes (metatarsophalangeal hyperextension with toe flexion) is most commonly associated with a cavus or calcaneocavus deformity. Neither of these foot deformities is prominent in cerebral palsy, being more often seen in conditions with flaccid paralysis (spina bifida, Charcot–Marie–Tooth syndrome). In cerebral palsy, toe clawing associated with calcaneus might result from excessive weakening of the triceps sura, and resultant overpull of the long and short toe flexors attempting to compensate for the weakened triceps in the presence of active long toe extensors. Alternatively, if the tibialis anterior is absent, the long toe extensors, in an attempt to substitute for it, might produce clawing if the toe flexors are intact.

Indications for treatment of clawing are primarily to relieve painful callosities, either under the metatarsal heads of the plantar surface or dorsal to the interphalangeal joints, where shoeing may be difficult. Treatment of claw toes in cerebral palsy must involve restoration of the muscle balance which was disturbed to allow the metatarsophalangeal hyperextension to begin in the first place. The accompanying calcaneus deformity is often very debilitating, owing to pressure concentration on the heel and to crouch gait (Perry et al 1974, Bleck 1987). Specific surgery on the toes is designed to remove the hyperextension force by transferring the toe extensors proximal to the metatarsal necks, or by producing proximal phalangeal flexion dynamically by either tenodesis or transfer.

The Jones transfer (Jones 1916b) originally described for clawing of the great toe, removes the hyperextension pull of the long toe extensors and elevates the metatarsal head. It is useful to counteract cavus, but because the

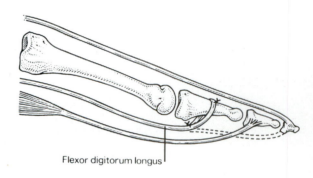

Figure 42

Flexor digitorum longus tenodesis for claw toe. The flexor digitorum longus is rerouted over the dorsum of the proximal phalanx to become a flexor of the metatarsophalangeal joint. Dorsal capsulotomy of the metatarsophalangeal joint may be necessary (after Parrish 1973)

long toe flexor is still undisturbed, interphalangeal fusion is often required to prevent flexion deformity. For this reason, tenodesis of the flexor tendon to the proximal phalanx in the great toe has been recommended by Sharrad as a simple procedure which produces active flexion at the proximal phalanx (Sharrard & Smith 1976). This counteracts the hyperextension deformity actively at the metatarsophalangeal joint. The tendon is simply exposed and fixed to the base of the proximal phalanx under the appropriate tension to correct hypertension. Dorsal capsulotomy can be utilized at the same time to obtain this correct tension of the tenodesis if necessary (Sharrard & Smith 1976). For the lateral toes, transfer of the long flexor over the dorsum of the proximal phalanx, deep to the extensor hood, by detaching the flexor distally and looping the tendon split into two tails over the proximal phalanx, is indicated (Parrish 1973) (Fig. 42). This produces dynamic depression (flexion) of the proximal phalanx provided fixed contracture is not present. Dorsal capsulotomy is again used as needed. Interphalangeal fusion is not recommended at the time of initial surgery, but is reserved for later correction of persistent interphalangeal flexion. Parrish (1973) reported 87% good or excellent results on feet with 1- to 12-year follow-up. In particular, these feet had either improvement or total resolution of callosities to obtain these ratings.

A late presentation with fixed clawing will probably be associated with a severe cavus deformity requiring metatarsal elevation by bony surgery (metatarsal or midfoot osteotomy) and toe fusion. Such a foot may also require triple arthrodesis for calcaneocavus. The management of such a foot – more of a salvage venture which should rarely be necessary in feet seen and treated early – is covered under the chapter dealing with calcaneus and cavus deformities (V.1).

References

Adelaar R S, Danelly E A, Meunier P A, et al. 1976 A long term study of triple arthrodesis in children. Orthop Clin North Am 7: 895–908

Aiona M 1990 Triple arthrodesis in cerebral palsy: long-term result. Developmental Medicine and Child Neurology 32: 23

Baker L D 1956 A rational approach to the surgical needs of the cerebral palsied patient. J Bone Joint Surg 38A: 313–323

Baker L D, Hill L M 1964 Foot alignment in the cerebral palsy patient. J Bone Joint Surg 46A: 1–15

Banks H H 1975 The Foot and Ankle in Cerebral Palsy. Orthopaedic Aspects of Cerebral Palsy. J B Lippincott, Philadelphia

Banks H H 1983 Equinus and cerebral palsy: its management. Foot Ankle 4: 149–159

Banks H H, Panagakos 1966 Orthopaedic evaluation in the lower extremity in cerebral palsy. Clin Orthop 47: 117–125

Barasso J A, Wile P B, Gage J R 1984 Extra-articular subtalar arthrodesis with internal fixation. J Pediatr Orthop 4: 555–559

Barnes M J, Herring J A 1992 Combined split anterior tibial-tendon transfer and intramuscular lengthening of the posterior tibial tendon. Bone Joint Surg 73A: 734–738

Barto P S, Supinski R S, Skinner S R 1984 Dynamic EMG findings in varus hindfoot deformity and spastic cerebral palsy. Dev Med Child Neurol 26: 88–93

Bassett F H I, Baker L D 1966 Equinus deformity in cerebral palsy. In Adams J P (ed), Current Practice in Orthopaedic Surgery. C V Mosby, St Louis. pp 59–74

Bennett G C, Rang M, Jones D 1982 Varus and valgus deformities of the foot in cerebral palsy. Dev Med Child Neurol 24: 499–505

Bisla R S, Louis H J, Albano P 1976 Transfer of the tibialis posterior in cerebral palsy. J Bone Joint Surg 58A: 497–500

Blackman J A, Reed M D, Roberts C D 1992 Muscle relaxant drugs for children with cerebral palsy. In Sussman M D (ed) The Diplegic Child: Evaluation and Management. American Academy of Orthopaedic Surgeons, Rosemont, Illinois, USA. pp. 229–239

Blair E, Stanley F 1985 Interobserver agreement in the classification of cerebral palsy. Dev Med Child Neurol 27: 615–622

Blasco P A 1992 Pathology of cerebral palsy. In Sussman M D (ed) The Diplegic Child. American Academy of Orthopaedic Surgeons: Rosemont, Illinois, USA. p. 5

Bleck E E 1984 Forefoot problems in cerebral palsy: diagnosis and management. Foot Ankle 4: 188–194

Bleck E E 1987 Orthopaedic management of cerebral palsy. In Bleck E E (ed) Clinics in Developmental Medicine. J B Lippincott, Philadelphia

Bobath B 1967 The very early treatment of cerebral palsy. Dev Med Child Neurol 9: 373–390

Boss J, Guggenheim J J, Tullos H S, Dennyson F 1983 Subtalar arthrodesis: results in 50 feet. Orthop Trans 7: 446

Brann A W, Myers R E 1975 Central nervous system findings in the newborn monkey following severe *in utero* partial asphyxia. Neurology 25: 327–338

Bratberg J J, Scheer G E 1977 Extra-articular arthrodesis of the subtalar joint: a clinical study and review. Clin Orthop 125: 220–224

Brown A 1968 A simple method of fusion of the subtalar joint in children. J Bone Joint Surg 50B: 369–371

Butler P B, Thompson N, Major R E 1992 Improvement in walking performance of children with cerebral palsy: preliminary results. Dev Med Child Neurol 34: 567–576

Campbell S K 1990 Consensus conference on efficacy of physical therapy in the management of cerebral palsy. Pediatr Physical Ther 2: 123–125

Carpenter E B, Mikhail M 1972 The use of intramuscular alcohol as a diagnostic and therapeutic aid in cerebral palsy. Dev Med Child Neurol 14: 113–114

Carpenter E B, Seitz E G 1980 Intramuscular alcohol as an aid in management of spastic cerebral palsy. Dev Med Child Neurol 22: 497–501

Coffrey R J, Cahill D, Steers W, Park T S, Ordia J 1993 Intrathecal baclofen of intractable spasticity of spinal origin: results of a long-term multicenter study. J Neurosurg 78: 226–232

Coleman S S 1983 Complex Foot Deformities in Children. Lea & Febiger, Philadelphia

Craig J J, van Vuren J 1976 The importance of gastrocnemius recession in the correction of equinus deformity in cerebral palsy. J Bone Joint Surg 58B: 84–87

Davids J R, Holland W C, Sutherland D H 1993 Significance of the confusion test in cerebral palsy. J Pediatr Orthop 13: 717–721

Delpech M J 1823 Tenotomie du tendon d'Achilles dans Chirurgie Clinique de Montpellier, ou observations et reflexions tirées des travaux de chirurgie clinique de cette école. Gabour, Paris p. 181

De Luca P A 1992 Cerebral palsy. In Drennan J C (ed) The Child's Foot and Ankle. Raven Press, New York

De Luca P A, Giachetto J, Gage J R 1988 Gait lab analysis of spastic equinus deformities: a new system of standardized assessment. Dev Med Child Neurol 30: 16–17

Dennyson W G, Fulford G E 1976 Subtalar arthrodesis by cancellous grafts and metallic internal fixation. J Bone Joint Surg 58B: 507–510

Dias L S, Marty G E 1992 Selective posterior rhizotomy. In Sussman M D (ed) Shriners Hospital for Crippled Children Symposium: The Diplegic Child. American Academy of Orthopaedic Surgeons, Rosemont, Illinois, USA. pp. 287–296

Dillin W, Samilson R L 1983 Calcaneus deformity in cerebral palsy. Foot Ankle 4: 167–170

Donovan E M, Aronson D D 1989 Serial casting for equinus contracture in children with cerebral palsy. Dev Med Child Neurol 31: 4

Dravaric D M, Schitt E W, Nakano J M 1989 The Grice extra-articular subtalar arthrodesis in the treatment of spastic hindfoot valgus deformity. Dev Med Child Neurol 31: 665–669

Drew A J 1951 The late results of arthrodesis of the foot. J Bone Joint Surg 33: 496–502

Duckworth T 1983 The hindfoot and its relation to rotational deformities of the forefoot. Clin Orthop 177: 39–48

Duncan J W, Lovell W W 1978 Hoke triple arthrodesis. J Bone Joint Surg 60A: 795–798

Duncan W R 1960 Tonic reflexes of the foot. Their orthopaedic significance in normal children and in children with cerebral palsy. J Bone Joint Surg 42A: 859–868

Duncan W R, Mott D H 1983 Foot reflexes and the use of the 'Inhibitive Cast'. Foot Ankle 4: 145–148

Dwyer F C 1959 Osteotomy of the calcaneum for pes cavus. J Bone Joint Surg 41B: 80–86

Dwyer F C 1960 Osteotomy of the Calcaneum in the Treatment of Grossly Everted Feet with Special Reference to Cerebral Palsy. Société Internationale de Chirurgie Orthopédique et de Traumatologie, Brussels. pp. 892–897

Engstrom A, Erickson U, Hjeknstedt A 1974 The results of extra-articular arthrodesis according to the Grice–Green method in cerebral palsy. Acta Orthop Scand 45: 945–951

Evans D 1975 Calcaneo-valgus deformity. J Bone Joint Surg 57B: 270–278

Evans E B 1975 The knee in cerebral palsy. In Samilson R L (ed) Orthopaedic Aspects of Cerebral Palsy. J B Lippincott, Philadelphia. pp. 173–194

Fisher R L, Shaffer S R 1970 An evaluation of calcaneal osteotomy in congenital clubfoot and other disorders. Clin Orthop 70: 141–147

Friedenburg Z B 1948 Arthrodesis of the tarsal bones. A study of failure of fusions. Arch Surg 57: 162–170

Gage J R 1991 Gait analysis in cerebral palsy. MacKeith Press, London

Garbarino J L, Clancy M 1985 A geometric method of calculating tendo-Achilles lengthening. J Pediatr Orthop 5: 573–576

Goldner J L 1981 Hallux valgus and hallux flexus associated with cerebral palsy: analysis and treatment. Clin Orthop 157: 98–104

Goldner J L 1982 Foot and ankle deformities in cerebral palsy (static encephalopathy). In Jahss M H (ed) Disorders of the Foot. W B Saunders, Philadelphia. pp. 282–334

Graham H K, Fixsen J A 1988 Lengthening of the calcaneal tendon in spastic hemiplegia by the white slide technique. J Bone Joint Surg 70B: 472–475

Grant A D, Feldman R, Lehman W B 1985 Equinus deformity in cerebral palsy: a retrospective analysis of treatment and function in 39 cases. J Pediatr Orthop 5: 678–681

Green N E, Griffin P P, Shiavi R 1983 Split posterior tibial tendon transfer in spastic cerebral palsy. J Bone Joint Surg 65A: 748–754

Grice D S 1952 An extra-articular arthrodesis of the subastragalar joint for correction of paralytic flat feet in children. J Bone Joint Surg 34A: 927–940

Grice D S 1959 The role of subtalar fusion in the treatment of valgus deformities of the feet. AAOS Instructional Course Lectures, Volume XVI. pp. 127–150

Gritzla T L, Staheli L T, Duncan W R 1972 Posterior tibial tendon transfer through the interosseous membrane to correct equinovarus deformity in cerebral palsy. Clin Orthop 89: 201–206

Gross R H 1976 A clinical study of the Batchelor subtalar arthrodesis. J Bone Joint Surg 58A: 343–349

Harris S R, Riffle K 1966 Effects of inhibitive ankle–foot orthoses on standing balance in a child with cerebral palsy. Phys Ther 66: 663–667

Hill N A, Wilson H J, Chevres R, Sweterlisch P R 1970 Triple arthrodesis in the young child. Clin Orthop 70: 187–190

Hoffer M M, Perry J 1983 Pathodynamics of gait alterations in cerebral palsy and the significance of kinetic electromyography in evaluating foot and ankle problems. Foot Ankle 4: 128–134

Hoffer M M, Garakat G, Koffman M 1985 10-year follow-up of split anterior tibial tendon transfer in cerebral palsied patients with spastic equinovarus deformity. J Pediatr Orthop 5: 432–434

Hoffer M M, Garrett A, Koffman M 1974 New concepts in orthotics of cerebral palsy. Clin Orthop Rel Res 102: 100–107

Hoffer M M, Reisweig J A, Garrett A M, Perry J 1974 The split anterior tibial tendon transfer in the treatment of spastic varus hindfoot of childhood. Orthop Clin North Am 5: 31–37

Hoke M 1921 An operation for stabilizing paralytic feet. J Orthop Surg 3: 494–505

Holstein A 1980 Hallux valgus: an acquired deformity of the foot in cerebral palsy. Foot Ankle 1: 33–38

Horstmann H M, Eilert R E 1977 Triple arthrodesis in cerebral palsy. Orthop Trans 1: 109

Hsu LC S, O'Brien J P, Yau A C M C, Hodgson A R 1976 Batchelor's extra-articular subtalar arthrodesis. A report of sixty-four procedures in patients with poliomyelitis deformities. J Bone Joint Surg 58A: 243–247

Hsu L C S, Yau A C M C, O'Brien J P, Hodgson A R 1972 Valgus deformity of the ankle resulting from fibular resection for a graft in subtalar fusion in children. J Bone Joint Surg 54A: 585–594

Hutton W C, Dhanendran M 1981 The mechanics of normal and hallux valgus feet: a quantitative study. Clin Orthop 157: 7–13

Ireland M L, Hoffer M 1985 Triple arthrodesis for children with spastic cerebral palsy. Dev Med Child Neurol 27: 623–627

Johnson W L, Lester E L 1989 Transposition of the posterior tibial tendon. Clin Orthop Rel Res 245: 223-227

Johnston C E I, Schutte J 1984 The Grice operation in cerebral palsy. Orthopaedics 7: 1223–1227

Jones R 1916a The soldier's foot and the treatment of common deformities of the foot. Part III: Hammertoe. BMJ 1: 782–785

Jones R 1916b The soldier's foot and the treatment of common deformities of the foot. Part II: Clawfoot. BMJ 1: 749–753

Kadaba M P, Wootten M E, Gainey J, Cochran G V B 1984 Repeatability of phasic muscle activity: performance of surface and intramuscular wire electrodes in gait analysis. J Orthop Res 3: 350–359

Kaufer H 1977 Split tendon transfers. Orthop Trans 1: 191

Keats S, 1974 Warning: serious complications caused by re-routing of the peroneus longus and brevis tendons in performing the Grice procedure in cerebral palsy. J Bone Joint Surg 56A: 1304

Keats S, Kouten J 1968 Early surgical correction of the planovalgus foot in cerebral palsy. Clin Orthop 61: 223–233

Kling T F J, Hensinger R N 1983 The results of split posterior tibial tendon transfer in children with cerebral palsy. Orthop Trans 7: 186–187

Knutson L M, Clark D E 1991 Orthotic devices for ambulation in children with cerebral palsy and myelomeningocele. Phys Ther 71: 947–960

Koman L A, Monney J F, Smith B, Goodman A, Mulvaney T 1993 Management of cerebral palsy with botulinum-A toxin: preliminary investigation. J Pediatr Orthop 13: 489–495

Koutsogiannis E 1971 Treatment of mobile flat foot by displacement osteotomy of the calcaneus. J Bone Joint Surg 53B: 96–100

Krebs D E, Edelstein J E, Fishman S 1985 Reliability of observational kinematic gait analysis. Phys Ther 65: 1027–1033

Kuban K C K, Leviton A 1994 Cerebral palsy. N Engl J Med 330: 188–195

Lahdenranta U, Pylkkanen P 1972 Subtalar extra-articular fusion in the treatment of valgus and varus deformities in children. Acta Orthop Scand 43: 438–460

Langenskiold A 1967 Pseudoarthrosis of the fibula and progressive valgus deformity of the ankle in children: treatment by fusion of the distal tibial and fibular metaphysis. Review of three cases. J Bone Joint Surg 49A: 463–470

Lapidus P W 1940 Dorsal bunion: its mechanics and operative correction. J Bone Joint Surg 22: 627–637

Lee L C, Bleck E E 1980 Surgical correction of equinus deformity in cerebral palsy. Dev Med Child Neurol 22: 287–292

Majestro T C, Ruda R, Frost H M 1971 Intramuscular lengthening of the posterior tibialis muscle. Clin Orthop 79: 59–60

Malekafzali S, Rosenthal R K 1981 Triple arthrodesis in cerebral palsy. Orthop Trans 5: 192

Mann R A 1980 Surgical implications of biomechanics of the foot and ankle. Clin Orthop 146: 111–118

McKay D W 1983 Dorsal bunions in children. J Bone Joint Surg 65A: 975–980

McKeever D C 1952 Arthrodesis of the first metatarsophalangeal joint for hallux valgus, hallux rigidus and metatarsus primus varus. J Bone Joint Surg 34: 129–134

Medina P A, Karpman R R, Yeung A T 1989 Split posterior tibial tendon transfer for spastic equinovarus foot deformity. Foot Ankle 10: 65–67

Miller G M, Hsu J D, Hoffer M M, Rentfro R 1982 Posterior tibial tendon transfer: a review of the literature and analysis of 74 procedures. J Pediatr Orthop 2: 363–370

Minear W L 1956 A classification of cerebral palsy. Pediatrics 18: 841

Mital M D, McCarthy J 1982 Experience with split tibialis anterior transfer in treatment of foot varus in spastic neuromuscular conditions. Orthop Trans 6: 119

Mitchell G P 1977 Posterior displacement osteotomy of the calcaneus. J Bone Joint Surg 59B: 233–235

Moreland J R, Westin G W 1986 Further experience with Grice subtalar arthrodesis. Clin Orthop Rel Res 207: 113–121

Mosca V S 1995 Calcaneal lengthening for valgus deformity of the hindfoot. Results in children who had severe, symptomatic flatfoot and skewfoot. J Bone Joint Surg 77A: 500–512

Mossberg K A, Linton K A, Friske K 1990 Ankle–foot orthoses: effect on energy expenditure of gait in spastic diplegic children. Arch Phys Med Rehabil 71: 490–494

Mott D H, Yates L 1981 An appraisal of inhibitive casting as an adjunct to the total management of the child with cerebral palsy. In American Academy of Cerebral Palsy and Developmental Medicine. Detroit

Mowery C A, Roach J W, Herring J A 1988 Long term followup of bunionectomy in children and adolescents. Orthop Trans 12: 714

Mutch L 1992 Cerebral palsy epidemiology: where are we now and where are we going. Dev Med Child Neurol 34: 547–555

Nakano J S, Schmitt E W J 1983 The Grice extra-articular subtalar arthrodesis in spasticity. Orthop Trans 7: 188–189

Nather A, Fulfort G E, Stewart K 1984 Treatment of valgus hindfoot in cerebral palsy by peroneus brevis lengthening. Dev Med Child Neurol 26: 335–340

Nelson K B, Ellenberg J H 1982 Children who "outgrew" cerebral palsy. Pediatrics 69: 529–536

Nelson K B, Ellenberg J H 1986 Antecedents of cerebral palsy. N Engl J Med 315: 81–86

Olney B W, Williams P F, Menelaus M B 1988 Treatment of spastic equinus by aponeurosis lengthening. J Pediatr Orthop 8: 422–425

Oppenheim W L, Staudt L A, Peacock W J 1992 The rationale for rhizotomy. In Sussman M D (ed) Shriners Hospital for Crippled Children Symposium: the Diplegic Child. American Academy of Orthopaedic Surgeons, Rosemont, Illinois, USA. pp. 271–285

Otis J C, Root L, Kroll M A 1985 Measurement of plantar flexor spasticity during treatment with tone-reducing casts. J Pediatr Orthop 5: 682–686

Palmer F B, Shaprio B K, Wachtel R C 1988 The effects of physical therapy on cerebral palsy: a controlled trial in infants with spastic diplegia. N Engl J Med 31: 803–808

Paluska D J, Bount W P 1986 Ankle valgus after the Grice subtalar stabilization: the late evaluation of a personal series with a modified technique. Clin Orthop 59: 137–146

Parrish T F 1973 Dynamic correction of clawtoes. Orthop Clin North Am 4: 97–102

Patterson R L J, Parrish F F, Hathaway E N 1950 Stabilizing operations on the foot. A study of the indications, techniques used, and end results. J Bone Joint Surg 32A: 1–26

Peacock W J, Arens L J 1982 Selective posterior rhizotomy for the relief of spasticity in cerebral palsy. S Afr Med J 62: 119–124

Penn R D 1992 Intrathecal baclofen for spasticity of spinal origin: seven years of experience. J Neurosurg 74: 236–240

Penn R D, Kroin J S 1985 Continuous intrathecal baclofen for severe spasticity. Lancet 2: 125–127

Penn R D, Savory S M, Corcos D 1989 Intrathecal baclofen for severe spinal spasticity. N Engl J Med 320: 1517–1521

Perry J 1992 Gait Analysis: Normal and Pathologic Function. Slack Publishing, Thorofare, New Jersey, USA

Perry J, Hoffer M M 1977 Preoperative and postoperative dynamic electromyography as an aid in planning tendon transfers in children with cerebral palsy. J Bone Joint Surg 59A: 531–537

Perry J, Antonelli D, Ford W 1975 Analysis of knee-joint forces during flexed-knee stance. J Bone Joint Surg 57A: 961–967

Perry J, Hoffer M, Antonelli D J P, et al 1976 Electromyography before and after surgery for hip deformity in children with cerebral palsy. J Bone Joint Surg 58A: 201–208

Perry J, Hoffer M, Giovan P, Antonelli D, Greenberg R 1974 Gait analysis of the triceps surae in cerebral palsy. J Bone Joint Surg 56A: 511–520

Phillips G E 1983 A review of elongation of os calcis for flat feet. J Bone Joint Surg 65B: 15–18

Pierrot A H, Murphy O B Heel cord advancement. A new approach to the spastic equinus deformity. Proc Am Foot Soc 5: 117–126

Pollock J H, Carrell B 1964 Subtalar extra-articular arthrodesis in the treatment of paralytic valgus deformities. A review of 112 procedures in 100 patients. J Bone Joint Surg 46A: 533–541

Rang M 1990 Cerebral palsy. In Morrissy R T (ed) Lovell and Winter's Pediatric Orthopaedics. J B Lippincott, Philadelphia. pp 465–506

Renshaw T S, Sirkin R B, Drennan J C 1979 The management of hallux valgus in cerebral palsy. Dev Med Child Neurol 21: 202–208

Ricks N R, Eilert R E 1993 Effects of inhibitory casts and orthoses on bony alignment of foot and ankle during weight-bearing in children with spasticity. Dev Med Child Neurol 35: 11–16

Root L, Kirz P 1982 The results of posterior tibial tendon surgery in 83 patients with cerebral palsy. Orthop Trans 6: 118–119

Rose S A, DeLuca P A, Davis R B, Ounpuu S, Gage J R 1993 Kinematic and kinetic evaluation of the ankle after lengthening of the gastrocnemius fascia in children with cerebral palsy. J Pediatr Orthop 13: 727–732

Rosenthal R K 1984 The use of orthotics in foot and ankle problems in cerebral palsy. Foot Ankle 4: 195–200

Rosenthal R K, Candage R C 1983 Extra-articular subtalar arthrodesis in cerebral palsy. Orthop Trans 7: 189

Ross P M, Lyne E D 1980 The Grice procedure. Indications and evaluation of long-term results. Clin Orthop 153: 194–200

Ruda R, Frost H M 1971 Cerebral palsy. Spastic varus and forefoot adductus treated by intramuscular posterior tibial tendon lengthening. Clin Orthop 79: 61–70

Rush G A I 1983 Split anterior tibial tendon transfer. Contemp Orthop 7: 51–57

Ryerson E W 1923 Arthrodesing operations on the feet. J Bone Joint Surg 5: 453–471

Samilson R L 1976 Crescentic osteotomy of the os calcis for calcaneocavus feet. In: Bateman J E (ed) Foot Science. W B Saunders, Philadelphia. pp. 18–25

Samilson R L, Hoffer M M 1975 Problems and complications in orthopaedic management of cerebral palsy. In Samilson R L (ed) Orthopaedic Aspects of Cerebral Palsy. J B Lippincott, Philadelphia. pp. 258–281

Schneider M, Balon K 1977 Deformity of the foot following anterior transfer of the posterior tibial tendon and lengthening of the Achilles tendon for spastic equinovarus. Clin Orthop 125: 113–118

Scrutton D, Gilbertson M 1975 The physiotherapist's role in the treatment of cerebral palsy. In Samilson R L (ed) Orthopaedic Aspects of Cerebral Palsy. J B Lippincott, Philadelphia. pp 98–111

Seaquist J L, Hoffer M M, Koffman M 1977 Surgical correction of hallux valgus in cerebral palsy. Orthop Trans 1: 237

Segal L S, Sienko Thomas S E, Mazur J M, Mauterer M 1989 Calcaneal gait in spastic diplegia after heelcord lengthening: a study with gait analysis. J Pediatr Orthop 9: 697–701

Seitz D G, Carpenter E B 1974 Triple arthrodesis in children: a ten-year review. South Med J 67: 1420–1424

Seymour N, Evans D K 1968 A modification of the Grice subtalar arthrodesis. J Bone Joint Surg 50B: 369–371

Sharrard W J, Bernstein S 1972 Equinus deformity in cerebral palsy: a comparison between elongation of the tendo calcaneus and gastrocnemius recession. J Bone Joint Surg 54B: 272–276

Sharrard W J W, Smith T W D 1976 Tenodesis of flexor hallucis longus for paralytic clawing of the hallux in childhood. J Bone Joint Surg 58B: 224–226

Silfverskiold N 1924 Reduction of the uncrossed two-joint muscles of the leg to one-joint muscles in spastic conditions. Acta Chir Scand 56: 315–330

Silver C M, Simon S D 1959 Gastrocnemius-muscle recession (Silfverskiold operation) for spastic equinus deformity in cerebral palsy. J Bone Joint Surg 41: 1021–1028

Silver C M, Simon S D, Litchman H M 1974 Long term follow-up observations on calcaneal osteotomy. Clin Orthop 99: 181–187

Silver C M, Simon S D, Spindell E, Litchman H M, Scala M 1967 Calcaneal osteotomy for valgus and varus deformities of the foot in cerebral palsy: a preliminary report on twenty-seven operations. J Bone Joint Surg 49A: 232–246

Simon S R, Deutsch S D, Nuzzo R M, et al 1978 Genu recurvatum in spastic cerebral palsy. Report on findings by gait analysis. J Bone Joint Surg 60A: 822–894

Skinner S R, Lesater D K 1985 Dynamic EMG findings in valgus hindfoot deformity in spastic cerebral palsy. Orthop Trans 9: 91

Skinner S R, Antonelli D, Perry J, Lester D K 1985 Functional demands on the stance limb in walking. Orthopedics 8: 355–361

Smith J B, Westin G W 1968 Subtalar extra-articular arthrodesis. J Bone Joint Surg 50A: 1027–1035

Smith T W D, Baker R H, Heaney S H, Leysham A 1976 The course of treated and untreated equinovalgus deformity of the foot in cerebral palsy. J Bone Joint Surg 58B: 133–134

Snyder M, Kkumar S J, Stecyk M D 1993 Split tibialis posterior tendon transfer and tendo-Achillis lengthening for spastic equino-varus feet. J Pediatr Orthop 13: 20–23

Southwell R B, Sherman F C 1981 Triple arthrodesis: a long term study with force plant analysis. Foot Ankle 2: 15–23

Staheli L 1977 The prone hip extension test. Clin Orthop 123: 12–15

Stayer L M 1958 Gastrocnemius recession. Five-year report of cases. J Bone Joint Surg 40: 1019–1030

Strecker W B, Via M W, Oliver S K, Schoenecker P L 1990 Heel cord advancement for treatment of equinus deformity in cerebral palsy. J Pediatr Orthop 10: 105–108

Sussman M D 1983 Casting as an adjunct to neurodevelopmental therapy for cerebral palsy. Dev Med Child Neurol 25: 804–805

Sussman M, Cusick B 1979 Preliminary report. The role of short-leg tone-reducing casts as an adjunct to physical therapy of patients with cerebral palsy. Johns Hopkins Med J, 145: 112–114

Tachdjian M O 1972 Pediatric Orthopedics. W B Saunders, Philadelphia. pp. 788–799

Tenuta J, Shelton Y A, Miller F 1993 Long-term follow-up of triple arthrodesis in patients with cerebral palsy. J Pediatr Orthop 13: 713–716

Throop F B, De Rosa G P, Reech C, Waterman S 1975 Correction of equinus in cerebral palsy by the Murphy procedure of tendo calcaneus advancement: a preliminary communication. Dev Med Child Neurol 17: 182–185

Tohen A C J, Chow L, Rosas J 1969 Extra-articular subtalar arthrodesis: a review of 286 operations. J Bone Joint Surg 51B: 45–52

Tohen F A, Cameron F J, Barrera J R 1966 The utilization of abnormal reflexes in the treatment of spastic foot deformities. Clin Orthop 47: 77–84

Trieshmann H, Millis M, Hall J, Watts H 1980 Sliding calcaneal osteotomy for treatment of hindfoot deformity. Orthop Trans 4: 305

Turner J W, Cooper R R 1972 Anterior transfer of the tibialis posterior through the interosseous membrane. Clin Orthop 83: 241–244

Vaughn C L, Nashman J H, Murr M S 1992 What is the Normal Function of Tibialis Posterior in Human Gait? American Academy of Orthopaedic Surgeons, Rosemont, Illinois, USA

Wasylenko M, Skinner S R, Perry J, Antonelli D J 1983 An analysis of posture and gait following spinal fusion with Harrington instrumentation. Spine 8: 840–845

Watkins M B, Jones J B, Ryder G T, Brown T H 1954 Transplantation of the posterior tibial tendon. J Bone Joint Surg 36A: 1181–1189

Watt J E A 1986 A prospective study of inhibitive casting as an adjunct to physiotherapy for cerebral-palsied children. Dev Med Child Neurol 28: 480–488

Westin G W, Dye S 1983 Conservative management of cerebral palsy in the growing child. Foot Ankle 4: 160–163

White J W 1943 Torsion of the Achilles tendon: its surgical significance. Arch Surg 46: 784–787

Williams P F 1976 Restoration of muscle balance of the foot by transfer of the tibialis posterior. J Bone Joint Surg 58B: 217–219

Willis C A, Hoffer M M, Perry J 1988 A comparison of foot-switch and EMG analysis of varus deformities of the feet of children with cerebral palsy. Dev Med Child Neurol 30: 227–231

Wilson F C J, Fay G F, Lamotte P, Williams J C 1965 Triple arthrodesis: a study of the factors affecting fusion after three hundred and one procedures. J Bone Joint Surg 47A: 340–348

Wiltse L L 1972 Valgus deformities of the ankle. A sequel to acquired or congenital abnormalities of the fibula. J Bone Joint Surg 54A: 595–606

Winters T F, Gage J R, Hicks R 1987 Gait patterns in spastic hemiplegia in children and young adults. J Bone Joint Surg 69: 437–441

Ziv I, Blackburn N, Rang M, Koreska J 1984 Muscle growth in normal and spastic mice. Dev Med Child Neurol 26: 94–99

IV.5 Tendon Transfer

Charles S B Galasko

Orthopaedic surgery has changed markedly during the past 30 years. However, tendon transfer has stood the test of time during this period. In many instances the same tendons are transferred and the same technique of transfer is used, but transfers are much less commonly performed. This is probably because of the virtual elimination of poliomyelitis and its sequelae in the developed world. As a result, many orthopaedic trainees today obtain very little practical experience in tendon transfer during their orthopaedic training.

Tendon transfer is a procedure by which the tendon is detached from its normal attachment and transferred to another location so that its muscle action may be substituted for another muscle. Tendon transfer is different to tendon transplantation, which refers to excision of all or part of a tendon as a free transplant to be used elsewhere. Recent advances in microvascular and microneurological surgery have allowed transfer of muscle and tendon units from one limb to another, re-establishing vascular and neurological continuity of remarkable success in some instances. However, this is not a tendon transfer.

Hundreds of different procedures have been described. It is not possible, within the confines of this chapter, to describe all the variations or to give details of any particular surgical procedure; however, the principles will be described.

In many instances the tendon transfer is part of a more complex operation. For example, severe rigid equinus in some neuromuscular disorders may be best treated by a combination of elongation of the Achilles tendon, tenotomy of extensor hallucis longus and flexor digitorum longus, and posterior ankle and subtalar capsulotomies, in addition to transfer of the tibialis posterior tendon. A tendon transfer may also be used to maintain the position after a deformity has been surgically corrected by soft tissue release, osteotomy, or wedge tarsectomy. If the deformity was secondary to muscle imbalance, correction of the deformity will not stop it from recurring unless the muscle pull across the joint is also balanced.

Tendon transfers are not limited to any age group. In young children, if complete stabilization is not obtained by redistributing the muscle pull, deformity may be preventable by using orthoses until the patient is old enough for arthrodesis.

The loss of original function resulting from tendon transfers must be balanced against potential gains. For example, an injudicious tibialis anterior transfer in a patient with functioning peroneal muscles may result in an iatrogenic planovalgus deformity.

Surgery only forms part of the management of foot deformity, particularly in patients with neuromuscular disorders, and tendon transfer only forms part of the surgical procedures required. However, the procedure may restore both balance and function.

Indications

Restoration of function following a ruptured tendon where repair of the tendon is not possible

For example, it may not be possible to repair an attrition rupture of tibialis posterior, which will result in a progressive valgus deformity. Normally the muscle inverts the foot during plantar flexion. The long flexors are unable to prevent the valgus deformity because of their lateral position. Since most of the functions of the foot are carried out during plantar flexion, loss of the tibialis posterior is a severe impairment. It is also the principal support for the arch of the foot, as its tendon divides and inserts into the navicular, the second, third and fourth metatarsals, the medial and intermediate cuneiforms and the sustentaculum tali. When the support is lost the arch collapses, the valgus deformity gradually increases and this may be painful.

A number of tendon transfers have been described to restore the function of the tibialis posterior, including transfer of flexor digitorum longus or flexor hallucis longus (see Chapter V.2). The additional use of an orthosis may be helpful in protecting the transfer.

Provision for deficient motor function following paralysis of a particular muscle or muscle group

Damage to the lateral popliteal nerve may result in a foot drop. Transfer of the tibialis posterior tendon may restore active dorsiflexion and avoid the necessity for an orthosis. It removes a dynamic deforming force and aids in active dorsiflexion, but active dorsiflexion may not be restored satisfactorily by this transfer alone.

Correction of muscle imbalance

There are several causes for the deformity that frequently occurs in patients with neuromuscular disease. Probably the most important cause is muscle imbalance, the joint being pulled in the direction of the more powerful muscle. Initially, this deformity is purely muscular, but if it is allowed to persist for any length of time the soft tissues on the contracted side of the joint thicken and a secondary soft tissue contracture occurs. Whereas initially it may be possible to correct the deformity by re-balancing the muscles, once a secondary soft tissue contracture has developed it must be released prior to rebalancing the muscle actions across the joint.

In a growing child, the bone can also be deformed if the tendons are attached distal to a growth plate. Not only is the joint pulled in the direction of the more powerful muscle, but the bone is also moulded in that direction. Under these circumstances a corrective osteotomy is required before rebalancing the muscles.

Although deformity tends not to occur when muscles are balanced, whether they be the hypertrophied muscles of a body builder, normal muscles, or weakened muscles, if the muscles are very weak gravity may cause deformity. For example, equinus and equinovarus deformities occur commonly in individuals with virtually flail feet, where the feet are not adequately supported by the footplates of their wheelchair.

In patients with flail feet, the weight of the bed clothes may be sufficient to produce an equinus deformity. This can be prevented by an ankle–foot orthosis (AFO) used to hold the foot and ankle in a neutral position.

Abnormal muscle may not grow at the same rate as the adjacent bone. This may explain the high rate of recurrence of deformity in growing children following correction of the deformity, e.g. recurrence of equinus following elongation of the Achilles tendon.

Movement is produced by coordinated muscle activity. The plantar flexor muscles are the triceps surae, tibialis posterior, flexor hallucis longus, flexor digitorum longus, peroneus longus, and peroneus brevis. The dorsiflexors are the tibialis anterior, extensor hallucis longus, extensor digitorum longus, and peroneus tertius. Inversion is produced by tibialis posterior, tibialis anterior, and flexor hallucis longus. Eversion is produced by peroneus longus, peroneus brevis, extensor digitorum longus, and peroneus tertius.

Muscle transfer is carried out to prevent development of contracture, to achieve balance between dorsiflexion and plantar flexion, as well as between inversion and eversion, and to re-establish a walking pattern that is as normal as possible. Bony procedures are generally delayed until the patient reaches approximately 12–15 years, when foot growth is adequate. These procedures are carried out to prevent or correct deformity, or to achieve stability.

When one muscle is paralysed, the other muscles in the group become over-reactive. For example, in paralysis of the tibialis anterior, the long toe extensors, which normally function as auxiliary dorsiflexors, become over-reactive during the swing phase, resulting in hyper-extension at the metatarsophalangeal joints with depression of the metatarsal heads. An anterior transfer of the peroneus longus to the base of the second metatarsal with suture of the peroneus brevis to the distal stump of the peroneus longus in order to preserve the activity of the peroneus longus on the first metatarsal and prevent formation of a dorsal bunion, may rebalance the foot. Alternatively, the extensor digitorum longus may be transferred to the dorsum of the mid-foot to supply active dorsiflexor power.

Surgery and anaesthesia are not without their risks, particularly in this group of patients, and therefore there must be definite indications for surgery.

Deformity interfering with movement

Probably the commonest indication for surgery in this group of patients is a deformity that interferes with locomotion. Patients with neuromuscular disease are weaker than their normal peers. Their gait is frequently not as good and in many conditions they may have great difficulty with independent ambulation. The development of an equinus deformity may make the difference between a patient being independently mobile or not. It is much more difficult to balance on one's tiptoes than to walk with plantigrade feet.

Pain

Some of the deformities are painful.

Pressure areas

Pressure areas may produce local discomfort, pain or tenderness; sometimes the pressure is sufficient to produce a pressure sore.

Quality of life

Some deformity interferes with the quality of life. For example, many patients with Duchenne dystrophy develop equinovarus deformities once they go off their feet and are confined to a wheelchair. In most patients this can be controlled with the use of an AFO, but sometimes the deformity becomes so severe that no shoes or boots can be fitted, including bespoke footwear. Under these circumstances, correction of the deformity may be required to allow the fitting of shoes that are comfortable, without which the patient may feel very self-conscious and may even refuse to go out of doors in his wheelchair. See Fig. 1.

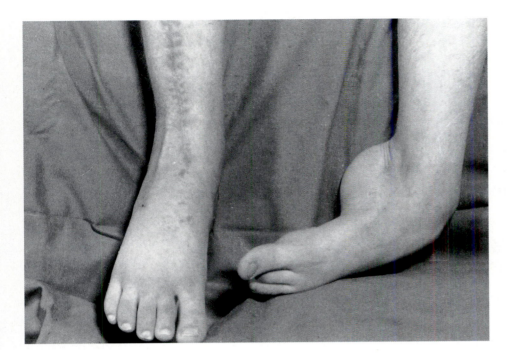

Figure 1
Patient with Duchenne muscular dystrophy when he was admitted for corrective surgery to his left foot. He had a severe equinovarus deformity and 3 months previously had undergone corrective surgery on the right side with elongation of the Achilles tendon, division of the flexor hallucis longus and flexor digitorum longus, posterior capsulotomies of the ankle and subtalar joints, and transfer of the tibialis posterior tendon through the intermuscular septum. The active tendon transfer can be seen, under the skin, when he was asked to dorsiflex his right ankle

Correction of deformity

Mobile clawed toes may be corrected by a flexor to extensor transfer. A mobile hyperextended great toe may be corrected by a Jones procedure, whereby the tendon of extensor hallucis longus is transferred to the first metatarsal, and the interphalangeal joint of the great toe is either arthrodesed or tenodesed (if the growth plate is still open).

Creation of a plantigrade foot in a patient with loss of sensation

Patients with spina bifida and some forms of hereditary motor sensory neuropathy (including the so called 'congenital insensitivity to pain') may develop deformity as well as anaesthesia. The combination may result in the development of trophic ulcers over prominent bones. It may not be possible to prevent recurrence of trophic ulceration without correcting the deformity, balancing the foot, and creating a plantigrade foot.

Stabilization of a joint

Tendon transfers may be used to stabilize a joint; the use of peroneus brevis for chronic lateral collateral instability of the ankle is one example of this. Several techniques have been described, including the

Watson–Jones and Evans procedures. The Watson–Jones procedure uses the tendon of peroneus brevis to reconstruct the anterior talofibular and calcaneofibular ligaments; the Evans technique reconstructs only the calcaneofibular ligament. In both these procedures, the tendon is divided at the musculotendinous junction, the severed end of the muscle belly is sutured to the adjacent peroneus longus tendon, and the freed tendon of peroneus brevis is passed through tunnels drilled in the fibular and talus (Watson–Jones), or the fibular only (Evans) before being sutured to itself and periosteum on the lateral malleolus (Watson–Jones), or soft tissue at both ends of the tunnel (Evans). In both procedures, the aim of the operation is to produce a tenodesis and not an active functioning musculotendinous unit.

Maintenance of position after correction of a deformity

The tendon transfer may be part of a more major operation, which may include bony procedures. Peabody (1938) examined 215 patients who had undergone a tendon transfer 3–10 years previously. He found a strong functioning transfer in 90%. He also concluded that it was essential to determine whether the deformity was static or dynamic. When the deformity was dynamic, arthrodesis alone would not prevent its recurrence in a growing child, and some form of muscle balancing procedure had to be carried out also. If the deformity was static (e.g. an almost flail planovalgus deformity), recurrence was unusual after fusion or a blocking procedure. Frequently, both elements were present – for example, in a planovalgus deformity with strong peroneal muscles, if the dynamic element was overlooked the deformity may have recurred following arthrodesis.

When the deformity is dynamic, the muscle imbalance must be corrected.

Temporizing procedure in a growing child

A tendon transfer may be used as a temporizing procedure in a growing child when the more definitive procedure may affect the growth of the foot. For example, patients with hereditary motor sensory neuropathy frequently develop a pes cavus deformity. Once growth has ceased, a severe fixed pes cavus deformity is probably best treated by a triple arthrodesis. Such an operation carried out in childhood is likely to have a significant effect on the growth of the foot. A soft tissue procedure including a Steindler release of the plantar structures, a Jones procedure to the first ray with transfer of the tendon of extensor hallucis longus to the first metatarsal and tenodesis of the interphalangeal joint of the great toe, and transfer of extensor digitorum longus into the forefoot, or transfer of tibialis posterior may be sufficient to correct the deformity (providing it is still mobile), and to maintain the correction for some years. However, the cavus deformity may recur with growth, and a subsequent triple arthrodesis may still become necessary.

Principles of technique

1. Absence of joint contractures. It is an essential prerequisite of tendon transfer that the joint to be moved by the transferred musculotendinous unit should have a free range of passive movement. Any fixed deformity of the joint must be corrected before transfer. This may require soft tissue release, osteotomy or wedge tarsectomy. A transferred muscle cannot be expected to correct a fixed deformity. Satisfactory function across a reasonably normal joint is all that can be expected.
2. Sufficient power and cross-sectional area in the transferred muscle to perform its expected function. The muscle to be transferred must have sufficient power to carry out the intended function. Muscles usually drop one MRC grade of power following the transfer. Therefore, the minimum power in the transferred muscle should be Grade 4 on the MRC scale. A muscle of power of Grade 3 or less may act as a

tenodesis after it is transferred but will not act as an active transfer. The muscle to be transferred must be strong enough to do reasonably well what the paralysed muscle did, or to supplement the power of a partially paralysed muscle. However, the transfer may fail or the muscle may only function for a short time and then, because of overstretching, lose its power.

The ideal muscle for a tendon transfer would be equal in strength and cross-sectional size to the paralysed muscle.

3. The amplitude of the pull of the transferred tendon should be about that of the tendon replaced.
4. The excursion of the transferred musculotendinous unit should be adequate and it should have no scarring or adhesions.
5. The tendon to be transferred should have, whenever possible, a range of excursions similar to the one it is reinforcing or replacing.
6. Whenever possible the line of pull of the transferred tendon should be straight. Power is lost by routing tendons around pulleys or angles.
7. The transferred tendon should pass in a direct line through subcutaneous fat or through a tendon sheath, in order to maintain mobility and to minimize the risk of adhesion. If it is left in normal muscle planes it may become adherent, leading to limited excursion.
8. Whenever possible phasic muscle should be transferred, since nonphasic muscles usually function as tenodeses. Dynamic electromyography has highlighted those muscles that act synchronously during movement. Gait analysis, with dynamic electromyography, has helped us understand much more about the phasic activities of muscles. For example, in the swing phase of walking, the foot and ankle dorsiflexors and evertors fire together while the calf is electrically quiet. It has been suggested that any muscle to be transferred should act phasically with the one whose action is to be supplemented. In general terms, the anterior muscles of the leg are predominantly swing-phase muscles, and the posterior muscles (flexors) are stance-phase muscles. Phasic transfers retain their preoperative phasic activity, and regain their preoperative duration of contraction. Nonphasic transfers (muscles transferred from stance-phase to swing-phase functions or *vice versa*) retain their preoperative phasic activity and may fail to assume the action of the muscles for which they are substituted. Some nonphasic transfers are capable of phasic conversion and careful postoperative rehabilitation is essential in these patients. However, an antiphasic transfer often functions only as a tenodesis.

A mixture of phasic and nonphasic transfers dooms the latter to failure of phasic conversion unless the transfer is done as a separate second procedure.

Postoperative bracing, which may be helpful in retaining physiological length of the muscle, has no effect on phasic conversion.

9. Ideally, the transfer should cross only one joint. Occasionally, however, it may have to cross more than one joint.

10. The musculotendinous transfer should only be asked to perform one function.

11. The unit should be attached under appropriate tension. The amount of tension is important and should be at least equivalent to an MRC Grade 4. It requires considerable judgement to find the optimal tension. As a general rule, tautness of a flexor tendon should be such that the joint lies in the neutral position, whereas an extensor tendon should be stretched tight. If the tension is insufficient, energy will be used in taking up the slack in the musculotendinous unit rather than in producing the desired effect.

12. The best results are achieved when the tendon is inserted directly in bone through a drill hole. Subperiosteal attachment is also satisfactory. When the transfer is sutured to another tendon, stretching may occur.

13. The freed end of the transferred tendon should be attached close to the insertion of the tendon whose muscle function is to be undertaken.

14. The transferred tendon should retain its own sheath.

15. The nerve and blood supply to the transferred muscle must not be impaired or traumatized in making the transfer.

16. Transfers through interosseous membranes should be avoided, but occasionally they are essential if the line of the pull is to be as direct as possible (e.g. transfer of the tibialis posterior to create a dorsiflexor of the ankle). The window resected in the interosseous membrane must be large enough to allow the tendon to glide without bending and to allow muscle fibres, rather than tendon, to be in contact with the interosseous membrane. These transfers may function as a tenodesis rather than as an active transfer. Routing a tendon through tunnels in fascia or bone is not usually wise because scar tissue and adhesions will rapidly form. Tendons passed under deep fascia retinacula frequently become adherent and function only as passive tenodeses.

17. Accurate preoperative evaluation is essential in the selection of an appropriate transfer. The advantage of the transfer and effective removal of a deforming force must be balanced against the loss of the original function.

18. Care must be taken not to produce the reverse deformity. Removal and transfer of a deforming force on one side of a joint may produce the reversed deformity, especially in cerebral palsy. For example, combined elongation of the Achilles tendon and tibialis posterior transfer for an equinus deformity may result in a calcaneus deformity. The aim is to balance the muscle action.

19. The removal of a muscle without consideration of the strength of its antagonist may lead to the development of a secondary iatrogenic deformity. The transfer of peroneus longus in the presence of a strong anterior tibialis results in a dorsal bunion as the foot supinates. It must therefore be combined with a lateral transfer of the tibialis anterior to the base of the second metatarsal.

20. The tendon transfer should be immobilized for a minimum of 3–4 weeks with the joint held in a slightly overcorrected position, followed by 3 weeks of carefully guarded motion before protective functional activity is allowed. The limb is supported by a bivalved plaster or orthosis except during exercise periods until there is no tendency towards recurrence of the deformity. The cast or orthosis is then discontinued gradually during the day, but prolonged use of an orthosis is advisable to prevent contracture. Exercises against resistance are initiated when the transfer attains the normal range of movement and fair strength. The final stage of training is the incorporation of the transfer into a functional pattern, such as gait. An orthosis should be used until the transfer has achieved adequate muscle power to assume its intended function.

21. Careful re-education of the transplanted muscle is important.

22. The tendon-balancing operation may be combined with fusion at a single operation.

23. If the deformity is primarily static, tendon transfers alone will be insufficient and a fusion is also required. However, a static deformity may be controlled mechanically without transfers until arthrodesis is feasible.

24. A tendon need not be transferred in its entirety. For example, a split anterior tibial tendon transfer is usually successful for paralysis of the peroneal muscles. One half of the tendon, or slightly more in severe cases, is detached distally, the tendon is split virtually to the musculotendinous junction, the separated half of the tendon is rerouted and fixed to the lateral tarsus at the insertion of the peroneus brevis tendon with the foot in a slightly overcorrected position.

25. In general, the results of tendon transfers are better in patients over 10 years. However, surgery should not be delayed and deformity must be corrected before irreversible secondary skeletal changes develop. When tendon transfers and bone stabilization are combined at the same operation, the latter is carried out first. When there is any significant muscle imbalance in a paralytic disorder, the transfer of even a single tendon is frequently preceded or accompanied by foot stabilizations. To balance the muscle power about a foot accurately with tendon transfers alone may be impossible in a child

because even the slightest imbalance, when combined with a long period of growth, frequently results in recurrent and progressive deformity.

26. The underlying disorder must be taken into consideration. For example, a calcaneus deformity in a paralytic disorder may be best treated by a posterior transfer of the tibialis anterior through the interosseous membrane into the os calcis. If there is a calcaneovalgus deformity, the peroneal tendons are transferred to the os calcis, in addition to the tibialis anterior transfer, and for a calcaneovarus deformity the tibialis posterior and flexor hallucis longus tendons may be transferred in addition to the tibialis anterior. If the calcaneus deformity is longstanding, tendon transfer alone is not likely to suffice, and it may need to be combined with a triple arthrodesis.

However, transfer of the tibialis anterior is less effective in children with myelomeningocele. Their most common form is a calcaneovalgus deformity caused by the active anterior leg muscles and inactive posterior muscles. Spasticity of the evertors and dorsiflexors may cause the deformity in children with high level lesions. Untreated calcaneus deformity produces a bulky prominent heel that is prone to pressure sores and that makes shoe wear difficult. Muscle imbalance can be corrected early by simple tenotomy of all the ankle dorsiflexors and tenotomy of the peroneus brevis and peroneus longus, without the necessity for a tendon transfer.

Illustrative examples

A few illustrative examples of tendon transfers are described. Although the results of specific tendon transfers may be excellent, this is not the case for all procedures. Reidy et al (1952) evaluated 125 tendon transfers about the foot and ankle that had been carried out for paralytic disorders. About one third of the transfers were rated as failures, one third as fair, and one third as good to excellent. Transfers carried out under the age of 11 were frequently unsuccessful. In 60% of these patients, reoperation was required. In properly selected patients, tendon transfers improved the results of arthrodesis by reinforcing the power of dorsiflexion or plantarflexion. Anterior transfers to reinforce dorsiflexion were generally more successful than posterior transfers to reinforce plantarflexion.

Clawing of great toe

Clawing of the great toe may be associated with insufficiency of the plantar flexors of the ankle. Persistent dynamic clawing of the great toe, after appropriate

surgery to restore plantar flexion to the ankle, may be best treated by transferring the flexor hallucis longus from the distal to the proximal phalanx and arthrodesing the interphalangeal joint. When clawing of the great toe is caused by insufficiency of the ankle dorsiflexors and contraction of the Achilles tendon, a Jones procedure is indicated. The tendon of the extensor hallucis longus is inserted into the neck of the first metatarsal via a drill hole and, depending on the age of the patient, the interphalangeal joint is either arthrodesed, or the distal stump of the tendon is used to tenodese the joint.

Pes cavus

There are multiple causes for a pes cavus, but almost always the deformity is secondary to muscle imbalance, irrespective of the underlying muscle disorder. Secondary clawing of the toes develops. For the moderately severe deformity, or for a severe deformity in a patient too young for tarsal reconstruction, a Steindler plantar release may be indicated. If the dorsiflexors of the foot are weak or there is dorsiflexion of the metatarsophalangeal joints, this may be supplemented by a Jones transfer of the extensor hallucis longus tendon or the Hibbs (1919) transfer of the extensor digitorum longus tendons (Fig. 2). Hibbs advised transfer of the tendons of the extensor digitorum longus as a group into the lateral cuneiform with a modified Jones procedure, whereas Frank & Johnson (1966) preferred transfer of the extensor tendons to the metatarsals. If there is an associated varus deformity of the heel, a Dwyer (1959) osteotomy of the os calcis should also be carried out.

Severe deformities in skeletally mature feet are complicated by structural changes in the tarsal bones. When the hindfoot is not deformed, a dorsal tarsal wedge resection is indicated, often combined with a Steindler release. When there is a varus deformity of the heel, a triple arthrodesis may be required; this can be combined with a plantar release. Often, 4–6 weeks later the tibialis posterior tendon is transferred to the dorsilateral aspect of the tarsus and, if necessary, deformities of the toes are corrected.

A fixed deformity requires a dorsal wedge tarsectomy usually combined with a Steindler release, correction of heel varus by triple arthrodesis, or Dwyer osteotomy or a triple arthrodesis. Drennen (1983) preferred a lateral incision for a plantar release, as there was less skin tension following correction of the deformity. Transfer of the tibialis posterior through the interosseous membrane may help maintain the correction and has been used in conjunction with triple arthrodesis.

Rochelle et al (1984) recommended a Steindler plantar release in the flexible cavus foot, a Steindler release with a dorsal wedge osteotomy for fixed mid-foot cavus with flexible heel varus, and triple arthrodesis and plantar release supplemented at times by a second stage anterior

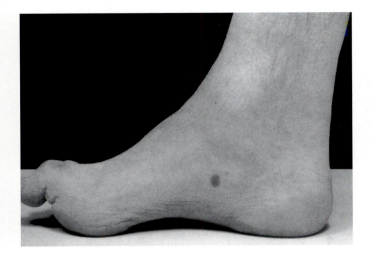

Figure 2a

Patient with bilateral pes cavus: medial view of right foot. He had previously undergone corrective surgery on the left and the photograph was taken when he was admitted for surgery to the right foot

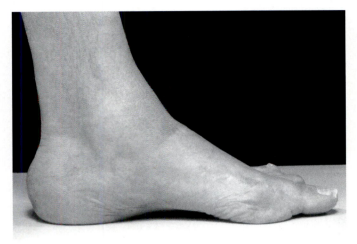

Figure 2b

Medial view of left foot. The left foot was treated by combined dorsal wedge tarsectomy, Jones procedure to the great toe with transfer of the tendon of extensor hallucis longus into the first metatarsal and fusion of the interphalangeal joint, and transfer of the tendons of extensor digitorum longus into the forefoot

transfer of the tibialis posterior tendon through the interosseous membrane for severe fixed cavovarus feet. Flexible claw toes were treated by transfer of the long toe flexors into the extensor expansions, and the fixed great toe was treated by a Jones procedure.

Levitt et al (1973) reported that a cavovarus deformity in hereditary motor sensory neuropathy or Friedreich's ataxia recurred after soft tissue or bony procedures exclusive of a triple arthrodesis. None of the other procedures was satisfactory over time. Levitt et al recommended that the other soft tissue and bony procedures be done as a first stage, followed by a triple arthrodesis at a later time.

However, Wetmore & Drennan (1989) reported 23.4% good results, 30% fair results and 46.6% poor results following triple arthrodesis in 16 patients with Charcot–Marie–Tooth disease. Degenerative disease of the ankle and progressive muscular imbalance resulted in recurrent cavovarus foot deformities in the majority of the patients they reviewed. They concluded that a triple arthrodesis was indicated only as a salvage procedure and should be limited to those patients with a severely rigid foot. Roper and Tibrewal (1989) reviewed 10 children at an average age of 14 years after soft tissue procedures alone had been carried out to correct the foot deformities. No patient had required a triple arthrodesis and the overall results in appearance, symptoms and function were satisfactory in all patients.

This brief review of the treatment of the cavovarus foot illustrates that in such complex deformities tendon transfer may be very useful as a supplement to bony procedures or other soft tissue procedures, but that they are not indicated on their own.

Calcaneal deformity

Calcaneal deformity can occur as a result of triceps surae paralysis. The tibialis anterior may be transferred posteriorly. This can be carried out as an isolated procedure if the lateral stabilizers are balanced and the strong toe extensors can be utilized for dorsiflexion. The toe extensors may require transfer to the metatarsal heads together with interphalangeal fusions to prevent the development of a claw toe. The tibialis anterior tendon is transferred through a window in the interosseous membrane and is attached to the tuber of the os calcis and distal Achilles tendon, which may require shortening.

The foot in cerebral palsy

Preoperative assessment in patients with cerebral palsy may be helped by gait analysis, including ambulatory electromyography. Transfer of the tibialis posterior tendon allows the muscle to assist in dorsiflexion, and removes a dynamic invertor and plantarflexor. Bisla et al (1976), Williams (1976), and Gritzka et al (1972) have all reported 80% or more excellent or good results after this procedure for equinovarus deformity, whereas

Turner & Cooper (1972) found good or excellent results in only 21%. Root (1984) suggested that the failures of this operation were due to unrecognized fixed varus deformity that could not be corrected by a tendon transfer alone, simultaneous lengthening of the Achilles tendon, which can result in a calcaneus deformity (see above), or transplanting the tendon too far laterally, which may lead to excessive valgus or inadequate attachment of the tendon to bone.

Varus deformity may be correctable by a split tendon transfer of tibialis posterior or tibialis anterior, depending on which muscle is the major deforming force. When the tibialis posterior muscle is the principle deforming force, its tendon is prominent subcutaneously through the distal part of its course, and there is adduction of the forefoot, varus of the heel, and metatarsal plantar flexion. When the tibialis anterior is the deforming force, the heel is in varus, the forefoot is adducted, the tibialis anterior tendon is prominent in the subcutaneous tissues, the forefoot is supinated, and the metatarsals are in less plantar flexion.

For a split tibialis posterior tendon transfer, the plantar half of the tendon is detached from its insertion, the tendon is split proximally to the musculotendinous junction, is re-routed posterior to the tibia, and is sutured to the tendon of peroneus brevis or is fixed to the cuboid. The tension should be sufficient to allow the foot to rest in a neutral position when unsupported. Any fixed deformity must be corrected before or during the tendon transfer. Kling et al (1985) reported excellent or good results in 34 of 37 cerebral palsy patients who had undergone this operation. Similar results were reported by Green et al (1983). The development of a calcaneus deformity does not appear to be a complication of this procedure.

The split tibialis anterior tendon is usually transferred to the cuboid.

For equinovarus deformity, Tohen et al (1966) suggested transfer of the extensor hallucis longus and tibialis anterior tendons to the dorsum of the foot at either its centre or lateral side.

A calcaneus deformity in cerebral palsy is usually secondary to excessive lengthening of the Achilles tendon, but it may develop as a primary deformity when the dorsiflexors of the foot are spastic and the triceps surae is weak. Surgical correction is usually unsatisfactory. If the dorsiflexors are spastic, the tibialis anterior tendon can be transferred to the Achilles tendon, which is shortened at the same time. If this does not restore muscle balance, the peroneus longus and tibialis posterior tendons can both be inserted into the Achilles tendon to further strengthen plantarflexion.

Tendon transfer as part of salvage

Tendon transfer alone or in combination with other procedures is not always successful or indicated in some deformities. For example, one of the most rigid defor-mities is talipes equinovarus in arthrogryposis. The deformity is usually severe and associated with limited ankle and tarsal motion. Surgical correction should be carried out before the child begins to walk – the objective is to convert a stiff, deformed foot into a stiff, plantigrade foot. Posteromedial release, tendon transfer and tenotomy may be ineffective and talectomy may be required at the age of 12–18 months.

Congenital convex pes valgus (congenital vertical talus) is treated by a combination of tendon lengthenings, tenotomies and soft tissue releases. Tendon transfer is usually not required as part of the correction, except in patients with myelomeningocele.

Ankle valgus in spina bifida may best be treated by tenodesis of the Achilles tendon to the fibular in patients under the age of 8 years (Dias, 1978), rather than by using tendon transfers.

Tendon transfer in spina bifida

Most patients with myelomeningocoele have foot deformities, usually secondary to muscle imbalance. Treatment is aimed at obtaining plantigrade, braceable feet. Muscle balance must be obtained in order to avoid recurrence or development of a secondary iatrogenic deformity. Ideally, plantigrade feet should be obtained before the child begins to stand. The feet are small relative to the size of the child, become even more disproportionately small, since the foot does not grow in parallel with the increasing weight and size of the child, and are insensate. Vasomotor instability, decreased amounts of subcutaneous tissue, and increased capsular fibrosis also make management difficult.

Failure to achieve a plantigrade position in an anaesthetic foot can lead to the development of trophic ulcers, secondary infection, osteomyelitis, and even the need for an amputation. Tendon transfer forms only part of the treatment required to obtain plantigrade feet. Tendon transfer should be delayed until neurological function is stabilized; this occurs at approximately 1 year of age (Brocklehurst et al 1967).

Equinovalgus deformity can result from overactivity of the peroneus muscles and shortening of the Achilles tendon. In this instance, the tendon of peroneus longus can be transferred through a subcutaneous tunnel deep to the Achilles tendon, and inserted into the navicular insertion of tibialis posterior. This is combined with suture of peroneus brevis to the distal stump of peroneus longus and elongation of the Achilles tendon. Calcaneus deformity in myelomeningocele may be treated by transfer of tibialis anterior and peroneus tertius, at about the age of 1 year, through the interosseous membrane to the os calcis. Additional tenotomies of the long toe extensors and occasionally capsulotomy of the anterior joint may be necessary. Shortening of the Achilles tendon may also be required.

In myelomeningocele, transfer of the tibialis anterior into the talar neck is often required as part of the correction of a congenital convex pes valgus (congenital vertical talus) deformity. This is carried out as part of a one-stage procedure that combines soft tissue releases, tenotomies and tendon transfers. The peroneus longus tendon may also need to be transferred to the insertion of the tibialis posterior.

Tendon transfer after stroke

More recently, Morita et al (1994) have described the results of transfer of flexor hallucis longus and flexor digitorum longus through the interosseous membrane to the fourth metatarsal, combined with elongation of the Achilles tendon for the treatment of equinovarus deformity following a cerebrovascular accident. They reviewed 29 patients more than 2 years after surgery and found that 21 were able to walk without an orthosis. Equinovarus deformity had recurred in six patients and hammer toes in 11 patients, but walking ability without bracing was still better in seven of these. They also found that the results were improved by release of the short toe flexors.

Summary

Tendon transfer still plays an important role in the management of foot deformity, particularly in patients with neuromuscular disease. Careful preoperative assessment is required before embarking upon such surgery, the aim of which is to balance the foot. The surgeon must ensure that the loss of function as a result of a tendon transfer is not likely to cause a greater handicap than the deformity that has been corrected. Careful attention to detail is required. Tendon transfer is frequently not an isolated procedure but forms part of a more complex operation that may include soft tissue releases and bony procedures. Careful postoperative management is required and surgery may form only part of the progressive management of the deformity.

References

Bisla R S, Louis H J, Albano P 1976 Transfer of tibialis posterior tendon in cerebral palsy. J Bone Joint Surg 58A: 497–500

Brocklehurst G, Gleave J R, Lewin W S 1967 Early closure of myelomeningocele with especial reference to leg movement. Dev Med Child Neurol Suppl 13: 51–56

Dias L S 1978 Ankle valgus in children with myelomeningocele. Dev Med Child Neurol 20: 627–633

Drennen J F 1983 Orthopaedic Management of Neuromuscular Disorders. J. B. Lippincott, Philadelphia, p. 28

Dwyer F C 1959 Osteotomy of the calcaneum for pes cavus. J Bone Joint Surg 41B: 80–86

Frank G R, Johnson W M 1966 The extensor shift procedure in the correction of claw toe deformities in children. South Med J 59: 889–896

Green N E, Griffin P P, Shiavi R 1983 Split posterior tibial-tendon transfer in spastic cerebral palsy. J Bone Joint Surg 65A: 748–754

Gritzka T L, Staheli L T, Duncan W R 1972 Posterior tibial tendon transfer through the interosseous membrane to correct equinovarus deformity in cerebral palsy. An initial experience. Clin Orthop 89: 201–206

Hibbs R A 1919 An operation for 'claw foot'. JAMA 73: 1583–1585

Kling T F Jr, Kaufer H, Hensinger R N (1985) Split posterior tibial-tendon transfers in children with cerebral spastic paralysis and equino-varus deformity. J Bone Joint Surg 67A: 186–194

Levitt R L, Canale S T, Cooke A J Jr, Gartland J J 1973 The role of foot surgery in progressive neuromuscular disorders in children. J Bone Joint Surg 55A: 1396–1410

Morita S, Yamamoto H, Furuya K 1994 Anterior transfer of the toe flexors for equinovarus deformity due to hemiplegia. J Bone Joint Surg 76B: 447–449

Peabody C W 1938 Tendon transposition: an end-result study. J Bone Joint Surg 20: 193

Reidy J A, Broderick T F Jr, Barr J S 1952 Tendon transplantations in the lower extremity: a review of the end results in poliomyelitis: Part 1. Tendon transplantations about the foot and ankle. J Bone Joint Surg 34A: 900–908

Rochelle J, Bowen J R, Ray S 1984 Pediatric foot deformities in progressive neuromuscular disease. Contemp Orthop 8: 41

Root L 1984 Varus and valgus foot in cerebral palsy and its management. Foot Ankle 4: 174–179

Roper B A, Tibrewal S B 1989 Soft tissue surgery in Charcot–Marie–Tooth disease. J Bone Joint Surg 71A: 17–20

Tohen Z A, Carmona P J, Barrera J R 1966 The utilization of abnormal reflexes in the treatment of spastic foot deformities: a preliminary report. Clin Orthop 47: 77–84

Turner J W, Cooper R R 1972 Anterior transfer of the tibialis posterior through the interosseous membrane. Clin Orthop 83: 241–244

Wetmore R S, Drennan J C 1989 Long-term results of triple arthrodesis in Charcot–Marie–Tooth disease. J Bone Joint Surg 71A: 417–442

Williams P F 1976 Restoration of muscle balance of the foot by transfer of tibialis posterior. J Bone Joint Surg 58B: 217–219

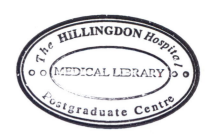
IV.6 Juvenile Arthritis

Barbara M Ansell and Malcolm Swann

Introduction

Chronic arthritis in childhood is rare. Persistent inflammation of the synovial membrane can lead to destruction of joints, and it can also cause alterations in growth of epiphyses, which leads to developmental abnormalities. The synovial sheaths of the tendons may be affected. From a prospective computerized study of patients seen within the first year of onset of disease, the ankle was affected in 40%, the subtalar and midtarsal joints in 27%, and the metatarsophalangeal joints in only 9% (Ansell & Wood 1976). The most frequently involved tarsal joints are the talonavicular and talocalcaneal (subtalar). By the 15-year follow-up, although some 50% had involvement of ankles or feet, only 0.9% considered these as their major limiting disability. Growth defects of toes or slight loss of function of the hindfeet were rarely commented on by patients.

Patterns of disease

There are still no consistent internationally accepted diagnostic labels for childhood arthritis (Cassidy 1993, Southwood & Woo 1993, Prieur 1993). A possible pattern is suggested in Table 1. By far the commonest pattern of disease is seronegative juvenile chronic arthritis. This is further divided by its mode of onset into three main groups: systemic and polyarticular (more than four joints involved in the first three months), and pauciarticular (fewer than four joints); further subdivision according to age is usual.

Systemic-onset disease

In systemic-onset disease, which commonly begins before the fifth birthday and affects boys and girls equally, there is recurrent high swinging fever associated with a maculopapular rash of coppery hue, generalized lymphadenopathy and often hepatosplenomegaly, pericarditis and occasionally myocarditis and liver dysfunction; there may be only arthralgia at this stage and established arthritis may take months to develop. In at least 50% a prolonged course with years of persistent disease activity occurs, often requiring corticosteroid therapy because of the severity of the systemic features such as pericarditis. It is among such patients that overall growth, including the feet, is retarded, both because of their disease and because of the corticosteroid therapy.

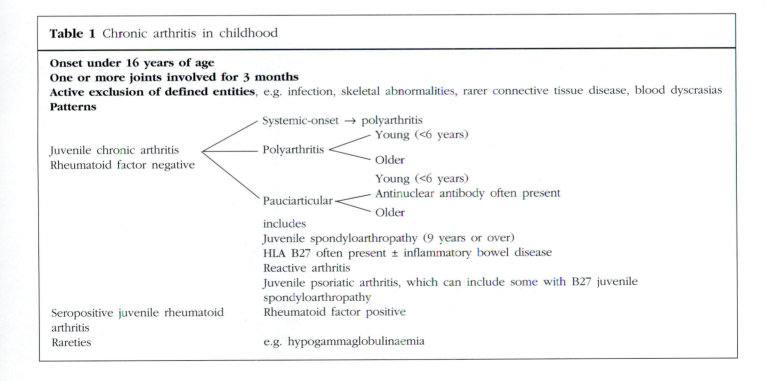

Table 1 Chronic arthritis in childhood

Onset under 16 years of age
One or more joints involved for 3 months
Active exclusion of defined entities, e.g. infection, skeletal abnormalities, rarer connective tissue disease, blood dyscrasias
Patterns

Juvenile chronic arthritis
Rheumatoid factor negative

- Systemic-onset → polyarthritis
- Polyarthritis
  - Young (<6 years)
  - Older
- Pauciarticular
  - Young (<6 years) — Antinuclear antibody often present
  - Older

includes
Juvenile spondyloarthropathy (9 years or over)
HLA B27 often present ± inflammatory bowel disease
Reactive arthritis
Juvenile psoriatic arthritis, which can include some with B27 juvenile spondyloarthropathy

Seropositive juvenile rheumatoid arthritis — Rheumatoid factor positive

Rareties — e.g. hypogammaglobulinaemia

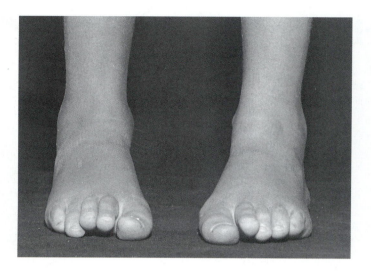

Figure 1

The feet of a child with still persistent disease activity six years after systemic-onset disease that requires high-dose corticosteroid therapy. Note the failure of overall growth, varus deformity of the forefoot with early hallux valgus on the left, and growth defects of the second and third metatarsals on one side and the second on the other with some clawing of the other toes

Involvement of the midtarsal joints is the third commonest presenting site of arthritis in systemic disease. Symmetrical involvement of the ankle can also occur early. Persistence of disease not only causes damage to ankle and tarsal joints, but can lead to metatarsophalangeal joint involvement, often in an asymmetrical fashion. This gives rise to a small foot with some toes elongated and others shortened (Figs. 1 and 2).

In systemic disease, there is a risk of intercurrent infections early in the course of the disease, and amyloidosis, the one potentially fatal complication of juvenile chronic arthritis, may occur later. Although many patients will eventually go into remission, residual deformity depends not only on the disease process but also on the care with which these patients have been managed in the early stages of the disease, particularly when general illness has required periods of bed rest. In addition, contractures of the calf muscle and Achilles tendon can cause dropped feet in children who have been confined to a wheelchair, either because of involvement of other lower limb joints or because of the severity of their disease (Fig. 3).

Polyarticular-onset disease

In polyarticular-onset juvenile chronic arthritis, the majority do not carry IgM rheumatoid factor. With persistent polyarthritis, ankle and hindfoot involvement is common; dependent to some extent on the age of presentation, any conceivable combination of deformities including growth anomalies of the toes can occur (Rana 1982, Truckenbrodt & Hafner 1991). Initially there is soft tissue thickening and limitation of movement of the ankle, marked spasm and loss of movement of the hindfoot, with a tendency to valgus deformity which is often associated with a compensatory varus at the midtarsal joint. The forefoot frequently widens and hallux valgus and clawing of the toes is common. In such children, measurement of the force distribution under the foot has been used to assess the effect of these deformities on foot function as compared to normal children. In general, those with arthritis have significantly reduced loading

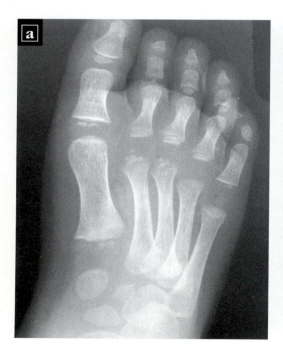

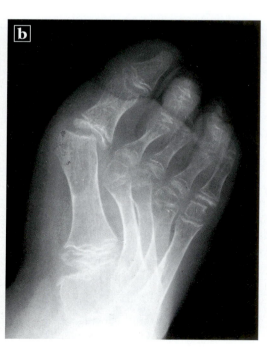

Figure 2

The sequential radiological state of a boy with systemic onset disease requiring high-dose corticosteroids (a) shortly after foot involvement; (b) six years into the disease. Note the destructive process, particularly in the first metatarsophalangeal joint, and the change in shape of all the epiphyses with varying growth defects at metatarsophalangeal level

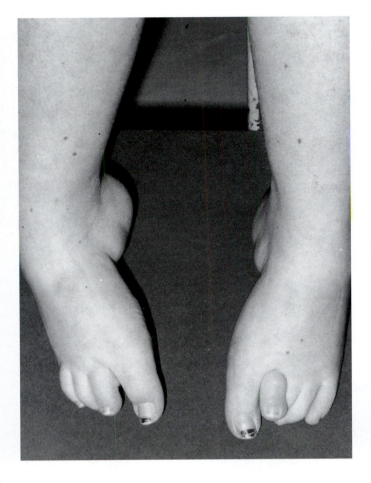

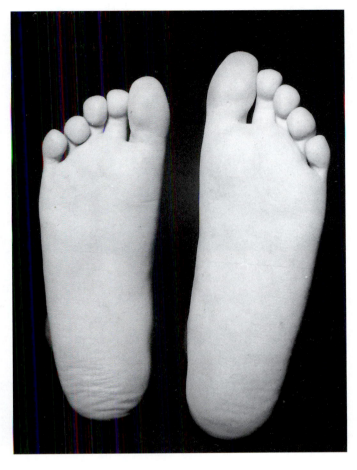

Figure 3

Dropped feet due to contractures of calf muscle and Achilles tendon with other growth anomalies due to severe foot involvement

Figure 4

Several years after persistent disease activity, failure of growth of the affected foot

under all the toes and the two medial metatarsal heads, but increased contact time for the heel (Dhanendran et al 1980). In seronegative arthritis, the overall prognosis for life is good, but the joint disease may persist for many years.

Pauciarticular disease

Pauciarticular disease is subdivided by age of onset. Those under six years are usually girls and often have chronic iridocyclitis and positive antinuclear antibody. The ankle is the second commonest site of presentation (after the knee), and this is frequently associated with hindfoot involvement. An affected foot rapidly assumes an abnormal posture with loss of movement, particularly at the tarsal joints. In older children overgrowth of the tarsal epiphyses is common. With persistence of disease activity, overall growth failure of the affected foot is common (Fig. 4). In older onset pauciarticular disease, the main group is that of spondyloarthropathy, but it

must be remembered that reactive arthritis following dysenteric infections frequently presents with asymmetrical involvement of a toe, ankle, or hindfoot; any age can be affected, but it is particularly common aged 10 or over, and these patients often carry HLA B27. A more transient synovitis of the ankles may also be seen in association with erythema nodosum or inflammatory bowel disease, but persistence from any cause can lead to unilateral overgrowth.

Spondyloarthropathy

Juvenile spondyloarthropathy affects predominantly boys aged eight to nine years or over and is characterized by a lower limb arthropathy, with the ankles the third commonest site of presentation. Other features include plantar fasciitis, which presents as heel pain and can cause prolific calcaneal spurs, and chronic Achilles bursitis (Jacobs & Johnson 1982) (Fig. 5). Tendon sheath involvement is frequent, often causing severe spasm so

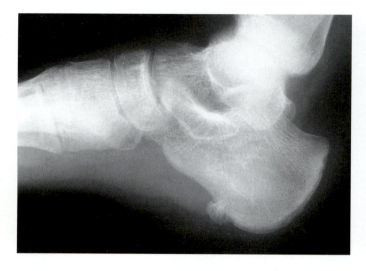

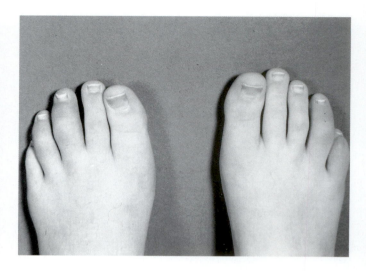

Figure 5

Calcaneal spur and early erosion of os calcis due to involvement of plantar fascia and Achilles tendon in an adolescent with juvenile spondylitis

Figure 6

Sausage toe as a presenting feature of juvenile psoriatic arthritis

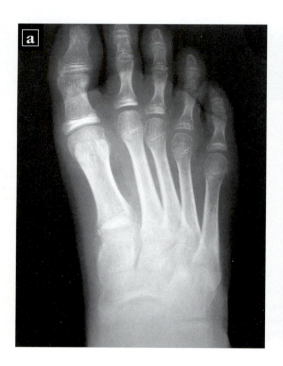

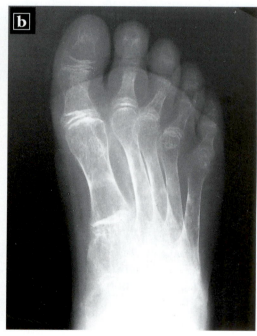

Figure 7

Seropositive juvenile rheumatoid arthritis (a) at presentation with foot involvement; (b) radiological progression over five years

that the adolescent can present as a peroneal spastic flatfoot, and only later develop further joint involvement. Midtarsal involvement has been a particular problem in adolescents, causing bony overgrowth and deformity (Levi et al 1990). Metatarsophalangeal joint involvement can be severe, is often asymmetric, and occurs early in some 10%. HLA B27 is usual, as is a strong family history of ankylosing spondylitis or acute uveitis, while the ultimate development of sacroiliitis some 5–10 years later is usual (Ansell 1980).

Psoriatic arthritis

Juvenile psoriatic arthritis, which can develop at any age, may start with a single swollen toe caused by involvement of all its joints and the tendon sheath; the sausage toe is not uncommon as a presenting feature (Fig. 6). A finger may be similarly affected. Although usually pauciarticular at onset, some 80% of patients will ultimately become polyarthritic, but even with a spreading arthritis the asymmetric pattern with growth anomalies persists (Shore & Ansell 1982, Southwood et al 1989).

Seropositive juvenile rheumatoid arthritis

Seropositive juvenile rheumatoid arthritis most frequently affects girls from about the age of 10 years. It is characterized by early bilateral symmetrical erosive disease affecting all the metatarsophalangeal joints (Fig. 7), with hindfoot involvement occurring later (Ansell 1983). The subsequent deformities are similar to adult rheumatoid arthritis; however, in the younger onset of seropositive disease (i.e. below nine), early hindfoot involvement is more usual. With the use of slow-acting rheumatic drugs, healing of erosions can occur.

In the arthritis of hypogammaglobulinaemia the possibility of infection with unusual organisms needs to be considered.

Assessment

A child with a foot problem requires an overall appraisal. This will include the pattern of disease present, its activity and duration, as well as the general state of the child. Examination of the lower limbs allows assessment of the likelihood of problems in other joints altering the forces on the feet. It is important to see the child stand (Fig. 8) and, whenever possible, walk. Deformity can result from active synovitis in one or many of the multiple articulations of the foot, and sometimes from tendon sheath involvement. Muscle spasm, which may be either voluntary or involuntary, will inevitably produce deformity and later stiffness. Secondary changes occur, with loss of joint space, contracture of capsules, and later distortion of growth.

The epiphyses in the foot as elsewhere must be singled out for their considerable contribution to deformity. They may be stimulated by hyperaemia causing excessive growth, with enlargement of bone which is sometimes asymmetrical. Conversely, premature fusion of an epiphysis will lead to stunted development of a bone. A joint unaffected by the disease itself may become involved by adaptive or secondary deformity, which, if left unattended, can become established by contracture. Valgus deformity of the knee is very common in these children, and in order to maintain a plantargrade foot, subtalar and midtarsal joints may become fixed in varus even though not directly involved in the inflammatory process. Normal function and development of the foot depends on the stimulus of weight bearing, and the child with chronic arthritis may be literally 'off its feet', not only because of disease within the feet or other lower limb joints, but also because of general illness. Thus deformity is compounded by many of the factors associated with a growing skeleton and will become irreversible if bony fusion is occurring. Clinical photographs are an excellent way of recording stance, and the use of a machine to assess pressure on the sole of the foot may be helpful. Good radiographs are essential. These should include a PA of the ankle and forefoot;

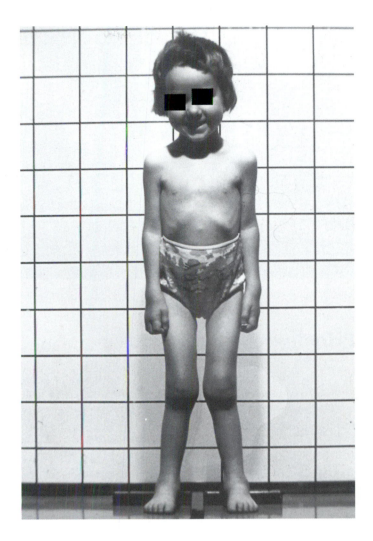

Figure 8

Nine years after a polyarthritic onset, there is widespread joint involvement; note the flexed hips, valgus knees and varus feet

a lateral X-ray of the foot and the ankle, taken when standing in full dorsiflexion and full plantar flexion, will confirm the amount of movement at the ankle. Video recordings are invaluable in assessment and as a record to monitor the effects of treatment. Clearer definition of the epiphyses can sometimes be obtained by an oblique view. Minor changes in epiphyseal growth are noted early; this is particularly easy to spot in unilateral cases in young children. There may be overgrowth, which can affect the ankle and tarsal bones (particularly the navicular bone), narrowing of joint space, and ultimately fusion (Fig. 8). The metatarsal heads can show irregular development accompanied by destruction of the joint.

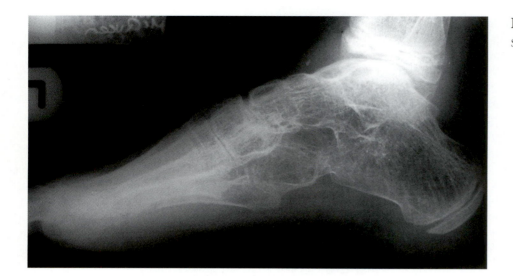

Figure 9
Spontaneous fusion of tarsal bones

Principles of treatment

The aim of treatment is to produce a normal-looking, mobile, painless, plantargrade foot. Unfortunately the multiplicity of synovial targets within the foot means that active disease lasting several years will inevitably defy these ideals. The position of the foot must take precedence over mobility, and a plantargrade foot must be attained at all costs. Periods spent in plaster or splints will mitigate against mobility, but as yet it is not possible to deal directly with the destructive nature of the disease and joint contracture, fibrosis, or even ankylosing that may occur unchecked.

The ankle

This joint is rarely involved in isolation although the patient or the parents often refer to the ankle, meaning in fact the hindfoot. An affected ankle tends to be stiff and painful and possibly deformed, but not usually unstable. Sometimes the talus undergoes avascular necrosis. Although there may be no deformity to correct, four weeks spent in a walking plaster may suffice to tide a patient over a painful period. This may be preceded by intra-articular steroid if active synovitis is present. The rarely used surgical alternatives are to fuse or to replace a destroyed ankle. In the light of present experience, fusion must remain the method of choice, although if bone stock is sufficient and the rest of the foot is stiff, the retention of only a few degrees of ankle movement is invaluable.

The hindfoot and midfoot

This includes the subtalar, midtarsal, intertarsal and tarsometatarsal joints. These are considered together, as involvement of one or several of them will have the same consequence and in particular lead to loss of inversion and eversion.

A valgus hindfoot from eversion of the os calcis at the subtalar joint may be associated with a pronated forefoot, and this association or the reverse may become fixed. This must be appreciated, as attempts to correct the position of the os calcis will in turn supinate the forefoot and result in the patient walking on the outer side of the foot. It is sometimes impossible to be sure at which site or sites a problem has arisen, and the ankle joint itself may also be affected concurrently. If pain rather than deformity is the dominant factor demanding attention, it is important to identify the site accurately. The use of targetted local anaesthetic can provide useful information in this respect.

In juvenile chronic arthritis there is no other region which will respond so readily to early correction of deformity using conservative methods. Serial correction using below-knee walking plasters may suffice to bring this about. If pain and spasm prevent ready correction of deformity, then a light general anaesthetic should be given, and the foot may be gently manipulated before the plaster is applied. No force must be used because the bones may be porotic and easily damaged. At the same time, an intra-articular injection of triamcinolone hexacetonide helps to damp down inflammation (Mavidrou et al 1991). The plaster is kept on for about six weeks and this is followed by a caliper when walking and a night splint in order to prevent recurrence. Rydholm (1990) has described the use of intravenous water soluble hydrocortisone below a tourniquet for multiple sites of inflammation.

A mobile but excessive valgus heel should be controlled with a simple heel cup and this often helps with the correction of an associated mobile pes planus. A well moulded ankle–foot orthosis may serve to control a deformity, but insoles that add bulk to the inside of the shoe are painful and unhelpful in most instances.

Surgery to the hindfoot and midfoot must be deferred as long as possible in order to allow growth and ossification to proceed. However on occasions, patients who are referred later or in whom treatment has been ineffective will present with a fixed deformity. A number of conventional orthopaedic procedures are appropriate (Swann 1978).

An isolated varus or valgus deformity of the hindfoot (os calcis) may be corrected by an osteotomy. Varus deformity may be corrected by closing an outer wedge (Dwyer 1959), and valgus by closing an inner wedge or by opening and grafting an outer wedge. Skin closure in the latter case may be difficult. Mobile lateral subluxation and valgus drift of the subtalar joint can be controlled by a Grice procedure (Grice 1955) if the joint fails to stabilize with conservative measures and the patient wishes to be rid of appliances.

Deformity at any site can be corrected by suitable bone surgery. Normal joints should not be sacrificed, but rather the correction obtained by taking suitable wedges through bone. If, however, the joint is the focus of pain from active disease, then this can be dealt with by wedge correction and fusion.

The range of surgery extends from a limited operation, such as talonavicular fusion, to a wedge tarsectomy or triple arthrodesis. Good bone apposition must be obtained because porosis will prevent the use of staples and other fixation devices.

Forefoot and toes

Synovitis of the interphalangeal and metatarsophalangeal joints induces clawing of the toes. While the clawing is passively correctable, physiotherapy will help and the patient should also have a good supportive shoe with adequate room in the toecap. Intra-articular hydrocortisone into the toes joints can be used, given under a light general anaesthetic.

If the clawing does not respond to these simple measures, selective tenotomy followed by intensive exercises is undertaken. Flexor and extensor transplant operations, practised in other conditions where clawing is passively correctable, is not appropriate here. Interphalangeal joint fusion may be required, particularly in the great toes. Minor growth anomalies in the toes may cause localized pressure and can be dealt with on an individual basis by trimming the bone or by other appropriate measures.

The metatarsophalangeal joints are commonly affected, particularly in seropositive disease. Joint erosions are noted early; this is proliferative and symmetrical, leading to early dislocation; the exception is the big toe, which tends to develop hallux valgus with varus drift of the first metatarsal. The principles of treatment must remain and an endeavour made to prevent dislocation and deformity by conservative means. Intrinsic foot exercises are practised daily and it is sometimes necessary to increase analgesia at this time in older patients to overcome painful inhibition of toe function. Metatarsal insoles are forbidden as they only serve to add bulk to the content of the shoe under circumstances when the foot and toes are already swollen. The addition of a metatarsal bar under the sole of the shoe can be helpful.

When the dislocations are extensive and irreducible, surgery may be necessary. It is recalled that the epiphyses are distal in the metatarsals, except in the first where it is basal; the phalangeal epiphyses are all basal. Account must be taken of this growth arrangement when planning surgery that may involve excision of bone.

It is uncommon to find one joint affected in isolation, although the degree to which adjacent joints are eroded or dislocated will vary. In the rare event of a single metatarsophalangeal dislocation, the Helal osteotomy is appropriate (Helal 1975).

Most seropositive juveniles are approaching skeletal maturity when the feet demand surgical attention and it is therefore satisfactory to perform an excision arthroplasty (Fowler 1959). Meticulous technique is necessary to leave a symmetrical fan shape to the metatarsal stumps. If any remnant of an active epiphyseal plate is left behind, irregular growth may continue, thus spoiling the intended pseudoarthrosis.

The destruction of the metatarsophalangeal joint of the big toe is less of a problem, although hallux valgus frequently develops. Conventional osteotomies, such as those described by Wilson (1963), have been used. Occasionally, the displacement of the first ray is so great and the erosions so severe that Mayo's operation (Mayo 1908) is preferred. This procedure gives an excellent result, and at the same time spares the growth plate of the proximal phalanx. Keller's operation (Keller 1904) is clearly inappropriate until growth has ceased.

The sesamoid joints are not troublesome in isolation, but when they cause pain due to synovitis, a local injection of hydrocortisone can help. No sesamoids have been removed in these children, although it is conceivable that an indication could arise.

Surgery of the soft tissues

A number of powerful tendons run around the foot before their insertion, notably the Achilles, tibialis posterior, and the peronei. Their superficial portions render them conspicuous when inflammation affects the synovial lining – such changes in other deeper tendons in the sole may go unnoticed. Tender, boggy swellings appear and, at first sight, may be mistaken for swollen joints. Their involvement contributes greatly to the pain, stiffness, and deformity of the child's foot. A local corticosteroid injection followed by a period of immobilization is often beneficial. Only rarely is it necessary to do a tenosynovectomy.

Summary

In juvenile chronic arthritis, the foot can be involved to a variable extent, depending on many factors. The natural course of the disease is variable and unpredictable in a particular patient. However, in patients with persistent disease activity, it is usually possible to modify this with a range of drugs, such as methotrexate in young polyarthritic patients and sulphasalazine in the spondyloarthropathy subgroup. Continuous supervision is necessary to try to prevent the establishment of fixed deformities and to maintain a plantigrade foot with as much painless mobility as can be achieved.

References

Ansell B M 1980 Juvenile spondylitis and related disorders. In: Moll J M H (ed) Ankylosing Spondylitis. Churchill Livingstone, Edinburgh. 120–136

Ansell B M 1983 Juvenile chronic arthritis with persistently positive tests for rheumatoid factor (sero-positive juvenile rheumatoid arthritis). Ann Pediatr (Paris) 30: 545–550

Ansell B M, Wood P H 1976 Prognosis of juvenile chronic polyarthritis. Clin Rheum Dis 2: 397–412

Cassidy J T 1993 What's in a name? Nomenclature of juvenile arthritis. A North American view. Perspect Pediatr Rheumatol 20: 4–8

Dhanendran M, Hutton W C, Klenerman L et al 1980 Foot function in juvenile chronic arthritis. Rheumatol Rehabil XIX: 20–24

Dwyer F C 1959 Osteotomy of the calcaneus for pes cavus. J Bone Joint Surg 41B: 80–86

Fowler A W 1959 A method of forefoot reconstruction. J Bone Joint Surg 41B: 507–513

Grice D S 1955 Further experience with extra-articular arthrodesis of the subtalar joint. J Bone Joint Surg 36A: 246

Helal B 1975 Metatarsal osteotomy for metatarsalgia. J Bone Joint Surg 57B: 187–192

Jacobs J C, Johnson A D 1982 HLA B27-associated spondyloarthritis enthesopathy in childhood: clinical, pathologic and radiographic observations in 58 patients. J Pediatr 100: 521–528

Keller W L 1904 Surgical treatment of bunions and hallux valgus. N Y State J Med 80: 741–742

Levi S, Ansell B M, Klenerman L 1990 Tarsometatarsal involvement in juvenile spondyloarthropathy. Foot Ankle 11: 90–92

Mavidrou A, Klenerman L, Swann M et al 1991 Conservative management of the hindfoot in juvenile chronic arthritis. Foot 1: 139–140

Mayo C H 1908 The surgical treatment of bunions. Ann Surg 4B: 300–302

Prieur A M 1993 What's in a name? Nomenclature of juvenile arthritis. A European view. Perspect Pediatr Rheumatol 20: 9–11

Rana N A 1982 Juvenile rheumatoid arthritis of the foot. Foot Ankle 3: 2–11

Rydholm U 1990 Surgery for juvenile chronic arthritis. Wallin & Dalholm, Oftoldm, Sweden. pp. 57–60

Shore A, Ansell B M 1982 Juvenile psoriatic arthritis – an analysis of 60 cases. J Pediatr 100: 529–535

Southwood T R, Petty R E, Malleson P N et al 1989 Psoriatic arthritis in children. Arthritis Rheum 32: 1007–1013

Southwood T P, Woo P 1993 Childhood Arthritis: The name game. Br J Rheumatol 32: 421–423

Swann M 1978 The Foot. In: Arden G P, Ansell B M (eds) Surgical Management of Juvenile Chronic Polyarthritis. Academic Press, London. p. 185–199

Truckenbrodt H, Hafner R 1991 General and local growth disorders in chronic arthritis in childhood. Schwiez Med Wochenschr 121: 608–620

Wilson J N 1963 Oblique displacement of osteotomy for hallux valgus. J Bone Joint Surg 45B: 552–556

V.1 Static Deformities

Paul P Griffin and Frank Rand

Flexible pes planovalgus (flatfoot)

Flatfoot is a descriptive term of broad usage that describes a foot in which the height of the longitudinal arch is diminished or absent. The term does not indicate what pathological anatomy is present. Pes planovalgus may be secondary to muscle imbalance, arthritis, tarsal coalition, and many other conditions. Specific etiologies must be excluded before one can make a decision on management of a flat foot. This section will discuss the flexible flat foot secondary to ligamentous laxity.

Pathological anatomy

In a flexible flat foot there may be a single area of collapse of the arch or a combination of several changes. The common findings are a sag of the naviculocuneiform joint, sag of the talonavicular joint, excessive plantar flexion of the talus, decrease in the pitch of the calcaneus, abduction of the navicular on the talus with abduction of the forefoot, and divergence of the talus and calcaneus in the horizontal plane (Fig. 1). Schwartz believed the major cause of the pronated calcaneus was a collapse of the calcaneocuboid joint (Schwartz & Heath 1949). In most flat feet the calcaneus is in pronation; this causes a change in its weight bearing axis. The lateral rotation of the anterior end of the calcaneus allows the talus to plantarflex and the talonavicular joint to collapse.

The pathological changes in the relationship of the bones of the foot can best be measured on standing anteroposterior and lateral radiographs.

Muscle forces about the foot have little effect in supporting the arch in stance. Basmajian (Basmajian & Stecko 1963) found through electromyographic recording that the intrinsic and extrinsic muscle were silent during stance. That muscles do not support the arch can be appreciated by the lack of change in the structure of the foot of a mature person with a complete resection of the sciatic nerve. However, muscle imbalance in the foot will cause a deformity, such as the valgus deformity that develops following paralysis of the posterior tibialis muscle in the presence of normal peroneal muscle (Schwartz & Heath 1949).

Clinical features

The flexible flatfoot can be appreciated by its flexibility and by the absence of muscle weakness. When

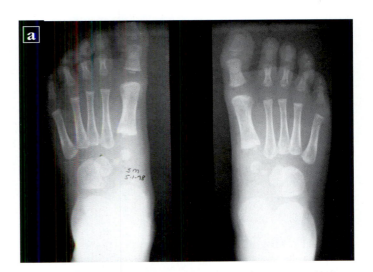

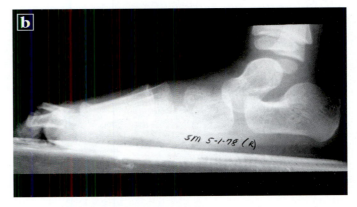

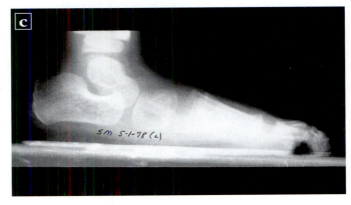

Figure 1

Standing X-rays of a 4-year-old patient showing all the features of a severe flat foot. The anteroposterior view (a) shows divergence of the talus and calcaneus with the long axis of the talus medial to the first metatarsal. The lateral view (b, c) shows collapse of the talonavicular joint. The navicular is not ossified, but the position of the cuneiform suggests that the cuneiform–navicular joint is also collapsed. Kite's angle is increased non-weight-bearing, the arch of the foot appears normal, only to disappear partially or completely on standing. When the standing patient raises the heel off the floor and stands on tiptoes. the arch is restored. The heel cord is frequently tight and dorsiflexion to neutral may be impossible unless the foot is allowed to go into valgus.

Although pain is rare in young children with flexible flat feet, teenagers occasionally have foot pain during and after standing for a long period or when running. Some children complain of leg pain and easy fatigability. This is more frequently seen in obese children, or in children with external rotation contractures of the hip or excessive external tibial torsion. Many of these children dislike physical activity. Whether or not this dislike is related to the weakness in the foot is uncertain. However, after successful treatment most children will increase their physical activity and have no pain.

Treatment

Asymptomatic pes planus

The management of asymptomatic flatfoot in children is controversial. In one survey, orthopaedic surgeons were evenly divided between those who recommended medial heel wedges and arch support and those who recommended no treatment for the asymptomatic flatfoot (Staheli & Griffin 1980). Wenger (Wenger et al 1986) found no difference between a matched group of children treated with special shoes or inserts and a group of children not treated.

Bleck & Berzins (1977) treated and followed 71 children with flat feet. His treatment was the use of a University of California Biomechanics Laboratory (UCBL) insert or a Helfet heel cup (Henderson & Campbell 1967, Helfet 1956). These children had increased plantar flexion of the talus greater than 25°, with excessive divergence of the talus and calcaneus of more than 18°. In the follow-up, 32% of the feet were normal, 48% were improved, and 20% unchanged. These figures are impressive but the question as to the number of patients who would have spontaneously improved with growth remains unanswered. We know of no comparative series that shows the change in the planovalgus foot that takes place with growth and development. Until this evidence is available, the treatment of asymptomatic flexible flatfoot will remain controversial.

We use the clinical appearance and the reported level of activity as guides to treatment of the asymptomatic flatfoot. The child of 3–8 years of age with a flexible flat foot with a prominent head of the talus, abduction of the mid- and forefoot (Fig. 2) and valgus of the heel should probably be treated. On observation of the barefoot gait, the patient who needs treatment will be seen to push off from the medial side of the foot. Usually the family will report that the child does not like to walk

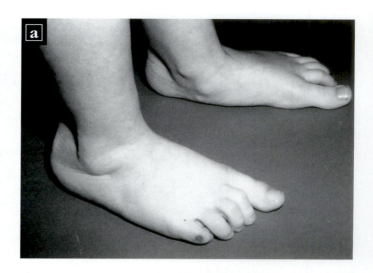

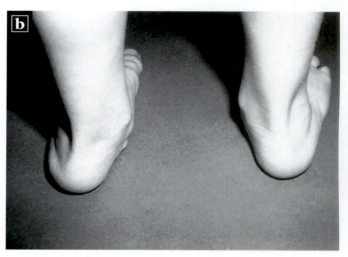

Figure 2

X-rays showing loss of longitudinal arch, prominent head of the talus, abduction of the forefoot and heel valgus in 4-year-old patient; (a) side view, (b) rear view

and that he runs poorly compared to other children. The patient whose radiograph is shown in Fig. 3 was such a patient. He had no pain but refused to walk more than short distances. Conservative treatment with a UCBL insert improved his level of activities. Correction of a flatfoot by supportive inserts is usually lost after the insert is discontinued (Mereday et al 1972).

We recommend that the severe flatfoot be treated with a UCBL orthosis (Fig. 4) for approximately three years in the child who is between 3 and 8 years of age. Older children are so unlikely to improve that it is not worth the expense and trouble of treatment unless they have pain. The Helfet heel cup may be used in the less severe deformity. Helfet reported good results in most patients (Helfet 1956). Bleck & Berzins (1977) suggested that

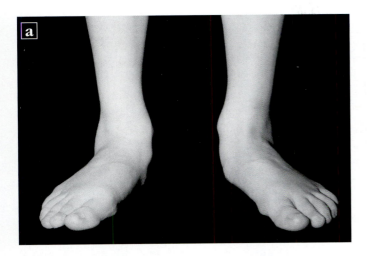

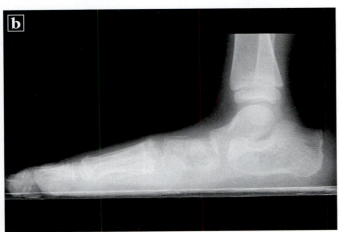

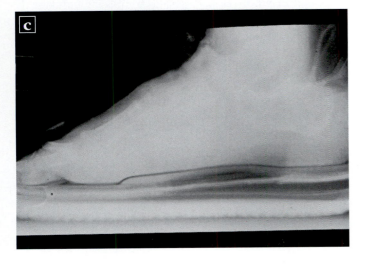

Figure 3

An 8-year-old with asymptomatic flexible flat foot: (a) severe valgus; (b) standing lateral; (c) standing view wearing UCBL

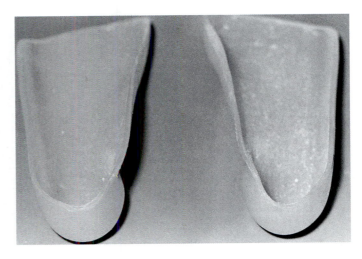

Figure 4

UCBL orthosis

Symptomatic flatfoot

Painful flat feet are very rare in children under 12 years of age and are not common even in teenagers. Specific disease or abnormalities such as juvenile arthritis, bone tumors, infections, tarsal coalitions, and traumatic arthritis may cause the foot to be flat. Motion in these conditions is limited either by pain or structural changes, or by both. Treatment should address the specific condition that is responsible for the symptoms.

The flexible flatfoot with pain usually has the more severe radiographic abnormalities and clinical appearance described above. The heel cord is frequently contracted and dorsiflexion of the ankle to neutral is possible only if the foot is allowed to go into valgus as the ankle dorsiflexes. If the foot is held with the subtalar joint in neutral or slight inversion, dorsiflexion is limited. The tight heel cord, if present, must be stretched either with passive exercise or by repeated manipulation and immobilization in a cast. It is important that the foot be held in slight varus when the cast is applied to prevent increasing the valgus deformity.

The appliance chosen for treatment must be capable of maintaining the calcaneus in a position where its weight-bearing axis is parallel to the long axis of the tibia or in slight varus. A medial heel wedge and rigid orthopaedic shoe and 'cookie' (support along the longitudinal arch) cannot achieve this goal. We are not confident that the classic type of arch pad, even if custom made, can hold the calcaneus in the proper position. However, treatment with a steel shank shoe and custom-made arch pads were reported by Basta et al (1977) to be uniformly effective in relief of pain in flexible flatfeet. We have not found the rigid shoe and arch pad to be effective and prefer a UCBL orthosis (see Fig. 4) or Helfet heel cup (Fig. 5). The Helfet cup has to be worn in a

radiographs be taken before treatment. For patients with a plantarflexed talus between 35 and 45° off the horizontal, they used the Helfet heel cup. If the plantar flexion of the talus was over 45°, they recommended the UCBL orthosis.

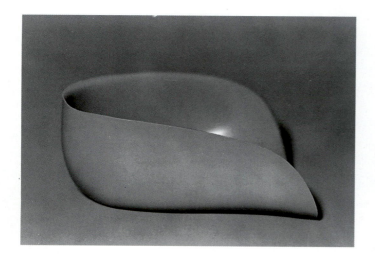

Figure 5

Helfet heel cup

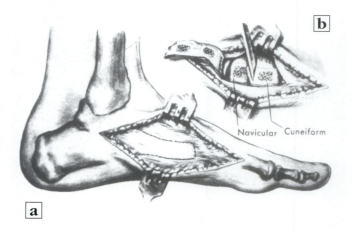

Figure 6

Miller operation: the outline for making the osteoperiosteal flap that includes the tibialis posterior and removal of the navicular–cuneiform cartilage after the flap is elevated (a); the advancement and suturing of the flap (b)

shoe that has a firm counter, but the UCBL orthosis can be used with a soft shoe.

Surgical treatment

Many painful flexible flatfeet respond to conservative measures, but those that do not can usually be relieved by surgical measures. Various osteotomies, arthrodesis and soft tissue procedures have been described for treatment of painful flexible feet (Dall 1978, Evans 1975, Haraldsson 1962, Jack 1953, Miller 1927, Seymour 1967). We have preferred the realignment of the calcaneus by a medial displacement osteotomy, or advancement of the insertion of the posterior tibialis tendon and arthrodesis of the cuneiform–navicular joint similar to the operation reported by Miller in 1927. For feet with excessive abduction of the mid- and forefoot, the Evans lengthening osteotomy of the calcaneus is preferred to correct the deformity (Evans 1975). The Miller procedure is seldom used today because the calcaneal osteotomy does not limit motion and gives good correction. In the pes planus foot with the primary deformity a collapse of the talocalcaneal joint with mild abduction of the navicular on the talus, the calcaneal medial slide gives good correction of the deformity and relief of pain. The Evans procedure is best for the foot with severe abduction of the navicular. In this type of foot, the anterior end of the talus is well forward of the anterior end of the calcaneus.

The Miller procedure (Fig 6) is done via an incision on the medial side of the foot extending from the medial malleolus to the base of the first metatarsal. The posterior tibialis tendon is dissected freely from the surrounding tissues from the malleolus to the insertion on the navicular. A 1.5 cm wide strip is outlined, extending from the navicular to the distal end of the cuneiform and including the insertion of the posterior tibialis tendon. The strip should be placed inferiorly enough to include a section of the spring ligament. An osteoperiosteal flap is then elevated along the outlined strip, including the navicular insertion of the posterior tibialis. Cartilage is denuded from the navicular–cuneiform joint. The osteoperiosteal strip with the posterior tibialis tendon and a portion of the spring ligament are advanced distally and firmly sutured superiorly and inferiorly along the entire course of the strip while the foot is held in a corrected position of slight inversion of the hindfoot, plantarflexion, and adduction of the forefoot. If the ankle will not dorsiflex to neutral with the foot held in the corrected position, the heel cord must be lengthened. We do not arthrodese the cuneiform first metatarsal joint, as Miller recommended. The foot is immobilized in a cast for 12 weeks, and the patient uses a UCBL insert for 6 months. If the heel cord is tight and dorsiflexion to neutral is not possible, the result will be unsatisfactory. This procedure should be done in feet that are flexible and that are corrected by Jack's test (Jack 1953). Jack's test is performed by asking the patient to extend the great toe passively while standing. If the loss of the arch is due to collapse of the navicular–cuneiform joint the arch will be restored. If on extension of the toes the arch does not improve, the Miller procedure should not be used (Fig. 7).

The medial displacement osteotomy of the calcaneus restores the weight-bearing axis of the calcaneus as related to the weight bearing axis of the tibia and increases the support of the arch (Fig 8). The procedure is performed through a lateral incision in line with and

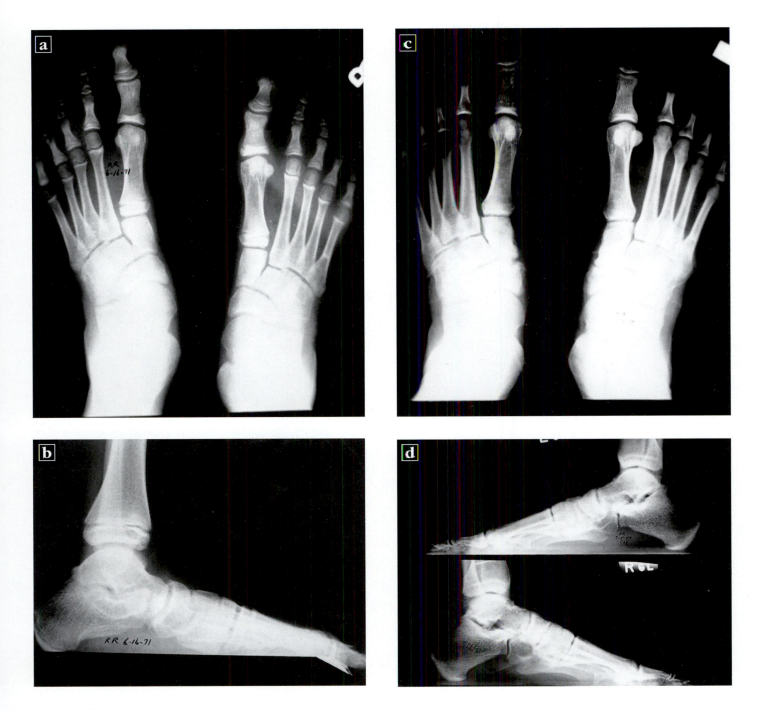

Figure 7

A 13-year-old boy. Painful flexible flat foot on left: (a) preoperative anteroposterior view; (b) preoperative lateral view; (c), (d) postoperative X-rays showing advancement of tibialis posterior and arthrodesis of navicular–cuneiform joint shows correction of collapse of the navicular–cuneiform joint of the left foot

just posterior to the peroneal tendons. The osteotomy is oblique from superior to inferior and oblique from posterior lateral to anterior medial. The posterior fragment is then displaced medially about half the width of the calcaneus. The position is maintained by a large Steinmann pin inserted anterior lateral to posterior medial. The foot is immobilized in a cast for 6 weeks or until the

osteotomy is healed. Figure 9 shows the preoperative flat foot and the postoperative correction of a 10-year-old boy. Preoperatively he denied pain but refused to play athletic games or to walk for any distance. Postoperatively he was fully active and pain-free.

The lateral column of the foot may be lengthened by a lateral opening osteotomy with either a triangular or

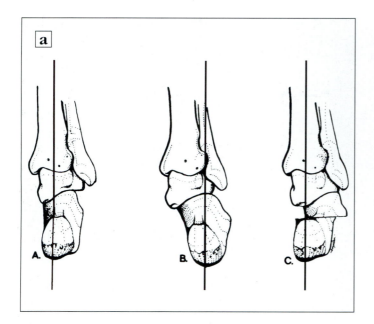

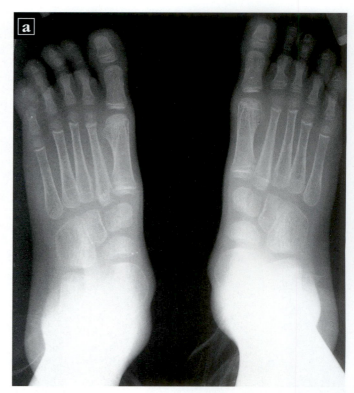

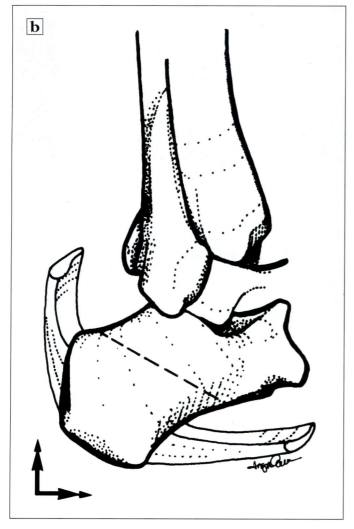

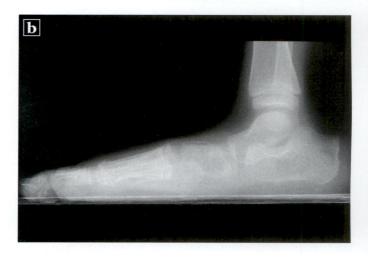

Figure 8

Medial displacement osteotomy of the calcaneus: (a) the
posterior segment of the calcaneus is displaced medially to
restore weight bearing axis; (b) the osteotomy is oblique
from posterior superior to anterior inferior

a rectangular graft. The osteotomy should be between
the medial and anterior facets, a point 6–10 mm from
the calcaneal–cuboid joint. Dall (1978) has reported on
his experience with an opening lateral wedge
osteotomy of the calcaneus with good results. He
recommends that this procedure be done before 12
years of age. If the heel cord is tight and prevents dorsiflexion to neutral it must be lengthened in all operations for flatfeet.

The extra-articular subtalar arthrodesis that has been so
beneficial in the neurological pes valgus is not recommended for the idiopathic flatfoot. It can successfully
restore the arch and correct the plantarflexed talus, but the

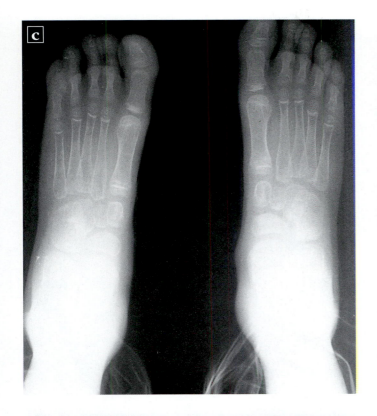

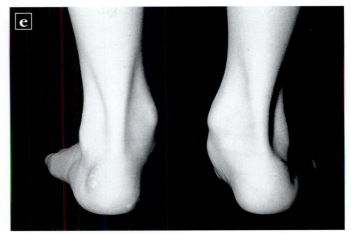

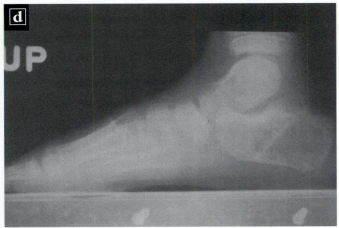

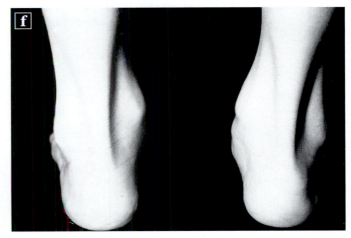

Figure 9

(a), (b) Anteroposterior and lateral views show the typical deformity of a flexible flat foot; (c), (d) anteroposterior and lateral views of the foot after a medial displacement osteotomy of the calcaneus; (e), (f) appearance of foot preoperatively and postoperatively

price of loss of motion is probably not a fair trade-off for the correction. The calcaneal osteotomies can be used in the paralytic foot although Evans recommended it be used only in feet with normal muscles.

An alternative method to correct the flexible flatfoot is the STA Peg procedure: this is an arthroereisis of the subtalar joint by the implantation of the polyethylene peg into the dorsal surface of the calcaneus just anterior to the posterior facet. The peg blocks subtalar lateral rotation and eversion. It has been used in children as young as 3 years of age (Lepow & Smith 1989). E A Millar has used it successfully in young patients who have cerebral palsy (personal communication).

Congenital convex pes valgus

The deformity present in a congenital convex pes valgus was described by Henken in 1914. However, it was first named properly by Lamey & Weissmann in 1939 in an article that reviewed the world literature on this subject. They correctly labeled it as congenital convex pes valgus. The most obvious radiological feature in this deformity is the vertical orientation of the talus, hence the more commonly used name of congenital vertical talus. It is unfortunate that it is referred to as a vertical talus, for the vertically oriented talus is only one of the features of this condition. The talus is vertically oriented (plantarflexed) in other conditions such as congenital pes calcaneovalgus and spastic cerebral palsy. The emphasis placed on the vertical attitude of the talus has led to inappropriate treatment both of this deformity and of other conditions with a similar radiographic appearance.

Convex pes valgus occurs in three patterns. It may be present as an isolated condition, or in association with other joint abnormalities, or in congenital neuromuscular disease (Ogata et al 1979). It is evenly distributed between males and females and about 50% of cases are bilateral.

The etiology of the primary isolated form is unknown. It is probably an embryological fault occurring in the first trimester. There is a familial relationship but the inheritance pattern is not clear (Herndon & Heyman 1963). It also occurs in certain chromosomal abnormalities, such as trisomy 18.

Pathology

The pathological anatomy was best described by Patterson et al (1968) from their dissection of a 6-week-old female with the classical deformity who died of a congenital heart disease. They found abnormalities in the tendons, joints and bones. Contractures of the tendons of the anterior tibialis, extensor hallucis longus, extensor digitorum communis and peroneus brevis are present and contribute to the difficulty in correcting the deformity. A significant feature is the dorsal dislocation of the navicular on to the neck of the talus. The calcaneus is in equinus and is rotated laterally. It is in valgus and displaced posteriorly so there is no support for the talar head from the anterior part of the calcaneus. There is a lateral and dorsal subluxation of the cuboid on the calcaneus. The changes in the calcaneus, besides its malposition as related to the subtalar joint, are an absence of the anterior facet, hypoplasia of the middle facet, and an abnormal shape to the posterior facet. The head of the talus is oval or pointed, and has a decreased circumference of the neck. The length of the talus is excessive for the size of the foot. This is not significant in the infant but becomes a major problem in reduction of the navicular in the older child if the treatment is delayed or unsuccessful.

Clinical features

The rigidity and the rocker-bottom appearance of the sole of the foot are the two most significant clinical features. In the older infant these two characteristics are easily appreciated. However in the newborn the rigidity is not so profound and the rocker appearance not so

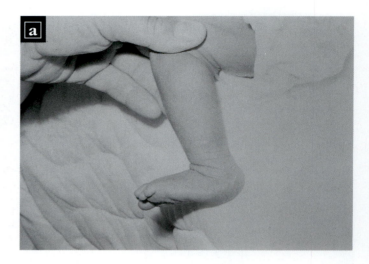

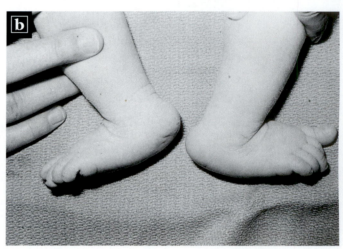

Figure 10

(a) Newborn with positional calcaneovalgus; (b) newborn with vertical talus

obvious. A severe talipes calcaneovalgus foot can be mistaken for a convex cavus pes valgus and vice versa. In the newborn the calcaneovalgus deformity is the most difficult differential (Fig. 10). To add to the confusion, the talus in a severe calcaneovalgus foot may be plantarflexed as seen on a lateral radiograph, but there are other radiographic and physical findings that will differentiate the two.

In convex pes valgus, the hindfoot is in equinus and valgus, and the midfoot and forefoot dorsiflexed and abducted. The equinus of the hindfoot may be severe and easily recognized but recognition of the equinus is difficult when it is less severe. If on examination one can demonstrate without doubt that on dorsiflexion of the forefoot the hindfoot remains in equinus, the diagnosis of congenital convex pes valgus can be made. This is not always easy to do. A maneuver we have used is to maximally plantarflex, adduct and supinate the foot, and while palpating the talus and calcaneus with the thumb and fingers of one hand dorsiflex the foot with the other hand. The failure of the talus and calcaneus to dorsiflex is further confirmatory evidence of this serious deformity. In some cases this position of the foot may prevent dorsiflexion of the forefoot to its resting position. These two physical findings do not occur in talipes calcaneovalgus.

Radiographic features

The main pathognomonic of congenital convex pes valgus is the dorsal dislocation of the navicular on to the neck of the talus. Since the navicular is not ossified until 3 years of age, radiographs will not show the dislocation. There are, however, diagnostic features present on appropriately taken radiographs. The anterior–posterior view shows the extreme divergence of the long axis of the talus and calcaneus. A Harris view with the foot dorsiflexed shows the medial rotation of the talus (Fig. 11). On the lateral view the calcaneus and talus are plantarflexed in relation to the forefoot. The lateral views should be taken with the foot held first in plantarflexion and then in dorsiflexion. The relationship of the talus and calcaneus changes very little in these two views. Of more importance is that a line along the long axis of the first metatarsal will pass anterior to the head of the talus in both views (Fig. 12). In the normal foot and in the calcaneovalgus foot, the line along the long axis of the first metatarsal will bisect the head of the talus when the foot is plantarflexed. With plantarflexion and dorsiflexion of the normal foot, the talus will change its relationship to the tibia and to the calcaneus. These normal findings should also be present in talipes calcaneovalgus if the lateral film is made with the foot held in a position of neutral valgus-varus. The talus in the severe spastic foot associated with cerebral palsy and other neuromuscular disease where the heel cord is tight may be plantarflexed and resemble the talus of the convex pes valgus foot. The difference, however, is that in these feet the navicular is always in contact with the articular surface of the talus. A lateral radiograph taken with the foot plantarflexed will show the cuneiform and first metatarsal to be in line with the head of the talus.

Treatment

Treatment is most successful when started early. This is true even when the final treatment is open reduction. It seems that preliminary stretching of the tight tendons and ligaments makes the reduction easier with less tendon lengthening.

There are those who believe that manipulation and casting in the corrected position is generally successful

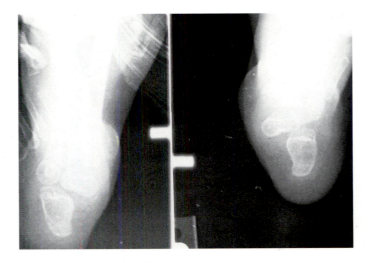

Figure 11

Harris view of the foot with the foot dorsiflexed

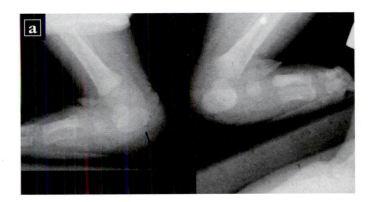

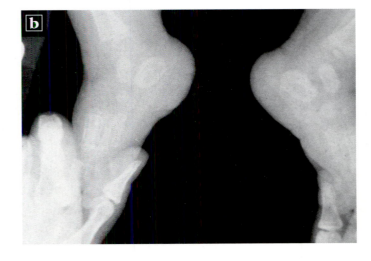

Figure 12

(a) A lateral view dorsiflexed; (b) plantarflexed view. The axis of the first metatarsal is anterior to the head of the talus on the right foot but is aligned with the talus on the left. The left foot corrected with cast treatment, the right did not

(Becker-Anderson & Reimann 1974, Giannestras 1973). Very detailed and elaborate descriptions of the technique are given by those who report success with non-operative treatment (Fitton et al 1979, Giannestras 1973). The radiographs of the feet that were successfully treated with plaster in these publications all had a vertically oriented talus, but the calcaneus did not appear to be in equinus. There were no lateral radiographs made with the foot plantarflexed to ascertain whether or not the first metatarsal cuneiform and navicular would come appropriately in line with the head of the talus. These feet could have been severe talipes calcaneovalgus.

Treatment should begin as early as possible. The goals are to stretch the tendons of the anterior tibialis, extensor hallucis longus, extensor digitorum communis and peroneus brevis, by plantarflexing the forefoot while attempting to prevent further plantarflexion of the hindfoot. The navicular has to be reduced on to the head of the talus by pushing the head of the talus upward as the midfoot and forefoot are plantarflexed and adducted. Pressure over the lateral surface of the calcaneus is applied to reduce the anterior part of the calcaneus beneath the talus. Giannestras (1973) described a technique in which the foot is manipulated and a slipper type cast is applied. The foot is then dorsiflexed in the slipper to stretch the heel cord and the cast extended up to the thigh.

Open reduction

Many authors believe that non-operative treatment of a convex pes valgus will always fail, and advise open reduction (Fitton et al 1979, Herndon & Heyman 1963, Ogata et al 1979). We have seldom completely corrected a convex pes valgus without surgery.

The surgical approach to the feet may be through whatever incision or incisions one prefers. It is essential that the talonavicular, calcaneocuboid, and talocalcaneal joints should be reduced. Equally important is the prevention of loss of correction by adequate correction of the deforming forces.

We prefer a one-stage correction through an oblique medial–posterior and dorsal–lateral incision. Fitton et al (1979) recommended an anterior transverse and posterior incision. Through the medial–posterior incision the navicular is identified and the talonavicular capsule is opened after removing the tibialis posterior. Open the capsule without removing the spring ligament. To open the dislocated talonavicular joint, the tibionavicular ligament is divided. This ligament is a deterrent to the adequate reduction of the talonavicular joint. After the head of the talus is well exposed, remove the elongated spring ligament from the navicular. Label it well so it can later be reattached distally. Dissect the tibialis anterior and lengthen it by Z-plasty tenotomy. Through a lateral incision the toe extensors and peroneus brevis are exposed and lengthened and the calcaneocuboid capsule divided superiorly and laterally.

At this point the talonavicular and subtalar joints should be reduced. At times the calcaneus may not rotate beneath the talus, and will not reduce until the posterior subtalar joint is opened. Occasionally the talocalcaneal interosseous ligaments may need to be divided before the talocalcaneal subluxation can be reduced. When the reduction has been accomplished, pass a Kirschner wire across the talonavicular joint and two wires across the subtalar joint from the plantar surface. The dislocated joints are now reduced and the foot will be in equinus.

Through the medial–posterior incision, lengthen the heel cord with a Z-plasty and open the ankle joint posteriorly. This may have to be done before the subtalar joint can be correctly repositioned and before the fixation wires are passed. Make sure this capsule is completely divided from the medial malleolus to the lateral malleolus. Avoid excessive lengthening of the heel cord, as one of the most frequent problems encountered has been the weakness of the gastrocsoleus muscle with persistent limited plantarflexion. Reattach the spring ligament to the navicular or cuneiform. It is important that the ligament should be taut. Close the talonavicular capsule medially and inferiorly, reefing it as much as possible.

The tibialis posterior is important in preventing the subluxation of the subtalar joint. Its reattachment must be secure to either the navicular or the cuneiform. If the posterior tibialis is found to be displaced anteriorly on the medial malleolus, an attempt should be made to reroute it behind and beneath the malleolus. Repair the heel cord so it is snug with the foot at neutral dorsiflexion and finish the operation by suturing the other lengthened tendons. Postoperatively the foot is immobilized for 6 weeks in plaster. It is possible to obtain correction of moderate or mild deformities without lengthening the anterior tibialis and toe extensors, but recurrence of the deformity is more likely if they are not lengthened.

In older children it may be impossible to reduce the talonavicular joint. This is because the talus becomes too long and there is not enough space in the medial column to accommodate both the talus and the navicular. In this situation the navicular can be excised; however, the release as described above must still be done for success. In children over 3 years of age a subtalar extra-articular arthrodesis should be done to prevent recurrence of the deformity. This can be done at the time of the initial correction or as a secondary procedure, though it is preferably done at the initial operation if the child is over 3 years of age.

In children 12 years of age and older, the function of the foot can be improved, pain relieved, and appearance made more normal by a triple arthrodesis.

Metatarsus adductus

Metatarsus adductus encompasses a considerable spectrum of deformity. At one end of the spectrum is the newborn with a supple mild adducted forefoot with a neutral heel that requires no treatment. At the other end of the spectrum is the older child with a ball and socket ankle joint, internal tibial torsion, valgus at the heel and a supinated adducted forefoot that is rigid (Lloyd-Roberts & Clark 1973). The latter child will require an operative procedure on both the forefoot and hindfoot for correction. Metatarsus adductus has been called by many names and clinical definitions over the years, including metatarsus varus, metatarsus adductovarus, metatarsus adductocavovarus, metatarsus et supinatus, hooked forefoot, metatarsus internus and pes adductus. The descriptive term metatarsus adductus is used to denote a foot with an adducted forefoot or adducted and supinated forefoot with a neutral heel (Henke 1863). Skew foot will be applied to a similar forefoot deformity in association with heel valgus (Peterson 1986, McCormick & Blount 1949).

Clinical features

With respect to the leg, some authors state that some degree of internal tibial torsion is always present (Bankart 1921), while others fail to recognize any abnormal torsion through the tibia (Ponseti & Becker 1966, Bleck 1983). There is universal agreement that the hindfoot is never in varus or equinus. The ankle may have limited plantarflexion. The hindfoot is described as being in neutral by some authors, while other authors state that there is valgus (Kendrick et al 1970, Kite 1950, Ponseti & Becker 1966). The valgus of the hindfoot seen clinically is apparent in radiographic examination. There is an increase in the talocalcaneal angle on the anterior posterior and lateral views of the foot. By definition,

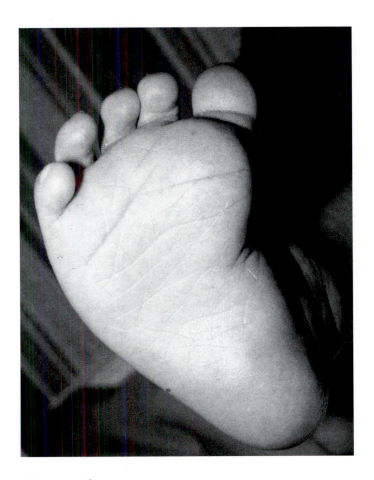

Figure 14

The typical plantar appearance of metatarsus adductus is a convex lateral border and a deep transverse molded crease with adducted forefoot

however, metatarsus adductus has a neutral heel and skew foot describes a similar forefoot deformity in association with a valgus heel. The medial cuneiform is misshapen, it ossifies late, and according to one report it is replaced by a fibrocartilagenous disk (Bankart 1921). The cuneiforms are rotated medially (in a varus position) on the hindfoot. The base of the first metatarsal articulates with the medial aspect of the first cuneiform. There is a medial angulation at the tarsometatarsal joints that is greatest at the first and least at the fifth (Fig. 13). Some authors have stated that the metatarsals have a dorsal and lateral bow while others believe that the bowing is a result of parallax on the anteroposterior radiograph, giving the appearance of bowing owing to the varus attitude of the metatarsal and the normal dorsal convexity (Kite 1967). The bases of the fifth metatarsal and cuboid are prominent, and the lateral border of the foot is convex. There is a crease across the medial border of the foot at the midtarsal joint (Fig. 14). The forefoot appears adducted and in a variable amount of supination (or varus) relative to the hindfoot. The arch of the foot is higher than normal and the first web space is frequently wide.

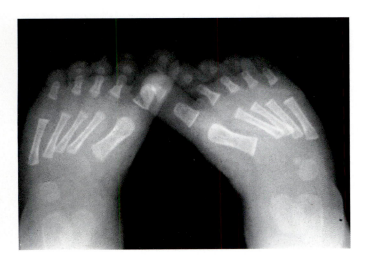

Figure 13

Anteroposterior radiograph showing the metatarsal adducted. The hindfoot is in a neutral position

Etiology

Several different theories have been advanced to explain the cause of metatarsus adductus. Bankart (1921) felt that the deformity was secondary to a deficiency of the medial cuneiform. Others have stated that it is secondary to muscle imbalance with abnormal insertion and action of the tibialis anterior (Peabody & Muro 1933). Abnormal insertion of the tibialis posterior tendon has also been thought to be important (Browne & Paton 1979). Evidence of the deformity being secondary to muscle imbalance is the occasionally reported late diagnosis of metatarsus adductus (Ponseti & Becker 1966), the imbalance presumably becoming more obvious as the child grows. In an effort to understand the forces involved in the development of metatarsus adductus, Reimann & Werner (1975) attempted to produce the deformity in stillborns by positioning the foot. They noted that, with the foot in maximal dorsiflexion and after capsulotomies of the tarsometatarsal and intratarsal joints, it was possible to position the foot in the deformed position.

Multiple series have shown few anomalies associated with metatarsus adductus, though an association with congenital hip dysplasia does exist. Males affected with metatarsus adductus slightly outnumber females, and it is more common than not to have bilateral involvement. Frequently, however, in cases with bilateral involvement, the two feet are not equally affected.

In order to decide who needs treatment, one should understand what is known about the natural history of this deformity. In 1978, Rushforth published a series of 130 feet in 83 children who were followed without treatment for 7 years. At follow-up, 86% were normal or had mild deformity, 10% were considered moderately deformed, and only 4% remained with a rigid deformity. It was not possible to differentiate early in life between those children who would go on spontaneously to resolve their deformity from those who would not. Of note is that Rushfort did not report any foot that became progressively worse without treatment and it has been stated by Bleck (1983) that metatarsus adductus does not predispose to hallux valgus or bunion deformities.

In 1966, Ponseti & Becker published the Iowa experience. While they state that the deformity is often not recognized in the first 3 months of life, fully two-thirds of their patients had the diagnosis made at birth. They stated that the heel is in moderate to severe valgus and that varying degrees of forefoot and hindfoot deformity are present. Therefore, they combined metatarsus adductus and what should be called a skew foot deformity when they reported on the results of their treatment. Of 379 patients who presented with metatarsus adductus, only 12% were felt to need treatment. The deformity in the patients who were not treated was noted to progress slightly until 1–2 years of age and then regress spontaneously. Ponseti & Becker stated that once the deformity was 'well corrected' there were no recurrences. While they quantitated their results in terms of fifth metatarsocalcaneal angles and talocalcaneal angles, they did not state the numbers of patients that fell into each group. The average age at the time of the initial treatment was 6 months, and the average number of plaster casts was four with the first three worn for 2 weeks each and the final cast worn for 3 weeks. Only two patients in their series went on to surgery.

In 1983, Bleck reported a retrospective review of the patients who were referred to him over a 21 year period with metatarsus adductus. All of his patients had a neutral hindfoot. Bleck treated all patients with metatarsus adductus because of the 'obvious practical, ethical and legal problems associated with not treating' patients with this deformity. In the 13–37-month-old age group that received manipulations and plaster cast treatment, he reported a failure rate of up to 70%. He introduced the concept of the heel bisector as a method of grading the severity of the deformity. The heel bisector is a line along the long axis of the heel pad. This line is projected onto the forefoot to determine which toe is intersected. If the heel bisects or intersects the second web space, the foot is normal; intersection of the third toe defines a mild deformity; and intersection of the fourth web space defines a severe deformity. Kite (1950) used a similar method but measured the angle between a line projected proximally along the axis of the forefoot. Bleck (1983) states that he assessed mild deformities as normal when he graded his results at follow-up. He reports that better results were obtained in the group of patients in whom treatment was begun before 8 months of age, and that this difference was statistically significant compared to those patients in whom treatment was begun after they were 8 months of age. However, if one eliminates the mild cases and reevaluates the data, there is no statistically significant difference in outcome between the two groups. Therefore from Bleck's data one cannot differentiate the patients that may require treatment according to the severity or the flexibility of the deformity or the age when treatment was initiated.

McCauley et al (1964), in a series of patients from New York University Medical Center pointed out that a high complication rate and high recurrence rate can be associated with the care of this deformity. Overall, 47% of the feet treated had some residual deformity, and 32% had recurrence. They felt that patients would have fewer recurrences if they were held in a corrected position for some time once the correction was achieved.

Peabody & Muro (1933) reviewed the literature and reported 14 cases of their own. Their cases, however, were fairly equally divided between what would be considered metatarsus adductus and skew foot deformities, and insufficient follow-up was recorded to assess results of their treatment.

Kite (1950, 1967) described metatarsus adductus in quite clear terms. He defined what is here designated metatarsus adductus as a forefoot deformity with a neutral heel and reported 300 and then 2818 cases. He differentiated patients with metatarsus adductus from a much smaller group of nine patients who had a fixed valgus deformity of the heel (skew foot), and stated that these patients have a different pattern of inheritance and different response to therapy. In his experience, patients with metatarsus adductus responded well to serial manipulations and plaster cast applications, and with this treatment recurrence was not a significant problem.

Therefore, from the reports that are currently in the literature, there is considerable variability in the ease with which correction of this deformity can be achieved. There are no clinical or radiographic clues as to which patients might benefit from treatment, and the best time to initiate treatment is unknown. Clearly the series reported by Rushforth (1978) and Ponseti & Becker (1966) have the best overall results. Ponseti & Becker used manipulation and cast treatment in only 12% of the patients who presented with metatarsus adductus. Their only indication for treatment was a deformity that could not be passively corrected.

Undertaking a manipulation and serial cast program followed by a post-cast splinting program on all patients who present with metatarsus adductus, when perhaps as few as 4% will have persistent severe deformity, hardly seems justified. It has never been proven that plaster cast treatment improves upon the natural history. It is possible that cast treatment or treatment with reversed last shoes and a Denis–Browne bar may produce a flat foot. It is to be recommended that patients with flexible metatarsus adductus (i.e. passively correctable) do not require any treatment other than observation. Those with more rigid forefoot adduction, and limited plantarflexion should be treated. It may be that those patients in whom the navicular is laterally displaced on the head of the talus do not spontaneously correct. Since the navicular is not ossified until the fourth year of life, this group has never been singled out and observed.

Treatment

Treatment should consist of serial manipulations and the application of plaster casts. However, a period of observation, perhaps with a supervised exercise/stretching program may be warranted, because there is no evidence that the deformity is progressive, and because cast treatment is not without complications. A period of observation would allow one to identify those patients who are not improving spontaneously.

Prior to the application of a cast, the foot is gently manipulated by abducting the forefoot with the foot in slight equinus. Counter pressure is placed over the calcaneus and cuboid to keep the hindfoot out of valgus. The cast is applied and molded, with the same forces being applied while the plaster sets. We use a short leg cast, but it is not unreasonable to use a long leg cast.

The surgical management of metatarsus adductus is reserved for those older patients in whom the deformity is considered significant. These children are generally 3 years

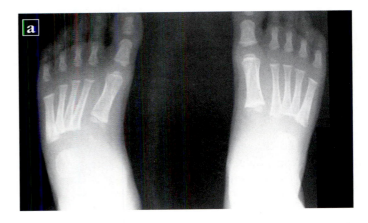

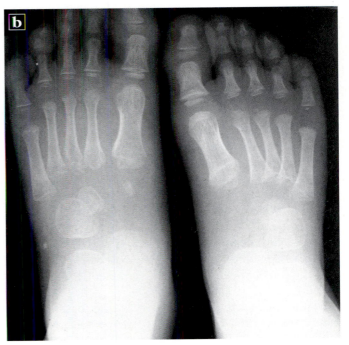

Figure 15

(a) This 3-year-old child had metatarsus adductus with hindfoot valgus that had not responded well to cast treatment earlier; (b) after tarsometatarsal capsulotomy

of age or older and have either failed to correct spontaneously or have failed serial manipulation and cast management. While no definite disability has been associated with uncorrected metatarsus adductus, some children complain of a generalized fatigue in their feet more readily than normal children after walking or standing for prolonged periods. Difficulty with footwear may also be a problem.

Recommended surgical procedures have varied. They have included excision of the cuboid, wedge resection of the cuboid, resection of the bases of all the metatarsals, excision of the abductor hallucis muscle or section of its tendon, osteotomies of the metatarsal shafts, excision of the bases of the central three metatarsals combined with subcutaneous osteotomy of the fifth metatarsal with reduction of the luxation of the first metatarsocuneiform joint, and triple arthrodesis (Bankart 1921, Peabody & Muro 1933).

Heyman et al (1958) reported on a soft tissue procedure that involved mobilization of the tarsometatarsal joint capsules so that the forefoot could be corrected (Fig. 15). A follow-up paper gave refinements of the procedure (Kendrick et al 1970). The Heyman–Herndon capsulotomy is performed through either a transverse incision or two axial incisions over the tarsometatarsal joints. A careful release of the tarsometatarsal joint capsule is carried out. The lateral portion of the plantar joint capsule is preserved to give stability and to prevent dorsal subluxation of the metatarsals. We find the tarsometatarsal joints can more easily be identified by beginning the dissection between the metatarsals. The growth plate of the first metatarsal must not be injured by the dissection. Following this release, the foot is corrected and the position held by Kirschner wires directed from the first and fifth rays into the tarsal bones. The patient is then placed in a plaster cast for 6 weeks. This procedure is recommended for children up to 6–8 years of age, but we have found that in children over 4 years of age, correction is better with a combination of capsulotomies of the first and fifth tarsometatarsal joints and osteotomy of the second, third and fourth metatarsals. As some incongruity of the joint surfaces occurs with the correction obtained with tarsometatarsal capsulotomies, this procedure may produce early degenerative arthritis in the older child in whom less potential for remodeling exists. Indeed, asymptomatic osteoarthritis has been reported at follow-up (Kendrick et al 1970).

In the older child, osteotomy of the bases of the metatarsals is our procedure of choice to correct the forefoot. Berman & Gartland reported their experience in 1971. They recommended the same incision as Heyman & Herndon but performed dome-shaped osteotomies, convex proximally, of the metatarsal bases with care being taken to avoid the growth plate at the base of the first metatarsal.

Skew foot

Skew foot is a rare foot deformity that is defined as an adduction deformity of the forefoot combined with a valgus heel and abduction of the navicular on the talus. X-rays show adduction of the metatarsals, lateral sublux-

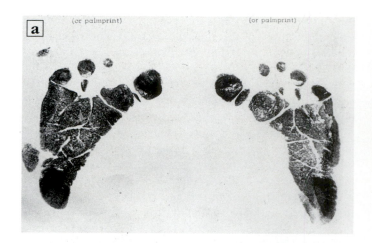

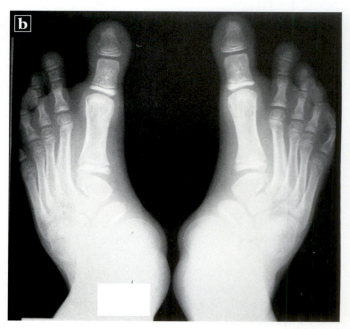

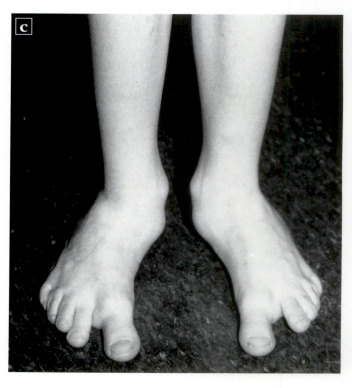

Figure 16

(a) Footprint of infant adducted forefoot: (b), (c) the same patient at 10 years of age. The metatarsals are adducted, the cuneiform short and oblique, the navicular displaced laterally and the hindfoot in valgus

ation of the navicular on the head of the talus and an increase in the talocalcaneal angle on both the antero-posterior and lateral films. The metatarsus adductus that fails to correct or recurs after cast treatment is very likely to have hindfoot valgus. It may well be that a subgroup of the patients with recurrent or resistant metatarsus adductus in fact represent skew foot deformities.

Peterson (1986), in a recent review of the literature, noted that less than 50 cases of skew foot have been reported to date. In the early literature the cases of skew feet were not clearly differentiated from metatarsus adductus. Kite (1967) reported 12 cases of skew foot deformity along with 2818 cases of metatarsus adductus and states that he felt these rarer cases had a different inheritance pattern, and that they generally required operative intervention for correction.

The etiology of skew foot deformity is unknown. Some have stated that it develops secondary to poor cast management of metatarsus adductus, and some of the case reports seem to bear this out (Peterson 1986). However, the precast X-rays are not always available from these cases and precast heel valgus may already have been present. Evidence for a congenital etiology is shown in the case presented in Fig 16. The patient shown in Fig. 16 had no treatment prior to these radiographs. Further evidence for this being a congenital deformity is presented by Peterson (1986), and in a case reported from Nové-Josserand and Fancillon (Peabody & Muro 1933).

Treatment

The natural history and treatment of the skew foot deformity are clearly not known, since they have not been studied or reported in any organized fashion. Peterson (1986) cites one case in which cast treatment was successful. One has to wonder, however, whether or not this case in many clinics would have fallen into the group of patients successfully managed by serial manipulations and application of plaster casts, and carried a diagnosis of metatarsus adductus. Cases with mild heel valgus and adducted forefeet represent skew feet by definition, but are probably often included with cases of metatarsus adductus. In the older child with an established skew foot, surgery remains the mainstay of therapy. These patients present with complaints related to the appearance of their feet and problems with footwear, and occasionally with pain.

Most authors teach that both a forefoot and hindfoot bony procedure are necessary to correct the deformity. Whether these should be staged or could be performed at one sitting depends on the procedure and the surgeon. In the younger child a forefoot procedure, either capsulotomies of the tarsometatarsal joints or metatarsal osteotomies combined with a medial slide osteotomy of the calcaneus is indicated. In the older child a triple arthrodesis to correct the hindfoot and laterally displaced navicular and osteotomies of the metatarsals is the procedure of choice.

Tarsal coalition

The coalition of tarsal bones was described nearly 150 years ago, but it is only in this century that these coalitions have been found to be of clinical significance. Although a coalition may exist between any tarsal bones and may be multiple, the two most common types are the calcaneonavicular (CN) and the talocalcaneal (TC). Coalitions between the talus and navicular and the calcaneus and cuboid are rare.

Etiology

The etiology of the coalition may be multiple, but two concepts prevail. Sloman (1920) gave credit to Pfitzner for describing a gradual union of the os calcaneus secundaris to either the navicular or the calcaneus, or to both. Harris & Beath believed that the TC coalition resulted from fusion of an accessory os sustentaculi to the talus and calcaneus. In the ossification of the talocalcaneal coalition there may be a pattern that suggests Harris & Beath were correct (Fig. 17). However, this may represent a secondary ossification center within the cartilaginous coalition.

A more accepted theory is that the coalition is the result of a segmentation defect of the mesenchyme. According to Sloman (1921), Holl (an anatomist from Vienna) described a CN coalition in a newborn. We have dissected a newborn foot with a cartilaginous coalition between the calcaneus and the navicular. This cartilaginous mass had the same configuration as that seen in the coalition in older patients. It appears that coalitions are cartilaginous at birth, gradually ossify, and eventually become completely osseous. In the adolescent there is usually a cartilaginous segment in the bar that becomes completely osseous at maturity.

There is a genetic aspect to this condition (Leonard 1974, Wray & Herndon 1963), the inheritance pattern appearing to be autosomal dominant. Leonard (1974) found a 39% incidence of coalition in first-degree relatives. A family tree of grandfather, father and child was described by Wray & Herndon (1963).

Clinical features

The features most commonly associated with tarsal coalition are flat rigid feet with apparent spasm of the peroneal tendons. Although pes valgus is common, the appearance of the foot may be normal, or there may be a cavus and varus deformity. Motion is limited in the subtalar complex. The limitation of motion is easier to appreciate when passive motion is painful, since the protective action of the muscles further limits motion. In the CN foot, there is talocalcaneal motion but it is limited, whereas in the TC foot there is no subtalar motion. The peroneal muscles are usually the prominent protector of the painful subtalar joint – hence the name 'peroneal spastic flatfoot'. These muscles are not spastic but are contracted and overactive as a protector. In some patients, the anterior tibialis is contracted and over-responsive to passive subtalar motion. In the asymptomatic foot, these muscles are neither contracted nor overactive during passive motion.

Pain in the foot with a coalition is seldom present until early adolescence. The pain is located around the midfoot and is usually dorsal and lateral. It is aggravated by activity but is most severe during the first few minutes of walking after resting for several hours. Periodically the patient has an antalgic gait. There is usually atrophy of the calf muscles.

Diagnosis

The clinical features are usually suggestive and radiographs confirmatory of the diagnosis but other conditions have to be ruled out. In the occasional patient no cause for the painful rigid foot can be identified.

The CN coalition that is either partially or completely osseous can always be seen on the oblique view of the foot (Fig. 18). The TC coalition of the middle facet can usually be seen in a properly made Harris view (Conway & Cowell 1969, Harris & Beath 1948). To be helpful, the tilt of the X-ray beam for the Harris view must be parallel to the posterior facet, which is also parallel to the middle facet. The angle for directing the X-ray beam is determined by the angle of the posterior facet as measured on the standing lateral radiograph of the foot.

When these two radiographic views do not show the suspected coalition, a study of the foot with computerized axial tomography should be done. To detect a TC coalition, the study is best carried out with the patient supine, the knees flexed, and the feet flat on the table (Stoskopf et al 1984). A computerized tomogram (CT) in the longitudinal direction with the patient supine, knees straight and the ankle dorsiflexed to neutral can demonstrate a CN coalition. The advantage of CT is that one can see the width of the coalition (Zuckerkandl 1877).

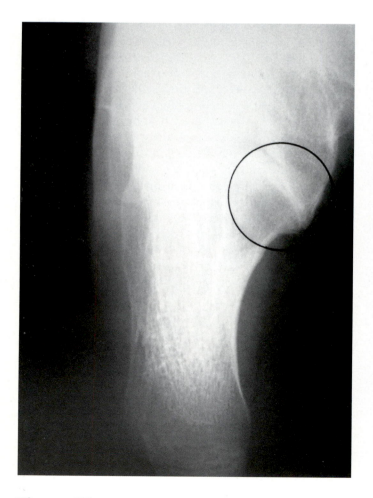

Figure 17

Harris view with talocalcaneal coalition

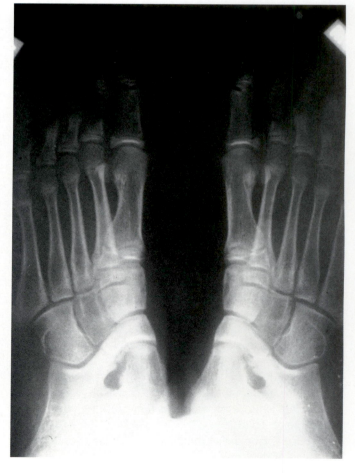

Figure 18

Oblique view with calcaneonavicular coalition

The differential diagnosis of the rigid painful foot includes juvenile rheumatoid arthritis (JRA), tumors, infection, and fractures. Monarticular JRA may affect only the subtalar joint. In the absence of radiographic demonstration of an abnormality a rheumatoid evaluation to include antinuclear antibodies, and HLA (human lymphocyte antibody) typing should be done. If symptoms last for more than 6–8 weeks, a slit lamp eye examination should be done. A bone scan should be part of the evaluation when the radiograph and CT scan of a painful foot with limited motion are normal. The bone scan would probably demonstrate increased activity if there had been a recent fracture or if there was a tumor or infection. Some increase in activity in the early phase of the study may be present with JRA. Increased activity in the late phase would be likely in osteomyelitis, fracture, or tumor.

Lateral tomography has been used to show a TC coalition at the anterior facet. The exact technique for this study was described by Conway & Cowell (1969). The foot should lie on the table in an absolutely lateral position. Measure the width of the foot at the sustentaculum. Four cuts are made from this position, at 1 cm, 1.5 cm, and 2 cm less than the width of the foot, and at half the width of the foot. The 1.0 cm cut bisects the middle TC facet, the 1.5 and 2 cm cuts bisect the anterior facet, and the fourth cut bisects the posterior facet. Centering is over the sustentaculum, and a 50° arc is used.

Occasionally, all studies in a patient with a painful rigid foot will be normal. These patients should be treated by 4 weeks of immobilization in a short leg cast that maintains the foot in a neutral position. This should be followed by the use of a well-made arch pad.

Calcaneonavicular coalition

The first description of a CN coalition was by Cruveilhier (1829). Sloman was the first, however, to associate a CN with a painful rigid flat foot (Sloman 1921). He was also the first to demonstrate the coalition by radiographs. Although Sloman did not excise the coalition, he suggested that excision was a possibility. Badgley (1927) was the first to report surgical excision of the CN coalition. The addition of the imposition of the extensor communis brevis was reported by Bentzon in 1928. Forty years later this procedure became a well-established technique for treatment.

Successful results from the surgical treatment of a CN coalition can be expected in the majority of patients (Andreasen 1968, Mitchell & Gibson 1967). Those with the best prognosis are patients under 14 years of age with no secondary changes in the TN joint who still have a cartilage segment in the coalition.

CN coalitions are commonly classified as fibrous, cartilaginous or osseous. The cartilaginous and osseous types are reflections of age, for all osseous coalitions were cartilaginous at one stage. We have never confidently identified a fibrous coalition although we have seen a number of painful feet with limited motion when all laboratory tests, radiographs, CT, and bone scans were normal. Some of these responded to treatment with casts and arch support, others have been relieved only after triple arthrodesis. According to Conway & Cowell (1969), if a fibrous coalition is present, the dense cortical surface of the navicular and calcaneus will be indistinct and irregular, and the head of the talus hypoplastic.

Treatment

The nonoperative treatment for a symptomatic CN coalition is a 4–6-week period of immobilization in a cast followed by the use of arch pads. The results are mostly unsatisfactory, but it is worth the effort, particularly if the coalition is completely osseous.

To excise the coalition, make an oblique incision over the sinus tarsus. The origin of the extensor communis brevis is carefully dissected free to expose the anterior part of the calcaneus, the calcaneocuboid joint, and the coalition. Two osteotomy cuts are made through the coalition. The anterior one is made just plantar to the head of the talus and directed plantarwards and medially. Care should be taken not to injure the head of the talus or to disrupt the talonavicular capsule. The second osteotomy is directed horizontally across the calcaneal end of the coalition. The entire width of the coalition must be removed. After removal of the coalition is complete, the raw bone surfaces should be cauterized and the extensor communis brevis muscle pulled between the calcaneus and navicular by means of an absorbable suture that is passed through the skin on the plantar medial surface and tied over a well-padded button.

Postoperatively the foot is placed in a cast that holds the foot in slight varus. After 3 weeks, the cast is bivalved and an active range of motion exercises for the ankle and subtalar joint is begun. At 6 weeks, partial weight bearing can be allowed with progression to full activity as tolerated.

Older patients with a complete osseous coalition and those with secondary degenerative changes in the subtalar joint such as narrowing of posterior facet or the talonavicular joint have such a high incidence of unsatisfactory results that a triple arthrodesis should be considered as the treatment of choice if conservative treatment fails.

Talocalcaneal coalition

The coalition at the middle facet of the talus and calcaneus was described in 1877 by Zuckerhandl. Harris & Beath (1948) first associated this coalition with the painful rigid foot. They discovered the coalition while approaching the subtalar joint medially to arthrodese the talonavicular and talocalcaneal joint in a rigid painful valgus foot. It was their impression that the coalition resulted from a fusion of an os calcaneus secundaris with the talus and calcaneus. We believe that this coalition is the result of a segmentation defect that leaves a cartilaginous segment intact between the talus and calcaneus. This cartilaginous segment gradually ossifies. The progression of the ossification may be from the talus or from the calcaneus. The direction of the cartilaginous bar as seen on a CT scan reflects the direction of the ossification pattern. If it flows from the calcaneus towards the talus, the cartilaginous bar is horizontal, and if the flow is from the talus towards the calcaneus, the bar is tilted plantarwards.

Treatment

Conservative treatment of the symptomatic foot with a TC coalition is not frequently satisfactory but should be tried just as in the CN coalition. For the failed conservatively treated foot the most common surgical treatment is a triple arthrodesis, but excision of the coalition can be successful. When there is either a severe valgus deformity or secondary joint changes with narrowing of the talonavicular joint, subtalar joint excision of the bar will not be satisfactory. The talar beaking so frequently present is not a sign of degeneration. It is the result of limited and abnormal motion of the subtalar complex where the navicular moves laterally and dorsally and elevates the talonavicular capsule and periosteum of the talus that responds by bony proliferation.

Excision of a TC coalition is possible in selected patients. The coalition should be relatively narrow and the deformity of the foot mild (Fig 18). A foot that has a severe valgus deformity is not likely to respond satisfactorily with excision of the coalition alone. If a severe valgus deformity is present, a calcaneal medial shift osteotomy should also be done. In one case where the coalition was too large to excise and a valgus deformity was present, we did a medial displacement osteotomy of the calcaneus, with relief of the pain.

The excision of a TC coalition at the level of the sustentaculum is approached through a medial incision. Identify the posterior tibialis tendon and release its sheaf sufficiently to retract the tendon for easy exposure of the anterior part of the subtalar joint. Open the subtalar capsule and identify the coalition at the sustentaculum. Continue the capsulotomy posterior to the sustentaculum to determine the posterior border of the coalition. Introduce a flat probe into the joint both anterior and posterior to the coalition to show the limits of the coalition. Use a dental bur to remove the coalition carefully and completely but without injuring the articular cartilage beyond the limits of the coalition. At completion, the space between the talus and calcaneus should be about 3 mm. Cauterize the raw bone surfaces and place a piece of fat into the area. Postoperatively, immobilize the foot in plaster for 1 week, after which motion

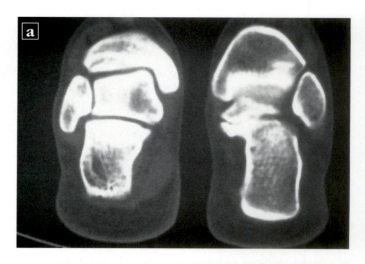

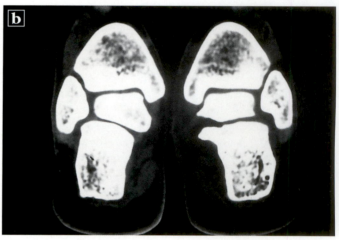

Figure 19

(a) Computerized tomography appearance of a talocalcaneal coalition; (b) after excision of the bar

exercises and partial weight bearing should be started. Protected weight bearing should be done for at least 12 weeks or until there is no pain on weight bearing.

References

Andreasen A 1968 Calcaneonavicular coalition: Late results of resection. Acta Orthop Scand 39: 424–432

Badgley C E 1927 Coalition of the calcaneus and the navicular. Arch Surg 15: 75–88

Bankart A S B 1921 Metatarsus varus. BMJ II: 685

Basmajian J R, Stecko G 1963 The role of muscles in arch support of the foot. An electromyographic study. J Bone Joint Surg 45A: 1184

Basta N W, Mital M A, Bonadio O, Johnson A, Kang S Y, O'Connor J 1977 A comparative study of the role of shoe, arch supports and navicular cookies in the management of symptomatic mobile flat feet in children. Int Orthop 1: 143

Becker-Anderson H, Reimann I 1974 Congenital vertical talus. Acta Orthop Scand 45: 130–144

Bentzon P G K 1928 Coalitio Calcaneonavicularis mit besonderer Bezugnahine auf die operative Behandlung des durch diese Aunomalie Bedingten Plattfusses. Verh Dtsch Orthop Ges 23: Kongress 269

Berman A, Gartland J J 1971 Metatarsal osteotomy for the correction of adduction of the forepart of the foot in children. J Bone Joint Surg 53A: 498

Bleck E, Berzins U 1977 Conservative management of pes valgus with plantar flexed talus, flexible. Clin Orthop 122: 85

Bleck E E 1983 Metatarsus adductus: classification and relationship to outcomes of treatment. J Pediatr Orthop 3: 2

Browne R S, Paton D F 1979 Anomalous insertion of the tibialis posterior tendon in congenital metatarsus varus. J Bone Joint Surg 61B: 74

Conway J J, Cowell H R 1969 Tarsal coalition: clinical significance and roentgenographic demonstration. Radiology 92: 799–811

Cruveilhier J 1829 Anatomie pathologique du corps humain. Tome I. J B Baillière, Paris

Dall G 1978 Open lateral wedge osteotomy of the calcaneum for severe postural pes valgus in children. S Afr Med J 53: 531

Evans D 1975 Calcaneo-valgus deformity. J Bone Joint Surg 57B: 270–278

Fitton J M 1979 The treatment of congenital vertical talus. J Bone Joint Surg 61B: 481–483

Giannestras N S 1973 The congenital rigid flatfoot. Orthop Clin North Am 4: 49–66

Haraldsson S 1962 Operative treatment of pes planovalgus staticus juvenilis. Acta Orthop Scand 32: 492

Harris R I, Beath T 1948 Etiology of peroneal spastic flat foot. J Bone Joint Surg 30B: 624–634

Helfet A J 1956 A new way of treating flat feet in children. Lancet I: 262

Henderson W H, Campbell J W 1967 UCBL shoe insert: casting and fabrication. The Biomechanics Laboratory, University of California at San Francisco and Berkeley Technical Report. p 53

Henke W 1863 Contracteur des metatarsus. Z Rat Med 17: 188

Henken R 1914 Contribution à l'étude des formes osseuses du pied valgus congénital. Thèse de Lyon. In: Tachdjian M O 1985 The Child's Foot. Saunders, Philadelphia: 2557

Herndon C H, Heyman C H 1963 Problems in the recognition and treatment of congenital convex pes valgus. J Bone Joint Surg 45A: 413–429

Heyman C H, Herndon C H, Strong J M 1958 Mobilization of the tarsometatarsal and intermetatarsal joints for the correction of resistant adduction of the forepart of the foot in congenital clubfoot or congenital metatarsus varus. J Bone Joint Surg 40A: 299

Jack E A 1953 Naviculocuneiform fusion in the treatment of flat foot. J Bone Joint Surg 35B: 75

Kendrick R E, Sharma N K, Hassler W L, Hernden C H 1970 Tarso metatarsal mobilization for resistant adduction of the forepart of the foot. J Bone Joint Surg 52A: 61–70

Kite J H 1950 Congenital metatarsus varus. Report of 300 Cases. J Bone Joint Surg. 32A: 500

Kite J H 1967 Congenital metatarsus varus. J Bone Joint Surg. 49A: 388–397

Lamey L, Weissman L 1939 Congenital convex pes valgus. J Bone Joint Surg. 21: 79–91

Leonard M A 1974 The inheritance of tarsal coalition and its relationship to spastic flatfoot. J Bone Joint Surg 56B: 520–526

Lepow GM, Smith SD 1989 A modified subtalar arthroereisis implant for the correction of flexible flatfoot in children. The STA Peg procedure. Clin Podiatr Med Surg 6: 585–590

Lichtblau S 1975 Section of the abductor hallucis tendon for correction of metatarsus varus deformity. Clin Orthop 110: 227

Lloyd-Roberts G C, Clark R C 1973 Ball and socket ankle joint in metatarsus adductus varus (S shaped or serpentine foot). J Bone Joint Surg. 55B: 193–196

McCauley J Jr, Lusskin R, Bromley J 1964 Recurrence in congenital metatarsus varus. J Bone Joint Surg 46A: 525

McCormick D W, Blount W P 1949 Metatarsus adductovarus 'Skewfoot'. JAMA 141: 449

Mereday C, Dolan C M E, Lusskin R 1972 Evaluation of the University of California Biomechanic Laboratory shoe insert in flexible pes planus. Clin Orthop 82: 45–58

Miller O C 1927 A plastic flat foot operation. J Bone Joint Surg. 9: 84–91

Mitchell G P, Gibson J M C 1967 Excision of calcaneonavicular bar for painful spasmodic flatfoot. J Bone Joint Surg 49B: 281–287

Ogata K, Schoenecker P L, Sheridan J 1979 Congenital vertical talus and its familial occurrence: an analysis of 36 patients. Clin Orthop 139: 128–132

Patterson W R, Fitz D H, Smith W S 1968 The pathologic anatomy of congenital convex pes valgus. J Bone Joint Surg 50A: 458–466

Peabody C W, Muro F 1933 Congenital metatarsus varus. J Bone Joint Surg 15: 171

Peterson H A 1986 Skewfoot (forefoot adduction with heel valgus). J Pediatr Orthop 6: 24

Ponseti I V, Becker J R 1966 Congenital metatarsus adductus: The results of treatment. J Bone Joint Surg 48A: 702

Reimann I, Werner H H 1975 Congenital metatarsus varus. A suggestion for possible mechanism and relation to other foot deformities. Clin Orthop 110: 223

Rushforth G F 1978 The natural history of hooked forefoot. J Bone Joint Surg 60B: 530

Schwartz R P, Heath A L 1949 Conservative treatment of functional disorders of feet in adolescents and adults. J Bone Joint Surg 31A: 501

Seymour N 1967 The late results of naviculo-cuneiform fusion. J Bone Joint Surg 49B: 558

Slomann H C 1921 On coalition calcaneo-navicularis. J Orthop Surg 19: 586–602

Staheli L, Griffin L 1980 Corrective shoes for children: a survey of current practice. Pediatrics 65: 13–17

Stoskopf C A, Hermandez R J, Kelikian A, Tachdjian M O, Dias L S 1984 Evaluation of tarsal coalition by computed tomography. J Pediatr Orthop 4: 365–369

Wenger D R, Mauldin D, Speck G, Morgan D, Lieber R L 1989 Corrective shoes and inserts as treatment for flexible flatfoot in infants and children. J Bone Joint Surg 71A: 800–810

Wray J B, Herndon C N 1963 Hereditary transmission of congenital coalition of the calcaneus to the navicular. J Bone Joint Surg 45A: 365–372

Zuckerkandl 1877 Ueber einen tall von Synostose zwischen Talus und Calcaneus. Allg Wein Med Zeitung 22: 293

V.2 Tibialis Posterior Tendon Disorders

Nigel Cobb

The functioning of any tendon about the hindfoot may be impaired by disease or injury. For a long time acute rupture of the Achilles tendon was regarded as the most common tendon disruption in the area. Today the foremost contender is tibialis posterior with an insidious process of disorder that leads ultimately to its rupture and as a consequence to the acquired unilateral flat foot of later adult life.

Anatomy

Tibialis posterior is the most deeply placed muscle at the back of the leg. It takes origin from adjacent areas on the upper two thirds of the tibia and fibula, from the interosseus membrane between them and from adjacent intermuscular septae. Its tendon inclines medially, deep to the tendon of flexor digitorum longus, into a groove at the back of the medial malleolus, where it occupies a separate synovial sheath. Passing forwards deep to the flexor retinaculum, across the deltoid and below the calcaneonavicular or 'spring' ligament, it inserts principally into the tuberosity of the navicular and the medial cuneiform bone. Strong slips of attachment are sent forward to the bases of the central metatarsals, laterally to the other cuneiform bones and the cuboid, and backwards to the sustentaculum tali.

Tibialis posterior is a powerful muscle with a strong tendon that passes the furthest away medially from the axis of the subtalar joint (Fig. 1). This affords lever arm advantage in serving its main function as a hindfoot sling to invert the subtalar joint and adduct the forefoot (Duchenne 1949). When a person rises onto the toes, tibialis posterior contracts first to initiate inversion and to stabilize the subtalar joint. The gastrosoleus can then contract to plantar flex the foot at the ankle. Later, by virtue of its line of insertion moving medially, the gastrosoleus becomes a secondary and probably a more powerful invertor.

The longitudinal arch of the foot is normally maintained by the shape of the bones and the integrity of ligamentous structures (Basmajian & Stecko 1963). When tibialis posterior fails, its principal antagonist, peroneus brevis, acts unopposed to evert the subtalar joint and abduct the forefoot, which stretches the ligamentous structures and causes a flat foot deformity.

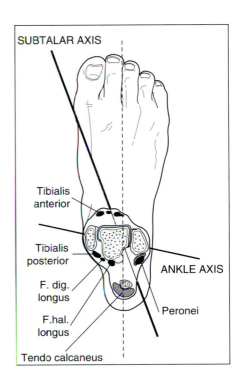

Figure 1

The line of action of the tibialis posterior tendon, being the furthest medial from the subtalar axis, gives that muscle the greatest mechanical advantage when acting as an invertor of the hindfoot

Aetiology and pathology of tibialis posterior tendon disorders

Clinically apparent tibialis posterior tendon dysfunction progresses through a phase of tenosynovitis to eventual rupture. Once looked upon as being something of a curiosity, spontaneous rupture of this tendon is today recognized to be more frequent than the better-known rupture of the Achilles tendon.

In 1936, Kulowski first referred to tenosynovitis in the sheath of the tibialis posterior tendon; other reports followed (Lipscomb 1950, Lapidus & Sedenstein 1950, Ghormley & Spear 1953, Fowler 1955, Williams 1963,

Jamieson 1964, Cozen 1965, Langenskiöld 1967, Norris & Mankin 1978, Trevino et al 1981). In 1953, Key describes partial rupture of the tibialis posterior tendon. At operation he removed a loose tab of tendon to achieve significant improvement, probably through incidental decompression of the tendon sheath; again, other reports followed (Kettelkemp & Alexander 1969, Goldner et al 1974, Trevino et al 1981, Jahss 1982, Fredenburg et al 1983). After Goldner et al (1974) drew attention to the association between rupture of the tibialis posterior tendon and the acquired painful flat deformity in adults, the frequency of this syndrome gradually came to be recognized (Henceroth & Deyerie 1982, Gould 1983, Mann 1983, Mueller 1984, Mann & Thompson 1985, Funk et al 1986).

The reason why tibialis posterior develops the initial tenosynovitis is not immediately apparent. Other tendons, such as the flexors hallucis and digitorum longus, follow a very similar route but they are not similarly affected. Trauma does not appear to play any significant role except for a few clear-cut cases of direct injury or previous surgery (Holmes & Mann 1992). The granulation tissue that forms about the affected tendon has a gross resemblance to rheumatoid disease but only very rarely are the typical histological changes of rheumatoid disease seen.

In 1933, McMaster, conducting experimental studies on tendon rupture, demonstrated that:

1. An intact normal tendon doesn't rupture even when subjected to severe strain;
2. With normal activity, the tendon ruptured only after at least 75% of the fibres had been divided; and
3. Obstruction of the blood supply leads to aseptic necrosis with consequent rupture of the tendon.

In 1990, Frey et al injected the vessels of cadavaric limbs with India ink and gelatine to demonstrate a zone of hypovascularity in the tibialis posterior tendon at a point about 40 mm proximal to its insertion into the navicular. As others before them (Cozen 1965, Jahss 1982), they noted that the tendon of tibialis posterior hugs the under-surface of the medial malleolus and curves more sharply than other tendons that run along the medial aspect of the ankle. The inference is that vessels of the area may be wrung out in a manner similar to that described by Rathbun & Macnab (1970) in their paper on the microvascular pattern of the rotator cuff.

Today, the most plausible explanation would seem to be that local vascular impairment causes necrosis and weaking of the tendon. A reactionary tenosynovitis then increases tension within the fibrous tendon sheath to embarrass further the blood supply, thereby setting up a vicious cycle that leads first to lengthening and then to rupture of the tendon. Because tibialis posterior is a powerful muscle with a short range of action, any lengthening of its tendon is immediately reflected in a clinically apparent loss of function well before the tendon finally ruptures.

Acute injuries to the tibialis posterior tendon usually occur in association with a fracture dislocation of the ankle. In these circumstances, displacement of the tendon has long been recognized, but more recently de Zwart & Davidson (1983) drew attention to a rupture of the tendon that could easily be overlooked as both ends might not be visible, the distal end being hidden in its sheath and the proximal end being retracted.

Clinical features

Presentation

Posterior tibial tendon dysfunction afflicts predominantly women of later middle age, of whom 75% have a significant identifiable systemic or local vascular risk, such as obesity, hypertension, diabetes, previous surgery or the administration of steroids. In younger patients, 50% have had previous surgery, notably excision of an accessory navicular carried out as an adult (Holmes & Mann 1992).

The onset of symsptoms is insidious, though about half of the patients recall an initial minor twisting injury to the foot or ankle. Usually only one foot is affected. The symptoms are discomfort, deformity and loss of function.

The discomfort is more commonly an ache than a pain; it is associated with local tenderness in the line of the tibialis posterior tendon, just distal to the medial malleolus (Fig. 2). Often this ache is so mild that it is largely dismissed by the patient or her physician as 'foot strain'. Sometimes it is more pronounced, and it may radiate proximally into the calf and, very occasionally, distally to the first metatarsal. Local pain may be provoked if the patient can be persuaded to adduct her plantarflexed forefoot strongly against the examiner's hand or if the foot is forcefully everted and dorsiflexed.

When the tendon ruptures, the discomfort on the medial side of the hind foot is often temporarily relieved, only to return later in a more diffuse form, of lower intensity, as the deformity increases and stretches the soft tissues. With the same increase in deformity, pain may appear on the lateral side of the hindfoot, in the region of the sinus tarsi. This may be due to the anterior process of the posterior talar articular facet impinging on the superior surface of the calcaneum.

The first deformity to appear is distension of the tibialis posterior tendon sheath. In some instances this is very noticeable but at other times, particularly with the obese patient, it isn't readily seen. As the hindfoot sling function of tibialis posterior fails so the heel drifts into valgus, the plantar arch is lost and the forefoot becomes abducted to produce a typical flat foot deformity.

The loss of function is often expressed as 'tiredness' of the foot that not only reduces the patient's capacity for outdoor leisure pursuits but also inhibits walking in

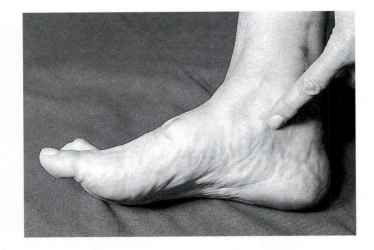

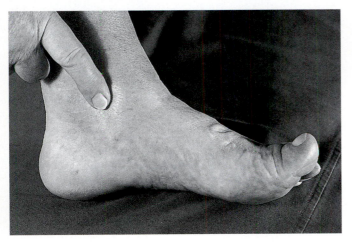

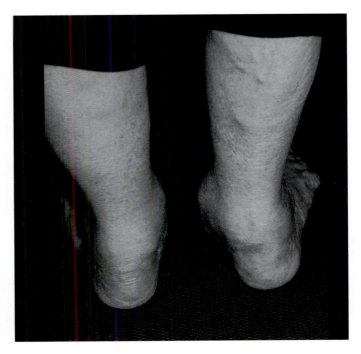

Figure 3

Tibialis posterior dysfunction in the right hindfoot. Note the increased valgus of the heel, the swelling behind and below the medial malleolus and abduction of the forefoot, producing the 'too many toes' sign

Figure 2

Patients indicating the site of their maximum discomfort

general, particularly when hurrying, going up slopes or negotiating stairs.

Examination

The hind foot valgus and forefoot abduction are best judged by looking at the patient from behind as she stands facing squarely forwards. The abnormal inclination of the heel is immediately apparent, as often is the swelling of the tendon sheath where it passes behind and below the medial malleolus (Fig. 3). Viewed from a distance, the degree of forefoot abduction is reflected in the number of toes visible beyond the outer side of the affected leg compared with the normal side – the 'too many toes' sign (Johnson 1983) (see Fig. 3). Loss of the tibialis posterior tendon function is best evaluated by the 'single heel rise' test (Johnson 1983). The patient stands close to a wall or by a desk so that she can balance

herself with her hands. Then, with the affected foot lifted from the floor, the patient is asked to stand tip toe on the normal foot. This action is achieved by first contracting tibialis posterior to stabilize the hind foot in varus before the gastrosoleus contracts to raise the heel. The test is then repeated with the affected foot, and it becomes apparent that the initial action of tibialis posterior to invert the heel does not occur; the patient then has difficulty raising the heel, and as she does so the valgus often increases. Most patients will complain of some discomfort at this stage. The functional effect of the test may be confirmed by asking the patient to repeat the tiptoe action. She may be able to demonstrate eight or ten rises on the normal side but only two or three on the affected side.

Radiographs

As the stabilizing effect of tibialis posterior is lost the calcaneonavicular complex, with the attached distal bones, rotates laterally away from beneath the talus. The effects of this are to be seen in the weight bearing dorsoplantar projection radiograph, in which firstly there is an increase in the angle between the axes of the talus and

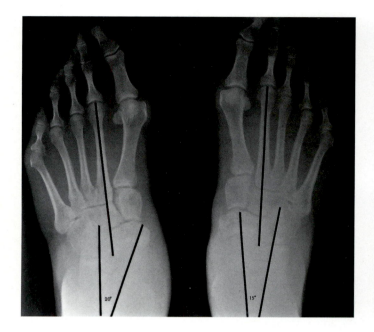

Figure 4

Dorsoplantar radiographs of the feet with the axes of the calcaneum, the talus and the second metatarsal marked on each axis. In the normal right foot, the metatarsal axis bisects the angle formed by the axes of the hindfoot bones. In the left foot, the tibialis posterior tendon has ruptured, allowing the hindfoot angle to increase and the second metatarsal axis to deviate and angulate laterally

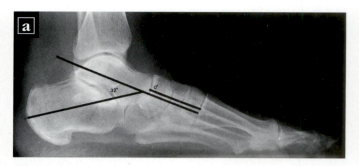

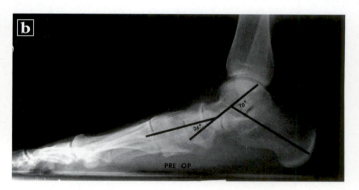

Figure 5

(a) Lateral radiograph of a normal foot, showing the angle formed between the axes of the calcaneum and the talus, and the alignment of the talus with the bones of the midfoot and the first metatarsal shaft; (b) where the tibialis posterior tendon has ruptured, the inclination of the talus relative to the calcaneum increases and the alignment of its axis with the midfoot and forefoot is lost

the calcaneum and secondly the axis of the second metatarsal is displaced laterally. In a normal foot, the metatarsal axis bisects the angle between the axes of the calcaneum and the talus; as the foot rotates into pronation and abduction, this metatarsal axis deviates and angulates laterally (Fig. 4).

As the midfoot complex together with the sustenaculum tali drifts laterally, support for the talar head is lost, allowing the bone to fall into flexion. The effect of this is seen on the weight bearing lateral projection as an increase in the angle between the longitudinal axis of the calcaneum and the talus. At the same time the normal axial alignment of the talus, navicular, medial cuneiform and the first metatarsal is seen to be broken, principally at the talonavicular joint but also at the cuneonavicular and tarsometatarsal joints (Fig. 5).

Where the diagnosis is in doubt a tenogram may very occasionally be helpful, though usually equivocal clinical features are matched by equivocal findings on the tenogram (Jahss 1982). More recently, magnetic resonance imaging (MRI) has been used to evaluate the soft tissues; sometimes it demonstrates an enlarged, abnormal or an absent tendon.

None of these investigations matches the cardinal value of careful clinical examination.

Management

Conservative management

During the early stages, when tenosynovitis is causing local discomfort and there may be swelling of the synovial sheath but good tendon function is retained, it is sufficient to advise a restriction in physical activities, to prescribe oral anti-inflammatory and analgesic medication, and to suggest that an elastic ankle support be worn during the day and that the foot of the bed be raised by 5.0–10 cm in order to allow the inflamed area to drain more effectively at night. Some local release of tension may be achieved with a soft arch support worn inside the shoe and a medial heel–sole wedge on the outside. Rest may be more effectively achieved through a below-knee walking cast retained over a matter of weeks.

It is very tempting to consider injecting steroid locally. Correctly placed this can have a most dramatic palliative effect, which sometimes persists for several weeks to a few months. It is a procedure not without risk, as local microvascular attenuation has been shown to result from such injections (Kennedy & Willis 1976). The literature abounds with reports of tendons rupturing following injections directly into their substance, so if steroid is used, it is best confined to the synovial sheath. This can be accomplished by first localizing the tendon a few centimetres above the medial malleolus just posterior to the tibial border. A needle is inserted obliquely and distally, bevel uppermost, along the course of the tibialis tendon gently injecting local anaesthetic at intervals. Once the needle has entered the tendon sheath, the anaesthetic may be felt or seen to distend it. If a sufficiently large needle has been used then a fine plastic tube can be passed through into the tendon sheath; otherwise the steroid is then injected, very gently and for as long as there is no resistance that might indicate the needle had penetrated the tendon.

Surgical management

If the condition fails to respond to conservative management or the patient first presents after several months of tenosynovitis, then the area should be surgically explored.

Through an incision directly over tibialis posterior, beginning a few centimetres proximal to the medial malleolus and continuing to the base of the great toe metatarsal, the full length of the sheath is opened and both surfaces of the tendon are carefully inspected down to its insertion. Various gross pathologies have been described, from the simple presence of granulation tissue (Fig. 6) through the formation of a longitudinal cleavage tear (Fig. 7), flaps and lengthening to a frank disruption. If the integrity of the tendon is sound then nothing further need be done. The simple decompression can be sufficient to halt the progress toward tendon degeneration and rupture (Lipscomb 1950, Lapidus & Sedenstein 1950, Ghormley & Spear 1952, Fowler 1955, Williams 1963, Langenskiöld 1967, Trevino et al 1981, Jamieson 1964). Some authors recommend removing granulation tissue and repairing the longitudinal tears. This is a matter of individual preference. The tendon sheath is very loosely approximated (Fig. 8) and a soft dressing applied. The patient is instructed to exercise the foot, gently as far as discomfort will permit, but she should not be encouraged to bear full weight for about 6 weeks.

Where the tendon appears to be separating, or has parted from its attachment to the inferior aspect of the navicular, reattachment has been recommended. This may be accomplished by drawing the tendon through a hole made in the navicular from dorsomedial to plantarmedial (Fig. 10) and then fixing it under tension as the foot is held in plantarflexion, inversion and adduction. Such a re-attachment could be reinforced using the flexor digitorum longus in side-to-side tenodesis.

The tendon usually ruptures just a few centimetres distal to the medial malleolus. In the early stages, when

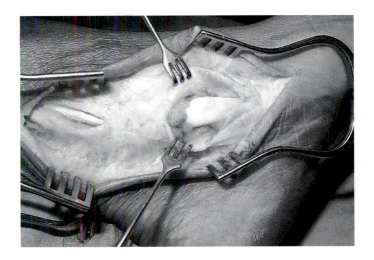

Figure 6

Granulation tissue surrounding the distal part of the tendon

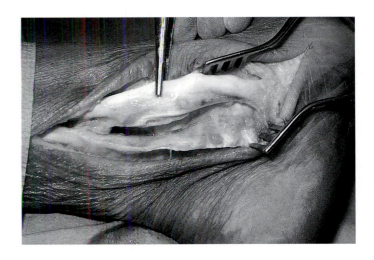

Figure 7

Tibialis posterior tenosynovitis: longitudinal splitting in the distal part of the tendon

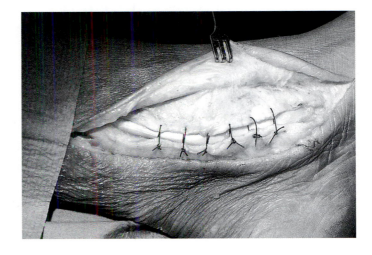

Figure 8

Following simple decompression, the cut edges of the tibialis posterior tendon sheath are loosely approximated

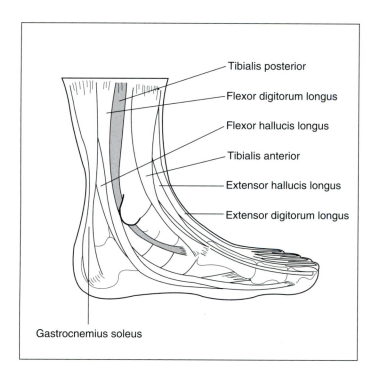

Figure 9

Relationship of the tibialis posterior tendon to other tendons on the medial aspect of the ankle

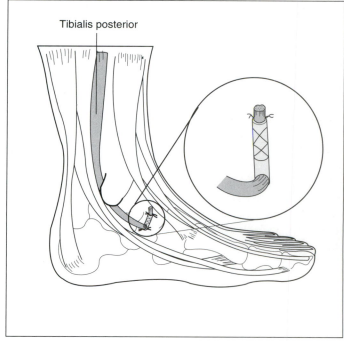

Figure 10

Reattachment of the avulsed tibialis posterior tendon to its insertion on the undersurface of the navicular

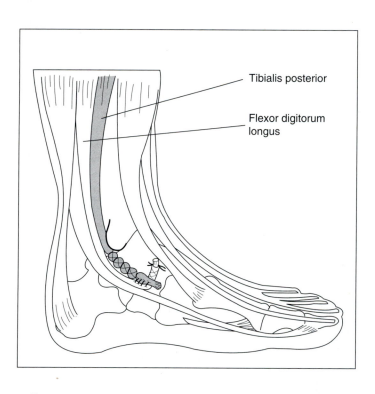

Figure 11

Repair of the avulsed tibialis posterior tendon with reinforcement using the flexor digitorum longus tendon

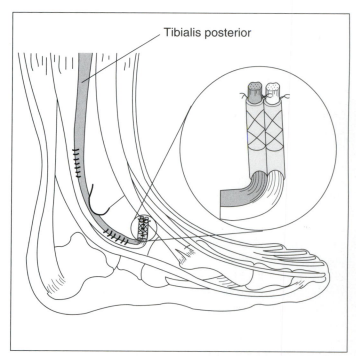

Figure 12

Reattachment of the avulsed tibialis posterior tendon to the navicular using the flexor digitorum longus tendon as reinforcement

rupture is incomplete or the ends not far separated, it may be possible to reconstruct the affected section using a Kessler or a Bunnell type suture. It is probably advisable that such a repair should be reinforced with a transfer of flexor digitorum longus tendon to the under surface of the navicular (Fig. 11). When the tendon appears to be grossly abnormal, it should be excised, a tendon transfer carried out and its proximal stump sutured to the transferred tendons.

Where there has been complete disruption, it is usual to find the area densely scarred and the tendon ends concealed. The remains of tibialis posterior tendon sheath can be identified just in front of the flexor digitorum longus tendon. Each end of tibialis posterior can then be defined; the distal end, rounded, apparently enlarged and 2–3 cm in length remains attached to the under surface of the navicular, whilst the proximal end, less easily defined, is found above and behind the medial malleolus. In this situation a tendon transposition is required to bridge the defect.

In 1974, Goldner et al reported having used the flexor hallucis longus or flexor digitorum longus either as a tendon reinforcement or as a complete motor unit substitution. In 1982, Jahss described the use of the flexor digitorum longus tendon in continuity, attaching the ends of tibialis posterior tendon proximally and distally by side-to-side suturing. In the same year, Mann & Specht recommended the use of flexor digitorum longus by attaching its tendon through a hole in the navicular.

A well-tried and commonly practised method uses the flexor digitorum longus tendon, detaching it distally and then passing the tendon through a dorsoplantar tunnel in the navicular (Johnson & Strom 1989, Thordarson 1993) (Fig. 12). If the muscle belly of tibialis posterior is sufficiently mobile it can be then sutured side to side proximally against the flexor digitorum to reinforce muscle action through the new attachment. The distal flexor digitorum longus tendon can be attached to the flexor hallucis tendon, but this is not necessary as the short plantar muscles seem to be strong enough to operate the lesser toes effectively.

Tibialis anterior tendon transposition

In 1923, as an adjunct to corrective osteotomy and arthrodesis for the correction of severe flat foot, Lowman re-routed the intact tibialis anterior tendon to act as a sling beneath the navicular. In 1939, Young employed the intact tibialis anterior in a similar manner, re-routing it through a keyhole slot in the navicular as an entirely soft tissue correction for pes planus.

Since 1979, the author has utilized tibialis anterior in a different manner, transferring part of its tendon to act along the line of tibialis posterior and then suturing it under tension to the proximal tibialis posterior stump. A curvilinear incision is made along the line of tibialis posterior, beginning 10–12 cm proximal to the ankle, continuing below the medial malleolus and forward to

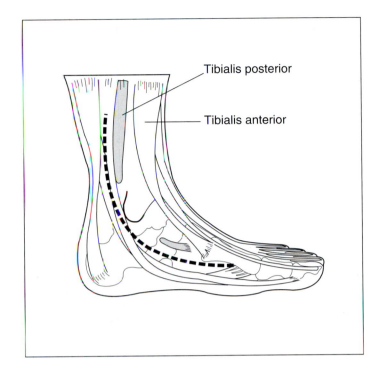

Figure 13

The incision along the line of tibialis posterior

the mid-part of the first metatarsal shaft (Fig. 13). The sheath of the tibialis posterior is identified in front of the flexor digitorum longus tendon and then cleared of all debris. The short distal stump of tibialis posterior is cut away at its insertion and the position marked. The proximal stump is usually retracted in the lower calf and most easily identified by blunt dissection with the finger. A toothed tissue clamp is attached to the tip and the muscle is pulled down hard, at the same time being mobilized by clearing it from adhesions for as far as blunt dissection can reach. Usually it is only possible to bring the tendon down by a centimetre or so. A 10 cm incision is then made, opening the anterior compartment to identify and mobilize the proximal end of the tibialis anterior tendon. The anterior half of the tendon can be traced for a few centimetres proximally into the substance of the muscle, in order to secure a greater length of tendon for transfer; it is then detached and split cleanly away from the posterior half of the tendon down to the distal part of the wound.

Returning to the primary wound, the upper skin flap is then dissected forward to expose the insertion of tibialis anterior and its distal tendon. A thin, curved tendon passer is eased alongside the tibialis anterior tendon and passed proximally into anterior wound to grasp the detached part of the tendon (Fig. 14). Because the tendon fibres of tibialis anterior run parallel, it is usually easy to draw the cut end back into the primary wound and then strip it firmly down to its insertion

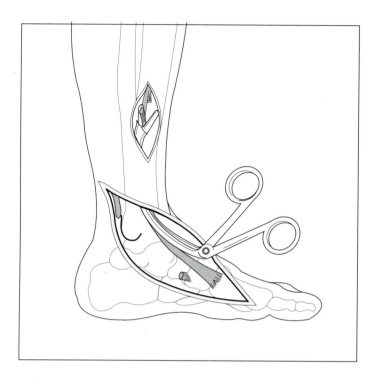

Figure 14

The tendon passer grasps the detached part of the tibialis anterior tendon

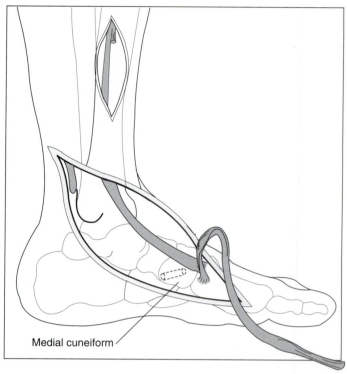

Medial cuneiform

Figure 15

A tunnel is formed through the medial cuneiform from the medial aspect distally to the inferolateral aspect proximally

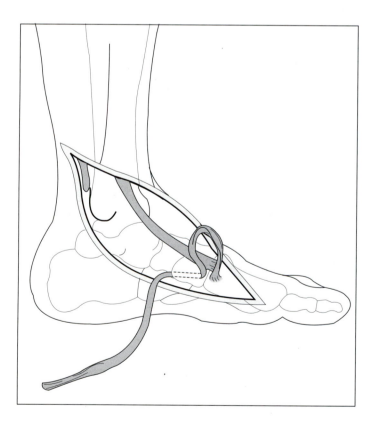

Figure 16

The tendon transfer is drawn proximally through the bony tunnel

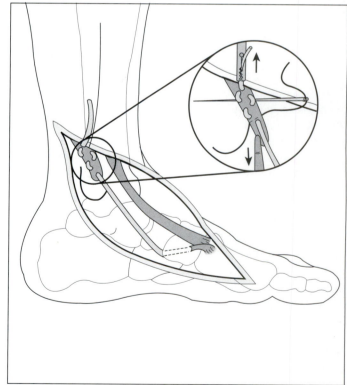

Figure 17

The tendon transfer is laced into the substance of the tibialis posterior stump. (Inset) The clamps are used to tension the transfer

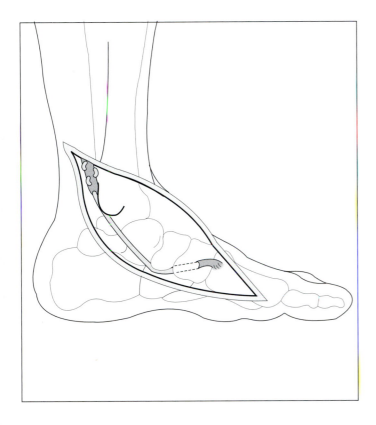

Figure 18

The tendon transfer is snapped into the groove of the tibialis posterior tendon

(Fig. 15). A hole is drilled obliquely downwards, laterally and posteriorly through the medial cuneiform from a point close by the insertion of tibialis anterior to one immediately lateral to the cleared attachment of tibialis posterior under the foot. The tendon transfer is then drawn proximally through the bony tunnel (Fig. 16). The anterior skin flap is then dissected further forward to expose the whole of the medial malleolus. The tendon transfer is passed proximally across the front of the medial malleolus and laced into the substance of the tibialis posterior stump (Fig. 17). The distal part of the stump should be avoided as it is very possibly avascular and nonviable.

The tibialis posterior stump is again grasped with a strong tissue clamp and now pulled both distally and anteriorly. Another tissue clamp is attached to the end of the tibialis anterior transfer where it emerges proximally from the tibialis posterior stump. As one assistant twists the plantar flexed foot into inversion and adduction, another grasps each clamp and pulls them forcefully apart in order to tension the transfer along a line that passes in front of the medial malleolus (Fig. 17 inset). The surgeon then fixes the laced tendon to the proximal tibialis posterior stump with a series of transverse sutures. The crushed ends of tendon are excised. The secured tendon graft is then 'thumbed', or eased,

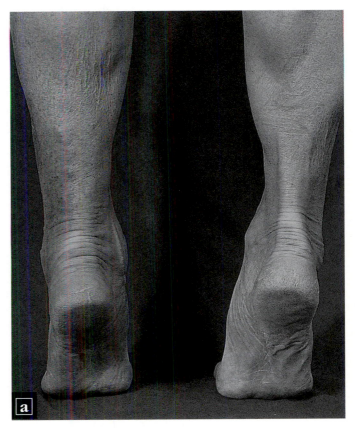

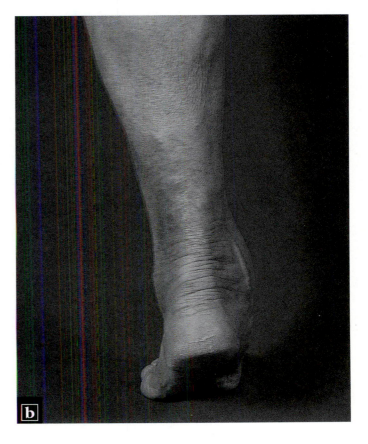

Figure 19

(a) A patient standing on tiptoe after a successful tibialis anterior transposition in the left foot; (b) the same patient standing on tiptoe on the left foot alone

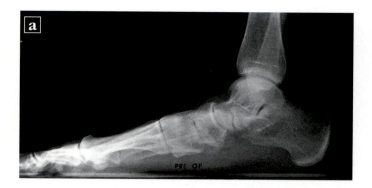

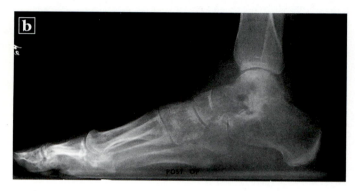

Figure 20

(a) Lateral radiograph of a foot showing the osseous displacements resulting from a tibialis posterior tendon rupture; (b) restoration of the normal alignment following a subtalar arthrodesis

backward over the medial malleolus to snap firmly into the groove previously occupied by tibialis posterior (Fig. 18).

Postoperatively, the patient remains non-weight-bearing for 6 weeks with the foot supported by a cast moulded into plantar flexion, inversion and adduction. The casting is then changed at intervals of about 2 weeks as the foot is eased back toward the plantargrade position. This is usually achieved within 8–10 weeks, and during this time the patient can bear some weight through a Böhler iron attachment to the cast.

Once the postoperative induration has subsided, it is often possible to confirm that the transferred tendon is working. The author has on one occasion taken the opportunity to inspect an established transfer and found a smooth tendon, smaller than the normal tibialis posterior, moving freely within a synovial sheath.

This procedure has the advantages of not sacrificing the function of any other muscle and of utilizing the strength of a natural tendon attachment to bone; it is usual for the shape of the foot to be improved and its function so far restored (Helal 1990) that some patients have been able to return to field sports and gymnastics (Fig. 19).

Before any tendon transfer is attempted, it is important to ensure that the foot is still supple and that full passive correction remains possible at both the subtalar and the mid-tarsal joints. In cases when the condition is long established and there is a fixed secondary deformity of the joints, or when the patient is over 70 or is obese and seeks only a modest level of activity, then an arthrodesis is to be preferred. As the primary deformity is rotation of the calcaneum away from beneath the talus, the logical least measure would seem to be a subtalar arthrodesis, sparing the mid-tarsal joint (Fig. 20); this often permits younger patients to return to former athletic recreations. Where the fixed deformity is more marked it may be necessary to combine subtalar fusion with talo-navicular fusion and sometimes with calcaneo-cuboid fusion to ensure a fully corrected stable hindfoot. The loss of movement necessarily limits the scope for recovery but the patient can usually walk for pleasure, ride a bicycle and play golf.

Conclusion

Once hardly regarded, tibialis posterior tendon dysfunction is now known to be a common source of hindfoot pain and the principal reason for the unilateral flat foot deformity and secondary hindfoot pathology of later adult life. The condition is progressive and disabling, but once considered it can be recognized and should be rectified.

References

Basmajian V J, Stecko G 1963 The role of muscles in arch support of the foot: an electromyographic study. J Bone Joint Surg 45A: 1184

Cozen L 1965 Posterior tibial tenosynovitis secondary to foot strain. Clin Orthop 42: 101–102

Duchenne G B A 1949 Physiology of Motion. Kaplan E B (translator and editor). W B Saunders; Philadelphia

Fowler A W 1955 Tibialis posterior syndrome (abst). J Bone Joint Surg 37B: 520

Fredenburg M, Tilley G, Yagoobian E M 1983 Spontaneous rupture of the posterior tibial tendon secondary to chronic non-specific tenosynovitis J Foot Surg 22: 198–202

Frey C C, Greenidge N C, Sereff M 1990 Vascularity of the posterior tibial tendon. J Bone Joint Surg 72A: 884–888

Funk D A, Cass J R, Johnson K A 1986 Acquired adult flat foot secondary to posterior tibial tendon pathology. J Bone Joint Surg 68A: 95–106

Ghormley R K, Spear I M 1953 Anomalies of the posterior tibial tendon: a cause of persistent pain about the ankle. Arch Surg 66: 512–516

Goldner J L, Keats P K, Bassett F H III, Clippinger F W 1974 Progressive talipes equinovalgus due to trauma or degeneration of the posterior tibial tendon and medial plantar ligaments. Orthop Clin North Am 5: 39–51

Gould N 1983 Evaluation of hyperpronation and pes planus in adults. Clin Orthop 181: 37–45

Helal B 1990 Cobb repair for tibialis posterior tendon rupture. J Foot Surg 29: 349–352

Henceroth W D II Deyerle W M 1982 The acquired unilateral flat foot in the adult: some causative factors. Foot Ankle 2: 304–308

Holmes G B Jr, Mann R A 1992 Possible epidemiological factors associated with rupture of the posterior tibial tendon. Foot Ankle 13: 70–79

Jahss M H 1982 Spontaneous rupture of the tibialis posterior tendon: clinical findings, tenographic studies, and a new technique of repair. Foot Ankle 3: 158–166

Jamieson E S 1964 Chronic tenosynovitis (abst). J Bone Joint Surg 46B: 570

Johnson K A 1983 Tibialis posterior tendon rupture. Clin Orthop 177: 140–147

Johnson K A, Strom D E 1989 Tibialis posterior tendon dysfunction. Clin Orthop 239: 196–206

Kennedy J C, Willis R B 1976 The effects of local steroid injections on tendons: a biomechanical and microscopic correlative study. Am J Sports Med 4: 11–21

Kettelkamp D B, Alexander H H 1969 Spontaneous rupture of the posterior tibial tendon. J Bone Joint Surg 51A: 759–764

Key J A 1953 Partial rupture of the tendon of the posterior tibial muscle. J Bone Joint Surg 35A: 1006–1008

Kulowski J G 1936 Tendovaginitis (tenosynovitis): general discussion and report of one case including posterior tibial tendon. J Missouri Med Assoc 33: 135–137

Langenskiöld A 1967 Chronic non-specific tenosynovitis of the tibialis posterior tendon. Acta Orthop Scand 38: 301–305

Lapidus P W, Sedenstein H 1950 Chronic non-specific tenosynovitis with effusion about the ankle: report of three cases. J Bone Joint Surg 32A: 175–179

Lipscomb P R 1950 Tendons: number 1. Non suppurative tenosynovitis and paratendinitis. Instr Course Lect 7: 254–261

Lowman C L 1923 An operative method for the correction of certain forms of flat foot. JAMA 81: 1500–1502

Mann R A 1983 Acquired flat foot in adults. Clin Orthop 181: 46–51

Mann R A, Specht L H 1982 Posterior tibial tendon ruptures – analysis of eight cases (abst). Foot Ankle 2: 350

Mann R A, Thompson F M 1985 Rupture of the posterior tibial tendon causing flat foot: surgical treatment. J Bone Joint Surg 67A: 556–561

McMaster P E 1933 Tendon and muscle ruptures. Clinical and experimental studies on the causes and locations of subcutaneous ruptures. J Bone Joint Surg 15: 705–722

Mueller T J 1984 Ruptures and lacerations of the tibialis posterior tendon. J Am Podiatr Assoc 74: 109–119

Norris S H, Mankin H J 1978 Chronic tenosynovitis of the posterior tibial tendon with new bone formation. J Bone Joint Surg 60B: 523–526

Rathbun J B, Macnab I 1970 The microvascular pattern of the rotator cuff. J Bone Joint Surg 52B: 540–553

Thordarson D B 1993 Surgical reconstruction of the posterior tibial tendon. Tech Orthop 8: 50–54

Trevino S, Gould N, Korson R 1981 Surgical treatment of stenosing tenosynovitis at the ankle. Foot Ankle 2: 37–45

Williams R 1963 Chronic non-specific tendovaginitis of tibialis posterior. J Bone Joint Surg 45B: 542–545

Young C S 1939 Operative treatment of pes planus. Surg Gynecol Obstet 68: 1099–1103

de Zwart D F, Davidson J S A 1983 Rupture of the posterior tibial tendon associated with fractures of the ankle. J Bone Joint Surg 65A: 260–262

V.3 Hallux Valgus and Rigidus

Derek W Wilson

Hallux valgus

Hallux valgus may be defined as 'a lateral deviation of the big toe toward the middle line of the foot at the metatarsophalangeal joint' (Elmslie 1926). The pathological changes in the metatarsophalangeal joint in hallux valgus were described accurately and completely 140 years ago (Broca 1852) and with the exception of replacement arthroplasty, the principles and the practice of surgical treatment were known by the turn of the century and most of their variations introduced before World War II.

The disease is very common (Creer 1938a, 1938b, Winner 1945, Mouchet 1992).

Pathological anatomy

The essential lesion is a stretching of the medial capsule and ligaments of the first metatarsophalangeal joint, which allows the phalanx to fall laterally into valgus and subsequently allows the metatarsal head to fall medially off the sesamoid platform.

Thereafter several changes are seen in the metatarsal head. The medial parts of the distal and plantar articular cartilage of the metatarsal head become atrophied into a groove (Broca 1852). Modes (1939) called this the 'fossa nudata'. This groove forms within the outline of the metatarsal head (Fig. 1), is continuous below with the area for the medial sesamoid and leaves on its medial side an apparent prominence which represents the original medial margin of the bone. While there may be some small osteophytes along the edge of the original medial margin of the metatarsal, there is little real new bone formation or exostosis (Lane 1886/7, Silver 1923, Stein 1938, Haines & McDougall 1954).

Broca noted that 'outside from the groove, the cartilaginous surface, still continuing in its movement, remaining in conformity with the phalanx, preserves longer its structure and its normal aspect', and that 'the skin compressed between the footwear and the underlying bone surface becomes the site of a small swelling designated by the name *oignon*' (bunion). 'Beneath it is there is constantly a mucous bursa, 1 to 2 cm in size, whose deep face rests on the medial collateral ligament of the joint... This mucous bursa comunicates with the joint synovium through a perforation in the capsule' (Broca 1852). On the inferior aspect of the metatarsal head there is early erosion of the articular cartilage of

the facet for the medial sesamoid (Haines & McDougall 1954).

As the condition progresses and the phalanx deviates more to the lateral side of the metatarsal head, the ligaments on the dorsimedial, medial and inferomedial sides of the head, especially the sesamoid ligament, become progressively stretched. These ligaments are the sole medial support of the metatarsal head and their incompetence allows the metatarsal head to escape from the upper surface of the sesamoids and to move medially. Note, with Volkmann (1856), that the deep transverse ligament of the sole does not connect the metatarsal heads themselves, but only the plantar pads and (in the great toe) the sesamoids. Thus there is the *appearance* of lateral migration of the sesamoids, with the medial lying under the ridge in the centre of the

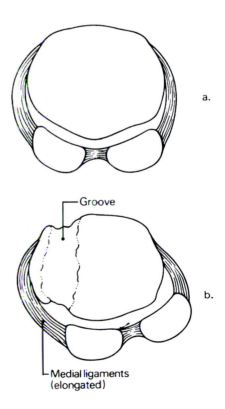

Figure 1

a: Normal transverse section through the metatarsal head.
b: In hallux valgus, showing the groove (erosion) on the medial part of the head, delimiting the pseudoexostosis and medial displacement of the head off the sesamoid platform, with stretching of the medial ligaments.

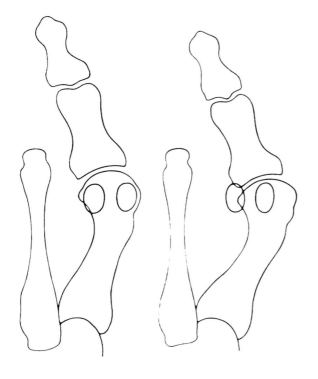

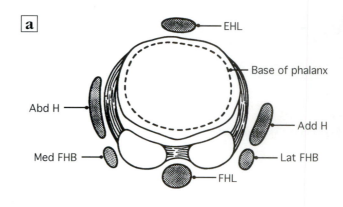

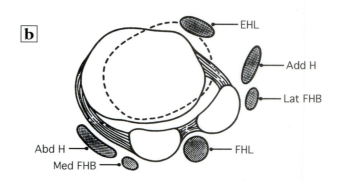

Figure 2

a: The normal disposition of the bones. b: Medial displacement of the metatarsal head from the sesamoids, giving the appearance of 'lateral subluxation' of the sesamoids. Note the constant distance of the lateral sesamoid from the second metatarsal.

Figure 3

a: Normal disposition of the intrinsic and extrinsic tendons. b: Displacements of the tendons in hallux valgus (after Miller 1975). The dotted outline represents the base of the phalanx, becoming internally rotated.

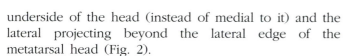

underside of the head (instead of medial to it) and the lateral projecting beyond the lateral edge of the metatarsal head (Fig. 2).

The medial sesamoid lies under a flat surface and the lateral bone lies beside the metatarsal head in the first intermetatarsal cleft (Haines & McDougall 1954). The first metatarsal undergoes 'a deviation which is precisely the reverse of the deviation of the phalanx; whereby it is inclined outward'. The extensor hallucis longus tendon, being placed now further from the bone surface, gains increased leverage and often pulls the toe off the ground to lie on the dorsum of the second toe. This destroys any weight-bearing function of the pulp of the great toe. Together with migration of the first metatarsal head off the sesamoids, which reduces the effective plantar prominence of the first ray, this loss of toe function contributes to the onset of lateral metatarsalgia.

Abductor hallucis and flexor hallucis brevis are carried further under the metatarsal head, losing any vestige of abductor action. The alterations of muscle pulls set up the imbalance which is associated with medial rotation

deformity of the proximal phalanx of the great toe (Fig. 3). This rotation becomes significant when the hallux valgus angle exceeds 35° (Hardy & Clapham 1951).

Aetiology

Any theory concerning the aetiology of hallux valgus must explain known facts about the condition.

Age

Hardy & Clapham (1951) noted that, of 52 patients with hallux valgus, in 24 (46%) the age of onset was under 20 years and in 16 (31%) under 15 years. Otherwise, they found a low correlation of hallux valgus with age (r = 0.1) and Shine (1965) reported no such correlation. Kilmartin et al (1991) discovered 96 cases of genuine hallux valgus,

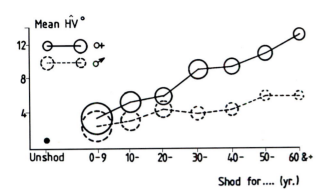

Figure 4
Relation of hallux valgus angle to the time for which shoes had been worn. (711 men; 903 women; area of circles proportional to number of persons). From Shine (1965).

defined as having a radiological toe angle greater than 14.5°, among 6000 children aged 10 years who were screened for the complaint, an incidence of 1.6%.

Heredity

Hardy & Clapham (1951) found a positive family history of hallux valgus in 63% of 91 patients and Glynn et al (1980) in 68% of 41 patients. Bonney & Macnab (1952) noted that affected subjects with a positive family history of hallux valgus showed an earlier than average age of onset.

Sex

All authors quote a higher proportion of females affected by hallux valgus than males and analysis of the figures of Shine (1965) shows a statistically highly significant divergence between shod men and women (p<0.001; Fig. 4).

Shoe wearing

Many studies have demonstrated the association of shoe wearing and hallux valgus (Hoffman 1905, Engle & Morton 1931, James 1939, Sim-Fook & Hodgson 1958), but especially Shine (1965), who showed that the incidence of hallux valgus was linearly related to the length of time for which shoes had been worn, rather than to age (Fig. 4). Also, Kato & Watanabe (1981) claimed that hallux valgus was not seen in Japan until

the traditional clog was abandoned in favour of European shoes.

Gottschalk et al (1979, 1980) and Noakes (1981) disagreed with this view.

High intermetatarsal angle

After examining 1851 normal British children aged up to 15 years, Hardy & Clapham (1952) noted an increase in hallux valgus with age, although the intermetatarsal angle remained constant at a mean of 7.5°.

After this modest early increase in hallux valgus (from 10° to 15°) without change in the intermetatarsal angle, the subsequent development of hallux valgus is then associated with an increase in intermetatarsal angle, with a normal adult value of 9°. In patients awaiting bunion surgery, a mean hallux valgus angle of 32° was associated with a mean intermetatarsal angle of 14°, with a strong positive correlation between the measurements (r = 0.71).

Metatarsus primus varus

In 1925, Truslow introduced the concept that the primary deformity in hallux valgus was varus (medial) deviation of the first metatarsal. He attributed the initial metatarsus primus varus to obliquity either of the medial cuneiform or of the base of the first metatarsal at the first cuneiform–metatarsal joint or to the pressure of an intermesial bone. Lapidus (1940) claimed a hereditary predisposition to the metatarsus varus and stated that the deformity appeared in early youth — a view which conflicts with that of Hardy & Clapham (1952) (see above). The concept gained support after 1950, and metatarsal osteotomy in the correction of hallux valgus increased in popularity.

Haines & McDougall (1954) claimed that the articular surface of the cuneiform was more medially directed than usual and that the base of the first metatarsal also was more oblique in cases of hallux valgus. Nevertheless they concluded that 'There is no convincing evidence of any primary lesion of the joint that could be regarded as a cause and not as a result of hallux valgus'. Durman (1957a, 1957b) found abnormalities in the first cuneiform–metatarsal joint in 43% of 418 feet with hallux valgus in persons under the age of 19 years.

Kilmartin et al (1991), in a statistical study of 10-year olds, found a slightly but significantly greater intermetatarsal angle in the affected feet of unilateral cases than in the unaffected feet (average difference 1.2°; p<0.01). However, other aspects of their studies led them to conclude that the 'alignment of the first metatarsal is clearly not determined by that of the metatarsocuneiform joint' and that neither splaying of the cuneiforms themselves nor a general metatarsus adductus nor disturbed growth of the metatarsal shaft could be shown to cause an increase in the varus angle of the first metatarsal.

Stability of the first ray

There is a clinical impression of a difference in the stability of the first ray at angles of hallux valgus above and below about 35°. This difference is embodied in the 'concertina test'. The tip of the toe is grasped by the thumb and forefinger of the examiner and a modest force directed proximally parallel to the axis of the *foot* (i.e. parallel to the second metatarsal), but not in the line of the proximal phalanx. The test is abnormal (positive) if the first ray collapses in its long axis, bulging medially at the level of the metatarsophalangeal joint (Fig. 5). Commonly the test is negative at hallux valgus angles below 35° and positive at angles above, suggesting that at about this degree of hallux valgus the medial capsule of the metatarsophalangeal joint has become weaker.

Miller (1975) noted that medial rotation of the toe in hallux valgus was associated with plantarward migration of the tendon of abductor hallucis with consequent weakening of the medial soft tissue support of the toe. Hardy & Clapham (1951) noted that, in those cases of hallux valgus in which the great toe was rotated on its long axis, the average hallux valgus angle was 36°, while in those without rotation the mean angle was 19°. Piggott (1960) reported that rotation of the toe was commoner (38%) in his more severe (subluxated) group than in the less severe deviated group (11%). Mygind (1954) says that at a valgus angle exceeding 35° the sesamoid is tilted and that the great toe is turned on its long axis into pronation.

Muscle imbalance

In his studies of acquired (iatrogenic) hallux varus, Miller (1975) demonstrated that dynamic hallux varus was due to muscle imbalance (favouring the abductor hallucis). Conversely, in hallux valgus he notes plantar displacement of and weakening of the action of abductor hallux, in favour of the adductor. Scranton & Rutkowski (1980) state that the action of the adductors 'is to stabilize the sesamoids and the insertion of flexor hallucis brevis during the later stages of foot flat and early push-off'. They note that the sesamoids do not migrate laterally after being released from the proximal phalanx as in the Keller operation, suggesting that there is no strong lateral pull from adductor hallucis and that such a pull could not contribute to the high intermetatarsal angle known to be associated with hallux valgus.

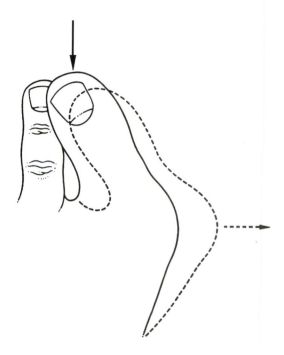

Figure 5

The 'concertina test'. A force is applied to the tip of the toe in a line parallel to the second metatarsal and neither in the axis of the phalanx nor at right angles to it. An incompetent joint allows the first ray to fold up like a concertina.

Other foot deformities

Other static deformities of the foot have been blamed as predisposing to hallux valgus, and Stein (1938) lists almost all the common lower limb deformities. Hiss (1931) noted that in 1812 patients with 3092 bunions, 60% had everted feet and 32% had a low medial arch. Elmslie (1926) suggested the sequence of flat foot, valgus position, weight bearing on the inner edge of the foot and pressure on the medial aspect of the great toe as causing hallux valgus.

Some modern groups ascribe hallux valgus to the biomechanical effects of that type of flat foot which is associated with inversion of the forefoot in relation to the hindfoot. This is not supported by Stott et al (1973) who state that, in established hallux valgus, less weight is born by the big toe, or by Grundy et al (1975) who showed that the line of weight bearing in hallux valgus remains roughly in the long axis of the foot (MT2 and MT3) and does not progress medially and distally to the pulp of the great toe as in the normal unshod foot.

Gottschalk et al (1980) found the commonest foot type to be a squared foot with index minus (i.e. great and second rays equal in length, but MT1 shorter than MT2). They failed to confirm others' contention that one type of foot shape is associated with hallux valgus. Harris &

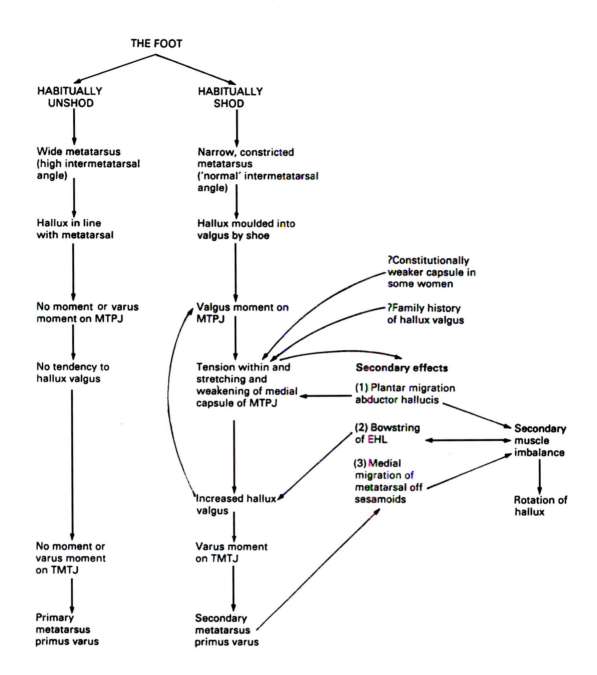

Figure 6

The 'hallux hypothesis'. A scheme of the suggested mechanism of the production of the deformity.

Beath (1949) found no correlation between a short first metatarsal and disturbances of weight bearing or function.

result in restoration of the toe to its normal position'. The author agrees with this concept of a *secondary* lateral displacement of extensor hallucis longus, which then becomes an aggravating influence.

Bowstringing of the extrinsic tendons

Fowler (1889) remarked that it was unlikely that extensor hallucis longus alone was to blame for the valgus as 'tenotomy of this structure in advanced cases does not

Weakness of the medial supporting structures

Stamm (1957) suggested that stretching of the medial capsule of the first metatarsophalangeal joint and volar

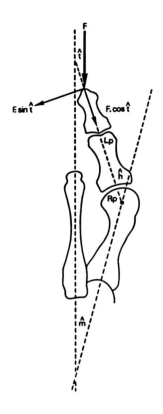

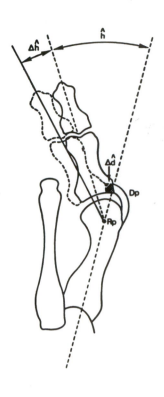

Figure 7

The turning moment on the phalanges of the great toe. The force 'F' on the tip of the toe, acting at angle '$\angle t$' to the axis of the phalanges, sets up a turning moment at the centre of rotation of the MPJ.

$$M_p = F.\sin \angle t \ (L_p + R_p)$$

where L_p = length of the two phalanges; R_p = radius of metatarsal head. Note that, by geometry,

$$\angle h = \angle t + \angle m$$

displacement of the abductor hallucis tendon created a weakness which allowed the first metatarsal head to migrate medially. This is in accord with the observations of Thomson (1960) and Miller (1975) (see p. 306) and with the opinions of Syms (1897), Fowler (1889) and Haines and McDougall (1954).

The hallux hypothesis

D W Wilson (1980) presented an hypothesis concerning the aetiology of hallux valgus based on the concept that the primary lesion in this condition was a weakness of the medial capsule of the metatarsophalangeal joint (Figs. 6, 7 and 8).

Bare feet show a larger intermetatarsal angle than shod feet. Conversely, in shod feet the great toe is moulded into increased valgus. The normal foot (epitomized by that of the normal, unshod child) is triangular and not

Figure 8

Tension in the medial capsule of the metatarsophalangeal joint. The turning moment (see Fig. 7) is opposed by a tension 'T_p' in the medial joint capsule, so that:

$$T_p R_p = F. \sin \angle t \ (L_p + R_p) \quad \text{or} \quad T_p = \frac{(F. \sin \angle t \ (L_p + R_p))}{R_p}$$

The stretch produced in the medial capsule 'Δd' will depend on the original length of the capsule 'D_p'; the modulus of elasticity of the capsule and the cross sectional area of the capsule 'A_p'.

The modulus of elasticity would be given by the equation:

$$E = \frac{T_p/A_p}{\Delta d/D_p} = \frac{T_p.D_p}{A_p.\Delta d} \ Nm$$

By geometry:

$$\Delta d = \frac{2\pi R_p \Delta \angle h}{360} \ \text{metres}$$

Therefore the increase in hallux valgus angle '$\Delta \angle h$', produced by the force 'F' is:

$$\Delta \angle h = \frac{180.T_p.D_p}{\pi.R_p.A_p.E} \ \text{degrees}$$

Values used in the calculation of tensions in Fig. 10 were:

Force on tip of toe (f) = 70 N; L_p = 0.05 m; length of metatarsal of great toe (L_m) = 0.06m; R_p = 0.01 m; radius of distal cuneiform surface (R_m) = 0.02m

the rounded kit shape of the common adult shoe. A foot never shod has the proximal phalanx of each toe in the line of its respective metatarsal (James 1939, Sim-Fook & Hodgson 1958). At toe-off in walking the final force falls on the pulp of the great toe and is of the order of 70 N (Stott et al 1973, Grundy et al 1975, Grieve, personal communication).

When walking shod this force lies more laterally than when walking barefoot (Grundy et al 1975). Figure 7 shows how a force F on the tip of the toe acting in or parallel to the long axis of the foot (taken as the axis of the second metatarsal), produces a resultant force, F. sin $\angle$t, which exerts a turning moment in a valgus direction at the centre of rotation of the metatarsophalangeal joint. By convention a force acting in a valgus direction is regarded as positive and vice versa.

The magnitude of this turning moment is

F. sin$\angle$t (Lp + Rp) Nm.

This moment will set up and be opposed by a tension, Tp, in the medial capsule of the metatarsophalangeal joint (see Fig. 8), such that

Tp.Rp = F. sin $\angle$t (Lp + Rp).

Fig. 10 shows the results of calculations of the theoretical tensions in the medial capsule for each of various combinations of hallux valgus and intermetatarsal angles, assuming an applied force of 70 N and the bone dimensions quoted.

Note that, for any given intermetatarsal angle, the tension in the capsule is directly related to the hallux valgus angle. For hallux valgus angles up to 50° or 60° this roughly linear relationship lies on the near-straight intermediate section of a sine curve, which bends over at higher values. Note also that an increase in the intermetatarsal angle *decreases* the tension set up in the medial capsule for any individual hallux valgus angle. Theoretically this makes it unlikely that a *primary* increase in an intermetatarsal angle would predispose to the occurrence of hallux valgus. Note also that, at hallux valgus angles equal to the intermetatarsal angle, the capsular tension falls to zero and that, at hallux valgus angles less than the intermetatarsal angle, the moment on the toe is negative (i.e. varus).

Continuing the analysis proximally, when any slack in the metatarsophalangeal joint is taken up and its medial capsule is elongated to the limit allowed by its elasticity, the same force continues to act, but at the next most proximal level (the medial cuneiform–first metatarsal joint).

Figure 9 illustrates the analysis at this level and Fig. 10 illustrates the calculations at both levels. It may be seen that the turning moments on the metatarsal at the tarsometatarsal joint are in a varus direction (negative), are proportional to the hallux valgus angle and are smaller than those acting on the metatarsophalangeal joint. Note also that an increase in the intermetatarsal angle produces a *greater* tension in the lateral capsule of the tarsometatarsal joint. This situation reflects the less extreme angles involved (the intermetatarsal angle

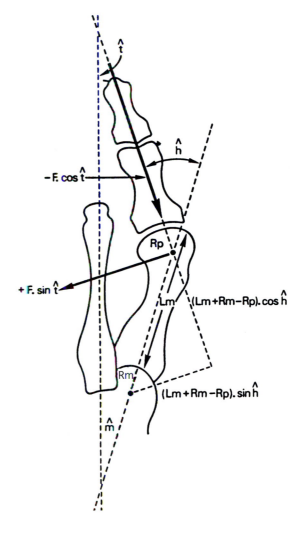

Figure 9

The turning moment on the metatarsal. The force +F.sin $\angle$t acts in a valgus direction at a distance L. cos $\angle$h from the centre of rotation. The force –F. cos $\angle$t acts in a varus direction at a distance L. sin $\angle$h, where 'L' is the effective length of the metatarsal segment and equal to

$$L_m + R_m - R_p$$

The net moment is therefore given by:

$$M_m = (F. \sin \angle t. L. \cos \angle h) - (F. \cos \angle t \, L. \sin \angle h)$$

and the tension developed in the lateral capsule of the tarsometatarsal joint is given by:

$$T_m = \frac{M_m}{R_m} N$$

I am indebted to Professor D Grieve (Dept. of Biomechanics, Royal Free Hospital School of Medicine, London) for his help with this anaylsis.

seldom exceeds 20°), the shorter lateral ligament of the tarsometatarsal joint and its better mechanical advantage, lying further (20 mm) from the centre of rotation at the tarsometatarsal joint than at the metatarsophalangeal level (10 mm). Thus the proximal joint is more resistant

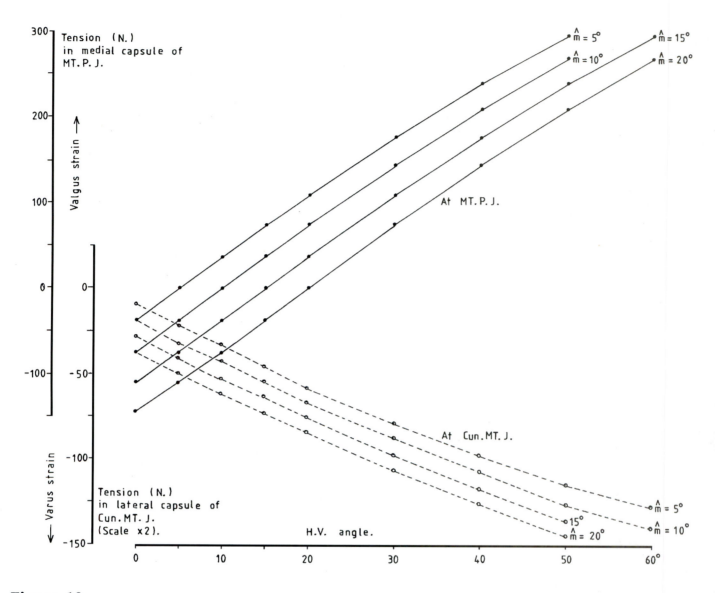

Figure 10

Theoretical capsular tensions at the joints of the first ray. The solid lines and dots show the tension in the medial capsule of the metatarsophalangeal joint when a force of 70 N. is applied to the tip of the toe. Note that the tension is *decreased* as $\hat{m}$ (the intermetatarsal angle) is increased. The broken lines and open circles show similar calculations for the lateral side of the cuneiform–metatarsal joint. Note that the tension is consistently varus (negative by the convention used) and is *numerically increased* as m rises. Note that the scale here has been doubled for the sake of clarity.

than the distal one and, presumably, develops deformity more slowly. Trimmings & Wilson (1988) showed that the medial capsular structures of the metatarsophalangeal joint obeyed Hooke's Law, in that the angular deviation of the intact toe was proportional to the tension developed in the medial capsule by a laterally directed force applied to the toe; also that in a group of women with bilateral hallux valgus, both the medial *and the lateral* capsular structures of the first metatarsophalangeal joint were significantly (p<0.001) more extensible than in any other group.

This evidence suggests some inherent defect in all the capsular tissues in these female subjects with clinical

hallux valgus, which might provide a logical basis for the observed familial and female incidence of the complaint.

Assessment and investigation

Apart from weight bearing X-rays there are few special investigations used in the assessment of hallux valgus. Forefoot pressure studies by both static and dynamic pedobarography may become more popular in the future. They provide an assessment of the weight bearing function of the great toe and of the lesser rays. Perhaps selection of the particular operative procedure should be more influenced by maldistributed weight bearing than it is at present (see p. 314 et seq).

Clinical assessment

(i) The hallux valgus deformity itself is usually recorded as the angle between the axes of the proximal phalanx and the metatarsal and may be measured (both clinically and radiologically) with a goniometer.

(ii) Assess the status of the first metatarsal at the tarsometatarsal joint, and record the intermetatarsal angle and the mobility of the ray in the dorso-plantar and mediolateral planes. Examine the foot with the patient standing, when both the hallux valgus and the metatarsal splay may be worse. Note if there is callosity under the first metatarsal head or if the skin there is soft and obviously not taking proper load.

(iii) Note the presence or absence of toe rotation.

(iv) Look for bony osteophyte formation (especially dorsally and laterally) around the metatarsophalangeal joint in association with degenerative changes.

(v) Uncommonly the interphalangeal joint is the level affected (hallux valgus interphalangeus) and the deformity is assessed as the angle between the axes of the two toe segments.

(vi) Examine the soft tissue on the medial side of the metatarsophalangeal joint for evidence of shoe pressure (redness, thickening, keratinization), for bursal swelling with fluid (see Fig. 35) and for infective bursitis or sinus formation.

(vii) Inspect the remainder of the foot for deformities of the lesser toes, bunionette over the lateral side of the fifth metatarsal, or any abnormalities of the arch or of the hindfoot. In particular look for *and record* evidence of metatarsalgia in the form of callosities or tenderness under the lesser metatarsal heads. Palpate the dorsum of the metatarsus to detect the common dorsal, degenerative dislocation of the lesser metatarsophalangeal joints (usually the second or third). Look for evidence of Morton's metatarsalgia (interdigital tenderness with referred pain to a toe tip, sensory disturbance of the toes, or pain or clicking on compressing the metatarsus from side-to-side).

(viii) Record passive movements of both joints of the great toe. Assess also the range of *active* flexion of the whole toe – the angle between the dorsum of the distal toe segment and the dorsum of the first metatarsal (ignoring the proximal phalanx) is convenient. Note if the pulp of the great toe reaches the ground in relaxed standing. In general

active dorsiflexion and active abduction (if possible) are not especially useful in assessment. Note if passive movements of the joints are painful, suggesting inflammation or degenerative disease.

(ix) Note the stability of the first ray in response to the 'concertina test' (see p. 306 and Fig. 5).

(x) Examine joint movements at the remainder of the foot and at the ankle.

(xi) Examine the vascular state of the foot and leg (colour, temperature, cutaneous nutrition and hyperkeratosis, hair preservation, etc) and palpate the pulses. Note any sensory disturbance. Look for any septic or fungal lesions around the foot, toes, nails or interdigital clefts.

(xii) Examine the shoes for suitability and for wear (for example, weight bearing and wear may be predominantly on the lateral edge of the shoe if the first ray is stiff and painful as in hallux rigidus).

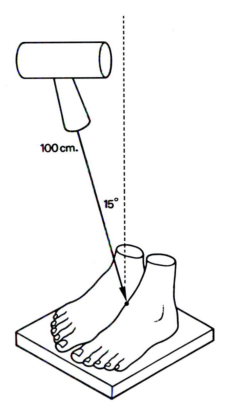

Figure 11

Dorsoplantar (anteroposterior) weight bearing X-rays.

Radiological assessment

The technique recommended here for securing standardized X-rays is similar to that of Venning & Hardy (1951) and Hardy & Clapham (1951):

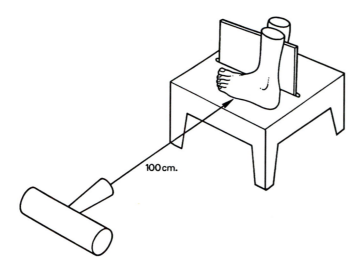

Figure 12

Lateral weight bearing X-rays.

(i)   Dorsoplantar (anteroposterior) weight bearing views are obtained by standing the patient, feet together, on a shallow, inverted, wooden tray just big enough to contain and protect the grid cassette, placed on the floor. With a source to film distance of 100 cm, the ray is directed 15° backward toward the hindfoot and is centred midway between the navicular bones (Fig. 11). The inclination of the beam avoids overshadowing of the foot by the tibia.

(ii) Weight-bearing lateral (lateromedial) views are taken with the patient standing on a raised stool whose top contains a slot in which the cassette may stand upright. Each foot is examined separately. The beam is directed horizontally from 100 cm at the base of the fifth metatarsal (Fig. 12). The diaphragm of the tube is opened enough to include the ankle joint in the field of view.

(iii) Non-weight-bearing oblique views are produced with the patient sitting on the standard couch with the foot rolled 15° inward (i.e. lateral border higher) and the vertical X-ray beam directed at the centre of the cuboid from a distance of 100 cm.

(iv) Sesamoid skyline views are taken by a suitable technique (see Chapter V.5).

Measurements and assessments from X-rays

From the standard films many measurements can be made, but the most commonly recorded are the hallux valgus angle (MT1 and PP1), the intermetatarsal angle (MT1 and MT2), the degree of metatarsosesamoid incongruity (either descriptively or numerically by the system of Hardy & Clapham (1951) for the *medial* sesamoid only) and the angle of metatarsus primus varus (MT1 and axis medial cuneiform – see Houghton & Dickson 1979, and Fig. 13).

Scott et al (1991) showed that of the possible measurements which could be made to assess varus of the first metatarsal, the most sensitive was the intermetatarsal angle, as this differed by the greatest amount between controls and affected cases. This was justified further as it was shown that the alignment of the second metatarsal (the medial angle between the axis of the second metatarsal and the transverse tarsal line) was more or less fixed, differed little between controls (mean 96°; range 86 to 120°) and those with hallux valgus (95°; range 87 to 108°; p>0.1) and was not significantly correlated with either the hallux valgus angle or the intermetatarsal angle in either controls or cases of the deformity. Thus it provided a stable reference point for measurement.

The method of measuring and the significance of relative metatarsal lengths is controversial. Hardy & Clapham (1951), using measurements in arcs centred on the transverse tarsal line (Fig. 13), found that the first metatarsal was significantly longer than the second in hallux valgus (+4 mm) than in controls (+2 mm). Bonney & Macnab (1952) found only six of 33 (18%) feet with hallux valgus and a low (under 10°) intermetatarsal angle to have the first metatarsal longer than the second, although in hallux rigidus 22 of 53 feet (42%) showed the first metatarsal the longer by 5 mm or more.

Radiological classification

The best classification of hallux valgus is that of Piggott (1960) in that it allows determination of prognosis. The scheme is based on a clinical and radiological survey of 113 patients, initially under the age of 21 years, presenting 216 feet, all with hallux valgus over 15°. The patients were re-examined after an average lapse of five years.

On standard X-rays the axes of the first metatarsal and the proximal phalanx were drawn by bisecting the diameters of their bases and joining the central points. Venning & Hardy (1951) showed that such measurements are consistent within 1°.

Normal
The normal arrangement is illustrated in Fig. 14a. There is slight valgus alignment due to slight tilting of the articular surfaces of both metatarsal and phalanx in relation to their respective shafts. At the joint the transverse diameters are parallel, the articular surfaces are concentric and the centres of their diameters are opposite each other.

Three types of hallux valgus deformity were defined on radiological grounds:

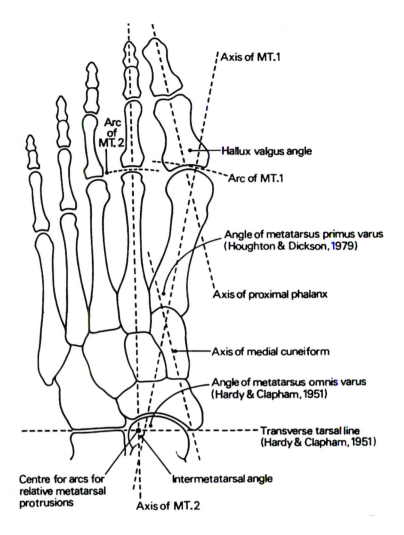

Axis of MT.1

Arc of MT. 2

Hallux valgus angle

Arc of MT.1

Angle of metatarsus primus varus
(Houghton & Dickson, 1979)

Axis of proximal phalanx

Axis of medial cuneiform

Angle of metatarsus omnis varus
(Hardy & Clapham, 1951)

Transverse tarsal line
(Hardy & Clapham, 1951)

Centre for arcs for
relative metatarsal
protrusions

Intermetatarsal angle

Axis of MT.2

Figure 13

Axes and angles of the forefoot bones and relative metatarsal protrusion.

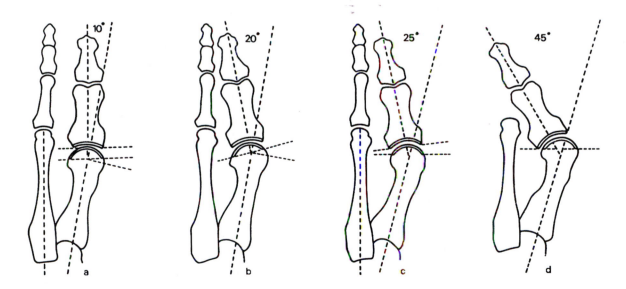

10° 20° 25° 45°

a b c d

Figure 14

The classification of Piggott (1960)

a: Normal situation. b: In congruous hallux valgus the distal articular surface of the metatarsal is tilted, but the joint is otherwise normal. c: In deviated hallux valgus the base of the phalanx remains in contact with the metatarsal articular cartilage, although the joint is deviated into valgus. d: In subluxated hallux valgus the joint is deviated far enough for the lateral side of the phalanx to overhang the end of the metatarsal.

Congruous (9%)

In this type the normal tilt of the articular surfaces is greater than average, producing a hallux valgus angle above 15°. Otherwise, the joint is entirely normal. The deformity is in the *bone* (Fig. 14b).

Deviated (38%)

In these toes the distal articular surface is deviated laterally on the proximal, exposing the medial edge of the latter (Fig. 14c). The transverse diameters of the articular ends of the bones are no longer parallel and their centres no longer opposite each other. The deformity is at the *joint*.

Subluxated (53%)

In this group, the lateral margin of the base of the proximal phalanx is subluxated from the edge of the metatarsal head (see Fig. 14d). Of 27 individual feet with good radiological data, 13 (48%) showed progression and the group as a whole showed an upward trend in the hallux valgus angle with time.

More complicated assessments have been suggested (Spinner et al 1984), but they seem to be more detailed than the accuracy of current operative treatments can equal.

Non-operative management

The main problem for the patient with hallux valgus (pain and bursitis on the medial side of the joint and displaced lesser toes) may be handled conservatively (making footwear to fit the deformed foot) or by operation. The cosmetic blemish is amenable only to surgical treatment.

Groiso (1992) published results of the treatment of juvenile hallux valgus with a custom-made thermoplastic night splint, remade periodically, and a regimen of exercise. He claimed that the hallux valgus angle was improved in 28 of 48 feet (58%) by an average of 6° (range 2 to 19°) over a follow-up period of 2 to 6 years, and that the intermetatarsal angle improved by a mean of 3° (range 2 to 7°) in 12 of 37 feet (32%). However, most surgeons seem to reserve splintage for a post-operative role. Insoles may be useful for associated problems such as metatarsalgia or flat foot.

In moderate degrees of hallux valgus and bunion formation, an appliance fitter may be able to stretch the upper of the shoe over the pressure area. If standard shoes cannot be fitted, individually made shoes or especially commodious stock shoes must be supplied. The former are more expensive, but are more acceptable cosmetically than the latter and more likely to be worn (Hughes & Klenerman 1985).

Surgical treatment of hallux valgus

Indications for operation

(i)   Pain due to shoe pressure over the medial side of the first metatarsophalangeal joint.
(ii)   Bursitis with pain, fluid accumulation or sepsis.
(iii) Increasing hallux valgus deformity.
(iv)   Excessive width of the foot and difficulty in fitting shoes.
(v)   Secondary deformities of the lesser toes.
(vi)   Cosmetic appearance.
(vii) Pressure on the inner edge of the nail due to medial rotation deformity of the toe (Mikhail 1960).

Contraindications to operation

(i)   Poor peripheral arterial circulation is an absolute contraindication.
(ii)   Current sepsis. (This must have been quiescent for a minimum of three months before operation is attempted under antibiotic cover.)
(iii) Uncontrolled diabetes.
(iv)   Peripheral neuropathy is a relative contraindication. Thought should be given to any possible secondary effects of an operation on the weight-bearing properties of the forefoot, lest secondary ulceration be precipitated.

There are seven groups of surgical procedure which may be used in hallux valgus:

(i)   Bunionectomy with medial capsulorrhaphy
(ii)   Arthroplasties: Phalangeal excision
                       Metatarsal excision
                       Prosthetic replacement
(iii) Tendon transfer procedures
(iv)   Osteotomies: Distal metatarsal varus without capsulorrhaphy
                    Distal metatarsal displacement with capsulorrhaphy
                    Proximal metatarsal valgus with capsulorrhaphy
                    Basal phalangeal varus
(v)   Arthrodesis
(vi)   Combined procedures
(vii) Cuneiform procedures

Arthroplasties

Phalangeal excision arthroplasty

Technique: Keller's (1904, 1912) prescription (Fig. 15) was for an incision in skin and capsule along the medial

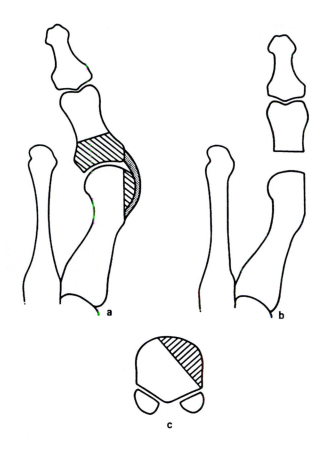

Figure 15

Excision arthroplasty. The technique of Davies-Colley (1887) and Keller (1904, 1912). Excision of the base of the phalanx and (c) excision of the medial side of the metatarsal head, taking more bone dorsally.

edge of the joint, clearance and disarticulation of the base of the phalanx and the excision of enough bone to enable the toe to straighten, and removal of the 'exostosis' on the head of the metatarsal.

Authors differ in what proportion of the proximal phalanx it is best to excise. Amounts from one-third (Holden 1954), through one-half (Cleveland & Winant 1950) or two-thirds (Galland & Jordan 1938, Schein 1940) to total removal (Alsberg 1924) have been advocated. Excessive bone removal is associated with marked weakness and a tendency for the residual toe to ride on the dorsum of the metatarsal head as a useless remnant. Too little removal may cause inadequate correction of valgus and stiffness of the pseudarthrosis.

Modifications to the procedure have been introduced at various times. Bearing in mind the importance of avoiding dorsal contracture of the pseudarthrosis, some advocate division of the tendon of extensor hallucis longus. There is little doubt that this addition avoids the tendency of the soft tissues to draw the truncated toe proximally, dorsally and into valgus.

In an attempt to increase the gap between the bones at the pseudarthrosis and to control the position of the stump of the proximal phalanx, it has been suggested that a longitudinal Kirschner wire be placed down the toe for 10 days (W Fitzgerald 1950) to six weeks after operation. However, Sherman et al (1984), in 51 Keller operations among 35 women, demonstrated that the use of a longitudinal Kirschner wire for two and a half weeks postoperatively did not improve results or the residual gap at the pseudarthrosis at follow-up. Indeed, there was a significant reduction in interphalangeal joint movement and an increase in radiological abnormalities at this joint.

The aftercare of the Keller arthroplasty is critical. While plaster of Paris fixation is not generally necessary, it is important to control the position of the toe with secure bandages or splints and to bring the toe into slight plantar flexion (to avoid dorsal contracture) and slight valgus (to avoid infolding the medial skin between the bone ends).

This type of operation is indicated for the older patient, with local joint troubles (eg, bursitis) with moderate deformity (hallux valgus angle under 40° and intermetatarsal angle under 20°, ie, without gross forefoot splay) and who will make low demands upon the use of the foot.

The anatomical correction after the operation is seldom full, but often the subjective satisfaction is better. Bonney & Macnab (1952) recorded only 41% of cases with correction to a hallux valgus angle under 20° and 75% under 30°, while Rogers & Joplin (1947) quoted improvement on the preoperative angle in only half their cases. On the whole, metatarsus primus varus is not improved by the operation. There is some fall-off in the results with time (Barnard 1930, Bonney & Macnab 1952).

The amount of bone excised has an influence on the result. If more is taken, the toe is shorter and weaker, but more mobile, and vice versa. Cleveland et al (1944) found that only 32% of their army personnel returned to full duties after operation. While Bonney & Macnab (1952) did not show much better results if the final postoperative width of the pseudarthrosis was over 3 mm, Henry & Waugh (1975) found that the average range of dorsiflexion after operation improved from 40° when one-third of the phalanx was excised to 60° when more than one-third was removed.

Conlan & Gregg (1991) found that the optimum managment of the overriding second toe in association with Keller's operation was proximal hemiphalangectomy of the lesser toe (with no recurrent overriding) rather than interphalangeal joint fusion in the second toe (with 38% recurrence of varus position).

In patients over 30, Turnbull & Grange (1986) found that those having metatarsal osteotomy had significantly less residual hallux valgus (average of 12° compared with 21° in the Keller group), better restoration of sesamoid anatomy (to neutral in 66% of osteotomies, unimproved with the arthroplasty) and less lateral metatarsalgia. Conversely, Kreiblich et al (1992), in

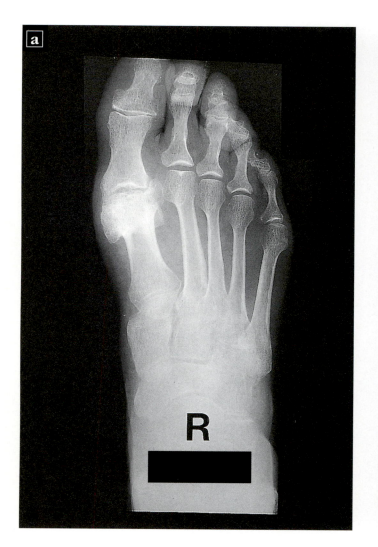
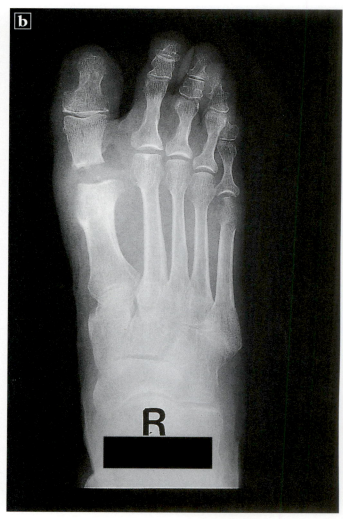

Figure 16

Longstanding stiff and uncomfortable Mayo arthroplasty (a), converted to a Keller type (b).

patients aged over 60 years, found little difference in results between distal metatarsal osteotomy and the Keller operation in respect of mean angular correction of hallux valgus or of postoperative metatarsalgia. Similarly, Ivory & Gregg (1993) found no difference between two groups, both over 45 years of age, one having first metatarsophalangeal joint fusion and the other Keller's operation, when assessing pain relief, cosmesis, the ability to wear shoes or subjective satisfaction (90% in both groups).

Secondary metatarsalgia poses a major problem after any forefoot operation. After the Keller procedure, because of the proximal shift of the phalangeal stump, there is proximal displacement of the sesamoids, which come to lie under the metatarsal neck rather than under its head (Fig. 16a). This decreases the plantar prominence of the region of the first metatarsal head and, together with the weakening of the toe itself, predisposes to an increase in the loading of the lesser metatarsals, especially the second and third. Gilmore & Bush (1957) found callosities present in 16 of 29 (55%) subjects of Keller's operation and Rix (1968) in 40% after Mayo's operation. Schein (1940) and Holden (1954) noted this complication as a factor in their less satisfactory cases.

Metatarsal excision arthroplasty

Resection of the first metatarsal head to correct hallux valgus was first advocated by Heuter in 1871. The procedure is now linked with the name of Mayo (1908) who reported on 65 cases over an eight-year period.

The operation seems to have fallen into disuse in the 1930s and the author has heard the view expressed that it may be regarded as negligent to perform it. In this climate of opinion any modern prospective evaluation of its worth or otherwise is difficult.

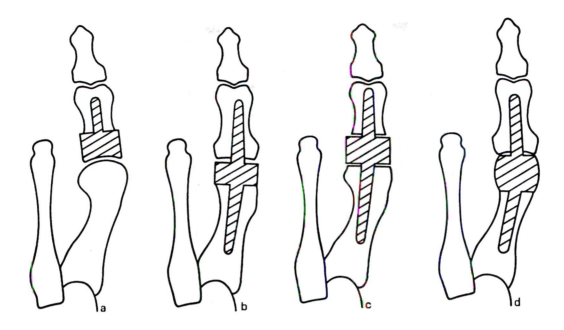

Figure 17

Replacement arthroplasty. Silicone elastomer prosthetic techniques: a: Swanson single-stem (1972); b: Swanson double-stem (1979); c: Wenger & Whalley (1978); d: Helal & Chen (1982).

However, a recent long-term retrospective review (at an average of 33 years) by Galloway and Majkowski (1992) of 35 feet having the Colley–Keller procedure and 46 feet the Hueter–Mayo operation, showed little difference between the two groups. Both had residual pain in under 5% and the difference in the incidences of metatarsalgia was not significant (40% after Keller and 45% after Mayo).

Historically, its indications were similar to those of phalangeal excision arthroplasty (see pp. 314–16).

In theory, the Mayo operation disturbs the relationship of the metatarsal head to the sesamoids less than the Keller (see Fig. 16a). The occasional stiff and painful Mayo result may be converted to a Keller type arthroplasty (Fig. 16b).

Replacement arthroplasty

Swanson, having tried to develop a metallic prosthesis for the first metatarsal head in 1952, from 1962 used instead a silicone elastomer replacement of the base of the proximal phalanx (Swanson 1972, 1975, Sethu et al 1980). The operation was done in hallux valgus, hallux rigidus, rheumatoid disease and cases of failed excision arthroplasty. With medial capsulorrhaphy, release of lateral capsule and adductor hallucis and with the elongation of extensor hallucis longus, one-third of the phalanx was excised and replaced by one of five sizes of silicone elastomer disc, secured by a simple intramedullary stem (Fig. 17a).

Later Swanson et al (1979) reported the use since 1974 of a double-stemmed silicone elastomer replacement, by

a similar technique, except that bone was removed from both sides of the joint. The authors stressed the need to preserve a portion of the metatarsal head for weight bearing, taking bone from the proximal phalanx if a larger gap was needed (see Fig. 17b).

Accounts have appeared of the development of foreign body reactions to particulate silicone elastomer abraded from prostheses in fingers and toes. Clinically this 'detritic synovitis' takes the form of painful swelling, redness and stiffness, settling if the device is removed. Bone lesions (Gordon & Bullough 1982) and lymphadenopathy (Christie et al 1977) have been reported, but both complications seem uncommon, bearing in mind the very large number of these prostheses which have been inserted. Histologically, particles indistinguishable from silicone elastomer have been found in synovium (Lemon et al 1984) and marrow spaces, in giant cells and in lymph glands. The changes have been reproduced experimentally in the knee joints of rabbits (Worsing et al 1982).

Helal & Chen (1982) reported favourably on use of the ball-spacer in great toes. Broughton et al (1987) published results of silicone elastomer ball arthroplasty in 62 feet (48 hallux valgus and 14 hallux rigidus) of 39 women, with a 77% excellent or good outcome. However, they found that of 53 feet without preoperative metatarsalgia, 14 (26%) developed it and of 9 feet affected by metatarsal head pain only 4 (44%) were improved.

Vlatis & Anderson (1990) in a retrospective study of 54 feet from 49 patients found subjective satisfaction in 90% and objective result at excellent or good in 75%. They noted persistent swelling in several patients.

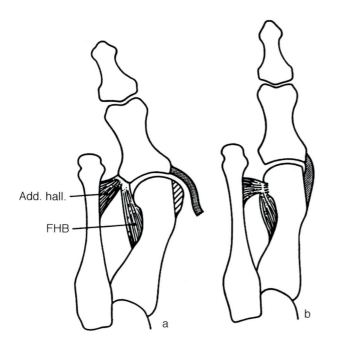

Figure 18

Tendon transfer. The operation of McBride (1928).

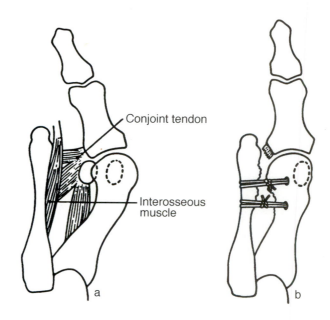

Figure 19

Soft-tissue operation. The operation of Botteri & Castellana (1961).

In a small personal series of 48 implants, reviewed by T.F. Sibley, the author found that in hallux valgus, 52% of toes showed deformity of 30° or over at review, that 75% lost significant joint movement and that there was poor satisfaction with the cosmetic result. The incidence of metatarsalgia was improved from 79% preoperatively to 37% postoperatively in hallux valgus sufferers.

Silicone elastomer replacement arthroplasty cannot any longer be regarded as filling a therapeutic lacuna between the younger patient who is best treated by metatarsal osteotomy or the McBride procedure and the older patient for whom the well-established excision arthroplasty may be appropriate. Anderson's criteria (1986, and 1990 with Vlatis) are for a patient over 55 years of age, with hallux valgus under 45° in an arthritic joint and with low demands on the feet. The author would now agree with this more limited selection of patients.

Selection of the correct type of patient (avoiding those with gross forefoot splay) and careful technique (which should include the excision of enough bone from each side of the joint, but not too much from the metatarsal head to retain some sesamoid articulation and a full lateral soft-tissue release) are essential if disappointment is to be avoided in hallux valgus. Double-stemmed prostheses have now superseded single-stemmed types.

Careful aftercare is important, with splintage of the toe against recurrent valgus for at least three weeks and concentration upon regaining adequate plantar flexion range and power.

Soft-tissue operations and tendon transfers

In 1928, McBride described what has now become the classic tendon transfer procedure for hallux valgus. He based the operation on what is now thought of as a misconception, that the sesamoids were displaced laterally by contracture of the adductor group of intrinsic muscles (Figure 18). Nevertheless the operation is effective in correcting medial metatarsal drift (Mann 1982).

For hallux angles over 40° or intermetatarsal angles of 15° or over, Mikhail (1960), Gibson et al (1972) and Mann (1982) added a metatarsal osteotomy to the soft-tissue procedure (see p. 326).

Krida (1939) used fascia lata and Joplin (1950, 1964) used the extensor tendon of the fifth toe to bind together the metatarsal heads, the latter adding a transfer of adductor hallucis to the first metatarsal. Botteri & Castellana (1961) and Pagella & Pierleoni (1971) achieved narrowing of the intermetatarsal angle by osteosynthesis between the first and second metatarsals, secured with two suture loops, and claimed that hallux valgus was automatically corrected (Fig. 19).

Operations of the McBride type may be used in patients with moderate (under 40°) hallux valgus and moderate forefoot splay (under 15° intermetatarsal angle) and would seem to be an alternative to distal varus or displacement osteotomy. Indeed, the principles of both types of operation may be combined (see pp. 325–6).

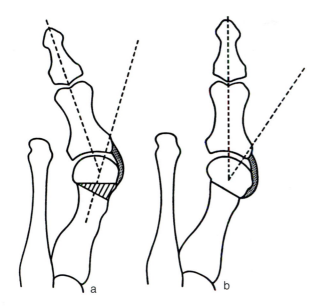

Figure 20

Metatarsal osteotomy. The distal varus osteotomy of Reverdin (1881, 1918), Barker (1884) and Hohmann (1923). Note that the joint alignment (dotted lines) is unchanged.

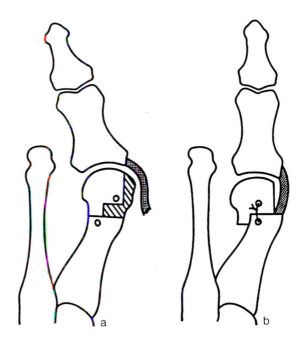

Figure 22

Metatarsal osteotomy. The distal displacement of Hawkins, Mitchell and Hendrick (1945).

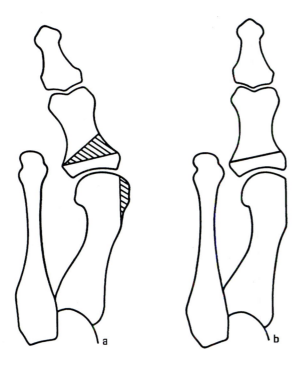

Figure 21

Phalangeal osteotomy. Proximal varus osteotomy of the phalanx, with bunionectomy (Akin 1925, Allan 1940)

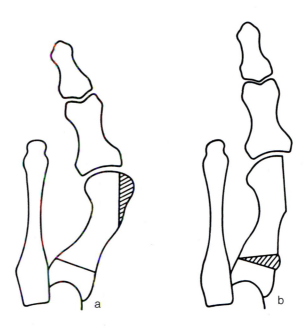

Figure 23

Metatarsal osteotomy. Basal valgus osteotomy with inserted wedge of bunion bone (Trethowan 1923).

Overcorrection to hallux varus would seem to be the most important complication (about 8% of cases) and may be managed by excision of the base of the phalanx, which removes the insertions of the unbalanced intrinsic musculature.

Metatarsal and phalangeal osteotomy

There are two separate principles embodied in osteotomy operations: first, that of tilting either the distal metatarsal on its shaft or the proximal phalanx on its base in the opposite sense to that of the hallux valgus,

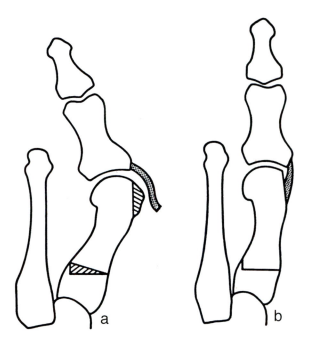

Figure 24

Metatarsal osteotomy. Basal valgus osteotomy with excised wedge (Golden 1961)

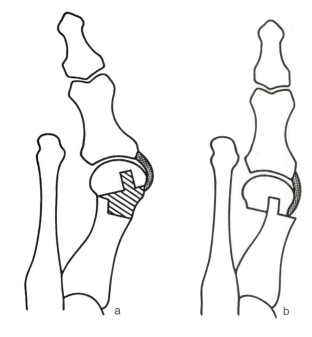

Figure 25

Metatarsal osteotomy. The distal varus and displacement osteotomy of Mygind (1952) and Thomasen

producing a second (varus) deformity to correct the primary one (see Figs 20 and 21). Adductor hallucis tenotomy is usually added. Second, that of dividing the metatarsal and displacing its head laterally (to narrow the forefoot, to reduce the bony prominence of the metatarsal head and to lower the intermetatarsal angle). This can be achieved distally (at the metatarsal neck or shaft) by lateral displacement of the head (Fig. 22) or proximally (just distal to the tarsometatarsal joint) by lateral (valgus) angulation of the whole shaft (Figs. 23 and 24). The hallux valgus deformity itself must be corrected by medial capsulorrhaphy. Some operations combine both principles (Figs. 25 and 26).

Each of the two main groups has its peculiar advantages and disadvantages. The first is suitable only for the milder cases of hallux valgus (say to 30°), but entails less disturbance of the metatarsophalangeal joint as no capsulorrhaphy is involved. Correction of intermetatarsal angle and forefoot narrowing is achieved only by those techniques which add displacement to varus (e.g. the Mygind–Thomasen procedure). The second can be applied to more severe cases, with higher valgus angles and with displacement of the metatarsal head medially off the sesamoid platform, since more drastic bone rearrangements are involved.

However, detachment of the medial capsule and excision of the medial aspect of the metatarsal head create a raw area to which the medial capsule is reapplied and to which it adheres. This shortens the

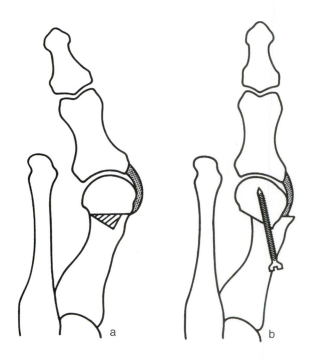

Figure 26

Metatarsal osteotomy. The distal varus and displacement technique of Pelet (1981) and Magerl

length of the capsule (which normally swings alongside the distal half of the medial side of the metatarsal head) and predisposes to joint stiffness after operation. Also the joint is realigned by drawing back the base of the phalanx into relation with the degenerate cartilage on the medial half of the articular surface of the metatarsal head.

By appropriate choice of technique, both groups of osteotomy permit correction in the dorsiplantar plane, particularly with plantar displacement of the metatarsal head or with volar tilt of the metatarsal as a whole. This aids in compensating for any first metatarsal shortening by increasing the plantar prominence and weight-bearing abilities of the first metatarsal head, important in relation to secondary metatarsalgia (Merkel et al 1983, Goddard & Wilson 1986).

A proximal metatarsal osteotomy is indicated in the pronated (flat) foot as a modest compensatory plantar flexion of the medial border of the forefoot may be produced.

It is not good practice to perform one favoured operation indiscriminately in all cases. A repertoire of osteotomy techniques is required, at least one from each of the three broad groups (distal varus, distal displacement and proximal valgus osteotomies). The basic group of operation selected depends on the patient's characteristics, while the exact method employed within each group may depend on the surgeon's preference.

Even after correct preoperative assessment accuracy of technique is of paramount importance. These operations should not be undertaken by unsupervised junior surgical staff. A period of apprenticeship is needed before independent performance is allowed. More judgment and skill are needed for these operations than for some other 'more major' ones.

To obtain a satisfactory result and to content the patient, certain criteria should be fulfilled:

(i)   The hallux valgus deformity must be adequately corrected, say to an angle of 10–15°. However, hallux varus must not be produced or shoe fitting will be made difficult.

(ii)   The forefoot should be narrowed and bunion pressure relieved.

(iii) Correction of displacement of the metatarsal head from the sesamoids should be achieved. If possible sesamoidectomy should be avoided.

(iv)   Undue shortening of the first ray should be avoided or compensated by volar displacement.

(v)   Soft tissue relaxation about the joint must be achieved, either by limited bone shortening or by appropriate *safe* capsulotomies. With a distal metatarsal osteotomy, capsulotomy on the lateral side must not be combined with capsulorrhaphy on the medial aspect, lest the head be devitalized.

(vi)   Dorsal displacement or angulation of the distal fragment of an osteotomy must be avoided.

(vii) An extended posture at the metatarsophalangeal joint must be prevented. Too much plication of the

easy dorsimedial part of the medial capsulorrhaphy over the more difficult plantar-medial aspect may predispose to this.

(viii) While certain techniques produce good stability at the osteotomy site (either by the peg-and-socket method or by internal fixation), a capsulorrhaphy needs to be supported either in a plaster cast or with a splint. Unstabilized osteotomies require plaster fixation for six weeks and a delay in weight bearing of two weeks.

(ix)   Avoid accidental section of the dorsimedial cutaneous nerve of the great toe, which gives rise to a troublesome neuroma.

(x)   Avoid forcible retraction, especially with bone levers, or skin-edge necrosis may delay wound healing. Similarly, keep subcutaneous dissection around the bunion area to a minimum.

(xi)   Institute a programme of physiotherapy to restore metatarsophalangeal joint motion, active plantar flexion as well as passive dorsiflexion, as soon as splintage is removed. Encourage the patient to bear weight on the medial ray of the foot when splintage is discarded.

(xii) Treat lesser toe deformities concurrently.

(xiii) Inculcate in the patient a reasonable expectation of footwear styles for postoperative wear.

In the older patient (50 to 67 years), Das De & Hamblen (1986) found good results after distal metatarsal osteotomy in only 57% of cases and advised caution in the use of this technique.

Tibrewall & Foss (1991) performed Wilson's osteotomy on a day-care basis, finding this satisfactory in patients under 55 but a struggle for those older than this.

The osteotomy catalogue

Innumerable osteotomies are described; the list below is not exhaustive, but is reasonably representative. Only important points of technique are mentioned in each case and appropriate aftercare is taken for granted.

Distal varus osteotomies without capsulorrhaphy
Reverdin (1881, 1918) and Barker (1884) independently described simple excision and closure of a medially-based wedge from the neck of the first metatarsal but the operation has come to be associated with the name of Hohmann (1922/3, 1924, 1925) (see Figure 20).

Mygind (1952, 1953) modified the technique to secure the osteotomy by a peg-and-socket method. After transverse osteotomy of the metatarsal neck, a peg of about 5 mm square is fashioned on the plantar and lateral corner of the proximal fragment, using nibblers and cutters. Bone is removed in such a way that a medially-based, trapezoidal wedge is excised, providing the necessary varus tilt. It is essential that the 'shoulders' of the peg be square and not sloping, or disimpaction may occur. The method automatically displaces the head

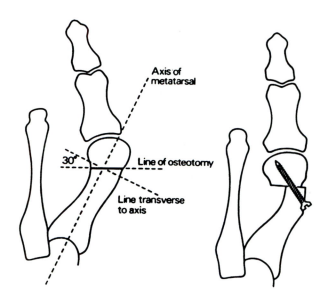

Figure 27

Metatarsal osteotomy. The distal displacement osteotomy of
Lindgren & Turan (1983).

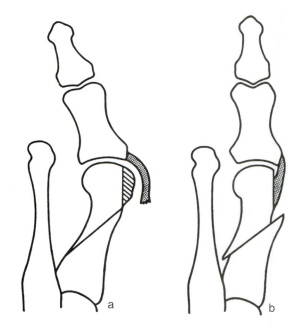

Figure 28

Metatarsal osteotomy. The technique of J Wilson (1963) for
oblique osteotomy of the distal shaft.

volarward, helping to compensate for the metatarsal
shortening, which is of the order of 1 cm (see Figure
25). The method is suitable for young patients with good
quality cancellous bone to give a firm grasp on the peg.

Lindgren & Turan (1983) described a simple oblique
osteotomy without capsulorrhaphy, allowing displacement laterally and only slightly proximally (in contrast
with the similar osteotomy of J Wilson, 1963, see page
324), the cut being more nearly transverse to the
metatarsal axis (Figure 27). Instability due to the
relatively transverse division was counteracted by internal fixation with a screw. The medial spike on the proximal fragment was trimmed.

Proximal phalangeal varus osteotomy

Akin (1925), Butterworth & Clary (1963) and Giannestras
(1972) treated hallux valgus by bunionectomy, medial
capsulorrhaphy and lateral muscular release, combined
with varus osteotomy of the proximal phalanx, excising
a medially-based wedge of bone 0.5 cm distal to the joint
and securing the closed osteotomy with a longitudinal
Kirschner wire (see Figure 21). The capsule was sutured
with the toe in up to 5° of varus and extensor hallucis
longus was lengthened or pulled across to a mid-line
position.

Giannestras (1972) reported 73% excellent or good
results from 92 operations, with cosmetic correction
comparable with other techniques and painless
movement preserved in all but four cases. However,
Colloff & Weitz (1967) in their 40 cases noted some interphalangeal joint stiffness in 30%.

Distal displacement osteotomy with capsulorrhaphy

Three types of osteotomy may be included within this
category: the transverse osteotomy of the metatarsal
neck, typified by the Hawkins–Mitchell–Hendrick operation (1945), the chevron osteotomy of Austin and
Leventen (1981) and the oblique osteotomy of the distal
shaft (as in the Ludloff 1918 or J Wilson 1963
techniques).

The first of these three is unstable and needs some
form of internal fixation, the second is stable and the
third may be made so by proper design and splintage.
In all these operations a bunionectomy is included and
correction of hallux valgus is by medical capsulorrhaphy.

Miller (1974) noted that 'the Mitchell osteoteomy-
bunionectomy was good middle-of-the-road procedure
for many patients with symptomatic bunion' (see Figure
22) and the same may be said of the J Wilson procedure (Figure 28). Certainly cases with deformity too great
for the distal varus osteotomy without capsulorrhaphy
may be tackled by these techniques. However, Miller
(1974) felt that certain cases were better treated by a
modified technique or by combining the Mitchell and
Keller principles (see page 325) 'because of inability to
obtain complete bunion correction by the Mitchell procedure alone in severe primary deformities, as well as in
recurrent deformities after standard procedures'.

Blunden (1968) cautioned against the procedure in
osteoarthritic joints or in feet with metatarsalgia and
Miller (1974) against its use in both osteoarthritic and
rheumatoid cases or in those with an excessive intermetatarsal angle (over 23°). The complications were

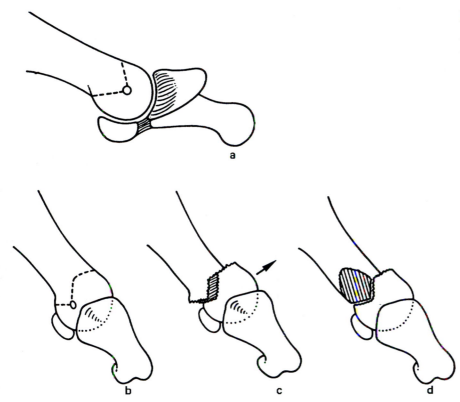

Figure 29

Metatarsal osteotomy. The 'chevron' method
of Austin & Leventen (1981).

discussed in detail by Mitchell et al (1958), Gibson et al (1972) and Miller (1973, 1974).

In common with all metatarsal osteotomies, exact technique is essential. Allowing dorsal angulation, failure to secure slight plantar displacement or inclination, or excessive bone shortening predispose to secondary metatarsalgia. Incomplete correction follows failure to secure sufficient displacement (which should be by one-quarter to one-half of the diameter of the bone, depending on the intermetatarsal angle) or poor medial capsular repair. Aseptic necrosis of the metatarsal head may be caused by interference with the lateral joint capsule. Stress fractures of the lesser metatarsals occasionally follow the operation (Miller 1974 reports an incidence of 0.75%).

The chevron osteotomy was introduced in the early 1960s by Austin (Austin & Leventen 1981) and other reports on its use have followed by Corless (1976), Johnson et al (1979), Shepherd & Guitronich (1982), and Turner & Todd (1984).

The technique called for bunionectomy followed by a horizontally directed, V-shaped osteotomy of the head and neck of the first metatarsal, begun with a central, medial to lateral 2 mm (5/64 in) drill hole and completed with a motor saw. Displacement is from 5 mm to half the width of the head and stability is by cancellous impaction. The medial residual prominence of the blunt wedge of the distal shaft is trimmed or rasped away (Figure 29).

After release of lateral structures (done across the joint), a medial U-shaped capsular flap, fashioned during the exposure of the metatarsal head, is resutured to drill holes in the bone. The technique usually provides stable control of position after operation and minimal metatarsal shortening, but occasional instability may be secured by the wire loop technique of Turner & Todd (1984).

Pring et al (1985) compared the operation with the J Wilson procedure. They concluded that it was a stable osteotomy (requiring no cast fixation), with a quicker recovery period, with better great toe weight-bearing characteristics, and with less metatarsal shortening, but that correction of the original deformity was inferior to the J Wilson operation.

Similarly Meier & Kenzora (1985) compared the chevron and Mitchell operations. Osteonecrosis occurred in only one case (8%) after the Mitchell procedure, but in 12 cases (20%) of the chevron, the incidence rising to four of ten (40%) in whom a lateral capsular release had been performed. The eight unsatisfactory results (11%) were associated with damage to the dorsal digital nerve, osteonecrosis or with preexisting osteoarthritis in the metatarsophalangeal joint.

Mann (1982) pointed out the disadvantages of the chevron procedure, quoting osteonecrosis, malalignment, excessive metatarsal shortening and hallux varus. Kinnard & Gordon (1984) in a similar comparison concluded that there was no major difference between the two operations, but that the Mitchell was 'more versatile and to allow better correction of the painful hallux'.

Horizontal, oblique osteotomy of the distal shaft was designed by Ludloff (1918) and a similar technique reported by Wilhelm (1934), but sagittal oblique osteotomy is associated with J Wilson (1963) (see Figure 28). The latter technique called for the raising of a medial capsular flap, trimming of the medial side of the metatarsal head and an oblique osteotomy at 45° to the axis of the bone, directed from medial and distal to lateral and proximal. Soft-tissue at the lateral end of the osteotomy must be divided to enable sufficient displacement, which is lateral and proximal and which is stable with the great toe overcorrected into varus. The angle of 45° is optimum; too transverse an osteotomy is unstable and too oblique a one is difficult to displace.

Proximal valgus osteotomy
Golden (1961) popularized one of the more common basal osteotomies. Through a dorsal incision, a medial capsular flap is raised and the medial aspect of the head excised sparingly. Tenotomy of adductor hallucis and lateral capsulotomy are performed. At the base of the first metatarsal a transverse osteotomy is made, incomplete on the lateral side where a spur of bone is left intact for stability. A laterally and volar-based wedge is excised from the distal fragment, allowing the metatarsal to swing into valgus and plantar flexion as the wedge is closed. Medial capsulorrhaphy corrects the hallux valgus deformity.

Reviewing 149 feet in 85 patients, postoperatively he recorded 60% cases with hallux valgus under 10°, 88% with more than 45° range of motion (34% with 80° or over), 72% with normal toe plantar flexion power and 94% with no more than slight pain in the metatarsophalangeal joint region. Eleven feet (7%) had hallux varus, of which seven (5%) were symptomatic.

Metatarsal osteotomy and metatarsalgia
No procedure is exempt, but in general metatarsalgia is a commoner problem if the first metatarsal head is elevated or tilted dorsally (usually a technical fault) or recessed by shortening of the shaft (usually inherent in the technique adopted). As the metatarsal shaft is at an angle of 15–25° to the floor in the standing position, a reduction in its length produces relative elevation. This can be compensated only by deliberate depression of the head. Theoretically 5 mm (8%) recession in a bone inclined at these angles to the horizontal would cause a 1.3 to 2.0 mm elevation of the head. Shortening of this order is caused in the Mygind–Thomasen and Mitchell procedures and about twice as much by the J Wilson osteotomy (Pring et al 1985).

Arthrodesis of the first metatarsophalangeal joint
Arthrodesis of the first metatarsophalangeal joint is done most often for hallux rigidus, but is suitable for severe hallux valgus (McKeever 1952, Marin 1960, MacDonald 1973, Mann 1982), for hallux valgus with metatarsalgia (Raymakers & Waugh 1971) and as a salvage procedure

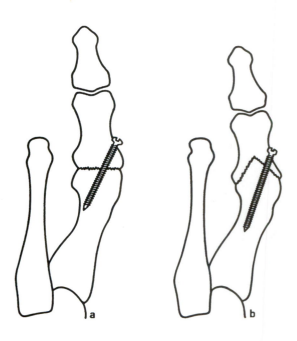

Figure 30

Arthrodesis. The methods of (a) Smith (1952) and (b) Marin (1960)

(Thompson & McElvenny 1940, Marin 1960, Mann 1982). There are a variety of methods described (Figure 30), but most techniques give a fusion rate of 94/97%. Methods of internal fixation listed include: screws, Kirschner wires, wire loops and Rush nails (C Wilson 1958). Alternatively an external fixation clamp may be used (Hulbert 1955). Many surgeons condemn this operation. It is claimed to be unpopular with women as the heel height is restricted to one level, but Johannson & Barrington (1984) found only three women among their 51 patients who experienced difficulties with shoe fitting.

Ivory & Gregg (1993), in a series of 80 feet in 57 patients over 45 years of age, found the procedure no better than the Colley–Keller excision arthroplasty, except in patients with pre-existing metatarsalgia.

However, there can be considerable benefits. There is no limit to the degree of hallux valgus which may be corrected; provided bony fusion is obtained, the correction is permanent; it reduces metatarsus primus varus by restabilizing the metatarsophalangeal joint (so that valgus forces on the tip of the toe are retransmitted directly to the tarsometatarsal level). Raymakers & Waugh (1971) noted a reduction in intermetatarsal angle in all their patients, with a significant reduction in forefoot width (averaging 6 mm) in 90%.

Currently, an angle of extension of 20–30° is considered optimum (Raymakers & Waugh 1971, Lahz 1973, Mann 1982).

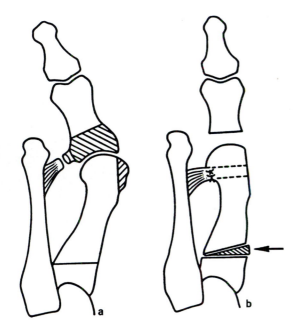

Figure 31

Combined operation. The technique of Stamm (1957), combining the Keller arthroplasty, the McBride transfer and a basal valgus osteotomy with wedge insert

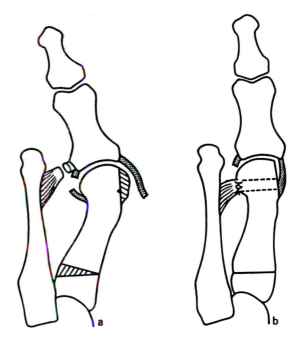

Figure 32

Combined operation. The method of Simmonds & Menelaus (1960) which combines a basal, valgus, closing wedge osteotomy with the McBride procedure.

In the anteroposterior plane, most recommend angles of 10–20° of valgus. Rotation of the toe in its long axis should be in neutral position.

The author holds the view that the optimum position is secured by holding the sole of the foot at 90° to the tibia and then placing the pulp of the toe in line with the sole of the foot in the lateral plane and comfortably alongside the second toe in the anteroposterior plane. Rotation should be neutral, as judged by the nail position.

Excessive angles of extension destroy the weight-bearing function of the great toe (predisposing to metatarsalgia and to feelings of instability) and make shoe fitting difficult, as does excessive varus or even the neutral (straight) posture. Fusion in the overflexed position leaves the patient with a feeling of the toe 'digging into the ground'. Fusion in too much valgus crowds the lesser toes and fusion in malrotation predisposes to pressure on the edge of the toe nail and on the plantar 'corner' of the interphalangeal joint.

The interphalangeal joint shows evidence of degenerative change after arthrodesis of the metatarsophalangeal joint in 25% (J Fitzgerald 1969) to 40% of cases (Mann 1982), with pain in 10–15% (Moynihan 1967) and arthritic changes in the interphalangeal joint are increased 2.5 times if the fusion angle of the metatarsophalangeal joint falls much below 20° of valgus (J Fitzgerald 1969).

Henry and Waugh (1975) showed with footprint studies that the great toe bore weight in 80% of cases after arthrodesis, compared with 40% after the Keller operation. They noted that preexisting metatarsalgia was not relieved if the great toe did not bear weight. If the toe took weight (102 cases), 16% had metatarsalgia, but if it did not (68 cases) then 43% had metatarsalgia.

Combined operations

These are procedures which combine two or more of the techniques discussed above, usually osteotomy with either arthroplasty or tendon transfer (of the McBride type) or both. They are major operations with a prolonged recovery period.

These more extensive procedures are indicated as salvage methods after unsatisfactory previous surgery (Miller 1974) or for severe cases (especially those with a splayed forefoot and a high intermetatarsal angle). Mann (1982) recommended an operation consisting of a McBride tendon transfer with a shaft osteotomy of the first metatarsal if the hallux valgus angle exceeded 40° and the intermetatarsal angle 15°, while Miller (1974) combined the Mitchell and Keller procedures for cases of severe hallux valgus with an intermetatarsal angle over 23°.

Stamm (1957) described the archetype operation which in its entirety or in part only goes by his name in the United Kingdom. In full, it consists of a proximal phalangeal excision arthroplasty, a bunionectomy, a

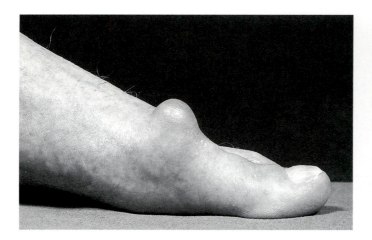

Figure 33

Typical dorsal bunion in hallux rigidus. Contrast Fig. 34.

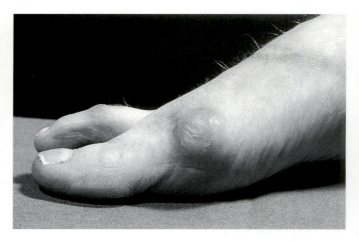

Figure 34

Typical medial bunion in hallux valgus. Contrast Fig. 33.

basal valgus metatarsal osteotomy (with a medial inserted wedge fashioned from the excised bone from the phalanx or metatarsal head), transfer of adductor hallucis to the first metatarsal and a medial capsulorrhaphy at the first metatarsophalangeal joint (with resiting of abductor hallucis medial to the joint) (Figure 31).

Evans (1957) reported on the results of 60 such operations noting cosmetic improvement in all, but a year-long period of postoperative discomfort, commensurate with the magnitude of the procedure. Mikhail (1960), Gibson et al (1972), Helal (1981) and Mann (1982) all combined the McBride tendon transfer with osteotomy of the neck or shaft of the first metatarsal. For cases of hallux valgus with a bunion and a wide intermetatarsal angle Mikhail excised an obliquely lying trapezium of bone from the distal metatarsal shaft, tilting the head into valgus, and secured the fragments with a Rush nail. He adduced a transfer of adductor hallucis to the metatarsal head. Gibson et al, to avoid excessive metatarsal shortening, substituted a simple oblique osteotomy with lateral displacement for the trapezoidal excision of bone and secured the bones with a pin.

Simmonds & Menelaus (1960) combined bunionectomy, lateral capsulotomy, medial capsulorrhaphy, the McBride transfer and basal valgus metatarsal osteotomy, with excised wedge (Figure 32). Their cases had an average preoperative hallux valgus angle of 29°, an ugly foot at presentation or evidence of progression of deformity, pain (24 of 33 cases: 73%) and shoe fitting difficulties. Helal (1981) reported on their technique in 35 feet. Mann et al (1992) gave results of a combination of the McBride procedure and crescentic basal first metatarsal osteotomy in 109 feet of 75 subjects.

Tarsometatarsal region and cuneiform procedures

Butson (1980) reported on 119 modified Kleinberg–Lapidus operations in 78 patients with 110 (92%) excel-

lent or good results and no non-unions at the basal fusion. He considered the procedure indicated for hallux valgus over 15° with symptomatic bunion, with moderate to severe metatarsus primus varus and with a minimum movement at the metatarsophalangeal joint of 30°, all in patients under 65 years of age.

Hansen (1993) recommended a similar operation with screw fixation of the basal arthrodesis for the unstable first ray in hallux valgus.

Hallux valgus interphalangeus

In 1935, Daw noted that 'there is another type of valgus deformity of the big toe where the deflection occurs at the interphalangeal joint'. He called it hallux valgus interphalangeus and reported two symptomless cases treated for cosmetic reasons.

Theander & Danielsson (1982) considered that this uncommon deformity was 'only rarely acquired', but that it was 'a malformation resulting from skew development of one or both phalanges'.

However, J Fitzgerald (1969) did note acquired interphalangeal deformity and degenerative change after metatarsophalangeal joint arthrodesis and 31% of cases had a minimum of 5° increase in the valgus angle of the interphalangeal joint. The incidence of osteoarthritis was nearly trebled by fusion of the metatarsophalangeal joint at an angle less than 20° of valgus. Occasionally, young patients present with the interphalangeal deformity, either because of the cosmetic blemish or because of pressure symptoms and callosity formation on the plantar and medial aspect of the joint.

Such cases may be managed by distal osteotomy of the proximal phalanx, excising a medially-based wedge of bone (if skeletally immature) or by excision and

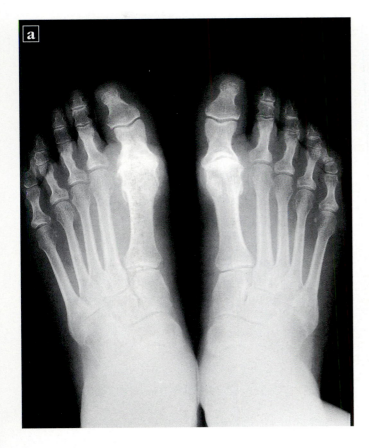

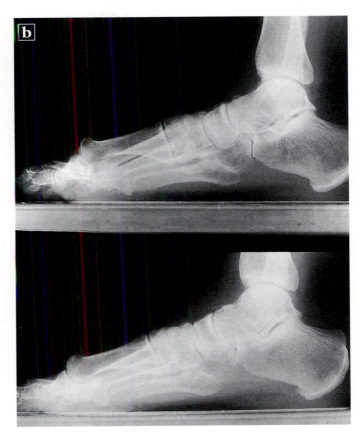

Figure 35

a: Typical hallux rigidus; b: Note the elevation of the first metatarsal and flexed posture of the toe

arthrodesis of the interphalangeal joint, correcting the deformity in the process (in adults or those with degenerative changes). For arthrodesis of this joint, internal fixation may be with an axial lag screw or with two longitudinal Kirschner wires.

Hallux rigidus

In juveniles the complaint is of the spontaneous onset of swelling and pain, worse on walking (especially in the toe-off phase of gait when the metatarsophalangeal joint is forced into passive extension). Adults also suffer from pressure over osteophytes, often on the dorsal and lateral sides of the metatarsal head (Figures 33 and 35; contrast Figure 34).

Movement is selectively restricted in early cases, with loss first of extension and later occasionally the development of flexion contracture, while plantar flexion remains free. In late cases the squared-off metatarsal head and the development of plane (rather than concentric) joint surfaces produces the fully developed picture of the rigid toe. There is a tendency for the patient to

limp, walking on the outer border of the foot in an attempt to spare the painful medial ray from passive extension during toe-off in walking.

Bingold & Collins (1950) noted the typical shoe wear pattern of hallux rigidus: the outer side of the heel, the outer side of the middle of the sole and under the pulp of the great toe itself. This pattern would arise from excessive pressure under the pulp of the flexed hallux and from transfer of weight to the lateral border of the foot, because of pain medially.

Some adult patients suffer from pressure over a dorsal osteophyte without any pain from a joint which is very rigid (due to fibrous ankylosis without actual fusion by bone). This is an important group to recognize from the point of view of treatment (see page 329).

Aetiology

While such generalized diseases as rheumatoid arthritis can give rise to stiffness and pain in the metatarsophalangeal joint of the great toe, these are excluded from discussion here (see Chapter VI.3). Notably a valgus element may be associated with rheumatoid arthritis, but is conspicuously absent in ordinary hallux rigidus.

Nilsonne (1930) suggested that there were two types of hallux rigidus, a primary type and 'ordinary' osteoarthritis. The age and sex associations of the disease tend to support this contention. Unselected by age, there is a slight preponderance of women in hallux rigidus, Bonney & Macnab (1952) finding that 68% of 44 patients and Hardy & Clapham (1951) 58% of 19 patients were female. However, in younger patients (aged 20 years and under) there is a marked preponderance of females (say 5:1 compared with males) and, in older age groups, a more even distribution between the sexes.

Osteochondritis dissecans

While Kessel & Bonney (1958) considered some of their cases of juvenile hallux rigidus to be due to this condition, the concept that the disease in the younger age groups was based on a post-traumatic osteochondral fracture (osteochondritis dissecans) of the metatarsal head was due to Goodfellow (1966) and McMaster (1978).

Goodfellow traced five likely stages in the progression of the disease and correlated these with the radiographic appearances. If the joint was explored in the earliest phase, a loose flap of articular cartilage was found on the metatarsal, between the apex of the dome and the dorsal margin of the head (Goodfellow 1966, McMaster 1978). Biopsy of underlying bone revealed dead trabeculae. At this stage the lesion was very difficult to visualize on X-rays.

A year or so later, progression of the lesion made radiological recognition easier, with the usual appearances of osteochondritis dissecans (a lucent pit with or without a central denser area). By about the second year, the typical appearances were obliterated first by filling-in of the depression in the head and eventually by the generalized secondary osteoarthritic changes of the adult.

Avascular necrosis

Changes in the basal epiphysis of the proximal phalanx were mentioned by Kingreen (1933), but the concept was refuted by Bingold & Collins (1950) who showed that increased density and division of the proximal epiphysis of the phalanx was seen also in the normal foot of unilateral cases of juvenile hallux rigidus and in controls.

Elevation of the first metatarsal

Lambrinudi (1938), Jack (1939/40), Lapidus (1940) and Bonney & Macnab (1952) noted the association of an extended posture of the first ray at the tarsometatarsal joint

with flexion deformity of and degeneration in the first metatarsophalangeal joint in approximately 65% of cases.

McKay (1983) described this deformity in children as a complication of surgery for poliomyelitis or congenitala talipes equinovarus.

Lapidus (1940) felt that one type of elevated first metatarsal and hallux flexus associated with dorsal prominence of the first metatarsophalangeal joint ('dorsal bunion') was *secondary* to hallux rigidus, for which he proposed another aetiology.

Kessel & Bonney (1958) considered this first ray posture to be a significant factor, noting that any metatarsal disposition carried with it a corresponding arc of metatarsophalangeal joint motion. They reported two cases of iatrogenic metatarsus primus elevatus, after metatarsal osteotomy or triple fusion, which were both associated with painful hallux flexus and one case of iatrogenic metatarsal depression associated with limitation of plantar flexion at the metatarsophalangeal joint.

Disparity in metatarsal lengths

Several authors (Cochrane 1927, Nilsonne 1930, Monberg 1935, Jack 1940, Bingold & Collins 1950) have ascribed metatarsophalangeal joint damage to an overlong first metatarsal or first ray as a whole.

Shoe wearing

Several authors considered the wearing of too short a shoe to be a significant cause of hallux rigidus (Davies-Colley 1887, Elmslie 1926, Bingold & Collins 1950), again presumably due to chronic strain or trauma to the joint.

Other causes

Some authors thought that hallux rigidus could follow any soft tissue contracture around the joint, due to immobilization (Monberg 1935) or 'synovitis' (Jack 1939/40, Bingold & Collins 1950). Cochrane (1927) suggested a plantar soft tissue release operation to correct this supposed contracture.

Osteoarthritis of the sesamometatarsal joint

Helal (Chapter V.5) speculates that some cases of hallux rigidus arise from degenerative disease (chondromalacia) of the sesamoid articulation.

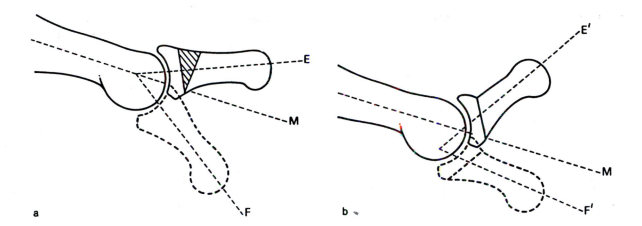

Figure 36

Phalangeal osteotomy. The principle of extension osteotomy in juvenile hallux rigidus.

Pathological function and anatomy

In 1887, Davies-Colley noted a transverse furrow in the articulate cartilage in cases of hallux flexus, corresponding to the edge of the proximal phalanx.

Early changes attributable to osteochrondritis dissecans are discussed on page 328, but it is generally noted that in established, yet not grossly advanced cases, articular cartilage erosion is seen in three sites. These are the dorsal lip and the centre of the articular surface of the proximal phalanx (Jack 1939/40, Bingold & Collins 1950) and the dorsidistal aspect of the metatarsal head (Goodfellow 1966, McMaster 1978). The proponents of the theory that juvenile hallux rigidus is due to traumatic osteochondritis dissecans hold that it is impaction of the dorsal lip of the proximal phalanx against the dorsidistal part of the metatarsal head during acute or repetitive traumatic (stubbing) episodes that sites the lesion.

Management

The mainstay of conservative treatment for painful hallux rigidus is alteration of the footwear. A convex rocker sole can be fitted to most modern glued composition soles except corrugated latex rubber. It should be about 1 cm (3/8 in) thick just behind the metatarsal heads and should taper away to nothing at the tip of the shoe and under the arch.

If there is a large dorsal bunion, the fitting of custom-made surgical shoes with a bulge to accommodate the abnormal bump may secure comfort. Such shoes may incorporate a rocker sole if indicated.

Operative treatment falls into various groups:

(i) Bunionectomy (exostectomy) and cheilectomy
(ii) Osteotomy of the proximal phalanx
(iii) Arthroplasty – phalangeal excision
        metatarsal excision
        prosthetic replacement
(iv) Arthrodesis
(iv) Others – operations for metatarsus primus elevatus
        soft-tissue release

Bunionectomy (exostectomy)

Medial bunion formation is not often a problem. Baker (1953) advocated trimming dorsal osteophytes in hallux rigidus and the author has found this to be a very satisfactory procedure for the adult (often elderly) patient who is bothered by shoe pressure, but who has a metatarsophalangeal joint virtually ankylosed and painless. Usually it is dorsal and lateral bony prominences which need to be planed flat. Little special after-care is needed, apart from that to secure wound healing. Hallux valgus does not develop postoperatively, as the arthritic joint is stable.

Cheilectomy

Thompson & Mann (1986) and Mann & Clanton (1988) advocated the cheilectomy operation of DuVries in the surgical management of hallux rigidus.

Through a dorsal incision, the joint is exposed and the margins of the bones freed from the capsule. All osteophytes are trimmed away and the dorsal 'corner' of the metatarsal head excised to allow 60 to 80° of passive dorsiflexion at the time of operation. Postoperatively, physiotherapy is arranged to maintain as much joint movement as possible.

The author has used this procedure in a small number of juvenile cases, which had proved resistent to conservative measure, with successful relief of symptoms. Enough bone must be excised from the dorsal lip of the metatarsal to permit passive extension; a mere sliver of damaged articular cartilage is not sufficient. Mann & Clanton recommended excision of 'the dorsal one-quarter to one-third of the metatarsal head'.

Mann & Clanton (1988) found that most improvement had occurred by three months, with 71% obtaining complete relief of symptoms, although some slow change for the better could occur up to 12 months.

Extension osteotomy of the proximal phalanx

Bonney & Macnab (1952), Kessel & Bonney (1958), Heaney (1970) and Moberg (1979) reported satisfactory results with this procedure. Citron & Neil (1987) reported universal early pain relief after the operation, with permanent relief in 50% at very long follow-up.

The operation takes advantage of the early preservation of plantar flexion in juvenile cases with painful limitation of extension (dorsiflexion). By excising a dorsally-based wedge from the proximal phalanx immediately distal to its basal epiphysis and bending the bone dorsally, the available range of motion is shifted from the flexed side to the extension extreme (Figure 39). Kessel & Bonney had nine cases out of ten pain-free after operation.

Arthroplasty

Several authors, especially Bonney & Macnab (1952), have expressed reservations about the results of the familiar Colley–Keller operation in hallux rigidus, and the commonest arthroplasty for hallux rigidus is now silicone elastomer replacement and generally this gives better results in hallux rigidus than in hallux valgus

In a small personal series the author found 80% of satisfactory cases after silicone elastomer replacement with either the Swanson finger prosthesis or the Helal ball-spacer, by the criteria of freedom from pain and from secondary metatarsalgia. However, in common with cases of hallux valgus, postoperative motion was disappointing, total range averaging 34°.

May et al (1991) reported on silicone elastomer ball replacement for hallux arthriticus (hallux rigidus or hallux valgus with degenerative joint changes) in 51 joints. They found 88% to be pleased and 68% totally pain free, but only 23% of the hallux rigidus patients had improvement

in their range of joint movement, and mobile joints in hallux valgus cases lost motion. Kampner (1984) reviewed a twelve year experience of silicone double-stemmed arthroplasties in 103 great toes and found results generally good, but better in osteoarthritis (hallux rigidus) than in rheumatoid arthritis.

Replacement arthroplasty is probably the operation of choice in women with hallux rigidus. In cases with bony ankylosis of the sesamometatarsal articulation, no attempt should be made to restore motion by excision and replacement, but arthrodesis should be advised.

Arthrodesis

The advantages and disadvantages of this procedure have been discussed on page 324. Many authors have recommended the operation for hallux rigidus (Thompson & McElvenny 1940, Smith 1952, Fitzgerald 1969, Marin 1960, Moynihan 1967).

Bonney & Macnab (1952) considered arthrodesis the operation of choice for the adult man with hallux rigidus, but without metatarsus primus elevatus. The author would agree with this view. Arthrodesis gives a durable result, a strong, weight-bearing first ray, freedom from secondary metatarsalgia and (at least in men who wear sturdy shoes which protect the interphalangeal joint) gives rise to few adverse sequelae.

As in all foot operations, technical precision is essential. The author favours the cutting of plane cancellous surfaces at the joint with a toe position determined by the system outlined on page 325 and with internal fixation with an oblique compression cortical screw. However, any method which secures bony fusion in optimum alignment will suffice and the procedure adopted is a matter of personal experience and preference.

References

Akin OF, 1925 The treatment of hallux valgus — a new operative procedure and its results. Med Sentinel 33: 678

Allan FG, 1940 Hallus vulgus and rigidus. Br Med J 579–581

Alsberg A, 1924 Zur Operationen des Hallux valgus. Zentrabl Chir 51: 2302–2303

Anderson EG, 1986 Hallux valgus: A rationale for treatment. J Bone Joint Surg (Br) 68: 844

Austin DW, Leventen EO, 1981 A new osteotomy for hallux valgus. Clin Orthop 157: 25–30

Baker LD, 1953 Diseases of the foot. Instruction Course Lecture X: Ch. XIV The Foot No. 1. 327–343

Barker AE, 1884 An Operation for hallux valgus. Lancet i 655

Barnard L, 1930 End results of bunion surgery. Ann Surg 91: 937

Bingold AC, Collins DH, 1950 Hallux rigidus. J Bone Joint Surg (Br) 32: 214–222

Blunden RE, 1968 Hallux valgus in the adolescent. J Bone Joint Surg (Br) 50: 677

Bonney G, Macnab I, 1952 Hallux valgus and hallux rigidus. J Bone Joint Surg (Br) 34: 366–385

Botteri G, Castellana A, 1961 L'osteodesi distale dei due primi metatarsi nella cura dell' alluce valgo. La Clin Ortop XIII: 39–46

Broca P, 1852 Des difformitiés de la partie antérieure du pied produite par l'action de la chaussure. Bull Soc Anat Paris, 27 année, 3e serie, Tome VII 60–67

Broughton NS, Doran A, Meggitt BF, 1987 Silastic ball spacer in the first metatarsophalangeal joint. J Bone Joint Surg (Br) 69: 678

Butson ARC, 1980 A modification of the Lapidus operation for hallux valgus. J Bone Joint Surg (Br) 62: 350–352

Butterworth RD, Clary BB, 1963 A bunion operation. Virginia Med Monthly 90: 11–14.

Carr CR, Boyd BM, 1968 Correctional osteotomy for metatarsus primus varus and hallux valgus. J Bone Joint Surg (Am) 50: 1353–1367.

Christie AJ, Weinberger KA, Dietrich M, 1977 Silicone lymphadenopathy and synovitis. JAMA 237: 1463–1464

Citron N, Neil M, 1987 Dorsal wedge osteotomy of the proximal phalanx for hallux rigidus. J Bone Joint Surg (Br) 69: 835–837

Cleveland M, Winant EM, 1950 An end result study of the Keller operation. J Bone Joint Surg (Am) 32: 163–175

Cleveland M, Willian LJ, Doran PC, 1944 Surgical treatment of hallux valgus in troops in training at Fort Jackson during the year of 1942. J Bone Joint Surg 26: 531–534

Cochrane WA, 1927 An operation for hallux rigidus. Br Med J i 1095–1096

Colloff B, Weitz EM, 1967 Proximal phalangeal osteotomy in hallux valgus. Clin Orthop 54: 105–113

Conlan D, Gregg PJ, 1991 The treatment of hallux valgus with overriding second toe. J Bone Joint Surg (Br) 73: 519–520

Corless JR, 1976 A modification of the Mitchell procedure. J Bone Joint Surg (Br) 58: 138

Creer WS, 1938a The feet of the industrial worker. Lancett ii 1480–1486.

Creer WS, 1938b Common foot ailments. Br Med J ii 5–9

Das De S, Hamblen DL, 1986 Problems of distal metatarsal osteotomy for hallux valgus in the middle-aged patient. J Bone Joint Surg (Br) 68: 667

Davies-Colley N, 1887 On contraction of the metatarsophalangeal joint of the great toe (hallux flexus). With cases. Clin Soc Trans XX: 165

Daw SW, 1935 An unusual type of hallux valgus (two cases). Br Med J ii 580

Dooley BJ, 1968 Osteotomy of the metatarsal neck for hallux valgus. J Bone Joint Surg (Br) 50: 677

Durman DC, 1957a Metatarsus primus varus and hallux valgus. Arch Surg 74: 128

Durman DC, 1957b Metatarsus primus varus and hallux valgus. J Bone Joint Surg (Am) 39: 221

Elmslie RC, 1926 The treatment of hallux valgus and hallux rigidus. Lancet ii 665–666

Engle ET, Morton DJ, 1931 Notes on foot disorders among natives of the Belgian Congo. J Bone Joint Surg 13: 311–318

Evans DK, 1957 The operative treatment of hallux valgus. A review of a 'radical' operation. Guy's Hosp Rep 106: 280

Fitzgerald JAW, 1969 A review of long-term results of arthrodesis of the first metatarsophalangeal joint. J Bone Joint Surg (Br) 51: 488–493

Fitzgerald W, 1950 Hallux valgus. J Bone Joint Surg (Br) 32: 139

Fowler GR, 1889 Partial resection of the head of the first metatarsal bone for hallux valgus. Med Record 36: 253–255

Galland WI, Jordan H, 1938 Hallux valgus, Surg Gynecol Obstet 66: 95–99

Galloway S, Majkowski RS 1992 Excision arthroplasty for hallux valgus in the elderly – A comparison between the Keller and Mayo operation. J Bone Joint Surg (Br) 74 (Suppl II): 143–144

Giannestras NJ, 1972 Modified Akin procedure for the correction of hallux valgus. Instr Course Lect XXI 254–261

Gibson MM, Corn D, Debevoise NT, Mess CF, 1972 Complications of Mitchell bunionplasties with modification of indications and technique. J Bone Joint Surg (Am) 54: 1564–1565

Gilmore GH, Bush LF, 1957 Hallux valgus. Surg Gynecol Obstet 104: 524

Girdlestone GR, Spooner HJ, 1937 A new operation for hallux valgus and hallux rigidus. J Bone Joint Surg 19: 30–35

Glynn MK, Dunlop JB, FitzPatrick D, 1980 The Mitchell distal metatarsal osteotomy for hallux valgus. J Bone Joint Surg (Br) 62: 188–191

Goddard NJ, Wilson DW, 1986 The avoidance of metatarsalgia as a complication of surgery for hallux valgus. Paper read at the Orthopaedic Section of the Royal Society of Medicine, London 1986.

Golden GN, 1961 Hallux valgus — The osteotomy operation. Br Med J: 1361–1365

Goodfellow J, 1966 Aetiology of hallux rigidus. Proc R Soc Med 59: 821–824

Gordon M, Bullough PG, 1982 Synovial and osseous inflammation of failed silicone–rubber prostheses. J Bone Joint Surg (Am) 64: 574–580

Gottschalk FAB, Sallis JG, Solomon L, Beighton PH, 1979 Comparison of the prevalence of hallux valgus in three South African populations. J Bone Joint Surg (Br) 61: 254–255

Gottschalk FAB, Sallis JG, Beighton PH, Solomon L, 1980 A comparison of the prevalence of hallux valgus in three South African populations. S Afr Med J 57: 355–357

Groiso JA 1992 Juvenile hallux valgus. J Bone Joint Surg (Am) 74: 1367–1374

Grundy M, Tosh PA, McLeish Rd, Smidt L, 1975 An investigation of the centres of pressure under the foot while walking. J Bone Joint Surg (Br) 57: 98–103

Haines RW, McDougall A, 1954 The anatomy of hallux valgus. J Bone Joint Surg (Br) 36: 272–293

Hamilton FH, 1873 Bunion and valgus of the great toe — resection. Med Record 8: 376–377

Hansen ST 1993 Reconstruction of the forefoot. J Bone Joint Surg (Br) 75 (Suppl I): 5

Hardy RH, Clapham JCR, 1951 Observations on hallux valgus. J Bone Joint Surg (Br) 33: 376–391

Hardy RH, Clapham JCR, 1952 Hallux valgus — predisposing anatomical causes. Lancet i 1180–1183

Harris RI, Beath T, 1949 The short first metatarsal. J Bone Joint Surg (Am) 31: 553–565

Hawkins FB, Mitchell CL, Hendrick DW, 1945 Correction of hallux valgus by metatarsal osteotomy. J Bone Joint Surg 27: 387–394

Heaney SH, 1970 Phalangeal osteotomy for hallux rigidus. J Bone Joint Surg (Br) 52: 799

Helal B, 1981 Surgery for adolescent hallux valgus. Clin Orthop 157: 50–63

Helal B, Chen SC, 1982 Arthroplastik des Großchengrundgelenks mit einer neuer Silastik-Endoprothese. Orthopädie 11: 200–206

Henry APJ, Waugh W, 1975 Use of footprints in assessing the results of operations for hallux valgus. J Bone Joint Surg (Br) 57: 478–481

Heuter C, 1871 Specielle Pathologie der Gelenkkrankheiten. Die Zehengelenke. In: Klinik der Gelenkkrankheiten 1 Ed. FCW Vogel, Leipzig pp 339–351

Hiss JM, 1931 Hallux valgus — Its cause and simplified treatment. Am J Surg 11: 51–57

Hoffman P, 1905 Conclusions drawn from a comparative study of the feet of barefooted and shoe-wearing peoples. Am J Orthop Surg 3: 105

Hohmann G, 1922/3 Über Hallux valgus und Spreizfuß, ihre Entstehung und physiologische Behandlung. Archiv für Orthopädische und Unfallchir 21: 525

Hohmann G, 1924 Zur Hallux valgus — Operationen. Zentrabl Chir 51: 230

Hohmann G, 1925 Der Hallux valgus und die übrigen Zehenverk rümmungen (Hallux valgus and the other bent toes). Ergebnisse der Chirurgie und Orthopädie 18: 308–376

Holden NT, 1954 The operative treatment of hallux valgus — a review of the Keller procedure. Guy's Hosp Rep 103: 274

Houghton GR, Dickson RA, 1979 Hallux valgus in the younger patient. The structural abnormality. J Bone Joint Surg (Br) 61: 176–177

Hughes J, Klenerman L, 1985 A study of the use of extra-depth footwear at Northwick Park Hospital. Paper read to the British Orthopaedic Foot Surgery Society

Hulbert KF, 1955 Compression clamp for arthrodesis of first meta-tarsophalangeal joint. Lancet i 597

Ivory JP, Gregg PJ 1993 A prospective trial of surgical treatment of the painful first metatarsophalangeal joint in the older patient. J Bone Joint Surg (Br) 75 (Suppl II): 135

Jack EA, 1939/40 The aetiology of hallux rigidus. J Bone Joint Surg 27: 492–497

James CS, 1939. Footprints and feet of natives of the Solomon Islands. Lancet ii 1390–1393

Johannson JE, Barrington TW, 1984 Cone arthrodesis of the first metatarsophalangeal joint. Foot Ankle 4: 244–248

Johnson KA, Cofield RH, Morrey BF, 1979 Chevron osteotomy for hallux valgus. Clin Orthop 142: 44–47

Joplin RJ, 1950 Sling procedure for correction of splay-foot, meta-tarsus primus varus and hallux valgus. J Bone Joint Surg (Am) 32: 779–785

Joplin RJ, 1964 Sling procedure for correction of splay-foot, meta-tarsus primus varus and hallux valgus. J Bone Joint Surg (Am) 46: 690–693

Kampner SL, 1984 Total joint prosthetic arthroplasty of the great toe – A 12 year experience. Foot Ankle 4: 249–261

Kato T, 1993 Treatment of hallux valgus in Japan. J Bone Joint Surg (Br) 75 (Suppl II): 135

Kato T, Watanabe S, 1981 The etiology of hallux valgus in Japan. Clin Orthop 157: 78–81

Keller WL, 1904 The surgical treatment of bunions and hallux valgus. NY Med and Philadelphia Med J 80: 741

Keller WL, 1912 Further observations on the surgical treatment of hallux valgus and bunions. New York Med J 95: 696

Kessel L, Bonney G, 1958 Hallux rigidus in the adolescent. J Bone Joint Surg (Br) 40: 668–673

Kilmartin TE, Barrington RL, Wallace WA, 1991 Metatarsus primus varus. A statistical study. J Bone Joint Surg (Br) 73: 937–940

Kingreen O, 1933 Zur Ätiologie des Hallux flexus. Zentrabl Chir 60: 2116–2118

Kinnard P, Gordon D, 1984 A comparison between Chevron and Mitchell osteotomies for hallux valgus. Foot Ankle 4: 241–243

Kreiblich DN, Porter BB, Epstein HP, 1992 Distal metatarsal osteotomy and Keller's arthroplasty: A comparison of the long-term results of two procedures for hallux valgus in patients over 55 years. J Bone Joint Surg (Br) 74: Suppl. II, p. 144

Krida, A, 1939 A new operation for metatarsalgia and splay-foot. Surg Gynecol Obstet 69: 106

Lahz JC, 1973 Metatarso-phalangeal arthrodesis for hallux valgus. J Bone Joint Surg (Br) 55: 220–221

Lambrinudi C, 1938 Metatarsus primus elevatus. Proc R Soc Med 31: 1273

Lane WA, 1886/7 The causation, pathology and physiology of several of the deformities which develop during young life. Guy's Hosp Rep 44: 241–333

Lapidus PW, 1940 'Dorsal bunion': Its mechanical and operative correction. J Bone Joint Surg 22: 627–637

Lemon RA, Engber WD, McBeath AA, 1984 A complication of silastic hemiarthroplasty in bunion surgery. Foot Ankle 4: 262–266

Leventen EO, 1975 Optical sound movie — 'Bunion surgery' J Bone Joint Surg (Am) 57: 138

Lindgren U, Turan I, 1983 A new operation for hallux valgus. Clin Orthop 175: 179–183

Lloyd EI, 1935 Prognosis of hallux valgus and hallux rigidus. Lancet ii 263

Logroscino D, 1948 Il trattamento chirurgico dell'alluce valgo. Chir Organi Mov 32: 81–96

Ludloff K, 1918 Die Beseitigung des Hallux valgus durch die schräge planta-dorsale Osteotomie des Metatarsus I (Erfahrungen und Erfolge). Archiv für klin Chir von Langenbeck 110: 364

McBride ED, 1928 A conservative operation for bunions. J Bone Joint Surg 10: 735–739

MacDonald D, 1973 Splaying of the first metatarsal space in common foot disorders. J Bone Joint Surg (Br) 55: 221

McKay DW, 1983 Dorsal bunions in children. J Bone Joint Surg (Am) 65: 975–980

McKeever DC, 1952 Arthrodesis of the first metatarsophalangeal joint for hallux valgus, hallux rigidus and metatarsus primus varus. J Bone Joint Surg (Am) 34: 129–134

McMaster MJ, 1978 The pathogenesis of hallux rigidus. J Bone Joint Surg (Br) 60: 82–87

Mann RA, 1982 Foot problems in adults. Part II Hallux valgus. Instr Course Lect XXXI 180–200

Mann RA, Clanton TO, 1988 Hallux rigidus: Treatment by cheil-ectomy. J Bone Joint Surg (Am) 70: 400–406

Mann RA, Rudicel S, Graves SC, 1992 Repair of hallux valgus with a distal soft tissue procedure and proximal metatarsus osteotomy. J Bone Joint Surg (Am) 74: 124–129

Marin GA, 1960 Arthrodesis of the first metatarsophalangeal joint for hallux valgus and hallux rigidus. Guy's Hosp Rep 109: 174

Matzen PF, 1983 Fragment fixierung bei hohmannscher Hallux-valgus Operationen. Zentrabl Chir 108: 425–427

Mauclaire, 1924 Ostéoplasties, arthroplasties et transplantations tendineuses combinée pour traiter l'hallux valgus. Rev D'Orthop 11: 305–313

May PC, Kurkup JR, Togantzi M, Granitzas N, 1991 Helal arthroplasty for hallux arthriticus. J Bone Joint Surg (Br) 73 (Suppl II): 174–175

Mayo CH, 1908 The surgical treatment of bunion. Am Surg XLVIII: 300

Meier PJ, Kenzora JE, 1985 The risks and benefits of distal first metatarsal osteotomies. Foot Ankle 6: 7–17

Merkel KD, Katoh Y, Johnson EW, Chao EYS, 1983 Mitchell osteotomy for hallux valgus: Long-term follow-up and gait analysis. Foot Ankle 3: 189–196

Mikhail IK, 1960 Bunion, hallux valgus and metatarsus primus varus. Surg Gynecol Obstet 111: 637–646

Miller JW, 1973 Distal first metatarsal displacement osteotomy — Its place in the scheme of bunion surgery. J Bone Joint Surg (Am) 55: 427

Miller JW, 1974 Distal first metatarsal displacement osteotomy. J Bone Joint Surg (Am) 56: 923–931

Miller JW, 1975 Acquired hallux varus: A preventable and correctable disorder. J Bone Joint Surg (Am) 57: 183–188

Mitchell CL, Fleming JL, Allen R, Glenny C, Sanford GA, 1958 Osteotomy-bunionectomy for hallux valgus. J Bone Joint Surg (Am) 40: 41–60

Moberg E, 1979 A simple operation for hallux rigidus. Clin Orthop 142: 55–56

Modes E, 1939 Zum Vorkommen echter Synovialgruben (Fossae nudatae) bei Meusch, Wiederkäuern und Pferd. Virchow's Arch Path Anat 303: 603

Monberg A, 1935 On the treatment of hallux rigidus. Acta Orthop Scand 6: 239–247

Mouchet A, 1992 Pathogénie et traitement des difformités du gros orteil. Rev d'Orthop 9: 583–637

Moynihan FJ, 1967 Arthrodesis of the metatarsophalangeal joint of the great toe. J Bone Joint Surg (Br) 49: 544–551

Mygind HB, 1952 Operations for hallux valgus. J Bone Joint Surg (Br) 34: 529

Mygind HB, 1953 Operativ Behandling af Hallux valgus, Ugeskrift for Laeger 115: 236

Mygind HB, 1954 Some views on the surgical treatment of hallux valgus. Acta Orthop Scand 23: 152

Nilsonne H, 1930 Hallux rigidus and its treatment. Acta Orthop Scand 1: 295–303

Noakes TD, 1981 The aetiology of hallux valgus. S Afr Med J 59: 362

Pagella P, Pierleoni GP, 1971 Hallux valgus and its correction. Lo Scalpello 1: 55–64

Pelet D, 1981 Osteotomy and fixation for hallux valgus. Clin Orthop 157: 42–46

Piggott H, 1960 The natural history of hallux valgus in adolescence and early adult life. J Bone Joint Surg (Br) 42: 749–760

Pring DJ, Coombes RRH, Klosok JK, 1985 Chevron or Wilson osteotomy: A comparison and follow-up. J Bone Joint Surg (Br) 67: 671–672

Raymakers R, Waugh W, 1971 The treatment of metatarsalgia with hallux valgus. J Bone Joint Surg (Br) 53: 684–687

Reverdin J, 1881 Sitzungsber d Genfer, Ges 4

Reverdin J, 1918 De la déviation en dehors du gros orteil (hallux valgus, vulg. 'oignon', 'bunions', 'Ballen') et de son traitment chirurgical. Int Med Congress 2: 408–412

Rix RR, 1968 Modified Mayo operation for hallux valgus and bunion — A comparison with Keller procedure. J Bone Joint Surg (Am) 50: 1368–1378

Rogers WA, Joplin RJ, 1947 Hallux valgus, weak foot and the Keller operation: An end result study. Surg Clin N Am 27: 1295

Schein AJ, 1940 The Keller operation — partial phalangectomy in hallux valgus and hallux rigidus. Surgery 7: 342

Scott G, Wilson DW, Bentley G, 1991 Roentgenographic assessment in hallux valgus. Clin Orthop 267: 143–147

Scranton PE, Rutkowski R, 1980 Anatomic variations in the first ray: Part I — Anatomic aspects related to bunion surgery. Clin Orthop 151: 244–255

Sethu A, D'Netto DC, Ramakrishna B, 1980 Swanson's silastic implants in great toes. J Bone Joint Surg (Br) 62: 83–85

Shepherd BD, Guitronich L, 1982 Correction of hallux valgus. Medical Journal of Australia 1: 131–133

Sherman KP, Douglas DL, Benson MKDA, 1984 Keller's arthroplasty: Is distraction useful? J Bone Joint Surg (Br) 66: 765–769

Shine IB, 1965 Incidence of hallux valgus in a partially shoe-wearing community. Br Med J i 1648–1650

Silver D, 1923 The operative treatment of hallux valgus. J Bone Joint Surg 5: 225

Sim-Fook L, Hodgson AR, 1958 A comparison of foot forms among the non-shoe and shoe-wearing Chinese population. J Bone Joint Surg (Am) 40: 1058

Simmonds FA, Menelaus MB, 1960 Hallux valgus in adolescents. J Bone Joint Surg (Br) 42: 761

Smith NR, 1952 Hallux valgus and rigidus treated by arthrodesis of the metatarsophalangeal joint. Br Med J ii 1385–1387

Soresi AL, 1931 The radical cure of hallux valgus (bunion). Subarticular resection of the head and metatarsal bone. Surg Gynecol Obstet 52: 776–777

Spinner SM, Lipsman S, Spector F, 1984 Radiographic criteria in the assessment of hallux abductus deformities. J Foot Surg 23: 25–30

Stamm TT, 1957 The surgical treatment of hallux valgus. Guy's Hosp Rep 106: 273

Stanley LL, Breck LW, 1935 Bunions. J Bone Joint Surg 17: 961

Stein HC, 1938 Hallux valgus. Surg Gynecol Obstet 66: 889–898

Stott JRR, Hutton WC, Stokes IAF, 1973 Forces under the foot. J Bone Joint Surg (Br) 55: 335–344

Swanson AB, 1972 Implant arthroplasty for the great toe. Clin Orthop 85: 75–81

Swanson AB, 1975 Silicone implant resection arthroplasty of the great toe. J Bone Joint Surg (Am) 57: 1173

Swanson AB, Lumsden RM, Swanson G de G, 1979 Silicone implant arthroplasty of the great toe. Clin Orthop 142: 30–43

Syms P, 1897 Bunion: Its aetiology, anatomy and operative treatment. New York Med J LXVI: 448–451

Theander G, Danielsson LG, 1982 Ossification anomaly associated with interphalangeal hallux valgus. Acta Radiol Diagnosis 23: 301–304

Thompson FM, Mann RA, 1986 Surgery of the Foot. Ed. RA Mann. CV Mosby Co, 5th edn. pp 163–165

Thompson FR, McElvenny RT, 1940 Arthrodesis of the first metatarsophalangeal joint. J Bone Joint Surg 22: 555–558

Thomson SA, 1960 Hallux valgus and metatarsus varus. Clin Orthop 16: 109–118

Tibrewall SB, Foss MVL 1991 Is day surgery of Wilson's osteotomy safe? J Bone Joint Surg (Br) 73: 340

Trethowan WH, 1923 In: CC Choyce (ed) A System of Surgery. Cassel & Co Vol. III pp 1046–1049

Trimmings NP, Wilson DW, 1988 The behaviour of the collateral structures of the hallux. J Bone Joint Surg (Br) 70: 855

Truslow W, 1925 Metatarsus primus varus or hallux valgus. J Bone Joint Surg 7: 98

Turnbull T, Grange W, 1986 A comparison of Keller's arthroplasty and distal metatarsal osteotomy in the treatment of adult hallux valgus. J Bone Joint Surg (Br) 68: 132–137

Turner JM, Todd WF, 1984 A permanent internal fixation technique for the Austin osteotomy. J Foot Surg 23: 199–202

Venning P, Hardy RH, 1951 Sources of error in the production and measurement of standard radiographs of the foot. Br J Radiol 24: 18–26

Vlatis G, Anderson EG, 1990 The Swanson double stem silastic arthroplasty for hallux valgus and hallux rigidus. J Bone Joint Surg (Br) 72: 530

Volkmann R, 1856 Ueber die sogenannte Exostose der grossen Zehe. Virchow's Arch Path Anat Physiol Klin Med 10: 297–306

Wenger RJJ, Whalley RC, 1978 Total replacement of the first metatarsophalangeal joint. J Bone Joint Surg (Br) 60: 88–92

Wilhelm R, 1934 Ein einfaches Operationsverfahren bei Hallux valgus. Zentralbl Chir 61: 2424–2425

Wilson CL, 1958 A method of fusion of the metatarsophalangeal joint of the great toe. J Bone Joint Surg (Am) 40: 384–385

Wilson DW, 1980 Treatment of hallux valgus and bunions. Br J Hosp Med 24: 548–559

Wilson JN, 1963 Oblique displacement osteotomy for hallux valgus. J Bone Joint Surg (Br) 45: 552

Winner A, 1945 Social medicine in women's services. Lancet ii 371–372

Worsing RA, Engber WD, Lange TA, 1982 Reactive synovitis from particulate silastic. J Bone Joint Surg (Am) 64: 581–585

V.4 The Lesser Rays

David L Grace

The lesser toes

There persists in some countries a cavalier attitude towards the loss of toes and the use of amputation as a quick method of resolving the problem of deformed and painful digits. Removal of all the toes (Pobble operation, after Edward Lear's poem about 'the Pobble' who had no toes) has been recommended in the past for multiple toe deformities such as occur in rheumatoid disease (Fig. 1). Major defunctioning operations such as proximal phalangectomy achieve the same biomechanical effect, and are akin to 'amputating the toe but leaving it behind'. This attitude to toes has arisen because they are often thought to exercise little or no function in humans, with a consequent failure to appreciate their role in foot biomechanics.

Unfortunately, studies of the non-weight-bearing foot have caused confusion in the past. When the foot is on the ground, the muscles acting on the toes do not move them, but plant them firmly to establish a base from which their owner can be propelled forwards. Their function is leverage, hence they also raise the metatarsal arch.

It used to be thought that toes were rather like fingers. Although some individuals can exercise marvellous control over their toes, being able to fan them out actively and, in some cases, to undertake skilful activities such as oil painting, their true function is to press against the ground (Lambrinudi 1932). The flexors do not flex but simply press the pulps down whilst the intrinsic muscles also do this by flexing the proximal phalanges. The extensors provide the pull that moves the body forward. In this, Ellis (1894) was well supported by Jones (1949) who said, 'To liken the action of the muscles of the foot to that of the hand is to abandon all hope of understanding the ordinary mechanics of standing and walking.'

Hence, defunctioning a toe by amputation, phalangectomy or diaphysectomy is generally bad practice. Such procedures can be made cosmetically acceptable by syndactyly to maintain toe length, but this nevertheless upsets the mechanics of the forefoot. The bad outcome of these procedures may take time to develop and we are now seeing forefoot problems produced by thoughtless procedures carried out a decade or more ago.

These so called 'minor' foot operations have previously been considered simple and straightforward. As such, they have often been relegated to the end of operating lists in some countries to be performed by inexperienced and unsupervised surgeons, and this has resulted in an unacceptably high percentage of unsatisfactory results. This yields a correspondingly high incidence of medical negligence claims (Glyn Thomas 1991). The truth is that many of these procedures are far from simple and the small size of the toes makes surgery difficult and fiddlesome, so that great precision is required to achieve the desired result.

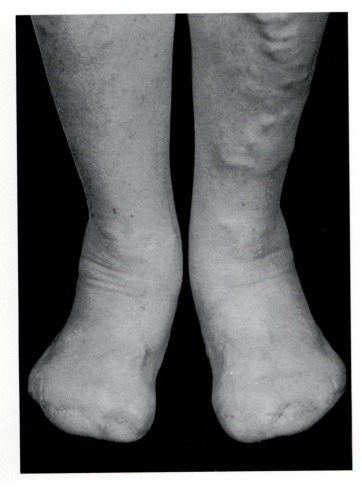

Figure 1

Amputation of all five toes (Pobble operation) for the treatment of severe multiple painful toe deformities in rheumatoid arthritis. This is seldom undertaken these days

Range of movements

Typical passive ranges of movements in the joints of the adult second toe are as follows:

Table 1 Differences between hammer and claw toes		
	Claw	*Hammer*
Extension deformity at MTPJ	Usually more severe	Less severe
PIPJ Position	Flexed	Flexed
DIPJ Position	Flexed	Extended
Neurological cause	Common	Rare
Hereditary predisposition	Common	Rare
Toes affected	Any toe	Usually second and third
Co-existent claw foot	Frequent	Rare

Metatarsophalangeal joint (MTPJ) dorsiflexion 90°, plantarflexion 70°.
Proximal interphalangeal joint (PIPJ) dorsiflexion 0°, plantarflexion 80°.
Distal interphalangeal joint (DIPJ) dorsiflexion 10°, plantarflexion 40°.

Lesser toe deformities

The common toe deformities are depicted in Fig. 2. The differences between hammer and claw toes are further explained in Table 1.

Aetiology

Idiopathic
This is by far the biggest group. Footwear is frequently to blame. Hammer toes, most commonly present in the second and third toes, may be due to a hereditary predisposition, but the commonest cause is the prolonged wearing of ill-fitting shoes. These may be too narrow or too short. If too narrow, the toes become crowded and the hallux usually underrides the second toe, which pops up, especially if it is too long already (Fig. 3). Similarly, if the shoe is too short or if it is a slip-on style with no constraint at the ankle, the foot is free to piston up and down within the shoe, with the result that an overlong second toe may buckle into flexion at the proximal interphalangeal joint and become hyperextended at the distal joint.

Congenital causes
There are numerous skeletal variations of the toes (Pfitzner 1896). The fifth toe frequently has only two phalanges, with the middle and distal phalanges being

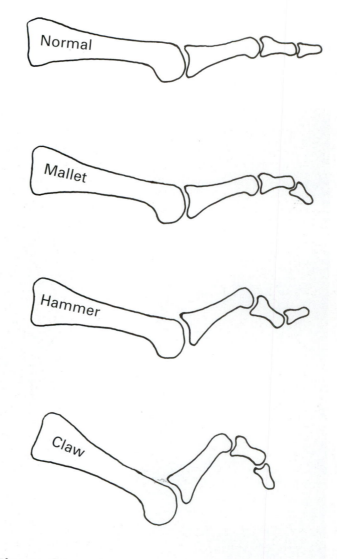

Figure 2

The common lesser toe deformities

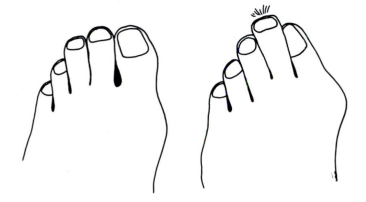

Figure 3

(Left) Normal foot showing an even curve of the tips of the toes. (Right) Uneven arc due to long second toe, hallux valgus or both. Painful rubbing may occur at the tip

fused together. This is encountered more frequently in females and occasionally also occurs in the third and fourth toes. The middle phalanx often lacks an epiphysis. Some individuals possess fourth and fifth toes that are rather more clawed than usual, and these are really normal variants unless they become painful. Very often the little toe is also excessively supinated or in varus (or both) so that it comes to lie more underneath the fourth toe, but again this can really only be considered abnormal if pain and callosities are present. In general the wearing of tight shoes will accentuate these minor deformities.

The classification of more major congenital disorders comes under the following seven headings:

1. Failure of formation of parts.
2. Failure of differentiation of parts.
3. Duplication.
4. Undergrowth.
5. Overgrowth.
6. Constriction bands.
7. Generalized skeletal abnormalities.

Toes may be totally or partially absent and an example of this is the lobster claw foot. These conditions are dealt with in Chapter IV.2.

Neurological causes

Toe clawing may occur in a wide variety of neuromuscular disorders, such as myelodysplasia, cerebral palsy, head or spinal cord injuries, poliomyelitis, stroke, Friedreich's ataxia, Charcot–Marie–Tooth disease and its variants, and multiple sclerosis. Loss of intrinsic tone or activity may occur from any one of these or indeed from other causes. The extrinsic tendons pull the toe into a clawed position. A full neurological and muscle investigation is carried out as a routine in cases of severe toe clawing or if there is an associated pes cavus.

Arthritic causes

Systemic arthropathy such as rheumatoid arthritis can lead to hammer and claw deformities in the toes, owing to joint destruction and soft tissue imbalance. Post-traumatic synovitis, sometimes unrecalled by the patient or following only trivial trauma, may lead to subluxation and sometimes frank dislocation at the second MTPJ, resulting in a painful hammer toe.

Iatrogenic causes

Surgical procedures that shorten the first ray, especially when the second toe is already overlong, can produce longitudinal pressure on the tip of the second toe, particularly if the shoe is too short. Operations on any of the lesser toes may result in an adjacent operated or unoperated toe being left too long or too dorsally-displaced relative to its neighbours. This may subsequently lead to pressure problems usually at the tip or the PIPJ (Fig. 4).

Fractures

Toe deformities may follow fractures of the phalanges or metatarsals. More proximal injuries such as os calcis fractures or fractures of the tibial shaft can produce claw toes secondary to plantar muscle scarring from increased compartmental pressures (Mittlmeier et al 1991). Claw toes may also follow tibial fractures, either because of tethering of the long toe flexors in the calf or because of intrinsic muscle imbalance.

Clinical features

Lesser toes subjected to decades of pressure from a succession of tight toeboxes inevitably become deformed and stiff. Deformed toes *per se* are not necessarily painful. Very often, they find their own 'niche' and become faceted like gallstones or teeth. This moulding phenomenon can also include the nail plates as well (Fig. 5). If a toe becomes protruberant, either through being too long or too dorsiflexed, it may become painful, owing to rubbing or shear forces from the shoe. Soft corns may develop over adjacent bony prominences between the toes (usually the condyles of the interphalangeal joints). The commonest points of pressure occur over the dorsal aspect of the PIP joints, at the tips of the toes and under the metatarsal heads. Painful hyperkeratoses develop at these pressure points and in severe deformities there is dorsal subluxation or dislocation at the MTPJ, producing dorsal discomfort here as well.

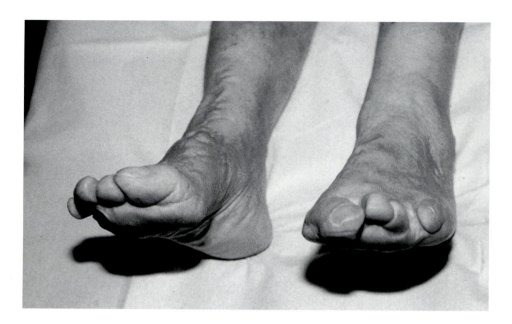

Figure 4

This elderly female patient had no fewer than 14 operations on the toes of both feet. Small differences in toe length and shape after each procedure resulted in transfer lesions, which took an average of two years to become painful. Note the different toe lengths, and absent digits

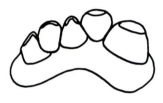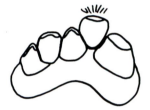

Figure 5

(Left) Prolonged wearing of ill-fitting shoes causes 'facets' of the toes (and nails). (Right) Dorsal displacement of the second toe causes pain over the PIPJ

Treatment

Nonoperative treatment

This is appropriate for minor deformities that are not producing much discomfort. For elderly patients who are unfit for surgery, regular chiropody is the best bet. Patients are advised to wear spacious hosiery, and to wear flat shoes that are fully lace-up and that have a wide toebox. There is virtually no deformity that cannot be accommodated either in a shoe modified by an orthotist or in a surgical shoe made from a last. A single cocked-up toe can be 'housed' by localized stretching of the leather upper, or by fitting a balloon patch in which the toe can comfortably fit. Dorsal corns can be protected by corn plasters or foam sleeves. Soft corns between the toes can be managed conservatively by keeping the toes apart using small silastic foam spacers, which can be individually moulded to the affected toe cleft. Plantar callosities can be partially off-loaded by the appropriate positioning of an anterior metatarsal pad, which may need special shaping if more than one metatarsal head is to be protected. The correct positioning of such a device needs to be extremely accurate. The shoe may need extra depth in the forefoot in order to accommodate any inserts (Cracchiolo 1982).

Operative treatment

This is reserved for patients in whom conservative management has failed or who have significant deformities. The main indication for surgery is pain. Informed consent is of paramount importance because of the relatively high incidence of medical negligence claims following toe surgery (Glyn Thomas 1991).

It is not so important to discuss precise details of surgical technique with the patient beforehand, but it is important to discuss the limitations of surgery and the possible complications, together with a general appraisal of the potential risks and benefits of the procedure and the likely recovery period. The success rate is often best expressed in betting terms such as, for example, a 'nine out of ten chance of success'. Patients also need to be warned that it is possible to be worse off after surgery. The commoner complications of recurrent deformity, delayed wound healing, prolonged swelling, infection and reflex sympathetic dystrophy require specific mention. It is important for the patient to have a realistic expectation of what surgery can achieve.

Hammer and claw toes

The choice of surgical procedure will depend on the degree of passive correctability of the PIPJ and MTPJ. In children or in mild mobile claw toes, flexor-to-extensor tendon transfer (Taylor 1951) with or without soft tissue release of the PIPJ will suffice.

Through a mid-lateral incision on the lateral side of the toe, the flexor digitorum longus tendon is identified within its sheath close to its insertion. It is then freed from its sheath as far back as the proximal third of the proximal phalanx. It is then brought dorsally across the centre of the proximal phalanx and there firmly sutured to the extensor tendon with enough tension to hold the toe straight. Before the incision is closed it is important to check that the deformity has been fully corrected, and if the position of the toe is not entirely satisfactory, bony surgery will be required. Plaster of Paris or Collodion splintage is unnecessary. When the PIPJ deformity is fixed, as it usually is in adults, either an arthrodesis or an excision arthroplasty are favoured (Fig. 6).

Arthrodesis

Through a transverse elliptical skin incision over the PIPJ, the articular surfaces are exposed and the articular cartilage is removed with a fine bone cutter or nibbler (or alternatively using powered burrs). A smooth Kirschner wire is passed distally through the base of the middle phalanx to emerge centrally at the apex of the toe and is then driven back proximally to enter the proximal phalanx. This is greatly facilitated by using a powered wiredriver, and the stoutest K wire compatible with the size of the bone should always be used. An alternative is to employ two parallel K wires to control rotation. The PIPJ should be transfixed in a small degree of flexion and the K wire (or wires) should not transgress the MTPJ. The protruding tip of the K wire is bent over to a right angle in order to prevent migration into the toe, and it is padded with a piece of tape to prevent it snagging on hosiery and bedclothes, etc. The wire remains *in situ* for 6 weeks, at which time fibrous union or bony fusion will have taken place. Once the immediate postoperative swelling has abated, the patient can be ambulant in an open toed shoe or sandal.

Excision arthroplasty

This is a simpler alternative to arthrodesis, and relies upon the formation of a stable pseudarthrosis. The distal one-third of the proximal phalanx is excised. This shortens the toe and allows the redundant proximal part of the extensor tendon to be coiled up within the joint as an interposition arthroplasty (see Fig. 6). By suturing the extensor tendon quite tightly, flexion deformity at the PIPJ is corrected. If the MTPJ is still dorsiflexed, it can be released by a more proximal extensor tenotomy, combined with dorsal capsulotomy and lateral collateral ligament release if necessary. If a claw toe has significant fixed flexion deformities at both proximal and distal interphalangeal joints, then both of these can be fused using the K wire technique (Lambrinudi 1927).

Table 2 lists the options available, depending upon the degree of deformity and fixation. These options illustrate the author's preferred procedures, which generally involve correction of the PIPJ first and the MTPJ second.

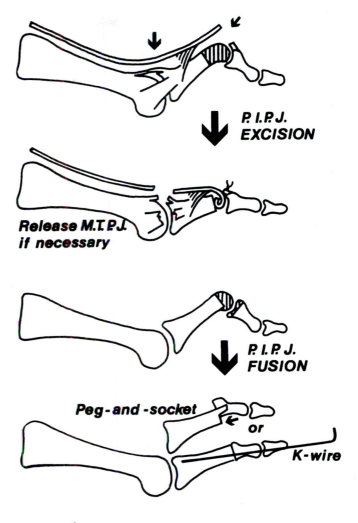

Figure 6

Common methods of hammer toe or claw toe correction by fusing or excising the PIPJ and releasing the MTPJ if necessary

Myerson & Shereff (1989), however, have proposed a sequence for the soft tissue correction of hammer and claw toes beginning with the dorsal soft tissues at MTPJ level, followed by tenotomy of extensor digitorum longus and brevis, dorsal capsulotomy and collateral ligament release at the MTPJ, and, i

f necessary, division of the plantar portion of the collateral ligaments. If the deformity remains uncorrected, then one or both interossei are divided, followed by excision of the distal one-third of the proximal phalanx. They recommend that in mild claw toes a simple soft tissue release of the PIPJ is all that is necessary without dividing flexor digitorum longus.

Whatever procedure is undertaken, the tips of all the toes should form a smooth curve to prevent a single overlong toe from being subjected to further pressure. This sometimes means operating on a painless toe in order to shorten it. Just as orthodontists and dental

Table 2 Options available for the surgical correction of hammer/claw toes (author's preferred procedures)

Deformity	Recommended procedure
1. PIPJ – mild, mobile MTPJ – normal	Flexor to extensor tendon transfer a. Single toe b. Multiple toes
2. PIPJ – fixed MTPJ – mild, mobile	Fusion or excision PIPJ plus percutaneous extensor tenotomy at MTPJ
3. PIPJ – fixed MTPJ – fixed (subluxed)	Fusion or excision PIPJ plus open extensor tenotomy, dorsal capsulotomy and collateral ligament release of MTPJ
4. PIPJ – fixed, severe MTPJ – fixed, severe (dislocated)	Either: 1. Fusion or excision PIPJ plus double-stemmed silastic implant at MTPJ *Advantage:* Toe length and function preserved *Disadvantage:* Technically difficult with greater risk of complications or: 2. Excision proximal half of proximal phalanx *Advantage:* Quick and simple *Disadvantage:* Toe often remains short and 'cocked up'

surgeons aim for a uniform array of teeth, so should foot surgeons achieve the same goal with the toes.

A common difficulty arises when the preoperative assessment reveals that a second hammer toe is underridden by a valgus big toe with the foot loaded. It may be clear that there is no space in which to correct the second toe. In elderly patients, the simplest solution is to amputate the second toe through the MTPJ but in younger patients, hallux valgus surgery will be necessary to create enough space for the second toe. This requires careful consideration if the hallux valgus is painless.

Revision surgery
About one in 10 patients will have significant residual deformities following surgery to claw or hammer toes. The toe usually remains dorsiflexed at the MTPJ and requires further release here. Sometimes, a double stemmed silastic implant in the MTPJ is needed to help maintain position, and occasionally surgical syndactyly to an adjacent toe is necessary. Revision surgery is often complicated by prolonged swelling of the toe, especially if transverse incisions have been used, and the patient should be warned that the toe may look like a 'little chipolata' for some months.

Mallet toe
This can be treated by simply dividing the flexor tendon over the middle phalanx, or if the joint is stiff in flexion, by either K wire fusion or excision arthroplasty by excis-

ing the distal one third of the middle phalanx and repairing the extensor tendon as described for hammer toes.

Soft corns
These can usually be managed conservatively but, if this fails, a weight bearing anteroposterior radiograph both within and without a shoe should demonstrate which bony prominences are in contact, although this is usually clinically obvious. The joint condyles can be trimmed by nibblers or by small rotating burrs.

Metatarsalgia

Definitions

This is generally taken to mean pain across the forefoot in the region of the metatarsal heads. It is not a diagnosis in itself, and has many causes. Careful clinical evaluation coupled with special investigations and a knowledge of relevant anatomy and biomechanics can elucidate the cause of the problem. This can then be specifically treated as indicated by the severity of the symptoms, the patient's demands and the natural history of the condition.

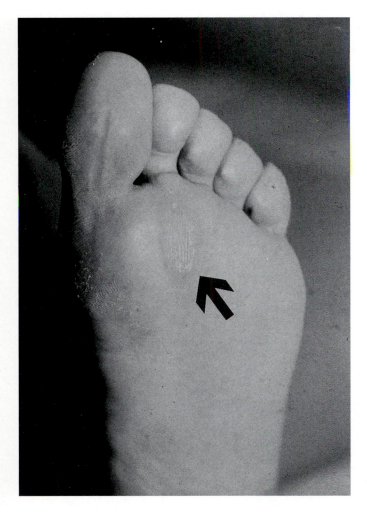

Figure 7
Plantar keratosis (callosity) under the second metatarsal head, indicative of excessive loading or shear forces

Anatomy and biomechanics

The five tarsometatarsal joints each allow a variable amount of dorsiflexion and plantarflexion during loading and unloading of the foot. This is dependent upon the shapes of their articular surfaces and on the elasticity of the soft tissue constraints. Each metatarsal is therefore 'independently sprung' to a variable degree, in order to allow each metatarsal head close contact with uneven ground. The second metatarsal is the least mobile in this respect, its base being recessed into the shallow mortice formed between the three cuneiforms. The fifth metatarsal has the maximum springing. Excessive splaying of the forefoot during loading is prevented by the firm attachments of the plantar intermetatarsal ligaments, which act as tie beams between the plantar plates of the MTP joints.

Both of the above mechanisms serve to dampen down impact loads during stance phase, which exceed body weight at either side of mid stance. These forces are greatly increased during running. Hence large forces are supported on the ball of the foot just after heel lift. The fibrofatty pads situated directly beneath each metatarsal head between the skin and flexor tendon sheath are highly adapted to absorbing impact loads. Their complex structure consists of large fat globules contained within 'cells' whose walls are composed of fibrous tissue containing abundant elastic-rich collagen. These cells are firmly attached superficially to the skin and deeply to the flexor sheaths and plantar plates. These pads are therefore extremely efficient at absorbing compression loads and dealing with shear forces. This effect has been likened to a tank track, since the metatarsal heads rotate within the envelope of skin and fibrofatty pads, whilst the skin surface remains stationary relative to the ground, owing to frictional forces.

Healthy tissues are capable of withstanding this degree of trauma but in elderly patients or those with abnormal foot shape, these shearing forces are increased. Excessive or repeated microtrauma causes hyperkeratosis of the skin in areas of greatest force concentration. Distal migration of the fat pad will cause loss of mobility of the metatarsal heads and increase frictional forces between the skin and the ground, resulting in painful callosities (Fig. 7). Each lesser metatarsal head and great toe sesamoid bears approximately one-sixth of the body weight, but there is a wide variation of normal in the weight bearing distribution between the metatarsal heads when standing on tiptoe.

Clinical evaluation

The history should include a detailed account of the precise location of pain plus any radiation into the toes or proximally up the foot and leg. Exacerbating and relieving factors and the effects of different footwear or inserts should be noted. Previous operations, occupation and recreational activities are also important. Medical clues as to the cause of the symptoms, such as the presence of systemic disease in rheumatoid arthritis, collagen disease or diabetes mellitus should be sought.

The clinical examination should include attention paid to the spine and lower limbs. The neurological status and peripheral circulation should be assessed in addition to the specific examination of the foot itself. Clinical analysis of gait and inspection of footwear are recommended.

Special investigations
Useful serological screening tests may include haemoglobin and full blood count, ESR, serum proteins, and electrophoretic strip, calcium, phosphate, alkaline phosphatase, uric acid, rheumatoid factor, and serologi-

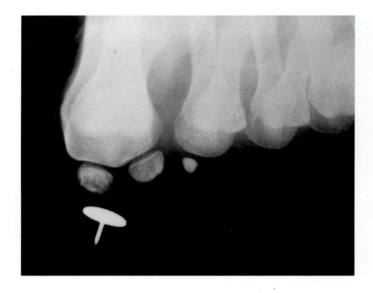

Figure 8

Skyline view of the metatarsal heads and sesamoid bones which are well shown in profile. This view may demonstrate the cause of plantar foot pain, and in this example, a metal marker has been taped to the skin at the point of pain

cal tests for *Treponema pallidum*, glucose, ASO, and antistaphylococcal titres.

The radiological investigations should include the standing anteroposterior and lateral X-rays. From these, congenital anomalies (tarsal coalition, short metatarsals), metabolic conditions (osteomalacia, hyperparathyroidism), erosions, and details of previous bony surgery as well as soft tissue anomalies may be apparent. Measurements of the intermetatarsal angle and the degree of hallux valgus can be made. The angle of inclination of the metatarsal bones with the horizontal can also be measured. A skyline radiograph of the metatarsal heads is also a useful investigation for forefoot pain (Fig. 8). Undue plantar prominence of individual lesser metatarsal heads may thus be demonstrated. The ankle and subtalar joints as well as the spine may also need to be X-rayed.

Technetium 99 bone scanning may demonstrate a stress fracture, osteomyelitis and some bone tumours. This is a nonspecific test, and it is positive in any condition that results in increased blood flow. A diffuse increase in uptake of the tracer may occur in reflex sympathetic dystrophy.

Pedobarography
This is dealt with in detail elsewhere (Chapter III.4). It can be a useful investigation if the cause of pain is unclear. It is especially useful in confirming the common type of 'idiopathic' metatarsalgia that is due to simple dropping of the metatarsal heads in the middle-aged and elderly. 'Hot spots' occur under those metatarsal heads

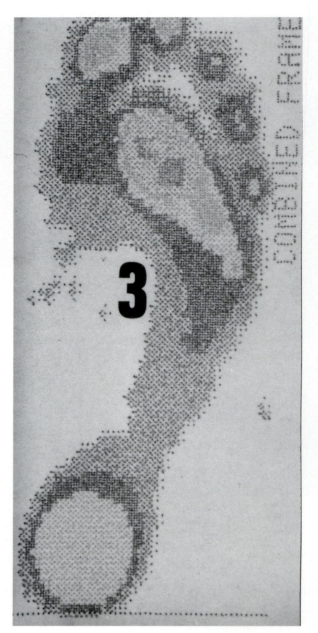

Figure 9

Glass plate dynamic pedobarograph gives a colour recording of pressure loading under the foot. A computer print-out can give precise values for these pressures under individual metatarsal heads

bearing the most pressure. The modern dynamic glass plate pedobarograph can yield very useful information in this way (Duckworth et al 1982) (Fig. 9), but there is still a place for the cruder grey-scale imprint recordings such as the Shutrak (Fig. 10).

Other investigations
Doppler or colour Doppler examinations and arteriography may be required to exclude vascular causes of pain. Nerve conduction studies may be indicated to exclude either posterior tibial nerve entrapment (tarsal tunnel syndrome)

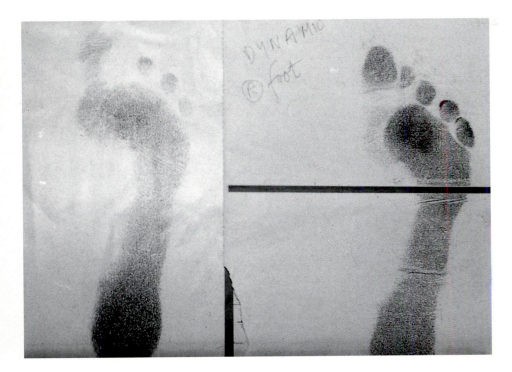

Figure 10

Shutrak, a more modern equivalent of the Harris and Beath ink mat, is quick and easy to use, providing a grey-scale reproduction for both static or dynamic footprints

or anterior tibial nerve entrapment. Magnetic resonance imaging (MRI) scans are valuable in detecting soft tissue tumours, tendon pathologies, and bone marrow abnormalities. Computed tomography (CT) scanning may demonstrate degenerative changes in joints, and ultra sound scans can be used to demonstrate Morton's neuromata.

Precise injection of small quantities of local anaesthetic may be injected into specific anatomical areas to help localize the source of pain in the forefoot. This can be a useful diagnostic procedure if one is stuck for a diagnosis.

Classification

Metatarsalgia may be classified into three types: primary, secondary, and a third category where symptoms are unrelated to disorders of weight distribution.

Primary metatarsalgia

In this group are found those patients with pain across the MTP articulations, with reactive plantar keratoses caused by chronic imbalance in weight distribution between the toes and the metatarsal heads, between individual metatarsal heads, and between the forefoot and hind foot. This can be either functional or structural, and in the latter instance may be iatrogenic following surgery to the foot.

Functional primary metatarsalgia

The human foot was never intended to walk on hard surfaces in tight, ill-fitting shoes. Without external constraints, the pulps of all the toes would be in contact with the ground during the push off phase of gait. The intrinsic muscles stabilize predominantly the proximal interphalangeal joints. In a constricting shoe, the toes can never flex properly at the MTP joints and the intrinsics fail, thus allowing splaying of the foot and curling of the toes. Adaptive shortening of the intrinsics occurs, and because their line of action is dorsal to the transverse axis of movement at the MTP joints, they act as extensors and perpetuate the deformity. Any weakness, whether congenital or acquired, will lead to this situation.

The brunt of the weight bearing forces lands on the central metatarsal heads. A tight toebox not only compresses the toes together, leading to moulding phenomena, but also causes the central metatarsal heads to become more prominent in the sole, producing transverse convexity in the forefoot. (This is the opposite to the normal situation in which the metatarsal heads form a transverse concave arch.)

Lack of shoe support at the ankle causes the foot to piston up and down inside the shoe, causing excessive shear forces under the now-prominent metatarsal heads. This is compounded by attenuation and atrophy of the fibrofatty pads which occurs with increasing age. Obesity and lack of padding within the insole of many slip-on fashion shoes and high-heeled shoes further aggravates the condition, leading to an irreversible sequence of events.

Table 3 Structural causes of primary metatarsalgia
Overload and insufficiency syndromes Long first metatarsal Short first metatarsal Metatarsus primus varus Length discrepancy between metatarsals Pes cavus Toe abnormalities

Table 4 Causes of secondary metatarsalgia
Rheumatoid arthritis Sesamoiditis Post traumatic Stress fractures Gout Short ipsilateral lower limb Freiberg's disease

Structural primary metatarsalgia

There is a spectrum of normal and anatomical variance which can sometimes become pathological entities. These are outlined in Table 3. Congenital anomalies, such as relative shortness of the first metatarsal (Morton's syndrome) (Morton 1935), or other length discrepancy between metatarsals may give rise to problems. Quantitative measurements in individual patients have only served to emphasize the difficulty in distinguishing mild cases from normal.

Viladot (1984) described three basic foot patterns, each exhibiting specific differences of comparative metatarsal length. Most of the population falls into one of these patterns:

1. Greek: 2 > 3 > 1 > 4 > 5
2. Egyptian: 1 > 2 > 3 > 4 > 5
3. Square: 1 = 2 = 3 = 4 > 5

He claimed that the Greek pattern of foot is the anatomical pattern most likely to predispose to metatarsalgia because of the relatively long second metatarsal.

Although the relationship between subtle variations in metatarsal anatomy and the development of metatarsalgia is often unclear, it is well accepted that surgical procedures can predispose to metatarsalgia or can aggravate pre-existing metatarsalgia. Virtually any operation on the first ray for hallux valgus can do this, especially those that defunction the great toe, such as excision arthroplasty of the first MTPJ. Elevation of the first metatarsal head by osteotomy of the metatarsal is well known as causing abnormal loading problems in the forefoot. Lesser metatarsal osteotomies performed on a single ray can offload stresses to their neighbours. Excision of a single lesser metatarsal head will overload both its neighbours.

Patients with pes cavus, especially if severe, fixed and related to an underlying neurological cause, will often develop anterior pressure metatarsalgia, partly because of defunctioning of the toes, but mostly because of the steeper angle of inclination with which the metatarsals strike the ground.

Secondary metatarsalgia

These patients have callosities, intra-articular pain and increased pressure under the metatarsal heads on force plate analysis. However, the cause is from factors other than the metatarsals (Table 4).

Rheumatoid disease
This has been dealt with elsewhere (Chapter VI.3). In most patients, minor surgery is likely to fail and those coming to surgery will require excision of the metatarsal heads in a smooth curve (Kates et al 1967). Some success has been reported with telescoping metatarsal osteotomy (Helal & Greiss 1984).

Sesamoid disease
Again this is dealt with elsewhere (Chapter V.5). The causes of sesamoid pathology are outlined in Table 5.

Post-traumatic malunion of metatarsal fractures
Any malunited fracture may disturb the pattern of forefoot loading in the long term, although it is surprising that one does not see long-term problems developing as often as one would expect.

Stress fractures
Otherwise known as march fractures, the topic has been fully described by Devas (1975). Usually, the middle or distal diaphysis of the second or third metatarsal shaft is involved. Although classically described in army recruits subjected to long walks with a heavy backpack, it is more likely to be seen in civilian practice. It is as likely to occur in the middle-aged individual as in a young person who has recently embarked upon a training programme or road running. Swelling and tenderness occur over the affected metatarsal and radiographs become positive after the first 2 or 3 weeks by showing a blob of callus, or a radiolucent line across the bone. It is simply treated by limiting physical activities and wearing soft-soled shoes such as trainers until the pain abates.

Rarely, a stress fracture affects the base of the first metatarsal, and it can occur in the proximal shaft of the fifth metatarsal in patients with pes varus from a neurological cause.

Table 5 Sesamoid pathologies
Subluxation
Dislocation
Fractures (various)
Chondromalacia
Osteoarthritis and other arthritides
Osteomyelitis
Presesamoid bursitis
Tumour

Table 6 The different types of nonoperative treatment available for metatarsalgia

1. Shoe modifications
   Rocker bottom sole
   Anterior heel
2. Insoles
   Metatarsal pad
   Metatarsal bar
   Medial arch support
   Moulded orthosis (heat-moulded Plastazote)
3. New footwear
   Moulded Plastazote (space shoes)
   Surgical shoes (custom)
   Surgical shoes (off the shelf)
   Modern trainers
4. Silicone oil injections

Gout

During acute attacks rest, elevation and nonsteroidal anti-inflammatory drugs should be prescribed. If serum uric acid is elevated, allopurinol should be given long term.

Short limb

Habitual plantar flexion of the ankle to compensate for lower limb shortening can lead to pain and thickening of the skin under the metatarsal heads.

Metatarsalgia unrelated to disorders of weight distribution

Spine

This may arise from L5 or S1 root pathology. A history of back pain, and clinical findings of restricted straight leg raising with signs of nerve root tension and positive motor and sensory signs or an absent or diminished ankle jerk should suggest the correct diagnosis.

Tarsal tunnel syndrome

This is an entrapment neuropathy of the posterior tibial nerve as it passes beneath the lanciate ligament behind the medial malleolus. The patient complains of burning pain and paraesthesiae in the sole of the foot, which is often worse in bed at night. Tinel's test may be positive, and the diagnosis can be confirmed with EMG studies. The condition is treated by surgical release of the nerve.

Vascular insufficiency

In severe cases this may present with pain in the forefoot at rest. In the early stages of arteriosclerosis, pain may be felt in the arch of the foot after exercise, and it may be relieved by rest. The absence of peripheral pulses and a low Doppler pressure at the ankle will confirm the diagnosis. Hitherto unsuspected diabetic feet may have plantar ulcers and may demonstrate bone and joint abnormalities on the radiograph.

Treatment of metatarsalgia

It is worthwhile pursuing conservative management in the majority of patients, since the results of surgery in this condition are often unpredictable and disappointing. The treatment should be tailored to meet the needs of the individual patient, since an athlete who runs 50 miles a week will have different requirements and expectations compared to someone with severe rheumatoid disease who is confined to the house.

Modification of existing shoes may work in some cases but insoles fashioned for each patient generally meet with more success. These arch supports or anterior metatarsal pads need to be positioned and shaped appropriately, and patience is needed by the patient and orthotist since its success is often based on trial and error. A shoe with extra depth is required to accommodate these insoles. It is pointless to expect an insole to be effective in a high heel or slip-on shoe. In this respect, education of the patient is an important part of the treatment. Patients need to be told to purchase flat lace-up court shoes, or alternatively a modern trainer for maximum comfort. They also need to be told where they can purchase suitable shoes locally, and which retailers are best for specific shoe types. In the author's experience, trainers, or court shoes with metatarsal pads fitted into them have proved the most satisfactory. For severe pain and callosities, an insole manufactured from thermoplastic material is heat-moulded to the patient's foot. Table 6 summarizes all these options.

In more recalcitrant cases, injection of up to 2 ml of sterile silicone oil between the plantar callosity and the metatarsal head can be performed under local anaesthesia. The silicone fluid is quite viscous (200 centistoke viscosity) and requires heating to 200°C for 2 hours to

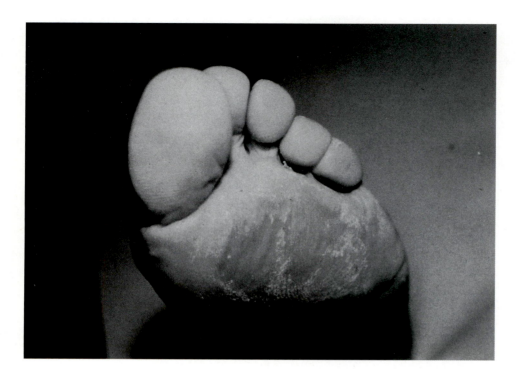

Figure 11

Thickening of the plantar skin in the middle of the tread with pain under the middle three metatarsal heads. This is sometimes an indication for osteotomy of the central three metatarsals

completely sterilize it. This provides an internal 'shock absorber' (Balkin 1975). This is particularly effective when there has been no previous surgery in the forefoot. The procedure is controversial and not very commonly employed; however, there have been no adverse systemic sequelae after follow-up of several hundred cases over many years, although the blob of silicone oil thus implanted has sometimes been found to migrate dorsally into the intermetatarsal spaces over a period of time. Infection and sinus formation appears not to be a problem. Balkin & Kaplan (1991) recommend repeated injections on several visits using small quantities of the oil.

Operative treatment

As stated earlier, this is best avoided at all costs unless the patient has persistent pain despite wearing sensible shoes over a period of time and having regular chiropody and insoles.

Surgical correction of hammer and claw toes will reduce the downward pressure of the proximal phalanx on the metatarsal head causing the metatarsalgia pain to improve. Bony procedures for persistent symptoms are usually necessary for rigid and fixed deformities. If there are painful callosities under the metatarsal heads (Fig. 11), some type of metatarsal osteotomy may be indicated.

Over the last 70 years there have been many procedures devised for relieving excessive localized metatarsal pressure. A critical review has been compiled by Greiss in 1981. These lesser metatarsal osteotomies to shorten or elevate the metatarsal may produce over- or under-correction, and this is the chief reason for their failure. It is difficult to estimate and quantify the precise amount of change in position that is necessary, and then to

achieve this precisely at surgery. Figure 12 shows the more commonly used operations, although modifications do exist. Thomas (1974) advocated basal closing wedge osteotomy of the lesser metatarsals. In theory the osteotomy could be secured by sutures, K wires, or screw or staple fixation.

An oblique, sliding distal lesser metatarsal osteotomy of the middle three metatarsals was described by Helal in 1975. The long-term follow-up of 508 feet in 310 patients showed a success rate of almost 90% after a mean follow-up of 4.3 years (Helal & Greiss 1984). The correct selection of patients, better choice of osteotomy site, adequate freeing of the metatarsal head from the plantar soft tissues, and the middle three metatarsal osteotomies being performed together are all important factors. Despite paying close attention to these recommendations, other studies have failed to achieve such a high success rate, and in a series of 124 feet followed up for 3.5 years, Winson et al (1989) reported less than 50% satisfactory results.

Closing dorsal wedge osteotomy through the neck of the metatarsal without internal fixation was described by Leventen & Pearson (1990). They reported that the procedure was simple to perform, was largely free of complications, and had a good success rate, but again stressed that the procedure should normally be done on more than one metatarsal. Dreeben et al (1989) reported complete relief of pain in 67% of 45 feet in which the second metatarsal was osteotomized in a similar fashion, with a greenstick fracture being made through the narrowest part of the neck, followed by immediate weight bearing without internal fixation.

Giannestras's (1973) stepcut diaphyseal shortening appears to be a rather complex and potentially compli-

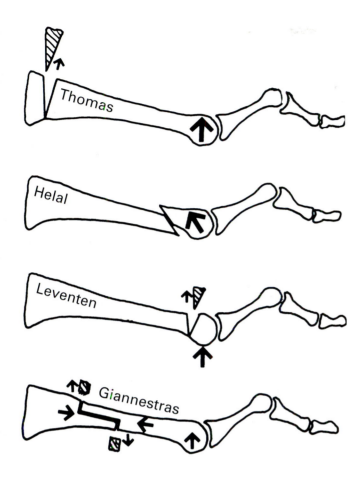

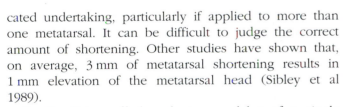

Figure 12

Different methods of treating metatarsalgia

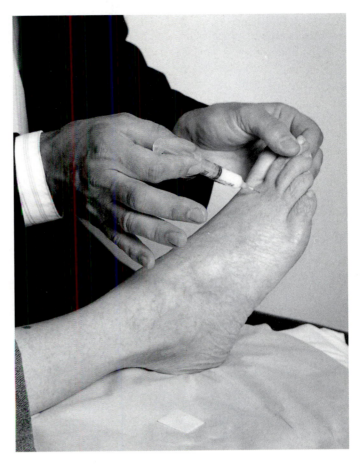

Figure 13

Diagnostic–therapeutic injection of local anaesthetic and hydrocortisone into the second MTPJ

cated undertaking, particularly if applied to more than one metatarsal. It can be difficult to judge the correct amount of shortening. Other studies have shown that, on average, 3 mm of metatarsal shortening results in 1 mm elevation of the metatarsal head (Sibley et al 1989).

Simply slicing off the plantar condyles of a single prominent metatarsal head, using a plantar incision, may have merit. However, whole-head removal of a single metatarsal is a poor choice as it leads to increasing loads on the remaining metatarsal heads. As stated earlier, when multiple, and combined with plantar fat pad repositioning (e.g. forefoot arthroplasty for rheumatoid disease), it is successful (Kates et al 1967). Some claw feet with metatarsalgia can be successfully treated by hindfoot surgery, such as plantar fascia release, mid-tarsal wedge osteotomies, calcaneal osteotomies or even triple arthrodesis.

Other causes of metatarsalgia

Traumatic synovitis of second MTPJ

This is a distinct entity that seems to affect both men and women of middle age, who present with pain in the region of the second MTPJ, usually without a history of antecedent trauma. Plantar plate injuries (usually degenerative tears) can lead to subluxation of the joint. In the early stages, clinical examination reveals a little tenderness and swelling with painful restriction of motion of the second MTPJ. At this stage, the radiographs are normal. If a little local anaesthetic is injected into the joint (Fig. 13) and pain is relieved, the diagnosis can be suspected. Cortisone can then be instilled.

The condition may progress to frank dislocation at the second MTPJ. This can take place rapidly over a period of months. If the condition is recognized early, before dislocation has occurred, an open synovectomy may be performed. Alternatively, the flexor digitorum longus tendon can be split longitudinally and wrapped around either side of the proximal phalanx and sutured into the extensor tendon, thus forming a 'loop' around the toe. This may serve to prevent future dislocation. Once dislocation has occurred, the base of the proximal phalanx can be excised, or a double stemmed silastic implant inserted.

Flexor synovitis
Patients complain of pain in a single metatarsophalangeal joint with tenderness just distal to this, the pain being under the proximal half of the proximal phalanx. It may be treated by cortisone injection.

Fibrofatty pad damage
This can become attenuated due to the effects of ageing, or sometimes following injury or injection of hydrocortisone, which can cause shrivelling of the tissues. It is best treated by a protective metatarsal pad or padded hosiery.

Morton's neuroma

This is an extremely common cause of forefoot pain and should be considered in all patients whose pain radiates into the toes, especially the third or fourth.

Early history

This is a unique disorder: it has no counterpart in the hand. The first account was given by Thomas G Morton of Philadelphia in 1876, whose patients described vivid accounts of their acute symptoms. In 1940, L O Betts of Adelaide confirmed that the source of pain was swelling of the interdigital nerve. Effective treatment was provided by excision of the lesion.

Pathogenesis

Ischaemia
This theory postulates that the intermetatarsophalangeal bursa balloons out distally with each step, and as a result, it stretches the communicating artery applied to its distal wall, thus exerting a traction effect on the main digital artery travelling adjacent to the interdigital nerve. This leads to ischaemic effects on the neural tissue. This theory is supported by the histological findings of resected specimens (Nissan 1948, Meachim & Abberton 1971).

Tethering of interdigital nerve
Betts (1940) knew that the nerve to the three–four cleft is usually formed by union of two branches that appear in the sole on either side of flexor digitorum brevis. He considered that contraction of the muscle caused the combined nerve to be stretched around the distal margin of the deep transverse ligament during toe extension.

It seems likely that a combination of peripheral entrapment, tethering, ischaemia and repetitive trauma combine to produce the lesion.

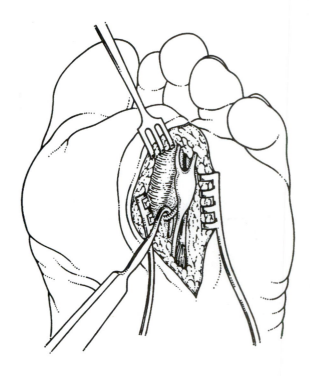

Figure 14

A typical fusiform lesion in the left 3/4 interspace has been widely exposed through an incision along the tread and through the thick protective fat body (Bojsen-Moller 1979) (reproduced by permission of Rob & Smith 1957)

Macroscopic & microscopic findings

In a classical case, the neurovascular bundle is fusiform and symmetrical in shape (Fig. 14). Bundles vary in size from 3 mm to more than 10 mm in diameter. Exceptionally large nodules are due to a great excess of loose-textured epineural fibrous tissue over a firm core. When the neuralgic pain has been concentrated in the fourth toe, marked asymmetry of a lesion in the three–four space is found. The neuroma itself is almost invariably adherent to the intermetatarsophalangeal bursa, and the digital artery is also firmly attached to the mass. Histological sections generally show three characteristic features (Bullough & Vigorita 1984)

1. End-arterial thickening of the digital artery with occasional thrombosis and occlusion of its lumen.
2. Extensive fibrosis both around and within the nerve, giving rise to demyelination and a marked depletion of axons within the digital nerve.
3. Evidence of Schwann cell and fibroblast proliferation.

Location
Three quarters of the lesions are found in the three–four

space and the remainder in the two–three space. Occasionally, two separate lesions are found in the same foot. Some patients have lesions in both feet, although a long interval, sometimes 30 years or more, may separate the onset of symptoms in each foot. A lesion in the four–five space is a rarity because of the small size of the interphalangeal component of the bursa or the large web space (Bossley & Cairney 1980). A genuine lesion probably never develops in the one–two space, where the entire bursa may be absent.

Clinical features

The patient is more often female than male, the ratio being about 5 to 1. The age of onset varies between 10 and 70 years, though the commonest ages of onset are between 20 and 50 years.

History
Many referrals to outpatients have been delayed by several years, owing to failure to make an early diagnosis. The intensity of pain varies greatly. Some patients use quite graphic descriptions which may suggest gross exaggeration to a sceptical clinician. Patients usually have two types of pain. The first is severe and acute, with sudden onset and radiation into the toes. It is usually precipitated by sudden direct pressure when the neuroma sustains a direct hit or is compressed. This pain usually lasts for 5–10 minutes, and for the next 2–3 hours the patient often complains of a dull ache. Pain occasionally disturbs sleep.

The usual location of the pain is in the middle of the tread, radiating into the third and fourth toes (Fig. 15). Pain in all three middle toes suggests a double lesion. Referred pain may extend proximally towards the knee. One fairly classical feature of the history is that pain is usually worse in tight or constrictive shoes, and patients often have no pain at all when walking bare foot or in soft slippers. The pain often brings the patient to a halt and forces her to sit down, remove the shoe, manipulate the forefoot and wait for relief. This sequence may be repeated several times during the day. There does not appear to be a single explanation for the variable timing of the pain, and as Klenerman et al (1983) suggested, abnormal impulses originating in small sprouting regenerating fibres may be implicated.

Clinical examination
When the patient is standing barefoot, the appearances are strikingly normal, with no spreading of the forefoot and no dorsal bulging of the intermetatarsophalangeal bursae. Almost invariably, however, the patient has localized tenderness on direct palpation with the tip of the index finger in the appropriate intermetatarsal space. This

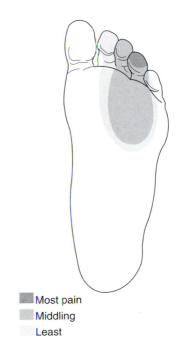

■ Most pain
■ Middling
□ Least

Figure 15
Location of pain with Morton's neuroma

is only present on the plantar aspect of the foot. With the index finger and thumb on the dorsal and plantar aspect of the relevant intermetatarsal space, the forefoot is compressed with the opposite hand by squeezing the metatarsal heads together. Larger neuromata can be felt at this point and can be 'balotted' in and out between the metatarsal heads. All but the smallest of neuromata produce a click at this point, often referred to as Mulder's click (Mulder 1951). This is almost pathognomonic of a neuroma. When adjacent normal intermetatarsal spaces are palpated in the same way, no click can be elicited. Approximately half of the patients will show signs of altered sensation in the adjacent halves of the affected toe cleft when tested with a pin prick.

Special investigations
Sensory nerve conduction tests are of limited value (Klenerman et al 1983) and X-rays of the foot are invariably normal. Rheumatoid factor may be worth checking. More recently, scanning methods, including ultrasound (Fig. 16) and MRI, have provided clinicians with more concrete evidence of the presence and location of neuromata where previously one had to rely purely on the clinical features.

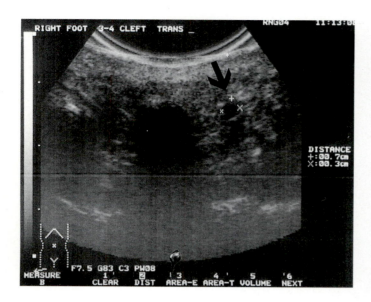

Figure 16

Ultrasound scan of the three–four intermetatarsal space shows spherical area of reduced signal (Morton's neuroma arrowed)

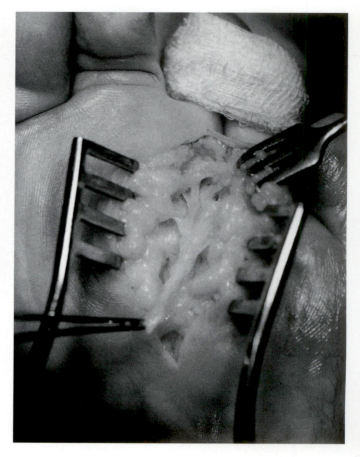

Figure 17

Resection of a Morton's neuroma through the plantar approach. The interdigital nerve has been divided at least 2 cm proximal to the lesion and is held with forceps prior to dissection distally

Treatment

There is no place for conservative management since the symptoms will persist and become worse in time as the neuroma enlarges. The best surgical procedure is resection of the lesion, and this is simple to undertake. In Great Britain the plantar approach described by Betts (1940) is more popular whereas in North America the dorsal approach advocated by McElvenny (1943) is preferred. A third approach directly in the web space itself has also been described. The operation is most easily done under general anaesthesia with a pneumatic tourniquet applied around the thigh following exsanguination of the limb. An alternative is to perform a local anaesthetic block at the level of the ankle together with an ankle tourniquet.

The plantar approach

The patient lies supine and the surgeon sits at the end of the operating table. An assistant grasps a gauze swab that has been applied as a loop around the third and fourth toes. The foot is held dorsiflexed and still. A longitudinal skin incision is then made in the affected cleft directly between the metatarsal heads so as to avoid the scar overlying bony prominences. The incision needs to be at least 5 cm in length. It is pointless making too short an incision because at least 2 cm of normal nerve trunk proximal to the lesion itself must be resected. Skin edges are held apart by a self-retaining retractor with sharp jaws to stretch the subcutaneous fibrofatty tissue. Transverse strands of fibrous plantar tissue require division with a scalpel or scissors, and when this has been accomplished, the neuroma should be evident between the metatarsal heads adherent to the inter-metatarsophalangeal bursa (Fig. 17). The mass is then pulled distally with forceps so that the nerve trunk can be divided as far proximally as possible with a pair of curved scissors. All of the distal branches are then dissected free and divided. The tourniquet is released and bleeding points are secured by diathermy. The subcutaneous tissue is left unsutured, with closure of the skin over a small suction drain. A firm wool and crepe bandage is applied, with strapping applied firmly between the relevant toes. The excised specimen is sent for histological examination.

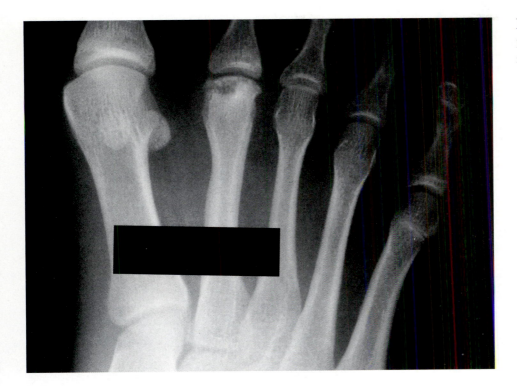

Figure 18

Freiberg's disease of second metatarsal head

The dorsal approach

This is more difficult than the plantar approach, and healing of the skin is not so good because it is so thin and poorly supported by the loose subcutaneous tissues. Nonetheless, it can be quite useful for exploring adjacent clefts if a double lesion is suspected as it avoids excessive dissection on the plantar surface of the foot. Gentle dissection between the metatarsal shafts is facilitated by using a separator such as a laminar spreader. The interosseus muscle and tendon is identified, and deep to this the transverse plantar intermetatarsal ligament has to be divided before the neuroma can be visualized. It is then resected in the same manner as described above. Division of the deep transverse ligament appears to be harmless. Indeed some authorities have suggested that simple division of this ligament combined with a neurolysis of the interdigital nerve and dissection of it free from the bursa may be all that is required to cure the condition.

Complications of surgery

Apart from wound healing problems and infection, the chief complication is recurrence of a stump neuroma at the distal end of the resected nerve. This can take several years to appear and it occurs in approximately 1 in 10 cases. Symptoms are similar to those at initial presentation, and maximum tenderness is usually found at the proximal end of the scar. On re-exploration, there may be either a discrete bulbous stump neuroma, or a series of fine nerve filaments up to 3 cm in length which have grown from the end of the nerve and have become embedded in scar tissue adherent to the skin. Following further resection, a second recurrence is most unusual. If it occurs, burial of the stump in bone solves the problem.

Other miscellaneous forefoot conditions

Freiberg's disease

Freiberg (1914) described six cases where the second metatarsal head appeared crushed. He described this process as an 'infraction'. The dictionary definition of an infraction is a violation, a break (of a law or an agreement, etc) or an infringement. This hardly seems a suitable medical term to describe a pathological process and it is of interest that this term has never been applied to similar pathologies at other anatomical sites. It is debated whether the condition is due to arterial insufficiency or trauma (Braddock 1959), but ischaemic necrosis of the metatarsal head is the most likely cause.

It most commonly affects the second metatarsal head but occasionally it affects the third. It is sometimes bilateral (Kohler 1923). Smillie (1957) described five stages in the evolution of the condition (Table 7). Basically, the metatarsal head becomes softened; this starts dorsally in the subchondral bone. Subsequent bony collapse occurs.

Table 7 The stages of Freiberg's disease
1. Fissure fracture 2. Bone absorption 3. Further absorption with sinking of central portion 4. Loose body separation 5. Flattening, deformity and arthrosis of the second metatarsophalangeal joint

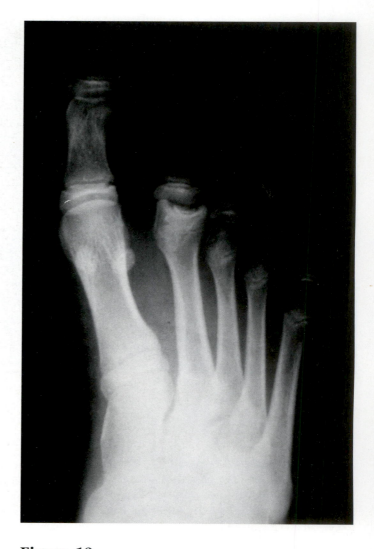

Figure 19

Advanced Freiberg's disease, showing expansion of the metatarsal head with a separated osteochondral fragment lying within a sizeable dorsal crater

Chondrolysis and dorsal cratering with expansion and flattening of the metatarsal head with secondary degenerative changes may occur rapidly.

The condition affects athletic adolescents, usually between the ages of 15 and 18. The pain begins insidiously so that at the time of presentation the disease is often well advanced. The sufferer complains of pain in the forefoot, and clinical examination shows swelling and tenderness over the affected MTPJ. Typical radiographic appearances are shown in Figs 18, 19. In some cases that present very early, there are no radiographic changes apparent and a diagnosis can then only be made by Technetium 99 bone scan or MRI scan.

Treatment

Sometimes the symptoms are so mild that it scarcely seems to justify surgery. A variety of procedures have been described, including bone grafting, removal of a loose body and trimming of the metatarsal head, osteotomy, excision of the metatarsal head, and silastic implantation. It is doubtful whether a bone graft, even if undertaken early in the course of the disease, can restore the blood supply across the epiphyseal plate. There may be some value in exploring the joint and excising inflamed synovium, trimming irregular joint margins and removing any loose bodies and loose flaps of articular cartilage.

An alternative to this is a dorsal closing wedge osteotomy through the neck of the metatarsal with K wire (Kanse & Chen 1989) or suture fixation (Figs 20, 21). This has the advantage that it can be undertaken at any stage of the disease (Kinnard & Lirette 1989) and is technically simple. It is effective for the following reasons:

1. It displaces the eroded cartilage from contact with the base of the proximal phalanx.
2. The fractional shortening that occurs reduces transarticular pressure across the joint.
3. Plantar pressure on the joint is reduced by dorsiflexing the metatarsal head, thus partially defunctioning the toe.

The condition can also be treated by shortening the metatarsal bone with internal fixation using a small T

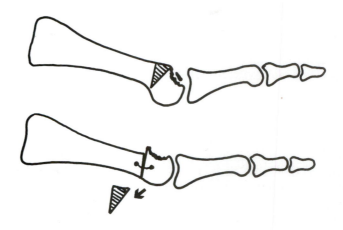

Figure 20

Dorsiflexion osteotomy of the metatarsal neck in the treatment of Freiberg's disease

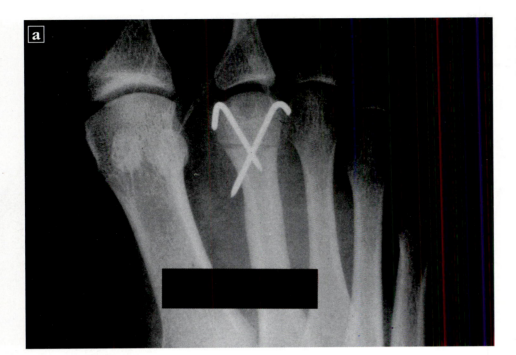

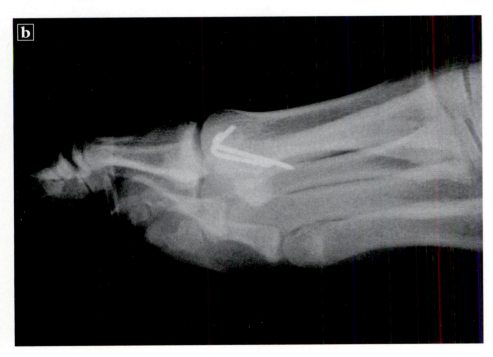

Figure 21

Postoperative X-ray demonstrating crossed K wire fixation of the osteotomy for Freiberg's disease

plate (Smith et al 1991).

In the very late stages of the condition, silastic replacement using a double-stemmed medical-grade high-performance silicone elastomer, such as the Swanson type, is preferable to simply excising the metatarsal head. This is because transfer metatarsalgia is less likely, and some toe function is preserved. The implant is simple to insert. About two-thirds of the metatarsal head together with its plantar condyles are resected with a micro-oscillating saw, and a thin shaving is also taken off the base of the proximal phalanx. The intramedullary canals are entered using a small bone awl, and these are enlarged using powered burrs until the holes are of sufficient size and shape to admit the rectangular shaped stems.

Bunionette

Since Davies (1949) first described the condition associated with prominence of the fifth metatarsal head and called it a tailor's bunion, opinions have differed as to its cause. Davies described a primary deformity with an increased fifth intermetatarsal angle caused by imperfect development of the transverse metatarsal ligament.

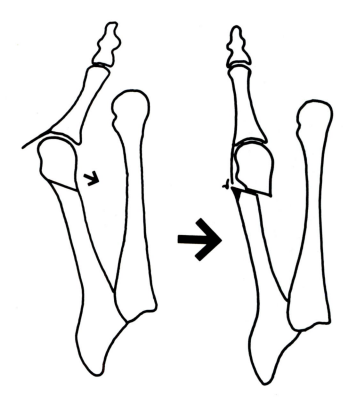

Figure 22

Distal, oblique sliding fifth metatarsal osteotomy with reattachment of the lateral capsule in the treatment of bunionette

However, the condition may also result from congenital widening of the fifth metatarsal head, from enlargement secondary to trauma or degenerative disease, or from acquired angulation of the metatarsal neck. It is almost invariably associated with hallux valgus and splay feet. There may be pain, caused by pressure from footwear, and despite conservative treatment, some patients may require operative intervention.

A variety of operations have been devised. These include simple exostectomy, fibular condylectomy, and fifth metatarsal head excision. Numerous osteotomies of the metatarsal neck or shaft have also been described. Theoretically, any of the commonly performed metatarsal osteotomies for correcting hallux valgus can be performed in 'reverse' or 'mirror image' to effect a cure. The osteotomy can be performed at the base of the metatarsal or in the distal shaft or neck. A current popular technique is an oblique sliding distal shaft osteotomy, which was described by Sponsel (1976); recent reports (Garlick & Chen 1993, Hansson 1989) have recommended it as a good procedure (Fig. 22). Distal neck osteotomy stabilized by manufacturing a 'peg and socket' has also recently shown an 86% success rate (Steinke & Boll 1989).

Congenitally adducted fifth toe

This common condition is present at birth. There are usually no associated deformities and it is often bilateral. Many adult patients who are seen to have this condition are never really bothered much by it. Nonetheless, it seems reasonable to offer surgical treatment but this can be delayed until the child is at least 5 or 6 years old. Again, a plethora of operative procedures have been recommended ranging from simple V–Y lengthening of the skin and extensor tenotomy to the most radical, namely amputation. McFarland (1950) and Kelikian et al (1961) advise excision of the proximal phalanx with syndactilization to the fourth toe. The Ruiz Mora procedure (Ruiz Mora 1954) involves excising an oval piece of skin on the plantar side of the proximal phalanx together with removal of the proximal phalanx. Lapidus (1942) described an extensor tendon transfer.

The Butler procedure described by Cockin (1968) is the author's preferred method. A circumferential 'racquet' incision around the base of the toe with a plantar extension to the incision ('racquet handle') is made. Extensor tenotomy and dorsal capsulotomy then brings the toe down into its corrected position within the racquet handle. The dorsal skin defect is sutured under tension such that the toe remains corrected without the need for a K wire or external splintage. This gives consistent results, although care must be taken to avoid damage to the neurovascular bundles. Gangrene of the toe is a rare but calamitous complication. Figure 23 shows an overlapped fifth toe before and after surgical correction.

Intermetatarsophalangeal bursitis

A remarkable degree of thickening of the walls of an intermetatarsophalangeal bursa may develop for no obvious reason. Sometimes this forms a soft swelling on the dorsum of the foot between the extensor tendons, and it can even cause the affected metatarsal heads and toes to spread apart on standing. The symptoms are similar to those of Morton's metatarsalgia, and the treatment is by excision of the bursa, with neurectomy when required.

Rheumatoid involvement of these bursae may be an early sign of the disease, with bursal distension due to effusion and synovitis causing separation of adjacent toes ('daylight sign').

Varus or valgus deformities

These are sometimes seen in association with valgus of the great toe or in rheumatoid disease of the foot. Soft tissue release at the metatarsophalangeal joint does not seem to be effective. They are best corrected by closing wedge osteotomies through the base of the proximal phalanx with K wire fixation.

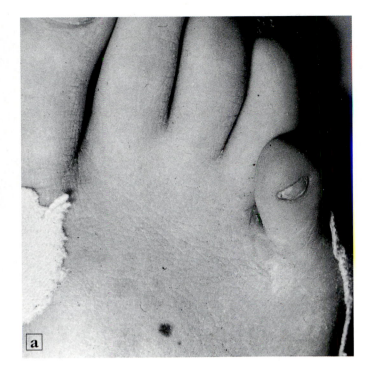

Figure 23
Overlapped little toe (a) before and (b) after correction

Trigger toes

These usually occur in the flexor apparatus of the great toe at sesamoid level and have been described mainly in ballet dancers. Decompression by division of the intersesamoid ligament and opening of the flexor sheath will effect a cure.

Nail deformities

These are dealt with in Chapter XI.1. If persistent, then usually partial or complete ablation of the nail growth is necessary, either by surgical excision of part or the whole of the base of the nail bed, or with phenolization, or both.

Curly toes

These have a varus–supination component as well as being clawed. In children, the vast majority can be left alone, and they usually improve with growth. If not, or if deformity is significant, they have traditionally been treated by flexor to extensor tendon transfer (Taylor 1951). However, a recent study demonstrated superior results after closing wedge osteotomy of the middle phalanx with axial K wire fixation (Zafiropoulos & Henry 1994).

References

Balkin S W 1975 Treatment of corns by injectable silicone. Arch Dermatol III. 1143–1145

Balkin S W, Kaplan L 1991 Injectable silicone and the diabetic foot: a 25 year report. Foot 2: 83–88

Betts L O 1940 Morton's metatarsalgia, neuritis of fourth digital nerve. Med J Aust I: 514–515

Bojsen-Moller G 1979 Anatomy of the forefoot, normal and pathologic. Clin Orthop 142: 10–18

Bossley C J, Cairney P C 1980 The intermetatarso-phalangeal bursa – its significance in Morton's metatarsalgia. J Bone Joint Surg 62B: 184–187

Braddock G T F 1959 Experimental epiphyseal injury and Freiberg's disease. J Bone Joint Surg 41: 154

Bullough P G, Vigorita V 1984 Miscellaneous orthopaedic conditions. In: Atlas of Orthopaedic Pathology. Gower Medical Publishing New York, London, pp 14.6–14.7

Cockin J 1968 Butler's operation for an overriding fifth toe. J Bone Joint Surg 50B: 78

Cracchiolo A 1982 Office practice: footwear and orthotic therapy.

Foot Ankle 2: 242–248

Davies H 1949 Metatarsus quintus valgus BMJ 1: 664–665

Devas M 1975 Stress Fractures. Churchill Livingstone, Edinburgh, pp 29–33

Dreeben S M, Noble P C, Hammerman S, Bishop J O, Tullos HS 1989 Metatarsal osteotomy for primary metatarsalgia: radiographic and pedobarographic study. Foot Ankle 9: 214–218

Duckworth T, Betts R P, Franks C I, Burke J 1982 The measurement of pressures under the foot. Foot Ankle 3: 130–141

Ellis T S 1894 The physiology of the foot. Lancet 1: 1113–1115

Freiberg A H 1914 Infraction of the second metatarsal bone. A typical injury. Surg Gynecol Obstet 49: 191–193

Garlick N I, Chen S C 1993 Correction of bunionette deformity by oblique fifth metatarsal osteotomy. Foot 3: 194–196

Giannestras N J 1973 Foot Disorders: Medical and Surgical Management. Lea and Febiger, Philadelphia, 2nd edn

Glyn Thomas T 1991 Medical litigation and the foot. Foot 1: 3–5

Greiss M E 1981 Pressure metatarsalgia and metatarsal osteotomy. MCh Thesis, Liverpool

Hansson G 1989 Sliding osteotomy for tailor's bunion – brief report. J Bone Joint Surg 71B: 324

Helal B 1975 Metatarsal osteotomy for metatarsalgia. J Bone Joint Surg 57B: 187–192

Helal B, Greiss M 1984 Telescoping osteotomy for pressure metatarsalgia. J Bone Joint Surg 66B: 213–217

Jones F W 1949 Structure and Function as Seen in the Foot. Ballière Tindall, London, 2nd edn

Kanse P, Chen S C 1989 Dorsal closing wedge osteotomy for Freiberg's disease. J Bone Joint Surg 71B: 889

Kates A, Kessel L, Kay A 1967 Arthroplasty of the forefoot J Bone Joint Surg 49B: 552–557

Kelikian H, Clayton L, Loseff H 1961 Surgical syndactylia of the toes. Clin Orthop 19: 208–231

Kinnard P, Lirette R 1989 Dorsiflexion osteotomy in Freiberg's disease. Foot Ankle 9: 226–231

Klenerman L, McClellan G E, Guiloff R J, Scadding J W 1983 Morton's metatarsalgia – a retrospective and prospective study. J Bone Joint Surg 65B: 220–221

Kohler A 1923 Typical disease of the second metatarsophalangeal joint. Am J Roentgenol 10: 705–710

Lambrinudi C 1927 An operation for claw toes. Proc R Soc Lond (Biol) 21: 239

Lambrinudi C 1932 Use and abuse of toes. Postgrad Med J 8: 459–463

Lapidus P W 1942 Transplantation of extensor tendon for correction of overlapping 5th toe. J Bone Joint Surg 24: 555–559

Leventen E O, Pearson S W 1990 Distal metatarsal osteotomy for intractable plantar keratoses. Foot Ankle 10: 247–251

McElvenny R T 1943 The etiology and surgical treatment of intractable pain about the fourth metatarso-phalangeal joint (Morton's toe). J Bone Joint Surg 25A: 675–679

McFarland B 1950 Congenital deformities of the foot. In: Platt H (ed) Modern Trends in Orthopaedic Surgery. P B Hoeber Inc, New York, pp 107–137

Meachim G, Abberton M J 1971 Histological findings in Morton's metatarsalgia. J Pathol 103: 209–217

Mittlmeier T, Machler G, Lob G, Mutschler W, Bauer G, Vogl T 1991 Compartment syndrome of the foot after intra-articular calcaneal fracture. Clin Orthop 269: 241–248

Morton D J 1935 The Human Foot. Columbia University Press, New York

Morton T G 1876 A peculiar and painful affection of the fourth metatarso-phalangeal articulation. Am J Med Sci 71: 37–45. (Reprinted in 1979, Clin Orthop 142: 4–9)

Mulder J D 1951 The causative mechanism in Morton's metatarsalgia. J Bone Joint Surg 33B: 94–95

Myerson M S, Shereff M J 1989 The pathological anatomy of claw and hammertoes. J Bone Joint Surg 71A: 45–49

Nissen K I 1948 Plantar digital neuritis, Morton's metatarsalgia. J Bone Joint Surg 30B: 84–89

Pfitzner W 1896 Bietrage zur Kenntniss des menschlichen Extremitätenskelets. In: Schwalbe G (ed) Morphologische Arbeiten, VI. Gustav Fisher, Jena, pp 245–527

Rob C, Smith R 1957 Operative Surgery: Fundamental Techniques. Butterworth, London

Ruiz Mora J 1954 Plastic correction of overriding fifth toe [Letter]. Orthop Surg: 60

Sibley F, O'Docherty D, Goddard N J, Grieve D W, Wilson D W (1989) Results of plantar displacement in first metatarsal osteotomy. J Bone Joint Surg 71B: 1–155

Smillie I S 1957 Freiberg's infraction. J Bone Joint Surg 39B: 580

Smith T W D, Stanley D, Rowley D I 1991 Treatment of Freiberg's disease. A new operative technique. J Bone Joint Surg 73B: 129–130

Sponsel K H 1976 Bunionette correction by metatarsal osteotomy. Orthop Clin North Am 7: 809–819

Steinke M S, Boll K L 1989 Hohmann–Thomasen metatarsal osteotomy for tailor's bunions (bunionette). J Bone Joint Surg 71A: 423–426

Taylor R G 1951 The treatment of claw toes by multiple transfers of flexor into extensor tendons. J Bone Joint Surg 33B 539–542

Thomas F B 1974 Levelling the tread. J Bone Joint Surg 56B: 314–319

Viladot A 1984 Patología del Antepie, 3rd edition. Ediciones Toray, Barcelona

Winson I G, Rawlinson J, Broughton N S 1989 Treatment of metatarsalgia by sliding distal metatarsal osteotomy. Adv Orthop Surg 12: 228–229

Zafiropoulos G, Henry A P J 1994 Wedge osteotomy for curly toes gave better results than tendon transfer. Foot 4: 20–24

V.5 The Accessory Ossicles and Sesamoids

Basil Helal

The accessory bones

The accessory ossicles are developmental anomalies, and are usually either a separated part of the main bone to which they are adjacent, or subdivisions of the main element (O'Rahilly 1953). They are frequently lined with hyaline or fibrocartilage where they abut against bone, sometimes forming a synovial joint, and may exhibit both macroscopically and microscopically the changes of chondromalacia; they may displace, suffer fractures of the avulsion or crushing type, become infected or involved in connective tissue disorders or osteoarthrosic changes, and may occasionally have to be excised to relieve symptoms (Fig. 1).

Os trigonum

This bone lies posterolaterally behind the talus and is a detached part of the posterolateral tubercle. It is present in some 5% of the population, and must be differentiated from a fracture of the trigonal process of the talus.

  The bone has been described as giving rise to symptoms particularly in ballet dancers (Quirk 1982) and in footballers (McDougal 1955) suffering the well-recognized posterior tibiotalar impingement syndrome of the trigonal process, and sometimes a fracture (Shepherd 1882). In the presence of persistent pain and limited plantar flexion of the ankle, the ossicle occasionally has to be excised to relieve symptoms and permit full plantar flexion of the ankle, especially in ballet dancers. Its union with the adjacent talus and calcaneum may be the cause of posterior talocalcaneal coalition (Pfitzner 1896).

Os tibiale (accessory navicular tibiale externum)

This lies posteromedial to the tuberosity of the navicular (Fig. 2). It varies in shape and is part of the tuberosity since it receives part of the insertion of the tibialis posterior. It is connected to the navicular by fibrous tissue or fibrocartilage, and occurs in about 5% of the population (Sarrafian 1983). The anatomical variations are well described. It generally gives rise to symptoms because of its prominence, inflammation of the overlying skin being caused by shoe pressure. Sometimes there is an overlying adventitious bursa.

Occasionally a synovial joint exists between this ossicle and the navicular, and pain may be due to distension of this joint and occasionally to a chondromalacia of the cartilage lining the joint. Zadek & Gold (1948) demonstrated variations in the type of joint and showed the synchondrotic type to have an incidence of union with the scaphoid.

If symptoms persist, the ossicle can be removed without any ill effect. Care must be taken in excising the ossicle in order to minimize damage to the posterior tibial tendon. Union of this bone with the adjoining navicular and talus may be the cause of the talonavicular synostosis. Kidner (1929) suggested a relationship between the presence of this ossicle and flatfoot. There is little support for this in subsequent literature or in the author's experience.

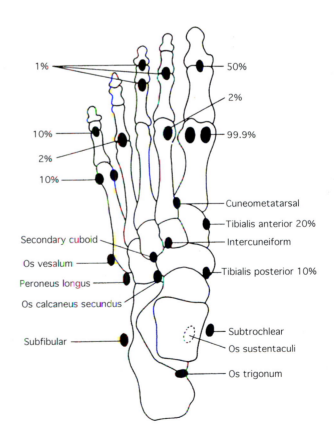

Figure 1

The sesamoids and accessory bones of the foot

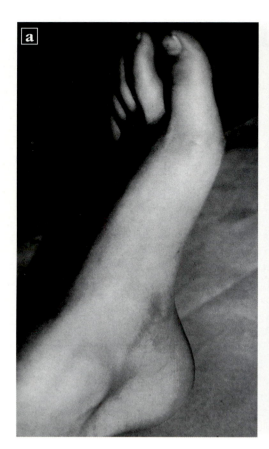

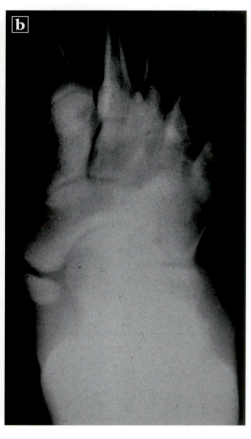

Figure 2

(a) Clinical appearance of the navicular ossicle; (b) radiograph

Os intermetatarseum

This bone lies between the bases of the first and second metatarsals and the medial cunciform proximally and was thought by Friedl (1924) to be a sesamoid in the first dorsal interosseus muscle. This author has never seen this bone give rise to a clinical problem. Henderson (1963) described four patients, three in one family with an ossicle and one with a spur at this site. All were associated with a varus first metatarsal and hallux valgus. He believed that resection of the ossicle produced a good correction of the metatarsus varus, and combined this procedure with an excision arthroplasty of the Keller type. He claims the results have produced a better correction than the Keller procedure alone.

Os sustentaculi

This bone has an incidence of 0.4–3% and is found at the posterior end of the sustentaculum tali, to which it is connected by fibrous tissue or fibrocartilage. It may be mistaken for a fracture. Union of this bone with neighbouring os calcis and talus results in medial talocalcaneal coalition.

Os calcaneus secundarius

This is a triangular or rounded piece of bone lying between os calcis, cuboid, navicular, and head of talus. Calcanconavicular coalition may be the result of union of this bone with the adjacent calcaneum and navicular bones.

Os cuboides secundarium

This bone is present on the plantar aspect between the cuboid, navicular, talus and os calcis.

Os talonaviculare dorsale (supranaviculare spurium)

This is dorsally placed on the talonavicular joint.

Os intercuneiforme

This bone is dorsally placed between proximal ends of the medial and middle cuneiforms.

Os cuneometatarsale plantare (pars peronica metatarsalis primi)

This is found on the plantar aspect between base of the first metatarsal and medial cuneiform.

Os vesalianum

This bone is found proximal to the tuberosity of the fifth metatarsal styloid. It has to be differentiated from ossification within the apophysis of the base of the metatarsal,

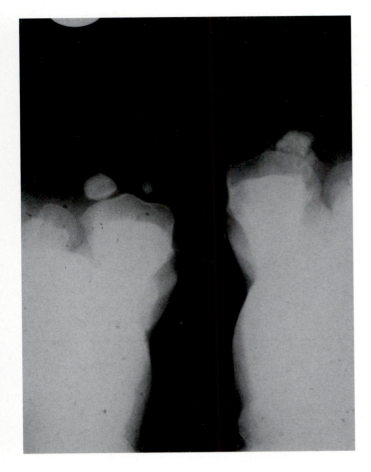

Figure 3
There is a congenital absence of the medial sesamoid on one side and a hypoplasia on the other

an ununited apophysis or fracture of the styloid. It has an incidence of 1%.

Os subtibiale and os subfibulare
These bones are found beneath the medial malleolus and the lateral malleolus. They are all of no particular clinical significance, but when they must be differentiated from fracture, they may achieve some medicolegal significance.

Tarsal coalitions and the accessory bones

The reported incidence of tarsal coalition averages about 0.5%. Pfitzner (1896) put forward the thesis that coalitions were due to fusions of accessory bones with their adjoining bones. This thesis received considerable support until Harris (1965) demonstrated the presence of

tarsal coalition in the fetus. Jack (1954) suggested that both metatarsal bones and accessory bones were different stages in the same process and both were genetically determined mesenchymal disorders.

Leonard (1974) carried out a population study in Edinburgh, UK, which showed that there was a pattern of inheritance as an autosomal dominant with almost full penetrance.

There was no genetic difference in the inheritance of different types of coalition, since 14% of relations were found to have a different form of coalition from the patient with a coalition under study.

The sesamoids

These small bones are generally found at specific sites (although several are not constantly present) and are usually embedded in a tendon. They form part of a gliding mechanism and generally are designed to withstand pressure. They tend to occur where there is a variation in directional pull on a tendon, particularly when this is in close contact with bone. The common sites are in the tendons of flexor hallucis brevis, the plantar plates of the metatarsophalangeal and interphalangeal joints, the tendons of the intrinsics to the lesser toes, the peroneus longus and the tibialis anterior and posterior tendons. The two sesamoids beneath the head of the first metatarsal are only rarely missing. Congenital absence of one or both is recorded (Fig. 3). The sesamoid beneath the interphalangeal joint of the great toe is inconstant.

Considerable variations in size and shape have been recorded, as has partition, which may be into two, three, four or more parts.

The complexity and balance of the sesamometatarsal articulation cannot be fully appreciated unless the attachments are noted. Thus to the lateral sesamoid are attached:

1. the lateral head of flexor hallucis brevis
2. oblique head of adductor hallucis
3. deep transverse metatarsal ligament
4. lateral metatarsosesamoid ligament
5. lateral side of fibrous flexor tunnel
6. intersesamoid ligament
7. the lateral longitudinal septum of the plantar aponeurosis to the great toe
8. the vertical and arcuate fibres of the deep fascia forming the tendon space of the flexors of the great toe
9. lateral sesamophalangeal ligament
10. a presesamoid bursa.

The medial sesamoid gives attachment to:

1. the medial head of flexor hallucis brevis
2. abductor hallucis tendon

3.   medial metatarsosesamoid ligament
4.   medial edge of fibrous tunnel for the flexor
      hallucis
5.   intersesamoid ligament
6.   medial septum of plantar apononeurosis to great
      toe
7.   the septal fibres from the preflexor tendon space
8.   presesamoid bursa.

The articular surfaces are concave and abut on and support the head of the great toe metatarsal, giving height to this ray (Fig. 4).

Lesser toe sesamoids
These are located in long flexors or intrinsic tendons.

Peroneus longus sesamoid
These are found where the tendon angulates to turn medially into the sole of the foot and articulates with the cuboid.

Tibialis posterior sesamoid
This is found where the tendon crosses the inferior calcaneonavicular ligament under the tuberosity of the navicular.

Tibialis anterior sesamoid
This is found near the tendon insertion on the outer inferior surface of the medial cuneiform.

Great toe sesamoids
It can be seen that these give height to the first metatarsal head. Their displacement not surprisingly produces a considerable biomechanical disturbance to the forefoot.

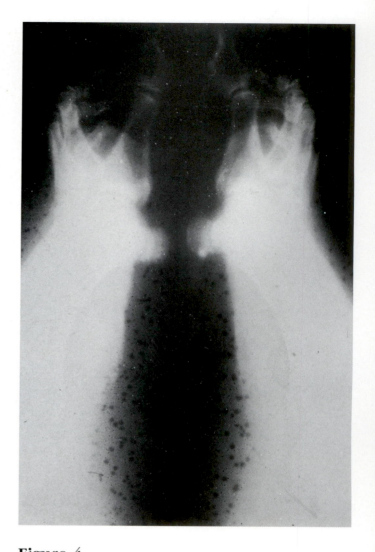

Figure 4

The sesamoids give considerable height to the first metatarsal head

History

Robert Nesbitt of London showed in 1736 that precursors of the sesamoids were present under the first metatarsal heads as early as the end of the first fetal trimester (Inge & Ferguson 1933). The first anatomic description was given by Placentini in 1656 (Kewenter 1936). Two sesamoid bones are constantly present under the heads of the first metatarsals: congenital absence is extremely rare (Inge 1936) although absence of the tibial sesamoid is described (Hubay 1949, Inge 1936). The author has seen one adult with congenital absence of both sesamoids.

Bizarro (1920) believed their presence to stem from phylogeny as well as function, for they are not residual primitive tarsal bones but are persistent structures in mammals. They form an integral part of the first metatarsophalangeal joint and around each of their facets there is the joint capsule. The plantar surfaces are enclosed by flexor hallucis brevis tendons, which proceed to be inserted into the base of the proximal phalanx and are joined together by a thickened portion of the capsule which forms an intersesamoid ligament. On its medial side, it receives part of the insertion of the abductor hallucis, and on its lateral aspect that of adductor hallucis: these insertions blend with the flexor hallucis brevis. There is a constant bursa on the plantar aspect of the sesamoid on the tibial side. The likeness to the patella and the knee is very striking and certain injuries as well as several disease processes are common to both.

Sesamoids appear where changes in direction in the pull of a tendon occur, providing protection for the tendon as well as giving a mechanical advantage. The great toe sesamoids also protect the long flexor tendon and give a lift to the metatarsal head, an important feature in the biomechanics of the forefoot. Ossification occurs at about the age of 8 years in girls and 10 in boys.

Developmental variations

Various incidences of partition are quoted in the literature. Kewenter (1936) found a 34% incidence with only 2% in the lateral sesamoid: others ranged from 7% to 20% for the lateral sesamoid. Bipartite sesamoids are twice as common as the multipartite type (Fig. 5). Common patterns of sesamoid division are described frequently, the most authoritative based on large series published by Kewenter (1936) (800 cases), Inge & Ferguson (1933) (433) and others (Bizarro 1920, Hubay 1949, Resnick et al 1977, Stieda 1904). Saxby et al (1992) describe a case of coalition of the hallux sesamoids producing a dumb-bell shaped bone similar to that seen in the rabbits' sesamoids arrangement under the 5th metacarpophalangeal joint of the forefoot. Awareness of these variations helps to avoid confusion with fractures.

Symptoms and signs of sesamoid disorders of the great toe

Pain may be well localized to the affected sesamoid or sesamoids and difficulty in walking and local tenderness experienced. In inflammatory conditions and in recent injury or in involvement of the local presesamoid bursa swelling will appear.

Secondary involvement of the great toe metatarsophalangeal joint will result in aching, stiffness and swelling of the joint. If displacements occur and the foot is supinated to avoid direct weight bearing on the first ray, weight will be displaced laterally to the lesser metatarsals and pain will occur following the unusual loading and biomechanical disturbance (Fig. 6).

Displacements

Displacements generally occur in association with deformities such as hallux valgus, when the sesamoids prolapse laterally, and after excision arthroplasty involving removal of the base of the proximal phalanx, when they prolapse proximally. If the sesamoids are displaced from under the first metatarsal head, the head will shift plantarwards. A shift of weight to the lateral metatarsals will follow with consequent metatarsalgia or even stress fractures.

In the personal series of 200 Keller's excision arthroplasties followed as long as 8 years, 22% had some

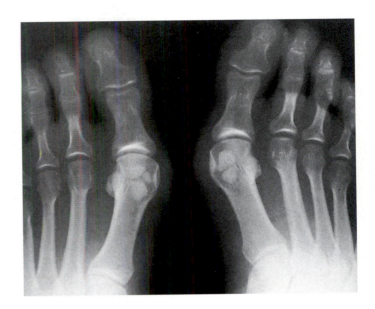

Figure 5
Multipartite medial sesamoid

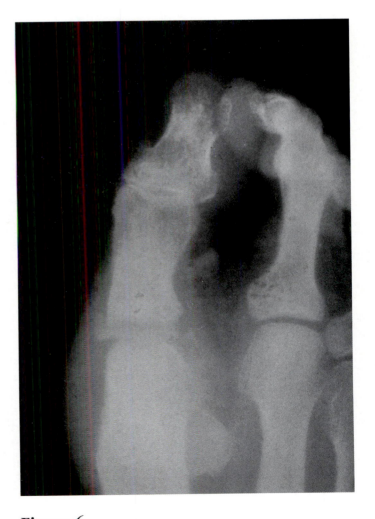

Figure 6
Detachment of sesamoids to proximal phalanx great toe causing proximal migration of sesamoids

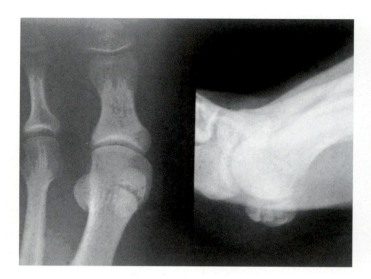

Figure 7

Comminuted fracture of medial sesamoid

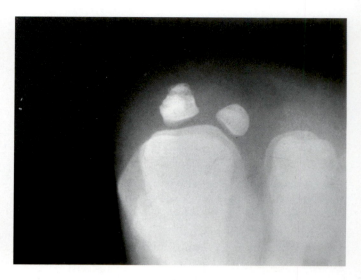

Figure 8

Crush fracture of sesamoid: a so-called 'toffee-paper' fracture, where the outline remains intact, like fragmenting a toffee in its wrapper

metatarsalgia, and 8% suffered stress fractures of one of the lateral metatarsals. In all but two of the latter cases there was complete proximal prolapse of the sesamoids from under the first metatarsal head.

Injuries to the perisesamoidal soft tissue are often clinically misdiagnosed. The soft tissue definition obtained by MRI makes accurate differentiation of these lesions possible. Rupture of the intersesamoid ligament can occur with divarication of the sesamoids and possible subluxation or dislocation. Rodeo, Warren, O'Brien, et al have reported four cases in footballers (quoted by Potter et al 1992). This condition is known as 'turf toe' and is a hyperextension injury. The mechanism is stress applied to a dorsiflexed toe when an opposing player falls on the opponent's leg, driving the joint into excessive extension. The greater hardness and diminished impact absorption of synthetic turf have been implicated in the predisposition to such injuries.

Fractures

The bulk of the literature on the great toe sesamoids is concerned with anatomic variations and fracture (Claustre & Simon 1978, Enna 1970, Hobart 1929, Hubay 1949, Inge & Ferguson 1933, Marx 1904, Stieda 1904). The author's personal records have been kept since 1965, and indicate 37 definite injuries to the sesamoids, 19 in athletes while indulging in their sport. Three types of injury have been

identified: two forms of fracture (Fig. 7; six of the avulsion type, two of which involved the lateral sesamoid), and the crushing type (Fig. 8) of which there were 28, all tibial sesamoids. The author has also seen two patients with dehiscence of the bipartite tibial sesamoid, as evidenced by localized pain and tenderness and a larger gap than on the uninjured side. The characteristic of an avulsion fracture with nonunion is a rounding off of the margins; roentgenograms at three week intervals may show an increase in the fracture gap (Fig. 9).

In general, if a stress fracture is suspected, MRI or a longitudinal computerized scan will reveal the injury in those cases where plain roentgenograms are unhelpful (Biedert 1993). A technetium scan will also be positive.

Osteochondritis

The characteristic feature of osteochondritis is the irregularity of the trabecular pattern giving a striped and stippled look to the bones on X-ray. This has been described as 'typical disease of the sesamoids', 'sesamoiditis', 'osteomalacia', 'osteitis fibrosa', 'juvenile necrotic osteopathy', 'traumatic osteitis', 'Kohler's or Schlatter's disease' of the sesamoids, 'sesamoid insufficiency', 'osteochondritis' and 'osteochondropathy' (Claustre & Simon 1978, Ilfeld & Rosen 1972, Inge & Ferguson 1933, Renander 1924). It is typically seen in the presence of bipartism. Apley's views are similar to

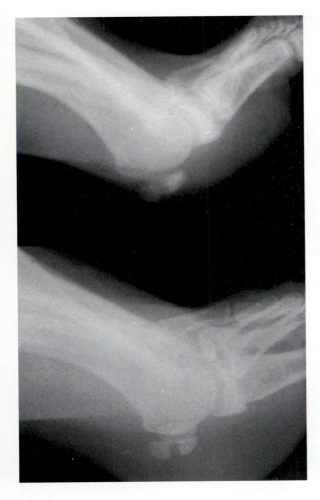

Figure 9

Typical avulsion fracture. A two-week period has elapsed between the upper and lower radiographs; in the interval the gap between the fragments has increased

indistinguishable from so-called osteochondritis. It is of some interest that Renander wrote in 1924, 'If the physiological solidity of a bone is reduced the result will, of course, easily be a spontaneous fracture and the above-mentioned compression of the sesamoid bones may be regarded as a depressed fracture'. Ilfeld & Rosen (1972) give a good description of the histology: 'The bone was irregularly osteosclerotic and marrow spaces between trabeculae were quite vascular and contained sparse fatty elements. Some marrow spaces were filled with loose collagenous stroma. Occasional osteoid seams and zones of new bone formation are seen. Orderly osteons were rare even in the cortex. Polarization revealed many scattered foci of uneven or fibrous bone with large osteocytes. Cartilagenous surfaces showed marked degenerative changes with clefting, fibrinoid change and microvillous pannus proliferation. There were many areas of cortical disruption and periosteal proliferation and chondroid metaplasia were seen'. This histology resembles that following a crush or stellate fracture. These authors comment that, since these patients were very young, it is unlikely that circulation of the sesamoid was involved. They reported good results after excision in three cases.

Chondromalacia

Apley first referred to chondromalacia in 1966, stating that it is not at all surprising that a condition so common in the patellofemoral joint should occur in the almost exactly analogous tibial sesamometatarsal joint. The condition seems to be confined to the medial sesamoid, developing most frequently in bipartite sesamoids (Fig. 11). The diagnosis is based on pain, almost invariably beneath the medial sesamoid and accurately localized, occurring only on weight bearing. The sign is tenderness on pressure over the bone although the radiograph appears quite normal. This condition has been seen in 14 patients, three of whom were affected bilaterally. In other words, it has occurred in 17 sesamoids in which this diagnosis has been made since 1966 (Helal 1977). All patients wore supports to remove pressure from the

the author's in this matter, namely, that no such condition exists and these are all forms of crush or stellate fracture (Fig. 10) (Apley 1966, Helal 1977).

An experiment was carried out on a cadaver in which such an injury was reproduced: the radiographs were

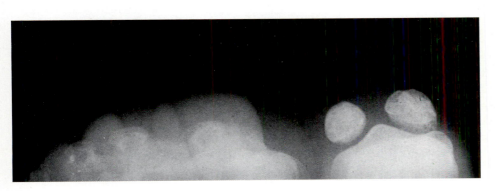

Figure 10

So-called 'osteochondritis' of medial sesamoid: this is a fragmentation of the trabecular type of crush fracture

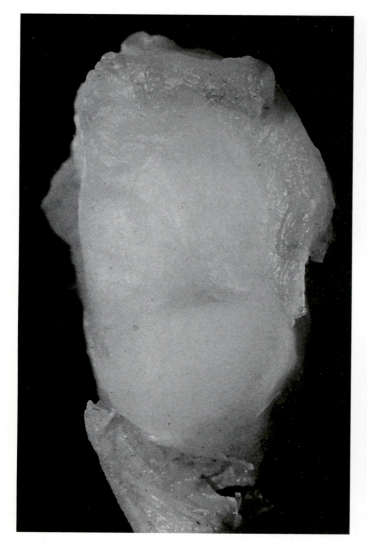

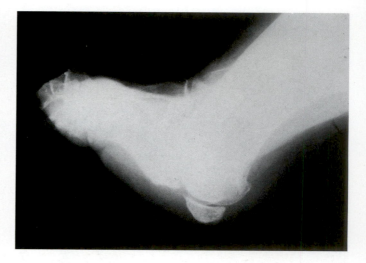

Figure 12

Osteoarthritis of the sesamometatarsal joint

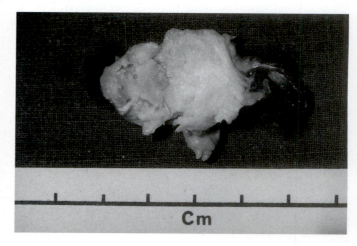

Figure 13

Osteoarthritic changes on the articular surface of a sesamoid

Figure 11

Bipartite sesamoid with chondromalacia of larger segment

sesamoid and those who came to surgery had taken a course of salicylates as well as one or more intra-articular steroid injections. Five medial sesamoids were removed: in one patient, the medial sesamoids of both feet were excised. All were relieved of their symptoms after surgery.

Bursae

The diagnosis of presesamoid bursae (Apley 1966, Helal 1977, 1979) is made by palpation when a tender soft tissue swelling is felt. The author has seen this as an isolated problem giving rise to symptoms in four patients: two required excision while the other two settled on conservative treatment. Six patients were seen (eight bursae) in which the bursal synovitis was a

manifestation of rheumatoid disease; one required surgical removal and the others settled on steroid injection and a protective insole.

Degenerative arthritis

The sesamoids may be involved in degenerative changes of the great toe metatarsophalangeal joint (Claustre & Simon 1978, Resnick et al 1977) (Figs 12, 13). There has never been any indication for their removal in our experience. They may possibly play some role in initiating hallux rigidus if chondromalacia (as in the patella) progresses to degenerative changes. Thus osteochondritis dissecans need not always be involved, although this speculation would be extraordinarily hard to confirm to scientific satisfaction.

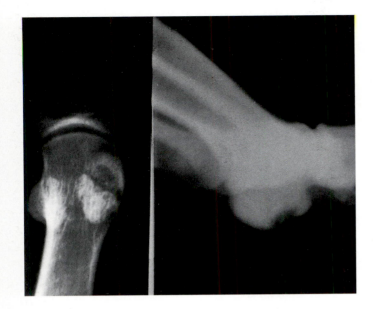

Figure 14

Gouty tophus notching sesamoid

Connective tissue disorders

The sesamoids have been involved (Claustre & Simon 1978) in rheumatoid arthritis, Reiter's disease (Doury et al 1979, Resnick et al 1977) and in gout (Fig. 14), but they have not presented as an isolated problem requiring local action. Osteomyelitis has been described frequently and with a variety of organisms (Colwill 1969, Seyss 1979, Stanley et al 1974).

In our unit, two patients, one of whom was a diabetic, presented with osteomyelitis (Fig. 15). Both conditions involved the tibial sesamoid and both required sesamoidectomy to effect a cure.

Conservative measures

Weight relief by suitable orthoses or a period of complete weight relief by using crutches, physiotherapeutic measures and local injections of steroid all may help depending upon the particular pathology.

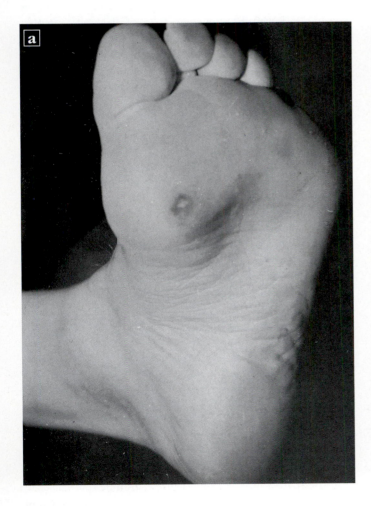

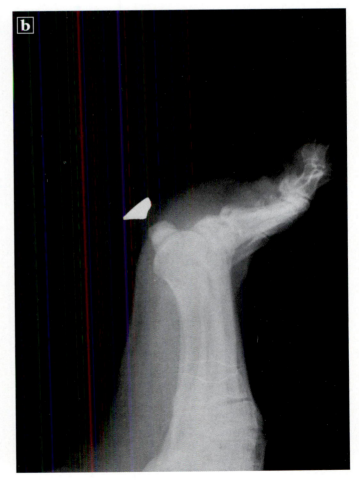

Figure 15

(a) Sinus leading to infected presesamoid bursa. There is early osteomyelitis of the underlying bone. (b) Radiograph

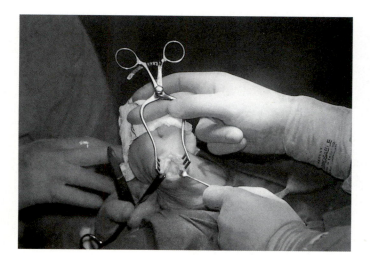

Figure 16

If the sesamoid has to be removed, a plantar approach is best. We have not encountered any problems with sole incisions in a weight-bearing area

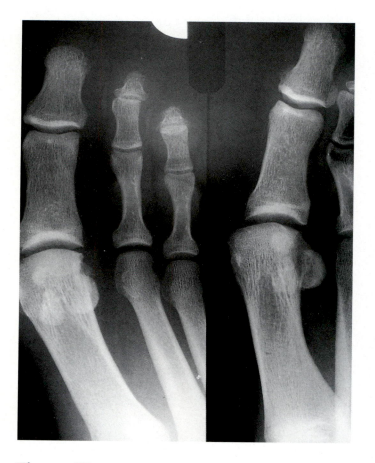

Figure 17

This patient has badly damaged both sesamoids. Both had to be replaced by silicone elastomer prostheses to maintain the height of the metatarsal head

Operation

Sesamoidectomy was first mentioned by Marx in 1904. Speed (1914) claimed that if excision was to be performed, then both bones should be removed, but this is wrong. The only case in my personal series with lateral metatarsalgia as a surgical complication was a patient in whom both had to be removed. In the best and most complete survey of the subject, Inge & Ferguson (1933) concluded that both sesamoids should not be removed if at all possible, stating that incisions should be kept free of weight-bearing surfaces and bony prominences against which the shoe will rub. Personal experience has shown that by far the best approach is through a longitudinal incision on the sole directly over the bone to be excised: rarely, if both need removal, the approach is through the midline between the two sesamoids.

Reduction of sesamoid prominence by partial resection of the plantar half is a bad operation and can result in avascular necrosis, as the arteries most often enter the plantar surface. This is evident when their blood supply is studied (Sobel et al 1992, Pretterklieber et al 1992).

It is now common knowledge that incisions on the sole are remarkably troublefree (Fig. 16). The bones should be carefully dissected free of the tendons that invest them. It is important not to divide flexor hallucis brevis, or a hammer deformity of the great toe will result. Replacements of the sesamoids (Helal 1979) were performed on two occasions, one in a cross-country runner who had to have lateral and medial sesamoids removed after injury to both in the right foot (Figs 17, 18). This was carried out as a prophylactic measure to avoid a plantar displacement of the first metatarsal head. The artificial bones were created out of a silicone rubber block. The patient has completed a second season of competition to his former standard and is completely free of symptoms. In the second patient the bones were excised for severe chondromalacia of both sesamoids.

Tumours of the sesamoids are extremely rare; the only reference in the literature was found in a report by Geschickter & Copeland (1931) referring to a xanthomatous tumour involving the sesamoid and also in close relation to the flexor tendon.

For four decades, orthopaedic surgeons have paid little attention to the sesamoids of the first metatarsals as a primary cause of pain, but recent active interest has led to closer observation and thus to the discovery of numerous problems directly related to these bones and their role as part of the first metatarsophalangeal joint. The sesamoids should always be kept in mind when pain occurs in this region or when examining the first metatarsophalangeal joint.

The sesamoids of the great toe are a source of symptoms and are involved in a number of disease processes. They suffer many of the diseases described in relation to their larger analogue, the patella (Fig. 19). These disorders include subluxations, dislocations,

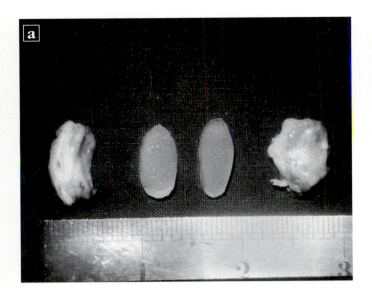

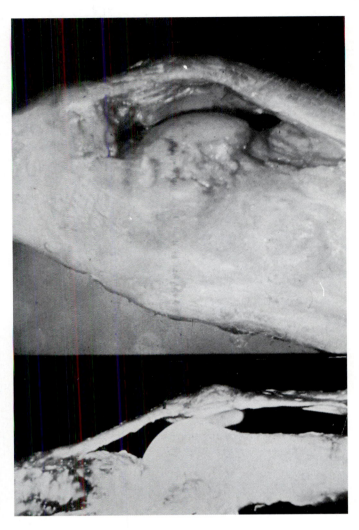

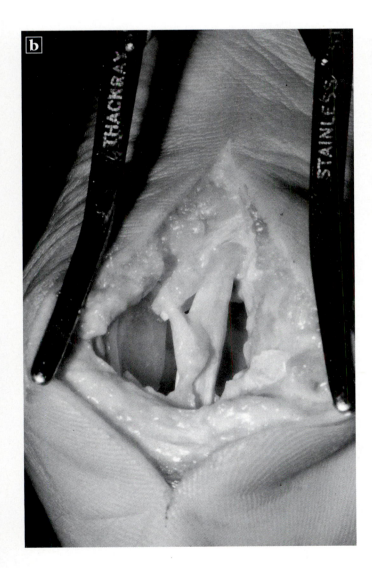

Figure 19

There are close similarities between the sesamoid (above) and the patella (below), including similar pathologies

various forms of fracture, chondromalacia and involvement in degenerative as well as other forms of arthritis, and there may be inflammation of the presesamoid bursa.

Figure 18

(a) Excised sesamoids with silicone elastomer sesamoids. (b) After removal of fractured medial and lateral sesamoids, artificial sesamoids are fashioned and inserted to maintain the height of the first metatarsal head

References

Apley A G 1966 Open sesamoid. Proc R Soc Med 59–120

Biedert R 1993 Which investigations are required in stress fracture of the great toe sesamoids? Arch Orthop Trauma Surg 112: 94–95

Bizarro E H 1920 On sesamoid and supernumerary bones of the limbs. J Anat 55: 26

Claustre J, Simon L 1978 Aspects de la pathologie sesamoidienne du premier metatarsien. Rev Rhum Mal Osteoartic 45: 479

Colwill M 1969 Osteomyelitis of the metatarsal sesamoids. J Bone Joint Surg 51B: 464

Doury P, Pattin S, Delahaye R P, Metges P J, Mine J, Casanova D 1979 Sesamoidite du gros orteil au cours d'un syndrome de Fiessinger-Leroy-Reiter. Rev Rhum Mal Osteoartic 46: 133

Enna C D 1970 Observations of the hallucal sesamoids in trauma to the denervated foot. Int Surg 53: 97

Friedl E 1924 Das Os Intermetatarsum und die Epiphysierbildung am Processus Trochlaris Calcanei. Dtsch Z Chir 61: 186

Geschickter C F, Copeland M M 1931 Giant xanthomatous tumours of the sesamoids. In: Tumours of bone. Am J Cancer. p 370

Harris R 1965 Retrospect peroneal spastic flat foot (rigid valgus foot). J Bone Joint Surg 47A: 1657–1667

Helal B 1977 Surgery of the forefoot. Br Med J 1: 276

Helal B 1979 Sesamoides du Pied du Sportif. Le Pied du Sportif. Masson et Cie, Paris. p 116

Henderson R S 1963 Os intermetatarseum and the possible relationship to hallux valgus. J Bone Joint Surg 45: 117

Hobart M 1929 Fracture of the sesamoid bones of the foot. J Bone Joint Surg 11: 299

Hubay C A 1949 Sesamoid bones of the hands and feet. Am J Roentgenol 61: 493

Ilfeld F W, Rosen V 1972 Osteochondritis of the first metatarsal sesamoid. Clin Orthop 85: 38

Inge G A L 1936 Congenital absence of the medial sesamoid of the great toe. J Bone Joint Surg 18: 188

Inge G A L, Ferguson A B 1933 Surgery of the sesamoid bones of the great toe. Arch Surg 27: 466

Jack E A 1954 Bone anomalies of the tarsus in relation to peroneal spastic flat foot. J Bone Joint Surg 36B: 530–542

Kewenter Y 1936 Die sesambiene des metatarsophalangelenks des menschen. Acta Orthop Scand (Suppl) 2: 521

Kidner F C 1929 The prehallux (accessory scaphoid) in its relation to flat foot. J Bone Joint Surg 11: 831–837

Leonard M A 1974 The inheritance of tarsal coalition and its relationship to spastic flat foot. J Bone Joint Surg 56B: 520

McDougal A 1955 The os trigonum. J Bone Joint Surg 37B: 257–265

Marx H 1904 Ein fall von sesambien fraktur. Muenchener Medizinische Wochenschrift (Munich) 38: 1688

O'Rahilly R 1953 A survey of carpal and tarsal anomalies. J Bone Joint Surg 35A: 626–642

Pfitzner W 1896 Die Variationen in Aufbar des Fussekelts Beitrage zur Kenntniss des Menschlichen extremitaten skelets. VII Morphol. Arbeit 6: 245

Potter H G, Pavlov H, Abrahams T G 1992 The hallux sesamoids revisited. Skeletal Radiol 21: 437–444

Pretterklieber M L, Wanivenhaus A 1992 The arterial supply of the sesamoid bones of the hallux: the course and source of the nutrient arteries as an anatomical basis for surgical approaches to the great toe. Foot Ankle 13: 27–31

Quirk R 1982 Talar compression syndrome in dancers. Foot Ankle 3 (2): 65–68

Renander A 1924 Two cases of typical osteochondropathy of the medial sesamoid of the first metatarsal. Acta Radiol 3: 521

Resnick D, Niwayama G, Feingold M L 1977 The sesamoid bones of the hands and feet. Participators in arthritis. Radiology 123: 57

Sarrafian S K 1983 Anatomy of the Foot and Ankle. J. B. Lippincott Co., Philadelphia. 84–98

Saxby T, Vandemark R M, Hall R L 1992 Coalition of the hallux sesamoids: a case report. Foot Ankle, 13: 355–357

Seyss R 1979 Periarthrose um die sesamknocken des grobzehengrundgelenks. Wien Klin. Wochenschr. 91: 276

Shepherd F J 1882 A hitherto undescribed fracture of the astragalus. J Anat Physiol 17: 79

Sobel M, Hashimoto J, Arnoczky S, Walther H O, Bohne M D 1992 The microvasculature of the sesamoid complex: its clinical significance, Foot Ankle 13: 359

Speed K 1914 Injuries of the great toe sesamoids. Ann Surg 60: 478

Stanley L G, Evans D, Greer R B 1974 Pseudomonas osteomyelitis of the metatarsal sesamoid of the great toe. Clin Orthop 99: 188

Stieda A 1904 Zur Kenntnis der Sesambiene der Finger und Zehen. Beitr Z Klin Chir 62: 237

Zadek I, Gold A M 1948 The accessory tarsal scaphoid. J Bone Joint Surg 30A: 957–968

V.6 Tendons and Bursae

David Prieskorn and Paul F Plattner

Introduction

Tendon injuries about the foot and ankle are much less common than ligament sprains, but they are not as rare as generally supposed (Gilcreest 1933, McMaster 1933, Haldeman & Soto-Hall 1935, Conwell & Alldredge 1937, Lipscomb 1950, Lipscomb & Kelly 1955, Anzel et al 1959, Griffiths 1965, Nicholas 1974, Scheller et al 1980, Wicks et al 1980, Floyd et al 1983). This chapter focuses only on the extrinsic tendons that cross the ankle. The literature is reviewed with regard to the cause, type, classification and anatomic distribution of and pathologic changes associated with tendon injuries.

Etiology of injuries to muscles and tendons

Many factors may be responsible for muscle and tendon dysfunction (Gilcreest 1933, Jahss 1982b) (Table 1). Most injuries are probably caused by a combination of these factors. A classification of injury is also important, and the scheme modified from Haldeman and Soto-Hall (1935) that is based on causative factors, contributing forces and relative frequency is most helpful (Table 2). Broadly, tendons may become inflamed (so-called tendinitis), rupture, and subluxate or dislocate.

Pathology of injuries to muscles and tendons

A knowledge of the anatomy and physiology of tendons, tendon sheaths and bursae is necessary for a clear concept of inflammatory processes involving these structures (Schatzker & Brånemark 1969, Hartmann 1981, Jahss 1982b). A tendon is connective tissue composed of closely packed collagen fibers and protein–mucopolysaccharide. These components are elaborated by a woven mesh of loose connective tissue, the endotenon. All of these bundles make up the tendon, which is also surrounded by a fine connective tissue sheath, the

---

* This revised and updated chapter is dedicated to the memory of Kenneth A. Johnson, whose enormous contributions to foot and ankle surgery will live on through his published works and through the lives of his students and colleagues, who all miss his wit, wisdom, and charm.

Table 1 Causes of muscle and tendon dysfunction

Aging and degeneration
Pathologic changes
  Peritendinitis
    Nonspecific
    Arthritic
    Infectious
    Neoplastic
  Myositis
  Calcinosis
  Vascular changes
Bony changes
  Fractures
  Rough bone
  Spurs, exostoses
Tethering
  Partial constriction
    Trigger toes, tarsal tunnel
    Peroneal constriction with a fractured os calcis
  Complete tethering
    Incarceration
    Adhesive, including checkrein deformity
Contractures
Occupation
Fatigue, stress
Trauma
  Direct
  Indirect
Iatrogenic conditions
Congenital conditions

---

epitenon (peritenon). The epitenon is continuous with the endotenon. The paratenon is loose, fatty areolar tissue that surrounds the entire tendon. In areas where the tendon is subjected to increased local pressure or friction, the paratenon is replaced by a synovial sheath or bursa. For the most part, true synovial sheaths are found only in the distal portions of the upper and lower extremities, especially where tendons lie contiguous to joints and motion is the chief function. The mesotenon, known as 'vinculum' in some areas, is a specialized mesentery-like structure on the nonfriction side of the tendons that carries blood vessels.

Tendons receive their blood supply at the musculotendinous junction, at the tendo-osseous junction, and along their length by means of the paratenon,

Table 2 Classification of muscle and tendon injuries
Direct injury
Laceration (open wound)
Blow or crush (closed wound)
Indirect injury
Stretching force applied to contracting muscle
Unusually forceful contraction
Spontaneous rupture (partial or complete)
Post-traumatic
Single injury (catastrophic failure)
Repetitive injury (fatigue failure)
Pathological (disease of tendon)
Degenerative
Dislocation or subluxation of tendons
Acute
Chronic
Iatrogenic (corticosteroids?) (Kleinman & Gross 1983)

Table 3 Sequential changes of tendon healing

Stage	Histologic change	Time (days)
1	Sparse inflammatory cellular infiltrate	0–1
2	Diffuse infiltration of leukocytes	1–4
3	Abundant granulation tissue	4–14
4	Formation of undifferentiated connective tissue	>14

mesotenon, and tendon sheath. These specialized structures are responsible for most of the segmental blood supply to most tendons (Lagergren & Lindholm 1958–1959, Schatzker & Brånemark 1969, Stein & Luekens 1976a).

A standard sequence of histologic changes occur after a tendon injury. The inflammatory process is the response of the body to tissue injury. This process involves neurologic, vascular, humoral and cellular reactions at the site of injury. The factors that influence the characteristics of this inflammatory response depend on the intensity and duration of insult, the type of injury (e.g. mechanical, bacterial, chemical or immunologic), the amount of cell degeneration and death (which ultimately influence the extent and progress of the inflammatory response), and the kinds of cells and tissues involved.

In acute inflammation, the dominant histologic changes are vascular and exudative with the emigration and accumulation of leukocytes. Chronic inflammation is characterized by proliferative changes as tissue attempts repair and healing (Allenmark 1992). The undifferentiated connective tissue that is formed may have changes of mucoid, fatty, hyaline, myxoid or fibrinoid degeneration, cartilage metaplasia, calcification, or bone metaplasia (Arner et al 1958–1959b, Lipscomb & Wakim 1961a, 1961b, Davidsson & Salo 1969, Fisher & Woods 1970, Burry & Pool 1973, Fox et al 1975, Clancy et al 1976, Puddu et al 1976, Gould & Korson 1980, Trevino et al 1981, Clancy 1982, Leadbetter 1992). Kannus & Jozsa 1991 assessed the pathologic changes noted in 891 spontaneously ruptured tendons. They noted hypoxic degenerative tendonopathy, mucoid degeneration, tendolipomatosis and calcifying tendonopathy. Arner et al (1958–1959b, 1959) described this orderly sequence of histologic changes in their classification of healing after rupture of the Achilles tendon (Table 3).

More recently Clancy et al (1976, 1982) used clinical findings to classify the inflammatory response as acute, subacute or chronic on the basis of temporal considerations, as follows: acute – symptoms present for less than 2 weeks; subacute – symptoms present for longer than 2 weeks but less than 6 weeks; and chronic – symptoms present for 6 weeks or longer.

Peritendinitis

There is much confusion in the literature regarding the proper terminology for inflammation about tendons. Puddu et al (1976) argued that the connective tissue of tendons, being dense and fibrous with little inherent vascularity, is not predisposed to inflammatory processes; hence, use of the term 'tendinitis' was inappropriate. Inflammatory processes can take place in the vascular peritendinous tissue. Lipscomb (1950) defined 'paratendinitis' as an inflammatory process about tendons or portions of tendons that possess no sheath; he used 'tenosynovitis' to refer to inflammatory processes about tendons with sheaths and used 'peritindinitis' as an inclusive term to denote either tenosynovitis or paratendinitis. Puddu et al (1976) introduced the term 'tendinosis', which they defined as degenerative lesions in tendon tissue with no evidence of alteration of the peritenon. Therefore, tendon disease could be manifested by pure peritendinitis, peritendinitis with tendinosis, or tendinosis alone. Peritendinitis with tendinosis or tendinosis alone may eventually result in rupture (Table 4).

Inflammatory processes involving tendons about the ankle are commoner than is generally believed. Lipscomb (1950) analysed 651 cases of nonspecific peritendinitis at the Mayo Clinic between 1935 and 1948. He described various types of peritendinitis (Table 5). Forty-eight percent of his cases involved the forearm, wrist and hand, 36% involved the ankle and foot, and 6% involved the long head of the biceps. The anatomic distribution of the involved tendons in the lower extremity was as follows: tibialis anterior, 24%; Achilles tendon,

Table 4 Classification of tendon inflammation

Peritendinitis: an inflammatory process involving
peritendinous structures
Paratendinitis: no synovial sheath
Tenosynovitis: synovial sheath
Peritendinitis with tendinosis: an inflammatory process
involving peritendinous structures with a
degenerative lesion of tendon tissue
Tendinosis: an asymptomatic degenerative process of
tendon tissue without inflammation

Table 5 Types of peritendinitis

Nonspecific	Infectious
Stenosing	Suppurative
Crepitans	Nonsuppurative
Hypertrophica	Tuberculous
Serosa chronica	Fungal
Arthritic	Syphilitic
Hypertrophic	Gonococcal
Rheumatoid	Neoplastic
Sarcoid	Xanthomatous
Gout	Lipomatous
Reiter's syndrome	Hemangiomatous
Collagen-vascular disease	Neurofibromatous
Scleroderma	

Table 6 Location of 143 tendon disruptions in the lower extremity

Muscle/tendon	Number	Percentage
Quadriceps	54	38
Achilles tendon	22	15
Triceps surae	21	15
Extensors of the toes	16	11
Tibialis anterior	10	7
Tibialis posterior	3	2
Flexor hallucis longus	3	2
Peroneus longus	2	1.5
Peroneus tertius	2	1.5
Others	10	7
TOTAL	143	100

20%; tibialis posterior, 16%; peroneals, 16%; and others, 24%.

The distribution and type of injuries that are occurring are changing as more people participate in jogging. Brody (1980) stated that 30% of the running-associated injuries he treated involved the knee, 20% involved the Achilles tendon, 15% were shin splints and stress fractures, and 10% were plantar fasciitis.

Rupture

McMaster's (1933) classic experiments with the tendons of rabbits showed that rupture does not occur when a normal muscle–tendon system is subjected to severe strain. Rupture occurred at one of four sites: tendon insertion into bone, musculotendinous junction, muscle belly, or tendon origin from bone. Approximately half of the fibers of a tendon had to be severed to permit immediate rupture when subjected to severe strain. Even when 75% of the fibers were severed, normal activity did not cause rupture. He concluded that true rupture of normal tendon does not occur and that rupture can take place only through diseased tendon substances.

When disease is mild, microscopic changes are minimal. More extensive inflammation may lead to gross thickening of the peritendinous sheath and enlargement and fraying of tendon. The final event in this process may result in a degenerated, fibrotic tendon that ultimately ruptures. Clancy et al (1976, 1982) classified these chronic inflammatory changes as interstitial microscopic failure, central necrosis, frank partial rupture, and acute complete rupture.

Microscopic damage to portions of the vascular supply of the tendon substance likely is an important factor in pathologic ruptures (Lagergren & Lindholm 1958–1959, Schatzker & Brånemark 1969). Other factors such as aging, degeneration and recurrent microtrauma are also contributory (Davidsson & Salo 1969). Clancy et al (1976, 1982) thought that repetitive mechanical stress results in disruption of the collagen fibrils and that subsequent chronic inflammatory changes permanently alter the capacity of fibroblasts to synthesize collagen; a vicious cycle is set up, and rupture finally ensues.

Anzel et al (1959) analysed 1014 disruptions of muscles or tendons in 781 patients from 1945 to 1954 at the Mayo Clinic. They found an incidence of approximately 70 disruptions per 100 000 patients per year. The upper extremity was involved six times more often than the lower extremity. The average age of the patients was 40.5 years. Males were affected more often than females for each type of injury.

Of the 1014 disruptions, approximately 60% were due to lacerations and 40% were due to all other causes (direct closed injury, stress rupture, and 'normal' activity). The anatomic distribution of the 143 injuries to the lower extremity is shown in Table 6.

As has been shown, tendon lesions about the foot are quite common but often present diagnostic problems. Swelling about a tendon may result from various pathologic conditions and even masquerade as neoplasm. Many times these 'pseudotumors' are unsuspected ruptures caused by underlying tendinosis and associated peritendinitis (Webster 1968, Jahss 1972, 1974, Fitzgerald & Coventry 1980). With increased awareness and recognition, the diagnosis of peritendinitis, rupture, and dislocation or subluxation will be more obvious.

Bursae

Anatomy

Synovial bursae are potential spaces with a secretory endothelial-type lining. These bursae are usually associated with joint cavities and are present at birth. They reduce friction and are usually located between the skin and bony projections (superficial or subcutaneous) and between tendons and the prominences over which they must move (deep or subfascial) (Kaplan & Ferguson 1937, Cherry & Ghormley 1941, Bywaters 1965).

Adventitial bursae are acquired, and they form in unusual locations after birth in response to repeated trauma (friction) to soft tissue over a bony prominence. These bursae have no true endothelial lining but rather seem to be a myxomatous or mucoid change of connective tissue. When a well-formed cyst is present, histologic study usually shows flattened fibroblastic cells rather than the secretory endothelial cells of synovial bursae (Kaplan & Ferguson 1937, Buck et al 1943, Kuhns 1943).

Jahss (1982b) classified bursae according to location and type (Table 7). Sarrafian (1983) and Hartmann (1981) provided excellent anatomic depictions and descriptions of the numerous bursae about the foot.

Bywaters (1965) stated that synovial bursae were a neglected class of anatomic structures of considerable importance 'subject to the same ills that joints are heir to'. This statement is probably most true for bursae about the foot and ankle, where Roberts (1929a, 1929b) believed that bursitis was a neglected cause of disability. Affliction of the various bursae about the foot was amply described in the early literature (Hertzler 1926; Roberts 1929a, 1929b) but it seems less well recognized in recent publications.

Bursitis

Various etiological classifications of bursitis have appeared in the literature. Meyerding (1938) thought that bursitis could be classified as acute or chronic, traumatic

---

Table 7 Types of bursae

Anatomic
    Subfascial
        Between tendon and bone
        Between tendon or muscle and a bony prominence
        Between tendons
    Between tendons and ligaments
    Subcutaneous
Adventitial
    Usually subcutaneous

Table 8 Classification of bursal irritation

Noninflammatory
    Pressure-induced
    Traumatic
    Spontaneous
Inflammatory
    Gout
    Rheumatoid arthritis
Suppurative
Calcified or ossified

---

or infectious, syphilitic, gouty, or malignant. He also mentioned tuberculosis, gonorrhea, and rheumatism as etiologic factors. Jones (1930) noted that when bursae become distended they are called bursal cysts or hygromas. Cherry and Ghormley (1941) modified and expanded on Meyerding's classification for further clarity. Jahss (1982b) also outlined a simple, workable classification of pathologic bursae (Table 8).

Any bursa about the foot can become inflamed by the mechanisms described above. Probably the commonest cause of chronic bursitis about the foot and ankle is increased pressure or friction over a bony area that leads to an adventitial bursa. Ill-fitting shoes often result in such a finding. This condition has been referred to eponymically as 'last bursitis' (Layfer, 1980). The bony prominences and tendons in and about the calcaneus, malleoli, metatarsophalangeal and interphalangeal joints, and dorsal and plantar surfaces of the foot are particularly susceptible to this condition. In most instances, symptomatic relief can be obtained by removing the pressure. Nonoperative means usually consist of modifications of footwear, such as a wider and deeper toe box, stretching the shoe at localized areas, softer heel counters, or various foot orthoses and pads.

Aspiration of an inflamed bursa may sometimes be helpful in decompressing the area and ruling out metabolic, rheumatoid or infectious causes (Nielson 1921, Patterson & Darrach 1937, Meyerding 1938, Sarma 1940). Corticosteroids can be injected locally when not contraindicated (such as in cases of sepsis) (Altman 1966, Helfand et al 1971).

Surgical measures usually relieve pressure by removing underlying exostoses or bony prominences or correcting an underlying deformity. An example of such a procedure is the removal of the medial eminence and connection of the metatarsus primus varus by means of a metatarsal osteotomy for bursal inflammation of a hallux valgus deformity. Surgery is usually performed only after failure of nonoperative methods.

Two bursal areas about the foot deserve special mention because the literature deals with them most extensively: bursa associated with the insertion of the Achilles tendon into the calcaneus and intermetatarsal bursa.

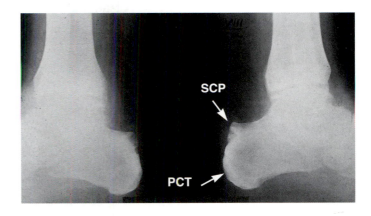

Figure 1

Radiograph of posterior calcaneus shows superior calcaneal prominence (SCP) and posterior calcaneal tuberosity (PCT)

Bursitis at the posterior part of the heel

Anatomy

Two separate bursae flank the Achilles tendon at its insertion: the superficial, subcutaneous bursa of the Achilles tendon and the deep, subfascial, retrocalcaneal bursa. The former is an adventitial bursa that forms in response to chronic trauma. This bursa lies superficial to the insertion of the Achilles tendon and is frequently, although not always, present. The deep, subfascial retrocalcaneal bursa is a synovial-lined structure that is constantly present; it is situated between the posterosuperior end of the calcaneus and the deep surface of the Achilles tendon.

Achilles tendon bursitis and retrocalcaneal bursitis

The clinical entity that manifests as irritation at the posterosuperior aspect of the heel may have various causes and has been variously referred to in the literature. It is important to distinguish anatomically between inflammatory lesions involving the subcutaneous and subfascial bursal structures at the insertion of the Achilles tendon (bursitis) and those of the peritendinous lining of the Achilles tendon (peritendinitis).

If the superficial, subcutaneous, adventitial bursa of the Achilles tendon is inflamed, tenderness will be palpable directly over the calcaneus at the tendon insertion. A noticeable bursal thickening may be present over the bony prominence lateral to the tendon attachment. This condition has been referred to as a 'pump bump' by some authors. Women are affected more often than men (Keck & Kelly 1965, Dickinson et al 1966). The formation of superficial bursitis of the Achilles tendon seems to be related to mechanical factors (i.e. chronic irritation from friction between the shoe and a prominence of the posterosuperior aspect of the calcaneus). This superficial

adventitial bursitis of the Achilles tendon is commoner than deep, subfascial retrocalcaneal bursitis (Keck & Kelly 1965).

If the deep, subfascial, synovial retrocalcaneal bursa is inflamed, tenderness is less well localized but it is usually anterior (deep) to the tendon. Frey et al (1992) have recommended retrocalcaneal bursograms to assist in the diagnosis and treatment of bursitis. Men are affected more often than women (Keck & Kelly 1965). Because of the synovial origin of this bursa, inflammation may be a prodrome of rheumatoid arthritis or one of its variants, such as Reiter's syndrome (Bywaters 1954, Keck & Kelly 1965, Brahms 1967, Palmer 1970, Weston 1970, Pavlov et al 1982, Canoso et al 1984, Heneghan & Pavlov 1984). Lateral radiographs of the calcaneus must be critically assessed for the presence of erosions suggestive of an inflammatory articular disorder. No conclusive evidence implicates a prominence of the superior portion of the calcaneal tuberosity as a major factor in producing retrocalcaneal bursitis (Keck & Kelly 1965).

Numerous authors have postulated that a prominent posterosuperior surface of the calcaneus may be a factor predisposing to bursal inflammation at the insertion of the Achilles tendon (Haglund 1928, Zadek 1939, Fowler & Philip 1945, Nisbet 1954, Steffensen & Evensen 1958, Fuglsang & Torup 1961, Keck & Kelly 1965, Dickinson et al 1966, Miller & Buhr 1969, Ruch 1974, Pavlov et al 1982, Heneghan & Pavlov 1984) (Fig. 1). This condition is particularly exacerbated by wearing high-heeled shoes or shoes with a closely contoured, rigid heel counter. Various angles, ratios, or other radiographic relationships, such as the parallel pitch line of Pavlov (Fig. 2), have been presented and are said to correlate with bursal abnormalities (Fowler & Philip 1945, Ferguson & Gingrich 1957, Steffensen & Evensen 1958, Pavlov et al 1982, Heneghan & Pavlov 1984).

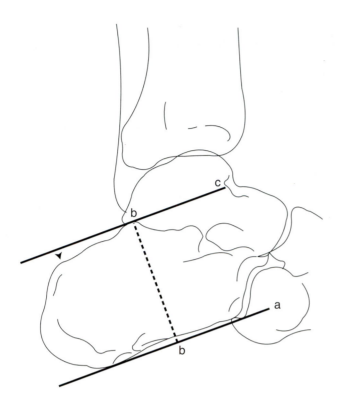

Figure 2

Parallel pitch line of Pavlov (c–b) is derived from inferior calcaneal pitch line (a–b). When superior calcaneal prominence (arrowhead) is superior to line c–b, a predisposition to retrocalcaneal bursitis is thought to exist

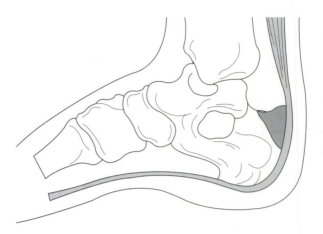

Figure 3

A large portion of the calcaneus needs to be excised surgically or symptoms will recur. (From Jahss 1991a with permission)

Pavlov et al (1982) and Heneghan and Pavlov (1984) radiographically characterized Haglund's syndrome by the presence of four features: retrocalcaneal bursitis; Achilles peritendinitis; superficial bursitis of Achilles tendon (pump bump); and cortically intact but prominent bursal projection of the posterosuperior aspect of the calcaneus, as seen on lateral radiographs. Although all four of these conditions may coexist, this is not always so.

Treatment

When superficial bursitis of the Achilles tendon is associated with a prominence of the superior part of the tuberosity of the calcaneus and is unresponsive to conservative measures, excision of the prominence may be necessary (Haglund 1928, Zadek 1939, Fowler & Philip 1945, Nisbet 1954, Steffensen & Evensen 1958, Fuglsang & Torup 1961, Keck & Kelly 1965, Dickinson et al 1966, Miller & Buhr 1969, Ruch 1974, Berlin et al 1982, Jones & James 1984) (Fig. 3). Keck and Kelly (1965) were cautious about recommending surgical resection of a calcaneal prominence in cases of retrocalcaneal bursitis because they thought that the bursitis may be a forerunner of rheumatoid arthritis. Nesse and

Finsen (1994) reported persistent heel pain in 12 of 35 heels treated with surgical resection. Injection of corticosteroids into the deep bursa, heel elevation, rest, and nonsteroidal anti-inflammatory drugs often provide relief. Occasionally, surgical extirpation of the bursa is necessary (Ippolito & Ricciardi-Pollini 1984).

Two basic types of surgery have been described. Haglund (1928) recommended resection of the most prominent portion of the posterosuperior aspect of the calcaneus. This can be combined with removal of the superficial or deep bursa. Zadek (1939) described a dorsally based wedge resection of the calcaneus in order to leave the posterior surface of the calcaneus intact. The surgical method for the posterior calcaneus may be either a medial or a lateral para-Achilles tendon approach or a direct posterior approach through the Achilles tendon (Fowler and Philip 1945). The foot is usually splinted for 2–4 weeks in a walking cast until healing is complete (Fig. 4).

Bursitis associated with intermetatarsophalangeal bursae

Anatomy texts do not devote much attention to the bursae associated with the web spaces of the foot. The intermetatarsophalangeal bursa lies between the metatarsophalangeal joints and is dorsal to the transverse metatarsal ligament, whereas the neurovascular bundle lies plantar to the ligament and courses dorsally as it passes distally to the end of the ligament. Bursae in the first, second and third web spaces are constant, whereas the bursa in the fourth web space is missing in 80% of cases (Hartmann 1981). Bossley and Cairney (1980), in a cadaveric and clinical study, found that the intermetatarsal bursa in the second and third web spaces extended 1 cm (1/3 inch) distally to the transverse

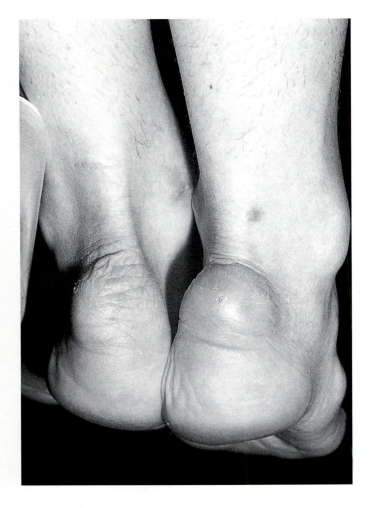

Figure 4
Inflammation secondary to pressure over posterosuperior prominence of calcaneus.

metatarsal ligament, whereas it lay at the same level as the distal margin of the transverse ligament in the fourth web space.

Intermetatarsal bursitis
Inflammation of the intermetatarsophalangeal bursa from any cause can be a source of pain in the forefoot in the region of the metatarsal heads. Classic Morton's metatarsalgia has been described as a clinical syndrome of pain under the metatarsal heads that often radiates to the toes and is sometimes associated with numbness (Scranton 1980). Symptoms are often exacerbated by walking in close-fitting shoes and are lessened when walking barefoot.

As pointed out by Bossley and Cairney (1980), because of the close proximity of the plantar digital nerve and the intermetatarsal bursa in the second and third web spaces, the classic symptoms of Morton's metatarsalgia could be caused not only by a neuroma but also by an intermetatarsophalangeal bursitis with pressure on a normal nerve.

Bursal swelling can often be detected clinically and radiographically by divergence of the toes bordering the affected web space (Shephard 1975). Lateral compression of the metatarsal heads squeezes the inflamed bursa, reproduces pain, and may cause a click. Because the intermetatarsophalangeal bursa is of synovial origin, its inflammation may be one of the first manifestations of rheumatoid arthritis in the foot (Palmer 1970; Shephard 1975). Radiographs should be closely inspected for any evidence of erosions of the metatarsophalangeal heads. The intermetatarsophalangeal bursa in patients with rheumatoid arthritis is often thick walled with lymphocytic infiltration, villous proliferation, fibrinoid necrosis, and the presence of 'rice bodies' (Jones 1930, Shephard 1975, Bossley & Cairney 1980).

Injection of hydrocortisone into the bursa often gives relief. Occasionally, surgical extirpation of the bursa is necessary.

Achilles tendon

The Achilles tendon (Fig. 5) will serve as the prototype for discussing peritendinitis and rupture. These two pathological processes can affect any tendon about the ankle. The peroneal tendons will serve as the prototype for discussing subluxation and dislocation, processes that seem to affect these tendons most often.

Peritendinitis and rupture

Pain in the Achilles tendon is a common problem, especially in runners (Snook 1972, Clancy et al 1976, Galloway et al 1992, Gould & Korson 1980, Kvist & Kvist 1980, Leach et al 1981, Ljungqvist & Eriksson 1982, Leach et al 1992). Disease of the Achilles tendon is likely to be a spectrum of manifestations on a continuum from peritendinitis to tendinosis to rupture (Clancy et al 1976, Puddu et al 1976, Gould & Korson 1980, Leach et al 1981, Clancy 1982). It is important to distinguish between bursitis at the posterior part of the heel, Achilles peritendinitis, and Achilles peritendinitis with tendinosis and partial rupture if one is to prevent partial rupture from becoming complete (Ljungqvist 1968, Snook 1972, Puddu et al 1976, Clancy et al 1976, Gillström & Ljungqvist 1978, Denstad & Roaas 1979, Gould & Korson 1980, Kvist & Kvist 1980, Leach et al 1981, Skeoch 1981, Clancy 1982, Ljungqvist & Eriksson 1982).

The diagnosis of acute, complete rupture should not be difficult because the history is very characteristic. Most published series, however, estimate that the diagnosis of complete rupture is missed in 20–25% of cases (Lawrence et al 1955, Arner & Lindholm 1959, Ralston & Schmidt 1971, Nillius et al 1976). This occurs because complete rupture, although not rare, is unfamiliar to

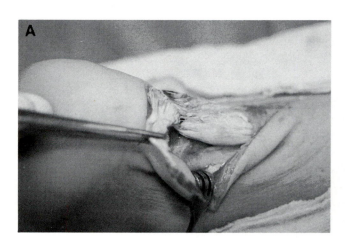
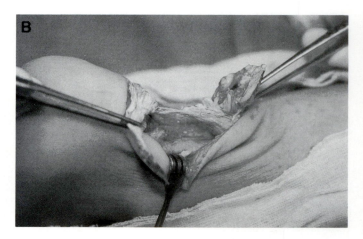
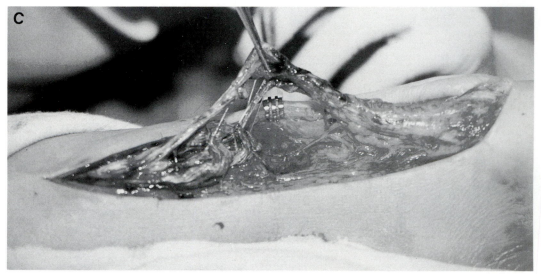

Figure 5

Examples of acute Achilles tendon ruptures. (a) Complete rupture with minimal fraying of the tendon. (b) Separation of the fragments, demonstrating lack of fraying of the tendon. (c) Achilles tendon rupture with marked fraying of the tendon

Table 9 Differentiating factors of peritendinitis, peritendinitis with tendinosis and partial rupture, and tendinosis with acute, complete rupture

Factor	Peritendinitis	Peritendinitis with tendinosis and partial rupture	Tendinosis with acute, complete rupture
Symptoms	Acute	Subacute, chronic	Immediate
Audible snap	No	Maybe	Yes
Weakness	Yes	Yes	Yes
Limp	Yes	Yes	Yes
Swelling	Yes	Yes	Yes
Tenderness	Yes	Yes	Yes
Defect in tendon	No	Maybe	Yes
Crepitus	Maybe	Maybe	No
Passive dorsiflexion	Decreased	Decreased	Increased
Thompson test	Negative	Negative	Positive
Atrophy	No	Yes	Proximal calf belly retraction
Ability to stand on tiptoes	Probably	Possibly	No

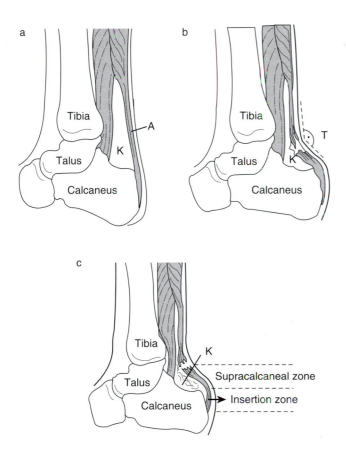

Table 10 Types of nonoperative treatment of peritendinitis

Patient education
    Proper warm-up, cool down
    Reduction or cessation of athletic activity
        No running on hills
        No interval training
        Avoidance of training on hard surfaces
Proper equipment
    Good running shoes (flexible, cushioned soles)
    Orthoses (heel lifts, University of California
    Biomechanics Laboratory [UCBL] inserts, inlays)
Physical therapy
    Massage
    Stretching exercises
    Ultrasound, heat, ice
Immobilization
    Taping
    Crutches
    Casting
Medication
    Nonsteroidal anti-inflammatory drugs
    Corticosteroid injections? (Kleinman & Gross 1983)

Figure 6

(a) Illustration of a lateral view of the ankle. Kager's triangle, K; the Achilles tendon, A. (b) Toygar's angle (T) has decreased and is less than 150°, which is characteristic of a ruptured Achilles tendon. Kager's triangle and the Achilles tendon are marked with K and A respectively. (c) Illustration of positive Arner's sign in a total Achilles tendon rupture. In the insertion zone of the Achilles tendon, the anterior contour of the ruptured tendon curves away from the calcaneus. Proximal to the upper part of calcaneus (the supracalcaneal zone), the anterior contour of the tendon shows a forward deviation and a nonparallelism of the tendon and the skin surface. Achilles tendon (A). Kager's triangle (K). (Taken from Cetti & Anderson 1993, with permission)

many physicians. Patients may minimize their symptoms after the acute pain, which is often associated with a 'snap'. Active plantar flexion is maintained because of the combined action of the peroneus longus, tibialis posterior, and long toe flexors. If a patient presents late, swelling and haemorrhage into the site of disruption may obscure the discontinuity at the rupture site (Lawrence et al 1955, Hooker 1963, Ralston & Schmidt 1971). The rupture usually occurs 2–6 cm (¾ –2⅓ inches) proximal to the insertion of the Achilles tendon, where vascularity has been shown to be decreased (Håstad et al 1958–1959, Lagergren & Lindholm 1958–1959) (Fig. 6). As the rupture becomes chronic, the defect in the tendon

becomes more difficult to palpate, but irregularity of the tendon can often be noted. Weakness in plantar flexion is the one constant finding, owing to lengthening of the tendon. Table 9 summarizes some of the differentiating findings of peritendinitis, partial rupture and complete rupture.

The Thompson calf squeeze test is very useful for the diagnosis of complete rupture (Thompson 1962, Thompson & Doherty 1962). If the calf muscles are squeezed just distal to their maximal girth, the foot invariably plantarflexes unless the soleus is detached from the Achilles tendon. A positive reaction, then, is no plantar movement of the foot, which indicates the complete rupture of the heel cord.

Some authors have suggested that a lateral radiograph or xerogram of the soft tissue may reveal subtle findings. Kager (1939) and Toygar (1947) analyzed the reliability of these techniques. Kager described what has been called Kager's triangle. This space is filled with fatty tissue bounded by the margins of the Achilles tendon, the calcaneus, and the deep flexors. When the Achilles tendon is ruptured, the triangle loses its regular configuration. Toygar suggested the value of measuring the angle of the posterior skin surface as visualized on the roentgenogram because the ends of the tendon are displaced anteriorly after rupture; the angle becomes 130–150°. This angle and the decrease of Kager's triangle were considered virtually diagnostic by Toygar.

In their series of 39 patients, Arner et al (1958–1959a) found that deformation of Kager's triangle was very nonspecific and that Toygar's sign rarely was positive (Fig. 6). Cetti & Anderson (1993) found Kager's triangle to be positive in 60 consecutive patients with operative verification of complete Achilles tendon ruptures. Hattrup & Johnson (1985) found these tests to be useless and considered X-ray studies as only of secondary importance to physical examination for the diagnosis of Achilles tendon rupture. Bursography, electromyography and computed tomography may be helpful for the diagnosis of partial ruptures (Ljungqvist & Eriksson 1982, Frey et al 1992). Although Kalebo et al (1992) found that ultrasound had a specificity of 0.94, a sensitivity of 1.00, and an overall accuracy of 0.95, this author has found the usefulness of ultrasound to be highly technician-dependent. Magnetic resonance imaging scans have demanded recent attention as the most useful means by which partial Achilles tendon ruptures can be graded (Weinstable et al 1991, Ferkel et al 1991).

Treatment

Peritendinitis

The initial treatment of inflammatory lesions should be nonoperative (Table 10). Operation is generally indicated only in a patient who is unresponsive to nonoperative treatment for several weeks or months (Snook 1972, Clancy et al 1976, Denstad & Roaas 1979, Kvist & Kvist 1980, Lea 1981, Leach et al 1981, Skeoch 1981, Clancy 1982). Surgical treatment usually consists of exploration and excision of the diseased peritendinous structures and resection of any diseased or degenerated tissue. The latter method may require some form of surgical reconstruction of the tendon.

Rupture

More than 400 articles have been published about rupture of the Achilles tendon (Barfred 1973). A great area of controversy is the proper treatment of this condition (Lancet Editorial, 1973). Some investigators favor surgical repair and postoperative casting (Jessing & Hansen 1975, Inglis et al 1976, Percy & Conochie 1978, Jacobs et al 1978, Schedl & Fasol 1979, Scott et al 1979, Edna 1980, Rubin & Wilson 1980, Leach 1982), surgical repair and postoperative functional bracing (Carter et al 1992), and others favor casting alone (Lea & Smith 1968, 1972, Gillies and Chalmers 1970, Nistor 1976, 1981, Stein & Luekens 1976a, 1976b, Lea 1981). For years, casting in an equinus position to minimize tension at the site of injury was the accepted treatment; now, this approach has come into question. Häggmark & Eriksson (1979) described selective atrophy of the soleus muscle if tension is not kept on the musculotendinous unit during healing.

Table 11 Considerations in the choice of treatment of acute rupture of the Achilles tendon

Consideration	Type of treatment	
	Nonoperative (casting alone)	Operative (operation and casting)
Morbidity	Decreased	Increased
Surgical risk	None	Increased
Hospital stay (cost)	Decreased	Increased
Dynametric data	Inferior	Superior
Rerupture	10%	2%
Compliance with rehabilitation	Less	More

Proponents of closed treatment state that the underlying reason for the success of this method is the ability of the Achilles tendon to reconstitute itself when severed. This trait has been shown both experimentally and clinically (Lipscomb & Wakim 1961a, 1961b, Saunders et al 1978, Lennox et al 1980, Taylor 1981). They also claim that the functional differences in strength, power and endurance are not statistically significant between patients treated operatively and those treated nonoperatively (Lea and Smith 1972, Lea 1981, Nistor 1981). The nonoperative approach avoids the risks of anesthesia and the complications of open operation. Nistor (1981) reviewed 25 reports, with a total of 2647 ruptures, in which surgical complications were recorded. The following major complications were noted: fistulas, 3%; necrosis of skin and tendon, 2%; rerupture, 2% and deep infection, 1%. Minor complications included haematoma, superficial infection, granulomas, and skin adhesions, and occurred in 5% of the cases. Although rare, death from pulmonary embolus has been reported after surgical repair (Arner & Lindholm 1959). The major drawback of the closed technique is a reportedly higher incidence of rerupture and questionably inferior dynametric data (Inglis et al 1976, Jacobs et al 1978, Shields et al 1978, Scott et al 1979, Edna 1980, Brown et al 1981, Nistor 1981, Taylor 1981).

The nonoperative technique is uncomplicated (Lea & Smith 1968, 1972, Lea 1981). It consists of gravity equinus casting for 8–12 weeks with cast changes at monthly intervals to gradually increase the amount of dorsiflexion. Casting is followed by heel elevations and possibly a double upright ankle–foot orthosis with a stop at the neutral position for an additional 4–8 weeks (Taylor 1981).

Advocates of open surgical treatment have a sound biomechanical rationale. An immediate repair that allows

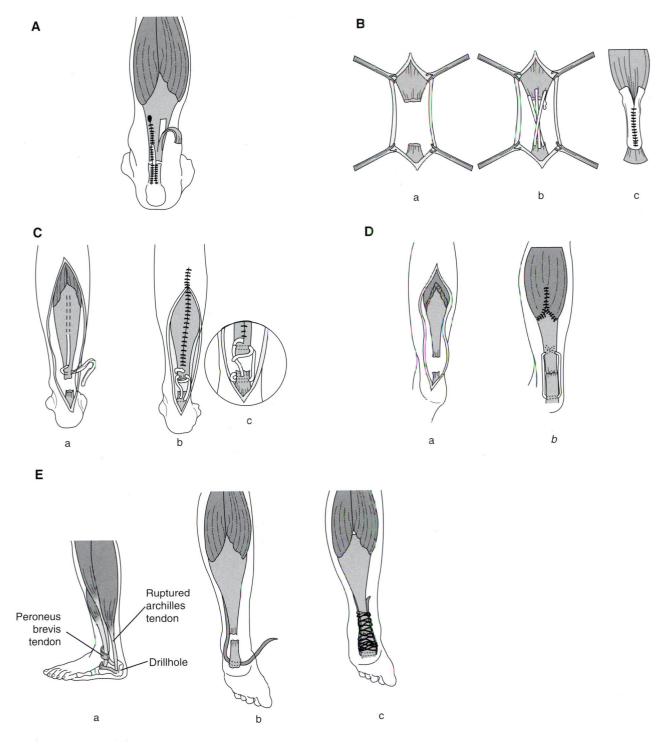

Figure 7

Various methods of reconstruction for untreated Achilles tendon ruptures. (A) One or two strips of fascia from the gastrocnemius–soleus complex may be turned down and used to reinforce the repair. (B) Repair utilizing fascia lata strips (a). Rupture with gap; (b) three fascial strips used to bridge the gap; (c) a sheet of fascia used to cover and reinforce the repair. (C) Repair utilizing fascial strip from proximal gastroc–soleus complex. (a) Distally based fascial strip is passed transversely through proximal tendon fragment. (b) The strip is woven across the gap. (c) Enlarged diagram of (b). (D) Repair using V–Y gastroplasty. (a) A V-shaped incision is made in the aponeurosis. The limbs of the V should be one and a half times longer than the width of the gap in the Achilles tendon. (b) The intermediate segment is advanced distally and the gap is closed and repaired. The proximal incision is closed as a Y in the lengthened position. (E) Repair utilizing peroneus brevis tendon. The peroneus brevis is isolated and detached from its insertion into the fifth metatarsal. (a) A transverse drill hole is placed in the calcaneus. (b) The peroneus brevis is transferred through the drill hole. (c) The tendon is sutured to itself and to the Achilles tendon proximally and distally. (Taken from Mann & Coughlin 1993, with permission. B redrawn from Bugg & Boyd 1968; C redrawn from Bosworth 1956; D redrawn from Abraham & Stirnaman 1975)

closure of the gap will keep the musculotendinous unit at its proper physiological length:tension ratio (Ma & Griffith 1977, 1981). Theoretically, this treatment should provide better strength than the scar tissue that forms if the gap is not closed. This added strength should ultimately lead to a decreased rate of rupture.

The advantages of operation in patients with a delay in diagnosis are less clear (Lennox et al 1980). Owing to retraction of the proximal stump, the gap often cannot be closed without lengthening the tendon (Abraham & Pankovich 1975, Fish 1982). In such cases, the biomechanical advantage of immediate repair is lost. Rather than performing a repair procedure in such cases, one is sometimes faced with a rather difficult reconstruction to close the gap (Bosworth 1956, Arner & Lindholm 1959, Lindholm 1959, Bugg & Boyd 1968, Goldman et al 1969, Teuffer 1974, Quigley & Scheller 1980, Taylor 1981). The literature abounds with methods of repair (Lynn 1966, Ma & Griffith 1977, 1981, Schedl & Fasol 1979, Cetti & Christensen 1983) and reconstruction (Bosworth 1956, Arner & Lindholm 1959, Bugg & Boyd 1968, Goldman et al 1969, Teuffer 1974, Abraham & Pankovich 1975, Quigley & Scheller 1980, Taylor 1981, Fish 1982).

Several prospective studies assess the results of surgical and nonsurgical treatment of ruptured Achilles tendons. Nistor (1981) concluded that nonoperative treatment offers advantages over operative treatment (Table 11). Wills et al (1986) reviewed the literature, comparing surgical treatment with nonoperative management and found a 1.54% rate of rerupture (12 out of 777) for surgically treated patients versus a 17.7% (40 out of 226) rate of rerupture for nonoperatively treated patients. These authors concluded that the difference in cost between surgical and nonoperative treatment, including the cost of rerupture treatment, may not be significant.

Cetti et al (1993) randomly assigned 111 patients to groups for operative (56 patients) or nonoperative (55 patients) treatment. In the operative group, he noted three reruptures and two deep infections. In the nonoperative group, there were seven reruptures, one second rerupture, and one extreme residual lengthening of the tendon. In addition, he noted a higher rate of resuming sports activities, less calf atrophy and better ankle motion in the operative group.

The ultimate decision as to which form of treatment is used must be individualized and depends on the physician, the patient and the circumstances. Probably, the persons who benefit most from operative treatment are high performance athletes.

Surgical treatment for acute, complete injuries is best treated by direct suturing with buried stitches. If the rupture occurs near the calcaneal attachment, the use of a pullout wire may be helpful (Mann & Coughlin, 1993). A percutaneous method of repair in which the strength of the repair compares favorably with the standard open repair has been described (Ma & Griffith 1977). This technique attempts to bridge the gap between non-

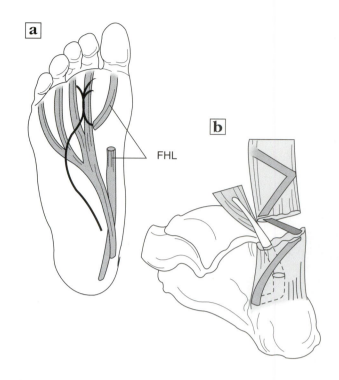

Figure 8

Autogenous tendon graft for treatment of ruptured Achilles tendon. (a) The distal portion of the flexor hallucis longus (FHL) is anastomosed into the flexor digitorum longus tendon. The proximal portion is then freed up of any interconnections and retracted from the posterior incision. (b) A drill hole is placed just deep to the Achilles insertion and directed plantarward. A second drill hole is made from medial to lateral to intersect the first drill hole midway through the posterior body of the calcaneus. These are then interconnected using a towel clip. The flexor hallucis longus tendon is transferred from proximal to distal

surgical and surgical treatment. In a series of 18 patients, minor wound infection developed in only two patients and there were no reruptures. This procedure has received enthusiastic reports; however, some investigators who have attempted to duplicate this procedure have met with technical difficulties, and one report had a 12% rerupture rate (Bradley & Tibone 1990). FitzGibbons et al (1993) reported comparable cybex assessments in 14 patients following percutaneous repair. They noted no infections, no delayed wound healing, and no reruptures, but one sural nerve was injured. Aracil et al (1992) reported one sural nerve injury and two early reruptures in five patients treated by the Ma & Griffith technique. They concluded that since the tendon is not fully visualized, inadequate opposition may result. The results of percutaneous repair are acceptable, with recovery of motion and strength essentially equal to open surgery. The rate of rerupture is higher than with open procedures, but probably better than with closed treatment.

For neglected or undiagnosed ruptures of the Achilles tendon, various methods of reconstruction have been advocated to achieve tendon continuity and close any gap of scar tissue between ruptured tendon ends. End-to-end anastomosis is very difficult because of proximal muscle contraction. Various methods of reconstruction to span the gap between ruptured tendon ends have been described (Fig. 7). For uncomplicated reconstructions, a lengthening of the tendon at the musculotendinous junction in a V-Y manner, resection of the diseased tendon, and direct suturing is recommended. After operation the immobilization is similar to that used for the nonoperative approach.

For complicated chronic or neglected rupture of the Achilles tendon in a patient who presents with pain, weakness and significant gap between ruptured tendon ends, or previously failed surgery, an autogenous tendon graft to span the gap may be necessary. The author's preferred method requires the use of the flexor hallucis longus tendon as popularized by Wapner et al (1993) (Fig. 8). Complications following this type of reconstructive surgery may be higher than for primary repair of an acute Achilles tendon rupture because of the amount of scar tissue and the extensive dissection that is necessary. Sural nerve injury and wound-healing problems are commoner. However, the results can be gratifying because the marked lack of endurance and strength in patients with a neglected Achilles tendon rupture is usually unacceptable.

Tibialis posterior tendon

Anatomy

The tibialis posterior tendon passes in front of the flexor digitorum longus muscle in the lower one-quarter of the leg and then behind the medial malleolus under the flexor retinaculum, and it is the most anteromedial structure behind the malleolus. Just beyond the medial malleolus, the tendon changes direction acutely. It passes through a shallow groove in the medial malleolus that is not sufficient to keep the tendon from bowstringing. The flexor retinaculum serves as a tether that prevents subluxation of the tendon out of its groove behind the malleolus. The strong unyielding retinaculum blends with the tibialis posterior tendon sheath and superficial deltoid ligament. The tendon courses under the plantar calcaneonavicular ligament and inserts into the tuberosity of the navicular bone, the underside of the cuneiform bone and the bases of the second, third and fourth metatarsals. One expansion passes backward to the sustentaculum tali. The sheath of this tendon is 7–9 cm (2¾–3½ inches) long and extends about 6 cm (2⅓ inches) above the malleolus. There is an area of relative hypovascularity of the tendon posterior and distal to the

medial malleolus. This may contribute to degenerative changes and be a predisposing factor in attrition leading to rupture (Frey et al, 1990).

By virtue of its lever arm length from the axis of the talocalcaneal joint and its muscle strength, this muscle–tendon unit is the main dynamic stabilizer of the hindfoot against valgus (eversion) deformity (Kaye & Jahss, 1991). A tear of the tibialis posterior tendon therefore imposes excessive stress on the static ligament–bone hindfoot constraints. With loss of the muscle power, the soft tissue gradually elongates and pain develops.

Peritendinitis

Clinical Features
In 1936, Kulowski first mentioned tenosynovitis of the sheath of the tibialis posterior tendon. This condition was also noted by Lipscomb (1950), who stated that it occurred in about 16% of cases of tensynovitis and peritendinitis of the feet and ankles. Other sporadic reports have appeared in the literature (Ghormley & Spear 1953, Fowler 1955, Williams 1963, Cozen 1965, Langenskiöld 1967, Norris & Mankin 1978, Lipsman et al 1980, Trevino et al 1981, Fredenburg et al 1983).

Myerson et al (1989) described two discrete groups of patients with idiopathic inflammation or rupture of the posterior tibial tendon or both. The first group of patients were younger (mean age 39 years) and had multiple manifestations of inflammation at other sites of ligament and tendon attachment (enthesopathy). Other features of a systemic inflammatory disorder such as oral ulcers, conjunctivitis, colitis, and psoriasis were common in patients and their families. The second group consisted of predominantly elderly patients (mean age 64 years) with isolated dysfunction of the posterior tibial tendon, suggesting mechanical factors leading to attrition and degeneration of the tendon in its hypovascular bone.

Rupture
Rupture of the tibialis posterior tendon is a cause of the painful acquired flatfoot deformity in adults (Goldner et al 1974, Henceroth & Deyerle 1982, Gould 1983, Johnson 1983, Mann 1983, Mueller 1984, Mann & Thompson 1985, Funk et al 1986). Although rupture of the tibialis posterior tendon has been described previously, the frequency of this problem has become more evident in recent years (Kulowski 1936, Key 1953, Williams 1963, Langenskiöld 1967, Kettelkamp & Alexander 1969, Goldner et al 1974, Trevino et al 1981, Jahss 1982a, Mann & Specht 1982, Johnson 1983, Mann & Thompson 1985, Funk et al 1986, Johnson & Strom 1989). This deformity is commonly described as being traumatic (Giblin 1980, De Zwart & Davidson 1983), degenerative, or spontaneous in origin (Henceroth & Deyerle 1982). Possibly a combination (Kettelkamp & Alexander 1969) of all three factors results in the disruption. The peritendinitis that

Table 12 Changes associated with various stages of posterior tibial tendon dysfunction (from Johnson & Strom 1989)

	Stage 1	Stage 2	Stage 3
TPT condition	Peritendinitis and/or tendon degeneration	Elongation	Elongation
Hindfoot	Mobile, normal alignment	Mobile, valgus position	Fixed, valgus position
Pain	Medial: focal, mild to moderate	Medial: along posterior tibial tendon, moderate	Medial: possibly lateral, moderate
Single-heel-rise test	Mild weakness	Marked weakness	Marked weakness
'Too-many-toes' sign with forefoot abduction	Normal	Positive	Positive
Pathology	Synovial proliferation, degeneration	Marked degeneration	Marked degeneration
Treatment	Conservative, 3 months; surgical, 3 months with synovectomy, tendon debridement, rest	Transfer flexor digitorum longus for posterior tibial tendon	Subtalar arthrodesis

has been described (Kulowski 1936, Lipscomb 1950, Key 1953, Langenskiöld 1967, Trevino et al 1981) may be a secondary reaction to a tendon tear. Another possibility is that deformity causes tenosynovitis (Cozen 1965).

The etiology of posterior tibial tendon rupture remains unclear, but it has been associated with obese middle-aged women with a pre-existing tendency toward pes planus. An epidemiologic study by Holmes & Mann (1992) attempted to define associated or predisposing factors. The study substantiated the association with late middle-aged population (average age 57 years). Seventy-five per cent of patients had significant identifiable systemic or local vascular risk. Age, hypertension, obesity, diabetes, traumatic disruption of local blood supply (antecedent injury or surgery) and the administration of corticosteroids were factors that were felt to contribute to vascular compromise and subsequent tendon rupture.

The history, symptoms, and signs of rupture of the tibialis posterior tendon are so typical that, once understood, they allow the correct diagnosis to be made readily. Previous acute trauma of a substantial degree usually cannot be recalled by a patient although tendon rupture in such cases has been reported (Kelbel & Jardon 1982, De Zwart & Davidson 1983, Stein 1985, Schaffer et al 1987, Søballe & Kjaersgaard-Anderson 1988, Monto et al 1991, Woods & Leach 1991, Burton & Page 1992). The deformity of the foot gradually evolves and becomes painful. More females than males are affected, and patients are usually over 40.

Pain and tenderness are present but are only mild to moderate in degree. Early tenderness along the course of the tendon from just distal to the medial malleolus to its infranavicular insertion may predominate. The pain is

not incapacitating; rather, it is a chronic medial weight-bearing ache that limits activities. Later, as the deformity progresses into the foot, the discomfort also commonly involves the lateral tarsal region. Swelling just medial to the hindfoot is an early sign; it is most evident when viewed posteriorly and compared with the noninvolved foot.

Deformity is the hallmark of the rupture of the tibialis posterior tendon and it gradually increases over a few months to years. The concurrent development of hindfoot valgus and forefoot abduction produces the so-called flatfoot. The hindfoot valgus, which can be mild to marked, is best evaluated from the posterior view. Although best appreciated from a frontal view, the presence of forefoot abduction can be suspected and clinically quantitated from the posterior view by being aware of the 'too many toes' sign. When a patient faces directly away from the observer, too many toes will be visible lateral to the patient's heel area when forefoot abduction is present.

Loss of function of the tibialis posterior tendon is best evaluated by using the single heel-rise test. The tendon must be used to bring the hindfoot into a locked, stable varus position. This position is necessary before the patient can easily rise up on the ball of the foot with the power of the gastrocnemius–soleus muscle. The single heel-rise test on the affected side is positive when, with an attempt to go up on the ball of the affected foot with the contralateral foot raised, the hindfoot does not assume a stable varus position and only with difficulty can the heel be even slightly raised off the ground.

Dysfunction of the posterior tibial tendon evolves through a series of stages described by Johnson and Strom (1989) (Table 12). In stage 1 disease, the tendon length is normal and the primary manifestations of dysfunction relate to peritendinitis of the tendon as it courses around the medial malleolus. There is mild weakness without secondary foot deformity. In stage 2 disease, the tendon has elongated with the hindfoot mobile in a valgus position. Patients exhibit more physical findings with marked weakness, more deformity, and increased pain along the course of the tendon. In stage 3 disease, the elongated tendon has given way to complete rupture, resulting in a fixed hindfoot valgus deformity, which is the most prevalent change. The tendon itself may be less painful because of complete disruption, and symptoms may be noted laterally over the sinus tarsi area where impingement occurs as the hindfoot goes into eversion.

Radiographic findings

Routine lateral and anteroposterior radiographic views of the foot will show pronounced changes in cases of rupture of the tibialis posterior tendon in stage 3 disease. As the head and neck of the talus rotate medially and inferiorly off the calcaneus, the forefoot distal to the talus deviates laterally. Thus, the talocalcaneal angle is increased, and a break at the talonavicular articulation is seen on a lateral view. From an anteroposterior view, an increase of the talocalcaneal angle is evident, and subluxation at the talonavicular articulation is present.

Plain radiographs of the foot and ankle in stage 1 or 2 disease may not be helpful. Magnetic resonance imaging (MRI) is a very sensitive diagnostic technique, effective in assessing the integrity of tendons (Alexander et al, 1987). More recently a detailed classification of posterior tibial tendon rupture based on MRI findings has been presented (Conti et al 1992). The MRI classification system separated posterior tibial tendon degeneration into three grades, 1 to 3. Grade 1 had longitudinal splits without attenuation or intramural degeneration; grade 2 demonstrated splits, attenuation and intramural degeneration, and grade 3 showed diffuse swelling of the tendon, uniform degeneration and near-complete to complete rupture. In this study MRI classification correlated with duration of symptoms and degree of deformity and was more predictive of outcome in surgical reconstruction than surgical evaluation of tendon dysfunction at the time of surgery.

Treatment

As with many musculoskeletal conditions, rupture of the tibialis posterior tendon can be treated nonoperatively or operatively.

Nonoperative

Rest provided by crutches or a cast, anti-inflammatory agents, or shoe modifications such as inserts or heel and sole lifts, or splinting the ankle with a lightweight ankle foot orthosis (AFO) may all be used to palliate tears of the tibialis posterior tendon. Probably the only nonoperative method that is not indicated is an injection of corticosteroids into the tendon itself. In fact, however, these noninvasive means, while providing some relief, should be considered as non-treatment for moderate to severe deformity. Factors such as advanced age, other medical problems, a low level of activity, and only minimal discomfort may frequently make a nonoperative approach the most prudent.

Operative

If chronic synovitis is present and the tendon is not disrupted, then only a tenosynovectomy and sheath division may be necessary (Goldner & Irwin 1949, Cozen 1965, Langenskiöld 1967, Wrenn 1975).

In a paper presented by Teasdall et al (1993), surgical release, tenosynovectomy and debridement where appropriate for stage 1 posterior tibial tendon dysfunction appeared to interrupt the progression of posterior tibial tendon peritendinitis to stage 2 and 3 disease (Johnson classification, 1989). In their study, 84% of the patients reported subjective responses of being 'much better' and no patients reported being 'worse' after surgery. In the more frequent situation in which restoration of the function of the tendon or foot alignment (or both) is thought to be indicated, the operative procedure depends on the site and the extent of the tear, the duration and the severity of the deformity, and factors such as the expectations of the patient and physician. Different surgical procedures have been described in treating posterior tibial tendon dysfunction (Johnson 1989, Jahss 1991a, Mann and Coughlin 1993).

An end-to-end suture can be used when the tear involves a relatively short portion of the tendon, usually just distal to the medial malleolus (Goldner et al 1974). Although occasionally tendon reapproximation is all that may be necessary, augmentation with a tendon transfer as described below is usually performed (Johnson 1989). If the tear involves the tendon insertion to the underside of the navicular bone, then a reattachment (Goldner et al 1974) through a drill hole is more appropriate. During surgical exposure of the tendon, the surgeon may find an apparently intact tendon. If, however, the exposure is carried distally to the navicular attachment, the separation from the bone can almost invariably be seen. Reinsertion of this avulsed tendon detachment into the navicular generally does not result in improvement unless it is augmented by a tendon transfer as described below (Funk et al 1986, Johnson 1989).

Most commonly, however, the tear involves a long segment of degenerated tendon that cannot be brought together. In such cases, the gap can be bridged by tendon transfer (Key 1953, Fowler 1955, Kettelkamp & Alexander 1969). Because of its size, strength, and availability, the flexor digitorum longus rather than the flexor hallucis longus is used (Johnson 1983, Mann & Thompson 1985, Goldner 1985, Funk et al 1986, Wapner et al 1994). The segment of affected tendon is bridged, and function is restored. Although the flexor digitorum longus transfer was originally attached distally by a tenodesis to healthy tibialis posterior tendon, we now prefer to insert it directly into the navicular bone through a drill hole. The last step of tenodesis of the distal stump of the flexor digitorum longus to the adjacent flexor hallucis longus is optional, because lesser toe flexion will be provided to a degree by the intact flexor digitorum brevis and perhaps by the quadratus plantae as well as other intrinsic muscles of the foot.

A study by Conti et al (1992) suggests that higher grade lesions as documented by preoperative MRI may have greater risk of failure when treated by posterior tibial tendon reconstruction. Failure was defined as postoperative progression of pain and deformity which required subsequent arthrodesis. Surgical treatment of type 1 MRI lesions had an 87.5% success rate for tendon reconstruction at an average follow-up of 25.6 months. Conversely only 63.6% of MRI type 2 ruptures that were similarly treated were successful at an average of 19 months. Type 3 MRI tears usually presented with hindfoot deformities too advanced to warrant reconstruction. The overall trend appears clear. The long-term outlook is guarded with respect to transfer for posterior tibial tendon insufficiency in types 2 and 3 lesions. It appears that patients with early posterior tibial tendon dysfunction with a supple foot and minimal if any deformity would benefit from early synovectomy and tendon transfer (Conti et al 1992, Teasdall et al 1993).

If the foot deformity is severe, supporting tissues are stretched and secondary degenerative arthritic changes are evident, an arthrodesis is the only reasonable surgical procedure. The triple arthrodesis, which involves the talonavicular, calcaneocuboid and talocalcaneal joints, has been the traditional operative treatment of hindfoot deformity. A triple arthrodesis is indicated when there is a fixed valgus deformity of the subtalar joint, fixed abduction of the transverse tarsal joint or a fixed varus deformity of the forefoot. An isolated subtalar fusion is utilized when there is a fixed deformity of the subtalar joint and a supple, easily correctable transverse tarsal joint and no fixed forefoot deformity. A double arthrodesis (talonavicular and calcaneocuboid) may be utilized when the transverse tarsal joint is flexible and the forefoot can be brought back into a plantigrade position. Graves et al (1993) reported a higher incidence of arthrosis in adjacent joints following triple arthrodesis in adults. This study suggests caution and judicious restraint when performing this operation.

If surgical treatment is chosen, the specific procedure used will depend on the anatomic presentation of the tendon deficit and stage of disease. Unless a better soft tissue reconstruction is developed, arthrodesis may become the treatment of choice in the intermediate and late stages of disease. In more active patients, soft tissue procedures provide the best opportunity to return to previous level of function.

Dislocation

Although emphasis has been on peritendinitis and rupture, other reports involving cases of dislocation or subluxation of the posterior tibial tendon remind us that other pathology must be considered (Nova 1968, Langan & Weiss 1980, Larsen & Lauridsen 1984, Soter et al 1986, Stanish & Vincent 1989, Biedert 1992, Ouzounian & Myerson 1992, Waldrop et al 1992). Posterior tibial tendon dislocation occurs most commonly in younger patients. An injury precipitates dislocation in almost all reports with the exception of one patient treated with multiple steroid injections and another who had undergone a prior tarsal tunnel release. The diagnosis of posterior tibial tendon dislocation is not straightforward and is frequently delayed. In the seven cases reported by Ouzounian and Myerson (1992), five of the patients were treated for an ankle sprain. Although conservative treatment was attempted, none of the patients in this series responded. In most cases, the retinaculum was repaired and in some cases this repair was augmented or reinforced with local tissue. Dislocation of the posterior tibial tendon is infrequent compared with that of the peroneal tendons or posterior tibial tendon rupture, but the diagnosis should be considered in younger patients with persistent medial ankle pain following even minor trauma. MRI is helpful in documenting the dislocation and distinguishing this entity from rupture.

Peroneal tendons

Reports in the literature of peroneal involvement with peritendinitis, rupture, and dislocation are sparse. Peritendinitis and traumatic dislocation are thought to be commoner than recognized, and spontaneous rupture is rare. All of these entities may be causes for persistent lateral ankle pain and swelling, which are most commonly thought to be residual of disruption of the lateral ligaments and ankle instability (Sobel et al 1993).

Anatomy

The tendons of the peroneus longus and brevis enter a common synovial sheath 4 cm (1½ inches) proximal to the lateral malleolus. They pass under the superior retinaculum and behind the lateral malleolus within this common sheath. A fibro-osseous tunnel restrains these tendons posterior to the lateral malleolus. The most important restraining anatomic structure proximally is the superior retinaculum. Also present distally along the posterior lip of the lateral malleolus is a fibrocartilaginous ridge (Marti 1977). The retromalleolar sulcus was described in detail by Edwards (1928); in 82% of cases it is very shallow, and in 18% of cases there is no well-formed sulcus.

Proximal to the peroneal trochlea of the calcaneus, the tendons enter separate sheaths. Each sheath is covered by the inferior retinaculum, and extension of the cruciate crural ligament, at the level of the peroneal trochlea. The sheath about the peroneus brevis extends to within 1 cm (⅓ inch) of the insertion of the tendon into the tuberosity at the base of the fifth metatarsal. The other sheath, enveloping the tendon of the peroneus longus as it passes from the plantar aspect of the peroneal trochlea, ends as it glides to the undersurface of the cuboid. A second sheath envelops the peroneus longus as it emerges from the canal formed by the long plantar ligament and cuboid groove.

The anatomy of additional peroneal muscles (i.e. peroneus quartus, the peroneus accessorius, and the peroneus digiti minimi) is nicely described in the study by Sobel et al (1990). The most important of these is the peroneus quartus, present in 21.7% of cadaver specimens. The size, origin, and insertion of this muscle takes its origin from the muscular portion of the peroneus brevis in the lower third of the leg and inserts on the peroneal tubercle of the calcaneus. The clinical relevance of this tendon is that it can be used for reconstructive procedures about the lateral aspect of the ankle, such as in anterior dislocation of the peroneal tendons and reconstruction of the lateral ankle ligaments (Mick 1987). Its use in these applications can avoid problems related to sacrificing the peroneus brevis tendon, which can result in restricted inversion of the foot or compromised eversion of the foot associated with loss of the peroneus brevis muscle.

Peritendinitis

Several articles have addressed nonspecific and post traumatic peroneal tenosynovitis (Burman 1953, Parvin & Ford 1956, Webster 1968, Fitzgerald & Coventry 1980, Trevino et al 1981). The commonest type of tenosynovitis is stenosing tenosynovitis. The peroneal tendon may become stenosed at three anatomic sites (Burman 1953): posterior to the lateral malleolus (peroneal sulcus), at the peroneal trochlea (tubercle) of the calcaneus, and at the under surface of the cuboid bone.

Trauma is the major factor attributed to precipitating tenosynovitis about the peroneal tendon sheath. Lateral malleolar fractures and inversion ankle injuries, direct trauma to the peroneal tubercle, and calcaneofibular impingement of the peroneal tendon sheaths (Isbister 1974a, 1974b) have been associated with stenosing tenosynovitis.

Burman (1956) and Pierrson (1992) reported that a congenitally enlarged peroneal tubercle or a sesamoid bone in the peroneus longus could be inciting factors. Burman also believed that nontraumatic acquired lesions, such as compressive tenosynovitis or tenosynovitis as a manifestation of arthritis, were possible etiological factors.

Sobel et al (1994) reported 10 patients treated for plantar lateral foot pain. They used the term 'painful os peroneum syndrome' to describe the entity. They considered that attrition, partial rupture, frank rupture of the peroneus longus tendon or the presence of a gigantic peroneal tubercle were partially responsible for the pain.

Clinical features

Pain and swelling inferior to the lateral malleolus with point tenderness over the peroneal tendons at the inferior peroneal retinaculum are suggestive of peritendinitis. Symptoms are exacerbated by forced plantar flexion and inversion. A patient may relate a history of increased pain when walking barefoot or on rough terrain. Physical examination reveals an antalgic gait, limitation of subtalar motion, and point tenderness. The diagnosis of peroneal peritendinitis is enhanced if the pain is relieved by injections of local anesthetic into the tendon sheath. Peroneal tenography may show either complete block or constriction of the sheath at the inferior peroneal retinaculum (Fitzgerald & Coventry 1980, Teng et al 1984). Pseudotumor formation of the peroneal tendons may also be visible at the level of the inferior peroneal retinaculum. This finding should not be confused, however, with enlargement of the peroneus longus distally by the os peroneum.

Treatment

Treatment options are similar to those outlined for the Achilles tendon. Nonoperative measures consist of rest, anti-inflammatory agents, stretching exercises, physical therapy, and possibly injections of corticosteroids. A medial heel wedge, custom-made foot orthosis, or shoes with a rocker-bottom sole and cushioned heel may diminish calcaneofibular impingement of the peroneal tendon sheath. If these measures are unsuccessful, surgical exploration and tenolysis may be advisable. Subtalar arthrodesis is recommended if significant degenerative changes exist at the subtalar joint.

Rupture

Closed, subcutaneous rupture of one or both of the peroneal tendons is rare but has been reported (Burman 1956, Evans 1966, Munk & Davis 1977, Abraham & Stirnaman 1979, Tehranzadeh et al 1984) (Fig. 9). In most case reports, the patients have initially been treated nonoperatively with the measures outlined above including casting for 6–8 weeks. Because the chronic lateral ankle pain and swelling persisted despite an adequate trial of nonoperative treatment, the above authors recommend surgical intervention for a presumed diagnosis of chronic lateral ligamentous instability or tenosynovitis of the peroneal sheath. In either case, a partial or complete

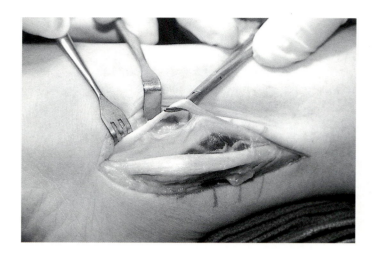

Figure 9

Longitudinal tear of peroneus brevis tendon where it changes direction inferior to lateral malleolus

rupture of the peroneal tendon(s) was discovered with pathological changes suggestive of peritendinitis, tendinosis, or both.

It is interesting to speculate as to how and why these tendons tend to develop longitudinal tears as they change direction around soft tissue or, more commonly, bony fulcrums. One idea is that the tendon does not compensate for the difference in the distance traveled in the outer compared with the inner tendon sides and so develops shear stress. Bassett (1993) reported impingement of the peroneus longus against the tip of the fibula in 15 cadaveric specimens when the ankle is plantar flexed 15–25° while held in inversion. It has been suggested that a zone of vascular compromise may result in the tendon as a result of compression loads near bony fulcrums. Sobel et al (1992) were unable, however, to demonstrate such zones.

Chronic longitudinal attrition or rupture of the peroneus brevis tendon at or distal to the fibular groove of the lateral malleolus is a commoner degenerative defect than previously recognized (Larsen 1987, Sammarco 1988, Sobel 1990, 1991). This lesion was noted in 11.3% of specimens and the longitudinal rupture averaged 1.9 cm (¾ inch) in length (Sobel 1990). The significance of this finding is that chronic lateral ankle pain disability may be related to attritional changes of the peroneus brevis tendon in the fibular groove. The etiology of this defect is probably secondary to the compressional wedge-like frictional force of the overlying peroneus longus tendon against the splayed-out peroneus brevis tendon as it passes around the lateral malleolus in the fibular groove with tendon excursion.

Diagnosis of peroneal tendon tears

In a clinical series of 47 ankle ligament reconstructions, peroneus brevis tendon lesions were observed in 11

ankles of 10 patients (Tudisco 1984). All patients had a history of chronic recurrent ankle sprains with symptoms of pain more disabling than instability. At the time of surgery there was gross evidence of chronic inflammation associated with through-and-through defects on the deep aspect of the tendon. None of the patients had any evidence of arthritis, steroid injections, infections, or connective tissue disorders. There was often a history of significant trauma to the ankle with abnormal repetitive stress to the peroneus brevis tendon over a long period of time.

The possibility of chronic longitudinal attritional rupture of the peroneus brevis tendon should be considered in patients with chronic lateral ankle pain, swelling, instability, or symptoms suggestive of stenosis. MRI is the diagnostic test of choice, both to assess longitudinal attrition of the peroneus brevis tendon and to identify the presence of the peroneus quartus tendon, which may be useful in lateral ankle ligament reconstruction (Sobel 1990).

Rupture of the peroneus longus tendon through a fracture of the os peroneum sesamoid or distal to the sesamoid bone adjacent to the cuboid tunnel has been surgically documented only a few times (Peacock 1986, Thompson 1989). Several mechanisms have been offered to account for this lesion: rupture of the tendon associated with peritendinitis, a crush injury due to a direct blow to the area of the os peroneum on the lateral aspect of the foot, pushing off with the foot in inversion, or increased stress where the tendon changes direction at the cuboid tunnel.

Careful examination of the radiographs with multiple views to distinguish an avulsion fracture of the cuboid from the os peroneum, as well as differentiate an os peroneum fracture from a congenitally multipartite os peroneum, is important. Serial radiographs, especially with opposite comparison views, are extremely helpful in identifying an abnormal position of the sesamoid bone or migration.

Treatment

Initially most patients with chronic lateral ankle pain and swelling are treated nonoperatively with nonsteroidal anti-inflammatory medication, restricted activity, and immobilization or strapping. If symptoms persist and are disabling enough in spite of casting for 6–8 weeks, surgical intervention may be suggested, as it has been for a presumptive diagnosis of chronic lateral ligamentous instability or tenosynovitis of the peroneal sheath.

In the cases described where surgery took place, either partial or complete rupture of the peroneal tendon(s) was discovered with pathologic changes suggestive of peritendinitis, tendinosis or both. Surgical repair consisted of tenolysis, excision of diseased tendon tissue, end-to-end repair if possible, or tenodesis of the peroneus longus and brevis tendons. Follow-up revealed satisfactory results.

Table 13 Gradations of dislocations of the peroneal tendons (from Ogden 1987 and Mann & Coughlin 1993)	
Type	Characteristics
1	The retinaculum is still attached to the periosteum on the posterior aspect of the fibula; however, the periosteum is elevated from the underlying malleolus by the dissecting tendons that are displaced anteriorly
2	The retinaculum is torn free from its anterior insertion on the malleolus, and the periosteum of the tendons dissects through at this level
3	The retinaculum is avulsed from the insertion on the malleolus with avulsion of a small fragment of bone
4	The retinaculum is torn from its posterior attachment as the tendon dissects through, with the retinaculum lying deep to the dislocating peroneal tendon

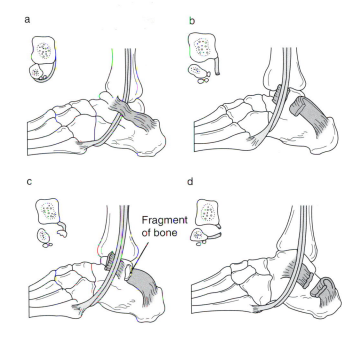

Figure 10

Gradations of dislocations of the peroneal tendons. (a) Retinaculum is still intact, although it is elevated from the underlying malleolus. (b) Retinaculum is torn from its anterior insertion on the malleolus, permitting dislocation of the peroneal tendons. (c) Retinaculum is avulsed from the insertion on the malleolus with a small fragment of bone. (d) Retinaculum is torn from its posterior attachment, permitting the tendon to dislocate over the retinaculum. (Redrawn from Ogden 1987)

These reports emphasize the importance of considering peritendinitis and rupture of the peroneal tendons in the differential diagnosis of any patient with chronic lateral ankle pain.

Traumatic dislocation

Dislocation of tendons about the ankle is uncommon. Although traumatic dislocation of the posterior tibial tendon is rare (Larsen & Lauridsen 1984), this injury may be commoner in the peroneal tendons than is recognized. It is usually associated with various athletic activities, most commonly skiing, soccer and ice skating, and less commonly basketball and the various codes of football (Murr 1961, Stover & Bryan 1962, Sarmiento & Wolf 1975, Marti 1977, Zoeliner & Clancy 1979, McLennan 1980, Savastano 1980, Cohen et al 1983). Inherent predisposition to peroneal tendon subluxation has been associated with the presence of an anomalous peroneus brevis muscle and osteochondromas (Mizuro 1991, Sobel 1992).

Peroneal dislocation is classified as acute or chronic. Acute injuries are often not recognized as anterior dislocations of the peroneal tendons and are misdiagnosed as 'ankle sprains'. If a patient is not examined when the tendons are dislocated and they have already returned to their retromalleolar groove, a missed diagnosis is common. Because the acute injury is often undiagnosed, lack of adequate treatment often results in chronic dislocations. Most of the literature deals with operations designed to treat patients with chronic dislocations (Kelly 1920, Jones 1932, Miller 1967, Platzgummer 1967, Sarmiento & Wolf 1975, Zoellner & Clancy 1979, Arrowsmith et al 1983, Poll & Duijfjes 1984, Pozo & Jackson 1984, Mann 1986).

Classification

In 1976, Eckert & Davis reported their surgical experience with 73 acute anterior dislocations of the peroneal tendon with injury to the peroneal retinaculum. They described three specific types of injury. Ogden (1987) modified the classification of Eckert & Davis by adding a rare type 4 tear of the peroneal retinaculum (Table 13 and Fig. 10).

Certain anatomic variants have been suggested to predispose the peroneal tendons to subluxation or dislocation (Stover & Bryan 1962). These variants include absence of the posterior fibular groove (11% of cases), convex surface to the posterior fibula (7% of cases), and laxity (either congenital or acquired) of the retinaculum (Edwards 1928). In Edwards' study (1928), 82% of the

178 fibulas that were examined had a groove, but it was usually very shallow – 2–3 mm in the dry, clean bone.

Clinical features

Most authors believe that this injury is the result of sudden, forceful, passive dorsiflexion of the inverted foot with reflex contraction of the peroneal tendons and plantar flexors (Murr 1961, Stover & Bryan 1962, Eckert & Davis 1976). This injury occurs if the ski tips dig in and the skier falls forward by deceleration. Escalas et al (1980) believed that the forceful contraction of the peroneal tendons as a skier digs the inner border of the ski into the snow when making turns also enhanced the risk of dislocating these tendons.

A history of a snapping sensation accompanied by pain in the posterolateral ankle is usually given (Eckert & Davis 1976). Characteristic swelling and tenderness occur posterior and superior to the lateral malleolus (Murr 1961, Eckert & Davis 1976, Escalas et al 1980, McLennan 1980, Savastano 1980, Arrowsmith et al 1983). The more common ankle sprain involving the anterior talofibular ligament manifests itself with swelling more distal and anterior to the lateral malleolus. Injury to the posterior talofibular ligament may elicit point tenderness similar to that of an acute dislocation. Stressing the retinaculum by eliciting dorsiflexion against resistance with the foot in plantar flexion and eversion causes retromalleolar pain and may result in dislocation. The findings of a grade 3 injury and a rim avulsion fracture of the lateral malleolus are considered pathognomonic of tendon dislocation (Mortiz 1959, Murr 1961, Stover & Bryan 1962). Of course, lateral ankle instability must be considered in the differential diagnosis for any patient with significant lateral ankle trauma, and stress views to determine the presence of talar tilt must be obtained when indicated. The combination of lateral ankle instability with peroneal tendon injury is rare but it has been reported. When it is present, use of the Christman–Snook procedure for lateral ankle instability with dislocation of the peroneal tendons has been reported (Sobel 1990).

Peroneal tenograms may show leakage of the contrast dye anteriorly. Computed tomography has also been reported to be of value for the evaluation of peroneal tendon dislocation (Szczukowski et al 1983). In the final assessment, however, unless the dislocation is seen when the patient is first examined or can be reproduced on examination, the diagnosis of acute anterior dislocation is uncertain and can only be suspected.

Chronic dislocation of the peroneal tendons should present less diagnostic difficulty. The history of a sense of uneasiness, giving way, or snapping at the ankle, especially when walking on uneven ground, is highly suggestive. Retinacular structures that are lax secondary to recurrent dislocations should be discernible on physical examination. Observation of the opposite uninjured ankle is helpful.

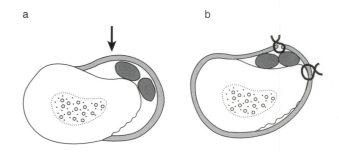

Figure 11

Diagram of a transverse section of the distal end of the left fibula viewed from above. (a) False pouch formed by stripping of the periosteum from the lateral malleolus in continuity with the superior peroneal retinaculum. Arrow denotes the site for incision in the retinaculum. (b) Normal anatomy is restored by obliteration of the false pouch and closing the incision in the peroneal retinaculum. (Redrawn from Das De & Balasubramanium 1985)

Treatment

Nonoperative treatment of the acute injury is controversial (Stover & Bryan 1962, Eckert & Davis 1976, Marti 1977, Escalas et al 1980, McLennan 1980, Savastano 1980, Arrowsmith et al 1983). Strapping techniques or well-molded, non-weight-bearing casts for 5–6 weeks are the usual methods. The rationale behind this is that holding the tendons reduced in an anatomic position heals the superior peroneal retinaculum by scarring. The ankle is replaced in mild plantarflexion to relax the tendons.

Stover & Bryan (1962) reported the results in 19 patients with acute injuries. Five of the 19 patients treated with non-weight-bearing casts had excellent results and no evidence of recurrent dislocation. Ten patients were treated with strapping techniques. Follow-up data were obtained for nine of these patients; six had recurrent dislocation, and four of the six had subsequent operations. They concluded that a well-molded, non-weight-bearing cast for 5–6 weeks was the initial treatment of choice. They thought that elastic strapping techniques were inadequate, especially if followed by early weight bearing.

Eckert & Davis (1976) stated that their experiences with closed treatment were disappointing. Hence, they treat all acute injuries operatively. They believe that if a lesion is determined to be grade I, closed treatment may be adequate. Oden et al (1987) believed that types 1 and 3 injuries should be treated with cast immobilization for 6 weeks to allow primary healing.

McLennan (1980) reported the results in a mixed series of acute and chronic dislocations. He concluded that the morbidity associated with nonoperative treatment is minimal and that this approach may be satisfactory in most cases (56%). He thought operative treatment may be indicated for acute injuries in athletes. Nonoperative

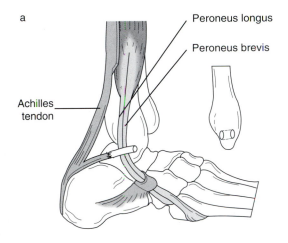

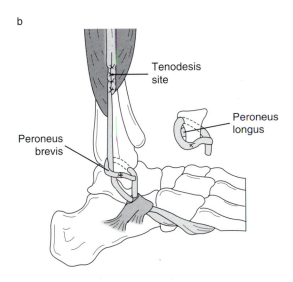

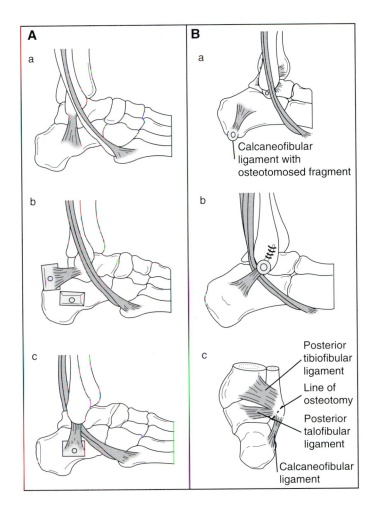

Figure 12

Reconstruction of peroneal retinaculum. (a) Ellis–Jones reconstruction of peroneal retinaculum employing the Achilles tendon. (b) Allmans' modification of the Evans lateral ankle reconstruction. (Redrawn from Arrowsmith et al 1983)

Figure 13

Techniques for rerouting the peroneal tendons under the calcaneofibular ligaments. (A) bone block from the calcaneus. (a) Tendons dislocated anteriorly. (b) Bone block mobilized from the calcaneus. (c) Tendons relocate with the ligament transposed over the tendons, and bone block fixed back in position. (Redrawn from Pöll & Duijfjes 1984.) (B) bone block from the fibular. (a) Diagram demonstrating the line of the osteotomy through the fibula. (b) Osteotomized fibular fragment attached to the calcaneofibular ligament. (c) Peroneal tendons are rerouted beneath the fibula and the osteotomized fragment reduced and internally fixed. (Redrawn from Pozo & Jackson 1984)

treatment seemed effective in cases that demonstrated stability against dislocation after an acute injury.

Most authors believe that recurrent, symptomatic, documented peroneal dislocations should be treated operatively (Kelly 1920, Jones 1932, Murr 1961, Miller 1967, Sarmiento & Wolf 1975, Zoellner & Clancy 1979, McLennan 1980, Arrowsmith et al 1983). Operation consists of soft tissue procedures to reconstruct the peroneal retinaculum, bony procedures to reconstruct the peroneal retinaculum, bony procedures to deepen the retromalleolar groove, or a combination of the soft tissue and bony procedures.

Techniques of surgical treatment for subluxing peroneal tendons include the following:

1. Direct repair or reattachment of the peroneal retinaculum (Fig. 11).
2. Reconstruction of the peroneal retinaculum (Fig. 12).
3. Bone block procedures.
4. Groove-deepening procedures with osteoperiosteal flaps.
5. Rerouting procedure of the peroneal tendons under the calcaneofibular ligaments (Fig. 13).

Extensor tendons of the foot and ankle

Peritendinitis

There are few reports of peritendinitis affecting the extensor tendons about the dorsum of the foot. In Lipscomb's review (1950), the tibialis anterior tendon was the most frequently involved, and the extensor digitorum longus was often affected. Tenosynovitis of these tendons is thought to be secondary to irritations by shoes, boots or skis. Rest, modification of footwear that impinges on the dorsum of the foot, and physical therapy usually suffice for treatment. Incision of the synovial sheath in front of the ankle is necessary only occasionally.

Rupture

Disruption of the extensor tendons about the dorsum of the foot and ankle is an infrequent injury, usually the result of an open wound or laceration (Lipscomb & Kelly 1955, Anzel et al 1959, Griffiths 1965, Floyd et al 1983). Closed subcutaneous rupture has been reported in the tibialis anterior tendon and extensor hallucis longus tendon, but this condition is much less frequent than the open lacerations involving the extensor tendons.

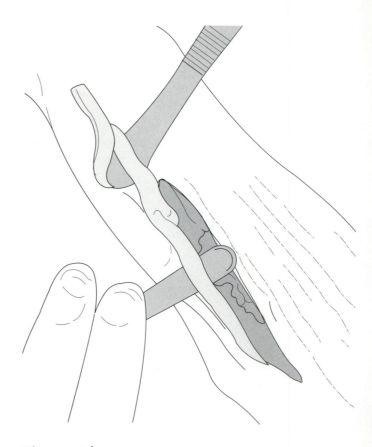

Figure 14

Turndown of portion of extensor hallucis longus to span gap

Tibialis anterior tendon

Closed subcutaneous rupture of the tibialis anterior tendon rarely appears in the literature (Burman 1934, 1943, Lapidus 1941, Moberg 1947, Mensor & Ordway 1953, Moskowitz 1971, Meyn 1975, Dooley et al 1980, Rimoldi 1991). The patients have almost always been men over 56. Rupture usually occurs after minimal or insignificant trauma that consists of forced plantar flexion against actively contracting dorsiflexors.

Clinical features

Patients often present with weakness of the ankle and swelling about the dorsum of the foot and ankle. If a patient presents late the pain is minimal, and the patient is left with minor degree of footdrop. Three cases of rupture of the tibialis anterior tendon have been reported in which the patient was thought to have an underlying neurological lesion: a peroneal palsy in two cases and an acute L5 radiculopathy the other (Moskowitz 1971, Meyn 1975).

Active dorsiflexion of the ankle may produce some eversion, and attempted inversion is weak. Discontinuity of the tendon may reveal a gap with no signs of a palpable tendon distally.

Treatment

The literature seems to favor surgical reattachment of closed rupture of the tibialis anterior tendon if a patient is active and presents within 3–4 months of the injury (Mensor & Ordway 1953, Dooley et al 1980). In patients who are treated nonoperatively, the tendon usually scars down more proximally and results in less ankle motion in dorsiflexion and less strength. However, in elderly patients who lead sedentary lives, the gait is almost always functionally normal and nonoperative treatment is thus justified (Meyn 1975, Dooley et al 1980).

Extensor hallucis longus and extensor digitorum longus

Incidence

In 1959, Anzel et al reported the incidence of tendon and muscle disruptions in a large series of patients examined at the Mayo Clinic. Disruptions of the toe extensors occurred in 16 patients and accounted for 11% of the 143 injuries to the lower extremity. All of these injuries were open lacerations. Griffiths (1965) described 20 patients with tendon injuries about the ankle. Nine patients had involvement of the extensor hallucis longus or extensor digitorum longus; only one patient had a closed disruption secondary to erosion by rheumatoid tissue. Floyd et al (1983) published a retrospective review of 80 patients with open injuries of various tendons about the foot and ankle. Of the 46 patients for whom follow-up data were obtained, 13 had laceration of the extensor hallucis longus and eight had lacerations of the extensor digitorum longus. Few reports have documented closed subcutaneous rupture or dislocation of the extensor hallucis longus or extensor digitorum longus (Sim & Deweerd 1977, Akhtar & Levine 1980).

Treatment

Generally, an aggressive surgical approach is advocated for open lacerations of tendons about the foot, especially in children (Lipscomb & Kelly 1955, Griffiths 1965, Wicks et al 1980, Floyd et al 1983). This treatment includes thorough debridement and exploration to define the extent of the injury, followed by anatomic restoration whenever possible. Griffiths (1965) alluded to the well-known tendency of the extensor tendons for spontaneous repair after tenotomy for clawtoe deformity. He therefore suggested that formal repair of the extensor hallucis longus may be unnecessary. This view is also shared by Wicks et al (1980). Floyd et al (1983), however, concluded that firm recommendations against repair of any specific tendon could not be supported by the literature and recommended surgical repair of both the extensor hallucis longus and the extensor digitorum longus, when possible. A turndown technique is possible if substance loss has occurred (Fig. 14).

Flexor hallucis longus

Several reports about lacerations of the flexor hallucis longus have been published, but until recently only a few reports have concerned other problems that affect this tendon (Reinherz 1984). The consensus regarding lacerations of the flexor hallucis longus is that they should be repaired primarily (Frenette & Jackson 1977, Yancey 1977, Wicks et al 1980, Floyd et al 1983). Frenette & Jackson (1977) also suggested that if both flexor hallucis brevis and flexor hallucis longus are divided and the proximal flexor portion of the longus could not be retrieved, the distal stump of the flexor hallucis longus could be sewn to the proximal stump of the brevis. Patients should be told that after repair of the flexor hallucis longus tendon, active flexion of the interphalangeal joint may not be possible. This does not seem to present any serious inconvenience or functional

problem. Although the studies are small and not conclusive in favor of either surgical or conservative treatment, attempts to repair the flexor hallucis longus tendon in cases of laceration or rupture seem justified.

Closed rupture of the flexor hallucis longus has been described, though it is distinctly uncommon. Sammarco & Miller (1979) described two cases of partial rupture of the central fibres of the flexor hallucis longus in classical ballet dancers. Krackow (1980) described one case of an acute, complete, traumatic rupture of the flexor hallucis longus in combination with a rupture of the Achilles tendon in a patient injured in a diving accident. Holt (1990) reported a complete rupture of the flexor hallucis longus tendon in a long-distance runner. All cases were surgically repaired. Thompson et al (1994) reported flexor hallucis longus rupture in a middle-aged women with no history of trauma or systemic disease. Repair in this case was achieved by tenodesis to the flexor digitorum longus above and below the fibroosseous tunnel.

Stenosing tenosynovitis

Several reports have described stenosing tenosynovitis of the flexor hallucis longus (Sammarco & Miller 1979, Gould 1981, Hamilton 1982, McCarroll et al 1983, Tudisco & Puddu 1984). Stenosing tenosynovitis occurs most often when a tendon with its surrounding peritendinous structures passes through or around a restricted fibro-osseous space. In the flexor hallucis longus, stenosis has been reported as occurring at three anatomic sites: within the flexor tendon sheath behind the medial malleolus; at the fibro-osseous tunnel on the posterior aspect of the talus between the medial and lateral tubercles; and distally as the tendon passes through the sesamoid bones and inserts into the terminal phalanx of the great toe. As a result of stenosis at each of these sites, 'triggering' can occur in the great toe.

Stenosis at the posteromedial ankle

Aetiology

Stenosis at the posterior process of the talus or sustentaculum tali of the calcaneus may result from fractures in this region, but it has more commonly been associated with ballet dancers (Sammarco & Miller 1979, Hamilton 1982), who, because of the unnatural position of the foot and ankle when in the *pointe* position, develop a tenosynovitis at the posteromedial ankle. McCarroll et al (1983) reported triggering of the great toe caused by entrapment of the flexor hallucis longus tendon within the flexor tendon sheath posterior to the medial malleolus. Moorman et al (1992) also attributed an aberrant flexor hallucis longus muscle within this sheath as a cause for triggering.

Clinical features

The symptoms may be similar to those described for posterior tibial peritendinitis. Pain, swelling, tenderness and crepitus may be present behind the medial malleolus. Triggering and locking of the great toe associated with a pop or snap in the posteromedial aspect of the ankle as the foot is brought into plantar flexion and the hallux is actively flexed are diagnostic of stenosing tenosynovitis of the flexor hallucis longus. If pain is present on forced plantar flexion of the foot and ankle, one must consider posterior impingement or block of the ankle joint caused by an os trigonum (Hamilton 1982, Howse 1982). The pain from this posterior impingement syndrome is most commonly posterolateral, but it should not be confused with peroneal peritendinitis (Burman 1953, 1956, Munk & Davis 1977, Fitzgerald & Coventry 1980, Trevino et al 1981). Lateral radiographs with the foot and ankle in maximal plantar flexion may reveal this abnormality.

Hamilton (1982) also described 'pseudohallux rigidus' and 'functional hallux rigidus'. In the former, the flexor hallucis longus becomes adhesive within its sheath, and movement of the hallux is restricted. In the latter, abnormal distal insertions of muscle fibres of the flexor hallucis longus become bound in the fibro-osseous tunnel at the posterior aspect of the talus and restrict dorsiflexion of the hallux when the knee is in full extension and the ankle is maximally dorsiflexed.

Stenosis at the great toe

Gould (1981) described nine patients with stenosis of the flexor hallucis longus as it passes through its sheath between the sesamoid bones of the great toe. This area is subject to repetitive impact loading, especially in runners, and may predispose to fractures or sesamoiditis. Laceration and subsequent scarring of the flexor hallucis longus can also occur in this area (Frenette & Jackson 1977). If the sheath of the flexor hallucis longus at the great toe is injured, it may heal in a constricted position and result in limited tendon excursion.

Clinical features

Pain in the sesamoid area and inability to flex the interphalangeal joint of the great toe actively when the metatarsophalangeal joint is stabilized in the neutral position are suggestive of stenosis in this area. Radiographs, including sesamoid views, may be helpful in ruling out fractures, cysts or arthritis.

Treatment

The considerations for treatment of peritendinitis of the flexor hallucis longus are the same as those described for peritendinitis of other tendons. The mainstays of nonoperative treatment are rest, stretching, physical therapy, nonsteroidal anti-inflammatory drugs and possibly corticosteroids. For stenosis distally, Gould (1981) described trying to break adhesions in the sesamoid area by inflating the tendon sheath with infiltration of 1% lidocaine. If an adequate trial of nonoperative treatment is unsuccessful, tenolysis, as described previously, may be used. Proximal lesions are usually approached from the posteromedial aspect of the ankle with a curvilinear incision.

References

Abraham E, Pankovich A M 1975 Neglected rupture of the Achilles tendon: treatment by V-Y tendinous flap. J Bone Joint Surg 57A: 253–255

Abraham E, Stirnaman J E 1975 Neglected rupture of the Achilles tendon. J Bone Joint Surg 57A: 253–255

Abraham E, Stirnaman J E 1979 Neglected rupture of the peroneal tendons causing recurrent sprains of the ankle: case report. J Bone Joint Surg 61A: 1247–1248

Akhtar M, Levine J 1980 Dislocation of extensor digitorum longus tendons after spontaneous rupture of the inferior retinaculum of the ankle: case report. J Bone Joint Surg 62A: 1210–1211

Albert E 1893 Achillodynie. Wiener Medizinische Presse 34: 41–43

Alexander I J, Johnson K A, Berquist T H 1987 Magnetic resonance imaging in the diagnosis of disruption of the posterior tibial tendon. Foot and Ankle 8: 144–147

Allenmark C 1992 Partial Achilles tendon tears. Clin Sports Med 11: 759–769

Altman D 1966 Managing bursitis in podiatry. J Am Podiatry Assoc 56: 408–410

Anzel S H, Covey K W, Weiner A D, Lipscomb P R 1959 Disruption of muscles and tendons: an analysis of 1,014 cases. Surgery 45: 406–414

Aracil J, Pina A, Lozano JA, Torro V, Escriba I, 1992 Percutaneous suture of Achilles tendon ruptures. Foot Ankle 13: 350–351

Arner O, Lindholm Å 1959 Subcutaneous rupture of the Achilles tendon: a study of 92 cases. Acta Chir Scand (Suppl) 239: 1–51

Arner O, Lindholm Å, Lindvall N 1958–1959a Roentgen changes in subcutaneous rupture of the Achilles tendon. Acta Chir Scand 116: 496–500

Arner O, Lindholm Å, Orell S R 1958–1959b Histologic changes in subcutaneous rupture of the Achilles tendon: a study of 74 cases. Acta Chir Scand 116: 484–490

Arrowsmith S R, Fleming L L, Allman F L 1983 Traumatic dislocations of the peroneal tendons. Am J Sports Med 11: 142–146

Barfred T 1973 Achilles tendon rupture: aetiology and pathogenesis of subcutaneous rupture assessed on the basis of the literature and rupture experiments on rats. Acta Orthop Scand (Suppl) 152: 1–126

Bassett F H, Speer K P 1993 Longitudinal rupture of the peroneal tendons. Am J Sports Med 21: 354–357

Berlin D, Coleman W, Nickamin A 1982 Surgical approaches to Haglund's disease. J Foot Surg 21: 42–44

Biedert R 1992 Dislocation of the tibialis posterior tendon. Am J Sports Med 20: 775–776

Bossley C J, Cairney P C 1980 The intermetatarsophalangeal bursa – its significance in Morton's metatarsalgia. J Bone Joint Surg 62B: 184–187

Bosworth D M 1956 Repair of defects in the tendo Achillis. J Bone Joint Surg 38A: 111–114

Bradley J P, Tibone J E 1990 Percutaneous and open surgical repairs of Achilles tendon ruptures: a comparative study. Am J Sports Med 18: 188–195

Brahms M A 1967 Common foot problems. J Bone Joint Surg 49A: 1653–1664

Brody D M 1980 Running injuries. Clin Symp 32(4): 2–36

Brown T D, Fu F H, Hanley E N Jr 1981 Comparative assessment of the early mechanical integrity of repaired tendo Achillis ruptures in the rabbit. J Trauma 21: 951–957

Buck R M, McDonald J R, Ghormley R K 1943 Adventitious bursas. Arch Surg 47: 344–351

Bugg E I Jr, Boyd B M 1968 Repair of neglected rupture or laceration of the Achilles tendon. Clin Orthop 56: 73–75

Burman M 1943 Subcutaneous strain or tear of the dorsiflexor tendons of the foot. Bull Hosp Jt Dis Orthop Inst 4: 44–50

Burman M 1953 Stenosing tendovaginitis of the foot and ankle: studies with special reference to the stenosing tendo-vaginitis of the peroneal tendons at the peroneal tubercle. Arch Surg 67: 686–698

Burman M 1956 Subcutaneous tear of the tendon of the peroneus longus: its relation to the giant peroneal tubercle. Arch Surg 73: 216–219

Burman M S 1934 Subcutaneous rupture of the tendon of the tibialis anticus. Ann Surg 100: 368–372

Burry H C, Pool C J 1973 Central degeneration of the Achilles tendon. Rheumatol Rehabil 12: 177–181

Burton P D, Page B J 1992 Fracture of the neck of the talus associated with a trimalleolar ankle fracture and ruptured posterior tibial tendon. J Orthop Trauma 6: 248–251

Bywaters E G L 1954 Heel lesions of rheumatoid arthritis. Ann Rheum Dis 13: 42–51

Bywaters E G L 1965 Bursae of the body (editorial). Ann Rheum Dis 24: 215–218

Canoso J J, Wohlgethan J R, Newberg A H, Goldsmith M R 1984 Aspiration of the retrocalcaneal bursa. Ann Rheum Dis 43: 308–312

Carter T R, Fowler P J, Blokker C 1992 Functional postoperative treatment of Achilles tendon repair. Am J Sports Med, 20: 459–462

Cetti R, Anderson I 1993 Roentgenographic diagnosis of ruptured Achilles tendons. Clin Orthop 206: 215–221

Cetti R, Christensen S E 1983 Surgical treatment under local anesthesia of Achilles tendon rupture. Clin Orthop 173: 204–208

Cetti R, Christensen S E, Ejsted R, Jensen N M, Jorgensen U 1993 Operative versus nonoperative treatment of Achilles tendon rupture. Am J Sports Med 21: 791–799

Cherry J H, Ghormley R K 1941 Bursa and ganglion. Am J Surg 52: 319–330

Clancy W G Jr 1982 Tendinitis and plantar fasciitis in runners. In: D'Ambrosia R, Drez D Jr (eds) Prevention and treatment of running injuries. Charles B Slack, Thorofare, New Jersey, pp 77–87

Clancy W G Jr, Neidhart D, Brand R L 1976 Achilles tendonitis in runners: a report of five cases. Am J Sports Med 4: 46–56

Cohen I, Lane S, Koning W 1983 Peroneal tendon dislocations: a review of the literature. J Foot Surg 22: 15–20

Conti S, Michelson J, Jahss M 1992 Clinical significance of magnetic resonance imaging in preoperative planning for reconstruction of posterior tibial tendon ruptures. Foot Ankle 13: 208–214

Conwell H E, Alldredge R H 1937 Ruptures and tears of muscles and tendons. Am J Surg 35: 22–33

Cozen L 1965 Posterior tibial tenosynovitis secondary to foot strain. Clin Orthop 42: 101–102

Das De S, Balasubramanian P 1985 A repair operation for recurrent dislocation of peroneal tendons. J Bone Joint Surg 67B: 585–587

Davidsson L, Salo M 1969 Pathogenesis of subcutaneous tendon ruptures. Acta Chir Scand 135: 209–212

Denstad T F, Roaas A 1979 Surgical treatment of partial Achilles tendon rupture. Am J Sports Med 7: 15–17

De Zwart D F, Davidson J S A 1983 Rupture of the posterior tibial tendon associated with fractures of the ankle: a report of two cases. J Bone Joint Surg 65A: 260–262

Dickinson P H, Coutts M B, Woodward E P, Handler D 1966 Tendo Achillis bursitis: report of twenty-one cases. J Bone Joint Surg 48A: 77–81

Dooley B J, Kudelka P, Menelaus M B 1980 Subcutaneous rupture of the tendon of tibialis anterior. J Bone Joint Surg 62B: 471–472

Eckert W R, Davis E A Jr 1976 Acute rupture of the peroneal retinaculum. J Bone Joint Surg 58A: 670–673

Edna T-H 1980 Non-operative treatment of Achilles tendon ruptures. Acta Orthop Scand 51: 991–993

Edwards M E 1928 The relations of the peroneal tendons to the fibula, calcaneus, and cuboideum. Am J Anat 42: 213–253

Escalas F, Figueras J M, Merino J A 1980 Dislocation of the peroneal tendons: long-term results of surgical treatment. J Bone Joint Surg 62A: 451–453

Evans J D 1966 Subcutaneous rupture of the tendon of peroneus longus: report of a case. J Bone Joint Surg 48B: 507–509

Ferguson A B Jr, Gingrich R M 1957 The normal and the abnormal calcaneal apophysis and tarsal navicular. Clin Orthop 10: 87–95

Ferkel R D, Flannigan B D, Elkins B S 1991 Magnetic resonance imaging of the foot and ankle: correlation of normal anatomy with pathologic conditions. Foot Ankle 11: 289–305

Fish J B 1982 Ruptured Achilles tendon: a method of repair. Contemp Orthop 5: 21–25

Fisher T R, Woods C G 1970 Partial rupture of the tendo calcaneus with heterotopic calcification: report of a case. J Bone Joint Surg 52B: 334–336

Fitzgerald R H Jr, Coventry M B 1980 Post-traumatic peroneal tendinitis. In: Bateman J E, Trott A W (eds) The foot and ankle: a selection of papers from the American Orthopaedic Foot Society Meetings. Brian C Decker, New York. pp 103–109

FitzGibbons R E, Hefferon J, Hill J 1993 Percutaneous Achilles tendon repair. Am J Sports Med 21: 724–727

Floyd D W, Heckman J D, Rockwood C A Jr 1983 Tendon lacerations in the foot. Foot Ankle 4: 8–14

Fowler A, Philip J F 1945 Abnormality of the calcaneus as a cause of painful heel: its diagnosis and operative treatment. Br J Surg 32: 494–498

Fowler A W 1955 Tibialis posterior syndrome (abstract). J Bone Joint Surg 37B: 520

Fox J M, Blazina M E, Jobe F W, Kerlan R K, Carter V S, Shields C L Jr, Carlson G J 1975 Degeneration and rupture of the Achilles tendon. Clin Orthop 107: 221–224

Fredenburg M, Tilley G, Yagoobian E M 1983 Spontaneous rupture of the posterior tibial tendon secondary to chronic non-specific tenosynovitis. J Foot Surg 22: 198–202

Frenette J P, Jackson D W 1977 Lacerations of the flexor hallucis longus in the young athlete. J Bone Joint Surg 59A: 673–676

Frey C, Rosenberg Z, Shereff M J, Kim H 1992 The retrocalcaneal bursa: anatomy and bursography. Foot Ankle 13: 203–207

Frey C, Shereff M, Greenide N 1990 Vascularity of the posterior tibial tendon, J Bone Joint Surg 72A: 884–888

Fuglsang F, Torup D 1961 Bursitis retrocalcanearis. Acta Orthop Scand 30: 315–323

Funk D A, Cass J R, Johnson K A 1986 Acquired adult flat foot secondary to posterior tibial-tendon pathology, J Bone Joint Surg 68A: 95–102

Galloway M T, Jokl P, Deyton D W 1992 Achilles tendon overuse injuries. Clin Sports Med 11: 771–782

Ghormley R K, Spear I M 1953 Anomalies of the posterior tibial tendon: a cause of persistent pain about the ankle. Arch Surg 66: 512–516

Giblin M M 1980 Ruptured tibialis posterior tendon associated with a closed medial malleolar fracture. Aust NZ J Surg 50: 59–60

Gilcreest E L 1933 Ruptures and tears of muscles and tendons of the lower extremity: report of fifteen cases. JAMA 100: 153–160

Gillies H, Chalmers J 1970 The management of fresh ruptures of the tendo Achillis J Bone Joint Surg 52A: 337–343

Gillström P, Ljungqvist R 1978 Long-term results after operation for subcutaneous partial rupture of the Achilles tendon. Acta Chir Scand (Suppl) 482: 78

Goldman S, Linscheid R L, Bickel W H 1969 Disruptions of the tendo Achillis: analysis of 33 cases. Mayo Clin Proc 44: 28–35

Goldner J L 1985 J Bone Joint Surg 67A: 1448 (letter to the editor)

Goldner J L, Irwin C E 1949 Paralytic equinovarus deformities of the foot. South Med J 42: 83–94

Goldner J L, Keats P K, Bassett F H III, Clippinger F W 1974 Progressive talipes equinovalgus due to trauma or degeneration of the posterior tibial tendon and medial plantar ligaments. Orthop Clin North Am 5(1): 39–51

Gould N 1981 Stenosing tenosynovitis of the flexor hallucis longus tendon at the great toe. Foot Ankle 2: 46–48

Gould N 1983 Evaluation of hyperpronation and pes planus in adults. Clin Orthop 181: 37–45

Gould N, Korson R 1980 Stenosing tenosynovitis of the pseudosheath of the tendo Achilles. Foot Ankle 1: 179–186

Graves S C, Mann R A, Graves K O 1993 Triple arthrodesis in older adults. Results after long term followup. J Bone Joint Surg 75A: 355–362

Griffiths D L L 1952 Tenosynovitis and tenovaginitis. Br Med J 1: 645–647

Griffiths J C 1965 Tendon injuries around the ankle. J Bone Joint Surg 47B: 686–689

Häggmark T, Eriksson E 1979 Hypotrophy of the soleus muscle in man after Achilles tendon rupture: discussion of findings obtained by computed tomography and morphologic studies. Am J Sports Med 7: 121–126

Haglund P 1928 Contribution to the diseased conditions of tendo Achilles (abstract). Acta Chir Scand 63: 292–294

Haldeman K O, Soto-Hall R 1935 Injuries to muscles and tendons. JAMA 104: 2319–2324

Hamilton W G 1982 Stenosing tenosynovitis of the flexor hallucis longus tendon and posterior impingement upon the os trigonum in ballet dancers. Foot Ankle 3: 74–80

Hartmann 1981 The tendon sheaths and synovial bursae of the foot. Foot Ankle 1: 247–2690

Håstad K, Larsson L-G, Lindholm Å 1958–1959 Clearance of radiosodium after local deposit in the Achilles tendon. Acta Chir Scand 116: 251–255

Hattrup S J, Johnson K A 1985 A review of ruptures of the Achilles tendon. Foot Ankle 6: 34–38

Hauser E D W 1956 Nonspecific tenosynovitis with effusion at the ankle. Postgrad Med 20: 365–369

Helfand A E, Hirt P R, Madresh A C, DeVincentis A 1971 Triamcinolone acetonide in the treatment of bursitis and other foot disorders. J Am Podiatry Assoc 61: 174–179

Henceroth W D II, Deyerle W M 1982 The acquired unilateral flatfoot in the adult: some causative factors. Foot Ankle 2: 304–308

Heneghan M A, Pavlov H 1984 The Haglund painful heel syndrome: experimental investigation of cause and therapeutic implications. Clin Orthop 187: 228–234

Hertzler A E 1923 Inflammation of the deep calcaneal bursa. JAMA 81: 8–9

Hertzler A E 1926 Bursitides of the plantar surface of the foot (painful heel, gonorrheal exostosis of the os calcis, metatarsal neuralgia). Am J Surg 1: 117–126

Holmes G B, Mann R A 1992 Possible epidemiologic factors associated with rupture of the posterior tibial tendon. Foot Ankle 13: 70–79

Holt K W G, Cross M J 1990 Isolated rupture of the flexor hallucis longus tendon: a case report. Am J Sports Med 18: 645–646

Hooker C H 1963 Rupture of the tendo calcaneus. J Bone Joint Surg 45B: 360–363

Howse A J G 1982 Posterior block of the ankle joint in dancers. Foot Ankle 3: 81–84

Inglis A E, Scott W N, Sculco T P, Patterson A H 1976 Ruptures of the tendo Achillis: an objective assessment of surgical and non-surgical treatment. J Bone Joint Surg 58A: 990–993

Ippolito E, Ricciardi-Pollini P T 1984 Invasive retrocalcaneal bursitis: a report of three cases. Foot Ankle 4: 204–208

Isbister J F St C 1974a Calcaneo-fibular abutment following crush fracture of the calcaneus (abstract). J Bone Joint Surg 56B: 567–568

Isbister J F St C 1974b Calcaneo-fibular abutment following crush fracture of the calcaneus. J Bone Joint Surg 56B: 274–278

Jacobs D, Martens M, Van Audekercke R, Mulier J C, Mulier Fr 1978 Comparison of conservative and operative treatment of Achilles tendon rupture. Am J Sports Med 6: 107–111

Jahss M H 1972 Unusual diagnostic problems of the foot. Clin Orthop 85: 42–49

Jahss M H 1974 Pseudotumors of the foot. Orthop Clin North Am 5(1): 67–87

Jahss M H 1982a Spontaneous rupture of the tibialis posterior tendon: clinical findings, tenographic studies, and a new technique of repair. Foot Ankle 3: 158–166

Jahss M H 1982b Disorders of the Foot, Vol 1. W B Saunders, Philadelphia. pp 828–868

Jahss M H 1991a Disorders of the Foot and Ankle: Medical and Surgical Management, 2nd edn. W B Saunders, Philadelphia. pp 1480–1509

Jahss M H 1991b Disorders of the Foot and Ankle Vol II. W B Saunders, Philadelphia. pp 1409–1414

Jessing P, Hansen E 1975 Surgical treatment of 102 tendo Achillis ruptures – suture or tenontoplasty? Acta Chir Scand 141: 370–377

Johnson K A 1983 Tibialis posterior tendon rupture. Clin Orthop 177: 140–147

Johnson K A 1989 Surgery of the Foot and Ankle. Raven Press, New York. pp 221–244

Johnson K A and Strom D E 1989 Tibialis posterior tendon dysfunction, Clin Orthop 239: 196–206

Jones D C, James S L 1984 Partial calcaneal ostectomy for retrocalcaneal bursitis. Am Journal Sports Med 12: 72–73

Jones E 1932 Operative treatment of chronic dislocation of the peroneal tendons. J Bone Joint Surg 14: 574–576

Jones H T 1930 Cystic bursal hygromas. J Bone Joint Surg 12: 45–89

Kager H 1939 Cited by Arner et al 1958–1959

Kalebo P, Allenmark C, Peterson L, Sward L 1992 Diagnostic value of ultrasonography in partial ruptures of the Achilles tendon. Am J Sports Med 20: 370

Kannus P, Jozsa L 1991 Histopathological changes preceding spontaneous rupture of a tendon. J Bone Joint Surg 73: 1507–1525

Kaplan L, Ferguson L K 1937 Bursitis. Am J Surg 37: 455–465

Kaye R A, Jahss M J 1991 Tibialis posterior: a review of anatomy and biomechanics in relation to support of the longitudinal arch. Foot Ankle 11: 244–247

Keck S W, Kelly P J 1965 Bursitis of the posterior part of the heel: evaluation of surgical treatment of eighteen patients. J Bone Joint Surg 47A: 267–273

Kelbel M, Jardon O M 1982 Rupture of the tibialis posterior tendon in a closed ankle fracture. J Trauma 22: 1026–1027

Kelly R E 1920 An operation for the chronic dislocation of the peroneal tendons. Br J Surg 7: 502–504

Kettelkamp D B, Alexander H H 1969 Spontaneous rupture of the posterior tibial tendon. J Bone Joint Surg 51A: 759–764

Key J A 1953 Partial rupture of the tendon of the posterior tibial muscle. J Bone Joint Surg 35A: 1006–1008

Kleinman M, Gross A E 1983 Achilles tendon rupture following steroid injection: report of three cases. J Bone Joint Surg 65A: 1345–1347

Krackow K A 1980 Acute, traumatic rupture of a flexor hallucis longus tendon: a case report. Clin Orthop 150:261–262

Kuhns J G 1943 Adventitious bursas. Arch Surg 46: 687–696

Kulowski J 1936 Tendovaginitis (tenosynovitis): general discussion and report of one case involving posterior tibial tendon. Journal of the Missouri Medical Association 33: 135–137

Kvist H, Kvist M 1980 The operative treatment of chronic calcaneal paratenonitis. J Bone Joint Surg 62B: 353–357

Lagergren C, Lindholm Å 1958–1959 Vascular distribution in the Achilles tendon: an angiographic and microangiographic study. Acta Chir Scand 116: 491–495

Lancet Editorial 1973 Achilles tendon rupture. 1: 189–190

Langan P and Weiss C A 1980 Dislocation of the tibialis posterior, a complication of tarsal tunnel decompression: a case report. Clin Orthop 146: 226–227

Langenskiöld A 1967 Chronic non-specific tenosynovitis of the tibialis posterior tendon. Acta Orthop Scand 38: 301–305

Lapidus P W 1941 Indirect subcutaneous rupture of the anterior tibial tendon: report of two cases. Bull Hosp Jt Dis Orthop Inst 2: 119–127

Lapidus P W 1953 Stenosing tenovaginitis. Surg Clin North Am October: 1317–1347

Lapidus P W, Seidenstein H 1950 Chronic non-specific tenosynovitis with effusion about the ankle: report of three cases. J Bone Joint Surg 32A: 175–179

Larsen E 1987 Longitudinal rupture of the peroneus brevis tendon. J Bone Joint Surg 69B: 340–341

Larsen E, Lauridsen F 1984 Dislocation of the tibialis posterior tendon in two athletes. Am J Sports Med 12: 429–430

Lawrence G H, Cave E F, O'Connor H 1955 Injury to the Achilles tendon: experience at the Massachusetts General Hospital, 1900–1954. Am J Surg 89: 795–802

Layfer L F 1980 "Last" bursitis – a cause of ankle pain (letter to the editor). Arthritis Rheum 23: 261

Lea R B 1981 Achilles tendon rupture: results of closed management. In: Moore M (ed) Symposium on trauma to the leg and its sequelae. C V Mosby, St Louis. pp 353–357

Lea R B, Smith L 1968 Rupture of the Achilles tendon nonsurgical treatment. Clin Orthop 60: 115–118

Lea R B, Smith L 1972 Non-surgical treatment of tendo Achillis rupture. J Bone Joint Surg 54A: 1398–1407

Leach R E 1982 Achilles tendon ruptures. In: Mack R P (ed) Symposium on the foot and leg in running sports. C V Mosby, St Louis. pp 99–105

Leach R E, James S, Wasilewski S 1981 Achilles tendinitis. Am J Sports Med 9: 93–98

Leach R E, Schepsis A A, Takai H 1992 Long term results of surgical management of Achilles tendinitis in runners. Clin Orthop 282: 208–212

Leadbetter W B 1992 Cell–matrix response in tendon injury. Clin Sports Med 11: 533–578

Lennox D W, Wang G J, McCue F C, Stamp W G 1980 The operative treatment of Achilles tendon injuries. Clin Orthop 148: 152–155

Lindholm Å 1959 A new method of operation in subcutaneous rupture of the Achilles tendon. Acta Chir Scand 117: 261–270

Lipscomb P R 1942 Non-suppurative tenosynovitis: a clinical and pathologic study. Thesis, Graduate School of the University of Minnesota

Lipscomb P R 1944 Chronic nonspecific tenosynovitis and peritendinitis. Surg Clin North Am August: 780–797

Lipscomb P R 1950 Tendons: Number 1. Nonsuppurative tenosynovitis and paratendinitis. Instr Course Lect 7: 254–261

Lipscomb P R, Kelly P J 1955 Injuries of the extensor tendons in the distal part of the leg and in the ankle. J Bone Joint Surg 37A: 1206–1213

Lipscomb P R, Wakim K G 1961a Regeneration of severed tendons: an experimental study. Proceedings of the Staff Meetings of the Mayo Clinic 36: 271–276

Lipscomb P R, Wakim K G 1961b Further observations in the healing of severed tendons: an experimental study. Proceedings of the Staff Meetings of the Mayo Clinic 36: 277–282

Lipsman S, Frankel J P, Count G W 1980 Spontaneous rupture of the tibialis posterior tendon: a case report and review of the literature. J Am Podiatry Assoc 70: 34–39

Ljungqvist R 1968 Subcutaneous partial rupture of the Achilles tendon. Acta Orthop Scand (Suppl) 113: 1–86

Ljungqvist R, Eriksson E 1982 Partial tears of the patellar tendon and the Achilles tendon. In: Mack R P (ed) Symposium on the foot and leg in running sports. C V Mosby, St Louis. pp 92–98

Lynn T A 1966 Repair of the torn Achilles tendon, using the plantaris tendon as a reinforcing membrane. J Bone Joint Surg 48A: 268–272

Ma G W, Griffith T G 1977 Percutaneous repair of acute closed ruptured Achilles tendon: a new technique. Clin Orthop 128: 247–255

Ma G W C, Griffith T G 1981 Percutaneous repair of acute closed ruptured Achilles tendon: a new technique. In: Moore T M (ed) Symposium on trauma to the leg and its sequelae. C V Mosby, St Louis, pp 358–370

McCarroll J R, Ritter M A, Becker T E 1983 Triggering of the great toe: a case report. Clin Orthop 175: 184–185

McLennan J G 1980 Treatment of acute and chronic luxations of the peroneal tendons. Am J Sports Med 8: 432–436

McMaster P E 1933 Tendon and muscle ruptures: clinical and experimental studies on the causes and location of subcutaneous ruptures. J Bone Joint Surg 15: 705–722

Mann R A 1983 Acquired flatfoot in adults. Clin Orthop 181: 46–51

Mann R A 1985 Biomechanics of the foot. In: American Academy of Orthopaedic Surgeons: Atlas of orthotics, 2nd edn. C V Mosby, St Louis. p 121

Mann R A (ed) 1986 Surgery of the foot 5th edn. C V Mosby, St Louis. pp 293–294

Mann R A, Coughlin M S (eds) 1993 Surgery of the Foot and Ankle, 6th edn. C V Mosby, St Louis. pp 767–780

Mann R A, Specht L H 1982 Posterior tibial tendon ruptures – analysis of eight cases (abstract). Foot Ankle 2: 350

Mann R A, Thompson F M 1985 Rupture of the posterior tibial tendon causing flat foot: surgical treatment. J Bone Joint Surg 67A: 556–561

Marti R 1977 Dislocation of the peroneal tendons. Am J Sports Med 5: 19–22

Mensor M C, Ordway G L 1953 Traumatic subcutaneous rupture of the tibialis anterior tendon. J Bone Joint Surg 35A: 675–680

Meyerding H W 1938 The treatment of bursitis. Surg Clin North Am 18: 1103–1117

Meyn M A Jr 1975 Closed rupture of the anterior tibial tendon: a case report and review of the literature. Clin Orthop 113: 154–157

Mick C A, Lynch F 1987 Reconstruction of the peroneal retinaculum using the peroneus quartus. J Bone Joint Surg 69A: 296–297

Miller B F, Buhr A J 1969 Pump bumps or knobbly heels. Nova Scotia Medical Bulletin 48: 191–192

Miller J W 1967 Dislocation of peroneal tendons – a new operative procedure: a case report. Am J Orthop 9: 136–137

Mizuno K, Ozaki T, Yamada M, Hirohata K 1991 Recurrent dislocation of the peroneal longus tendon as a complication of multiple osteochondromatosis. Foot Ankle 12: 52–54

Moberg E 1947 Subcutaneous rupture of the tendon of the tibialis anterior muscle. Acta Chir Scand 95: 455–460

Monto R R, Moorman C T III, Mallon W J, Nunky J A 1991 Rupture of the posterior tibial tendon associated with closed ankle fracture. Foot Ankle 11: 400–403

Moorman C T, Monto R R, Bassett F H 1992 So-called trigger ankle due to an aberrant flexor hallucis longus muscle in a tennis player. J Bone Joint Surg 74A: 294–295

Mortiz J R 1959 Ski injuries. Am J Surg 98: 493–505

Moskowitz E 1971 Rupture of the tibialis anterior tendon simulating peroneal nerve palsy. Arch Phys Med Rehabil 52: 431–433

Mueller T J 1984 Ruptures and lacerations of the tibialis posterior tendon. J Am Podiatry Assoc 74: 109–119

Munk R L, Davis P H 1977 Longitudinal rupture of the peroneus brevis tendon. J Trauma 16: 803–806

Murr S 1961 Dislocation of the peroneal tendons with marginal fracture of the lateral malleolus. J Bone Joint Surg 43B: 563–565

Murrell G A C, Phil D, Lilly E G et al 1993 Achilles tendon injuries: a comparison of surgical repair versus no repair in a rat model. Foot Ankle 14: 400–406

Myerson M, Solomon G, Shereff M 1989 Posterior tibial tendon dysfunction: its association with seronegative inflammatory disease. Foot Ankle 9: 219–225

Nesse E, Finsen V 1994 Poor results after resection for Haglund's heel. Analysis of 35 heels in 23 patients after 3 years. Acta Orthop Scand 65: 107–109

Nicholas J A 1974 Ankle injuries in athletes. Orthop Clin North Am 5(1): 153–175

Nielson A L 1921 Diagnostic and therapeutic point in retrocalcaneal bursitis. JAMA 77: 463

Nillius S A, Nilsson B E, Westlin N E 1976 The incidence of Achilles tendon rupture. Acta Orthop Scand 47: 118–121

Nisbet N W 1954 Tendo Achillis bursitis ("winter heel"). Br Med J 2: 1394–1395

Nistor L 1976 Conservative treatment of fresh subcutaneous rupture of the Achilles tendon. Acta Orthop Scand 47: 459–462

Nistor L 1981 Surgical and non-surgical treatment of Achilles tendon rupture: a prospective randomized study. J Bone Joint Surg 63A: 394–399

Norris S H, Mankin H J 1978 Chronic tenosynovitis of the posterior tibial tendon with new bone formation. J Bone Joint Surg 60B: 523–526

Nova B E 1968 Traumatic dislocation of the tibialis posterior tendon at the ankle: report of a case, J Bone Joint Surg 50B: 150–151

O'Brien T 1984 The needle test for complete rupture of the Achilles tendon. J Bone Joint Surg 66A: 1099–1101

Oden R F 1987 Clin Orthop 216: 63–69

Ogden R F 1987 Tendon injuries about the ankle resulting from skiing. Clin Orthop 216: 63–69

Ouzounian T J, Myerson M S 1992 Dislocation of the posterior tibial tendon, Foot Ankle 13: 215–219, 364

Palmer D G 1970 Tendon sheaths and bursae involved by rheumatoid disease of the foot and ankle. Australas Radiol 14: 419–428

Parvin R W, Ford L T 1956 Stenosing tenosynovitis of the common peroneal tendon sheath: report of two cases. J Bone Joint Surg 38A: 1352–1357

Patterson R L Jr, Darrach W 1937 Treatment of acute bursitis by needle irrigation. J Bone Joint Surg 19: 993–1002

Pavlov H, Heneghan M A, Hersh A, Goldman A B, Vigorita V 1982 The Haglund syndrome: initial and differential diagnosis. Radiology 144: 83–88

Peacock K C, Resnick E J, Thodes J J 1986 Fracture of the os peroneum with rupture of the peroneus longus tendon, Clin Orthop 202: 223–226

Percy E C, Conochie L B 1978 The surgical treatment of ruptured tendo Achillis. Am J Sports Med 6: 132–136

Pierson J L, Inglis A E 1992 Stenosing tenosynovitis of the peroneus longus tendon associated with hypertrophy of the peroneal tubercle and an os peroneum. J Bone Joint Surg 74A: 440–442

Plattner P F, Johnson K A 1988 Tendons and bursae. In: Helal B, Wilson D (eds) The Foot. Churchill Livingstone, London. pp 581–613

Platzgummer H 1967 Über in einfaches Verfahren zur operativen Behandlung der habituellen Peroneussehnen-luxation. Arch Orthop Unfallchir, 61: 144–150

Pöll R G, Duijfjes F 1984 The treatment of recurrent dislocation of the peroneal tendons. J Bone Joint Surg 66B: 98–100

Pozo J L, Jackson A M 1984 A rerouting operation for dislocation of peroneal tendons: operative technique and case report. Foot Ankle 5: 42–44

Puddu G, Ippolito E, Postacchini F 1976 A classification of Achilles tendon disease. Am J Sports Med 4: 145–150

Quigley T B, Scheller A D 1980 Surgical repair of the ruptured Achilles tendon: analysis of 40 patients treated by the same surgeon. Am J Sports Med 8: 244–250

Ralston E L, Schmidt E R Jr 1971 Repair of the ruptured Achilles tendon. J Trauma 11: 15–19

Reinherz R P 1984 Management of flexor hallucis longus tendon injuries. J Foot Surg 23: 366–369

Rimoldi R L, Oberlander M A, Weldrop J I, Hunter S C 1991 Acute rupture of the tibialis anterior tendon: a case report. Foot Ankle 12: 176–177

Roberts P W 1929a Bursitis of the foot: a neglected cause of disability. Am J Surg 6: 313–317

Roberts P W 1929b Fifty cases of bursitis of the foot. J Bone Joint Surg 11: 338–344

Rubin B D, Wilson H J Jr 1980 Surgical repair of the interrupted Achilles tendon. J Trauma 20: 248–249

Ruch J A 1974 Haglund's disease. J Am Podiatry Assoc 64: 1000–1003

Sammarco G J, Di Raimondo C V 1988 Chronic peroneus brevis tendon lesions. Foot Ankle 9: 163–170

Sammarco G J, Miller E H 1979 Partial rupture of the flexor hallucis longus tendon in classical ballet dancers: two case reports. J Bone Joint Surg 61A: 149–150

Sarma P J 1940 The injection treatment of ganglions and bursae: indications and limitations. Surg Clin North Am 20: 135–140

Sarmiento A, Wolf M 1975 Subluxation of peroneal tendons: case treated by rerouting tendons under calcaneofibular ligament. J Bone Joint Surg 57A: 115–116

Sarrafian S K 1983 Anatomy of the foot and ankle: descriptive, topographic, functional. J B Lippincott, Philadelphia. pp 251–259

Saunders D E, Hochberg J, Wittenborn W 1978 Treatment of total loss of the Achilles tendon by skin flap cover without tendon repair. Plast Reconstr Surg 62: 708–712

Savastano A A 1980 Recurrent dislocation of the peroneal tendons. In: Bateman J E, Trott A W (eds) The foot and ankle: a selection of papers from the American Orthopaedic Foot Society Meetings. Brian C Decker, New York. pp 110–115

Schaffer J J, Lock T R, Salciccioli G G 1987 Posterior tibial tendon rupture in pronation-external rotation ankle fractures. J Trauma 27: 795–796

Schatzker J, Brånemark P-I 1969 Intravital observation on the microvascular anatomy and microcirculation of the tendon. Acta Orthop Scand (Suppl) 126: 1–23

Schedl R, Fasol P 1979 Achilles tendon repair with the plantaris tendon compared with repair using polyglycol threads. J Trauma 19: 189–194

Scheller A D, Kasser J R, Quigley T B 1980 Tendon injuries about the ankle. Orthop Clin North Am 11(4): 801–811

Scott W N, Inglis A E, Sculco T P 1979 Surgical treatment of reruptures of the tendoachilles following nonsurgical treatment. Clin Orthop 140: 175–177

Scranton P E Jr 1980 Metatarsalgia: diagnosis and treatment. J Bone Joint Surg 62A: 723–732

Sever J W 1912 Apophysitis of the os calcis. New York Medical Journal 95: 1025–1029

Shephard E 1975 Intermetatarso-phalangeal bursitis in the causation of Morton's metatarsalgia. J Bone Joint Surg 57B: 115–116

Shields C L Jr, Kerlan R K, Jobe F W, Carter V S, Lombardo S J 1978 The Cybex II evaluation of surgically repaired Achilles tendon ruptures. Am J Sports Med 6: 369–372

Shoda E, Kurosaka M, Yoshiya S, Kurihara A, Hirohata K 1991 Longitudinal ruptures of the peroneal tendons. A report of a rugby player. Acta Orthop Scand 62: 491–492

Sim F H, DeWeerd J H Jr 1977 Rupture of the extensor hallucis longus tendon while skiing. Minn Med 690: 789–790

Skeoch D U 1981 Spontaneous partial subcutaneous ruptures of the tendo Achillis: review of the literature and evaluation of 16 involved tendons. Am J Sports Med 9: 20–22

Snook G A 1972 Achilles tendon tenosynovitis in long-distance runners. Med Sci Sports Exerc 4: 155–158

Søballe K, Kjaersgaard-Anderson P 1988 Ruptured tibialis posterior tendon in a closed ankle fracture. Clin Orthop 231: 140–143

Sobel M, Bohne W H O, Levy M E 1990 Longitudinal attrition of the peroneus brevis tendon in the fibular groove: an anatomic study. Foot Ankle 11: 124–128

Sobel M, Bohne W H O, Markisz J A 1991 Cadaver correlation of peroneal tendon changes with magnetic resonance imaging. Foot Ankle 11: 384–388

Sobel M, Bohne W H, O'Brien S J 1992 Peroneal tendon subluxation in a case of anomalous peroneus brevis muscle. Acta Orthop Scand 63: 682–684

Sobel M, Geppert M J, Warren R F 1993 Chronic ankle instability as a cause of peroneal tendon injury. Clin Orthop 296: 187–191

Sobel M, Levy M E, Bohne W H O 1990 Congenital variations of the peroneus quartus muscle: an anatomic study. Foot ankle 11: 81–89

Sobel M, Pavlov H, Geppert M J, Thompson F M, Di Carlo E F, Davis W H 1994 Painful os peroneum syndrome: a spectrum of conditions responsible for plantar lateral foot pain. Foot Ankle 15: 112–124

Sobel M, Warren R F, Brourmans 1990 Lateral ankle instability associated with dislocation of the peroneal tendons treated by the Christman–Snook procedure: a case report and literature review. Am J Sports Med 18: 539–543

Soter R R, Castany F J G, Ferret J R, Ramiro S G 1986 Traumatic dislocation of the tibialis posterior tendon at the ankle level. J Trauma 26: 1049–1052

Stanish W D, Vincent N 1989 Recurrent dislocation of the tibialis posterior tendon – a case report with a new surgical approach, Can J Appl Sport Sci 9: 220–222

Steffensen J C A, Evensen A 1958 Bursitis retrocalcanea Achilli. Acta Orthop Scand 27: 228–236

Stein R E 1985 Rupture of the posterior tibial tendon in closed ankle fractures – possible prognostic value of a medial bone flake: Report of two cases. J Bone Joint Surg 67A: 493–494

Stein S R, Luekens C A 1976a Methods and rationale for closed treatment of Achilles tendon ruptures. Am J Sports Med 4: 162–169

Stein S R, Luekens C A Jr 1976b Closed treatment of Achilles tendon ruptures. Orthop Clin North Am 7(1): 241–246

Steinbock G, Pinsger M, 1994 Treatment of peroneal tendon distraction by transposition under the calcaneofibular ligament. Foot Ankle 15: 107–111

Stiehl J B 1988 Concomitant rupture of the peroneus brevis tendon and bimalleolar fracture. J Bone Joint Surg 70A: 936–937

Stover C N, Bryan D R 1962 Traumatic dislocation of the peroneal tendons. Am J Surg 103: 180–186

Szczukowski M Jr, St Pierre R K, Fleming L L, Somogyi J 1983 Computerized tomography in the evaluation of peroneal tendon dislocation. A report of two cases. Am J Sports Med 11: 444–447

Taylor L W 1981 Achilles tendon repair: results of surgical management. In: Moore M (ed) Symposium on trauma to the leg and its sequelae. C V Mosby, St Louis. pp 371–384

Teasdall R D, Johnson K A, Donnelly R E 1993 The surgical treatment of stage 1 posterior tibial tendon dysfunction. American Orthopedic Foot and Ankle Society, 23rd annual meeting, San Francisco, CA, 21 February 1993

Tehranzadeh J, Stoll D A, Gabriele O M 1984 Open-quiz solution: case report 271. Skeletal Radiol 12: 44–47

Teng M M H, Destouet J M, Gilula L A, Resnick D, Hembree J L, Oloff L M 1984 Ankle tenography: a key to unexplained symptomatology. Part 1: Normal tenographic anatomy. Radiology 151: 575–580

Teuffer A P 1974 Traumatic rupture of the Achilles tendon: reconstruction by transplant and graft using the lateral peroneus brevis.

Orthop Clin North Am 5(1): 89–93

Thompson F M, Patterson A H 1989 Rupture of the peroneus longus tendon. J Bone Joint Surg 71A: 293–295

Thompson F M, Snow S W, Hershon S J 1993 Spontaneous atraumatic rupture of the flexor hallucis longus tendon under the sustentaculum tali: case report, review of the literature, and treatment options. Foot Ankle 14: 414–417

Thompson T C 1962 A test for rupture of the tendo Achillis. Acta Orthop Scand 32: 461–465

Thompson T C, Doherty J H 1962 Spontaneous rupture of tendon of Achilles: a new clinical diagnostic test. J Trauma 2: 126–129

Toygar O 1947 Cited by Arner et al 1958–1959

Trevino S, Gould N, Korson R 1981 Surgical treatment of stenosing tenosynovitis at the ankle. Foot Ankle 2: 37–45

Tudisco C, Puddu G 1984 Stenosing tenosynovitis of the flexor hallucis longus tendon in a classical ballet dancer: a case report. Am J Sports Med 12: 403–404

Waldrop J, Ebraheim N A, Shapiro P, Jackson W T 1992 Anatomical considerations of posterior tibialis tendon entrapment in irreducible lateral subtalar dislocation. Foot Ankle 13: 458–461

Wapner K L, Hecht P J, Shea J R, Allardyce T J 1994 Anatomy of second muscular layer of the foot: considerations for tendon selection in transfer for Achilles and posterior tibial tendon reconstruction. Foot Ankle Int 15: 420–423

Wapner K L, Pevlock G S, Hecht P J, Noselli F, Walther J 1993 Repair of chronic Achilles tendon rupture with flexor hallucis longus tendon transfer. Foot Ankle 14: 443–449

Webster F S 1968 Peroneal tenosynovitis with pseudotumour. J Bone Joint Surg 50A: 153–157

Weinstable R, Stiskal M, Wenhold A, Aamlid B, Hertz H 1991 Classifying calcaneal tendon injury according to MRI findings. J Bone Joint Surg 73B: 603–605

Weston W J 1970 The bursa deep to tendo Achillis. Australas Radiol 14: 327–331

White C S 1913 Retrocalcanean bursitis. New York Medical Journal 98: 263–265

Wicks M H, Harbison J S, Paterson D C 1980 Tendon injuries about the foot and ankle in children. Aust NZ J Surg 50: 158–161

Williams R 1963 Chronic non-specific tendovaginitis of tibialis posterior. J Bone Joint Surg 45B: 542–545

Wills C A, Washburn S, Caiozzo V et al 1986 Achilles tendon rupture: a review of the literature comparing surgical versus nonsurgical treatment. Clinical Orthop 207: 156–163

Woods L, Leach R E 1991 Posterior tibial tendon rupture in athletic people. Am J Sports Med 19: 495–498

Wrenn R N 1975 Isolated injuries of posterior tibial tendon (abstract). J Bone Joint Surg 57A: 1035

Yancey H A Jr 1977 Lacerations of the plantar aspect of the foot. Clin Orthop 122: 46–52

Zadek I 1939 An operation for the cure of Achillobursitis. Am J Surg 43: 542–546

Zoellner G, Clancy W Jr 1979 Recurrent dislocation of the peroneal tendon. J Bone Joint Surg 61A: 292–294

V.7 Plantar Fibromatosis

Andrea Cracchiolo III

Plantar fibromatosis is a benign tumour of the plantar fascia (Pedersen & Day 1954). It has been known for a long time, probably first being described by Sir Astley Cooper, but was best characterized by Dupuytren in 1832 when he mentioned foot lesions in two of his cases of classic contractures of the hand which bear his name (Meyerding & Shellito 1948). However, it was Madelung in 1875 who reported an isolated lesion in the foot. The condition consists of fibrous nodules which develop within the plantar fascia. They are usually found on the medial side of the fascia near the highest point of the longitudinal arch, but may of course occur anywhere. Classically the nodules extend out toward the skin but larger nodules also protrude toward the inner portion of the sole of the foot. In contrast to contractures of the fingers, seen in Dupuytren's of the hand, toe contractures are not seen (Stoyle 1964).

Anatomy

A review of the anatomy of the plantar aponeurosis shows that the main medial portion arises from a strong thick attachment on the medial tubercle of the calcaneus. The more pronounced medial band traverses the longitudinal arch attaching to the undersurface of the first metatarsal and also to the first cuneiform. At about midfoot, the aponeurosis divides into digitations which proceed toward the toe. Deeper fibres form transverse fasciculi between the longitudinally running bands (Hollishead 1964). Distal to the transverse fasciculi, the digital nerves and vessels lie within the connective tissue, and they continue forward to the toes. Across the metatarsal head area, the digitations are united by a thin band of transverse fibres, the superficial transverse metatarsal ligament. Distally the fascial digitations split to pass around the flexor tendons strengthening the sheaths. Lateral slips of the aponeurosis end in thin and somewhat insignificant digital extensions. For this reason, contractures of the toes almost never occur, and nodules are seldom seen on lateral bands (Curtin 1962). It is important to remember that the plantar aponeurosis sends septa from its deep surface to attach to the first and fifth metatarsal, dividing the foot into compartments.

The medial and lateral plantar nerves and blood vessels enter the foot together. They pass under the flexor retinaculum and traverse under the abductor hallucis where they separate. The lateral neurovascular bundle courses obliquely under the plantar structures, penetrating the lateral intermuscular septum lateral to the flexor digitorum brevis just underneath the plantar aponeurosis. The medial neurovascular bundle courses distally, penetrating the septum medial to the flexor brevis. At this point, at about the base of the metatarsals or at the midfoot, the nerves divide into their digital branches. Cutaneous branches of the lateral plantar nerve pierce the plantar fascia and supply the skin of the medial side of the foot. The common digital nerves lie immediately deep to the plantar aponeurosis. The lateral plantar nerve also gives off plantar cutaneous branches, which pierce the deep fascia and supply the lateral side of the sole. This nerve is somewhat analogous to the ulnar nerve in the hand: although it gives rise to fewer digital branches, it does supply most of the intrinsic muscles of the foot.

Clinical findings

Clinically the overlying skin may be unaltered, dimpled, fissured or fixed as a result of the underlying nodules. The best method of palpating and measuring the nodule is to dorsiflex the foot and the toes. This tenses the plantar fascia and one can measure the length and width of a nodule.

Patients usually present with nodules that are at least 1 cm in diameter. However smaller nodules can be palpated if one suspects their presence, such as when evaluating a patient with palmar fibromatosis. The nodules, even the larger ones, are usually non-tender and moveable within the confines of the plantar fascia.

No clear association has been established between Dupuytren's contracture of the hand and plantar fibromatosis (Allen et al 1955, Lund 1941, Meyerding & Shellito 1948, Pickren & Day 1954), although it is common to examine both areas if a lesion is seen in either.

Radiographs are usually negative, although calcifications in the area of a palpable mass suggest a diagnosis of juvenile aponeurotic fibroma (Keasbey 1953, Keller & Baez-Giangreco 1975). A plantar mass that also extends proximally into the tarsal canal is likely to be a more aggressive variant of fibromatosis or a desmoplastic fibroma (Lee et al 1993). Such lesions usually occur in younger patients and are quite large (Keasbey 1953).

Pathology

On gross examination the nodule is firm, solid and of a yellowish–orange colour when cut (Curtin 1962).

Microscopically the nodule consists of islands of proliferating fibroblasts on a relatively acellular collagenase background. On low power there is a nodular multicentric growth pattern. In Allen's (1955) series, inflammatory cells were seen in every case. Lymphocytes were seen in perivascular locations. The fibroblast nuclei are elongated fusiform, oval and contain scant chromatin material and one to two pale nucleoli.

It is well known that, unless he is supplied with the relevant clinical data, a pathologist reviewing the slide may entertain an erroneous diagnosis of fibrosarcoma. Both tumors lack encapsulation and spread diffusely (Curtin 1962). However, fibrosarcoma of the foot is an extremely rare tumour and malignant degeneration of a clinical plantar fibroma is not thought to occur.

Meyerding & Shellito (1948) attempted to stage the disease. They divided it into active disease and resting disease. The active stage is early, with the gross detection of nodules that might be tender or somewhat painful. During this stage there is increased fibroblastic activity and cellular proliferation with perivascular round cell infiltration. The resting stage is later in the disease with hard nontender nodules.

Enneking (1983) has more recently also staged these lesions. Stage I is a benign tumor, limited to one compartment or anatomical border: the usual clinical presentation. However, stage III is unusual and is a high-grade tumor with extracompartmental extensions and skip lesions. Most lesions are classified as stage II during the developmental phase when the fibromas are palpable within the plantar fascia. Attempted surgical excision of nodules at this stage may result in a rapid recurrence of the more aggressive stage III lesion.

The differential diagnosis can include: stage I fibrosarcoma, leiomyoma, chondroma, rhabdomyosarcoma, clear-cell sarcoma, synovial sarcoma, liposarcoma, lipoma, a ganglion, giant cell tumor of the tendon sheath, a rheumatoid nodule, granuloma annulare, neurofibroma, neurilemoma, sporotrichoses, and sweat gland carcinoma (Wu 1986).

Occurrence

The actual incidence of this condition has been difficult to estimate. Meyerding's comprehensive 20-year review was based on patients with Dupuytren's contractures of the hands or with plantar fibromatosis. He found only 24 patients with foot involvement and 12 patients (1.5%) with foot and hand involvement. It was noted that there may be many more cases of foot nodules, but in general the feet have not always been evaluated, particularly when the patients were being examined for contractures of the hand. Plantar fibromatosis is not common.

Allen et al (1955) reviewed a 50-year experience of soft tissue tumors of the foot at the Mayo Clinic. Sixty-nine had plantar fibromatosis and nine had malignant neoplasms. Jahss (1982) showed a slight male preponderance of 63% in his series, with 39% of cases being bilateral. There was an association with epilepsy in 7% of cases and the occurrence of Dupuytren's contractures of the hands in 37%.

There is a definite increase in Dupuytren's contractures of the hands and plantar fibromatosis in patients with epilepsy (Lund 1941). When 361 epileptics were studied, 50% of the males had Dupuytren's disease of the hand, as did 32% of the females. Plantar fibromatosis was seen in 25 patients. This was compared to 1021 control brewery workers, of whom only one had plantar fibromatosis (Allen et al 1955).

Pickren et al (1951) described 16 patients with this condition; six males and 10 females with an age range from 5 to 60 years old, though most were under 30. Four had bilateral involvement and five had pain. Two patients had associated epilepsy, and although the lesions were excised in 15, recurrence occurred in 11 patients. Pickern also reviewed the literature at that time and reported an equal distribution between men and women in 104 patients. Twenty-one had bilateral involvement and 49 had associated lesions in the palm. Twenty-five patients were epileptic, and only one had a penile contracture.

Aviles et al (1971) reported 22 patients, most having the onset of their disease after age 40. Five had bilateral involvement and only one had pain. Fourteen had simple excision of a nodule and of these eight had recurrence. Only one of the eight patients with wide radical excision had a recurrence.

The disease seems to increase with advancing age, although most patients are seen in the fourth or fifth decade. There seems to be no positive correlation with factors in the patient's history such as occupation, level of activity, possible trauma or family history of this condition.

Radiographically there may not be any changes, although at times a very large nodule can be seen in the soft tissue, especially in a tangential projection. Other conditions also present with distinct nodules in the palms and soles. Juvenile aponeurotic fibroma is one such condition seen in children and adolescents (Keller & Baez-Giangreco 1975). The tumors are small and painless, and lesions on the trunk have also been described. Microscopically a spotty calcification is seen in these tumors, which along with the low number of mitoses seen, leads to a correct diagnosis and differentiation from fibrosarcoma.

Diagnostic studies

Usually a history and physical examination are all that are needed for a diagnostic evaluation. Radiographs are usually negative. Probably the only study of any merit would be an MRI (magnetic resonance imaging); however, the routine use of this study is unnecessary as

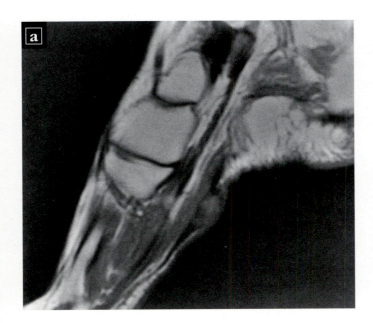
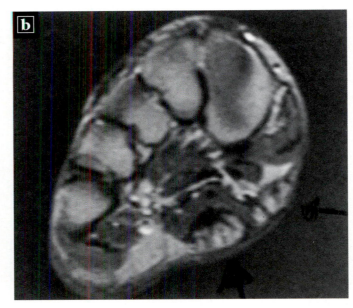

Figure 1

Sagittal and coronal MRI scans of a patient with a second recurrence of a plantar mass. The MRI signals are intermediate to low strength and indicate that the tumor is well confined and invades towards the dermis of the skin and that there is no extension dorsally towards the muscles or the metatarsal or tarsal bones. The two previous attempts at excision were made through a small incision without any attempt at radical excision of the plantar fascia. It is of course possible that recurrences could represent additional sites of this benign tumor

these lesions are benign and their size can usually be accurately measured by palpation. MRI is helpful in two circumstances.

When there has been a recurrence of a plantar fibroma, one should review the pathology report from the prior excision and determine if there may have been any doubts as to the microscopic findings (Fig. 1). It is also helpful to determine whether the mass has invaded the dermis, which usually indicates that a skin graft will be needed after excising all the involved skin, and to estimate the size of the mass, particularly if it has extended dorsally, and to appreciate the relationship of the mass to the neurovascular structures.

A plantar mass that appears to be atypical for a fibroma, either primary or recurrent, may also be an indication for obtaining an MRI. This may be particularly helpful if the tumor appears to be growing rapidly or if there is more than one palpable mass. Calcifications within the mass and a painful mass might also be better evaluated using an MRI.

Treatment

There is probably no indication to treat a patient with plantar fibromatosis unless the nodules are large enough to cause discomfort or disability. Initially it is probably best to observe the nodules on two or three separate occasions over a period of several months. The length and width of the nodules should be measured and this should be recorded so that the course of the disease can be evaluated. Frequently the nodules do not grow. However, if the patient is seen at an early stage, the nodules can increase in size and later other nodules, perhaps not previously appreciated, may be palpated.

Historically, radiation has been described as a treatment, but apparently it has had no effect on the lesions. Other non-operative treatments, such as local infiltration of hydrocortisone, local anesthetic or ultrasound treatments, are of no value. There is no reason to attempt to aspirate a nodule on the sole of the foot. The most obvious diagnosis should be a solid plantar fibromatosis and the pathologic anatomy of this area does not lead to the development of a cystic fluid-filled lesion such as a ganglion or a bursa. Early treatment should consist of modifying the patient's shoes to accommodate the nodules if they are tender. This can be done by excavating a portion of the inner sole and perhaps filling in with a softer lining material (Cracchiolo 1982).

The decision to excise nodules surgically should be based on the patient's discomfort. Obviously, large nodules that are causing significant discomfort should be excised. It is not necessary to biopsy these nodules, but a complete excision is indicated.

A recurrence rate of these nodules has been reported. Allen's study (1955) indicates that 15 of 28 (54%) recurred after a single excision. In seven cases two excisions were performed and in four of these there was recurrence. In three patients, three or more excisions were performed. Probably the explanation for recurrence is an incomplete removal of the nodule. Conservative excision such as resecting only the palpable nodule is not adequate, as other areas of involvement may exist.

At times, patients present with a single small palpable nodule, which may be symptomatic. Although it may be tempting to excise the small nodule, it can usually be treated conservatively. It is better to observe such a patient, as other nodules may become palpable and justify, both to the patient and the surgeon, the need to perform an adequate excision of the plantar aponeurosis.

One must appreciate the extensive involvement of this disease and the anatomy of the plantar fascia, which may extend deep within the sole of the foot toward the metatarsal shafts. It is not always appreciated that complete excision of the plantar fascia, particularly the medial band, is essential to prevent a recurrence (Curtin 1962). Reoperation on the foot, like the hand, leads to poorer results, owing to additional postoperative fibrosis. Therefore, in a primary case, it is best to excise the entire medial band of the plantar aponeurosis and one should avoid excising only the palpable nodule.

Operative treatment

Adequate exposure of the plantar fascia, particularly the medial band, is essential. The skin incision is critical and the plantar approach as devised by Curtin (1962, 1965) provides the optimal exposure for this operation (Fig. 2).

In the past, incisions on the plantar aspect of the foot were condemned. The common approach to the sole of the foot was through the medial incision of Henry (1963) who stated that 'incisions to the sole are best avoided'. He advocated approaching from the medial side of the arch, dividing the skin and superficial fascia on the inner side of the foot from the hallux metatarsal head to the heel. This would require extensive subcutaneous dissection of the lateral flap. Unfortunately, skin incisions placed high on the medial side of the longitudinal arch are precarious. The undermining necessary to expose even the medial band of the plantar fascia disrupts the arterial supply to the lateral plantar skin flap and also encourages venous congestion, which leads to skin necrosis (Curtin 1965).

It is preferable to place the patient in the prone position and to perform the operation under tourniquet control (Fig. 3). The skin incision is longitudinal and medial to the midline of the foot. The proximal and distal portions of the incision can be curved depending on the location of the nodule or nodules. A nodule closer to the heel might be better exposed by curving

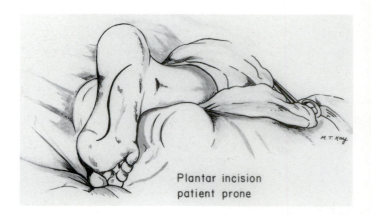

Figure 2

Plantar incision with the patient placed in the prone position. The portion of the incision toward the heel can either start on the medial or the lateral side depending on the area of tumor. In general, it is usually not necessary to cross the plantar fat pad either in the heel or under the metatarsophalangeal joints

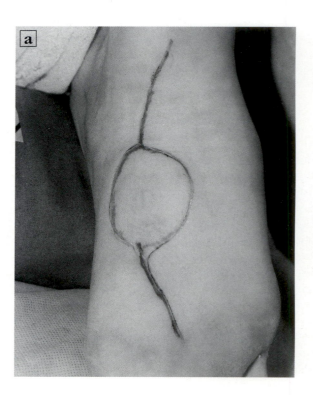

Figure 3

A 48-year-old woman with a painful large mass on the plantar aspect of her right foot which mostly involves the middle and medial side of the plantar aspect of the foot. She has had two previous attempted excisions through very small medial incisions and no attempt had been made to remove the entire plantar fascia or to include enough surrounding tissue to possibly prevent the development of adjacent fibromas.

(a) The patient is placed in the prone position for ease of performing the operation. The mass is encircled with a marking pen and the proximal and distal portions of the incision are outlined.

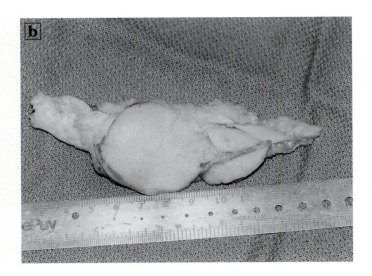

(b) Excision of all of the plantar fascia as well as the tumor and overlying skin which was quite involved with the mass of the tumor.

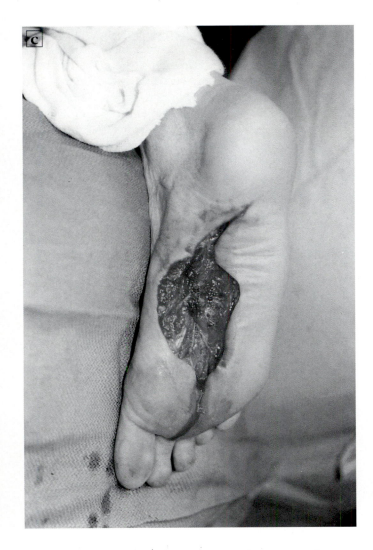

(c) The foot after removal of the tumor showing good underlying intrinsic muscles of the foot, which are intact and viable.

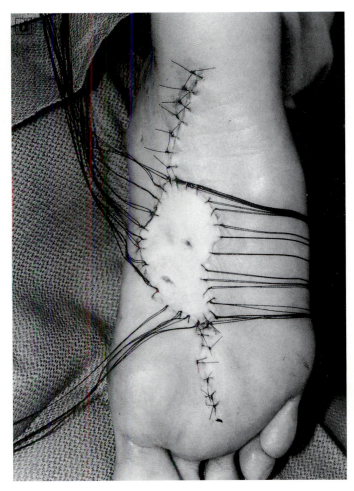

(d) Closure of the wound proximally and distally and application of the full thickness skin graft obtained by a plastic surgeon from the patients contralateral buttock. The graft and incision were covered with a compression dressing.

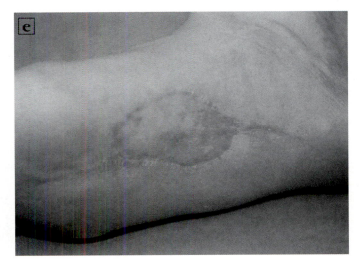

(e) The patient's foot 6 months later with a well-healed graft and no evidence of recurrence. Further follow-up for an additional year has shown no recurrence. The patient is asymptomatic

the posterior part of the incision medially. Conversely, if the nodule is located more toward the forefoot, the anterior portion of the incision can curve medially, just behind the head of the first metatarsal (Fig. 4). It is possible to avoid any potential weight-bearing surface that is under a bony prominence. The plantar fascia is exposed proximally and transected from its attachments to the calcaneus.

Distal dissection should be done carefully to avoid injury to the medial or lateral plantar nerve. Since the medial and lateral plantar nerves pass under the abductor hallucis proximally in the foot, care must be taken to avoid deep pressure or dissection in that area. Once the plantar fascia has been transected from the calcaneus, it can be held away from the underlying muscle belly of the flexor digitorum brevis. At about the midfoot these nerves may first be seen as they course on either side of the flexor brevis. More distal dissection brings the common digital branches into view; these lie just beneath the fascia, and care must be taken to avoid their injury. For all these reasons, it is easier and safer to begin the dissection proximally and proceed with care distally.

Most nodules are in the mid-portion of the medial plantar fascia, which is also in the area of the medial plantar nerve. At times, loop magnification is most helpful in performing a safe dissection. Dissection should be carried out to the metatarsal heads but should not proceed distally because of the lack of involvement of the fascial bands in the area of the toes. Excessive lateral excision of the fascia is usually unnecessary since most of the nodules have always been found within the medial portion of the fascia. Nodules that extend into the sole of the foot should be carefully dissected plantarward along the deeper fascial extensions to the metatarsals.

Meticulous hemostasis is necessary because skin flaps are usually present. The tourniquet should be deflated and hemostasis secured. Suction drainage is essential, particularly where large nodules or multiple nodules have been removed creating a dead space. A compression dressing should be kept in place for seven to 10 days. The patient should have bed rest, and get up only when indoors and using bilateral support such as crutches or a walker. Every precaution should be taken to ensure good wound healing. The wound should be inspected prior to discharge from hospital and at approximately 7–10 days later, and the interrupted sutures should probably be removed no earlier than 14 to 21 days postoperatively.

Another excellent alternative is to place the patient in a short leg non-weight-bearing cast. This immobilizes the hindfoot and ankle, gives excellent skin compression and is most helpful in achieving a well healed wound.

It is very important to assess the relationship of the nodule to the overlying plantar skin. In any nodule that is affixed to the dermis of the plantar skin, and in most recurrent nodules requiring surgical excision, it is usually necessary to resect the overlying plantar skin. Most of these cases will require a skin graft and several donor areas are available from the proximal posterior thigh or the buttock.

Summary

Plantar fibromatosis is a benign condition of the plantar fascia consisting of either a large single nodule or multiple nodules. The condition seems to be more common in patients with Dupuytren's contractures of the hands and in epileptic patients.

Treatment is frequently unnecessary. However, when significant pain and discomfort are caused by the nodule, a wide excision of the plantar fascia, particularly the medial band, is indicated. A careful clinical history is necessary so that a proper diagnosis can be made following microscopic examination of the specimen. This benign lesion should not be confused with a fibrosarcoma.

Proper surgical excision is accomplished through a plantar incision, which adequately exposes the plantar fascia. Recurrences will only occur if the fascia has been incompletely excised. Meticulous dissection and hemostasis as well as proper drainage and skin closure are necessary if wound healing is to be optimal. A proper compression dressing, with or without a short leg cast, as well as the avoidance of dependency and weight bearing aid in the healing process. At times, it is also necessary to excise the overlying skin, if involved, and to skin graft the defect.

References

Allen R A, Wollner L B, Ghormley R K 1955 Soft tissue tumours of the sole with special reference to plantar fibromatosis. J Bone Joint Surg 37A: 14–26

Aviles E, Arlen M, Miller T 1971 Plantar fibromatosis. Surgery 69: 117–120

Cracchiolo A 1982 Office practice: footwear and orthotic therapy. Foot Ankle 2: 242–248

Curtin J W 1962 Surgical therapy for Dupuytren's disease of the foot. Plast Reconstr Surg 30: 568–576

Curtin J W 1965 Fibromatosis of the plantar fascia: surgical technique and design of skin incision. J Bone Joint Surg 47A: 1605

Enneking W F 1983 Musculoskeletal Tumor Surgery. Churchill–Livingstone, New York. pp 747–775

Henry A K 1963 Extensile Exposure. Williams and Wilkins Co, Baltimore

Hollishead W A 1964 Anatomy for Surgeons. Volume 3. Harper and Row, New York

Jahss M H 1982 Disorders of the Foot. W B Saunders, Co., London. pp 841–842

Keasbey L E 1953 Juvenile aponeurotic fibroma (calcifying fibroma). Cancer 6: 338–346

Keller R B, Baez-Giangreco A 1975 Juvenile aponeurotic fibroma. Clin Orthop 106: 198–205

Lee T H, Wapner K L, Hecht P J 1993 Current Concepts Review. Plantar Fibromatosis. J Bone and Joint Surg 75A: 1080–1084

Lund M 1941 Dupuytren's contracture and epilepsy. The clinical connection between Dupuytren's contracture, fibroma plantae, periarthrosis humeri, helodermia, induratio penis plastica and epilepsy, with an attempt at a pathogenic evaluation. Acta Psychiatr Neurol 16: 465–492

Madelung O W 1875 Die Aetiologie und die operative Behandlung der Dupuytrenschein Fingerverhummung. Berlin Klin Wochenschr 12: 191–193

Meyerding H W, Shellito J G 1948 Dupuytren's contracture of the foot. J Int Coll Surg 11: 595–603

Pedersen H E, Day A J 1954 Dupuytren's disease of the foot. JAMA 154: 33

Pickren J W, Smith A G, Stevenson T W Jr, Stout A P 1951 Fibromatosis of the plantar fascia. Cancer 4: 846–856

Stoyle T F 1964 Dupuytren's contracture in the foot. J Bone Joint Surg 46B: 218

Wu K K 1986 Surgery of the Foot. Lea and Febiger, Philadelphia. pp 154–156

VI SYSTEMIC DISORDERS

VI.1 Systemic Disease

Colin G Barnes

Inflammatory arthropathies

The inflammatory arthropathies affect the joints of the feet and ankles in the vast majority of patients. These diseases may be classified in a simplified form as follows:

1. Rheumatoid arthritis
2. Seronegative spondarthritis
   a. ankylosing spondylitis
   b. psoriatic arthritis
   c. reactive arthritis
      i. sexually acquired (SARA), Reiter's syndrome
      ii. post-dysenteric
   d. colitic (enteropathic)
3. Associated with systemic connective tissue diseases, especially systemic lupus erythematosus
4. Postviral, e.g. rubella
5. Miscellaneous
   a. associated with erythema nodosum
   b. Behçet's syndrome
   c. anaphylactoid (Henoch–Schönlein) purpura
   d. Clutton's joints
   e. acne arthritis

Rheumatoid arthritis

Rheumatoid arthritis is considered in Chapter VI.3. It should be noted that the symmetrical small joint polyarthritis of rheumatoid disease usually involves the metatarsophalangeal joints but not the interphalangeal joints of the toes (Table 1). Metatarsal pain frequently is the presenting symptom of the disease.

Radiologically, erosions may be seen in the metatarsophalangeal joints earlier than in the small joints of the hands or wrists even if symptoms in the feet are mild or absent. Thus diagnostic radiographic investigation of a case of possible rheumatoid arthritis, or the assessment of progression of disease in an established case, requires posteroanterior films of both hands and feet as a minimum.

Seronegative spondarthritis/spondylarthropathy

The definition of inflammatory arthritis, which has negative tests for rheumatoid factor (seronegative), in

Table 1 Patterns of joint involvement

		Osteoarthritis	Rheumatoid arthritis[a] Systemic lupus erythematosus	Seronegative[b] Spondarthritis	Gout
Ankles	Subtalar		+	+	+
Feet	Midtarsal	+	+	+	+
	1st metatarsophalangeal	++		(+)	++
	2nd–4th metatarsophalangeal		+	+	(+)
	Interphalangeal			+	
Plantar fasciitis				+	
Achilles tendinitis					

[a]usually symmetrical involvement; [b]often asymmetrical involvement

Table 2 Seronegative spondarthritis

	Genito-urinary	Gastro-intestinal	Eyes	Skin/Mucosal	Nails	HLA-B27[†]
Ankylosing spondylitis	Prostatitis		Uveitis			90+%[1]
Psoriatic arthritis			Uveitis Conjunctivitis	Psoriasis	Pitting Hyperkeratosis and dystrophy	S: 50–100%[2] P: 9–28%
			Keratoconjunctivitis sicca			
Reactive arthritis SARA	Urethritis Cervicitis		Uveitis Conjunctivitis	Psoriasis/ skin rash Keratoderma Circinate balanitis Mouth ulcers (painless)	Hyperkeratosis and dystrophy	60–80%[3]
Post-dysenteric		Infective dysentry				
Colitic (enteropathic)		Ulcerative colitis	Uveitis	Erythema nodosum Pyoderma gangrenosum	Clubbing	UC: 19%[4]
		Crohn's		Mouth ulcers (painless)		Cr: 4% S: 33–91%[5] P: 5–29%

†   Normal ≤ 8% Caucasians
S   Sacroiliitis/spondylitis
P   Peripheral arthritis only
UC Ulcerative colitis only
Cr Crohn's disease only
[1] Brewerton et al (1973), Schlosslein et al (1973), Arnett (1979), Keat et al (1979)
[2] Brewerton et al (1974a,b), Masi (1979), Kammer et al (1979)
[3] Morris et al (1974), Harris et al (1975), Arnett (1979), Keat et al (1979), Masi (1979), Olhagen (1983), Aho et al (1983), Sheldon & Pell (1983)
[4] Dekker-Saeys et al (1978)
[5] Brewerton et al (1974a,b), Brewerton & James (1975), Masi (1979)

contrast to rheumatoid arthritis, in which 75% of patients are seropositive, does not depend solely on laboratory tests for rheumatoid factor. As shown in Tables 1 and 2, the pattern of joint involvement, the spectrum of extra-articular manifestations and the association with the histocompatibility antigen HLA B27 distinguishes this group from rheumatoid arthritis.

The term seronegative spondarthritis or spondyl-arthropathy emphasizes the frequent involvement of the sacroiliac joints and spine (spondylitis) in this group of diseases (Moll et al 1974). It has been shown that sacroiliitis and spondylitis are present more often than expected in patients with ulcerative colitis (Wright & Watkinson 1965, Macrae & Wright 1973), Crohn's disease (Haslock & Wright 1973–4) and psoriatic arthritis, but not

in those with psoriasis alone (Jajic 1968, Moll & Wright 1973a) or sexually acquired reactive arthritis (Reiter's syndrome) (Wright 1963, Lawrence 1974, Olhagen 1983).

Similarly, there is an increased prevalence of inflammatory bowel disease (Jayson et al 1970, Brewerton & James 1975), and prostatitis and urethritis (Mason et al 1958) in patients with ankylosing spondylitis. First degree relatives of patients also have an increased incidence of all these features.

This has led to the formulation of diagnostic criteria to classify spondylarthropathies and distinguish them from other forms of inflammatory arthritis.

The European Spondylarthropathy Study Group's preliminary classification criteria (Dougados et al 1991) are as follows:

Inflammatory spinal pain defined by four of the following:

- onset before age 45;
- insidious onset;
- improved by exercise;
- associated with morning stiffness;
- at least three months' duration (Calin et al 1977)

Or synovitis–asymmetrical or predominantly in the lower limbs plus one or more of the following:

- positive family history
- psoriasis
- inflammatory bowel disease
- urethritis or cervicitis (non-gonococcal), or acute diarrhoea within one month before arthritis
- buttock pain alternating between right and left gluteal areas
- enthesopathy
- sacroiliitis

Earlier classifications (Moll et al 1978, Wright et al 1983) also included the absence of serum rheumatoid and antinuclear factors, the absence of subcutaneous 'rheumatoid' nodules, clinical overlap between members of the group and significant association with the HLA B27 antigen (Ebringer & Shipley 1983).

Pattern of joint involvement

The pattern of peripheral joint involvement in the seronegative spondarthritides differs from rheumatoid arthritis, osteoarthritis and gout (see Table 1), and possible involvement of the sacroiliac joints as well as those of the hands and feet must be taken into account. The major differences in the pattern of joint involvement, therefore, are that in the seronegative group

- the terminal interphalangeal joints of the fingers and interphalangeal joints of the toes are often affected (Fig. 1);
- sacroiliitis is common (see above);
- asymmetrical or predominantly lower limb joint involvement is usual.

Nevertheless, the histological appearance of the synovium may be indistinguishable from rheumatoid arthritis, although rheumatoid factor is not present in the synovial plasma cells.

Although not strictly part of the pattern of joint involvement, plantar fasciitis and inflammation at the point of attachment of the Achilles tendon to the calcaneum are common, representing enthesopathies (see below).

Ankylosing spondylitis

Sacroiliitis and spinal involvement are characteristic of ankylosing spondylitis but peripheral joints may be affected in up to 50% (Sharp 1957), and may be the

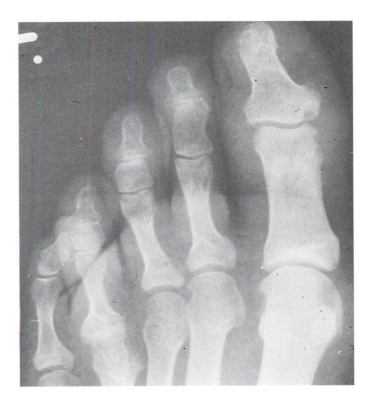

Figure 1

Involvement of the interphalangeal joints of the toes

presenting feature in 15% (Sharp 1965). The peripheral joints most commonly affected are the hips and knees, presenting as a monoarticular synovitis, but the interphalangeal joints of the toes, ankles and subtalar joints may also be involved.

Inflammation at the site of attachment of ligament or tendon to bone is characteristic and is known as an enthesopathy (Ball 1971, 1983). This leads to cortical erosion, new bone formation and ossification into the ligament and is typically seen in the development of spinal bony ankylosis, radiologically being seen as the 'bamboo spine' of advanced severe cases. Many other sites may be affected by this process, and in the foot this occurs at the attachment of the Achilles tendon and plantar fascia to the calcaneum, leading to pain and tenderness at these sites. Radiological erosion and new bone (spur) formation are seen. The latter has the fluffy appearance associated with inflammatory periostitis in contrast to well-corticated 'hard' calcaneal spurs, which are not of clinical significance (Fig. 2).

Psoriatic arthritis

The prevalence of skin psoriasis is approximately 2% of the population and the overall incidence of arthritis in these patients is approximately 5–7% (males 1.5–5.8%; females 4.1–7.9%) (Wright 1978, Kammer et al 1979, Espinoza et al 1992).

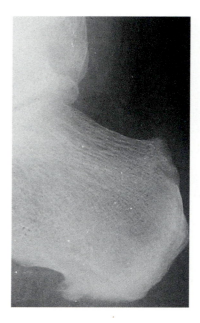

Figure 2

A 'fluffy' calcaneal spur due to periostitis in Reiter's syndrome

Moll & Wright (1973b) defined five clinical forms of psoriatic arthritis:

- involvement confined to the terminal interphalangeal joints of the hands and the interphalangeal joints of the toes (5%).
- severe deforming, destructive 'arthritis mutilans' affecting hands and feet with sacroiliitis (5%).
- symmetrical polyarthritis resembling rheumatoid arthritis but with negative serology (15%).
- asymmetrical oligoarthritis, pauciarticular, small joint involvement, with 'sausage' digits (70%).
- ankylosing spondylitis with or without peripheral arthritis (5%).

However, more recent studies suggest that a symmetrical polyarthritis resembling rheumatoid arthritis is the most frequent form of the disease (Gladman et al 1987; Helliwell et al 1991). Approximately 80% of patients with polyarticular and approximately 30% with oligoarticular disease have ankle and foot involvement, which is frequently the initial site of arthritis (Torre Alonso et al 1991; Hammerschlag et al 1991). Males and females are equally affected, with male predominance in patients with involvement of the distal joints of the digits and of the spine (Wright & Helliwell 1992).

The psoriasis may be detected as nail pitting alone, or be asymptomatic but present in the scalp, umbilicus or natal cleft. There is no direct relationship between exacerbations, or the severity, of skin disease and joint disease. Nail dystrophy (pitting, hyperkeratosis and ridging) is more common in patients with terminal interphalangeal joint involvement. Radiographic changes of peripheral joints include periarticular osteoporosis, loss

of cartilage joint space and erosive destruction of joints. The latter is frequently asymmetrical, as is the arthritis clinically, so that some joints are severely destroyed while others nearby remain normal.

Oligoarticular arthralgia and inflammatory arthritis affecting predominantly lower limb joints (knees and ankles) have been described as a rare association of severe acne (acne fulminans; acne conglobata) in male patients (Burns & Coleville 1959, Davis et al 1981, Clement et al 1982). This is now grouped with palmar–plantar pustulosis which, with involvement of the sterno-clavicular and manubriosternal joints, sternoclavicular and spinal hyperostosis and sterile multifocal osteomyelitis, form the SAPHO syndrome (Benhamou et al 1988, Kahn et al 1991). The SAPHO syndrome is now being considered as part of the clinical spectrum of psoriatic arthritis (Helliwell et al 1991).

A modified classification of psoriatic arthritis, therefore, is now being proposed (Espinoza et al 1992):

- peripheral arthritis resembling rheumatoid arthritis but including common involvement of the terminal interphalangeal joints, and also dactylitis and arthritis mutilans
- sacroiliitis and spondylitis
- SAPHO syndrome

Reactive arthritis

The term Reiter's syndrome, defined as the association of arthritis, conjunctivitis and urethritis, has largely been replaced by the term reactive arthritis. This may be defined as inflammatory arthritis following, or as a reaction to, infection at a distant site, often dysenteric or genital, the latter then acquiring the title of 'Sexually Acquired Reactive Arthritis' (SARA) (Keat et al 1979). In fact Reiter himself described the post-dysenteric rather than the sexually acquired form.

Infections commonly associated with arthritis are nongonococcal urethritis (Catterall 1983), with an association in a substantial proportion of cases with chlamydial infection, and infective enterocolitis (dysentery) due to *Shigella* species, *Yersinia* species and *Campylobacter jejuni* (Amor et al 1983, Good 1983, Aho et al 1983, Ford 1983a,b) in particular. Masi (1979) recorded an incidence of 1.7% of Reiter's syndrome in association with nongonococcal urethritis, 9% postdysenteric arthritis after *Salmonella* infection and 33% after *Yersinia* infection.

More recently reports have shown that about 2% of cases of *Salmonella* dysentery are associated with reactive arthritis and that approximately 4% of patients had chronic rheumatic disease after *Yersinia* or *Campylobacter* infections. (Bremell et al 1991; Lindholm and Visakorpi 1991; Mäki-Ikola et al 1991). *Chlamydia pneumoniae* has also been shown to be a cause of reactive arthritis (Saario and Toivanen 1993, Braun et al 1994).

The features of reactive arthritis are:

- it develops two to four weeks after an episode of infective enterocolitis or coincident with, or

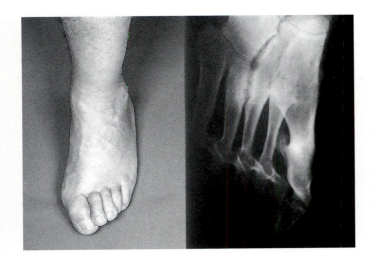

Figure 3

The rigid flat foot of Reiter's syndrome (by permission from Barnes 1980)

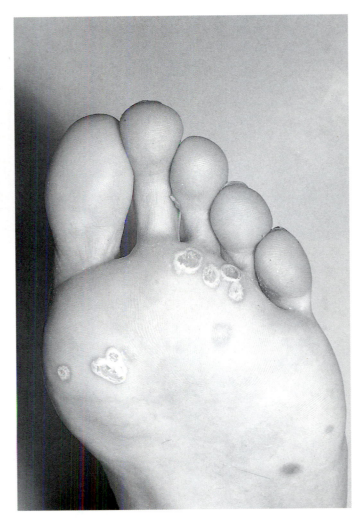

Figure 4

Keratoderma in Reiter's syndrome

preceded by, nongonococcal urethritis or cervicitis and/or conjunctivitis.

- an infective organism cannot be isolated from the blood. In postdysenteric forms, the organism cannot be isolated from joint fluid although *Chlamydia* has been isolated from the joint fluid of patients with SARA. However, lipopolysaccharide determinants from *Salmonella*, *Yersinia* and *Shigella* have been found in synovial cells or synovial fluids from patients with reactive arthritis triggered by these agents (Granfors 1992). *Salmonella* specific antibodies have also been detected in serum and synovial fluid (Mäki-Ikola et al 1992).

- the arthritis frequently resolves within six months although recurrent and chronic destructive forms occur.

Lower limb joint involvement is characteristic of this group of arthritides, and this leads to pain, swelling and stiffness of the interphalangeal joints of the toes, the metatarsophalangeal, midtarsal and subtalar joints and the ankles. Progressive joint destruction tends to lead to rigidity of the foot (Fig. 3). Thus the flat, immobile foot and toes, with severe limitation of the ankle and subtalar joints and valgus heel, occurs in severe, chronic and advanced cases. Achilles tendonitis and plantar fasciitis are common, as in ankylosing spondylitis.

While keratoderma (Fig. 4) and nail dystrophy are typical of sexually acquired reactive arthritis, they may also occur in the postdysenteric type.

Colitic (enteropathic) arthritis

Dekker-Saeys et al (1978) confirmed three patterns of joint involvement in patients with inflammatory bowel disease, in whom they found 13% to have a peripheral arthritis, 10% asymptomatic sacroiliitis and 3.7% classical ankylosing sponylitis. Peripheral arthritis has also been shown to occur in 12% of patients with ulcerative colitis and 22% of those with Crohn's disease (Haslock 1986). Although episodes of acute, nondestructive inflammation of large joints, usually the knees, are characteristic, very occasionally peripheral small joints are involved as in ankylosing spondylitis.

Pyoderma gangrenosum

Pyoderma gangrenosum (Fig. 5) is a condition of unknown cause with necrosis and ulceration of skin, usually affecting the lower legs and less frequently the thighs and rarely the arms. It may accompany inflammatory bowel disease, especially ulcerative colitis (Perry & Brunsting 1957), and thus may be associated with colitic arthropathy. It has also been recorded as occurring with typical rheumatoid arthritis and as being associated with a progressive erosive seronegative arthritis affecting mainly upper limb and sacroiliac joints (Holt et al 1980).

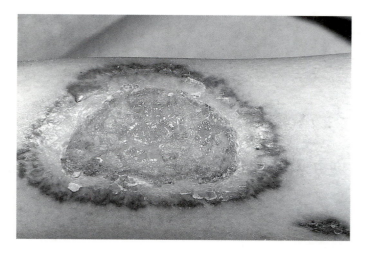

Figure 5

Pyoderma gangrenosum

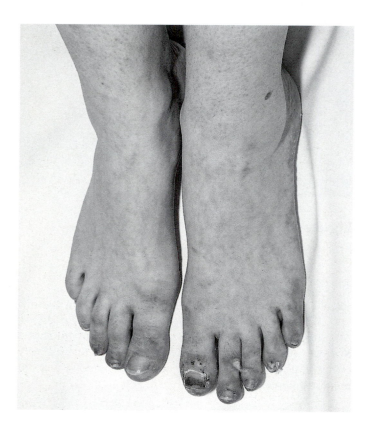

Figure 6

Vasculitis and arthritis in systemic lupus erythematosus

Systemic connective tissue diseases

A symmetrical inflammatory polyarthritis, resembling rheumatoid arthritis, may be the presentation of any of the systemic connective tissue diseases, especially systemic lupus erythematosus (SLE). Arthralgia often

Table 3 Major clinical features of the systemic connective tissue diseases

Systemic lupus erythematosus
   polyarthritis
   Raynaud's phenomenon
   skin rash (for example 'butterfly')
   renal involvement
   alopecia
   neuropsychiatric lesions
   leucopenia
   rheumatoid factor tests positive in approx. 30%
   positive antinuclear antibody and DNA binding tests
   absence of radiological erosions
Polyarteritis nodosa (classical)
   arteritis
   mononeuritis multiplex
   pulmonary involvement
      'asthma'
      pulmonary opacities
   abdominal pain
   hypertension
   haematuria
   leucocytosis
   eosinophilia (with pulmonary involvement)
Systemic sclerosis
   Raynaud's phenomenon
   skin involvement (scleroderma)
   telangiectasia
   polyarthritis
   subcutaneous calcinosis
   dysphagia
   hypertension
   fibrosing alveolitis
   renal involvement
   polymyositis
Dermatomyositis
   characteristic skin rash
   periorbital heliotrope rash
   facial oedema
   scaling erythema of face, trunk, arms and thighs
   which is irritating and burning
   'collodion' patches over the dorsum of finger joints
   telangiectasia around nail beds
   inflammatory proximal myopathy

exceeds objective signs of synovitis. The arthritis is mild and usually nondeforming and nondestructive. As in all cases of inflammatory arthritis, close enquiry and examination is required for evidence of associated systemic features (Table 3). Thus arthritis and vasculitis may both present in the feet (Fig. 6).

Rheumatoid factor tests are positive in approximately one-third of patients, antinuclear antibody tests in almost 100% of SLE and 30% of other conditions. DNA-binding assays are positive in SLE, in which leucopenia may also be present. A positive fluorescent antinuclear antibody test with a speckled pattern is the immunological marker of the so-called 'Mixed Connective Tissue Disease'. In these cases, DNA-binding assays are usually negative and extractable nuclear antibody (ENA) assays are positive with specificity for RNA. Whereas this was originally thought to represent a separate disease entity (Sharp et al 1972) it is now apparent that these patients usually follow the disease pattern of SLE, of systemic sclerosis or occasionally of rheumatoid arthritis.

Raynaud's phenomenon

Raynaud's phenomenon, while often benign and idiopathic in young females, is a prominent feature of the systemic connective tissue disorders with which they may present. Although this commonly affects the hands, involvement of the feet is not unusual, and in the most severe cases leads to ischaemic lesions of the tips of the fingers and toes.

The development of Raynaud's phenomenon in middle age must always be regarded as a possible onset of a connective tissue disorder, especially systemic lupus erythematosus or systemic sclerosis. The skin changes of systemic sclerosis (scleroderma) affect the feet less often than the hands.

Viral infections

Metatarsophalangeal joints and the ankles, together with the small joints of the hands, wrists and knees, may be involved in a symmetrical inflammatory synovitis in association with viral infections. The synovitis is usually mild and nondestructive but there is marked arthralgia. This may precede, be coincident with, or follow a few days after the development of other features of the infection. The arthritis resolves completely without residual joint damage in a variable time from a few days to a few weeks; during this time it may be migratory or persistent, and it is sometimes accompanied by myalgia, tenosynovitis and carpal tunnel syndrome.

This clinical picture has been described most commonly in young females in association with rubella (Chambers & Bywaters 1963) and after rubella immunization (Sprunance & Smith 1971). Rubella virus has been isolated from affected joints. Other infections associated with similar joint manifestations include infectious mononucleosis, mumps (Lass & Shepherd 1961, Ghosh & Reddy 1973), viral hepatitis (Schumacher & Gall 1974), influenza, chicken-pox (Friedman & Naveh 1971) and smallpox (Ansell 1986).

Erythema nodosum

Up to 75% of patients with erythema nodosum of any cause may experience arthralgia and a benign self-limit-ing symmetrical polyarthritis. The causes of erythema nodosum include streptococcal infections, sarcoidosis (Lofgren's syndrome), tuberculosis, Behçet's syndrome, ulcerative colitis, leprosy, meningococcal infections, fungal infections and sulphonamides (Blomgren 1974). Severe, often confluent, erythema nodosum around the distal part of the lower leg and ankle, with warmth, redness, tenderness, pain on movement and hence stiffness, may mimic a synovitis of the ankle.

Involvement of the ankles

A number of unrelated conditions may present as, or include, an inflammatory arthritis of the ankles; these rarely, if ever, involve smaller joints of the feet.

Palindromic rheumatism

Palindromic, or episodic, rheumatism presents attacks of acute joint inflammation lasting for up to seven days. These occur irregularly, affecting one or two joints at a time, commonly the ankles, knees, hands, wrists and elbows. The involved area is swollen, red, hot, stiff, painful and tender, the swelling and redness often being periarticular. There is nevertheless a true synovitis present (Wajed et al 1977). In approximately half of these patients, the disease progresses to a more typical continuous polyarticular pattern of rheumatoid arthritis. Positive tests for rheumatoid factor often develop during the palindromic phase.

Treatment of the acute attack requires full doses of anti-inflammatory analgesics, and, if the attacks are frequent, regular use of these drugs will prevent or alleviate such attacks. In those with very severe and acute attacks of palindromic rheumatism, in whom rheumatoid factor tests are positive, treatment with gold injections, penicillamine, or sulphasalazine is indicated, as in rheumatoid arthritis.

Clutton's joints

A nonspecific inflammatory synovitis, developing in children and young adults with congenital syphilis, characteristically affects the knees symmetrically and much less frequently the ankles and elbows (Gray & Philp 1963). The synovitis is nondestructive and self-limiting.

Vascular disease

Vasculitis

Vasculitis, classically polyarteritis nodosa, may be part of any of the systemic connective tissue diseases and may occur in rheumatoid arthritis. The vasculitides may be classified as follows (Chakravarty & Scott 1992, Lie 1994):

- primary (e.g. polyarteritis nodosa or Wegener's granulomatosis) or secondary to other diseases (e.g. connective tissue diseases or rheumatoid arthritis).
- by possible aetiopathogenesis:
    immune complex deposition
        systemic necrotizing vasculitis
        polyarteritis nodosa
        Churg–Strauss syndrome
    hypersensitivity
        serum sickness
        Henoch–Schönlein purpura
        connective tissue diseases
        associated with malignancy
    cell-mediated immunity
        giant cell arteritis (granulomatous)
            temporal (cranial) arteritis
            Takayasu
        Wegener's granulomatosis
    uncertain
        thromboangiitis obliterans (Buerger's disease)
        Kawasaki disease
        Behçet's disease etc
- according to the size of vessel involved (those with granulomatosis marked *)
    large vessels
        temporal arteritis
        Takayasu's arteritis
        aortitis in ankylosing spondylitis and rheumatoid arthritis*
    medium and small vessels
        polyarteritis nodosa
        arteritis of systemic lupus erythematosus and rheumatoid arthritis
        Wegener's granulomatosis*
        Churg–Strauss syndrome*
    small vessels (leucocytoclastic)
        Henoch–Schönlein purpura
        systemic lupus erythematosus and rheumatoid arthritis*
        drug induced*

Antinuclear cytoplasmic antibody (ANCA) with a cytoplasmic staining pattern directed against proteinase 3 is highly specific for Wegener's granulomatosis and is sometimes present in other vasculitides (Chakravarty & Scott 1992, Kallenberg et al 1992, Kallenberg 1994). The clinical features caused by the vasculitis depend on the effects of vascular occlusion that results from the inflammatory involvement of the vessel wall, intimal proliferation, and healing with fibrosis, each of which may result in thrombosis. The clinical features of the vasculitis are shown in Table 4. In the foot, this may present as skin necrosis (Fig. 7), arthritis or arthralgia, and the effects of a mononeuritis multiplex.

Table 4 Clinical features of vasculitis

Subcutaneous nodules	– along affected vessels
Skin	– necrotic lesions (Fig. 7)
	– livedo reticularis
	– nonthrombocytopenic purpura
Cardiovascular system	– hypertension
Gastrointestinal	– abdominal pain
	– intestinal infarction
	– mucosal ulceration
Renal	– hypertension
	– renal failure
Pulmonary	– asthma
	– radiological opacities and cavitation
Central nervous system	– cerebral infarction
	– epilepsy
Peripheral nervous system	– mononeuritis multiplex

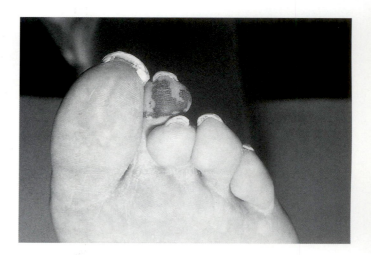

Figure 7

Skin necrosis in polyarteritis nodosa (by permission of the publishers and editor of Currey 1986)

Anaphylactoid (Henoch–Schönlein) purpura

Anaphylactoid purpura arises from vasculitis of small vessels (arterioles and capillaries), and histologically it may include a necrotizing arteriolitis (Gairdner 1948). The cause remains unknown, but an allergic response to streptococci (Bywaters et al 1957), various foods, insect bites, and drugs, especially penicillin (Casser 1956), has been incriminated. Levinsky & Barratt (1979) detected both circulating and skin-bound immune complexes, including IgA (Lie 1994).

Papular nonthrombocytopenic purpura develops on the buttock and legs, typically on the soles of the feet,

and occasionally on the upper half of the body.
Widespread ecchymoses and skin necrosis may develop.

Henoch originally described the gastrointestinal lesions
of haemorrhage and oedema of the intestinal wall, with
colicky abdominal pain, intestinal haemorrhage or intus-
susception (Allen et al 1960).

Medium and large joints are the site of inflammatory
synovitis of the ankles, knees and hips in the lower
limbs, and less commonly the wrists and elbows.

Additional features may include acute proliferative or
focal glomerulonephritis, which may become chronic
and hypertension, and renal failure, as well as intracranial and ocular haemorrhage (Derham & Rogerson 1956,
Lewis & Philpott 1956, Bywaters et al 1957, Vernier et
al 1961).

Thromboangiitis obliterans (Buerger's disease)

Acute inflammation with thrombosis of peripheral arteries
and veins characterizes Buerger's disease. Men between
the ages of 20 and 40 years are affected almost exclusively. The cause remains unknown but cigarette smoking
is closely related to the clinical manifestations of intermittent claudication, Raynaud's phenomenon and peripheral gangrene affecting the feet more than the hands.

Hypertrophic osteoarthropathy

Clubbing of the nails (Fig. 8), swelling of joints with local
pain and tenderness most commonly involving the
ankles and wrists, and radiological periostitis are the
characteristic features of hypertrophic osteoarthropathy.
The overlying skin is red, warm and oedematous, and
tenderness extends to the distal part of the long bones
of the forearm and lower leg. A mild synovitis of the
knees may also be present, although the synovial fluid
does not contain the high cell count characteristic of an
inflammatory condition.

A narrow band of periosteal new bone is present
radiologically, especially at the distal ends of the radius
and ulna and the tibia and fibula, but this may also affect
the bones of the hands and feet, and the vertebrae and
clavicles (Yacoub & Simon 1966, Greenfield et al 1967).

Formerly the condition was known as hypertrophic
pulmonary osteoarthropathy since it is most commonly
secondary to pulmonary pathology, especially bronchial
carcinoma. However, many causes that are not primarily pulmonary have been identified, leading to the
omission of the word pulmonary from the name of the
disease. Causes identified are listed in Table 5. From this
it will be seen that the majority of primary pathologies
are pulmonary or gastrointestinal, and the report of
hypertrophic osteoarthropathy in cystic fibrosis (Wasser

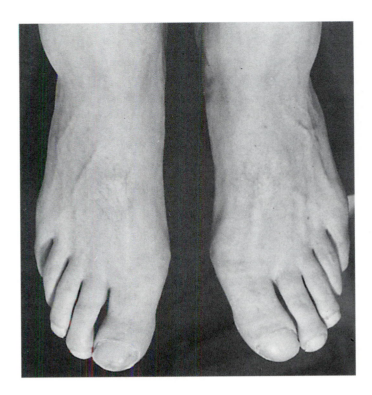

Figure 8

Hypertrophic osteoarthropathy – clubbing of the toe nails

et al 1982) interestingly links these two systems. A
coincidence of both hypertrophic osteoarthropathy and
metastatic synovial and bony deposits from a bronchial
neoplasm has been reported (Fam & Gross 1979).
Nevertheless, the pathogenesis is unknown. It has been
suggested that periostitis is responsible for the clinical
manifestations and that this may be dependent on vagal
stimulation (Dixon 1963). It has been demonstrated that
the rheumatological manifestations may regress after
vagotomy (Flavell 1956, Yacoub 1965, le Roux 1968) or
after parasympathetic blockade (Lopez-Enriques et al
1980, Schwartz 1981) without removal of a primary
bronchial neoplasm. Removal of the primary cause will
lead to a resolution of hypertrophic osteoarthropathy,
and this has also been achieved by chemotherapeutic
treatment of neoplastic disease (Evans 1980).

Pachydermoperiostosis (Touraine–Solente–Gole syndrome)

This is a rare primary form of hypertrophic osteoarthropathy. It has been shown to be inherited by a
Mendelian dominant or sex-linked trait affecting males
(Fischer et al 1964, Rimoin 1965). Clubbing, periostitis, skin
and scalp thickening (pachydermia) and painful swelling
around the knees, wrists and ankles are characteristic.

Table 5 Causes of hypertrophic osteoarthropathy

Pulmonary – neoplastic[1]	bronchial carcinoma
	all primary lung neoplasms (except cylindromic adenoma)
	metastases from other sites
	pleural fibrosarcomata
– non-neoplastic[2]	bronchiectasis
	empyema
	tuberculosis
	aspergillosis
Congenital cyanotic heart disease[3]	
Gastrointestinal	biliary atresia[4]
	biliary cirrhosis[5]
	portal cirrhosis[6]
	intestinal lymphoma[7]
	ulcerative colitis[8]
	Crohn's disease[9]
	gastrointestinal neoplasms[10]
	pseudomembranous enterocolitis[11]
Hodgkin's disease[12]	
Cystic fibrosis[13]	
Thyroid acropachy	

[1] Flavell 1956, Stenseth et al 1967, Yacoub et al 1967, le Roux 1968
[2] Yacoub & Simon 1966
[3] McLaughlin et al 1967
[4] Cavanaugh & Holman 1965
[5] Mendlowitz 1942
[6] Buchan & Mitchell 1967, Han & Colins 1968, Epstein et al 1979
[7] Bakhshandeh et al 1971
[8] Honska et al 1957, Farman et al 1976
[9] Neale et al 1968, Fielding & Cooke 1971
[10] Hollis 1967
[11] Ueno et al 1981
[12] Mullins & Lenhard 1971
[13] Wasser et al 1982

Ankle swelling is due to the periostitis without synovitis (Calabro et al 1966). Bone marrow failure has been reported (Metz & Dowell 1965).

The disease usually presents at about the time of puberty and progresses for up to 5 years thereafter (Calabro et al 1966, Salfeld & Spalckhaver 1966).

Thyroid acropachy

Long-standing severe hyperthyroidism, often with pretibial myxoedema and exophthalmos, may rarely be associated with clubbing and periostitis. Periostitis leads to swelling of the hands and feet; the thickened, coarse and fissured skin that accompanies the swelling is possibly due to lymphatic obstruction (Scanlon & Clemett 1964, Williams 1967, Ford 1970, Bland et al 1979, Rothschild & Yoon 1982).

Metabolic and endocrine disorders

Hyperlipoproteinaemias

Five groups of hyperlipoproteinaemias have been identified (Fredrickson et al 1967, Rifkind 1970). Tendon xanthomata may occur in Types II and III, often in the Achilles tendon (Glueck et al 1968), and a polyarthritis may occur in Types II and IV. Large joints tend to be affected in Type II, the symptoms being migratory, lasting for up to one month in an individual joint. The ankles may be involved, and it is debated whether the swelling, redness and tenderness is due to a true synovitis (Glueck et al 1968) or a periarthritis (Rooney et al 1978). A histologically proven synovitis may cause a large and small joint polyarthritis in Type IV hyperlipoproteinaemia (Buckingham et al 1975).

Hyperuricaemia occurs in association with Types III, IV and V hyperlipoproteinaemia (hypertriglyceridaemias) with an increased incidence of gout, obesity and diabetes (Berkowitz 1964, 1966).

Hyperparathyroidism

Hyperparathyroidism may lead to five forms of rheumatic manifestations (Holt 1986a):
- bone pain resulting from fracture or trabecular collapse (which may involve metatarsal bones), from periosteal new bone formation or from osteomalacia. In osteomalacia, there is local bone tenderness, pain may arise from tendon insertions, and neuropathy and myopathy may also be present (Patten et al 1974).
- an erosive small and medium sized joint polyarthritis. Bywaters et al (1963) attributed the erosions to collapse of subchondral bone, although Resnick (1974) reported articular, without subperiosteal, erosions. Subchondral bone collapse may occur, usually at the tibial plateau, with an associated synovitis, all of which may be traumatic.
- chondrocalcinosis articularis and pyrophosphate arthropathy.
- secondary (renal) hyperuricaemia and gout.
- fusion of sacroiliac joints (Bunch & Hunder 1973) and tenderness at points of tendon attachment to bone, likened to ankylosing spondylitis and the associated enthesopathy (Ball 1971, 1983).

Thus, in the foot, hyperparathyroidism may present as a small joint polyarthritis, as a 'March' fracture or as (secondary) gout. Symptoms of the associated hypercalcaemia (polyuria, fatigue, weight loss, vomiting, depression) are likely to be more prominent than the rheumatological symptoms.

Acromegaly

Acromegaly may be associated with low back ache (Bluestone et al 1971), carpal tunnel syndrome, coarse crepitus with variable noninflammatory effusions of large joints without pain, entrapment neuropathies (especially carpal tunnel syndrome), and fatigue, sometimes with a mild proximal myopathy.

Thus, in the foot, the principal feature is a diffuse enlargement, as seen also in the hand. Radiologically, early widening of the cartilage joint space and late degenerative changes are seen. Prominent tufting of the terminal phalanx also develops; this is best seen in the fingers, but it may also be present in the toes (Bluestone et al 1971). Thickening of the soft tissue of the heel pad seen radiologically is a supporting diagnostic feature.

Hypothyroidism

Muscle cramps, entrapment neuropathies (carpal tunnel or tarsal tunnel syndromes (Frymoyer & Bland 1973) and tenosynovitis of the dorsum of the foot (Dorwart & Schumacher 1975) may all produce symptoms referable to the foot in hypothyroidism. Examination of the foot includes eliciting the ankle jerk which, with other reflexes, is characteristically slow in relaxation in hypothyroidism.

Hyperthyroidism

Thyroid acropachy is considered on page 416. In severe hyperthyroidism, proximal myopathy with weakness, and cramp (spreading distally in the most severely affected cases) may develop.

Diabetes mellitus

Five principal complications, or manifestations, of diabetes affect, and therefore may present in, the foot. These are neuropathic (Charcot's) joint disease, peripheral neuropathy, peripheral vascular disease and possibly Dupuytren's diathysis (Gray & Gottlieb 1976), each of which are considered separately within this chapter.

The fifth is gout, but there are doubts whether this is a true association. Obesity and hypertriglyceridaemia are associated with both hyperuricaemia and diabetes (Berkowitz 1966). Two large population studies (Mikkelson et al 1965, Hall et al 1967) failed to demonstrate a statistical clinical relationship between the two diseases.

Haematological disorders

Haemophilia

In patients with haemophilia (haemophilia A – factor VIII deficiency) or Christmas disease (haemophilia B – factor IX deficiency) 90% of haemorrhages occur in joints or muscles. Severe joint damage develops in those patients with less than 2 iu/dl (2% of normal) factor VIII or IX levels, resulting from frequent and apparently often spontaneous bleeding (Ahlberg 1967).

Chronic joint damage appears to result from several mechanisms, including synovitis, synovial fibrosis and cartilage destruction arising from mechanical, chemical and enzymatic processes (Stein & Duthie 1981). Knees, elbows and the ankle–subtalar joints are most commonly affected, followed by hips and shoulders; small joints of the hands and feet are rarely involved. The proportion of bleeds into joints decreases in lower limb and increases in upper limb joints during adolescence, but the overall number of haemarthroses usually falls rapidly in adult life (Aronstam et al 1979, Barnes & Colvin 1983). Chronic synovitis may also result from repeated haemarthroses.

Damaged joints are vulnerable to repeated haemarthroses, and severe local muscle wasting usually develops. Thus the final outcome is joint limitation and deformity. Radiologically the changes are those of severe degenerative joint disease with prolific new bone formation and, often, large bone cysts (Fig. 9).

It is essential that intravenous replacement of the missing factor is given immediately on development of a haemarthrosis. With modern treatment using concentrated preparations of factor VIII or IX and home treatment programmes, aspiration of affected joints is very rarely required. Long-term management of chronic joint damage requires a home programme of physiotherapy to maintain associated muscle power and prevention, or correction, of deformity. Lightweight plastic splints for the ankle–subtalar joints is appropriate for the most severely affected cases with gross joint damage, where the knees especially are not in themselves a limiting factor.

Leukaemia

Acute leukaemia in childhood may present with bone and joint pain and migratory synovitis, resembling

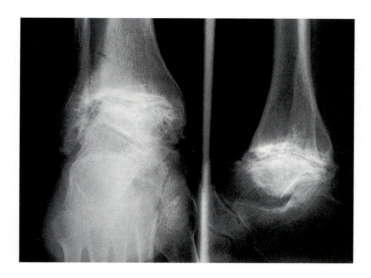

Figure 9

Haemophilia – chronic arthritis of the ankle

juvenile arthritis. Since the latter may include fever, weight loss, lymphadenopathy, splenomegaly, anaemia and leucocytosis, the differential diagnosis may be difficult (Holt 1986b).

Haemoglobinopathies

Bone and joint changes in sickle cell disease (Hb_{S-S}) and its variants (Hb_{A-S} Hb_{S-rhai}) include:

- pathological fractures due to cortical thinning, itself due to erythroid hyperplasia.
- bone infarction due to sickle cell crises. These crises are usually due to hypoxia, which leads to the formation of sickle cells in vivo because of a physio-chemical alteration of Hb_S. The sickle cells then form thromboses, and the patient presents with fever, abdominal pain, and joint or bone pain; bone pain is due to infarction. Joint pain may be associated with effusion, haemarthrosis, or haemorrhage into subchondral bone.
- dactylitis causing painful swelling of the hands and feet. Periostitis of metacarpals and metatarsals is present radiologically.
- septic arthritis and osteomyelitis with a high incidence of *Salmonella* infection of bone (Barrett-Connor 1971, Engh et al 1971).

Neurological disorders

Peripheral neuropathies

The causes of peripheral neuropathies have been outlined in Chapter III.5, where the electrodiagnostic

abnormalities have also been described; the causes are listed in Table 6. The majority of patients have 'cryptogenic' neuropathy thus implying an unknown cause.

Patients present with burning dysaesthesiae, numbness or paraesthesiae in the feet and toes, extending up into the lower legs in the more severe cases. In such cases peripheral weakness, for example foot drop, is also present.

The signs are those of a glove-and-stocking loss or diminution of sensation, peripheral weakness and absent peripheral tendon reflexes. Features of the possible cause need to be sought, and the diagnosis can be confirmed by nerve conduction studies.

Neuropathic arthropathy (Charcot's joints)

Loss of pain sensation has been regarded as the cause of joint destruction known as Charcot's joints. It is unlikely, however, that this is the true cause, as some patients with this condition do experience pain. However there is a combination of impairment of pain sensation and positional sense in most patients which, together with trauma, may lead to the joint destruction.

Table 6 Causes of peripheral neuropathy

Cryptogenic	cause unknown
Metabolic	diabetes mellitus (15%)
	diabetic amyotrophy
	porphyria
	amyloidosis
	uraemia
Toxic	arsenic
	lead
	mercury
	thallium
Vitamin deficiencies	vitamin B (including thiamine and B_{12})
	alcoholic
	pyroxamine
	pantothenic acid
In rheumatic diseases	rheumatoid arthritis
Drug induced	gold salts
	isoniazid
	metronidazole
	nitrofurantoin
	phenytoin
	vincristine
Neoplastic	bronchial
	lymphoreticular
	gastric
Genetic	Charcot–Marie–Tooth

The classical description by Charcot was of joint destruction in syphilitic tabes dorsalis. Other causes now identified include diabetes mellitus, syringomyelia, leprosy, congenital indifference to pain, Charcot–Marie–Tooth disease, paraplegia, meningomyelocele, subacute combined degeneration of the cord, and familial amyloid polyneuropathy.

Lower limb joints, including those of the foot, are involved, especially in tabes dorsalis, diabetes mellitus with painful involvement of the tarsus (Sinha et al 1972), paraplegia and Charcot–Marie–Tooth disease (Bruchner & Kendall 1969).

Joint destruction with hypertrophic bone formation is usual, although an atrophic resorptive radiological picture has been described in diabetes, affecting upper more than lower limb joints (Schwartz et al 1969).

Mononeuritis multiplex

A mononeuropathy implies a lesion of an individual nerve. Thus the symptoms and signs are those of motor and sensory deficit in the distribution of the affected nerve distal to the lesion. An isolated foot drop may thus develop. This may arise from mechanical injury or nerve entrapment. Multiple lesions due to vasculitis of the vasa nervorum affect a number of individual nerves, and summation of such lesions would lead to a symmetrical picture resembling a glove and stocking neuropathy. Such summation of nerve lesions is usually evident in a careful assessment of the patient's history. This occurs classically in polyarteritis nodosa but also in systemic lupus erythematosus and rheumatoid arthritis. It can also occur in diabetes mellitus, although then the cranial nerves are usually affected as well.

Acquired neurological disorders

Motor neurone disease and hereditary neuropathy (Charcot–Marie–Tooth disease) need to be considered in cases of acquired pes cavus, and in the development of foot drop and peripheral muscle wasting and weakness. Although abnormalities in the upper limb develop earlier than in the lower limb, the signs are those of combined upper and lower motor neurone lesions in motor neurone disease.

Multiple sclerosis may present in a number of apparently unrelated forms, arising from the dispersion of neurological lesions in time and space. Thus, presentation in the feet may be with isolated sensory symptoms, isolated peripheral nerve palsies, or with the development of upper motor neurone lesions leading to lower limb spasticity.

Cramps

Muscle cramp is usually a painful, involuntary contraction of muscle lasting for a few seconds to several minutes. Electromyographically, high frequency motor unit discharges are present with a repetition rate of 200–300 per second (Kimura 1983). It is extremely common, tends to increase in incidence and also in frequency in the individual patient with age, and often occurs at night.

Muscles of the lower leg and foot are most frequently involved, causing a 'spasm', for example with extreme extension and abduction of the hallux. Frequent and severe cramps may lead to a more persistent aching after the acute episode.

The majority of cases of cramp occur in otherwise healthy subjects, or follow periods of unaccustomed exercise. They occasionally result from peripheral ischaemia, hyponatraemia, hypokalaemia due to acute diarrhoea or the excessive use of diuretics, hypocalcaemia or hypothyroidism (Joekes 1979). Cramps may also occur in patients with peripheral neuropathy of any cause or in early cases of motor neurone disease.

Dupuytren's diathesis

Dupuytren's syndrome presents in the hands as a flexion deformity of the fingers resulting from thickening and contraction of the palmar fascia. This occurs in 1–3% of the population, men being affected more frequently than women. It is most common in Northern Europe and is rare in coloured peoples (Hueston 1962, 1968, Viljanto 1973). There is a strong inherited predisposition, which is expressed as a dominant inheritance in men (Early 1962).

Rarely, this is part of a wider spectrum of manifestations, which is then known as Dupuytren's diathesis or disease (Lynch & Jayson 1979). This includes nodules in the palmar and plantar fasciae, epilepsy, gum hypertrophy, stiff shoulders, Peyronie's disease and Garrod's pads (Lettin 1964, Hueston 1975). A high incidence of Dupuytren's syndrome has been reported in patients with diabetes mellitus (Lynch & Jason 1979, Noble et al 1984).

Fibrous nodules associated with proliferation and thickening of the plantar fascia (Gabbiani & Manjo 1972, Viljanto 1973) may thus produce severe discomfort on weight bearing and be the presenting symptom or the most prominent symptom, of the syndrome.

Paget's disease of bone

Paget's disease of bone is usually asymptomatic and monostotic. Its cause remains unknown and it is characterized by excessive resorption and deposition of bone.

This leads to the production of abnormal bone with characteristic radiological changes of loss of normal trabecular pattern, marked thickening of the cortex and expansion of the bone, and the presence of a coarse trabecular pattern. Abnormal bone is often sharply demarcated from normal bone, and fractures may occur at this junction (Brailsford 1954, Grainger & Laws 1957, Barry 1961).

Long bones, the pelvis, the vertebrae and the skull are most commonly affected; involvement of the small bones of the hands and feet is very rare with the exception of the occasional monostotic involvement of the calcaneum (Barry 1969). Thus, significant involvement of the bones of the feet is extremely rare, and it is usually a radiological incidental finding which does not require any treatment.

Pigmented villonodular synovitis

Pigmented villonodular synovitis presents as a swelling, which is often painless, of a joint or tendon sheath. Both sexes at any age may be affected, although Rao & Vigorita (1984) have reported a female:male ratio of 2:1 and a younger mean age in those with lower limb involvement compared with those with involvement of the hands.

Joints most commonly involved are those of the fingers and the knees (Granowitz & Mankin 1967, Rao & Vigorita 1984), but involvement of the hips, shoulders, elbows, wrists, ankles and toes is not unusual. Rao & Vigorita (1984) reported a 9% incidence in the toes and a 2.5% incidence in the ankles in a series of 81 patients, compared with 58% in the wrists and hands and 28% in the knees. In that series, pain was mild or absent when the ankles, toes or hands were involved, but mild to severe in the majority of involved knee joints. Tenderness is uncommon except in the knees.

Villous, nodular or villonodular lesions may be present in both joints and tendon sheaths, and localized nodular proliferation produces the clinical feature of a mechanical derangement. Aspiration of the affected joint reveals a heavily blood-stained fluid.

Radiologically, the early feature is the presence of soft tissue swelling while the adjacent bone and joint remains normal. Marginal erosion of juxta-articular bone, cystic changes, narrowing of the joint space representing cartilage erosion and localized osteoporosis develop as late radiological features (Breimer & Freiberger 1958, Smith & Pugh 1962, Schajowicz & Blumenfeld 1968, Pantazopoulos et al 1975, Rao & Vigorita 1984).

The differential diagnosis includes any cause of haemarthrosis, such as coagulation disorders, trauma, malignant tumours and synovial haemangioma, as well as synovial sarcoma and fibrous xanthomata. Fibrous xanthomata are especially likely when there is tendon sheath involvement (Jones et al 1969).

Histologically, the villi are covered by synovial lining cells and sheets of compact round and polyhedral cells, many of which are multinucleate, are present in the stroma of the synovium. Excessive amounts of haemosiderin are present in both the synovial lining cells and stroma. Foamy histiocytes, plasma cells and lymphocytes are present. The lesion may be encapsulated by fibrous tissue (Clark 1958, Nilsonne & Moberger 1969, Schumacher et al 1982, Rao & Vigorita 1984).

Complete excision of the lesion by synovectomy is the treatment of choice, although recurrences may occur for which radiotherapy has been advocated (Granowitz & Mankin 1967, Rao & Vigorita 1984).

The classification and aetiology of pigmented villonodular synovitis remains uncertain. The name was introduced by Jaffe et al (1941) as a description of the chronic proliferative synovium, which is dark brown because of the presence of haemosiderin. It has been classified as a benign haemangioma, a low-grade malignant tumour, an inflammatory granulomatous condition and a metabolic disease (Flipo and Delcambre 1993); it may also follow local trauma (Granowitz & Mankin 1967, Byers et al 1968, Bobechko & Kostvik 1968, Molnar et al 1971, Vilppula et al 1982). Despite the possible confusion with malignant neoplasia (single joint involvement, blood stained fluid, radiological bone destruction and increased number of mitoses), it is probably more accurate to classify the diffuse form as a chronic inflammatory granulomatous condition of unknown cause, although the nodular form probably represents a benign neoplastic proliferation of synovium. Metastasis does not occur.

References

Ahlberg S 1967 Treatment and prophylaxis of arthropathy in severe haemophilia. Clin Orthop 53: 135–146

Aho K, Ahvonen P, Juvakoski T, Kousa M, Leirisalo M, Laitinen O 1983 Immune responses in Yersinia-associated reactive arthritis. Ann Rheum Dis 38 (Suppl): 123–126

Allen D M, Diamond L H, Howell D A 1960 Anaphylactoid purpura in children (Henoch–Schönlein syndrome). Amer J Dis Child 99: 833–854

Amor B, Kahan A, Orfila J, Thomas D 1983 Immunological evidence of chlamydial infection in Reiter's syndrome. Ann Rheum Dis 38 (Suppl): 116–118

Ansell B M 1986 Infective arthritis. In: Scott J T (ed) Copeman's Textbook of the Rheumatic Diseases, 6th edn. Churchill Livingstone, Edinburgh. p 1150

Arnett F C 1979 Incomplete Reiter's syndrome: clinical comparisons with classical triad. Ann Rheum Dis 38 (Suppl): 73–78

Aronstam A, Rainsford S G, Painter M J 1979 Patterns of bleeding in adolescents with severe haemophilia A. Brit Med J 1: 469–470

Bakhshandeh K, Nasr K, Haghighi P, Haghshenas M 1971 Clubbing and osteoarthropathy associated with primary upper small intestinal lymphoma. J Trop Med Hyg 74: 117–119

Ball J 1971 Enthesopathy of rheumatoid and ankylosing spondylitis. Ann Rheum Dis 30: 213–223

Ball J 1983 The enthesopathy of ankylosing spondylitis. Brit J Rheumatol 22 (Suppl 2): 25–28

Barnes C G 1980 The Practitioner, 224: 45–57

Barnes C G, Colvin B T 1983 Haemophilia. Arthritis and Rheumatism Council Reports on Rheumatic Diseases 85

Barrett-Connor E 1971 Bacterial infection and sickle cell anaemia. Medicine (Baltimore) 50: 97–112

Barry H C 1961 Sarcoma in Paget's disease of bone in Australia. J Bone Joint Surg 43A: 1122–1134

Barry H C 1969 Paget's disease of bone. E & S Livingstone Ltd, Edinburgh

Benhamou C L, Shamot A M, Khan M F 1988 Synovitis acne pustulosis hyperostosis osteomyelitis syndrome (SAPHO). A new syndrome among the spondylarthropathies? Clin Exp Rheum 6: 109–112

Berkowitz D 1964 Blood lipid and uric acid inter-relationships. JAMA 190: 856–858

Berkowitz D 1966 Gout, hyperlipaemia and diabetes. JAMA 197: 77–80

Bland J H, Frymoyer J W, Newberg A H, Revers R, Normal R J 1979 Rheumatic syndromes in endocrine disease. Semin Arthritis Rheum 9: 23–64

Blomgren S E 1974 Erythema nodosum. Semin Arthritis Rheum 4: 1–24

Bluestone R, Bywaters E G L, Hartog M, Holt P J L, Hyde S 1971 Acromegalic arthropathy. Ann Rheum Dis 30: 243–258

Bobechko W P, Kostvik J P 1968 Childhood villonodular synovitis. Can J Surg 11: 480–486

Brailsford J F 1954 Paget's disease of bone. Br J Radiol 27: 435–442

Braun J, Laitko S, Treharne et al 1994 Chlamydia pneumoniae – a new causative agent of reactive and undifferentiated oligoarthritis. Ann Rheum Dis 53: 100–105

Breimer C W, Freiberger R H 1958 Bone lesions associated with villonodular synovitis. Am J Roentgen 79: 618–629

Bremell T, Bjelle A, Svedhem A 1991 Rheumatic symptoms following an outbreak of *campylobacter* enteritis: a five year follow-up. Ann Rheum Dis 50: 934–938

Brewerton D A, Caffrey M F P, Hart F D, James D C O, Nicholls A, Sturrock R D 1973 Ankylosing spondylitis and HL-A27. Lancet 1: 904–907

Brewerton D A, Caffrey M, James D C O 1974a The histocompatibility antigen (HL-A27) and its relation to disease. J Rheumatol 1: 249–253

Brewerton D A, Nicholls A, Caffrey M, Walters D, James D C O 1974b HL-A27 and arthropathies associated with ulcerative colitis and psoriasis. Lancet 1: 956–957

Brewerton D A, James D C O 1975 The histocompatibility antigen (HL-A27) and disease. Semin Arthritis Rheum 4: 191–207

Bruchner F E, Kendall B E 1969 Neuroarthropathy in Charcot–Marie–Tooth disease. Ann Rheum Dis 28: 577–583

Buchan D J, Mitchell D M 1967 Hypertrophic osteoarthropathy in portal cirrhosis. Ann Intern Med 66: 130–135

Buckingham R B, Bole G G, Bassett D R 1975 Polyarthritis associated with Type IV hyperlipoproteinaemia. Arch Int Med 135: 286–290

Bunch T W, Hunder G C 1973 Ankylosing spondylitis and primary hyperparathyroidism JAMA 225: 1108–1109

Burns R E, Coleville J M 1959 Acne conglobata with septicaemia. Arch Dermatol 79: 361–362

Byers P D, Cotton R E, Deacon O W, Lowy M, Newman P H, Sissons H A, Thompson A D 1968. The diagnosis and treatment of pigmented villonodular synovitis. J Bone Joint Surg 50B: 290–309

Bywaters E G L, Isdale I, Kempton J J 1957 Schönlein–Henoch purpura. Q J Med 50 (NS26): 161–175

Bywaters E G L, Dixon A St J, Scott J T 1963 Joint lesions of hyperparathyroidism. Ann Rheum Dis 22: 171–187

Calabro J J, Marchesano J M, Abruzzo J L 1966 Idiopathic hypertrophic osteoarthropathy (pachydermoperiostosis): onset before puberty. Arthritis Rheum 9: 496

Calin A, Porta J, Fries J F, Schurman D J 1977 Clinical history as a screening test for ankylosing spondylitis. JAMA 237: 2613–2614

Casser L 1956 Anaphylactoid purpura following penicillin therapy. J Med Soc N J 53: 133–134

Catterall R D 1983 Clinical aspects of Reiter's disease. Brit J Rheumatol 22 (Suppl 2): 151–155

Cavanaugh J J A, Holman G H 1965 Hypertrophic osteoarthropathy in childhood. J Pediatr 66: 27–40

Chakravarty K, Scott D G I 1992 Systemic vasculitis. Rheumatol Review 1: 81–99

Chambers R J, Bywaters E G L 1963 Rubella synovitis. Ann Rheum Dis 22: 263–268

Clark W S 1958 Pigmented villonodular synovitis. Bull Rheum Dis 8: 161–162

Clement G B, Vasey F B, Fenske N A, Bridgeford P, Germain B F, Espinoza L R 1982 Acne arthritis: clinical manifestations, human leucocyte antigens and circulating immune complexes. Arthritis Rheum 25 (Suppl): 51, Abstract 58

Currey H L F (ed) 1986 Clinical Rheumatology. Churchill Livingstone, Edinburgh

Davis D L E, Viozzi F J, Miller F, Vlodgett R 1981 The musculoskeletal manifestations of acne fulminans. J Rheumatol 8: 317–320

Dekker-Saeys B J, Meuwissen S G M, Berg-Loonen E M Van der, DeHaas W H D, Meijers K A F, Tygat G N J 1978 Ankylosing spondylitis and inflammatory bowel disease. Ann Rheum Dis 37: 30–41

Derham R J, Rogerson M M 1956 The Schönlein-Henoch syndrome with particular reference to renal sequelae. Arch Dis Child 31: 364–368

Dixon A St J 1963 Unusual effects of bronchial carcinoma and other lung tumours. Thorax 18: 197

Dorwart B B, Schumacher H R 1975 Joint effusions, chondrocalcinosis and other rheumatic manifestations in hypothyroidism. Am J Med 59: 780–790

Dougados M, Linden S van der, Juhlin R et al 1991 The European Spondylarthropathy Study Group preliminary criteria for the classification of spondylarthropathy. Arthritis Rheum 34: 1218–1227

Early P F 1962 Population studies in Dupuytren's contracture. J Bone Joint Surg 44B: 602–613

Ebringer A, Shipley M (eds) 1983 Pathogenesis of HLA-B27 associated diseases. Br J Rheumatol 22 (Suppl 2)

Engh C A, Hughes J L, Abrams R C, Bowerman J W 1971 Osteomyelitis in the patient with sickle-cell disease. J Bone Joint Surg 53A: 1–15

Epstein O, Ajdukiewicz A B, Dick R, Sherlock S 1979 Hypertrophic hepatic osteoarthropathy. Clinical, roentgenologic, biochemical, hormonal and cardiorespiratory studies, and review of the literature. Am J Med 67: 88–97

Espinoza L R, Cuéllar M L, Silveira L H 1992 Psoriatic arthritis. Curr Opin Rheumatol 4: 470–478

Evans W K 1980 Reversal of hypertrophic osteoarthropathy after chemotherapy for bronchogenic carcinoma. J Rheumatol 7: 93–97

Fam A G, Gross E G 1979 Hypertrophic osteoarthropathy, phalangeal and synovial metastases associated with bronchogenic carcinoma. J Rheumatol 6: 680–686

Farman J, Twersky J, Fierst S 1976 Ulcerative colitis associated with hypertrophic osteoarthropathy. Dig Dis 21: 130–135

Fielding J F, Cooke W T 1971 Finger clubbing and regional enteritis. Gut 12: 442–444

Fischer D S, Singer D H, Feldman S M 1964 Clubbing: a review, with emphasis on hereditary acropachy. Medicine (Baltimore) 43: 459–479

Flavell G 1956 Reversal of pulmonary hypertrophic osteoarthropathy by vagotomy. Lancet 1: 260–262

Flipo R M, Delcambre B 1993 La synovite villo-nodulaire pigmentée, affection tumorale ou métabolique? Rev Rheum 60: 861–864

Ford D K 1983a Yersinia-induced arthritis and Reiter's syndrome. Ann Rheum Dis 38 (Suppl): 127–128

Ford D K 1983b Cell-mediated immunity to *U. urealyticum* (Mycoplasma) in patients with Reiter's syndrome. Ann Rheum Dis 38 (Suppl): 129–130

Ford P M 1970 Thyroid acropachy. Proc R Soc Lond 63: 284–285

Fredrickson D S, Levy R I, Lees R I 1967 Fat transport in lipoproteins – an integrated approach to mechanisms and disorders. N Engl J Med 276: 34–44, 94–103, 148–156, 215–225, 273–281

Friedman A, Naveh Y 1971 Polyarthritis associated with chicken pox. Am J Dis Child 122: 179–180

Frymoyer J W, Bland J 1973 Carpal tunnel syndrome in patients with myxedematous arthropathy. J Bone Joint Surg 55A: 78–82

Gabbiani G, Manjo G 1972 Dupuytren's contracture: fibroblast contraction? An ultrastructural study. Am J Pathol 66: 131–147

Gairdner D 1948 The Schönlein-Henoch syndrome (anaphylactoid purpura). Q J Med NS 17: 95–122

Ghosh S K, Reddy T A 1973 Arthralgia and myalgia in mumps. Rheumatol Rehabil 12: 97–99

Gladman D D, Shuckett R, Russell M L, Thorne J C, Schachter R K 1987 Psoriatic arthritis: an analysis of 220 patients. Q J Med 62: 127–141

Glueck C J, Levy R I, Fredrickson D S 1968 Acute tendinitis and arthritis. JAMA 206: 2895–2897

Good A E 1983 Shigellae and Reiter's syndrome. Ann Rheum Dis 38 (Suppl): 119–122

Grainger R G, Laws J W 1957 Paget's disease – active or quiescent? Br J Radiol 30: 120–124

Granfors K 1992 Do bacterial antigens cause reactive arthritis? Rheum Dis Clin North Am 18: 37–48

Granowitz S P, Mankin H J 1967 Localized pigmented villonodular synovitis of the knee. J Bone Joint Surg 49A: 122–128

Gray M S, Philp T 1963 Syphilitic arthritis. Ann Rheum Dis 22: 19–25

Gray R G, Gottlieb N L 1976 Rheumatic disorders associated with diabetes mellitus. Semin Arthritis Rheum 6: 19–34

Greenfield G B, Schorasch H A, Shkolnik A 1967 The various roentgen appearances of pulmonary hypertrophic osteoarthropathy. Am J Roentgenol 101: 927–931

Hall A P, Barry P E, Dowber T R et al 1967 Epidemiology of gout and hyperuricaemia: a long-term population study. Am J Med 42: 27–37

Hammerschlag W A, Rice J R, Caldwell D S, Goldney J L 1991 Psoriatic arthritis of the foot and ankle: analysis of joint involvement and diagnostic errors. Foot Ankle 12: 35–39

Han S Y, Colins L C 1968 Hypertrophic osteoarthropathy in cirrhosis of the liver. Radiology 91: 795–796

Harris J R W, Gelsthorpe K, Doughty R W, Lee D, Morgan R S 1975 HL-A27 and W10 in Reiter's syndrome and non-specific urethritis. Acta Derm Venerol (Stockholm) 55: 127–130

Haslock I 1986 Enteropathic arthritis. In: Scott J T (ed) Copeman's Textbook of the Rheumatic Diseases, 6th edn. Churchill Livingstone, Edinburgh. p 806

Haslock I, Wright V 1973–1974 The arthritis associated with intestinal disease. Bull Rheum Dis 24: 750–754

Helliwell P S, Marchessoni A, Peters M, Barker M, Wright V 1991 A re-evaluation of the osteoarticular manifestations of psoriasis. Br J Rheum 30: 339–345

Hollis W C 1967 Hypertrophic osteoarthropathy secondary to upper gastrointestinal tract neoplasm. Ann Intern Med 66: 125–130

Holt P J L 1986a Endocrine disorders and metabolic bone disease. In: Scott J T (ed) Copeman's Textbook of the Rheumatic Diseases, 6th edn. Churchill Livingstone, Edinburgh. p 959

Holt P J L 1986b Arthritis and blood disease. In: Scott J T (ed) Copeman's Textbook of the Rheumatic Diseases, 6th edn. Churchill Livingstone, Edinburgh. p 1191

Holt P J L, Davies M G, Saunders K C, Nuki G 1980 Pyoderma gangrenosum. Clinical and laboratory findings in 15 patients with special reference to polyarthritis. Medicine (Baltimore) 59: 114–133

Honska W L, Strenge J, Hammarsten J F 1957. Hypertrophic osteoarthropathy and chronic ulcerative colitis. Gastroenterology 33: 489–492

Hueston J T 1962 Digital Wolfe grafts in recurrent Dupuytren's contracture. Plast Reconstr Surg 29: 342–344

Hueston J T 1968 Dupuytren's contracture and specific injury. Med J Aust 1: 1084–1085

Hueston J T 1975 Dupuytren's contracture selection for surgery. Br J Hosp Med 13: 361–370

Hughes R, Keat A 1992 Reactive arthritis – the role of bacterial antigens in inflammatory arthritis. Clinical Rheumatol 6: 285–308

Jaffe H L, Lichtenstein L, Sutro C J 1941 Pigmented villonodular synovitis, bursitis and tenosynovitis. Arch Pathol 31: 731–765

Jajic I 1968 Radiological changes in the sacro-iliac joints and spine of patients with psoriatic arthritis and psoriasis. Ann Rheum Dis 27: 1–6

Jayson M I V, Salmon P R, Harrison W J 1970 Inflammatory bowel disease in ankylosing spondylitis. Gut 11: 506–511

Joekes A M 1979 Cramp. Clin Rheum Dis 5: 873–881

Jones F E, Soule E H, Coventry M B 1969 Fibrous xanthoma of synovium (giant-cell tumour of tendon sheath, pigmented synovitis). A study of one hundred and eighteen cases. J Bone Joint Surg 51A: 76–86

Kahn M-F, Bouvier M, Palazzo E, Tebib J G, Colson F 1991 Sternoclavicular pustulotic osteitis (SAPHO): 20 year interval between skin and bone lesions. J Rheumatol 18: 1104–1108

Kallenberg C G M 1994 Anti-neutrophil cytoplasmic antibodies (ANCA): current perspectives. Rheum Eur 23 (Suppl 2): 5–6

Kallenberg C G M, Mulder A H, Tervaert J W 1992 Anti-neutrophil cytoplasmic antibodies: a still-growing class of autoantibodies in inflammatory disorders. Am J Med 92: 675–682

Kammer G M, Soter N A, Gibson D J, Schur P H 1979 Psoriatic arthritis: a clinical immunological and HLA study of 100 patients. Semin Arthritis Rheum 9: 75–97

Keat A C, Scott J T, Ridgway G, Maini R N, Pergrum G D 1979 Sexually acquired reactive arthritis. Ann Rheum Dis 38 (Suppl): 52–54

Kimura J 1983 Neuromuscular diseases characterised by abnormal muscle activity. In: Electrodiagnosis in Diseases of Nerve and Muscle: Principles and Practice. F A Davis, Philadelphia. p 549

Lass R, Shepherd E 1961 Mumps arthritis. Br Med J 2: 1613–1614

Lawrence J S 1974 Family survey of Reiter's disease. Br J Vener Dis 50: 140–145

le Roux B T 1968 Bronchial carcinoma with hypertrophic pulmonary osteoarthropathy. S Afr Med J 42: 1074–1075

Lettin A W F 1964 Dupuytren's diathesis: a case report. J Bone Joint Surg 46B: 220–225

Levinsky R J, Barratt T M 1979 IgA immune complexes in Henoch–Schönlein purpura. Lancet 2: 1100–1103

Lewis I C, Philpott M G 1956 Neurological complications of the Schönlein–Henoch syndrome. Arch Dis Child 31: 369–371

Lie J T 1994 Classification and histopathologic specificity of vasculitis. Rheum Eur 23 (Suppl 2): 4

Lindholm H, Visakorpi R 1991 Late complications after a *Yersinia enterocolitica* epidemic: a follow-up study. Ann Rheum Dis 50: 694–696

Lopez-Enriques E, Morales A R, Robert F 1980 Effect of atropine sulfate in pulmonary hypertrophic osteoarthropathy. Arthritis Rheum 23: 822–824

Lynch M, Jayson M I V 1979 Dupuytren's disease and contracture. In: Dixon A St J (ed) Soft Tissue Rheumatism. Clin Rheum Dis 5: 837–840

Macrae I, Wright V 1973 A family study of ulcerative colitis, with particular reference to ankylosing spondylitis and sacroiliitis. Ann Rheum Dis 32: 16–20

Mäki-Ikola O, Leirisalo-Repo M, Kantele A, Toivanen P, Granfors K 1991 *Salmonella*-specific antibidoes in reactive arthritis. J Infect Dis 164: 1141–1148

Mäki-Ikola O, Yli-Kerttula V, Saario R, Toivanen P, Granfors K 1992 *Salmonella* specific antibodies in serum and synovial fluid in patients with reactive arthritis. Brit J Rheum 31: 25–29

Masi A T 1979 Epidemiology of B27-associated diseases. Ann Rheum Dis 38 (Suppl): 131–134

Mason R M, Murray R S, Oates J K, Young A C 1958 Prostatitis and ankylosing spondylitis. Br Med J I: 748–751

McLaughlin G E, McCarty D J Jr, Downing D F 1967 Hypertrophic osteoarthropathy associated with cyanotic congenital heart disease. Ann Intern Med 67: 579–587

Mendlowitz M 1942 Clubbing and hypertrophic osteoarthropathy. Medicine (Baltimore) 21: 296–306

Metz E N, Dowell A 1965 Bone marrow failure in hypertrophic osteoarthropathy. Arch Intern Med 116: 759–764

Mikkelson W M, Dodge H Z, Valkenburg E 1965 The distribution of serum uric acid values in a population unselected as to gout or hyperuricaemia. Tecumseh, Michigan 1959–1960. Am J Med 39: 242–251

Moll J H M, Wright V 1973a Family occurrence of psoriatic arthritis. Ann Rheum Dis 32: 181–201

Moll J M H, Wright V 1973b Psoriatic arthritis. Semin Arthritis Rheum 3: 55–78

Moll J M H, Haslock I, Macrae I F, Wright V 1974 Associations between ankylosing spondylitis, psoriatic arthritis, Reiter's disease, the intestinal arthropathies and Behçet's syndrome. Medicine (Baltimore) 53: 343–364

Moll J M H, Haslock I, Wright V 1978 Seronegative spondarthritides. In: Scott J T (ed), Copeman's Textbook of the Rheumatic Diseases, 5th edn. Churchill Livingstone, Edinburgh. p 578

Molnar Z, Stein W H, Stolzner G H 1971 Cytoplasmic tubular structures in pigmented villonodular synovitis. Arthritis Rheum 14: 784–787

Morris R I, Metzger A L, Bluestone R T, Terasaki P I 1974 A useful discriminator in the arthropathies of inflammatory bowel disease. N Engl J Med 290: 1117–1119

Mullins G M, Lenhard R E 1971 Digital clubbing in Hodgkin's disease. Johns Hopkins Med J 128: 153–157

Neale G, Kelsall A R, Doyle F H 1968 Crohn's disease and diffuse symmetrical periostitis. Gut 9: 383–387

Nilsonne U, Moberger G 1969 Pigmented villonodular synovitis of joints. Histological and clinical problems in diagnosis. Acta Orthop Scand 40: 448–460

Noble J, Heathcote J G, Cohen H 1984 Diabetes mellitus in the aetiology of Dupuytren's disease. J Bone Joint Surg 66B: 322–325

Olhagen B 1983 Urogenital syndromes and spondarthritis. Br J Rheumatol 22 (suppl): 33–40

Pantazopoulos T, Stavrou S, Stamos C, Kehayas G, Hartofilaleidis-Gerofalidis G 1975 Bone lesions in pigmented villonodular synovitis. Acta Orthop Scand 46: 579–592

Patten B M, Bileyikian J P, Mallette L E, Prince A, Engel W K, Aurback G D 1974 Neuromuscular disease in primary hypoparathyroidism. Ann Intern Med 80: 182–193

Perry H O, Brunsting L A 1957 Pyoderma gangrenosum: a clinical study of 19 cases. Arch Dermatol 75: 380–386

Rao A S, Vigorita V J 1984 Pigmented villonodular synovitis (giant cell tumour of the tendon sheath and synovial membrane). J Bone Joint Surg 66A: 76–94

Resnick D L 1974 Erosive arthritis of the hand and wrist in hyperparathyroidism. Radiology 110: 263–269

Rifkind B M 1970 The hyperlipoproteinaemias. Br J Hosp Med 4: 683–692

Rimoin D L 1965 Pachydermoperiostosis (idiopathic clubbing and periostosis). Genetic and physiological considerations. N Engl J Med 272: 923–931

Rooney P J, Thind J, Madkour M M, Spender D, Dick W C 1978 Transient polyarthritis associated with familial hyperbetalipoproteinaemia. Q J Med 187 (NS47): 249–259

Rothschild B M, Yoon B H 1982 Thyroid acropathy complicated by lymphatic obstruction. Arthritis Rheum 25: 588–590

Saario R, Toivanen A 1993 Chlamydia pneumoniae as a cause of reactive arthritis. Br J Rheumatol 32: 1112

Salfeld K, Spalckhaver I 1966 Zur Kenntnis der Pachydermoperiostosis. Dermatol Wochenschr 152: 497–511

Scanlon G T, Clemett A R 1964 Thyroid acropachy. Radiology 83: 1039–1042

Schajowicz F, Blumenfeld I 1968 Pigmented villonodular synovitis of the wrist with penetration into bone. J Bone Joint Surg 50B: 312–317

Schlosslein L, Tevasaki P I, Bluestone R T, Pearson C M 1973 High association of an HL-A antigen, W27, with ankylosing spondylitis. N Engl J Med 288: 704–706

Schumacher H R, Gall E P 1974 Arthritis in acute hepatitis and chronic active hepatitis. Am J Med 57: 655–664

Schumacher H R, Lotke P, Akthreya B, Rothfuss S 1982 Pigmented villonodular synovitis: light and electron studies. Semin Arthritis Rheum 12: 32–43

Schwartz G S, Berenyi M R, Siegel N W 1969 Atrophic arthritis and diabetic neuritis. Am J Roentgen 106: 523–529

Schwartz J A 1981 Pro-banthine for hypertrophic osteoarthropathy. Arthritis Rheum 24: 1588 (letter)

Sharp G C, Irwin W S, Tan E M, Gould R G, Holman H R 1972 Mixed connective tissue disease. An apparently distinct rheumatic disease syndrome associated with a specific antibody to an extractable nuclear antigen (ENA). Am J Med 52: 148–159

Sharp J 1957 The differential diagnosis of ankylosing spondylitis. Br Med J I: 975–978

Sharp J 1965 Ankylosing spondylitis: a review. In: Dixon A St J (ed), Progress in Clinical Rheumatology. Churchill, London. p 180

Sheldon P J, Pell P 1983 Yersinia arthritis in the Midlands: clinical and immunological features in ten cases during 1980–1983. Br J Rheumatol 22 (Suppl 2): 46–49

Sinha S, Munichoodappa C S, Kozak G P 1972 Neuroarthropathy (Charcot joints) in diabetes mellitus. Medicine (Baltimore) 51: 191–210

Smith J H, Pugh D J 1962 Roentgenographic aspects of articular pigmented villonodular synovitis. Am J Roentgen 87: 1146–1156

Sprunance S L, Smith C B 1971 Joint complications associated with derivatives of HPV-77 rubella varus vaccine. Am J Dis Child 122: 105–111

Stein H, Duthie R B 1981 The pathogenesis of chronic haemophiliac arthropathy. J Bone Joint Surg 63B: 601–609

Stenseth J H, Clagett O T, Woolner L B 1967 Hypertrophic osteoarthropathy and pseudomembranous enterocolitis. J Rheumatol 8: 825–828

Torre Alonso J C, Rodriguez Perez A, Arribas Castillo J M, Ballina Garcia J, Riestra Noriega J L, Lopez Larrea C 1991. Psoriatic arthritis: a clinical immunological and radiological study of 180 patients. Br J Rheum 30: 245–250

Ueno Y, Cassell S, Barnett E V 1981 Hypertrophic osteoarthropathy and pseudomembranous enterocolitis. J Rheumatol 8: 825–828

Vernier R L, Worthen H G, Patersen R D, Colle E, Good R A 1961 Anaphylactoid purpura. Paediatrics 27: 181–193

Viljanto J A 1973 Dupuytren's contracture: a review. Semin Arthritis Rheum 3: 155–176

Vilppula A H, Yli-Kerttula U I, Aine R A T, Ojala A T 1982 Pigmented villonodular synovitis. Scand J Rheumatol 11: 145–149

Wajed M A, Brown D L, Currey H L F 1977 Palindromic rheumatism. Clinical and serum complement study. Ann Rheum Dis 36: 155–176

Wasser K B, Cohen A M, Yulash B S, Root J M, Vignos P J, Jones P K, Sorin S B 1982 Pulmonary hypertrophic osteoarthropathy in cystic fibrosis: a survey of 375 patients. Arthritis Rheum 25 (Suppl): F154, Abstract E94

Williams B L 1967 Acropachy in a case of thyrotoxicosis. Proc R Soc Med Lond 60: 899–900

Wright V 1963 Arthritis associated with venereal disease. Ann Rheum Dis 22: 77–89

Wright V 1978 Psoriatic arthritis. In: Scott J T (ed) Copeman's Textbook of the Rheumatic Diseases, 5th edn. Churchill Livingstone, Edinburgh. p. 537

Wright V, Watkinson G 1965 Sacroiliitis and ulcerative colitis. Br Med J ii: 675–680

Wright V, Helliwell P S 1992 Psoriatic arthritis. Arthritis and Rheumatism Council Reports on Rheumatic Diseases (Series 2): Topical Reviews No. 21

Wright V, Neumann R, Shinebaum R, Cooke E M 1983 Pathogenesis of seronegative arthritis. Br J Rheumatol 22 (Suppl 2): 29–32

Yacoub M H 1965 Cervical vagotomy for pulmonary osteoarthropathy. Br J Dis Chest 59: 28–31

Yacoub M H, Simon G 1966 Hypertrophic osteoarthropathy and intrathoracic inflammatory conditions. Brit J Dis Chest 60: 81–86

Yacoub M H, Simon G, Ohnsorge J 1967 Hypertrophic pulmonary osteoarthropathy in association with pulmonary metastases from extrathoracic tumours. Thorax 22: 226–231

VI.2 Skin Disorders

B Martina Daly

Introduction

There are two main types of skin, and both types are represented in the foot. The skin of the dorsum of the foot is hair bearing and sebaceous glands are present in the dermis. The skin of the sole is nonhairy skin (glabrous skin) and is characterized by a thickened epidermis which is grooved to produce characteristically unique dermatoglyphics.

Dermatitis

Dermatitis refers to a pattern of inflammation of the skin that may be induced by a variety of external and internal factors acting singly or in combination. In many cases, the cause is unknown. No universally accepted classification of dermatitis exists. Dermatitis can be simply divided into two main groups: exogenous, where an external cause can be identified, and endogenous, where there is no obvious aetiology (Table 1).

Incidence

It is difficult to determine the true incidence of dermatitis but studies suggest that 20% of patients seen in dermatology clinics in the UK present with dermatitis of some form (Bowker et al 1976).

Contact dermatitis

Contact dermatitis is caused by contact of the skin with either a substance that acts as a primary irritant (irritant contact dermatitis) or a substance to which the patient has become sensitized (allergic contact dermatitis). Allergic contact dermatitis is an example of delayed hypersensitivity (Type IV allergy) and there is a characteristic delay between induction of sensitivity and the development of dermatitis on re-exposure to the allergy. The distinction clinically is often blurred and histology may not help.

Clinical features

Irrespective of the cause, the clinical features of the dermatitic reaction are similar. The main symptom is itch, which may be severe. Erythema with papules and

Table 1 Categories of dermatitis	
Exogenous dermatitis	Contact dermatitis
	Irritant
	Allergic
	Infective dermatitis
	Asteotic dermatitis
	Stasis dermatitis
Endogenous dermatitis	Atopic dermatitis
	Nummular or discoid dermatitis
	Seborrhoeic dermatitis

vesicles is the initial change seen in acute dermatitis; this progresses to exudation and crusting. Dry scaling lichenified fissured plaques are seen in the chronic phase. Secondary hyperpigmentation occurs, owing to chronic inflammation and scratching.

On the palms and soles, where the stratum corneum is thick and resistant, the vesicles are deep-seated with minimal erythema. This pattern is called cheiropompholyx. Burning pain and not itch is the predominant feature in this situation. If the vesicles coalesce large bullae (up to 2 cm) develop; these may eventually rupture with deep fissure formation.

Irritant contact dermatitis

Primary irritant reactions on the feet are not common, but do occur in those engaged in wet work with inadequate protective footwear.

Allergic contact dermatitis (Fig. 1)

There are many factors which influence the development of allergic contact dermatitis of the foot. There is increased percutaneous absorption due to occlusion caused by footwear. Sweating may further irritate the skin and has the effect of leaching out chemicals like dichromate salts from leather. Friction plays a part in the development of allergic contact dermatitis by damaging the stratum corneum and increases the ease of penetration of the antigen.

There are three major groups of agents which commonly cause allergic contact dermatitis on the foot – footwear, medicaments and cosmetics, and foot appliances.

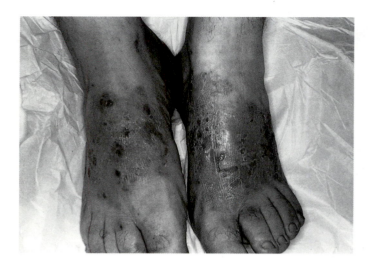

Figure 1

Allergic contact dermatitis

Shoe dermatitis

Shoe-induced contact dermatitis is not common and is frequently misdiagnosed (Fisher 1986a).

Clinical features of shoe dermatitis

The distribution of dermatitis may be useful in identifying the cause. Dermatitis of the dorsa of the feet and toes with sparing of the toe webs and soles implicates the upper shoe, whereas involvement of the weight-bearing areas of the sole of the foot with sparing of the instep suggests the sole. The straps of a sandal may produce an imprint of dermatitis on the foot.

Diagnosis

An accurate history, the presence and localization of the eruption, and a high index of suspicion help to make the diagnosis. Patch testing is necessary to help identify the putative allergen. It is important to patch test the constituents of all the patient's footwear, including bedroom slippers.

Rubber

The major group of footwear allergens is rubber accelerators and vulcanizers of the thiuram and mercaptobenzothiazole groups (Conde-Salazar et al 1993). These chemicals are most commonly found in the materials used to manufacture soles of shoes.

Leather

Chromium compounds and vegetable tannins used to tan leather are still important causes of shoe dermatitis. The hexavalent chromium salt is considered the most likely sensitizer. Sweat is known to leach out chromates from leather and hyperhidrosis is an important factor in the development of shoe dermatitis.

Dyes

Dyes in shoes rarely cause problems but if fabric shoes or redyed leather shoes are worn, allergy to the nonfast dyes may develop.

Other causes of shoe dermatitis

In patients who are sensitive to nickel, nickel-plated arch supports and eyelets may cause a foot dermatitis. Fungicides used as antimildews in shoes are a rare cause.

Stocking dermatitis

Dermatitis from stockings, socks or tights is uncommon in women and rare in men (Fisher 1986b).

Medicament dermatitis of feet

The present preoccupation with soft, sweet-smelling feet has led to a large variety of medicaments to achieve this aim. All of these have the ability to sensitize some patients. The incidence will increase if they are applied to already inflamed skin. Patch testing to constituents and preservatives of these medicaments is required to make the diagnosis. Occasionally, photosensitizing fungicides used for the treatment of athlete's foot may give rise to an allergic photo-contact dermatitis.

Treatment

Wet dressings using dilute solutions of potassium permanganate, silver nitrate or sodium hypochlorite applied three to four times daily will help to speed resolution of the acute phase. Potent corticosteroid creams with or without topical antibiotics will suppress inflammation. Corticosteroid ointments are suitable for dry scaling eruptions. As the condition resolves, weaker strength corticosteroids should be used. Tar combinations are useful for lichenified dermatitis. Oral corticosteroids are indicated for severe dermatitis, in widespread disease or in dermatitis not responding to topical therapy.

On recovery, open toed shoes or sandals are recommended until the skin hardens and complete resolution has taken place. Occlusive shoes and synthetic fibre socks should be avoided, and natural fibres are more comfortable. Control of hyperhidrosis using aluminium chloride may prevent relapse.

Alternative shoes

An allergen-free shoe probably does not exist. Rubber-sensitive patients should be advised to choose shoes with soles made of leather, crepe, polyurethane, polyvinyl chloride (PVC), ethylene vinyl acetate or thermoplastic rubber. Knitted shoes and welded plastic shoes should be free of all rubber chemicals. Leather-sensitive patients should be safe with all plastic or fabric shoes, while PVC sensitive patients can wear all leather or fabric shoes.

Asteotic eczema

Asteotic eczema (Fig. 2) is a dry scaling eczema. Many factors are required for its development; these include: a life-long tendency to dry and chapping skin; increasing age with reduction in skin surface lipids; malnutrition, illness and hormonal decline; low environmental humidity; excessive use of degreasing agents; and diuretic therapy.

Clinical features
The asteotic skin is dry and scaly with a characteristic crazy-pavement appearance in the lower legs. Some of the fissures may be haemorrhagic. Irritation may be intense and scratching aggravates the condition. A vesicular dermatitis may result.

Treatment
Rehydration of the skin by the substitution of aqueous cream or a bath oil for soap and a reduction in bathing is essential. Liberal amounts of emollients will help to keep the skin hydrated and to achieve normal suppleness. Topical corticosteroid ointments are indicated if marked inflammatory changes are present.

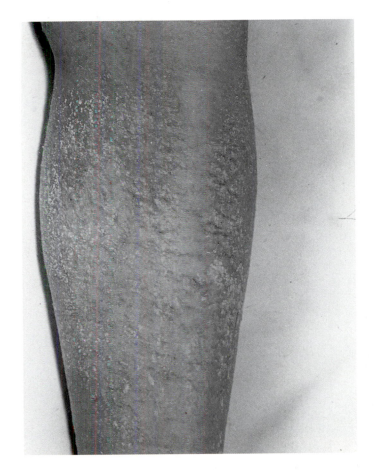

Figure 2

Asteotic eczema

Atopic dermatitis

Atopic dermatitis (Rajka 1989) is a chronic recurrent disease starting in infancy, which may be associated with other atopic disorders of asthma and hayfever. The prevalence of this disorder is estimated at between 1.1 and 4.3% of the general paediatric population.

Aetiology
A family history of atopy is obtained in about 70% of cases but the transmission is not that of a simple dominant trait. Several immunological abnormalities have been recognized in atopic patients. The most frequent is the high incidence of positive skin reactions to common allergens. Despite increasing knowledge of the physiological and immunological abnormalities, the basic process giving rise to the dermatitis is unknown.

Clinical features
The disease occurs from 2 months onwards. It may settle at the age of 2–3 years, only to recur later on in childhood, adolescence or adulthood. At different ages, varying patterns of dermatitis occur. In infancy, the face is usually the first area affected – the so-called teething eczema. As the infant starts to become mobile the rash spreads to the exposed surfaces of the ankles, knees and wrists. The dermatitis is usually red, moist and crusted. In later childhood, the characteristic flexural pattern develops involving the antecubital and popliteal fossae, around the ankles and in front of the wrists.

Atopic skin is sensitive to environmental changes – excessive atmospheric dryness, rough wool fabrics and sweating may irritate the skin and start the itch–scratch cycle with resultant deterioration in the patient's dermatitis.

Treatment
Management of atopic dermatitis is never easy. The parents must be involved, and the long-term objectives of treatment must be discussed. The fact that the diathesis is inherited and treatment is not going to cure this tendency must be emphasized at the outset.

Treatment is aimed at breaking the itch–scratch cycle. This can be achieved by rehydrating the skin, by careful avoidance of strong detergents on the skin, by reducing the number of baths and by the liberal use of non-perfumed emollients. The avoidance of friction from shoes or excess occlusion and the wearing of soft cotton

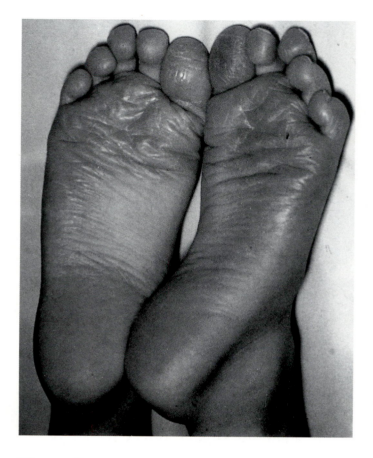

Figure 3

Juvenile plantar dermatitis

next to the skin will considerably improve the patient's comfort. Topical corticosteroids in an appropriate strength are extremely useful.

Prognosis

50% of infants are clear of dermatitis at 18 months and most children will be clear before puberty.

Juvenile plantar dermatitis

This is a scaling, fissuring dermatitis of the plantar surface of the forefoot of prepubertal children (Fig. 3).

Aetiology

The aetiology is obscure (Ashton & Griffiths 1986) and the condition was first described in 1968. Its appearance coincided with the increased use of synthetic materials in children's footwear and socks. This type of footwear is occlusive and interferes with sweating. There is marked sweat retention.

Most affected children are actively involved in sports and friction plays a role. There is a slight male predominance. Extensive allergy testing to various components of shoes and socks has failed to demonstrate footwear allergy. Reports of the incidence of atopy are conflicting and there is no clear evidence that this condition is more common in atopic children.

Clinical features

The skin changes are strikingly symmetric and mainly involve the anterior foot and toes. The skin texture is altered and the glazed sheen of the skin is characteristic. Scaling and fissuring is seen, especially on the plantar surface of the great toes and the pads of the other toes. There is sparing of the interdigital spaces, which helps to distinguish it from tinea pedis. Pain due to the deep fissuring is the main symptom and can make walking difficult.

Treatment

Treatment is unrewarding. A variety of topical emollients including white soft paraffin, urea preparations, Lassar's paste or tar are useful. Potent topical corticosteroids should be avoided as atrophy may develop and they do not significantly improve the condition. Changing to all-leather shoes and cotton socks should be encouraged as this may help a minority of children. Some dermatologists recommend wearing two pairs of socks or insoles made of cork or felt to increase sweat absorption.

Differential diagnosis

This condition is often misdiagnosed as fungal but the sparing of the webs and the age of the patient helps to rule it out. Fungal infections are uncommon in prepubertal children.

Prognosis

There is apparent spontaneous resolution at puberty.

Nummular dermatitis

Nummular dermatitis is characterized by oval or circular patches of dermatitis with a well-demarcated edge. It tends to involve the limbs more than the trunk. The cause is unknown but the role of trauma, infection and a tendency to dry skin have been stressed by some authors. It is relatively uncommon in children and more frequent in middle-aged men.

Clinical features

The characteristic coin-shaped lesions have a papulovesicular edge with central clearing; oozing and crusting is common, and itch may be intense. The individual lesions resolve, leaving dry scaling patches. Relapses and remissions over many years are a frequent feature of the condition, with dormant lesion flaring rapidly on cessation of therapy.

Treatment

Emollients and topical corticosteroids are useful. Tar preparations or a tar–corticosteroid combination are effective for long-term management.

Varicose dermatitis

Varicose dermatitis is a manifestation of prolonged venous hypertension and calf pump insufficiency, which gives rise to poor tissue perfusion and nutrition. It occurs more commonly in middle-aged obese women than in men. About one-third of patients give a past history of deep venous thrombosis, major trauma or prolonged periods of immobility.

Clinical features

Varicose dermatitis has a predilection for the gaiter area, which extends from the lower border of the malleolus to the bulge of the gastrocnemius. It is characterized by pigmentation, oedema and varicosities. As the disease progresses, induration and inflammation giving rise to fibrosis and scarring occurs. The clinical pattern is called lipodermatosclerosis. Ulceration may occur with further scarring. Pigmentation occurs early and is due to the deposition of haemosiderin following rupture of small venules. It starts as small light brown macules which enlarge and darken and may cover large areas of the lower leg and foot.

Erythema and oedema is usually accompanied by pruritus. Scratching causes lichenification and an exudative vesicular dermatitis. The injudicious use of topical preparations may worsen the situation by giving rise to a primary irritant or an allergic contact dermatitis. Local spread may be associated with a more widespread patchy dermatitis known as an 'id' (autosensitization) reaction. Secondary infection gives rise to considerable pain and increased oozing and crusting.

Prolonged oedema leads to progressive deterioration and eventually results in fibrosis which clinically is manifested by induration of the tissues. Ulceration occurs, usually following minor trauma. Ulcers may heal with scarring, or progress to involve large areas of the lower leg. An ulcer outside the gaiter area is extremely unlikely to be of venous aetiology. The edge of the ulcer is soft and irregular, with a necrotic base which may penetrate deeply to reveal underlying tendon and bones. Secondary bacterial infection usually gives rise to rapid expansion of the ulcer and considerable pain.

Recalcitrant ulcers are seen where there is significant fibrosis.

Management

Uncomplicated venous dermatitis requires treatment (Winter 1972) with emollients and topical steroids. Failure to respond to moderate potency topical steroids may be an indication of contact allergy and patch testing is necessary. Allergic contact dermatitis is a common complication and occurs in up to 70% of cases. Overnight elevation of the legs above the level of the heart is a useful way of reducing oedema. Compression bandaging should be applied while still in bed following prolonged elevation.

Ulceration

Despite the myriads of dressings available, none have been proven to enhance the healing rate of venous ulcers. Occlusive dressings have been shown in some studies to relieve pain. Gel and hydrocolloid dressings absorb exudate and protect the surrounding skin. The use of antiseptics such as sodium hypochlorite is controversial. The theoretical damage caused by these substances on fibroblasts must be balanced by the lack of healing which occurs when necrotic or infected tissue is present in a wound. Topical antibiotics should be avoided if possible and systemic antibiotics are only required for deeper infections. Grafting with 'pinch' grafts to the ulcer base of excision and split-thickness grafting may need to be considered.

Psoriasis

Psoriasis (Cram 1981) is a chronic inflammatory dermatosis characterized by reddish papules and plaques associated with fine silvery scaling. It has a predilection for extensor surfaces. There is epidermal hyperplasia and a two-fold increase in epidermal turnover rate in the active lesion. Psoriasis affects 2% of the population. It affects both sexes equally and may occur at any age. It is inherited as a simple autosomal dominant trait with incomplete penetrance. The basic defect in psoriasis is unknown.

Clinical features

The clinical lesion has three main features:

1. The lesion is thickened and clearly demarcated from normal skin.
2. The dull pink–red colour, often described as salmon pink, is especially helpful in diagnosing plantar lesions. The colour reflects the increased vasculature and dermal blood flow. Auspitz's sign is characteristic of psoriasis and is produced by blunt scraping of the scale revealing punctate bleeding points.

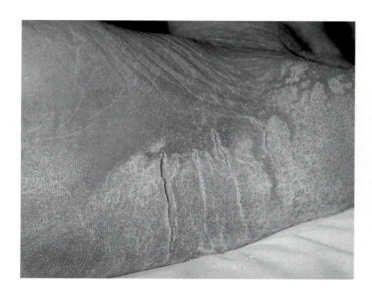

Figure 4

Psoriatic keratoderma

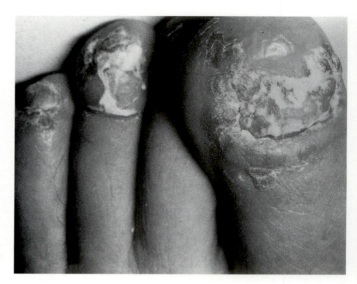

Figure 5

Psoriasis of nails

3. The amount of scaling is variable and is a fine loosely adherent silvery scale.

Psoriatic lesions are modified by site. The most common forms of psoriasis on the foot are plaque-type psoriasis, psoriatic keratoderma of the sole, interdigital psoriasis, psoriasis of nails, exfoliative and erythrodermic psoriasis, and pustular psoriasis of palms and soles.

Plaque-type psoriasis

Stable plaque-type psoriasis occurs on the feet and lower limbs as part of widespread psoriasis. Lesions tend to be symmetrical with well-demarcated scaling and erythematous plaques. Waxy yellow hyperkeratotic rupioid lesions occur alone or in association with pustules, especially on the sole. Similar but smaller lesions occur in Reiter's disease.

Psoriatic keratoderma

This presents as sharply marginated hyperkeratotic scaly plaques which are symmetrical and bilateral (Fig. 4). The plaques usually occur on the heels and beneath the instep. Deep painful fissures may occur, associated with the thickened yellow keratoderma. Palmar hyperkeratosis of varying degrees usually accompanies it. The absence of vesiculation is helpful in distinguishing this form of psoriasis from hyperkeratotic dermatitis.

Interdigital psoriasis

Psoriasis localized to the interdigital spaces has been referred to as 'white psoriasis'. It may occasionally occur in isolation, but it is usually accompanied by psoriatic changes in the toe-nails and psoriasis elsewhere. The lesions are characterized by thick white hyperkeratosis with ulceration and fissuring between the toes or at their bases.

Psoriasis of nails

Nail changes are present at some stage of the disease in almost all patients. Discrete punctate pits which occur in lines are characteristic but not specific to psoriasis (Fig. 5). Periungual changes, swelling, diffuse erythema and desquamation are frequent. Nail growth is increased, both in the affected and clinically normal nails.

Treatment

Topical preparations containing salicylic acid, dithranol, tar, or calcipitrol form the first line of treatment. This may be combined with ultraviolet light. Topical corticosteroids are used but the side effect of atrophy limits their use.

Systemic treatment is used for more severe psoriasis. Photochemotherapy is successful in inducing clearance of psoriasis and appears to be useful in maintenance of remission. A photosensitizing drug, usually 8-methoxypsoralen, is prescribed before exposure to ultraviolet light at 360 nm (UVA). Acetretin, a synthetic aromatic retinoid, has recently been introduced. It is used alone or in combination with PUVA. Side effects include teratogenicity and the long half life limits its usefulness.

Immunosuppressive and cytotoxic agents tend to be reserved for older patients with resistant psoriasis. Methotrexate, hydroxyurea and azathioprine are the main second-line drugs; their use is limited by their side effects, both short and long term.

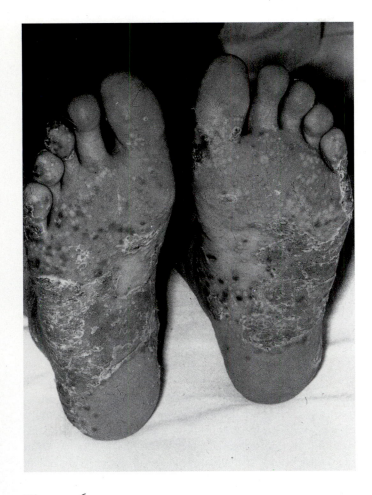

Figure 6
Pustular psoriasis

Pustular psoriasis

A localized pustular dermatosis (Fig. 6) involving the palms and soles occurs in middle-aged patients but its relationship to psoriasis is in some dispute. It is immuno-genetically distinct and the positive association of HLA-B27 and BW17 seen in psoriasis vulgaris is lacking.

Clinical features

The rash is usually bilateral and remarkably symmetrical. It starts on the instep of the plantar arch as showers of sterile pustules on erythematous plaques. This is often associated with a burning sensation or itch. The pustules dry out and form brown crusts, which gradually exfoliate to leave an erythematous base. Recurrent crops of pustules occur, so early pustules and exfoliating brown crusts are present in the same plaque.

Marked pain and disability occurs when the lesions extend on to weight-bearing areas. Nail changes with punctate stippling and onycholysis are very common.

Differential diagnosis

In the absence of psoriasis elsewhere, the disorder must be distinguished from chronic hyperkeratotic lichenified eczema, Reiter's disease, Bowen's disease, lichen planus and drug eruption.

Course

Psoriasis is unpredictable and undergoes spontaneous remissions and relapses. Guttate psoriasis following a sore throat tends to clear in several months. Generalized pustular and erythrodermic psoriasis are associated with appreciable morbidity and mortality.

Psoriatic arthropathy is of two forms:

1. a rheumatoid-like erosive peripheral arthropathy with a predilection for the distal interphalangeal joints which is seronegative for rheumatoid factor; and
2. ankylosing spondylotitis, which is associated with a high incidence of HLA-B27 especially in those patients with sacroiliitis.

Infection

The skin has a normal resident population of micro-organisms (Noble 1981), which probably do not invade into the intact stratum corneum but remain in the loose surface layer. The normal skin flora includes *Staphylococcus*, *Corynebacterium*, *Acinetobacter* and *Streptococcus*. There is 'normal' carriage of dermatophytes in patients who do not develop clinical disease: up to 9% of normal webs in one series had fungi isolated.

The degree of hydration of the stratum corneum has a very important influence on the skin flora. Increasing the quantity of water at the skin surface greatly increases the number of micro-organisms. This is of particular importance in the case of the feet, where occlusive footwear and sweating can so alter the flora that extensive dermatophytosis and bacterial infection may occur. Drying of the skin results in a reduction in the number of micro-organisms.

Dermatophyte infections

Athlete's foot (Leyden & Kligman 1978) is a term which is applied to the white macerated itchy disorders of interdigital spaces. It is important to realize that all interdigital infection is not fungal, and isolation of fungus from overt clinical ringworm is reported in less than 25% of cases.

Clinical features

The spectrum of tinea pedis in the interdigital webs ranges from minimal dry scaling to a highly inflammatory reaction (Fig. 7).

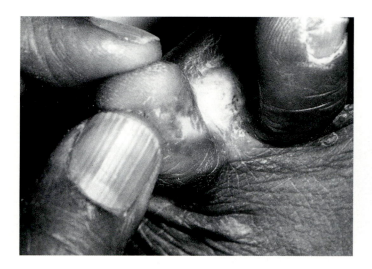

Figure 7
Tinea pedis

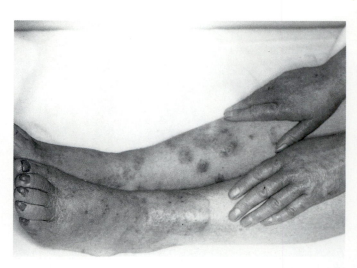

Figure 8
Tinea incognito

The change from mild disease to severe infection occurs with prolonged occlusion and sweating with superhydration of the stratum corneum. This allows bacterial invasion, and the fungus appears to be driven deeper into the stratum corneum. The main dermatophytes that cause interdigital ringworm are *Trichophyton rubrum*, *Trichophyton interdigitale* and *Epidermophyton floccosum*. These are anthropophilic species and humans are the primary host.

The main clinical variety is an itchy, peeling, inflamed, moist and fissured toe space. The fourth and fifth spaces are the most commonly involved. Extension to involve the other spaces, the dorsum and plantar surfaces gradually occurs. A widespread papular rash called a dermatophytide may be associated with highly inflammatory tinea pedis.

Tinea incognita

Tinea incognita is the term applied to a fungal infection inappropriately treated with topical corticosteroid cream. A widespread rash on the feet, hands and groins is common (Figure 8). The presence of a marginated edge helps make the diagnosis.

Diagnosis

This is made by identifying the causative organism. Skin scrapings from dry scaling interdigital webs are usually positive. The recovery rate of fungus is dramatically reduced in severe infection and increases when the secondary bacterial infection is treated.

Treatment

Topical antifungal agents, e.g. micronazole or clotrimazole, are useful for uncomplicated tinea pedis. Whitfield's

ointment (benzoic acid) is cheap but not always effective and can be an irritant to inflamed skin. Antibiotics, either local or systemic, will be necessary where bacterial infection complicates tinea pedis. Physical separation of the toes and the wearing of open shoes will reduce maceration.

Differential diagnosis

Erythrasma and occasionally *Candida albicans* may cause a clinical picture indistinguishable from tinea pedis. A macerated interdigital wart, soft corns or condylomata lata may present as athlete's foot. Eczema rarely affects the interdigital spaces and involves the medial rather than the lateral toe spaces.

Candidiasis

Candidiasis or moniliasis is caused by a yeast-like fungus (Ray & Wuepper 1976). It is an opportunistic pathogen and causes disease only in the presence of an underlying host defect, such as poorly controlled diabetes mellitus or prolonged antibiotic therapy. On the foot, candidiasis may present as interdigital infection, paronychia and onycholysis, and rarely as candida granuloma.

Interdigital candidiasis gives rise to eroded, macerated tissue with fissuring commonly affecting the fourth web space. Sweating, closely opposed toes, the wearing of tight occlusive socks which prevent evaporation of sweat all predispose to interdigital candidiasis.

Paronychia and onycholysis produced by *Candida* infections of the toe nails is much less common than in finger-nails. The skin surrounding the nail fold becomes red, swollen and tender.

Candida granuloma

Candida granuloma is regarded as a variant of chronic mucocutaneous candidiasis. Lesions on the feet, face and scalp are common. The nodules are multiple and break down to form a fungating crusted surface. There may be evidence of serious bacterial infection in these patients. Defects in delayed hypersensitivity are present in some but not all patients.

Bacterial diseases

Bacterial infections are common on the feet. They may occur on intact skin or as a secondary phenomenon on inflamed skin. *Staphylococcus aureus* and Group A beta-haemolytic *streptococcus* are the common pathogens in primary bacterial infection, while *Staphylococcus aureus* is the usual cause in secondarily infected skin.

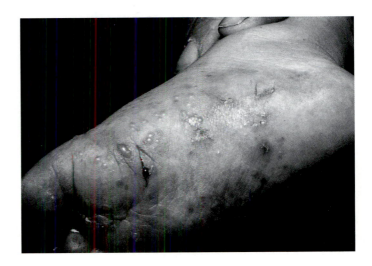

Figure 9
Bullous impetigo

Impetigo

Definition
Impetigo is a contagious, superficial pyogenic infection of the skin. Two forms present clinically: bullous impetigo caused by *Staphylococcus aureus*, and a non-bullous form caused by *Staphylococci*, *Streptococci* or a combination of both organisms.

Clinical features

Bullous impetigo
In bullous impetigo (Fig. 9) the vesicles are less easily ruptured and coalesce to produce bullae 1–2 cm in diameter, which persist for 2–3 days. A flat brown crust develops as the bullae rupture. Central healing and peripheral expansion gives rise to a characteristic annular lesion. The palms and soles may be affected and regional adenitis is uncommon.

Non-bullous impetigo
Non-bullous impetigo starts as a thin-walled vesicle on a synthetic base which ruptures to produce the characteristic yellow–brown crusted spreading lesions. The crusts eventually dry and separate to leave erythema, which fades without scarring in about 2–3 weeks. The face and limbs are commonly affected. In severe infection, regional adenitis with fever and constitutional symptoms develop.

Treatment
In mild and localized infections, topical application of Mupirocin or fusidic acid is as effective as oral erythromycin (Mertz et al 1989). An oral antibiotic is indicated if widespread disease or systemic symptoms develop.

Erythrasma
Erythrasma is a mild, chronic, localized, superficial infection of the axillae, groins and toe clefts, caused by a diptheroid bacteria (*Corynebacterium*). *Corynebacterium minutissimum* is frequently part of the normal flora of the clefts, and alteration in the normal host–parasite relationship induced by warm humid conditions is a predisposing factor in the development of clinical erythrasma.

Clinical features
Scaling, erythema, fissuring and maceration is the common clinical finding, but toe cleft infection is often asymptomatic. Wood's light examination reveals the classical coral-red fluorescence, which helps to distinguish erythrasma from candidal intertrigo, which it closely resembles clinically.

Treatment
Topical imidazole antifungal agents such as clotrimazole or topical fucidic acid are useful preparations if used for at least 2 weeks. Oral erythromycin may be required for extensive disease. Relapse is common and long-term use of drying agents such as povidone iodine may be useful.

Pitted keratolysis
This is a superficial infection caused by a corynebacterium which produces circular erosion of the skin (Zaias 1982).

Clinical features
Superficial erosions develop on the soles and plantar surfaces of the toes to give a honeycombed appearance

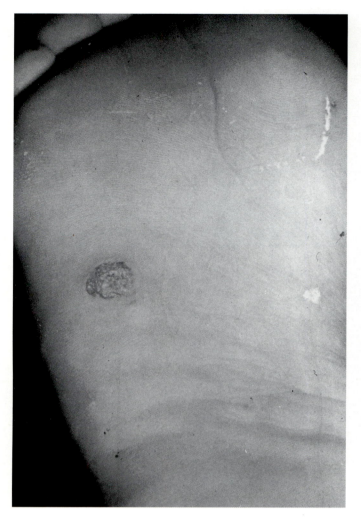

Figure 10
Plantar warts

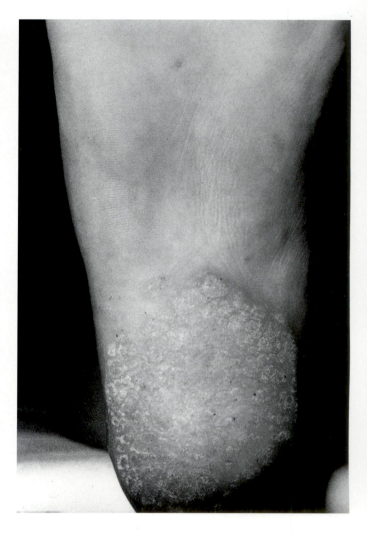

Figure 11
Mosaic warts

to the skin. This appearance is accentuated if the feet are soaked in water. Hyperhidrosis and a foul odour may be present but in most patients it is asymptomatic.

Treatment
Topical antibiotic such as fusidic acid, erythromycin and an imidazole such as clotriazole may be effective. Control of hyperhidrosis using 20% aluminium hexa-hydrate helps to keep the condition under control.

Warts

Warts are tumours caused by human papilloma viruses (HPV) (Bunney 1984). They are pleomorphic and can involve any skin site, but principally are found in the hands, feet and genital areas. Fifty-four different types of HPV have been identified by DNA hybridization. Different HPV types vary in this specificity for different sites, e.g. HPV 1 replicates best in the highly keratinized plantar and palmar skin.

Warts occur at any age but are commonest in the school child, incidence declines sharply by the age of 20. Warts are spread by direct or indirect contact. Trauma or maceration, singly or in combination, results in impairment of the epidermal barrier front and predisposes to inocculation of the virus.

Plantar warts or verrucae

Plantar warts (Fig. 10) are caused by HPV 1,2 or 4. The deep 'myrmecia' contain HPV 1; smaller ones are due to HPV 4; HPV 2 commonly causes mosaic warts. Most plantar warts are beneath pressure points on the heels or metatarsal heads. Warts may be single or multiple. Mosaic warts are plaques or closely grouped warts (Fig. 11).

Treatment

Treatments for warts abound and each culture and age has its own folk cures. Spontaneous remission occurs, and 67% will clear within 2 years. Spontaneous remission is often heralded by increasing pain and haemorrhage into the wart before it involves. Itching sometimes precedes resolution.

The response of warts to treatment is inversely proportional to their duration, the age of the patient, the number of warts and type. Mosaic warts tend to persist while single deep warts respond readily. Antiwart preparations act by destroying the virus infected cells physically or chemically. Salicylic acid, formaldehyde, and glutaraldehyde all cause keratolysis of the wart and the surrounding tissue when applied topically. This is a slow process and may take several weeks to months.

Podophyllin (15–25%) has a potent antimitotic effect and is be applied weekly. This drug is highly irritant and the normal skin should be protected. It should not be used in pregnancy. It is one of the more effective treatments of mosaic warts.

Cryotherapy is the most popular mode of treatment at present. Carbon dioxide and liquid nitrogen are the two freezing agents available, the latter being more efficient. It is widely used and may be applied using cotton buds or special delivery systems. It is not necessary to provoke blister formation. Excessive blistering may be rewarded by new wart formation at the periphery. Warts need to be treated at 3-week intervals or less. Longer intervals reduce the cure rate by half. Care must be taken to make sure that treatment does not end with scarring. Warts will eventually clear but a painful scar may be a permanent reminder. Carbon dioxide laser is less commonly used. Intralesional bleomycin results in a 70% cure rate in previously resistant warts.

Hand-foot-and-mouth disease

Hand-foot-and-mouth disease is a disease of childhood caused by the coxsackie viruses. It may occur as an epidemic disease where it is associated with coxsackie A16 or as sporadic cases associated with A5 and A9. A similar clinical picture occurs in infection with enterovirus 71.

Clinical features

It is characterized by the presence of small, painful, oral ulcers, usually lasting about 5–10 days. The vesicular stage is transient and the typical oral lesion is a shallow grey ulcer surrounded by an erythematous halo. The skin lesions, varying in number, appear either simultaneously with or shortly after the oral lesions. Involvement of the palms and soles is common. Each blister, which arises from an erythematous base, is greyish in colour and tends to be oval or linear running in or parallel to the skin creases. They may be painful, especially when on the soles of the feet, and they resolve in 7–10 days.

Treatment

There is no specific treatment but symptomatic relief may be obtained from analgesics or topical local anaesthetic in the mouth.

Mycobacterial infection

The mycobacteria (Cott et al 1967) are acid-fast bacilli which characteristically produce chronic granulomatous lesions which may ulcerate and disseminate. In man the most important are *Mycobacterium tuberculosis* and *Mycobacterium leprae*.

The other group of mycobacteria to cause human disease are the opportunistic or atypical mycobacteria. They are found in soil, water and excreta. They differ from mycotuberculosis in that they are nonvirulent in guinea pigs, able to grow at room temperature, resistant to pretherapy with isoniazid and unable to form nicotinic acid.

Mycobacterium marinum infection

A chronic granulomatous skin lesion produced by direct inoculation by *Mycobacterium marinum*. The organism's natural habitat is water and it is found in the crevices and grooves in the cement walls of swimming pools, which have been identified as the focus of outbreaks of the disease.

Clinical features

The lesions develop on traumatized skin and commonly on the dorsal aspects of the feet, the fronts of the knees and sometimes the elbows. It usually occurs in adolescents who forsake the steps or ladders of the pool and prefer to climb out onto the deck.

A small reddish papule develops at the site of inoculation after a 3–4 weeks' incubation period. The lesion enlarges to form a hard reddish-brown nodule which sometimes ulcerates and may be covered with a greyish exudate or becomes verrucous. Lymphangitis or regional adenopathy does not occur. In some instances satellite nodules may develop along the line of the lymphatics, resembling a sporotrichoid infection.

Spontaneous healing occurs with scarring within a year but persistence for up to 45 years has been recorded. The response to therapy with antituberculosis agents is variable and is only indicated for resistant or severe disease. Minocycline, tetracycline and cotrimazole have all been reported as successful but only in very small groups of patients. Skin testing with purified protein derivative (PPD) is positive.

Infection with other atypical mycobacteria
Cutaneous infection with atypical mycobacteria other than *Mycobacterium marinum* is rare. They produce lesions similar to those of *Mycobacterium marinum* but infection is not transmitted by water.

Bullous Disorders

Epidermolysis bullosa

Epidermolysis bullosa (EB) is a term applied to a large group of genetically determined disorders which are characterized by blistering of the skin and of mucosal membranes (Gedde-Dahl 1981). The blisters result from minor trauma and arise spontaneously. At least seven different forms have been identified; these are genetically distinct diseases mediated by different mechanisms.

Epidermolysis bullosa simplex (Weber–Cockayne type)

Epidermolysis bullosa simplex is the commonest type and is transmitted as an autosomal dominant trait. Bullae usually develop in the first year when the child begins to walk or crawl. Clear, tense bullae occur at sites of trauma, usually the hands and feet. They heal without scarring or milia formation, milia being small subepidermal keratin cysts 1–2 mm in size. When milia occur in the course of the blistering disorders they represent retention cysts. Heat increases the tendency to blister, particularly in patients with palmar–plantar hyperhidrosis. The condition may improve at puberty but tends to persist.

Recessive dystrophic epidermolysis bullosa

More severe and widespread blistering occurs in recessive dystrophic epidermolysis bullosa. Bullae appear at birth or in early infancy. They are large and flaccid, sometimes haemorrhagic, and may occur spontaneously. The bullae heal with milia formation and atrophic scarring. Pseudowebbing due to scar tissue covers the fingers and toes, producing gross deformities. Nails are shed early and sclerosis of the fingertips develops. Rarely, large eroded nonhealing areas occur on the extensor surface of the limbs.

The mucus membranes are usually involved, with oral bullae, erosions and ulcers complicating early feeding. Oesophageal casts may be shed and strictures occur in early childhood. These strictures interfere with adequate nutrition and chronic anaemia results. Aspiration pneumonia may occur and, in those who survive, carcinoma of the cardia.

Surviving children are usually physically retarded but mentally normal. Squamous carcinoma, sometimes multiple, have developed in the scarred atrophic skin, especially on the legs. Leukoplakia followed by carcinoma has also been reported in the mouth.

Treatment

This is unsatisfactory. In the milder forms, protection from trauma and the use of topical or systemic antibiotics if infection occurs is all that can be offered to these patients. Reduction in sweating improves blistering on the soles. Skilled nursing and control of infection improves survival in children with dystrophic types of EB. High doses of corticosteroids are no longer recommended. Plastic surgery is required repeatedly in order to maintain function of fingers and hands. Phenytoin with its effect on collagenase activity does not significantly alter the disease.

Prayer nodules

Hyperkeratosis of the lateral and anterior aspects of the ankles is common. The position adopted to induce these lesions is acute inversion of the foot so that the rim of the lateral talar condyle is being continually rubbed against the skin.

Piezogenic pedal papules

These are flesh coloured papules which appear on the medial aspects of the heels (Schlappner et al 1972). They are usually asymptomatic and are visible on weight bearing. They are often overlooked as most patients are examined recumbent. The papules are true herniations of subcutaneous fat through defects in connective tissue into the dermis. This extrusion of fat with its blood vessels and nerves could account for the pain on standing in some patients.

Treatment

Cushioning of the shoe or supportive orthopaedic devices may help to relieve pressure on the heel.

Calcaneal petechial 'black heel'

A speckled black lesion appears on the back or side of the heel just above the junction of the hyperkeratotic skin of the sole of the foot and the thinner skin. It occurs as the result of rupture of small papillary capilla because of a shearing force; it is commonly seen in adolescents involved in football, basketball and squash.

Clinical features

It is usually a painless condition which on closer examination is made up of closely grouped black dots caused by haemorrhage.

Diagnosis and treatment

Gentle paring of the skin reveals that the black pigment comes away in the horny layer. Treatment is not indicated but a softer heel piece in the shoe or a felt pad may help. The main importance of this condition is that it must be differentiated from malignant melanoma or a tattoo.

Subungual exostosis

In this condition, a bony lump appears below the nail. It is not a true exostosis as the tumour consists of normal mature bone. It occurs mainly in children and adolescents and is most commonly found in the great toe.

The lesion presents as a hard lump under the skin of the distal nail bed. The overlying portion of nail is often rubbed away by shoe pressure. Although it often resembles subungual warts or an ingrowing toe nail, ulceration does not occur. Confirmation of the diagnosis is by X-ray, which clearly demonstrates the bony lesion lying lateral to the distal phalanx.

Pyogenic granuloma (granuloma telangecticum)

This lesion usually occurs after trauma. It involves the hyponychium and enlarges to involve the nail bed. Removal of the nail and either surgical excision or electrodesiccation usually cures the lesion.

Fibromas

These occur in 50% of patients with tuberous sclerosis. They are usually periungual but may occur subungually. Grooving of the nail is a common manifestation. They occur after puberty, and stigmata of the disease are usually well established. Surgical excision will cure the lesion.

Junctional naevi

Linear pigmented bands are frequently seen in the nails of coloured races. Naevus cells in the matrix produce the pigmented bands which may vary in colour from light brown to black. A linear pigmented band in a white patient should be excised to exclude a subungual melanoma.

Glomus tumours

Glomus tumours are vascular tumours arising in the dermis of the nail bed. They are intensely painful when even the lightest pressure is applied. Removal of the nail plate and excision of the lesion results in a complete cure.

Eccrine poroma

This is a benign growth of the distal eccrine sweat duct (Heyman & Brownstein 1969).

Clinical features

The lesion occurs on the non-hair-bearing areas of the foot and occasionally the palm. It presents as a nontender smooth reddish tumour, which may protrude from a shallow cup-shaped depression forming the base. It bleeds readily and may vary in size from 2–12 mm in diameter. Although the lesions tend to be singular, multiple lesions do occur.

Incidence and treatment

This is an uncommon tumour and affects both sexes equally. It tends to be a disease of middle-age. Local excision is curative. Curettage with electrodesiccation of the base may be adequate.

Differential diagnosis

This lesion may simulate Kaposi's sarcoma, malignant melanoma, basal cell carcinoma or a pyogenic granuloma.

Malignant eccrine poroma or porocarcinoma

Malignant change may occur in an eccrine poroma of long duration or may arise *de novo*. It may present localized and indistinguishable from an eccrine poroma or as an ulceration nodule. Cutaneous and visceral metastases have been recorded as causing death.

Kaposi's sarcoma (multiple idiopathic haemorrhagic sarcoma)

Kaposi's sarcoma (KS) is a rare vascular tumour first reported by Kaposi in 1872 (Tappero et al 1993). KS occurs in four different settings: classic KS, African (endemic KS), iatrogenic KS and acquired immunodeficiency syndrome KS (AIDS KS).

Classic KS

Classic KS occurs in elderly men of Mediterranean, Eastern European and Jewish origin. It is a chronic disease, with patients surviving on average 10 to 15 years before dying of unrelated disease. It is predominantly a skin disease of the lower legs although visceral and lymph node disease may occur.

African endemic KS

African endemic KS has a high prevelance in sub-Saharan Africa and is not associated with immunodeficiency (Kestens et al 1985). It occurs in two distinct groups; young adults and children. It presents in four clinically distinct patterns:

1. benign nodular skin disease resembling classic KS;
2. aggressive localized cutaneous disease involving soft tissue and bone;
3. florid mucocutaneous and visceral disease; and
4. fulminant lymphadenopathic disease with little or no cutaneous disease; this pattern is fatal in 2–3 years.

Iatrogenic KS

Iatrogenic KS is a cutaneous complication of immunosuppressive drug therapy (Brooks 1986). Spontaneous remission occurs after cessation of immunosuppressive therapy.

AIDS KS

By 1989, KS was the primary AIDS–defining illness in 15% of all AIDS cases in the United States. AIDS KS is more common in homosexual men than in men with haemophilia. This suggests that both human immunodeficiency virus (HIV) and a second sexually transmitted cofactor play a role in the pathogenesis of AIDS KS. It usually presents after some degree of immune impairment. The activity or progression of AIDS KS roughly correlates with the overall health of the patient.

Clinical features

The initial lesions usually occur on the soles of the feet as bluish-red or black macules which spread and coalesce to form a large plaque. Rubbery angiomatous nodules with oedema may then develop. The nodules ulcerate and have a foul-smelling discharge. The disease slowly advances with more nodules developing and increasing lymphoedema.

In the early stages of the disease, spontaneous resolution of some or all of the nodules may occur, leaving atrophic hyperpigmented scars. Later on, macules,

patches and nodules appear on the face, ears, soft palate and the trunk. The disease becomes slowly progressive. Gangrene of the feet may occur. Involvement of bone and the small bowel is common and is indicative of disseminated disease. Once visceral involvement occurs death is rapid.

Diagnosis

The histological picture is variable. The early lesions resemble granulation tissue, while in the late phase, prominent endothelial cells are seen lining the vessels with spindle-shaped cells lying peripherally.

Treatment

Local therapy, including liquid nitrogen cryotherapy, irradiation and intralesional chemotherapy, allows for limited intervention. Systemic chemotherapy is useful in widespread classic KS and African endemic KS. Combined chemotherapeutic regimes have not to date resulted in the salvage of any patient with AIDS KS, as most patients will die of opportunistic infection rather than AIDS KS.

Verrucous squamous cell epithelioma (epithelioma cuniculatum plantare)

This rare tumour of the plantar surface of the foot is a variant of squamous cell carcinoma (Reingold et al 1978) (Fig. 12).

Clinical features

The exophytic tumour has a cauliflower-like or verrucoid ulcerating surface, which is often associated with a foul discharge. At first the lesion closely resembles a recalcitrant plantar wart. It is capable of great local destruction with deep penetration of the underlying fascia and it may destroy the metatarsal bones and go on to invade the skin on the dorsum of the foot. It has little tendency to metastasize, though the development of regional lymph node metastases has been documented.

Treatment

Local wide excision is important. Amputations may be necessary if bone is involved. Radiation should not be used as it has led in some instances to the development of metastatic squamous carcinoma.

Differential diagnosis

The diagnosis is often difficult and it must be distinguished from an intractable plantar wart, giant kerato-

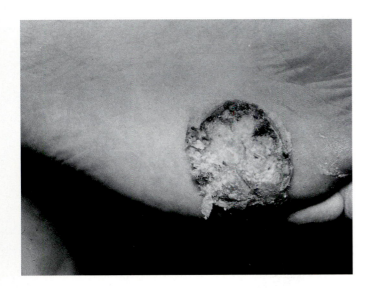

Figure 12
Verrucous squamous cell epithelioma

acanthoma, deep fungal infection and pseudo-epitheliomatous hyperplasia.

Malignant melanoma

This is an uncommon malignant tumour which arises from epidermal melanocytes (McGovern 1982). Cutaneous malignant melanoma (MM) are usually divided into four types:

1. Lentigo maligna melanoma (LMM)
2. Superficial spreading (SMM)
3. Acral lentiginous melanoma (ALM)
4. Nodular melanoma (NM)

In the first three types an early horizontal growth phase exists – melanoma *in situ*, where the tumour is confined to the epidermis. After a varying length of time an invasive or vertical growth phase occurs. Invasive melanoma arising from melanoma *in situ* tends to have a better prognosis than nodular melanoma arising *de novo*.

Acral lentiginous melanoma *in situ*

ALM *in situ* has only recently been recognized as a separate entity (Coleman et al 1980). Characteristically, it occurs on the hairless skin of the palms and soles and also in the subungual and periungual areas. Uneven pigmentation with an irregular, ill-defined edge is seen. If it occurs in the nail bed, matrix or nail, it presents as a pigmented longitudinal band.

Diagnosis of ALM *in situ* is difficult and may not be recognized clinically or histologically. Wide excision at this stage offers excellent prognosis.

Acral lentiginous melanoma (ALM)

ALM is the invasive form of ALM *in situ* (Paladuga et al 1983). The earliest lesions are irregular macular lesions with uneven pigmentation. They may be present for a considerable time – up to 7 years – and are usually ignored by the patient.

Itch is sometimes present even before any discernible change in pigmentation occurs. The skin surface markings are lost with the early pigmentary changes. Blue–black or pink nodules are often found within the tumour. Bleeding is a sinister sign and is often associated with ulceration and necrosis in the tumour.

No single sign is a specific indicator of malignancy, as all may occur simultaneously. However any previously uniform pigmented lesion on the sole of the foot which shows alteration in the pigment either centrally or peripherally, or which develops elevated nodules with an inflammatory edge, should be regarded with a high index of suspicion.

Incidence
There is a slight female predominance of 3:2 in most series. It has a peak incidence in the sixth decade for women and a decade later for men. There is considerable epidemiological evidence implicating the role of sunlight in the formation of malignant melanoma. It is obvious that sunlight is not the only factor in inducing melanoma on the foot, and the role of repeated trauma is difficult to assess.

Prognosis
Prognosis is poor for ALM as tumefaction, ulceration and metastases occur early. Prognosis is directly related to tumour thickness. Volar melanomas less than 1 cm deep and those in the horizontal growth phase have a better prognosis and usually only require local wide excision. The overall five year survival rate varies from 11–15%.

Foreign body reactions

Foreign bodies in the skin are a common problem. Granulomatous reactions may occur at the site of entry in the skin.

Silica granulomas

Silica in the form of glass, quartz, sand or flint may give rise to silica granuloma, which develop months or even years after the initial injury has healed (Epstein 1955). It is the conversion of silica to silica colloid in the tissues that is thought to account for the granuloma formation. The silicates in the spines of sea urchins may also produce a sarcoidal granuloma and even local osteitis. They present as red–brown or violaceous maculopapules. Ulceration is rare. The lesions may spontaneously remit but can be treated surgically or by local injection of corticosteroid. Foreign bodies may introduce micro-organisms into the skin. *Staphylococcal* and *streptococcal* infections may give rise to cellulitis. Sporotrichosis may be transmitted by infected thorns.

Hair

Hair acting as a foreign body results in a number of reactions. This usually depends on the site and depth of penetration. Mild erythema, abscess and sinus formation as well as chronic granuloma may all be associated with hair reactions.

Hair sinuses of the feet

A very characteristic syndrome occurs when a hair penetrates the skin of an interdigital web, usually the fourth (Price & Popkin 1976). This is often unsuspected and the patient may present with a long history of recurrent episodes of pain, swelling or cellulitis. Examination reveals oedema of the adjacent dorsal foot, with a pinhole sinus present in the base of the web. This is often hidden beneath an accumulation of macerated skin. Surgical excision of the sinus tract is curative.

Hair penetrating the foot is an occupational hazard of hairdressers and dog groomers. Hyperkeratotic tender nodules on the heels and toes and abscess formation on the toes have all been reported in hairdressers.

Granuloma annulare

This granulomatous condition of children and young adults may be an indicator of latent diabetes (Fig. 13). The aetiology is unknown. The histological features may merge into those of necrobiosis lipoidica. It is commoner in females than in males.

Clinical features

The lesions are commonly found on the extensor aspects of the hands, feet, arms and legs. The lesions are pink or flesh coloured papules or nodules which form rings and there is characteristic beading of the edge of the lesions.

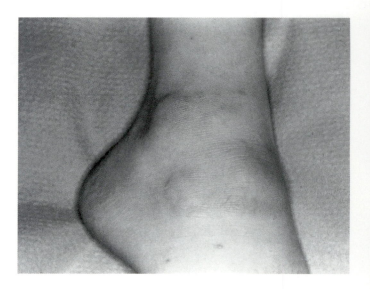

Figure 13
Granuloma annulare

Treatment

No treatment is necessary as the lesions resolve spontaneously, but its course may be influenced by local or intralesional corticosteroids.

For ainhum and pseudoainhum see Chapter VIII.1.

References

Ashton R E, Griffiths W A 1986 Juvenile plantar dermatosis – atopy or footwear. Clin Exp Dermatol 11: 529–534

Blair S D, Wright D D T, Backhouse C M, et al 1988 Sustained compression and healing of chronic venous ulcers. Br Med J 297: 1159–1161

Bowker N V, Cross K W, Fairburn E A et al 1976 Sociological implications of an epidemiological study of eczema in the city of Birmingham. Br J Dermatol 95: 137–44

Brooks J J 1986 Kaposi's sarcoma: a reversible hyperplasia. Lancet 2: 1309–1311

Bunney M H 1984 Viral Warts: their Biology and Treatment. Oxford University Press, Oxford.

Coleman W P III, Loria P R, Reed R J et al 1980 Acral lentiginous melanoma. Arch Dermatol 116: 773–776

Conde-Salazar L, del-Rio E, Guimaraens D et al 1993 Type IV allergy to rubber additives. J Am Acad Dermatol 29: 176–180

Cott R E, Carter D M, Sall T 1967 Cutaneous disease caused by atypical mycobacterium: review of two chromagen infections and review of the subject. Arch Dermatol 95: 259–269

Cram D L 1981 Psoriasis: current advances in etiology and treatment. J Am Acad Dermatol 4: 1–18

Epstein E 1955 Silica granuloma of the skin. Arch Dermatol 71: 24–35

Fisher A A 1986a Contact Dermatitis, 3rd edn. Lea and Febiger, Philadelphia. pp 316–337

Fisher A A 1986b Contact Dermatitis, 3rd edn. Lea and Febiger, Philadelphia. pp 309–313

Gedde-Dahl T Jr 1981 Sixteen types of epidermolysis bullosa, Acta Derm Venereol (Suppl) 95: 74–87

Heyman A B, Brownstein M G 1969 Eccrine poroma analysis of 45 new cases. Dermatologica 138: 29–38

Kaposi M 1872 Idiopathic multiple pigmented sarcoma of the skin. Arch Dermatol Syphil 4: 265–273

Kestens L, Melbye M, Bigger R J et al 1985 Endemic African Kaposi's sarcoma is not associated with immunodeficiency. Int J Cancer 36: 49–54

Leyden J J, Kligman A M 1978 Interdigital athlete's foot. The interaction of dermatophytes and resident bacteria. Arch Dermatol 114: 1466–1470

McGovern VJ, 1982 The nature of melanoma. A critical review. J Cutan Pathol 9: 61–82

Mertz P M, Marshal D A, Eaglstein W H et al 1989 Topical Mupirocin treatment of impetigo is equal to oral erythromycin therapy. Arch Dermatol 125: 1069–1073

Noble W C 1981 In: Microbiology of Human Skin. Lloyd–Luke, London. p 79

Paladuga R R, Winbeeg C D, Yonemoto R H 1983 Acral lentiginous melanoma. Cancer 52: 161–168

Price S M, Popkin G L 1976 Barber's interdigital hair sinus. A case report in a dog groomer. Arch Dermatol 112: 523

Rajka G 1989 Essential Aspects of Atopic Dermatitis. Springer-Verlag, Berlin.

Ray T L, Wuepper K D 1976 Experimental cutaneous candidiasis in rodents. J Invest Dermatol 66: 29–35

Reingold I M, Smith B R, Graham J H 1978 Epithelioma cuniculatum pedis, variant of squamous cell carcinoma. Am J Clin Pathol 67: 561–565

Schlappner O L A, Wood M G, Gerstein W, Gross P R 1972 Painful and non-painful piezogenic pedal papules. Arch Dermatol 106: 729–733

Tappero J W, Conant M A, Wolfe S F et al 1993 Kaposi's sarcoma. J Am Acad Dermatol 28: 371–395

Winter G D 1972 Epidermal regeneration studied in the domestic pig. In: Maibach H I, Rovee D T (eds) Epidermal Wound Healing. Year Book Medical Publishers, Chicago. pp 71–112

Zaias M 1982 Pitted and ringed keratolysis. J Am Acad Dermatol 7: 787–791

VI.3 The Rheumatoid Foot and Ankle

Introduction

Andrea Cracchiolo III

Rheumatoid arthritis is one of the few diseases that frequently involves the entire foot, producing painful deformities that can usually be treated. Since the pathology varies and can involve so many joints and soft tissues, a number of methods have been developed for the surgical correction of these deformities.

The rheumatoid patient usually has other pathology which limits their function and activity. Therefore the need has been to relieve pain, and restoration of 'normal' foot function is not usually a primary objective. For these reasons many widely differing procedures have been utilized over the past few decades by many excellent surgeons. Obviously, each has been greatly influenced by their training and experience, and since the rheumatoid patient is usually satisfied with pain relief, many if not most of these operations are considered to be successful. It would be impossible in a single chapter to cover all of these treatments and operations; therefore we will attempt to give you some perspectives which are obviously based on the authors' individual prejudices.

The forefoot

Foot involvement and pathology

Since there are many synovial-lined joints within the foot, active rheumatoid disease can produce widespread foot pain. Joint swelling is best seen in the forefoot in the metatarsophalangeal (MTP) joints. Although the exact incidence of rheumatoid arthritis involving the foot and ankle is unknown, it does appear to vary in various parts of the world. For example, involvement of the ankle has been reported to be as high as 68% in Europe, and as low as 10–15% in the USA (Tillmann 1979). Moreover, operations in patients with inflammatory joint disease are common and have been estimated to be between one-fifth and one-third of all operations performed (Tillmann 1979). Many more operations are carried out on the forefoot than the hindfoot or ankle, probably four to five times as many.

It is essential to remember that RA is a progressive disease. Once there is involvement of some of the forefoot, it is usual that all joints, especially the MTP joints, will become destroyed. Early in the disease, at 1–3 years from onset, synovitis occurs equally in the MTP

joints in 65% of patients (Spiegel & Spiegel 1982). This decreases with time so that by 10 years only 18% show synovitis in these joints. Conversely, joint deformity increases with the duration of the disease, so that by 10 years of disease 58% of RA patients will show some forefoot deformity. More specifically, Spiegel & Spiegel (1982) found that moderate to severe hallux valgus deformity was present in 40% of RA patients with disease for longer than 10 years, whereas only 6% had moderate deformity with disease of 1–3 years.

The classic findings of RA in the forefoot include hallux valgus, usually severe, with intra-articular degeneration of the MTP joints. Frequently, synovitis and erosions of the MTP joints are the presenting signs of early RA. Occasionally, degenerative joint changes are also present in the interphalangeal (IP) joint. The toes drift laterally and at first subluxate, and then dislocate dorsally. As this occurs, the metatarsal heads are pushed more plantarward, the toes develop a clawtoe deformity, and the weight bearing plantar fat pad is drawn further forward, losing its normal location underneath the metatarsal heads. Eventually destructive changes occur, mainly to the metatarsal heads. Large bursae with overlying calluses are frequent under the middle metatarsal heads, and at times, under the hallux. Web space pathology (Dedrich et al 1990), usually an intermetatarsal bursa, gives neuroma-like symptoms as an early sign of forefoot involvement (Auerbach et al 1982, Shephard 1975), and may be an early sign of RA.

A common skin problem in patients with RA is the ease with which it bruises and the development of ecchymosis. This can be seen about the lower leg, over the malleoli and on the dorsum of the foot. The skin is very thin and fragile. It can be damaged by the slightest injury, which may result in an ulcer that can take many weeks or months to heal. These problems are most likely due to the disease and the types of medications with which patients are treated.

Vasculitis is also a feature of RA. It usually involves the small vessels of the foot and lower leg. Vasculitic lesions are seen in the skin and appear as small brownish spots or splinter-shaped hemorrhages that are frequently found in the nail folds or in the digital pulp. The foot must be examined specifically for such lesions, which should be carefully evaluated by the rheumatologist. Vasculitic lesions may be a contraindication to elective surgical procedures. An uncontrolled vasculitis could produce delays in wound healing and thus jeopardize the surgical result (Spiegel & Spiegel 1982). It is unusual for rheumatoid disease to involve major vessels, but a neuropathy can be produced by the RA. In the foot it may appear as a peripheral sensory neuropathy, a sensorimotor neuropathy, or an entrapment neuropathy, though entrapment neuropathy is much more commonly seen in the medial nerve at the wrist than in the foot or ankle (Geppert et al 1992).

Radiographic evaluation

A standard set of radiographs should be obtained when evaluating any rheumatoid patient with significant involvement of the foot. These should include a weight bearing anteroposterior (AP) and lateral view of the foot. A weight-bearing AP view of the ankles is also important, especially if there is any ankle or hindfoot pathology. Although the forefoot is more commonly symptomatic than the hindfoot and ankle, it is important to evaluate the entire foot in all patients with RA.

Any patient with RA about to undergo an operation under either general or spinal anesthesia should have a medical evaluation. This should include a clinical and radiographic assessment of the cervical spine. Lateral radiographs of the cervical spine in neutral, flexion and extension are helpful to assess the stability of the neck. At times, odontoid views are also necessary.

Shoes

The most important aspect of nonoperative care is proper shoe wear in patients with rheumatoid disease (Cracchiolo 1979, 1982b, 1982c). A shoe must be selected or modified to fit the patient's deformity. Shoes do not correct deformities, rather they accommodate the deformities and thus reduce pain. Since the forefoot is a common area of symptoms and pathology, wearing a shoe with a wider and deeper toebox is important in rheumatoid patients. The most frequent shoe modification is a metatarsal pad, which should be placed with the apex of the pad just proximal to the area of maximum tenderness or callus formation, usually between the second and third metatarsal heads. The inner sole can also be excavated under painful calluses. The excavations can be filled in or covered with any material to line the sole and reduce shear pressures on the skin (Cracchiolo 1982c). Composites of various materials can be fabricated which give some support while cushioning the skin. Unfortunately, these materials do not last forever and most liners must be replaced or refurbished every 3–6 months, depending on the patient's weight and activity level.

The effect of medication on surgical procedures

One of the most important preoperative considerations should be the type of medications the patient is taking for the arthritis. Patients taking over 10 mg per day of prednisone are at high risk for failure of primary wound healing (Cracchiolo et al 1992) and the possibility of then developing an infection. Ideally it may be safest to reduce the oral prednisone dose to about 5 mg per day before undertaking major foot or ankle surgery. Methotrexate, in my experience, also delays wound healing and should, if possible, be discontinued about 1 week before the surgery and for about 2 weeks postoperatively.

Timing of operations on the rheumatoid foot

The forefoot is usually the most painful area and it is usually easy to determine whether an operation is indicated. However, there are some unusual factors that may first require surgical correction of another area.

1. In a patient with both forefoot and hindfoot deformity, both of which are painful, it may be best to correct the hindfoot deformity first. Forefoot deformities may recur in patients with significant pronation and valgus deformity of the foot.
2. At times, it may be necessary to perform a more minor procedure to allow for skin healing and to eliminate sepsis. This might be the treatment of an infected toenail or the excision of a proximal interphalangeal (PIP) joint to eliminate a dorsal corn that has ulcerated.

It is usually unwise to perform extensive bilateral forefoot surgery. Even in advanced deformity, the patient can better rely on the nonoperated foot to ambulate; this places less stress on the operated foot, pain is less and wound healing is improved. Operations on the ipsilateral forefoot and hindfoot should also be avoided as this may produce extensive swelling leading to problems with wound healing. Thus it is best and safer to proceed with a properly planned forefoot reconstruction unilaterally and then 4–6 weeks later, when it appears that wound healing has occurred, proceed with the opposite side.

I do not favor performing major hand or wrist reconstruction at the same time as performing a major foot operation. The upper extremity operation will usually impede the patient's ability to ambulate using crutches or a cane, and may restrict the patient's ability to attend the very important postoperative therapy required following major hand reconstruction. Obviously, I have been greatly influenced by the demand made on us in the USA to perform some of these operations as outpatients or to keep the patients in hospital for only a day or two.

Surgical procedures to correct rheumatoid deformities of the forefoot

The indication to perform a surgical procedure in the foot of a patient with rheumatoid arthritis is to relieve pain, and whenever possible to correct all forefoot deformities. In the past, the destroyed MTP joint has been excised in patients with rheumatoid arthritis. This operation has been performed for many years, and almost all conceivable varieties of excisional arthroplasty done through various dorsal and plantar incisions have been described (Fowler 1959, Amuso et al 1971, Faithful & Savill 1971, Lipscomb et al 1972, Barton 1973, Watson 1974, Vahvanen et al 1980, Craxford et al 1982, Mann & Thompson 1984, Hassalo et al 1987, Gainor et al 1988, McGarvey & Johnson 1988, Stockey et al 1989, Hughes et al 1991).

Clayton (1982) popularized excision of both the metatarsal head and the base of the proximal phalanx. The sesamoids were excised only if they were fused to the bottom of the metatarsal head or if they were grossly deformed. Clayton's observations, after extensive clinical experience, indicate that if one or two joints were relatively spared by the disease, they should also be excised so that in general all MTP joints should be included in the forefoot operation. He also emphasized that the postoperative results of these procedures on the rheumatoid forefoot, if the patient is followed long enough, will gradually deteriorate. Rheumatoid disease is progressive in most patients and if deformities increase in the remaining joints of the foot, particularly the hindfoot joints, then forefoot deformities may recur (Cracchiolo 1993).

One should avoid the indiscriminate resection of bone as the only method of correcting the forefoot deformity. It is as important to realign the soft tissue structures as it is to resect the bone.

McGarvey & Johnson (1988) reviewed 20 different series involving more than 1730 feet in which the RA forefoot had been reconstructed. Overall, they estimate an average 'success' of approximately 85% (range 55–100%). Most of these studies report 'success' using the patient's subjective response to the operation. Thus it is difficult to know which procedure is the best. In fact, when Barton (1973) reviewed three different types of excisional arthroplasty in 65 feet, he was unable to find major differences in their clinical results. Hassalo et al (1987) also followed 26 patients (45 feet) from 4 months to 15 years and were able to conclude only that forefoot surgery in RA was beneficial but the benefit may not be long-lasting (Amuso et al 1971, Craxford et al 1982, Hassalo et al 1987). Most series report satisfactory results in up to 85% of patients, and failures of less than 10% (Kates et al 1967, Amuso et al 1971, Faithful & Savill 1971, Watson 1974, Vahvanen et al 1980, Clayton 1982, Craxford et al 1982, Newman & Fitton 1983, Mann &

Thompson 1984, Morgan et al 1985, Reffior & Hoos 1987, Hughes et al 1991).

Factors associated with unfavorable results include:

Inadequate bony resection (Faithful & Savill 1971, Watson 1974, Vahvanen et al 1980).
Recurrent hallux valgus (Watson 1974).
Wound problems (Faithful & Savill 1971, Lipscomb et al 1972, Newman & Fitton 1983).
Disease progression (Hassalo et al 1987).
Neurovascular problems (Kates et al 1967, McGarvey & Johnson 1988).

Usually it is best to perform RA forefoot surgery under tourniquet control. A thigh-high tourniquet is preferred. Although not essential, the tourniquet allows the operation to be carried out without any bleeding, which greatly aids in performing an accurate dissection. A tourniquet is safe as long as it is not inflated to an excessive pressure (usually 300–350 mmHg is sufficient to control bleeding) and as long as it remains inflated continuously for no longer than about two hours. Most operations can easily be completed by this time. The tourniquet is placed as proximal as possible around the ipsilateral thigh. This area has considerable muscle and soft tissue bulk, which protects the neurovascular structures from the pressure. Also, in this area there are no muscles or tendons that insert on the foot or ankle. A tourniquet can be used just above the ankle. However, it potentially exerts more pressure on the neurovascular structures and binds all the tendons, making correction of soft tissue and bony deformities much more difficult. A tourniquet is contraindicated when there is evidence of vasculitis or peripheral vascular disease.

Correction of forefoot deformities is facilitated by operating on the four lateral MTP joints before operating on the hallux, since it is often difficult to gain full correction of the hallux MTP joint first when there is severe deformity of the second through fifth joints. Dorsal longitudinal incisions provide an excellent exposure to the MTP joints and usually heal well. Three incisions are usually required; the first two incisions are made in the second web space and in the fourth web space to expose the lateral four MTP joints. Lastly, a dorsal medial incision is made to expose the hallux MTP joint. A plantar approach to the MTP joints also gives a good exposure and is the easiest approach to the dislocated metatarsal heads (Kates et al 1967). The incision is transverse and is placed at the level of the metatarsal necks, to the heel side of the dislocated MTP heads.

Surgical correction of the lateral four metatarsophalangeal joints

The metatarsal head is most frequently resected because it is usually grossly destroyed and pushed plantarward by the dorsally dislocated toes. One must then decide whether to resect the base of the proximal phalanx. This is usually not necessary. However, excision of the proximal one-third usually results in a loss of control of the toe, and the toe may become floppy. Excision of the base of the proximal phalanx is probably best done in conjunction with syndactylization of the adjacent toes (Saltzman et al 1993). It is a most useful procedure to correct severely deformed toes or when revision forefoot operations are performed (Cracchiolo 1984).

Currently there are probably at least three surgical techniques for correcting the rheumatoid deformities in the lateral four metatarsophalangeal joints:

1. Excision of the metatarsal head through a dorsal approach.
2. Excision arthroplasty through longitudinal web space incisions along the lateral sides of the second and fourth toes and along the medial sides of the third and fifth toes.
3. A plantar approach, with resection of the metatarsal heads only.

Excision of the metatarsal heads through a dorsal approach: The lateral four MTP joints are approached in sequence (Cracchiolo 1988). If the joints are severely dislocated, it is best to perform both incisions and to release the extensor tendons, ligaments and capsules of all four joints before attempting to expose the metatarsal heads. It is important to excise the metatarsal head in an oblique direction, removing more bone from the plantar aspect of the distal metatarsal as plantar bone regrowth may occur and cause a painful callus. Sufficient bone should be excised and sufficient soft tissues released to allow a 1.5–2.0 cm space (about the width of the tip of the index finger) between the resected end of the metatarsal and the proximal phalanx. A small amount of the base of the proximal phalanx can also be resected, especially with a severe deformity. This frees the plantar plate, which can be placed over the resected end of the metatarsal and transfixed with a 0.062 inch K-wire passed retrograde through the toe and then across the plate and into the metatarsal shaft.

This procedure is called plantar plate arthroplasty and is mainly used to help centralize the flexor tendons under the involved ray (Clayton & Smyth 1992) (Fig. 1). This operation also enables the surgeon to determine if the tendon is intact (which is usually the case). If the base of the proximal phalanx does not need to be excised, then the plantar plate can be carefully dissected off its plantar insertion. The toe is flexed and, using a number 11 scalpel blade, the plate is detached from the plantar side of the proximal phalanx, care being taken not to cut the flexor tendon. It is best not to advance the wire across the base of the metatarsal as this then 'skewers' the toe, leaving it immobile and perhaps jeopardizing its vascular supply. The K wire should be passed only about 2 cm into the intramedullary canal of the metatarsal so that it stabilizes

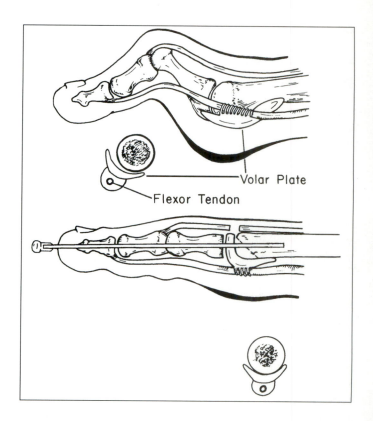

Volar Plate

Flexor Tendon

Figure 1

Plantar plate arthroplasty is helpful in that it realigns the flexor tendon under the involved ray. Note that the deformed metatarsal head is resected in an oblique fashion. At times the plantar plate has been destroyed, but it is always important to check for the flexor tendon and properly align the flexor tendon

the alignment of the ray (see Fig. 2C). Depending on the type of RA, the wires should stay in place for 3–6 weeks. Some patients have a 'stiff type' of rheumatoid disease, and the wires can be removed at about 3 weeks. Those with a 'loose type' should have the wires in place for about 5–6 weeks. I have not found it necessary to lengthen and then resuture the extensor tendons. However, it is important to close the skin incisions carefully since wound healing is always a concern. I no longer utilize any drains for these wounds. A sterile compression dressing is placed and then the thigh-high tourniquet is deflated. The combination of good wound closure and the dressing controls any wound hematoma.

Once the metatarsal heads are excised and before the K wire is passed, it is important to check for the presence of plantar bursae. These are usually present if significant plantar skin calluses are present. They can be pushed up into the dorsal incisions by digital pressure on the plantar surface and should be excised.

Excisional arthroplasty can also be performed through longitudinal incisions placed along the lateral side of the second toe, and the medial side of the third toe (also the same for the fourth and fifth toes), as described by Daly & Johnson (1992) and Saltzman et al (1993). The incisions are joined at the top of the web space and were originally described when excising the base of the proximal phalanx of the second and third toes. However, this approach also allows excision of the head of the metatarsal as well as the base of the proximal phalanx by extending the incision dorsally in the web space between the distal metatarsals. The toe incisions are then sutured so that a syndactylization is performed, which stabilizes the adjacent toes. This is an excellent method of stabilizing the lateral toes when the base of the proximal phalanx is excised. It is also excellent for revision operations on the rheumatoid forefoot.

A plantar approach to the dislocated MTP joints has been described by Kates et al (1967) with only the metatarsal heads being resected. This is described in this chapter by Tillmann. Excision of some of the redundant skin, as much as 2 cm from the proximal (calcaneal) side of the incision, helps to keep the fat pad more properly repositioned. I believe this incision should be used when the dorsal skin is poor, when the patient may have had previous operations with inappropriately placed dorsal scars, when there are multiple large plantar bursae, when the forefoot deformity is severe, and in revision operations on the rheumatoid forefoot. I prefer to use this incision to resect the lateral four metatarsal heads. However, with a little effort, the base of the proximal phalanx can be adequately exposed through this exposure. It is also possible, albeit a little difficult, to place K wires across the resected joints. I prefer to approach the hallux MTP joint through a longitudinal dorsal incision. For this reason, I operate with the patient in the supine position (the operating table can be tilted head down, and the foot elevated on towels to facilitate the plantar exposure) rather than in the prone position as described by Kates et al (1967). Fowler (1959) combined both the dorsal and plantar approaches to the rheumatoid forefoot. He performed most of his bony surgery through a dorsal incision and then used the plantar incision to excise an ellipse of skin and draw the toes into more plantar flexion.

Correction of toe deformities

The most common toe deformities are seen in the second and third toes, occasionally in the fourth and fifth toes. Claw toe deformities can be painful and are associated with a painful corn over the dorsum of the proximal interphalangeal joint (PIP). Occasionally there is a painful callus on the plantar tip of the toe, caused by the flexion deformity. Usually the toes deviate laterally. However, crossover deformities are seen and the fifth toe can be angulated medially (varus), being under or over the fourth toe.

Most of these deformities, and especially the angular deformities, are corrected by a surgical procedure to the MTP joints. Mild to moderate flexion deformities can be

manipulated straight especially if they are to be held by a K wire. Severe claw-toe deformity usually requires resection of the base of the proximal phalanx as well as the metatarsal head. Whether this is necessary can be determined after first resecting the metatarsal head – an insufficient space between the end of the metatarsal and the base of the proximal phalanx will mean that the claw toe deformity is unchanged, and the base of the proximal phalanx must be resected. Usually, however, this can be anticipated during the preoperative clinical assessment of the forefoot. In such feet it may be advisable to plan the skin incisions so that surgical syndactylization of the adjacent toes can be performed. Occasionally the toe deformity is a flexion deformity only of the PIP joint (like a hammertoe) and will not respond to a gentle manipulation. Such toes will require excision of the head of the proximal phalanx. This can be performed through a dorsal elliptical incision over the PIP joint or through a medial or lateral incision. Enough bone should be excised to straighten the toe, which is held over a K wire. It is usually unnecessary, but it is perfectly acceptable, to attempt to arthrodese the PIP joint.

The IP joint of the hallux is occasionally malaligned or even dislocated. It is usually sufficient to realign the joint and hold it with crossed K wires for about 3–4 weeks. Surgical arthrodesis of the joint is usually not necessary, particularly if an arthrodesis is being performed on the patient's hallux MTP joint.

Surgical procedures to the hallux metatarsophalangeal joint

Occasionally (perhaps rarely), the hallux metatarsophalangeal joint may be spared and is not destroyed. However, if there is significant synovitis, a synovectomy should be performed. If there is a significant hallux valgus deformity with near-normal joint surfaces, this must be corrected to accommodate the more normal realignment of the lateral four toes. However, in most cases, there is significant joint destruction with a severe valgus deformity. There are probably only three choices for treating this joint surgically:

1. Resection arthroplasty
2. Arthrodesis
3. Double stem silicone implant arthroplasty

The one selected should be performed after first correcting the lateral four MTP joints.

Resection arthroplasty of the hallux metatarsophalangeal joint
Resection arthroplasty of the hallux MTP joint has been commonly performed using a variety of techniques, and

appears to be much more popular in Europe than in the USA. Resection arthroplasty removes sufficient bone from the deformity to allow correction of the deformity. The various types of resection include:

1. Resection of the base of the proximal phalanx and the metatarsal head (Clayton 1982)
2. Resection only of the base of the proximal phalanx (Keller procedure)
3. Brandes procedure
4. Hueter–Mayo procedure
5. Modification of the Heuter–Mayo; technique of Tillmann (1979), described in this chapter.

Resection arthroplasty of the MTP joint is out of favor in some parts of the world, perhaps because subsequent problems with the hallux have been reported in several clinical series (Barton 1973, Hassalo et al 1987, McGarvey & Johnson 1988, Stockey et al 1989). Recurrence of deformity, pain, and patient dissatisfaction have been cited. There may be several reasons for these unfavorable results.

1. Resection arthroplasty was the earliest operation used in the hallux MTP joint.
2. Soft tissue reconstruction to stabilize the joint was not usually performed; the joint was simply excised and occasionally temporarily fixed with a K wire.
3. Many patients have such poor soft tissue, owing to their disease and their deformity, that any attempt at soft tissue stabilization of the joint may ultimately fail. Therefore, these factors perhaps can be addressed by performing a more definitive procedure to the hallux MTP joint such as an arthrodesis or silicone implant arthroplasty.
4. Patients with RA were not as mobile following lower extremity reconstructions until after the advent of total hip and knee replacement. Now that the hip and knee can be greatly improved with these implants, more is expected of the forefoot reconstruction.

Arthrodesis of the hallux metatarsophalangeal joint

Arthrodesis of the hallux MTP joint is done to correct the deformity, provide stability to the first ray and to prevent recurrence of deformity of the hallux. Arthrodesis is probably the best option when there is severe advanced deformity of the destroyed hallux MTP joint (metatarsal I–II angle of 15° or more, hallux valgus of 40° or more) or for revision operations.

There are many techniques that surgically fuse the hallux MTP joint. It may be best to create two flat surfaces so that there is some intrinsic stability to the arthrodesis site (Mann & Thompson 1984). However, all types of peg or ball-and-socket bony preparations are also utilized. The lateral rays will be shorter if all or part of the MTP joints have been excised; therefore, it is important to resect sufficient amounts of the metatarsal

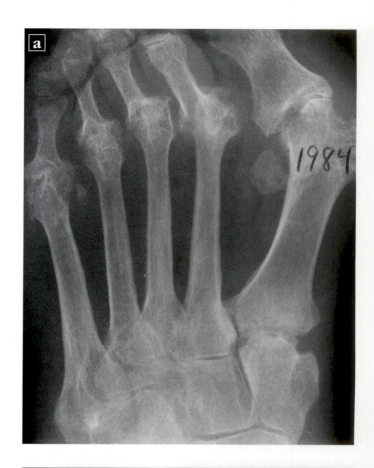

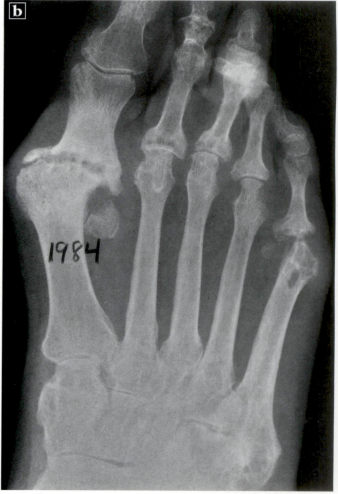

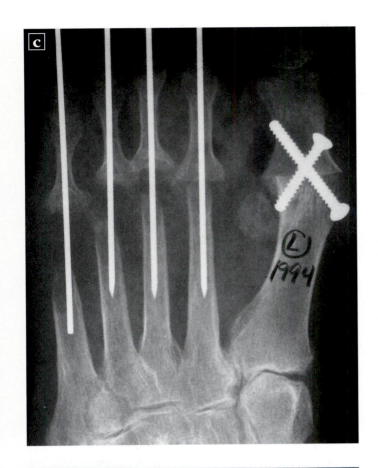

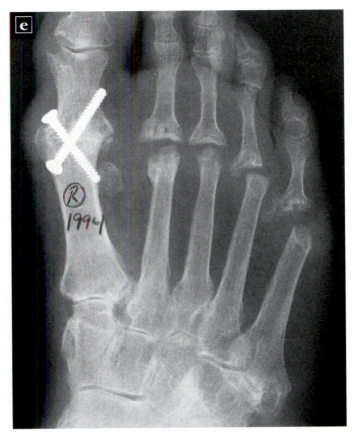

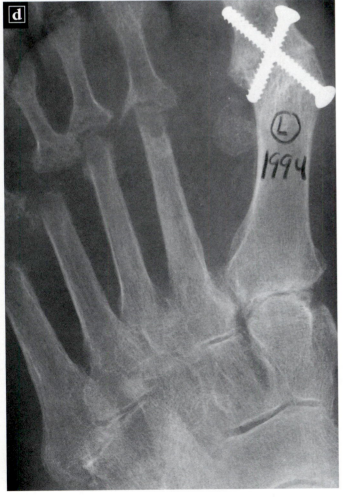

Figure 2

(a, b) Anteroposterior lateral weight bearing views of the feet of a 56-year-old woman with rheumatoid arthritis for 10 years. She had extensive deformity and considerable pain. She was no longer able to wear shoes because of this problem. (c) One can see the resectional arthroplasty of the lateral four metatarsophalangeal joints done approximately three weeks postoperatively. Two crossed screws were used to give good internal fixation for the hallux metatarsophalangeal joint fusion. Note the length of the K wires used to hold the lateral toes. (d, e) Approximately 2 months later there is a well-aligned foot and a good early arthrodesis of the hallux metatarsophalangeal joint of both feet.

head and the base of the proximal phalanx so that the first ray will not be overly long. The hallux should not protrude more than about 1 cm beyond the second toe at the end of the procedure. The final position of the hallux is also very important (Raunio et al 1987). Owing to a lateral drift of the toes with time, it may be best to fuse the hallux in 20–25° of valgus. About 15° of dorsiflexion as measured from the floor or about 30° as measured from the first metatarsal, is also adequate. There should be no rotation of the toe and the toenail should point directly dorsally. Internal fixation is accomplished using a variety of techniques. Multiple 0.062 inch K wires, either threaded or plain, have been used. Two 3.5 mm cortical screws placed as lag screws can be used if the quality of bone is adequate and if the medial flare of the proximal phalanx can be salvaged (Fig. 2). The screws seem to give sufficient internal fixation, and fusion occurs if there is no gross motion at the bone ends following their placement. These bones always have some degree of osteoporosis and the screws rarely provide the solid fixation seen in nonrheumatoid bone.

Recently, a five- or six-hole one-quarter tubular plate fixed with 3.5 mm cortical screws has been used dorsally to hold the bony surfaces together until arthrodesis occurs. The plate must be bent to allow the proper angle of dorsiflexion. Unfortunately, the dorsal position of the plate allows it to act only as a neutralizing force, so that the internal fixation may be suboptimal. All three of the above methods share the advantage of not crossing the interphalangeal joint. Mann & Thompson (1984) utilized two heavy [%₄ inch (3.6 mm) and ⅛ inch (3.2 mm)], double-ended threaded Steinmann pins to fix the arthrodesis site. These have the disadvantage of crossing the interphalangeal joint but they do not appear to cause further damage to the joint. The average time to radiographic fusion in their study was 97 days (range: 62–150 days). This is an excellent method and a solid arthrodesis can be achieved even in osteoporotic bone.

Postoperatively I prefer to place the foot in a short leg cast; a fiberglass cast is used because it is much lighter. At about 4 weeks, the cast is discontinued and the foot is supported in a wooden-sole postoperative shoe until there is some radiographic evidence of fusion, usually 2–4 weeks later. If Steinmann pins are used, I remove the pins one at a time, removing the second pin about 2 weeks after the first has been removed. Appropriate postoperative shoes can be fitted after the foot swelling recedes.

Implant arthroplasty of the hallux metatarsophalangeal joint

Implant arthroplasty of the hallux MTP joint is possible using a double-stem implant made of a high-performance silicon elastomer (Cracchiolo et al 1981, Swanson et al 1983). This procedure is indicated for the restoration of more normal alignment of the hallux with maintenance of some hallux motion and the provision

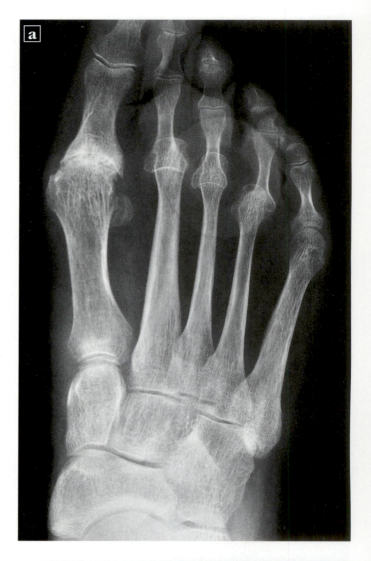

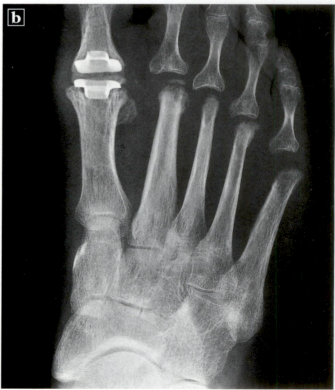

Figure 3

(a) Preoperative weight bearing radiograph of the right foot of a 52-year-old woman with rheumatoid arthritis for approximately eleven years. She was taking only 2 mg of prednisone per day and could no longer walk comfortably in her modified shoes. (b) The hallux metatarsophalangeal joint has been resected and has been replaced with a size 0 double-stem silicone implant made of a high-performance silicone elastomer. The implant is protected with titanium grommets. At 2 years there is no evidence of any damage to the implant and the proper alignment has been maintained

of stability to the first ray. An ideal candidate for this procedure is a rheumatoid patient who has a destroyed MTP joint with adequate bone stock and intact soft tissues but without evidence of sepsis or vascular insufficiency (Fig. 3). Implants should always be used as an alternative in patients who otherwise would have an excision of the joint or an arthrodesis. They can sometimes be used as salvage for patients with an unsatisfactory result following excision of the hallux MTP joint. Two long-term follow-up series have recently been reported, and both indicate excellent results can be obtained using the double-stem silicone implant in selected patients (Cracchiolo et al 1992, Moeckel et al 1992). Several features of this operation are important.

1. Prophylactic antibiotics should be given, and antibiotics should be continued orally for 2–3 postoperative days.
2. The operative procedure emphasizes soft tissue balancing with release of contracted tissues (usually on the lateral side of the joint), repositioning the sesamoids whenever possible, and careful closure of the capsule on the medial side to the distal phalanx when it has been detached, and always to the medial distal metatarsal. Capsular closure is best done by suturing the capsule directly to the bone through small 1.5 mm drill holes.
3. There is no need to excise extra bone in order to place a large implant. Usually a size 0, 1, or 2 double stem implant will be satisfactory.
4. Preparation of the intramedullary canals must be meticulous. I prefer using a hand broach initially, which compacts the cancellous bone, and then a pilot burr if necessary. All rough bone edges must be eliminated and trial reduction with a trial implant must show optimal correction of the hallux deformity.
5. Currently, I am utilizing titanium grommets to protect the silicone implant, but an experience with over 7

years of follow-up indicates that fracture of these implants, if the patient is properly selected, occurs infrequently, as does silicone synovitis, particularly in rheumatoid patients (Cracchiolo et al 1992, Moeckel et al 1992).
6. Meticulous wound closure is important.
7. One of the most important features of the operation is the postoperative care – the corrected position must be held by the dressings for at least 6 weeks. At about 2–3 weeks, motion of the joint can be started, but the time may vary depending on the condition of the wound and the patient.

The foot is placed in a standard, wooden-sole postoperative shoe, and patients are instructed to walk with most of their weight on their heel. Crutches, if the patient can use them, are helpful for the first 3 weeks. The foot can be placed into an inexpensive athletic shoe about two sizes larger than the patient's preoperative shoe, and a rubber spacer is placed between the hallux and the second toe. By this time, the K wires, which may have been placed in the lateral four toes, have been removed. The rubber spacer is maintained in place all the time for at least 6 weeks postoperatively. The foot can be placed in more appropriate shoes once swelling has diminished.

Summary

Forefoot reconstructive operations can provide the rheumatoid patient with relief of pain and improved ambulation and shoe wear. Proper patient selection and preparation is also important. However, it is always necessary to recall that rheumatoid patients have a chronic disease and deformities may be progressive. Therefore, proper patient assessment and follow-up are always indicated.

Rheumatoid Forefoot Surgery
Nelly De Stoop

The pathological observations of Fassbender (1975) show the systematic nature of RA – it is not confined to the bones and joints, rather it also affects the soft tissues (ligaments, muscles, nerves, vessels and skin). Vasculitis is invariably associated with the production of rheumatoid factor which suggests the presence of other autoimmune diseases. Functional status is an important issue of patient care.

Forefoot destruction occurs early and frequently in active RA. Longstanding disease commonly leads to a complete collapse of the forefoot with a rigid hallux valgus, fixed dislocations of the metatarsophalangeal joints and claw toes. Topographically, the forefoot is the most distal and caudal area of the human body. Biomechanically, it influences and is influenced by more proximal joints. Midfoot and hindfoot instability or a break in the talonavicular or naviculocuneiform joint, can cause or produce a recurrence of the rheumatoid forefoot deformities; prior stabilization of these more proximal segments can prevent many failures in forefoot surgery. The biomechanical influence of the forefoot extends proximally to the knee and the hip joint. A planovalgus rheumatoid foot will increase the medial load on the knee joint. Conversely, a valgus knee flattens the longitudinal arch of the foot. In severe rheumatoid arthritis, permanent recumbency and flexion contractures of the hips and knees contribute to an excessive load on the forefoot. The above-mentioned interrelations are serial and mutual. The symmetric nature of rheumatoid arthritis also causes a parallel effect on the extremities.

Tenosynovitis decreases the tensile strength of the tendons. In some cases, arthrodesis of a joint will be more appropriate than suturing of a ruptured and weakened tendon. Myopathy plays a central role in the pathogenesis of forefoot deformities of rheumatoid arthritis. Vasculitis presents a serious risk for performing elective surgery since an uncontrolled vasculitis can produce delays in wound healing, thus jeopardizing surgical results. Skin problems can be caused by steroid therapy. Osteoporosis, inherent to rheumatoid arthritis and worsened by steroid therapy or immobilization, should be taken into account.

Disease-modifying drugs are the therapeutic mainstay for active RA. They should be started before irreversible articular destruction occurs and before surgical correction becomes necessary. In order to avoid delayed wound healing, we limit their interruption to the strict perioperative period. It is our conviction that disease activity complicates the outcome of forefoot surgery in the short and long term. On the other hand, surgical intervention should not be restricted to burnt-out cases.

Optimal prospective planning of different surgical interventions of a varying disease course will be improved by a bidisciplinary team approach – 'rheumatopaedic and orthological'.

Some historical considerations
For almost half a century, surgery of the rheumatoid forefoot has not changed. The metatarsal heads were – and are – resected, regardless of the severity of their destruction. Insertion of a silastic prosthesis follows the same principle: a functional forefoot amputation with an acceptable cosmetic result. Many studies have been devoted to specific issues: plantar or dorsal exposure, longitudinal or transverse incision, and so on. The long-term results show a high rate of recurrence, reported by several authors (Tillmann 1979, Denis et al 1980, Viladot 1983, 1988a, 1988b); these authors also stressed the difficulty of revision (osteotomy or anatomical amputation).

I share the opinion of Valenti (unpublished discussion held at Montpelier, France in 1987 during the meeting *Actualités de Médecine et Chirurgie du Pied*) that conserving the metatarsal length prevents postoperative metatarsalgia. From this hypothesis, and, considering the poor results of the Lelievre procedures, we developed our own technique (De Stoop et al 1987), which conserves the metatarsal heads.

It preserves the length of the metatarsals and increases the weight bearing area. (Early progressive weight bearing limits osteoporosis caused by immobilization.) This rather conservative surgery relieves mechanical pain and does not preclude later revision by existing techniques.

Surgery of the big toe and the first metatarsophalangeal joint
A straight medial incision is centred over the first MTP joint. This joint is easily exposed by subperiosteal dissection. After an extensive synovectomy, a resection of the medial bunion and the base of the proximal phalanx of the big toe is performed. Through this medial incision, a lateral capsulectomy and a release of the phalangeal insertion of the adductor hallucis tendon is possible.

If the cartilage of the first MTP joint is preserved, a modified Regnauld procedure is performed. A cylinder with usable cartilage of the resected base of the proximal phalanx is selected. It is remodelled into a cone which is plugged into the remaining diaphysis of the proximal phalanx of the big toe (Fig. 4).

If the cartilage of the first MTP joint is destroyed or hallux rigidus occurs, a modified Keller procedure is

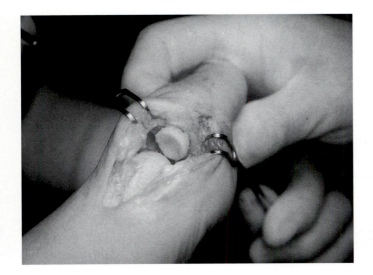

Figure 4

The remodelled base of the proximal phalanx

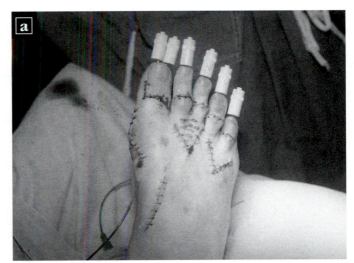

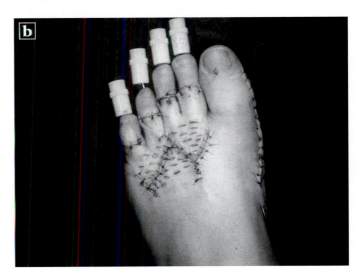

Figure 5

(a, b) Examples of postoperative appearance after reduction of longstanding dislocation of the toes

performed. Two transverse holes are drilled medially in the remaining proximal phalanx of the big toe and the metatarsal head of the first ray respectively. They serve as anchorpoints for a prebent K wire (of diameter 1.5 mm). This external spacer allows rotation around a transverse axis, with the pin pointing through the metatarsal head. After 4 weeks of progressive mobilization, the neoarticulation allows a painless mobility of the toe.

Lengthening of the extensor hallucis longus tendon may be necessary in order to prevent a cock-up deformity or a recurrent hallux valgus.

Surgery of the interphalangeal joint of the big toe

If there is a hyperextension of the interphalangeal joint of the big toe, an arthrodesis should be performed and fixed by staples, screws or crossed K wires. I prefer a dorsal extensile exposure, which also allows a medialization of the extensor hallucis longus tendon.

Surgery of the tarsometatarsal joint of the first ray

Pronounced metatarsus varus of the first ray is corrected by an arthrodesis of the medial metatarsocuneiform joint. I prefer a dorsal incision. The arthrodesis is fixed by staples or screws.

Surgery of the lesser toes

Two V-shaped dorsal incisions are made over the dorsum of the foot, the first starting between the second and the third toe and the second between the fourth and the fifth toe. These V-shaped incisions have an advantage over the longitudinal Z-incision as they permit lengthening of the skin, which is often necessary after reduction of a longstanding dislocation of the toes. Multiple transverse incisions allow a lengthening of the skin similar to a skin graft. This heals well within 2–3 weeks (Fig. 5a,b). Furthermore, if more exposure is needed, it can be lengthened into a Y-shaped incision.

Through these incisions, the extensors of the second to the fifth toes are divided. It is my belief that in rheumatoid arthritis, muscle imbalance is caused by neurogenic amyotrophy of the intrinsic muscles. In order to prevent recurrence of the dislocations, I prefer a tenotomy rather than a lengthening of the extensor mechanism (De Stoop et al 1987).

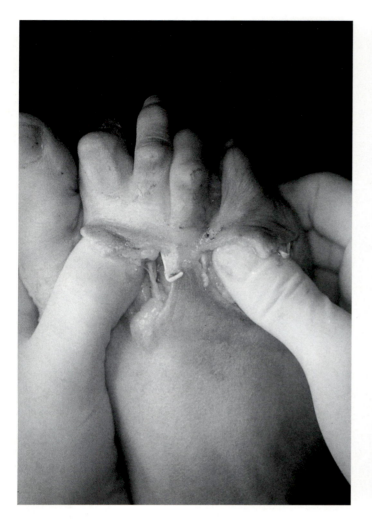

Figure 6

Reduction of the metatarsophalangeal dislocations by means of gentle but constant pressure

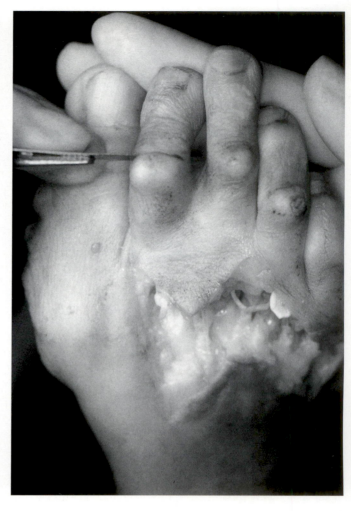

Figure 7

Inspection of the proper alignment. Note the damaged metatarsal heads

Surgery of the metatarsophalangeal joint capsule

Finally one proceeds to a capsulectomy and section of the collateral ligaments of the second to fifth MTP joints. This precedes their reduction. The reduction of the metatarsophalangeal dislocations is possible by gentle but constant pressure by the thumbs on the bases of the phalanges (Fig. 6).

Through transverse incisions over the PIP joints, the heads of the proximal phalanges and the bases of the middle phalanges are removed (Fig. 7). The aim is to arthrodese these joints to prevent recurrences of the claw toes and to act as levers for the flexors to keep the toes in place. This also removes the pressure on the metatarsal heads by shortening the toes. The toe is fixed by K wires through the phalanges and the metatarsal heads (Fig. 8).

Care must be taken to have a good alignment of the metatarsal heads in the sagittal and frontal plain (Fig. 9).

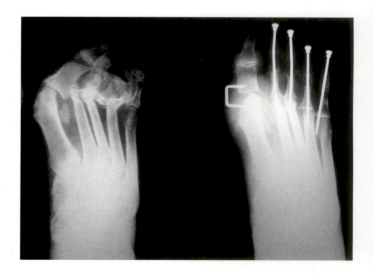

Figure 8

Reduction is possible at all stages of the disease

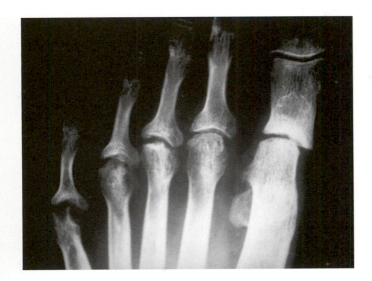

Figure 9

5 years postoperative asymptomatic foot, notwithstanding the severe damage to the metatarsal heads

If a malalignment exists, corrective osteotomies of the metatarsals should be performed.

Before closure the tourniquet should be deflated to assure good haemostasis as well as to allow prompt blood circulation into the toes. Often there is a reactionary constriction of the arteries. If the toe remains bloodless, the K wire should be placed to allow more dorsiflexion of the toe (not plantarflexion). This avoids circulation problems and the subsequent need for amputation of the toes.

A capsular repair is made over the first MTP joint and the abductor tendon is released from the plantar side to be sutured into the capsule. The skin is then closed over three drains. A non-weight-bearing plaster cast with the foot in dorsiflexion is used for 24 hours.

Mobilization of the big toe is started from the second postoperative day, and weight bearing is encouraged from the second postoperative day onward. In case of an arthrodesis of the first metacuneiform joint only partial weight bearing with the Barouk shoe is allowed.

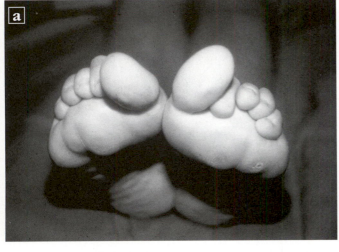

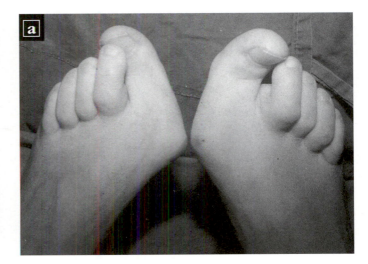

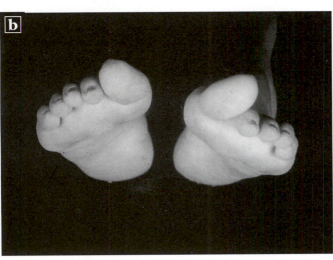

Figure 10

(a) Preoperative and (b) 5 years postoperative

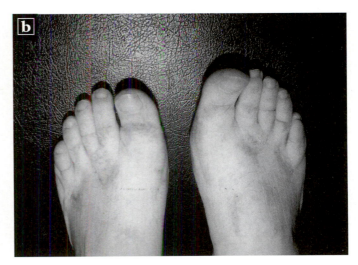

Figure 11

(a) Preoperative and (b) 3 years postoperative

Iodopodovine dressings for the wound are applied. After 14 days, the sutures are removed and physiotherapy is started. After 4–6 weeks, the wires are removed and mobilization of the MTP joints and rehabilitation of walking are started (Figs 10, 11).

Conclusion

The conservative surgical technique has several advantages:

It can be done at all stages of rheumatoid disease, although early surgery is advisable in order to avoid unnecessary pain and surgical risk.

During a 7-year follow-up, no recurrence of synovitis in the operated site has been noted despite disease progression in other joints.

Isolated dislocations of MTP joints can be corrected under local anaesthesia if necessary.

The same procedure can be repeated and, if required, more aggressive surgery such as resection of the metatarsal heads can be performed.

It is of the utmost importance that the hindfoot is stabilized before the forefoot surgery in order to avoid collapse of the correction through an overloading of the forefoot and the longitudinal arch.

Rheumatoid forefoot surgery

Karl Tillmann

If it could be more readily seen in its typical deformed shape, the rheumatoid forefoot could compete with the hand as a symbol of rheumatoid arthritis.

This may be amazing, for the origin of the deformities and the direction of the deviations are, to a large extent, identical with those that develop on a mechanical background (Hohmann 1951): splayfoot, hallux valgus, hammer toes of the lesser toes, lateral deviation of the lesser toes, and 'digitus V varus', resulting in a triangular form with an approximately cylindrical cross-section. Inflammatory swelling increases the callosities. Skin atrophy and ulcerations can be caused by vasculitis and by drug treatment, especially by steroids. Rheumatoid nodules may complete the characteristic appearance (Fig. 12).

Pathomechanics

There appear to be two mechanisms that produce forefoot deformities: the accelerating influence of the inflammation, and the splayfoot deformities.

In rheumatoid arthritis there is a mutual interplay of the frequently involved joints on the tibial side of the foot, especially of the talonavicular and the first metatarsophalangeal joint (Tillmann 1979, 1987). Unloading these joints because of pain must be the main reason for the lateral displacement of foot pressures found in pedographic studies (Hagena et al 1987, Hughes et al 1991). The corresponding clinical feature has been described by Vainio (1956) as 'metatarsus primus elevatus'. That means a supination of the forefoot and a flattening of the transverse as well as of the longitudinal arch. When this position becomes fixed, a plantigrade loading of the forefoot will force the hindfoot automatically into a valgus position. By this mutual interplay (Tillmann 1987) of fore- and hindfoot afflictions and deformities the 'pes antice supinatus, postice pronatus' develops (Hohmann 1951) (Fig. 13).

Forefoot deformities

The most common deformity of the hallux in rheumatoid patients is hallux valgus (Tillmann 1979). The incidence and severity increase with the duration of the disease. It occurs in females more often than in males. We see this deformity as a result of the varus and supination of the first metatarsal, and the valgus and pronation of the hallux. The inflammatory synovitis weakens the capsule and ligaments. There is a plantar displacement

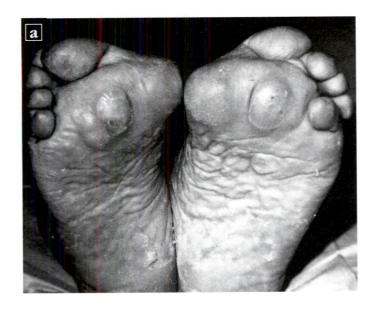

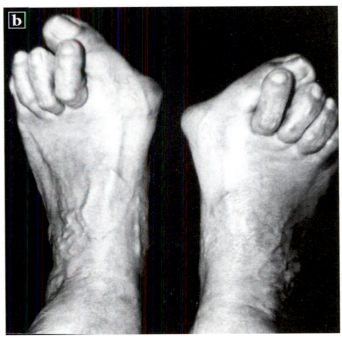

Figure 12

Typical appearance of the rheumatoid forefoot: (a) round rheumatoid foot; (b) triangular foot

of the abductor tendon and a fibular subluxation of the base of the proximal phalanx. The extensor and flexor tendons displace laterally, with the proximal phalanx increasing the deformity. Rigidity of the first MTP joint is a frequent functional disability in rheumatoid patients

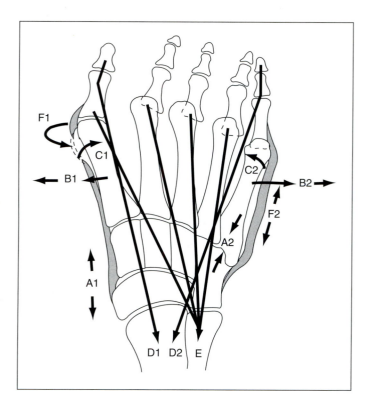

Figure 13

The most common pathomechanical pathways of rheumatoid foot deformities.

A1, Lengthening of tibial side of foot by flattening of longitudinal arc; A2, shortening of fibular side of foot by inflammation and destruction of fibular TMT joints. B1, Varization of first MT; B2, valgization of fifth MT. (B1/B2 are consequences of A1/A2 and of splayfoot deformity.) C1, Supination–rotation of first MT; C2, pronation–rotation of fifth MT. (C1/C2 are caused by flattening of transverse arc – splayfoot.) D1, Fibular pull of long extensor tendon of big toe (result of B1/C1); D2, tibial pull of extensor tendon of little toe (result of B2/C2). E, Fibular pull of short extensor tendons I–IV (result of A2/B2). F1, Plantarward tilting of abductor hallucis tendon (due to B1/C1); F2, slackening of abductor tendon V (due to A2/C2). Results: hallux valgus, fibular deviation of lesser toes II–IV, tibial deviation of little toe

(Tillmann 1979, Vainio 1956), whereas hallux varus is very rare. Limited dorsiflexion of the MTP joint is frequently combined with hyperextension and/or instability of the IP joint of the big toe.

In the lesser toes, the typical deformity is a hammer toe in combination with a fibular deviation. These deformities are correlated with the splayfoot and midfoot and forefoot abduction caused by flattening of the longitudinal arch. The pull of the short extensor tendons is translocated laterally, favouring lateral deviation of the toes, and in cases of ligamentous instability, lateral dislocation of the toes.

The hyperextension and dorsal dislocation of the base of the proximal phalanx of the lesser toes is mainly a result of weakening and later perforation of the plantar capsule by the synovitis from inside the joint, and of inflammatory plantar bursitis from outside the joint. Weakening of the plantar capsule leads to a malalignment of the flexor tendon, which also contributes to the hyperextension and dorsal dislocation of the lesser toes (Tillmann 1979). When the position of the flexor tendons migrates dorsal to the axis of the MTP joint, the deformity becomes fixed.

The fifth toe may develop a different deformity, owing to the resultant valgus position and pronation of the fifth metatarsal. The fifth toe does not have a short extensor tendon and may deviate in a tibial or varus direction. The 'digitus V varus rheumaticus' in our patients is more than twice as frequent as the fibular deviation of the little toe (Tillmann 1979). The latter deformity we saw predominantly in patients with an exaggerated longitudinal arch. In our experience flexion contracture of the PIP joints in RA is more of a secondary phenomenon caused by tendon imbalance rather than by local inflammation.

Soft tissue procedures

Synovectomy

Synovectomy of the MTP joints has not achieved any popularity, in contrast to synovectomy of the joints of the hand. According to Raunio & Laine (1970), Brattström (1973), Aho (1987) and Aho & Halonen (1991), the results are satisfying. Our own experience, which is limited to unusual cases, is very small. Because of the surgical approach, the removal of the synovium is limited to the dorsal part of the joint so that not all the synovium can be excised. We perform this procedure only in young patients, preferably those with juvenile chronic arthritis (Ansell 1978, Tillmann 1979, Tillmann et al 1993), and in patients who have failure of conservative treatment with only a single joint involved. When the joint is destroyed, we combine the operation with a partial resection and reshaping of the metatarsal head. In these cases pain relief can be expected, and this usually lasts until the neighbouring joints become involved and major surgery becomes necessary. So we see these operations more as temporary procedures.

Aho (1987) reported persistent pain relief for a mean of 7 years postoperatively in about half of the patients. If resection arthroplasty was necessary, it was performed 2–6 years later. Benjamin and Helal (1980), found 14 out of 18 feet free of pain for 5 years after synovectomy of the MTP joints. However, four feet underwent further surgery within 3 years.

Marmor (1967) suggested a combined procedure with a Z lengthening of the extensor tendon, transverse incision of the dorsal capsule and synovectomy of the MTP joint, and if necessary, excision of the dorsal callosities over the PIP joint by a longitudinal approach (see Fig. 14). Preston (1968) recommended subcutaneous tenotomies proximal to the short extensor insertion and, if necessary, a dorsal capsulotomy. Postoperatively, protection against recurrence of hyperextension by active physical therapy was considered mandatory. Theoretically, there is a risk of increasing fibular deviation, owing to the persistence of the short extensor tendons. Also, removal of callosities from both plantar and dorsal surfaces without shortening the ray, in our experience, gives a high risk of skin tension after closure of the tissues.

As far as is known, there are no valid controls of these soft tissue procedures.

Osteotomy

In addition to soft tissue procedures, distal metatarsal osteotomies offer another way of correcting forefoot deformities without sacrificing the joints.

Proximal osteotomies for correcting the varus position of the first metatarsal are not very popular in rheumatoid arthritis. They do not solve the MTP joint problems and they are usually too demanding for patients with severe or multiple handicaps, and these patients represent the majority of candidates for forefoot reconstruction. In contrast, distal metatarsal osteotomy, which has been popularized by Helal (1975) is usually performed through a distal longitudinal web space incision on the dorsum of the foot. The osteotomy is done in an oblique direction from proximal dorsal to plantar distal through the metatarsal necks without disrupting the MTP joints (Fig. 14). A few days after surgery, the patients are permitted (and are usually able) to bear weight. We provide them with a form-protecting elastic dressing, adding a small cushion pillow in the centre of the transverse arch in order to secure and enhance its remodelling. By loading the forefoot, the distal fragments with the metatarsal heads are pushed dorsal and proximal and thus unload and shorten the forefoot.

Benjamin & Helal (1980) also included an oblique osteotomy of the distal first metatarsal, from proximal fibular to distal tibial, to correct the valgus position of the big toe. An osteotomy was also performed in the reverse direction to correct the varus deformity of the fifth one.

According to Benjamin & Helal (1980), Helal (1975) and Helal & Greiss (1984), the effects of osteotomy are pain relief, correction of deformity, regression of rheumatoid synovial swelling, relative lengthening of contracted soft tissue and improvement in the X-ray appearance. The frequent suppression of inflammation of the MTP joints is desirable but unexplained. Distal metatarsal osteotomies are used for rheumatoid deformities of all toes with good success. The postoperative treatment is simple and the long-term results are good; less than 10% are poor (Helal & Greiss 1984, Wiasmitinow & Zollinger 1993).

In our hands osteotomies give good results, especially in rheumatoid patients with pronounced deformities of the second to fourth toes. In suitable cases, the support of the preserved first and fifth metatarsal heads can be maintained.

Resection arthroplasty

Resection arthroplasties are the most popular procedures for pain relief and correction of rheumatoid forefoot deformities. The rationale includes removal of destroyed bone, which is a cause of pain, and re-balancing of contracted and displaced soft tissues by surgical release and by shortening the total length of the deformed ray. The resection itself may be done on the proximal or the distal side of the joint, or both sides. The usual joint is the MTP joint, less frequently the PIP joints are resected; only occasionally are the DIP joints resected.

Metatarsal head resection

The hallux

At the first metatarsal head, the Hueter (1871) and Mayo (1908) procedures are well known and frequently used, especially for rheumatoid hallux valgus. Depending on the degree of the deformity (Tillmann 1979), we prefer a partial resection and a very meticulous remodelling of the remaining metatarsal head rather than the metatarsal index, in contrast to other authors (Gschwend et al 1977). The head is then covered with a proximally based flap from the tibial dorsal extensor hood. Depending on the destruction of the joint surfaces, the sesamoids may be excised. When we started with this modification about 25 years ago, we saw that leaving the sesamoids with their destroyed cartilage had been a frequent source of postoperative pain and a cause for reoperation. The resected portion of the short flexor tendon must be closed in order to avoid a mallet deformity of the big toe. The abductor tendon and the insertion of the fibular collateral ligament are released. The abductor tendon is shortened and repositioned. In case of excessive deformity (more than 60°), it may also be necessary to resect the base of the proximal phalanx to avoid excessive shortening of only the first metatarsal. Reattachment of the abductor tendon to the phalanx under proper tension must be performed (Fig. 15).

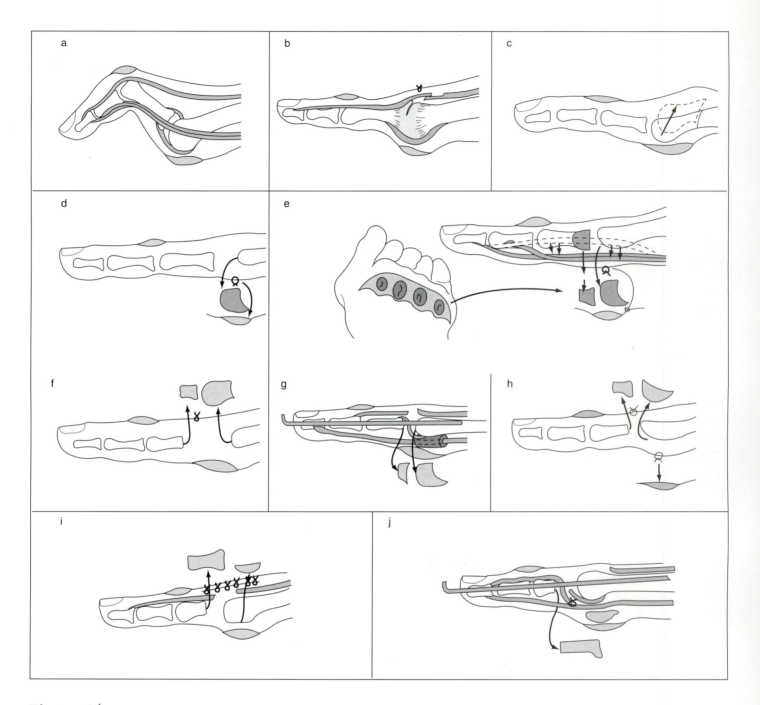

Figure 14

Some popular surgical procedures for (a) the correction of typical deformities of the lesser toes in RA according to (b) Marmor 1967, (c) Helal 1975, (d) Kates et al 1967, (e) Tillmann 1973, (f) Clayton 1960, and (g) 1992, (h) Fowler 1959, (i) Lipscomb et al 1972, (j) Stainsby 1992

The lesser toes

At the lesser toes, the Hoffman procedure (Hoffman 1911) – resection of the metatarsal heads in correct alignment – is the basic method we use. Kates et al (1967) performed this procedure from a plantar approach with excision of all callosities (see Fig. 14d); Tillmann (1973) modified the procedure using a plantar

transverse skin excision across the distal forefoot to produce a dermadesis (Figs. 14e, 16a). A tenolysis is performed and in case of ruptures a reconstruction of the flexor tendons is attempted. The metatarsal heads are resected, rounded and smoothed (Fig. 16b,c). The plantar capsule is reefed together on the tibial side for the second to fourth MTP joints, and on the fibular side

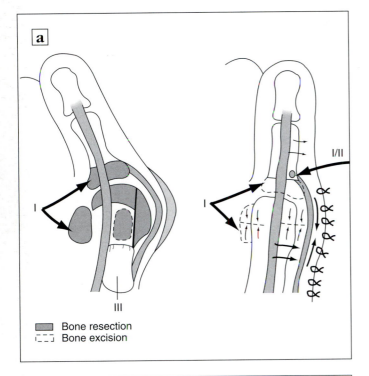

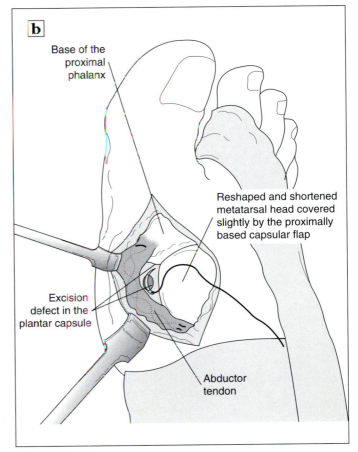

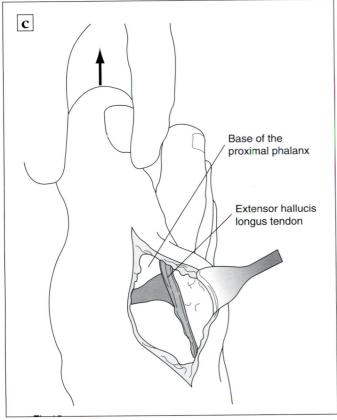

Bone resection
Bone excision

Base of the
proximal
phalanx

Reshaped and shortened
metatarsal head covered
slightly by the proximally
based capsular flap

Excision
defect in the
plantar capsule

Abductor
tendon

Base of the
proximal phalanx

Extensor hallucis
longus tendon

Figure 15

(a) Correction of typical deformities of the big toe in RA
(modified from Hueter 1971 and Mayo 1908). I, Optional
bone resection/excision (according to extent of deformity);
II, drill hole for refixation of abductor tendon (necessary in
case of base resection); III, proximally based dorsal flap of
extensor hood and periosteum (reflected) for covering the
reshaped MT head. (b) Reinforcement and shortening of
abductor tendon using a 2 mm unabsorbable suture weaved
through tendon from distal to proximal. (c) A distraction of
the joint space of about 8 mm should be possible without
any deterioration of the correct position. No additional
fixation is used

of the fifth MTP joint in cases of 'typical' deviation (Fig.
16d). By doing this, a correct position of the toes can
be achieved, so that K wires are seldom necessary (Fig.
17).

In general, we prefer the resection of the metatarsal
head, which is the main site of bone destruction and
pain during walking and standing.

The Keller procedure (Keller 1904) is also widely used
to correct hallux valgus in RA forefoot deformities. In
Germany, an excessive resection of the proximal two-
thirds of the phalanx (Brandes 1929) is very popular
even for non-inflammatory hallux valgus. In rheumatoid
arthritis we dislike this procedure. We have frequently
been in the unhappy situation of needing to perform a

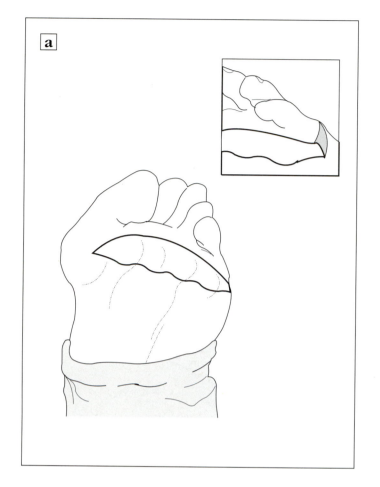

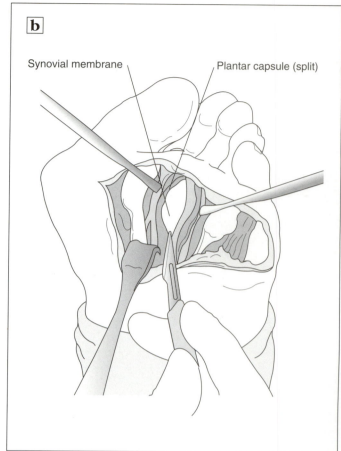

Synovial membrane

Plantar capsule (split)

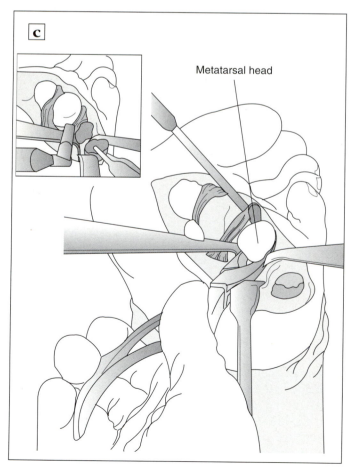

Metatarsal head

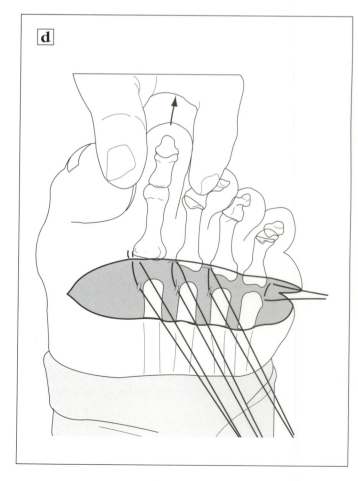

Figure 16

(a) Plantar approach and excision of skin and callosities: upon closure this will produce a dermadesis. (b) Exposure and mobilization of the long flexor tendons by dividing the (frequently displaced) tendon sheaths and dividing the plantar capsule longitudinally. Proliferative synovium is then excised. (c) A transverse osteotomy of the metatarsal neck is performed using an oscillating saw protected by two small Hohmann-elevators. With very poor quality, osteoporotic bone, the head can be removed using a bone cutter. After this a synovectomy of the dorsal part of the joint can be completed. The final step is rounding off and smoothing the metatarsal stumps in correct alignment. (d) Suturing of the plantar plate on the tibial side for the second, third and fourth MTP joints, using a purse-string like suture for the fifth toe (2 mm). Distraction of the joint space of about 6–8 mm should remain possible without loss of correction. The correcting effect of these sutures is usually striking.

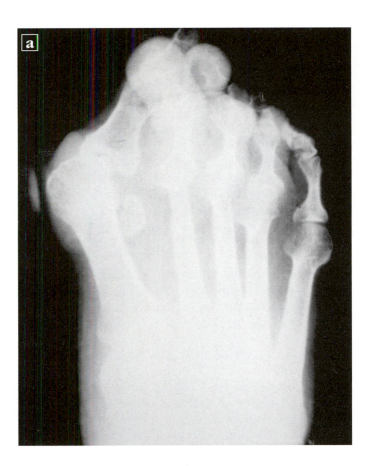

subsequent revision operation to resect the destroyed metatarsal head, thus ending up with a short and unstable big toe. Moreover, a biomechanical disadvantage results if the first metatarsal remains longer than the fibular ones. The first metatarsal head remains painful after a Keller procedure – this is the rule rather than the exception. In such a foot, the need for unloading the first metatarsal (Tillmann 1987) and correcting the forefoot supination as well as the convex deformation of the metatarsal arch becomes even more pronounced than before the operation. In our experience the fibular deviation of the lesser toes also increases.

The lateral metatarsals

For the lesser toes, resection of the proximal phalanges may make more sense, avoiding most of the above mentioned disadvantages. Lipscomb et al (1972) excised the base of the proximal phalanges and the plantar condyles of the metatarsal heads through a dorsal longitudinal incision. The extensor tendons were resected at the level of the joint space (Fig. 14). Stainsby (1992) also resects the base of the proximal phalanx in the same way, leaving the metatarsal heads untouched. The extensor tendons are divided at the level of the metatarsal necks and the distal stump is sutured plantarward to the flexor tendon. A Kirschner wire holds the alignment for two weeks (see Fig. 14). We use this procedure only in severe cases of claw toes in patients not having an inflammatory disease.

Resections of both sides of the MTP joints are used in two well-known procedures. Through a transverse dorsal incision, Fowler (1959) resected the base of the proximal phalanx of the lesser toes. Simultaneously through a plantar incision he resected the metatarsal heads and excised the plantar callosities (see Fig. 14). Clayton

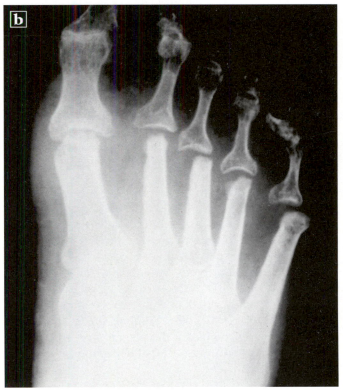

Figure 17

Rheumatoid forefoot deformity before (a) and after resection arthroplasty (b) of all MTP joints: correct alignment and proper suturing of the plantar capsule are preconditions for achieving and maintaining a good position

(1960), also through a transverse dorsal approach, excised the entire MTP joint of all toes including the first one, without any internal fixation. The result was good pain relief at the cost of the stability of the toes (Gschwend et al 1977) (see Fig. 14). Later, Clayton (1992) developed a new surgical technique using the plantar plate for interposition as a proximally based flap, suturing its distal margin to the dorsal side of the proximal phalanx. Simultaneously he performs a rerouting of the flexor tendons (see Fig. 14). He also releases the short extensor tendons. The results are amazingly good: 2–6 years after surgery, 92% of all patients are satisfied (Clayton ML, personal communication). The surgical technique has been explained in detail by Cracchiolo (1993).

The results of the different methods of resection arthroplasty are hardly comparable, mainly because of the different clinical status at the time of surgery. Regardless of the technique, these different operations and the different follow-up times have a success rate of about 70–80% (Fowler 1959, Clayton 1967, Kates et al 1967, Lipscomb et al 1972, Barton 1973, Gschwend et al 1977, Hansens et al 1987, Miehlke et al 1987, Salzmann et al 1987, Stockley et al 1989, Clayton 1992). We think that only in early cases it is possible to leave the metatarsal heads untouched. In late cases with gross destruction and severe deformities and dislocations, it seems more logical to sacrifice the destroyed metatarsal heads or to unload them by altering their position by an osteotomy. We feel that, regardless of the surgical technique, by resecting the metatarsal heads, pain relief, which is the aim of all these procedures, is about the same. There may be differences with respect to the cosmetic result and perhaps (though this is still unproven) the function of the toes. In our experience it is most important to achieve or to maintain the length of all toes. We strive for a good alignment of the metatarsals, and avoid excessive shortening of the first metatarsal.

The follow-up time for these operations is most significant. We found a loss of half our postoperative corrections after more than 10 years of follow-up in spite of a demanding postoperative physical therapy regime. We also lost some mobility of the reshaped first MTP joint over the years. But very good pain relief persisted (Hansens et al 1987). The superiority of a dorsal or plantar approach is still a matter of discussion. It seems that in spite of some critics (Barbier 1976) there is a tendency towards the use of the plantar incision (Hagena et al 1987, van Loon et al 1992, Richardson et al 1993).

Endoprosthetic replacement

Many attempts at replacement of the first MTP joint have been attempted, but only a few have become popular for rheumatoid joint destruction (Ferdini et al 1988).

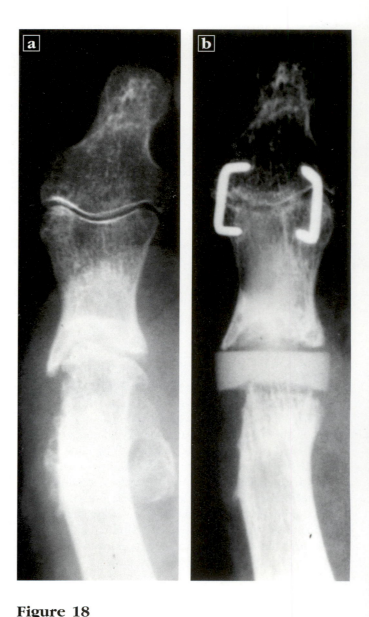

Figure 18

(a) Painful instability of the IP joint and painful stiffness of the MTP joint after Keller's procedure at the big toe in RA. (b) Arthrodesis of the IP joint (Shapiro staples) and salvage of the MTP joint using Swanson's single stem spacer

Swanson et al (1979) recommended a single-stem silicone spacer for replacement of the base of the proximal phalanx of the hallux (Fig. 18). A double-stemmed silicone implant for total replacement and stabilization of the first MTP joint has also been recommended (Swann 1978, Sethu & D'Netto 1980, Raunio et al 1987, Salzmann et al 1987, Stockley 1989, Swanson et al 1991, Cracchiolo et al 1992, Stainsby 1992, Richardson et al 1993, Swanson A.B. 1994, personal communication). Later, Swanson recommended the use of titanium grommets for the protection of the silicone implant (Swanson et al 1991). Helal & Greiss (1984) use a ball-like silicone endoprosthesis with thinner stems, reinforced by polyester fibre mesh, for the replacement of the painfully destroyed rheumatoid MTP joint of the big toe.

Less successful and much less popular have been several cemented designs, mainly metal or polyethylene endoprosthesis. Poor bone quality and a very high load on a small implant may have been the main reasons for the lack of success of these designs in rheumatoid patients.

There are several studies on the results of first MTP endoprostheses with different follow-up times, especially for Swanson's double-stem prosthesis (Swanson et al 1979, Delagoutte 1980, Swanson et al 1987, Granberry et al 1991, Cracchiolo et al 1992, Dennis & Clayton 1992, Moeckel et al 1992, Cracchiolo 1993, Freed 1993). The fracture rate seems to be quite different, but the clinical assessment is generally positive.

The results of Swanson's single-stem prosthesis in rheumatoid patients differ and the general experience seems to be less positive (Swanson et al 1979, Delagoutte 1980, Sethu & D'Netto 1980, Girlando & Berlin 1981, Breewood & Griffiths 1985, Krismer et al 1990). Swanson et al (1991) actually prefer an implant made of titanium which may result in less particulate debris. Perhaps the Helal design (Helal & Chen 1986) is mechanically more stable. The early results have been satisfying: about half of the pre-existing deformity was corrected, the mobility maintained, and 86% of the patients were pain-free. Metatarsalgia has not been influenced, either in a positive or in a negative sense (Helal & Chen 1986). The main concern has been a relatively high infection rate, which has resulted in the routine use of antibiotic prophylaxis (McAuliffe & Helal 1990).

For the MTP joints of the lesser toes, Swanson uses cylindrical silicone joint spacers (1994, personal communication). Pfeiffer et al (1992) reported the use of small hinged silicone double stem prostheses in the lesser MTP joints with good results after an average of 5.7 years follow-up. The fracture rate was lower (3%) compared to the first MTP joints (9.7%). However, the procedure as a routine was discontinued as there was no evidence of any superiority compared to resection procedures (Cracchiolo 1994, personal communication). We have used single stem silicone implants in several cases for replacement of a single destroyed metatarsal head (Tillmann et al 1989). We also saw no advantages compared to resection arthroplasties and abandoned this procedure.

Arthrodesis

For severe rheumatoid deformities of the first MTP joint, Vainio (1956) strongly recommended arthrodesis. The fusion was performed with the hallux in about 10–15° of valgus and about 30° dorsiflexion. In fact, more valgus is now recommended: about 15–25° (Cracchiolo 1993, Niskanen et al 1993) (Fig. 19). For internal fixation we

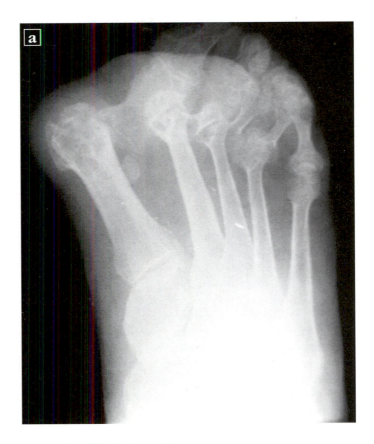

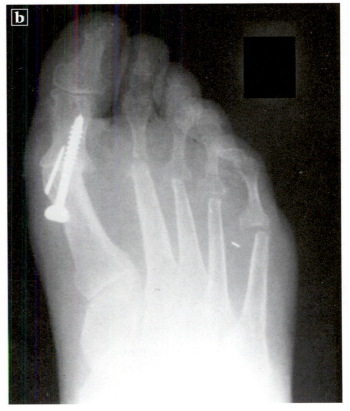

Figure 19

In case of (a) excessive rheumatoid hallux valgus deformity, (b) arthrodesis is the only safe way of correction and protection of the realigned lesser toes against recurrence of valgus deviation

use screws and power staples, mostly in combination. In addition we placed our patients in a cast for at least 8 weeks. Then we used a stable insole with an integrated protective splint for the big toe for at least another 2 months. In severely and multiply handicapped patients this proved to be very demanding, so that we used this procedure in only a few patients with excessive deformities (Tillmann 1979).

Results

The results of arthrodesis, especially of the first MTP joint, are probably best when patients have a severe deformity, especially a varus deformity (Vainio 1956). Fusion must be in the correct position for patients to have an excellent result (Niskanen et al 1993, Raunio et al 1987). Moreover, a fusion seems to protect and to secure the position of the lesser toes which have been simultaneously corrected by a resection arthroplasty. A precondition is an unaffected IP joint which we found only in about 50% of the advanced cases of RA deformity (Tillmann 1979). Our concern is the need for prolonged external fixation, which is intolerable for many severely and multiply handicapped patients. So the number of patients in whom we perform an arthrodesis remains limited. Moreover, the biomechanical effect of an arthrodesis of the first MTP joint in combination with corrections of the lesser toes seems to be inferior compared to an excision arthroplasty (Hughes et al 1991).

To correct painful fixed deformities of the interphalangeal joints of the hallux and the lesser toes, we aim to produce either a bony or a fibrous ankylosis in a correct position (Hohmann 1955). For the first IP joint we perform a compression arthrodesis with a central screw from distal to proximal (Tillmann 1986). A cast is usually not necessary, and the patient is permitted to bear weight after 2 weeks. Only in patients with very poor bone quality do we add power staples for internal fixation (see Fig. 18). In our experience arthrodesis of the IP joint of the big toe proved to be advantageous for the mobility of the first MTP joint when a simultaneous resection arthroplasty was performed.

For the correction of fixed flexion deformities of the proximal interphalangeal joints, we prefer the Hohmann (1951) technique with resection of the head of the proximal phalanx, and reefing the extensor hood. Frequently we add a central K wire for internal fixation for only 2 weeks. Alternatively small titanium power staples can be used when doing an arthrodesis. However, most of the deformities and contractures of these joints are secondary ones caused by the flattening of the transverse arch (Tillmann 1979) and the deformities and luxations of the MTP joints. In our experience they can be corrected merely by a blunt manipulation (Hansens et al 1987).

The rheumatoid hindfoot

Andrea Cracchiolo III

Pathology and evaluation

The hindfoot in the patient with RA is gradually involved by the disease process. However, the pathology may be subtle, though it can progress rapidly once it occurs, and frequently affects the forefoot. Swelling can be seen surrounding the tendon sheaths across the dorsum of the ankle, along the posterior tibialis tendon, and occasionally along the peroneal tendons. Hindfoot joint swelling is best seen medially at the talonavicular joint, and laterally over the sinus tarsi. Synovitis of the hindfoot joints, subsequent loss of articular cartilage, erosion of the talonavicular and subtalar joints, and possible posterior tibial tendon dysfunction, lead to a persistent valgus deformity of the hindfoot, which is seen in about 80% of patients with hindfoot involvement. The talonavicular joint becomes unstable with the head of the talus drifting medially and plantarward (Cracchiolo 1988, Elbaor et al 1976). The remainder of the midfoot and forefoot drifts into abduction (Fig. 20). The calcaneus drifts into valgus and may also abut against the distal fibula producing pain at the lateral malleolus (Cracchiolo et al 1990), and at times producing a stress fracture of the distal fibula. The posterior tibial tendon may rupture (Downey et al 1988), or if intact it may not function effectively as the medial stabilizer of the hindfoot, owing to the altered hindfoot mechanics. Only 8% of patients

with disease of less than 5 years' duration had moderate to severe hindfoot deformities. However, in patients with disease of more than 5 years' duration, 25% had abnormal hindfoot valgus on weight bearing (Spiegel & Spiegel 1982). Gschwend & Steiger (1987) report that at an average of 10 years of disease, the ankle and subtalar joints were involved in 52% of his RA patients.

Ankle pathology gives far fewer symptoms, and when patients complain of ankle pain, most may be actually experiencing hindfoot pain. Ankle instability can occur from erosions of the dome of the talus and ligament instability so that a valgus deformity may result from pathology within the tibiotalar joint rather than the hindfoot. It is essential to make this distinction between hindfoot and ankle pathology (Cracchiolo 1984, Cracchiolo 1990). However, a valgus deformity may involve both the hindfoot and ankle joint. The ankle joint also appears to be involved by the rheumatoid disease rather late in the course of disease. However, it may be that it is recognized only then. Radiographic changes occur usually after 7 or more years from the onset of RA (Vainio 1956).

Clinical and radiographic evaluation

Clinically, it may be difficult to determine whether a patient's hindfoot symptoms and deformity originate from either the hindfoot joints or the ankle joint or foot. It is probably more correct and safer to not separate this portion of the anatomy into hindfoot and ankle, but in fact to consider all these bones and joints together, so that the hindfoot can be considered to include the ankle joint. Physical examination may be difficult as patients may have difficulty standing, so one cannot accurately assess the degree of flatfoot and hindfoot valgus which may be present. Furthermore, because of the multiple foot deformities that are usually present and painful, assessment of tendon function may be difficult. Almost all patients will attribute their pain to the ankle joint as most patients and some physicians are unaware of the anatomy and the type of disease involvement that occurs in this part of the foot of a patient with RA.

Radiographic evaluation must include weight bearing views whenever possible, since non-weight-bearing views are inaccurate and may only show a fixed deformity. The lateral weight bearing view of the foot should also include the ankle joint. This view may demonstrate deterioration of the subtalar, talonavicular and calcaneocuboid joints. One can estimate the alignment of the hindfoot with the forefoot, as a line drawn through the

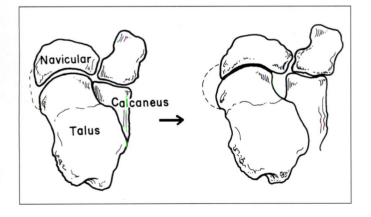

Figure 20

Drawing of the hindfoot deformity in rheumatoid arthritis with the head and neck of the talus rotating and drifting medial and plantarward and the remainder of the foot, the calcaneus, the midfoot and forefoot drifting into heel valgus, and abduction of the midfoot and forefoot

longitudinal axis of the talus should pass straight through the longitudinal axis of the first metatarsal (the talo-first metatarsal angle). If the lines diverge and form an angle pointing plantarward, this suggests a planovalgus deformity, which at times may appear identical to the deformity seen in patients who only have posterior tibial tendon dysfunction.

An anteroposterior weight bearing view of the foot may also show deterioration of the talonavicular and calcaneocuboid joints. The anteroposterior weight bearing view of the ankle joint can be used to evaluate the degree of intra-articular pathology in the ankle and to determine if a significant talar tilt is present – this may be the cause of the valgus deformity. Whenever there is hindfoot pathology it is important to determine, as accurately as possible, whether the tibiotalar joint is involved. Any talar tilt (even 5–10°) might indicate ankle joint pathology.

If one suspects instability of the ankle, stress views may be appropriate. Even following a successful triple arthrodesis, the ankle may deteriorate and therefore it is helpful to know whether there is ankle pathology before planning such an operation (Faithful & Savill 1971). Other studies are rarely useful. Occasionally, a technetium bone scan can determine the degree of inflammation that may exist in the joints or the tendons. Magnetic resonance imaging is occasionally useful in assessing the degree of tendon pathology. However, following some failed operations, especially to the joints, magnetic resonance imaging might be needed to assess the presence and degree of osteonecrosis, especially in the talus.

Treatment of the hindfoot

The most significant soft tissue involvement is seen in the tarsal tunnel with synovitis about the tendon sheath of the posterior tibialis, flexor digitorum longus, and flexor hallucis longus (Bluestone 1982, Cracchiolo 1982a). However, other tendons can be similarly involved, for instance the extensor tendons at the dorsum of the ankle and the peroneal tendons under the superior peroneal retinaculum. Initially, patients with this type of synovitis should have a thorough medical evaluation to establish a diagnosis as to their type of inflammatory arthritis. Although RA is the more common disease, Reiter's syndrome, infectious arthritis, and the arthritis associated with inflammatory bowel disease can all cause synovitis. Appropriate medical measures should be promptly utilized; these include drugs and physical modalities. However, it is important for the patient to be followed closely to determine if this regime is effective in controlling the synovitis.

Tendon rupture must be avoided and it may be necessary to be more aggressive if synovitis has not resolved in 2–3 weeks. Immobilization should be used early if

possible. Frequently, a short leg cast for about 3 weeks is all that is needed to control the synovitis (i.e. to eliminate the swelling and pain); however, recurrence may occur despite all these measures. Should non-operative treatment fail to control the synovitis, an operative decompression of the involved tendons, excising the proliferative synovium, should be performed as soon as possible to prevent tendon rupture. This is very important if the posterior tibial tendon is involved, since its rupture, which has been described in rheumatoid patients (Cracchiolo 1988), may lead to the planovalgus deformity which is seen in the hindfoot.

Shoes can also be helpful in treating the hindfoot deformities in patients with RA. The shoe should provide stability to the hindfoot, so the counter of the shoe must be stable to aid in supporting the calcaneus. A longitudinal arch support, an orthotic device, and one-quarter inch medial heel and sole wedges on the outside of the shoe may be useful in a patient with a flexible hindfoot deformity. At times, an ankle-foot orthosis is also useful, particularly if weakness is also present in the hindfoot. Stiffness can be helped by using a rocker bottom sole on the patient's shoe; the use of a cushion heel can also be helpful. Fixed deformities cannot be changed by any shoe modification. However, proper padding may reduce some of the pain.

Surgical treatment

Stabilization of the rheumatoid hindfoot is frequently necessary and should be performed early before the development of severe hindfoot valgus deformity. These patients rarely undergo a spontaneous fusion of any of their hindfoot joints.

The medications that the patient is taking to control RA should be evaluated. Patients taking in excess of 7.5 mg of prednisone orally appeared to have more postoperative complications including wound healing problems and non-unions (Cracchiolo et al 1992). Methotrexate also appears to delay wound healing and should be discontinued about 1 week before the operation and for about 2 weeks postoperatively. Nonsteroidal anti-inflammatory drugs should be curtailed about 5–7 days preoperatively if a procedure is being planned which might lead to significant blood loss (e.g. obtaining a large quantity of iliac bone graft for an arthrodesis). Simple analgesics are usually able to control the arthritic pain for short periods and may not contribute to increased bleeding as seen with some of the anti-inflammatory drugs.

The ultimate aim of a successful hindfoot arthrodesis is to have the foot in a plantigrade position with the metatarsals all level when the hindfoot is corrected to approximately 7° of valgus. The operative technique selected depends on the type of deformity. Various possibilities exist:

1. A hindfoot with no evidence of malalignment.
2. A hindfoot with a significant valgus deformity and this is by far the most common pathology and is more difficult to treat.
3. A varus malalignment usually associated with some cavus deformity, which is infrequent and more commonly seen in patients with juvenile rheumatoid arthritis.

In addition to the clinical examination, the radiographs assist in determining the type of operation that may be required.

The surgical exposure of the hindfoot joints requires two incisions:

1. A medial or dorsomedial incision is centered over the talonavicular joint to expose that joint.
2. If the hindfoot is in neutral or varus, an oblique incision centered over the sinus tarsi can be used to expose the subtalar and calcaneocuboid joints.

However, if there is a significant valgus deformity of the heel (10° or more), it will be difficult to close an oblique incision if the valgus deformity is corrected (which is preferable), or the wound may have difficulty healing. Therefore in almost all patients, I prefer the anterolateral approach, which is a longitudinal incision placed about 2 cm anterior to the fibula. It begins about 4 cm superior to the ankle joint and crosses the sinus tarsi, curving distally to end just distal to the calcaneocuboid joint (Fig. 21). Care must be taken to avoid entering the ankle joint

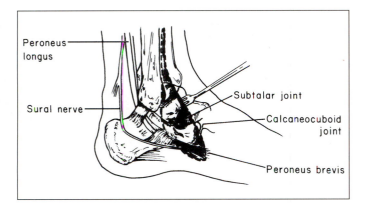

Figure 21

The lateral approach to the subtalar and calcaneocuboid joints for triple arthrodesis. This is particularly useful if there is a valgus deformity of the hindfoot. It is usually not necessary to expose or release the peroneal tendons, and the sural nerve is usually not damaged. This is also an excellent incision if one is going to operate on the ankle joint at the same time, and in fact one can perform an arthrodesis of the ankle and subtalar joint through this approach if indicated

or damaging the anterior talofibular ligament. This technique gives excellent exposure, and after correcting a valgus deformity it is relatively easy to close and heals well. I always make this incision first and prepare the posterior facet of the subtalar joint and the calcaneocuboid joints. The anterior and middle facets of the subtalar joint can also be freed through this incision using curved elevators. The talonavicular joint is then approached through a dorsomedial incision.

Operative technique for correction of a hindfoot in neutral alignment

Isolated talonavicular joint arthrodesis is performed in a hindfoot that is still flexible or is in neutral. Although the talonavicular joint is grossly destroyed, some narrowing of the other hindfoot joints is acceptable; early arthrodesis of that joint has been advocated. It is most unusual for these patients to require additional hindfoot fusions (Elbaor et al 1976). Such patients may, of course, represent a limited population whose other joints may have been spared anyway. Several techniques have been used to fuse the talonavicular joint. These include removing the surfaces and securing the joint with bone screws or staples (Feiwill & Cracchiolo 1994). In fusing only the talonavicular joint, I prefer to use either two 4.5 mm screws placed as lag screws (Fig. 22), or one screw and several power-driven titanium staples. Dowel grafting also can be utilized but it should be supplemented with some type of internal fixation; staples are the easiest to use as screws may disrupt the graft (Cracchiolo et al 1990, Ljung et al 1992).

Fixed hindfoot deformities or severe destruction of other hindfoot joints usually indicates the need to perform a triple arthrodesis. Arthrodesis of the hindfoot joints (usually a triple arthrodesis) can be accomplished by removing the articular surfaces and roughening the underlying subchondral bone. Internal fixation is required and this can be accomplished using a 6.5 mm cancellous bone screw across the subtalar joint (about 65 mm long), one 4.5 mm screw from the navicular into the talus (about 50 mm long – a 6.5 mm screw may fracture the navicular tuberosity) and a single screw across the calcaneocuboid joint (about 35 mm long). The calcaneocuboid joint can also be easily fixed using the powered stabilizer gun, which fires thin titanium staples across the joint.

Patients with a varus deformity are stabilized using a similar technique for fixation. The deformity is corrected by freeing up all three joints. It may be necessary to resect some bone from the subtalar joint, usually a small laterally based wedge.

Hindfoot stabilization in patients with significant valgus deformities

It is essential to attempt to correct the valgus deformity and not perform an arthrodesis that leaves the patient

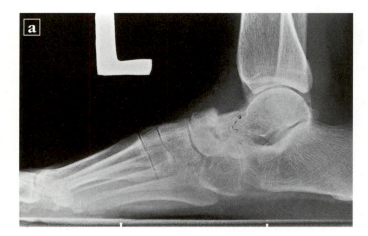

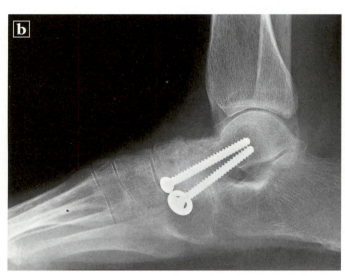

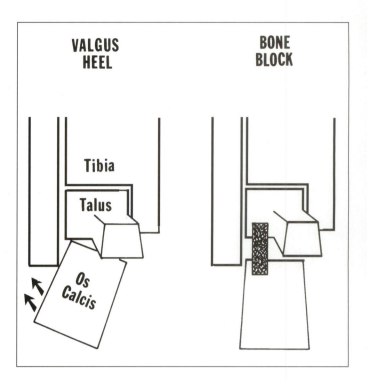

Figure 23

The heel can be in marked valgus, will touch the lateral malleolus and can cause a stress fracture of the distal fibula. At times, with a severe valgus deformity of the heel, it is essential to utilize bone graft in the posterior facet of the subtalar joint to correct this deformity. This can be done as a dowel graft, or as an in-lay graft

Figure 22

Lateral weight bearing radiograph of the foot of a 42-year-old woman. She has had rheumatoid arthritis which has been active for about nine years, and is currently treated with nonsteroidal anti-inflammatory medications. (a) The talonavicular joint had become very painful, but the remainder of her foot was stable and relatively uninvolved. (b) Arthrodesis was performed by removing the abnormal surfaces of the talonavicular joint and then using two 4.5 mm cortical screws for internal fixation. The joint is initially prepared and realigned and held temporarily with a 0.062 inch Kirschner wire. The first 4.5 mm screw is then placed as a lag screw starting the drill hole as close to the naviculocuneiform joint as possible. The Kirschner wire is then removed and a second screw is placed for additional stability. If there is any evidence of osteoporosis in the area of the drill hole, a washer should be used and this is very common in rheumatoid arthritis

with their original hindfoot deformity. Most deformities can usually be corrected by exposing the joints and by freeing the joint surfaces. It is occasionally necessary in some patients with a fixed valgus deformity to remove some of the head of the talus in order to be able to

correct the overall foot deformity. In a severe valgus deformity, correction usually leaves a gap across the posterior facet of the subtalar joint and this gap must be filled with some type of bone graft (Fig. 23). A dowel of bone from the ilium can be placed into a prepared dowel hole across the posterior facet of the joint (Cracchiolo 1984, Cracchiolo et al 1990). A tricortical graft from the iliac crest can be slotted into the joint, or the joint can be excised and filled with autogenous cancellous bone. A 6.5 mm cancellous bone screw can be used to fix the subtalar joint and is placed from the talus into the calcaneus, avoiding any solid portion of the graft. One should not overcorrect the hindfoot if there is a significant forefoot deformity as well. There usually is enough residual midfoot motion so that the forefoot can compensate even when a severely deformed hindfoot is corrected. However, it may be necessary to arthrodese the hindfoot in 10–12° of valgus in order to keep a plantigrade forefoot. After obtaining the desired correction, internal fixation should be utilized. It is usually best to first secure the subtalar joint, which has been bone grafted; the talonavicular joint is stabilized next and then the calcaneocuboid joint.

Postoperatively, patients are placed in a non-weight-bearing cast for about 5–6 weeks if possible and then a walking cast until they do not have any significant pain when fully weight bearing. If there is no pain, then there is probably enough clinical fusion to continue without a cast. Radiographs will usually not show a solid arthrodesis at this point. However, it is possible to place the patient in a shoe with a good longitudinal arch support. The average time of immobilization in our series was approximately 12 weeks (Feiwill & Cracchiolo 1994).

The rate of non-union in hindfoot fusion is variable. Painful pseudoarthroses of the talonavicular joint were seen in 3–5% (Elbaor et al 1976). After triple arthrodesis lack of radiographic bony union was seen in between 0% and 15% (Vahvanen 1967, Adam & Ranawat 1976, Cracchiolo et al 1990, Feiwill & Cracchiolo 1994). However, the majority of these patients were asymptomatic. This was also reported by Ljung et al (1992) in talonavicular joint fusions where a 37% non-union rate was seen radiographically, but all of these patients had either no pain or slight pain. They strongly recommended using internal fixation to augment their dowel graft technique. Moreover, their patients only were immobilized for 6–8 weeks (possibly a bit short) and weight bearing started at 3 weeks (possibly a bit early).

The ankle joint in rheumatoid arthritis

Persistent synovitis of the ankle resistant to non-operative treatment, and with no significant radiographic evidence of joint destruction, may be an indication to perform a synovectomy. A thorough lavage and debridement of the ankle using an arthroscopic technique may give significant relief of pain while retaining ankle joint motion. Open synovectomy of the ankle is also an option. As an alternative, intra-articular radiation treatment has been used to control the ankle joint synovitis. Gold-198 (^{198}Au) and Yttrium-90 (^{90}Y) have been used, but their relatively long half-lives (approximately 2.7 days) may result in a significant radiation dose to the tissues. Using a radionuclide with a shorter half-life (2.3 hours), dysprosium-165 (^{165}Dy) ferric hydroxide macro-aggregates, six of eight patients responded favorably when it was used to treat their ankle synovitis (Barnes et al 1994). However, very little is known of the effects of any method of ankle synovectomy, as few patients are candidates for this treatment.

Arthrodesis

The only reliable procedure to treat a painful destroyed ankle in rheumatoid arthritis continues to be ankle arthrodesis (Cracchiolo et al 1992). These patients usually have multiple deformities of other joints, either in the foot or in the lower extremity. Thus, ankle arthrodesis can probably only achieve pain relief and may not be able to improve function. A patient with intact transverse tarsal joints (talonavicular and calcaneocuboid) who also requires an ankle arthrodesis will usually have a better functional result. The transverse tarsal joints allow about 15° of plantar flexion motion if the hindfoot is in valgus. This motion acts as simulated ankle motion especially if the talus is fused in neutral or 5° of dorsiflexion. Such patients are unusual, since most RA patients have more hindfoot than ankle joint involvement. Many operations have been described for ankle arthrodesis and although they are different, there are several common features that place the various techniques into groups:

1. Compression arthrodesis using an external fixator is utilized as an adjunct to many arthrodesis techniques (Vahvanen 1967);
2. The fibula can be used as a strut or spike graft;
3. The anterior tibia may act as a donor bone graft by sliding a portion of the bone into the talus;
4. Recently, internal fixation with the use of a plate or rigid screw fixation (Morgan et al 1985) (Fig. 24) has been reported; however this may be insufficient fixation if moderate to severe osteoporosis is present.

Bone grafting is usually not necessary unless there is significant loss of the dome of the talus. This is seen infrequently in RA, but, of course, is most challenging in achieving fusion after removal of a failed ankle implant. Interpositional bone grafts are useful when the talus has been previously resected and they do provide some intrinsic stability to the ankle. However, when the dome of the talus has been eroded and has lost its normal height, a technique of posterior bone grafting through a posterior exposure is very useful (Russotti et al 1988). The grafts are placed to bridge across the tibia to the calcaneus. An external fixator probably provides the best form of stabilization when any of these grafting techniques are required. We recently reviewed our ankle fusions in all of our RA patients, including those with failed ankle prostheses, using either internal fixation or an external fixator. Fusion rates were 80% for each group, and the average time to fusion was 18 weeks (Cracchiolo et al 1992). Most of the failures were complicated by infection.

The final position of the foot as it relates to the leg is a significant factor in ankle fusions. The neutral position, no dorsiflexion or equinus, about 7° of hindfoot valgus, and 10° of external rotation, appears to give the best overall results (King et al 1980). Furthermore, it is important to keep the dome of the talus as far posterior under the resected surface of the tibia as possible. This will prevent the foot from acting as too great a lever when walking after achieving a solid arthrodesis. If there has been a previous triple arthrodesis or if the hindfoot is stiff, then it may be best to place the foot in about

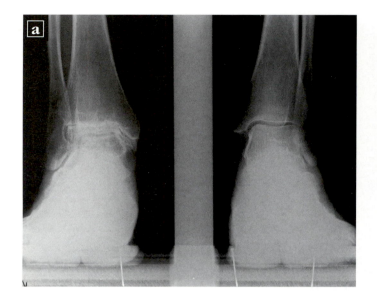

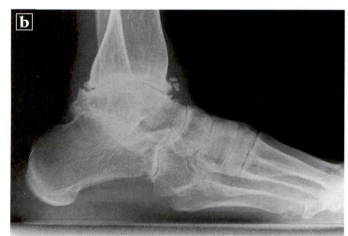

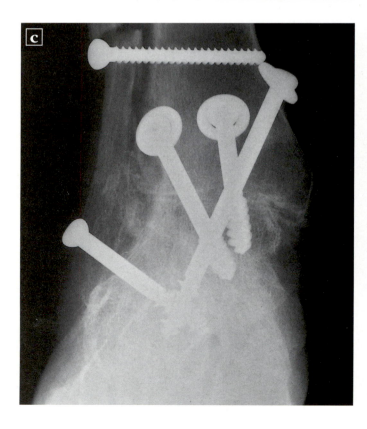

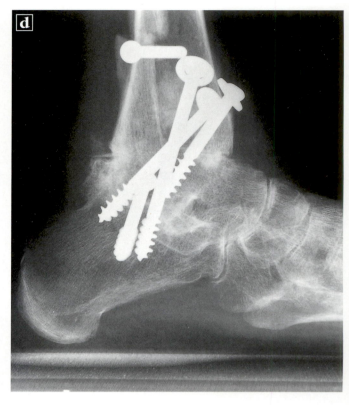

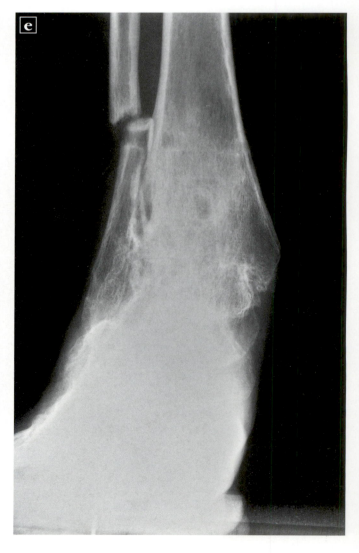

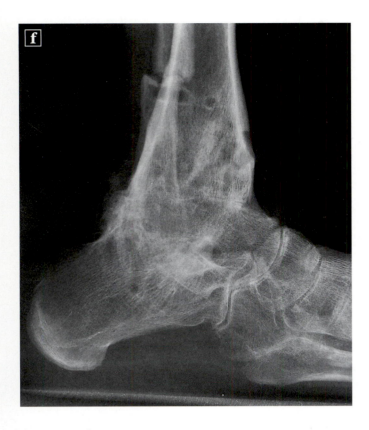

Figure 24

(a, b) Anteroposterior and lateral weight bearing radiographs of the patient's ankles. On the anteroposterior radiograph one can see that the left ankle has been spared and the right ankle has lost its joint space completely. Fortunately, the alignment is excellent. (b) Shows a lateral view with significant involvement of both the ankle joint and the subtalar joint. Fortunately, the remainder of the hindfoot appears to be spared. (c, d) Anteroposterior and lateral radiographs of this patient approximately 1 year following the surgery. The fibula has been utilized as a strut graft and is held in place proximally with a 4.5 mm cortical screw passed across both cortices of the tibia and the fibula. The distal screw is a short 6.5 mm cancellous bone screw. Washers are usually required as the distal tibia can be quite osteoporotic. This patient required approximately 14 weeks in a cast until her pain was relieved. (e, f) She has had an excellent result, however, due to some pain around the screws they were removed at 18 months

5° of dorsiflexion as this may make it easier for the patient to get out of a chair.

In some patients both the ankle joint and subtalar joint are arthritic and painful. Arthrodesis of both joints can be performed; however, the procedure is more complex and probably requires longer to heal (see Fig. 23).

Ankle arthroplasty

During the late 1970s and early 1980s, total ankle arthroplasty, using cemented implants of varying design, became popular. Although short-term follow-up studies showed favorable results with total ankle arthroplasty, longer evaluations indicate that the results were generally unfavorable (Kitaoka et al 1994, Unger et al 1988) (see Fig. 19). Stauffer & Segal (1981) initially reported excellent results in patients with RA at an average of 23 months follow-up. However, Kitaoka's study (1994) showed the long-term results to be much poorer. Newton's (1982) results in RA patients were so poor that he felt the procedure was contraindicated. Bolton-Maggs et al (1985) concluded that the Imperial College, London Hospital implant had such poor results that it should no longer be used. Unger et al (1988) followed patients with RA having an ankle replacement for an average of 5.6 years. Moreover, they followed a group of patients originally reported with excellent results but who only had an average follow up of 39 months (Lachiewicz et al 1984). They concluded that the results deteriorated with time, and that the radiographic analysis showed loosening of both components with time in the majority of patients. Their larger group now only showed excellent or good results in 65%. Because of the loosening of the implants they concluded that the revision rate would be unacceptably high.

Pahle et al (1987) reported that about 50% of patients had ankle and subtalar joint involvement. They performed more synovectomies than arthrodeses of these joints (3:1). After 1976 no ankle fusions were performed. It was his impression that the patient could tolerate considerable ankle joint destruction. His results with total ankle arthroplasty performed in the late 1970s and early 1980s, followed an average of 5 years, were good, and he recommended its use in patients with RA.

Kitaoka et al (1994) recently reviewed the experience with total ankle arthroplasty using the Mayo total ankle, and their large series of 174 patients with 214 ankle replacements was followed for an average of 9 years (range 2–17 years). Of significance was the fact that 98 patients with 125 treated ankles had a diagnosis of RA. Unfortunately, they used the subsequent removal of the implant as their failure end-point so that their data must represent the best possible results of total ankle arthroplasty. Even so, they noted a constant decrease in the cumulative rate of survival of the implants. At 5, 10 and 15 years the survival rate of the implant was, respectively, 79, 65 and 61%. They identified two independent variables that were associated with a significantly higher risk of failure: a previous operation on the ipsilateral foot or ankle and an age of 57 years or less. Therefore, their best results were achieved in patients over 57 years who had not had a previous operation on the ipsilateral foot or ankle. The probability of the implant being *in situ* at 10 years was 73%. However, we are not told of the condition of the arthroplasty. Conversely, the worst results were in patients less than 57 years old who had previous operative treatment. In this group the probability of retaining the implant for 10 years was only 42%. Interestingly, they report no significant difference between the 10-year cumulative rate of survival in patients with RA and survival in patients with osteoarthritis and traumatic arthritis. This was surprising, since many RA patients requiring ankle surgery are young and many RA patients have had more than one operation on their foot or ankle. The 10-year survival rates were 60% for the ankles affected by RA and 70% for the other ankles.

Thus it appears that the success enjoyed by replacing the hip joint and knee joint in the RA patient is not shared by the ankle joint. Unfortunately, the need to develop a successful ankle replacement is not so great as it was for the other joints – far fewer ankles are destroyed, patients seem to tolerate some degree of ankle pathology, and a successful arthrodesis gives good pain relief. Buechel et al (1988) have reported good early results with an ankle replacement implanted without cement and utilizing a polyethylene bearing. However, they only reported on 23 ankles with a mean follow-up of 35 months. Tillmann also continues cautiously to perform ankle replacements. Cemented ankle joint replacements like the prototype St Georg (1993) had a relatively high rate of loosening; about 12% of Tillmann's patients required reoperations an average of 8 years after implantation. Revision required an arthrodesis using voluminous bone grafts. Tillmann began in November 1990 using the New Jersey design ankle implant. Up to September 1994 he performed 53 uncemented ankle replacements (32 New Jersey and 21 STAR-Link implants). Three revision replacements of cemented ankle implants in two patients were also performed. To date there have been two loose implants in one woman with RA; one required removal and an arthrodesis was performed using allograft bone. This patient had severe osteonecrosis of the talus and probably was not a good candidate for ankle replacement.

The first 19 ankle replacements were reported at a meeting of the Rheumatoid Arthritis Surgical Society in England in 1992. This was a pilot study, since all had only a 1-year follow up. However, the uncemented implants seemed to give good pain relief, like the early results with the cemented ones. There was a bit less loss of preoperative motion (10° as compared with 20° for the cemented implant). This short experience seems to be encouraging (Tillmann & Straub 1993), but of course the final result will need many more years of clinical evaluation. Hopefully, future reconstructive techniques may allow us to achieve pain relief in these destroyed joints as well as providing motion and stability for a more normal joint.

References

Adam W, Ranawat C S 1976 Arthrodesis of the hindfoot in rheumatoid arthritis. Orthop Clin North Am 7: 827–840

Aho H 1987 Synovectomy of MTP joints in rheumatoid arthritis. A preliminary report. Rheumatology 11: 126–130

Aho H, Halonen P 1991 Synovectomy of MTP joints in rheumatoid arthritis. Acta Orthop Scand 61 (suppl 243): 1

Amuso S J, Wissinger H A, Margolis H M, Eisenbeis C H Jr, Stolzer B L 1971 Metatarsal head resection in the treatment of rheumatoid arthritis. Clin Orthop 74: 94–100

Ansell B M 1978 Introduction. In: Ansell B M, Arden G P (eds) Surgical Management of Juvenile Chronic Polyarthritis, Academic Press: London, Grune & Stratton: New York. pp 1–7

Auerbach M D, Shephard E, Vernon-Roberts B 1982 Morton's metatarsalgia due to intermetatarso-phalangeal bursitis as an early manifestation of rheumatoid arthritis. Clin Orthop 167: 214

Barbier M 1976 Vorfusskorrektur von dorsal oder plantar? Technische Probleme und Ergebnisse. Orthop Praxis 12: 533–538

Barnes C L, Shortkroff S, Wilson M, Sledge C B 1994 Intra-articular radiation treatment of rheumatoid synovitis of the ankle with Dysprosium-165 ferric hydroxide macroaggregates. Foot Ankle 15: 306–310

Barton N J 1973 Arthroplasty of the forefoot in rheumatoid arthritis. J Bone Joint Surg 55B: 126–133

Benjamin A, Helal B 1980 Surgical Repair and Reconstruction in Rheumatoid Disease. Macmillan Press, London, Basingstoke

Bluestone R 1982 Collagen diseases affecting the foot. Foot Ankle 2: 311–317

Bolton-Maggs B G, Sudrow R A, Freeman M A R 1985 Total ankle arthroplasty: a long-term review of the London Hospital experience. J Bone Joint Surg 67B: 785

Brandes M 1929 Zur operativen Behandlung des Hallux valgus. Zentralbl Chir 56: 2434–2440

Brattström H 1973 Synovektomien in Metatarsophalangealgelenken. Orthopäde 2: 81

Breewood A F M, Griffiths J C 1985 The long term results of a single stem silastic arthroplasty of the great toe, J R Coll Surg Edin 30: 159–161

Buechel F F, Pappas M J, Iorio L J 1988 New Jersey low contact stress total ankle replacement: biomechanical rationale and review of 23 cementless cases. Foot Ankle 8: 279–290

Clayton M L 1960 Surgery of the forefoot in rheumatoid arthritis. Clin Orthop 16: 136–140

Clayton M L 1967 Results of surgery in rheumatoid feet, Proceedings of the 4th Panamerican congress of rheumatology. Excerpta Medica Intern Congress Service 165: 107–115

Clayton M L 1982 Evolution of surgery of the forefoot in rheumatoid arthritis. J Bone Joint Surg 64B: 640

Clayton M L 1992 Management of the rheumatoid foot. In: Clayton M L, Smyth C J (eds) Surgery for Rheumatoid Arthritis. Churchill Livingstone, New York. pp 307–343

Clayton M L, Smyth C J 1992 Surgery for rheumatoid arthritis. Churchill Livingstone, New York

Cracchiolo A 1979 The use of shoes to treat foot disorders. Orthop Rev 8: 73

Cracchiolo A 1982a Arthritic diseases of the foot and ankle. Foot Ankle, 2: 309–341, 3: 2–44

Cracchiolo A 1982b Management of the arthritic forefoot. Foot Ankle, 3: 17–23

Cracchiolo A 1982c Office practice: Footwear and arthritic therapy. Foot Ankle 2: 242–248

Cracchiolo A 1984 Surgery for Rheumatoid Disease. AAOS Instruction. Course Lecture. Mosby Times Mirror. Vol 33, p 386

Cracchiolo A 1988 Rheumatoid arthritis of the foot and ankle. In: Gould J (ed.) The Foot Book. Williams and Wilkins, Baltimore. pp 239–267

Cracchiolo A 1993 The rheumatoid foot and ankle: pathology and treatment. Foot 3: 126–134

Cracchiolo A, Cimino W R, Lian G 1992 Arthrodesis of the ankle in patients who have rheumatoid arthritis. J Bone Joint Surg 74A: 903–909

Cracchiolo A, Swanson A, Swanson G D 1981 The arthritis great toe metatarsophalangeal joint: a review of flexible silicone implant arthroplasty from two medical centers. Clin Orthop 157: 64

Cracchiolo A, Pearson S, Kitaoka H, Grace D 1990 Hindfoot arthrodesis in adults using a dowel graft technique. Clin Orthop 257: 193–203

Cracchiolo A, Weltman J B, Lian G, Dalseth T, Dorey F 1992 Arthroplasty of the first metatarsophalangeal joint with a double stem silicone implant: results in patients who have degenerative joint disease, failures of previous operation in rheumatoid arthritis. J Bone Joint Surg 74A: 552–563

Craxford A D, Stevens J, Park C 1982 Management of the deformed rheumatoid forefoot: a comparison of conservative and surgical methods. Clin Orthop 166: 121–126

Daly P J, Johnson K A 1992 Treatment of painful subluxation or dislocation at the second and third metatarsophalangeal joints by partial proximal phalanx excision and subtotal webbing. Clin Orthop 278: 164–170

Dedrich D K, McCune W S, Smith W S 1990 Rheumatoid arthritis presenting as spreading of the toes. J Bone Joint Surg 1990 72A: 463–464

Delagoutte J P 1980 Les endoprosthèses dans la chirurgie du pied rhumatoide. Rev Rhumatisme 47: 135–137

Denis A, Huber-Levernieux C, Debeyre J, De Séze S, Ryckewaert A, Gontallier D 1980 Notre expérience de la chirurgie de l'avant-pied rhumatoide (150 interventions). Rev Rhum 47: 9–14

Dennis D A, Clayton M L 1992 Management of juvenile rheumatoid arthritis. In: Clayton M L, Smyth C J (eds) Surgery for Rheumatoid Arthritis. Churchill Livingstone, New York. pp 373–388

De Stoop N, Suykens S, Veys E 1987 Le pied psoriasique. In Claustre J, Simon L (eds) Actualitiés de médecine et chirurgie du pied. Masson, Paris, pp 44–49

De Stoop N, van Niewhuyse W, van Meirhaeghe J, Bongaerts W, Claessens H 1989 L'emploi de l'agrafe comme tuteur externe dans le traitement de l'hallux valgus. In Claustre J, Simon L (eds) Actualitiés de médecine et chirurgie du pied. Masson, Paris, pp 119–122

Downey D T, Simkin P A, Marc L A, Richardson M L, Kilcoyne R F, Hansen S T 1988 Tibialis posterior tendon rupture: a cause of rheumatoid flat feet. Arthritis Rheum 31: 441–446

Elbaor J E, Thomas W K, Weinfeld M S, Potter T A 1976 Talonavicular arthrodesis for rheumatoid arthritis of the hindfoot. Orthop Clin North Am 7: 827

Faithful D K, Savill D L 1971 Review of the results of excision of metatarsal heads in patients with rheumatoid arthritis. Ann Rheum Dis 30: 201–202

Fassbender H G 1975 Pathology of Rheumatic Diseases. Springer Verlag, Berlin. pp 245–258

Ferdini R, Schöpke K, Wölbert E 1988 Silikon-Implantate am Grosszehengrundgelenk. Eine kritische 10-Jahres-Studie, Z Orthop 126: 606–608

Feiwill L A, Cracchiolo A 1994 The use of internal fixation in performing triple arthrodesis in adults. Foot 4: 10–14

Fowler A W 1959 A method of forefoot reconstruction. J Bone Joint Surg 41B: 507–513

Freed J B 1993 The increasing recognition of medullary lysis, cortical osteophytic proliferation and fragmentation of implanted silicone polymer implants. J Foot Ankle Surg 2: 171–179

Gainor B J, Epstein R G, Henstorf J E, Olson S 1988 Metatarsal head resection for rheumatoid deformities of the forefoot. Clin Orthop 230: 207–213

Geppert M J, Sobel M, Bohne W H O 1992 The rheumatoid foot: Part I. Forefoot. Foot Ankle 13: 550–558

Girlando J, Berlin J St 1981 Complications of Keller bunionectomy and Keller with Swanson hemi-implant. J Foot Surg 20: 148–150

Granberry W M, Noble P C, Bishop J O, Tullos H S 1991 Use of a hinged silicone prosthesis for replacement arthroplasty of the first metatarsophalangeal joint. J Bone Joint Surg 73A: 1453–1459

Gschwend N, Steiger U 1987 Stable fixation in hindfoot arthrodesis. A valuable procedure in the complex RA foot. Rheumatology 11: 113–125.

Gschwend N, Barbier M, Dybowski W R 1977 Die Vorfusskorrektur.

Häufigkeit und Bedeutung der Zehen- und Metatarsalindices, Arch Orthop Traumatol Surg 88: 75–85

Hagena F W, Bracker W, Hoffmann T-F, Rosemeyer B, Zwingers T 1987 How do various operative procedures on the forefoot influence the rheumatoid foot. Rheumatology 11: 161–172

Hansens C, Horstmeyer M, Tillmann K 1987 Mittel- und langfristige Ergebnisse bei kompletten Vorfusskorrekturen nach Tillmann bei Patienten mit chronischer Polyarthritis. Akt Rheum 12: 222–225

Hassalo L G, Wilkens R F, Toomey H E, Darges D E, Hansen S T 1987 Forefoot surgery in rheumatoid arthritis: subjective assessment of outcomes. Foot Ankle 8: 148–151

Helal B 1975 Metatarsal osteotomy for metatarsalgia. J Bone Joint Surg 57B: 187–192

Helal B, Chen S C 1986 Arthroplasty of the metatarsophalangeal joint of the big toe using a new elastomer prosthesis. Med Chir Pied 7: 95–101

Helal B, Greiss M 1984 Telescoping osteotomy for pressure metatarsalgia. J Bone Joint Surg 66B: 213–217

Hoffmann P 1911 An operation for severe grades of contracted or clawed toes. Am J Orthop Surg 9: 441–449

Hohmann G 1955 Fuss und Bein – ihre Erkrankungen und deren Behandlung 5th edn. J F Bermann, Munich

Hueter C 1871 Klinik der Gelenkkrankheiten 1st edn Vol 1. F C W Vogel, Leipzig. pp 338–351

Hughes J, Grace D, Clarc P, Klenerman L 1991 Metatarsal head excision for rheumatoid arthritis. 4-year follow-up of 68 feet with and without hallux fusion. Acta Orthop Scand 62: 63–66

Kates A, Kessel L, Kay A 1967 Arthroplasty of the forefoot. J Bone Joint Surg 49B: 552–557

Keller W L 1904 The surgical treatment of bunions and hallux valgus. N Y Med J 80: 741–742

King H A, Watkins T B, Samuelson K M 1980 Analysis of foot position in ankle arthrodesis and its influence in gait. Foot Ankle 1: 44

Kitaoka H B, Patzer G L, Ilstrup D 1994 Survivorship analysis of the Mayo total ankle arthroplasty. J Bone Joint Surg 76A: 974–979

Krismer M, Eichenauer M 1990 Mittelfristige Ergebnisse mit dem Grosszehenimplantat nach Swanson. Z Orthop 128: 519–524

Lachiewicz P F, Inglis A E, Ranawat C S 1984 Total ankle replacement in rheumatoid arthritis. J Bone Joint Surg 66A: 340

Lipscomb P R, Benson G M, Sones D A 1972 Resection of proximal phalanges and metatarsal condyles for deformities of the forefoot due to rheumatoid arthritis. Clin Orthop 82: 24–31

Ljung P, Kaij J, Knutson K, Rydholm U 1992 Talonavicular arthrodesis in the rheumatoid foot. Foot Ankle 13: 313–316

van Loon P J, Aries R P, Karthaus R P, Steenaert B J 1992 Metatarsal head resection in the deformed, symptomatic rheumatic foot. A comparison of two methods. Acta Orthop Belg 58: 11–15

McAuliffe T B, Helal B 1990 Replacement of the first metatarsophalangeal joint with a silicone elastomer ballshaped spacer. Foot Ankle 10: 257–263

McGarvey S R, Johnson K A 1988 Keller arthroplasty in combination with resection arthroplasty of the lesser metatarsophalangeal joints in rheumatoid arthritis. Foot Ankle 9: 75–80

Mann R A, Thompson F M 1984 Arthrodesis of the first metatarsophalangeal joint for hallux valgus in rheumatoid arthritis. J Bone Joint Surg 66A: 687–692

Marmor L 1967 Surgery of Rheumatoid Arthritis. Lea and Febiger, Philadelphia

Mayo C H 1908 The surgical treatment of bunions. Ann Surg 48: 300–302

Miehlke R K, Blanke R, Stegers M 1987 Die Rekonstruktion des rheumatischen Vorfusses nach Tillmann: Bericht über 100 Fälle. Akt Rheum 12: 34–37

Moeckel B H, Sculco T P, Alexiades M M, Dossiek P H, Inglis A E, Ranawat C S 1992 The double stemmed silicone rubber implant for rheumatoid arthritis of the first metatarsophalangeal joint. Long-term results. J Bone Joint Surg 74A: 564–570

Morgan C D, Henke J A, Bailey R W, Kaufer H 1985 Long term

results of tibiotalar arthrodesis. J Bone Joint Surg 67A: 546

Newman R J, Fitton J M 1983 Conservation of metatarsal head in surgery of rheumatoid arthritis of the forefoot. Acta Orthop Scand 54: 417–421

Newton St E III 1982 Total ankle arthroplasty: clinical study of fifty cases. J Bone Joint Surg 64A: 104

Niskanen R O, Lethimäki M Y, Hämäläinen M, Törmälä P, Rokkanen P U 1993 Arthrodeses of the first metatarsophalangeal joint. Biodegradable rods and Kirschner-wires in 39 cases. Acta Orthop Scand 64: 100–102

Pahle J A, Teigland J C 1987 The complex foot. Rheumatology 11: 179–187

Pfeiffer W H, Cracchiolo A III, Grace D L, Dorey F J, van Dyke E 1992 Double-stem silicone implant arthroplasty of all metatarsal joints in patients with rheumatoid arthritis. Semin Arthroplasty 3: 16–24

Preston R L 1968 The Surgical Management of Rheumatoid Arthritis. Saunders, Philadelphia

Raunio P, Laine H 1970 Synovectomy of the metatarsophalangeal joints in rheumatoid arthritis. Acta Rheum Scan 16: 12–17

Raunio P, Lehtimäki M, Eerola M, Hämäläinen M, Pulkki T 1987 Resection arthroplasty versus arthrodesis of the first metatarsophalangeal joint for hallux valgus in rheumatoid arthritis. Rheumatology 11: 173–178

Refior H J, Hoos R 1987 Midterm results of arthroplasty of the forefoot by Clayton-Vainio in rheumatoid arthritis. Rheumatology 11: 131–135

Richardson E G, Brotzman S B, Graves S C 1993 The plantar incision for procedures involving the foot. J Bone Joint Surg 75A: 726–731

Russotti G J, Johnson K A, Cass J R 1988 Tibiocalcaneal arthrodesis for arthritis of the hind part of the foot. J Bone Joint Surg 70A: 1304–1307

Saltzman C L, Johnson K A, Donnelly R E 1993 Surgical treatment for mild deformities of the rheumatoid forefoot by partial phalangectomy and syndactylization. Foot Ankle 14: 325–329

Salzmann G, Sarfert D, Hardt T 1987 Die Korrektur der schweren Vorfussdeformität bei der chronischen Polyarthritis. Akt Rheum 12: 19–25

Sethu A, D'Netto D C D, Ramakrishna B 1980 Swanson's silastic implants in great toes. J Bone Joint Surg 62B: 83–85

Shephard E 1975 Intermetatarso-phalangeal bursitis in the causation of Morton's metatarsalgia. J Bone Joint Surg 57B: 115–116

Spiegel T M, Spiegel J S 1982 Rheumatoid arthritis in the foot and ankle – diagnosis, pathology, and treatment. Foot Ankle 2: 318–324

Stainsby G D 1992 A modified Keller's procedure for the lateral four toes. Paper read at the Annual Meeting of the British Orthopaedic Foot Surgery Society, Stanmore, 20 November

Stauffer R M, Segal N M 1981 Total ankle arthroplasty: four years' experience. Clin Orthop 160: 217

Stockley I, Betts R P, Getty C J, Rowley D I, Duckworth T 1989 A prospective study of forefoot arthroplasty. Clin Orthop 248: 213—218

Swann M 1978 The foot. In: Arden G P, Ansell B M (eds) Surgical management of juvenile chronic polyarthritis. Academic Press, London; Grune and Stratton, New York. pp 185–199

Swanson A B, deGroot Swanson G, Frisch E E 1983 Flexible (silicone) implant arthroplasty in the small joints of the extremities: Concepts, physical and biological considerations, experimental and clinical results. In: Rubin L R (ed) Biomaterials and Reconstructive Surgery. C.V. Mosby, St Louis. pp 595–623

Swanson A B, Lumsden R M, de Groot Swanson G 1979 Silicone implant arthroplasty of the great toe. Review of single stem and flexible hinge implants. Clin Orthop 85: 75–81

Swanson A B, de Groot Swanson G, Mayhew D E, Khan A N 1987 Flexible hinge results in implant arthroplasty of the great toe. Rheumatology 11: 138–152

Swanson A B, de Groot Swanson G, Maupin B K et al 1991 The use of a grommet bone liner for flexible hinge implant arthroplasty of the great toe. Foot Ankle 12: 149–155

Tillmann K 1973 Vorfusskorrektur. Orthopäde 2: 99–100

Tillmann K 1979 The Rheumatoid Foot. Georg Thieme, Stuttgart. pp 1–116.

Tillmann K 1987 The mutual interplay between forefoot and hindfoot affections and deformities in RA. Rheumatology 11: 97–99

Tillmann K, Straub M L 1993 Early experience with uncemented ankle joint replacements in rheumatoid arthritis (abstract). J Bone Joint Surg 75B: 293

Tillmann K, Küster R M, Rüther W 1993 Entzündliche Erkrankungen des kindlichen Fusses. In: Venbrocks R, von Salis-Soglio G (eds) Jahrbuch der Orthopädie 1993. Biermann: Zülpich. pp 73–79

Tillmann K, Rüther W, Kranz R, Koss W 1989 Der Ersatz rheumatisch zerstörter Mittelhandköpfchen mit einem einstieligen Implantat. Act Rheumatol 14: 259–266

Unger A S, Inglis A E, Mow C S, Figgie H E 1988 Total ankle arthroplasty in rheumatoid arthritis: a long term follow-up study. Foot Ankle 8: 173–179

Vahvanen V, Piirainen H, Kettunen P 1980 Resection arthroplasty of the metatarsophalangeal joints in rheumatoid arthritis: a follow-up study of 100 patients. Scand J Rheumatol 9: 257–265

Vahvanen V A 1980 Rheumatoid arthritis in the pantalar joints. A follow-up study of triple arthrodesis on 292 adult feet. Acta Orthop Scand (Suppl) 107: 3–137

Vainio K 1956 The rheumatoid foot. A clinical study with pathological and rheumatological comments. Ann Chir Gynaec Fenn 45: suppl 1

Vainio K 1956 The ankle joint. Ann Chir Gynaecol (Suppl) 45: 9

Viladot A 1983 Traitement chirurgical de l'avant-pied rhumatoïde. In: Le Pied en practique rhumatologique. Pathologie articulaire. Masson, Paris. pp 245–248

Viladot A 1988a La semelle antialgique de 'Denis'. Ses indications dans la pied rhumatoïde. Méd Chir Pied 4: 67–69

Viladot A 1988b La chaussure orthopédique de 'Dixon' dans la traitement du pied rhumatoïde. Méd Chir Pied 4: 70–72

Watson M S 1974 A long-term follow-up of forefoot arthroplasty. J Bone Joint Surg 56B: 527–533

Wiasmitinow N P, Zollinger H 1993 Osteotomien nach Helal. Med Orthop Tech 113: 292–296

VI.4 The Diabetic Foot

Bernard F Meggitt

Epidemiology

Continued advances in the medical treatment of diabetes mellitus have resulted in a significant decrease in the life-threatening metabolic disorders. There has, however, not been a parallel reduction in the main diabetic complications of retinopathy, nephropathy, vasculopathy, cardiac problems, and foot disorders. Many of these complications are particularly seen in the lower limbs, where the group of symptoms and signs resulting from neuropathies, angiopathies and infective lesions constitute the 'diabetic foot syndrome'. These progressive complications leave the diabetic patient at high risk for foot breakdown with deformities, ulceration, infection and gangrene. Such diabetic foot breakdowns have become major medical problems today. Studies of large populations in Europe have shown the prevalence in diabetics of the signs of neuropathy to be 23–33% and forefoot deformities 14–28%, and foot ulceration to be 3–7%. Amputation rates of 1–3% are reported (Neil et al 1989, Borssen et al 1990, Young et al 1993). Further reports demonstrate a 10% increase in lower limb diabetic amputations over a 10-year period, accounting for 21% of all lower limb amputations in 1983. In 1989 this incidence was 22%, with 60% over 60 years old (UK DHSS Amputation Statistics 1974–83, 1989). Similarly, there have been a number of reports from the USA of increasing admissions for diabetic foot breakdown in the 1980s with a 12% increase in 12 years in hospital admissions (Kozak & Rowbotham 1984). A large Community Hospital diabetic clinic study has indicated a 16% admission rate and 23% of all in-patient hospital days for diabetic foot breakdown (Smith et al 1987). The National Institute of Health in the USA estimates that 15% of diabetic patients in the USA will develop feet ulcerations at some time (Palumbo & Melton 1985). Between 5.1 and 8.6 per thousand diabetics will undergo at least one amputation per year, with 55% of the overall incidence of nontraumatic amputations being in diabetics (Most & Sinnock 1983).

This increase in diabetic complications is likely to continue unless a treatable cause is found. This is because the majority of cases of diabetes onset are age-related and thus they increase with the general population's improved life expectancy. The prevalence of diabetes in the UK is approximately 1.5%, with 80% presenting over the age of 40 in the population at large. The duration of diabetes is associated with the onset of complications (Young et al 1993, Moss et al 1992) and most diabetic feet show some changes of neuropathy or angiopathy after 10 years of known disease (Fagerberg 1959). These complications are progressive, with increasing and recurrent susceptibility to foot breakdown.

The cause of diabetes remains unknown but the previous simplistic concept that it was due to a single group of disorders resulting in degeneration of the pancreatic beta cells, associated with hereditary factors, is no longer accepted. Diabetes mellitus can probably be produced by nearly all the commonly recognized pathological processes, such as infections (particularly viral), toxins, immune reactions, specific genetic protein defects, as well as by secondary conditions involving inflammatory pancreatitis, haemochromatosis, acromegaly, and occasionally neoplasia. With this wide spectrum of aetiologies, diabetes has been loosely classified into groups:

(a) Juvenile-onset insulin-dependent diabetes (JOD, Type I)
(b) Maturity-onset diabetes of youth (MODY)
(c) Gestational diabetes
(d) Polyendocrine diabetes
(e) Maturity-onset diabetes (MOD, Type II)
(f) Secondary diabetes

More recently, specific research areas have focused on islet amyloid secretory and processing defects in Type II diabetes, a new immunogenic abnormal HLA-DQ molecule in Type I diabetes, new inhibitors to reduce peripheral insulin resistance, and studies in genetic susceptibility to Type I with imprinting and rearrangement of the insulin gene (International Diabetes Federation Congress, 1991).

Pathology in diabetic foot tissues

The classical triopathy of the diabetic foot syndrome is angiopathy, neuropathy and infection, either presenting alone or in combination. Neuropathy and infection underlie many diabetic foot problems, but it is the vascular tissue disease that produces the most destructive lesions.

Blood vessels

The increased incidence and severity of complications attributable to macrovascular arteriosclerotic disease such as myocardial infarction and gangrene, especially in the maturity-onset diabetic, have been long known. Somewhat later, arteriolar disease was appreciated, and more recently a microangiopathy involving the capillaries has been recognized. None of the vascular pathologies seen in diabetics is unique to diabetes mellitus: they are qualitatively similar to those occurring in nondiabetics.

Macroangiopathy

Macrovascular disease in the diabetic is arteriosclerotic in nature – that is, there is marked thickening and loss of elasticity of the arterial wall. Histopathologically three types of arteriosclerosis are seen: atherosclerosis, medial calcific sclerosis, and diffuse intimal fibrosis.

Atherosclerosis

This may occur in single, multiple or diffuse patterns in any of the lower limb muscular arteries. Development occurs from fatty streaks in the intima progressing to fibrolipid atheromatous plaques that extend into the media and cause destruction of the elastic fibres, replacing them with collagen. Large quantities of extracellular lipid and cholesterol are found and the plaques may calcify. Segmental stenosis, surface thrombosis and plaque emboli or arterial thrombosis may progress to produce distal ischaemia, infarction and gangrene. Qualitatively this atherosclerosis is similar in diabetics and nondiabetics, but in the diabetic group, the lesions occur more frequently (Strandness et al 1964) and appear to progress more rapidly (Warren et al 1966; Janlea et al 1980). More diffuse involvement of the medium and small arteries in the lower leg and foot occur in diabetes (Haimovici et al 1960, Ferrier 1965, Warren et al 1966). This produces the 'end-artery state' of the foot tissues with a limited number of patent supply vessels, loss of collateral circulation and a decreased vascular reserve. Further obstruction or sudden vascular demand can result in ischaemia and gangrene.

Medial calcific sclerosis (Monckeberg's sclerosis)

This involves a progressive calcification of the media of muscular arteries but, unlike atherosclerosis, it does not develop in the large elastic vessels. Calcification occurs around smooth muscle cells, forming plates, rings and finally pipe stems, but the intima is not involved and the lumen is not compromised. As is the case with atherosclerosis, medial calcific sclerosis involves diabetics more severely than non-diabetics. It occurs at an earlier stage and often in association with atherosclerosis.

Diffuse intimal fibrosis

This affects the larger arteries and, as it occurs throughout life, is considered to be part of the ageing process (Wilens 1951). Normal mechanical haemodynamic forces appear to stimulate fibromuscular proliferation producing the intimal thickening. It is not associated with any specific cell wall damage or luminal obstruction.

Microangiopathy

Small vessel disease involves the small arteries, arterioles and capillaries. It presents as a generalized hyalinization of the wall with intimal proliferation, hypertrophy and fibrosis. The capillary pathology of basement membrane thickening is seen throughout diabetic tissues but it is not pathognomonic of diabetes, as such thickening occurs as part of the ageing process in nondiabetics. The rate and quantity of this thickening, however, is much greater in the skin and muscle of diabetics (Kilo et al 1972, Siperstein et al 1968). This thickening has been shown by isotope clearance studies to cause increased permeability in skeletal muscles in diabetics (Trap-Jensen 1971), and it may also affect the normal inflammatory response with interference in healing and infections, though this has not been proven. This basement membrane thickening does not interfere with gaseous exchange, as demonstrated by measurements of transcutaneous oxygen tension in diabetic and nondiabetic patients (Wyss et al 1984).

Pathogenesis of diabetic vascular disease

The concept that the pathogenesis of vascular disease is similar in diabetics and non-diabetics, but accelerated in the diabetic, is currently accepted. The original 'response to injury hypothesis' has received more support, suggesting that the primary mechanism is damage and disruption of the arterial endothelium by mechanical, chemical or immune factors (Ross 1981).

Other research studies have shown abnormalities in platelet reactions (Cowell et al 1981, Peterson et al 1987) and in the low viscosity lipoproteins (Reckless et al 1978, Goldstein & Brown 1982, Lopez-Vivella et al 1982, Galle et al 1990) in diabetic patients that are capable of initiating endothelial damage. The significance of these changes as primary atherogenic agents is not certain, but their presence at a younger age and the acceleration effect on muscular damage would support their association with the more severe progression of atherosclerosis in the diabetic patient.

Furthermore, diabetics are susceptible to the common atherogenic factors seen in nondiabetic patients, including adverse family history, hypertension, smoking, obesity and hyperlipidaemia. A number of haematological changes have also been reported in diabetic patients involving hyperfibrinogenaemia, abnormal fibrinolysis and abnormal platelet function with increased prostaglandin secretion (Ganda 1980, Gough & Grant 1991).

Nerves

Diabetic neuropathy is a general term describing a group of disorders of the peripheral nervous system, though the aetiology remains uncertain. Two pathological groups have been suggested with a predominantly metabolic-induced neuropathy in one (Asbury et al 1978) and a vascular cause in the other (Raff et al 1968). These form the basis of a currently accepted classification of neuropathy (Sibley 1982):

1. Metabolic neuropathy
   (a) Chronic symmetrical distal polyneuropathy with sensory, motor and autonomic involvement
   (b) Acute symptomatic distal neuropathy
2. Vascular neuropathy
   Mononeuritis solitary and multiplex
   (i) Large nerve trunks
   (ii) Radiculopathy
   (iii) Cranial neuropathy
3. Nerve compression syndromes

Chronic symmetrical distal polyneuropathy

This forms the commonest diabetic neuropathy. It has a characteristic symmetry of overlapping nerve terminals most distant from the cell body. The correlation with poor hyperglycaemic control suggests a metabolic cause (Gregersen 1967). The neuropathy is not associated with the severity of the diabetes, but more with the degree of control. The mechanism of prolonged hyperglycaemic-induced neuropathy is uncertain. Abnormal endoneural capillary leakage, blood–nerve barrier defects, endoneural toxic oedema, perineural cell basement membrane thickening and, most recently, abnormal sorbitol and fructose accumulation, have all been reported and critically reviewed (Eliasson 1983). Recent studies of sensibility recovery after pancreas transplantation, with return of insulin hyperglycaemic control, support the metabolic induced concept of this peripheral neuropathy.

The main pathological change in this type of neuropathy appears as distal axonal degeneration with loss of the myelin sheath and disappearance of many of the axons (Thomas & Lascelles 1966). With decrease in motor axons, there is a widespread collateral sprouting of the residual intact ones with reinnervation of denervated muscle fibres. This is incomplete, leaving a peripheral motor neuropathy with wasting, weakness and contracture of the small muscles of the foot.

Involvement of the distal sensory nerves by these pathological changes produces a symmetrical neuropathy with loss of touch, pain, proprioception and temperature discrimination sensibility. Demyelination of the proprioceptor and mechanoreceptor nerves to the joints and bones leads to secondary intrinsic trophic changes of the Charcot type arthropathies and osteopathies. A similar diffuse degeneration occurs in the autonomic nerves producing the interference in sweating and vasomotor function in the foot.

Acute symptomatic distal neuropathy

This is now rare, having been reported in the past during periods of very poor diabetic control with excessive weight loss, and following rapid correction of diabetic acidosis with insulin or tolbutamide. The acute presentation and recovery suggested a metabolic neuropraxic lesion of motor and sensory nerves.

Mononeuritis – solitary and multiplex neuropathies

These are considered the result of vascular changes in the limb nerves with local ischaemic areas and micro-infarcts (Raff & Asbury 1970). Almost any nerve or nerve root may be involved, but the most common mononeuropathies involve the femoral, peroneal, oculomotor, abducens, median or ulnar nerves and the lower lumbar nerve roots. In some cases multiple nerve trunks or nerve roots are involved successively, producing the mononeuritis multiplex picture. Despite the severe incapacity, the pathological process appears to be reparative, often with good functional recovery.

Nerve compression syndromes

The nerve trunks of diabetic patients are more susceptible to compression and traction trauma from the latent diffuse neuropathy of metabolic, ischaemic or mixed pathologies (Mulder et al 1961). The posterior tibial nerve in the tarsal tunnel and the peroneal nerve at the fibula neck, the ulnar nerve at the elbow, and the median nerve at the wrist are at high risk of compressive neuropathies in diabetics.

Infection

There is very little epidemiological evidence to support any higher incidence of primary sepsis in the diabetic patient. However, with the greater frequency of breakdown, especially in the foot, secondary infection is much more common than in the nondiabetic (Pratt 1965, Bessman & Wagner 1975). Studies on humoral immunity reactions in both diabetic patients and experimental diabetic animals, both with infections, have shown no immunological incompetence (Lipcomb et al 1959, Dolkart et al 1971). However, many changes in cell-mediated immunity have been recorded and critically reviewed (Axtine 1982). Thus, impairment of leucocyte migration and mobilization, decreased granulocyte adherence and diminished leucocyte chemotaxis, phagocytosis and bacteriocidal activity, have all been implicated (Wilson 1986, Leslie et al 1989). Also, these abnormalities appear worse in the poorly controlled diabetic and in ketoacidotic states; there is usually marked improvement on insulin stabilization (Rayfield et al 1985).

The basic pathology of much of the diabetic foot infection follows on from ulceration due to local trauma and high loading in the presence of insensitive deformed feet and, at times, deficient vascularity. The loss of protective pain results in failure to reduce the higher and repetitive loads leading to underlying tissue damage, necrosis and ulceration (Brand 1978). Secondary infection may then follow at any stage, giving further and deeper tissue destruction; cellulitis, oedema, lymphangitis, abscess, septic arthritis and osteomyelitis are possible sequelae. Increased tissue pressure and septic thrombosis may obliterate the remaining 'end-artery vessels' with resulting distal gangrene. With slower arterial obstruction, a dry atrophic type of gangrene occurs; with a more acute blockage, oedema and infection following, giving the wet-type septic gangrene. The third, less common, type of 'central or core gangrene' may occur in the diabetic with infections involving the plantar spaces, producing obliterative septic thrombosis and extensive deep tissue necrosis. The skin and peripheral tissues may survive for a period.

Osteomyelitis and septic arthritis are serious lesions in the diabetic foot, accounting for over one-third of a large series of patients with bone infection (Waldvogel et al 1970). Most bone and joint infections in diabetic feet develop from chronic perforating ulcers and, less commonly, from direct penetrating wounds in the neuropathic foot. Osteomyelitis may be present in much higher proportions – up to 68% in foot ulcers – than is clinically apparent (Newman et al 1991). When deep chronic infection, recurrent ulceration or sinus formation persists, there is the ever-present danger of acute infection flare-ups.

The most common infective organisms in diabetic foot sepsis are streptococci, staphylococci, aerobic gram-negative bacilli and anaerobic bacteria (Louie et al 1976). Mixed facultative and obligatory anaerobes have been reported to be mainly responsible for the foul-smelling, gas-forming infections in the diabetic 'foetid foot' (Fierer et al 1979). Gas formation by non-clostridial organisms in soft tissue infections occurs more frequently in the diabetic patient and must be differentiated from true clostridial infections (see Fig. 17). These non-clostridial gas-forming infections are much more common, rarely progress rapidly and usually are systemically non-toxic, often being amenable to local treatment (Bessman & Wagner 1975).

Although the diabetic may suffer from the same types of infection as the nondiabetic, fungal infections of the skin and nails do seem to make up a greater proportion of infections in diabetics than they do in nondiabetics. These infections usually occur in moist areas of the foot and are often associated with poor general hygiene and a lack of patient education. The commonly involved fungal species are *Tricophyton rubrum*, *T. interdigitale* and *Epidermophyton flocculosum*.

Clinical presentation

The diabetic foot syndrome rarely presents as an isolated complication in the diabetic patient – it is usually seen with vascular, neurological or breakdown lesions. It forms part of a generalized disorder, most often associated with retinopathy, nephropathy and cardiovascular disease (Yamagata & Yamauchi 1969). In the absence of these foot changes, the other complications are much less common (Fagerberg 1959). Vascular lesions in the lower limb have been shown to be two to three times more frequently seen in association with a neuropathy,

which itself occurs in most patients with diabetes of more than 10 years. The presence of an autonomic neuropathy often precedes the somatic type, and may be an indicator of those patients at risk from diabetic foot breakdown (Dearfield et al 1980). Thus the diabetic patient may present with complications in the lower limbs arising from peripheral vascular disease, neuropathy, deformities and infection, often in combination.

Peripheral vascular disease

Atherosclerosis

Major vessel stenosis or obstruction presents with peripheral ischaemia in diabetics in a way similar to that seen in nondiabetic patients. Intermittent claudication occurs in the calves with increasing severity and decreasing walking tolerance. Night pains from nerve ischaemia progress to rest pain at any time and are often relieved by leg dependency because this increases tissue profusion. A severe sensory neuropathy, however, may result in little pain at all if severe ischaemia is present. With atherosclerosis, the main pulses at the foot and knee are often absent, associated with dependency rubor and elevation blanching with delayed venous filling time. Ischaemic skin changes present with shiny, cool, atrophic, hairless skin and with thickened, slow-growing nails. With severe chronic ischaemia, the subcutaneous tissues atrophy, particularly in the heel and metatarsal pads, and the skin appears tight. With critical ischaemia, minor trauma leaves ulcers, which become infected and, with insufficient healing potential, patchy or more diffuse gangrene then occurs.

The diabetic and nondiabetic atherosclerotic vascular disease may present with acute arterial obstruction from emboli or thrombosis. The clinical outcome depends upon the collateral circulation and the duration of the avascular episode before surgical relief. Irreversible changes of the most sensitive tissues, the muscles and nerves, occur after 4–6 hours. Acute arterial obstruction from a large embolus with little collateral circulation produces the acute severe pain and a pale wax-like extremity. With slower obstruction from arterial thrombosis, often of an atheromatous plaque, a more cyanotic distal limb occurs. In association with the pain, pallor and pulselessness, the arterial occlusion also produces the paraesthesiae from peripheral nerve ischaemia and paralysis from muscle infarction.

Small vessels

The nonatheromatous peripheral small artery hyalinization disease, common in the diabetic foot, produces the 'end-artery state'. With little collateral circulation, any single artery obstruction will result in distal avascular tissue. Thus small vessel disease may present with insidious gangrene involving skin patches, toe segments, complete toes or the whole forefoot area. With infected ulcers, septic obliterative arteritis or thrombosis produces spreading gangrenous areas.

Distal artery obstruction from penetrating infection in the toes or web spaces presents with progressive cyanosis, swelling and then gangrene of the toe. Obliteration of the transverse plantar metatarsal arterial arch may produce gangrene in the middle toes or the whole forefoot. The clinical presentation may often appear confused, with good pulsatile arterial vessels at the ankle, or even in some toes, in the presence of gangrenous areas in the foot unless this non-atheromatous peripheral small artery disease is understood.

Neuropathy

Sensory neuropathy

The sensory neuropathy in the diabetic foot presents symptomatically in two contrasting forms: one with pain and paraesthesiae and the other with numbness, giving loss of pain and temperature appreciation. The latter is much the more common type and some degree of overlap is occasionally seen. Clinical differentiation from ischaemic pain is made from the quality of the pain and the state of the peripheral circulation. The hyperalgesic neuropathy produces sharp stabbing or shooting pains that occur at any time and are often severe at night, appearing as 'pseudotabetic' in nature. The paraesthesiae is variable with tingling or burning, and often hyperaesthesic on contact. Radicular pain, from a mononeuropathy, appears to arise from the spinal roots, giving low back pain and variable radiation into the leg, and often being associated with dermatomal paraesthesiae, muscle weakness and decreased reflexes.

The second and main group of diabetic sensory neuropathies present only rarely with symptoms directly as there is decreased sensation to pain, temperature, vibration and proprioception. Feelings described as 'heavy legs' and 'walking on cotton wool' are the main common neuropathic complaints. The loss of superficial and deep pain sensibility produces two main clinical pictures – one of repeated trauma from mechanical, chemical or thermal injury giving ulceration and ensuing infection, the other of deformities and disorganization of the foot from Charcot's type osteoarthropathies, which may also produce ulceration over high pressure areas.

These characteristic neuropathic ulcers usually occur on the plantar surfaces, often with round punched-out appearances. They are described as 'mal-perforans, plantar, trophic, perforating and pressure ulcers'. The loss of deep sensibility may also present with painless deep infections involving soft tissue spaces, bone and joints, spreading insidiously from the penetrating ulcer in the unwary patient. Insensitive toes commonly produce breakdown lesions caused by extrinsic pressure from footwear, by foot warming devices and by minor mechanical trauma. Intrinsic pressure from nail ingrowths, and underlying prominent bone and toe deformities also produce breakdown and are often the first presenting sign of a sensory neuropathy.

Motor neuropathy

Motor neuropathy presents with weakness and atrophy, and later fibrous contracture, of the intrinsic foot muscles producing various forefoot deformities. The result is alteration of the normal foot compliance on weight bearing, with increased or repetitive high local pressures. Often associated with the sensory neuropathy, these deformity changes from the motor neuropathy give localized high pressure and further liability to ulceration and infection. The diabetic amyotrophy may present with wasting, weakness and contractures within the calf muscles, leading to deformities such as dynamic equinovalgus and pes cavus with abnormal gait and weight bearing.

Autonomic neuropathy

Autonomic nervous system involvement in diabetic neuropathy presents with loss of pseudomotor function, giving a dry, flaky skin. Cracks and fissures may be present with secondary infection. Loss of the skin thermoregulation, with vasomotor instability, may produce both vasodilation and vasoconstriction with decreased or increased foot temperatures. Loss of the small arterial and arteriovenous shunting control may cause local ischaemic areas in the skin and deeper tissues, with inability to divert the circulatory requirements to damaged new sites.

Deformities

Contractures

The deformities presenting in diabetic patients are similar to those in nondiabetics but they appear to occur more frequently and to progress more severely. These deformities present in the early phases with dynamic contractures from muscle weakness and atrophy, but later become fixed joint contractures. The forefoot deformities are the most common and are frequently associated with breakdown problems. Hammer, claw and angular deformities in the lesser toes and 'cock-up' claw toe and valgus deformities, most frequently in the hallux, commonly occur.

Further pressure from the contractures occurs over the medial side of the first metatarsal head, with a bunion bursitis reaction, and under the sesamoid bones. The hallux may underride the second toe, giving further clawing with plantar and dorsal pressure sites. Any adjacent toe contracture may produce nail pressure or a soft corn. Plantar callosities may develop under any of the metatarsal heads with dynamic or fixed depression secondary to the intrinsic muscle contracture.

Midfoot deformities occur with a forefoot plantaris associated with contracture of the plantar intrinsic and calf flexor extrinsic muscles. The resulting pes cavus gives the forefoot claw toes and hindfoot high pressure loads. Occasionally a pes planovalgus deformity may develop from invertor weakness and a dropped foot from dorsiflexion loss. Hindfoot deformities may present with prominence of the calcaneum on either the plantar surface, with atrophy of the heel pad, or posteriorly at the insertion of the Achilles tendon; they are often associated with a pes cavus contracture. Reactive hyper-keratosis of the heel, with secondary fissuring and breakdown from the increased pressure loads, also occurs.

Nail deformities

Deformities of the toe nails are common in the general population but appear to involve almost all patients with diabetes. These deformities are associated with atrophy, infection – both fungal and bacterial – local trauma, footwear pressure and poor nail hygiene. The common deformities producing a local pressure and infection are curved edges, giving the ingrowing toenail (onychocryptosis), the thickened horny nail (onychogryphosis), horny nail bed epithelial growth (onychophosis) and the thick-ened discoloured nail from fungal infection (onychomycosis). As the sensory neuropathy usually starts in the toes, these nail deformities may cause local skin break-down and infection in addition to the patient's footwear and increased pressure from trauma or deformities.

Osteoarthropathies

Deformities of the diabetic foot are also produced by structural changes resulting from Charcot's neuropathic joint (Charcot 1868, Jordan 1936, Heiple & Cammarn 1966). These changes are usually associated with a full sensory neuropathy and often follow foot trauma (Boehm 1962).

Osteoarthropathy may appear as an acute or chronic pathology. However, these probably represent different periods of the disease process, which has been described as falling into three stages (Eichenholtz 1966). The development stage involves the acute destructive period with a hot oedematous foot, widespread osteoporosis, joint destruction and subluxation, fractures and often ulceration. This phase is usually induced by minor trauma and further activated by continued weight bearing on an insensitive foot, with further breakdown. The second coalescence stage is a reparative phase with a reduction in the hyperaemia and oedema, stabilization of subluxed joints, healing of fractures and generally increased bone density. The third reconstruction stage shows further progress of repair and remodelling of soft tissues, bones and joints with the foot then stabilizing. As a result of this osteoarthropathy and osteopathy with subluxations, osteolysis, sclerosis, fragmentation and ectopic bone formation, the foot finally settles leaving the diabetic neuropathic deformed foot.

Various classifications have been reported on the patterns of bone and joint destruction in Charcot's diabetic neuropathic osteoarthropathy and osteopathy (Harris & Brand 1966; Cofield et al 1983; Brodsky et al 1987; Sanders & Frykberg 1991). These classifications involve localization of the site of the major deformity, although occasionally one or more sites are involved. Bone and joint destruction most commonly occurs in the forefoot of the metatarsal and phalangeal bones and joints (Fig. 1a) and is often associated with ulceration (Kelly & Coventry 1958; Cofield et al 1983). The second and most common site is the tarsometatarsal (Fig. 1b) and naviculocuneiform joints, and the third pattern involves the hindfoot – the subtalar joint, the talonavicular joint and the calcaneocuboid joint (Fig. 1c). The fourth pattern involves the ankle joint, and the fifth, the calcaneum with osteopathic fragmentation (Fig. 1d). The residual changes after consolidation may result in severe deformities, commonly with claw toes and pressure metatarsalgia in the forefoot, planus, adduction and varus or valgus of the hindfoot. The 'rocker bottom foot' results from collapse of the longitudinal arch and subluxation of the midfoot tarsus. These residual deformities present with high bony pressure areas in the usually insensitive foot with a high risk of ulcerative breakdown (see further Chapter VI.5.)

Infection

Infection of the diabetic foot often presents as the first sign of peripheral neuropathy or angiopathy. Three basic anatomical forms of the most common major foot infections have been described (Meade & Mueller 1968, Bose 1979):

- septic ulcer of the plantar surface (less commonly the dorsal surface);
- non-suppurative cellulitis of the dorsum of the foot; and
- abscess in the deep tissues, bone or joint.

Many of these lesions are progressive, starting with a superficial ulcer, proceeding to a deeper one and then developing an abscess formation in the tissues. If the circulation is compromised by the infection or pre-existing angiopathy, gangrenous lesions may develop as shown from a study of the natural history (Meggitt 1973, 1976).

Ulcers

These present most commonly in association with areas of high pressure or with friction over bony prominences. The commonest site is under the metatarsal heads (Fig. 2a) with toe deformities over the pulp and nail of the toe ends. Also, ulceration is common with high pressure

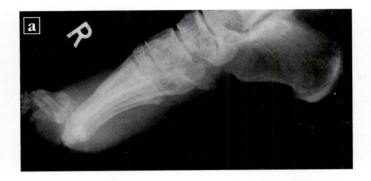

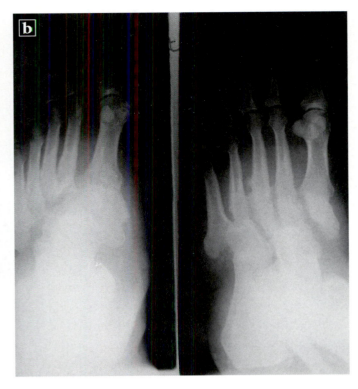

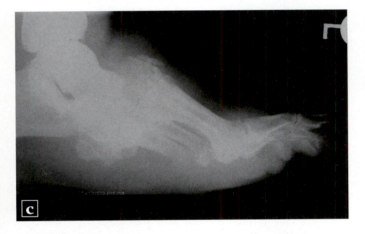

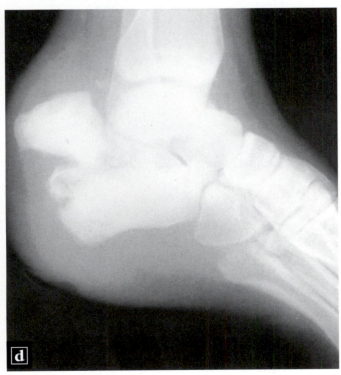

Figure 1

Diabetic neuropathic osteoarthropathies: (a) forefoot metatarsophalangeal joints dislocation; (b) metatarsotarsal joints subluxation; (c) midtarsal joints dislocations (rocker bottom foot); (d) calcaneum fracture

over residual deformities from Charcot's osteoarthropathy. Ulceration in the heel is less common than in the forefoot but this may similarly occur from footwear pressure, Charcot deformities and also from decubitus ulceration. Ulceration over the dorsum and side of the foot occurs; it commonly involves the first metatarsal bunion, fifth metatarsal bunionette and base of the fifth metatarsal styloid and is caused by shoe friction pressure.

These ulcerative lesions appear in two forms: with a corn or callus hyperkeratosis reaction, often with incomplete sensibility loss; or as a 'punched out' perforating ulcer with little reaction and usually in a fully insensitive area. The individual ulcers may present as a relatively clean lesion, with or without a necrotic base, or with an infected pus-discharging centre with surrounding cellulitis. Direct mechanical, thermal or chemical trauma to the neuopathic foot may also produce ulcers. Also, ischaemic ulcers may present spontaneously, with or without trauma. They occur mainly on the toes or dorsum of the foot with progress either to healing or to further breakdown depending upon the adequacy of the circulation.

Dorsal cellulitis

Spreading cellulitis and swelling may present on the dorsum of the foot and is usually secondary to surface infection in the nails, toes or web space (Fig. 2b). A systemic reaction with pyrexia is often present and a deeper abscess may occasionally develop.

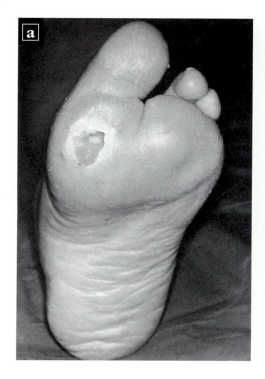

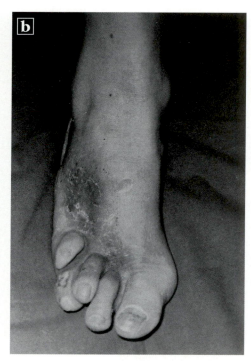

Figure 2

Diabetic foot infections: (a) deep plantar ulceration of the metatarsal head; (b) dorsal cellulitis from 4th toe abrasion; (c) medial plantar space abscess; (d) central plantar space abscess and heel necrosis; (e) septic arthritis and osteitis of the metatarsophalangeal joint (previous resection of the second metatarsal and third toe)

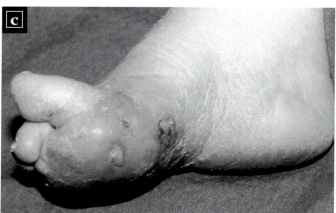

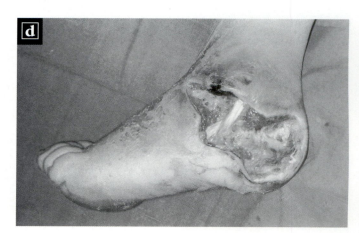

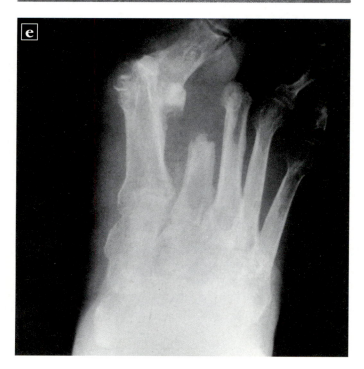

Abscess

The common sites for abscess formation are the toes, web spaces, flexor sheaths, the heel and the plantar spaces (lateral, medial and central) of the foot. The abscess often presents with little or no pain and the patient remains walking, thereby 'pumping' the infection widely. Loculated pus usually presents with deep extension of pyogenic infections from either an open surface ulceration, a previous closed lesion or a penetrating injury. Clinically, two forms of abscess occur: one involves an acute loculated infection with extensive foot swelling and systemic reaction, and the second is a more chronic abscess cavity with an open draining sinus or ulcer.

The toe abscess may present as a paronychia, or in the pulp, volar spaces or flexor tendon sheaths. The web space abscess presents with swelling and cellulitis extending to the adjacent toes and the dorsum of the forefoot.

Abscesses of the medial and lateral plantar spaces produce local swelling and dorsal oedema and are usually associated with infected ulceration over the first or fifth metatarsal heads (Fig. 2c). The now much less common central plantar space abscess occurs with severe swelling of the whole plantar area, rapidly spreading to the dorsum of the foot, together with loss of the longitudinal arch and skin creases, giving the 'flipper foot'. Further proximal spread along the flexor tendons and sheaths gives induration and necrosis around the ankle (Fig. 2d) and occasionally a higher calf abscess.

Osteitis

Diabetic osteomyelitis is often associated with local abscess formation and, less commonly, vascular deficiency. Most cases occur following deep chronic ulceration with sinuses and infected discharge. There is variable pain, depending upon the degree of sensory neuropathy, swelling and cellulitis as the local signs. The most common sites of osteomyelitis are associated with those of the ulcerations, mainly the toes, metatarsals and calcaneum. Septic necrosis, fragmentation and sequestrum formation may occur. A small surface sinus may communicate with a large abscess cavity, having infected bone within, and constitutes the 'volcano lesion', which may erupt into a full spreading abscess at any time. Sequestrated necrotic bone may appear in the deeper chronic abscess cavity and, at times, can be discharged.

Septic arthritis

This presents commonly underlying an infected penetrating ulcer in the interphalangeal or metatarsophalangeal joints giving swelling, stiffness and variable pain. In the acute form, loculation gives systemic reaction and, locally, subluxation or dislocation with contracture and recurrent episodes of swelling, cellulitis and a secondary discharging sinus. There may be associated infection spreading to adjacent bones or tissue spaces with further abscess formation (Fig. 2e). These chronic septic lesions involving joints carry a poor prognosis for healing and are at high danger of spreading (Margo 1967, Singer & Rossi 1968).

Imaging changes in the diabetic foot syndrome

Plain film radiographic examination of the foot provides diagnostic and progress monitoring of the often asymptomatic diabetic limb with neuropathic and infective abnormalities. The radiological features of the neuropathic and infective lesions in the foot have been reported (Schwartz et al 1969, Cofield et al 1983), but the differentiation between the two is often very difficult (Hodgson et al 1948, Whitehouse 1978). Also, major disorganization of the skeletal structures in the neuro-

pathic diabetic foot is not uncommon and may involve spontaneous fractures (Johnson 1967) and spontaneous dislocations (Newman 1979). Recent advances in imaging techniques have increased the accuracy of diagnosing and localizing acute and more chronic infective lesions, giving more detailed assessment of the neuropathic skeletal changes and in monitoring their recovery. Technetium 99 bone scans and magnetic resonance imaging (MRI) are both very much more sensitive in detecting early bone changes of osteomyelitis and Charcot joints than plain radiographs. MRI is significantly more sensitive than the bone scans and shows osteomyelitis earlier. The bone scan is still a valuable screening method where a negative bone scan result strongly excludes significant bone pathology, such as osteomyelitis; however, a positive scan is nonspecific, indicating only bone reaction (Berquist et al 1985, Yuh et al 1989). Computed tomography (CT) can give anatomical localization of infection, in both the deep soft tissues and the bone; however, it gives poor differentiation between normal and infected tissue and has now been superseded by MRI (Williamson et al 1989). MRI has been a major development in the diagnosis and treatment of the diabetic foot and can show early pathology in both the bone and soft tissues; it has, however, not yet been shown to differentiate between osteomyelitis and the marrow changes in Charcot joints. The dual scan, using technetium 99 to localize the bone and joint lesions, followed by indium-labelled white blood cells (WBC), is highly specific for diagnosis of osteomyelitis in bone or abscesses in the soft tissues. A negative indium WBC scan with a positive technetium 99 scan would be highly specific for a Charcot-type osteoarthropathy (Eymontt et al 1991, Keenan et al 1989).

Skeletal changes

Infection

Osteomyelitis is usually associated with soft tissue swelling, ulceration or abscess formation. These changes occur mainly in the forefoot, occasionally in the heel, and rarely in the midfoot bones. Radiographic changes may show very little in the first 14 days in the acute form, but local diffuse osteoporosis, periosteal reactions, cortical erosions and later cortical and medullary bone destruction, which may proceed to bone collapse with fragmentation and fractures, are seen after this.

Septic arthritis similarly may show few radiographic changes in the first 2 weeks, but then local osteoporosis becomes apparent with subchondral bone resorption and collapse of the articular surface with subluxation or dislocation of the joint. With more advanced infection, the bones adjacent to the joint may undergo osteolysis with further changes in the subperiosteal, cortex and medulla.

Diagnosis of the acute deep infection without radiographic changes can be undertaken using the isotope technetium diphosphonate scan and gamma camera screening. Although increased isotope uptake is useful in localizing early acute infections without radiographic changes, it is nonspecific in indicating any hyperaemia in the early pool phase or any increased bone metabolism in the delayed imaging. Technetium diphosphonate scans will localize bone reactive lesions, but they will not differentiate infection from neuropathic osteoarthropathy. The isotope gallium citrate localizes granulocytes and bacteria as well as areas of increased bone remodelling and thus is also nonspecific. Indium 111 leukocyte labelling does give a highly specific localization within areas of focal leukocyte sequestration and, in the absence of active marrow in the foot bones, is highly specific imaging for infection (Eisenberg et al 1989).

CT can give definitive imaging of bone and joint changes, particularly periosteal, cortical and subchondral articular changes that may indicate underlying bone infection. Abnormalities of the bone medullary space and areas of soft tissue can also be shown with CT scan. However, CT now seems to have been surplanted by MRI, which is much more sensitive in showing these various changes.

MRI has developed over the last 10 years and offers direct multiplanar imaging giving detailed and contrast anatomical screening that is superior to other imaging techniques. It depends upon screening the concentration of free protons in the tissues, which is proportional to the water content. With variation in the T_1-weighted images, these produce increased or decreased signals from the water and are very sensitive to focal bone marrow oedema, which is an indication of osteomyelitis. Local abscess formation can, in selected patients, be detected noninvasively with the appearance of focal pockets of fluid within the soft tissues and bone (Durham et al 1991).

Neuroosteopathy

Radiological appearances of diabetic neuropathic osteopathy show demineralization, osteolysis and often fractures. Osteolysis appears as localized bone resorption defects, most often involving the ends of the phalanges and distal metatarsals. Thinning of the shafts may produce the 'hour glass' deformity, whereas resorption of the head region produces the 'pencil-shaped' appearances which, if flattened, give the 'pestle and mortar' deformities. These bone changes may remain static, undergo slow progression or develop a massive acute osteolysis with extensive destruction. Spontaneous fractures may occur painlessly in the calcaneum (see Fig. 1d), metatarsals and phalanges, but these are far less common than the other bone changes. They are often associated with neuropathic joints and can themselves proceed to callus healing.

Differentiation of the acute neuropathic osteopathy from acute osteomyelitis can be difficult, as previously discussed. Both types of lesions produce bone destruction and pathological fractures, but the acute infection would also have all the local and systemic signs of a septic toxic lesion. Radiographs are usually sufficient for the diagnosis in the primary lesions but in those with previous problems, such as healed ulcers, then investigation with isotope scans and MRI may be needed to separate the neuropathic osteopathy from the septic one.

Neuroarthropathy

A wide spectrum of specific radiological changes present in the neuropathic joint from the acute swelling and osteoporotic demineralization of the bone, to periostitis and osteophytosis, through cartilage loss, joint collapse and fragmentation to subluxation and dislocation. Often multiple changes are present in various joints constituting the Charcot neuropathic osteoarthropathy picture. The five anatomical patterns involving the forefoot, midfoot, hindfoot, ankle and calcaneum (see above) are diagnosed by various plain radiographic views. Changes, often rapid in the acute phase, can also be monitored by serial radiographs. In the later stages, with stabilization of the foot, localization of high pressure areas with potential or actual ulceration can be identified with radio-opaque surface markers for consideration of reconstructive surgery.

In severe collapse, subluxation and dislocation, particularly of the midtarsal and hindfoot joints, CT and MRI scans are very helpful in identifying the resulting abnormal anatomy, again in order to plan stabilizing and reconstructive surgery.

As with the neuropathic osteopathy, the osteoarthropathy can present a confusing picture with destructive septic arthritis lesions. In the primary osteoarthropathy, the absence of the local and systemic infective reaction enables the radiographic diagnosis to be made. In those situations associated with previous or present breakdown, then differentiation is needed with the isotope bone scans and MRI investigations.

Soft tissue changes

These are shown radiologically as increased density with oedema, irregularity of the skin surface with ulceration, and subcutaneous cystic areas from gas formation (see Fig. 16A). Bone or calcific debris is seen adjacent to neuropathic joints, osteolysis or osteomyelitic lesions.

Vascular calcification in the foot arteries is commonly due to medial calcific sclerosis and may extend to the distal metatarsal and digital vessels (see Fig. 2e). Skin or subcutaneous calcification may be due to local ischaemia or calcified venous thrombosis. Occasionally foreign bodies such as needles, tacks or glass fragments are seen embedded in the foot, confirming the insensitive neuropathic foot.

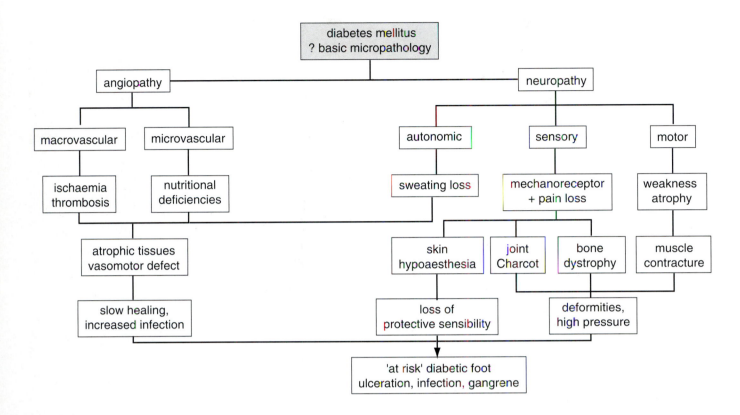

Figure 3

Pathogenesis of diabetic foot breakdown: 'at risk' concept

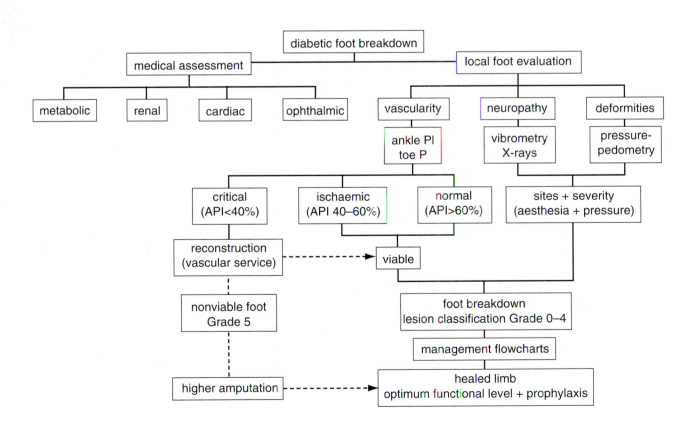

Figure 4

Diabetic foot breakdown: overview management flow chart

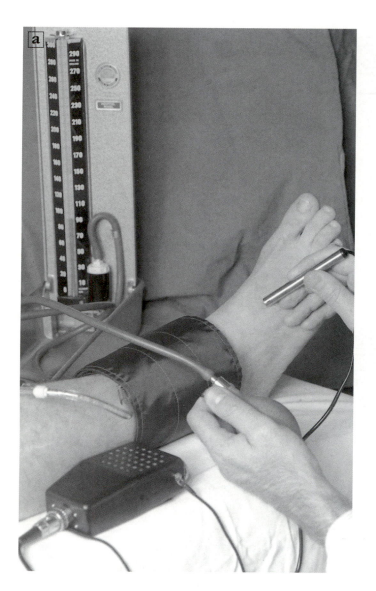

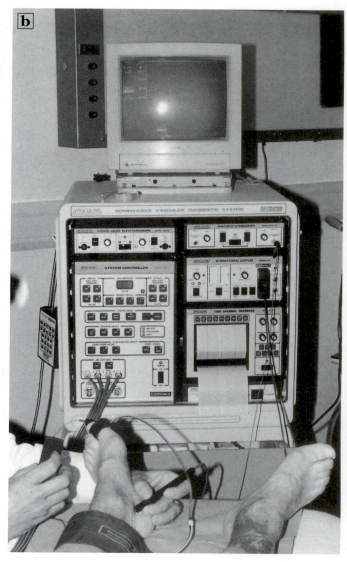

Figure 5

Foot vascularity pressure assessment: (a) Simpler Doppler probe, audio unit and sphygmomanometer; (b) Vasculab Doppler and toe photoplethysmograph; (c) Vasculab Doppler segmental pressures: computer printout with right arteriopathy

'At risk' diabetic foot concept

The concept of the 'at risk' diabetic foot (Meggitt 1976) is derived from a combination of the loss of protective sensibility, lowered resistance to infection with delayed healing, and the development of deformities with high pressure areas (Fig. 3). Early assessment of the severity of these complications with instigation of appropriate treatment is essential if the 'at risk' diabetic foot is not to be lost. Long term prophylactic treatment is then essential for both feet, because the 'at risk' status remains and may increase with time.

Assessment of the diabetic foot

As diabetes mellitus is a progressive multisystem disease, it is essential to have a full general medical assessment under the diabetic physician's care before undertaking a local evaluation of the diabetic foot condition. Thus the present metabolic state requires full investigation, and also other appropriate specialist's opinions, with involvement of renal, cardiovascular and ophthalmic services. Also, the patient's mental and physical status, and his or her occupation and mobility require assessment and consideration.

It is essential to have an overview of the local assessment of the diabetic foot severity, and these principles are shown in the management flow chart in Fig. 4.

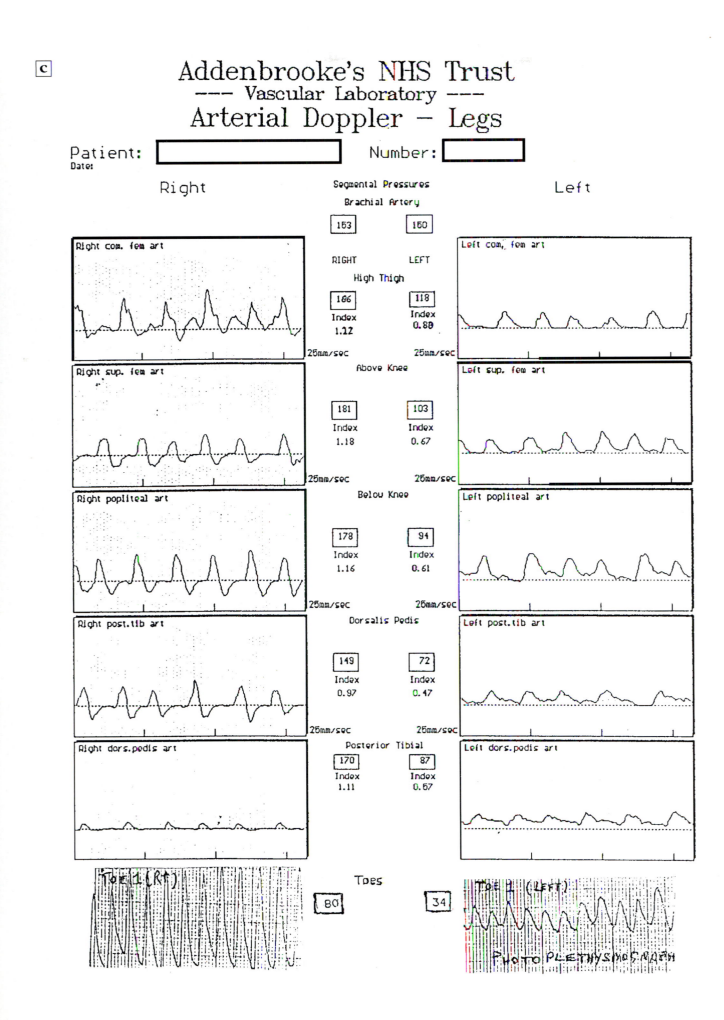

Addenbrooke's NHS Trust
--- Vascular Laboratory ---
Arterial Doppler – Legs

Patient:
Date:

Number:

Right	Segmental Pressures	Left
	Brachial Artery	
	163 160	
Right com. fem art	RIGHT LEFT	Left com. fem art
	High Thigh	
	186 118	
	Index Index	
	1.12 0.80	
	25mm/sec 25mm/sec	
Right sup. fem art	Above Knee	Left sup. fem art
	181 103	
	Index Index	
	1.18 0.67	
	25mm/sec 25mm/sec	
Right popliteal art	Below Knee	Left popliteal art
	178 94	
	Index Index	
	1.16 0.61	
	25mm/sec 25mm/sec	
Right post.tib art	Dorsalis Pedis	Left post.tib art
	149 72	
	Index Index	
	0.97 0.47	
	25mm/sec 25mm/sec	
Right dors.pedis art	Posterior Tibial	Left dors.podis art
	170 87	
	Index Index	
	1.11 0.57	
TOE 1 (RT)	Toes	TOE 1 (LEFT)
	80 34	
		PHOTOPLETHYSMOGRAPH

Vascularity assessment

Clinical assessment

Clinical parameters indicating a reduced arterial flow and poor tissue nutrition provide more of a qualitative diagnosis than a quantitative evaluation. In early major vessel disease, there are often few clinical signs; this is most likely to be due to an adequate collateral circulation. In more severe macrovascular disease, intermittent claudication and walking distance tolerance is a rough guide to the severity of the vascular disease. Palpable peripheral pulses indicate adequate circulation to at least the ankle level, and rapid blanching and filling on pressure release over the nails indicates reasonable toe circulation. Atrophic changes in the lower limb also give a qualitative assessment; these changes include loss of hair growth, thin inelastic skin, reduction in heel turgor and metatarsal pads, and defective nail growth.

Pressure index

Blood flow varies directly with the systolic blood pressure. This pressure, at a given level, may be used as an index of tissue perfusion to the local area supplied.

However, the noninvasive pressure index test has become a standard, more practical evaluation of the vascular status in the lower limb (Yao et al 1969, Yao 1970, Carter 1973). The segmental systolic pressure is accurately recorded using 12 cm cuffs placed on the upper and lower thigh, on the upper calf and above the ankle, using an audio signal with a Doppler ultrasound probe (10 MHz) at 45° over the artery below (Fig. 5a,b). The brachial artery pressure is also recorded and a pressure index is calculated using the leg pressure as a percentage of the arm pressure (Fig. 5c). The ankle pressure index (API) is a crude guide to the circulation in the hindfoot. The prognosis for healing after foot surgery and amputation has been variable, with good results in some series (Wagner & Buggs 1978) whereas other have found no correlation (Mehta et al 1980).

This lack of correlation is probably due to distal vessel obstruction beyond the ankle which led to the introduction of the toe pressure (TP) measurements using a small digital blood pressure cuff at the base of the first and second toes, and an infrared light transducer taped to the pulp recording the pulsatile microcirculation. This digital photoplethysmography pressure has been correlated with predictions for healing in the foot (Holstein et al, 1978, Barnes et al 1981, Bone & Pomajzl 1981). However, the API has been correlated with prediction of healing in the Syme amputation as a final foot salvage procedure (Wagner et al 1980). The lower limb Doppler segmental pressures and photoplethysmograph recordings can be undertaken manually in the ward or, more accurately by utilizing the advances in computerized equipment in the vascular laboratory (see Fig. 5). In the normal pattern, there is a steady decrease in the pressure index with each peripheral segment, and the high thigh pressure is approximately 1.3 times the brachial systolic pressure. A drop of 40 mmHg or more between two levels suggests a severe stenosis or obstruction. One problem in evaluation of the segmental pressures down to the foot is calcification, which occurs in higher frequency in the diabetic and which can prevent pressure cuff occlusion thereby giving high readings. However if there is a pulsatile flow occurring distally, there may still be adequate circulation for healing. The toe pressures in this situation are invaluable as a prediction for foot healing. Although the arterial pulsatile wave form is recordable, there has been little practical quantitative analysis obtainable and it only has qualitative elasticity value as the 'pulsatility index'.

These evaluations of the foot vascularity with the hindfoot inflow ankle Doppler pressure index, and the forefoot more accurate as absolute pressure from the photoplethysmography are then recorded and assessed in three groups for the prognosis for healing:

- critical ischaemia   API < 40%   TP < 30 mmHg
- viable ischaemia   API 40–60%   TP 30–60 mmHg
- normal range   API > 60%   TP > 60 mmHg

Regional tissue perfusion assessment

More direct techniques to measure the tissue blood flow have been developed. One group involves the use of isotope clearance following subdermal injection, but this technique requires a regular supply of isotopes (Xe^{33}, Tc^{99m}, I^{125}) and a nuclear medicine department setup.

Transcutaneous oxygen pressure ($tcpO_2$) can give an assessment of the local tissue perfusion in absolute numbers. The development of laser doppler velocimetry, used percutaneously to measure the mean velocity of red blood cells within the skin capillaries, gives an index of local tissue perfusion. Both the transcutaneous oxygen tension and the laser Doppler velocimetry measurements have been shown to have a high correlation in predicting healing of ischaemic forefeet ulceration and of amputations in diabetic and nondiabetic patients (Lee et al 1979, Radcliffe et al 1984, Karanfilian et al 1986). Thus, either of these tests or the toe pressure photoplethysmography would all seem to provide the most accurate monitoring for the local tissue perfusion and prediction for healing in the diabetic foot.

Contrast arteriography

This method is still the standard investigation for assessing the site, extent and degree of patency of the larger peripheral vessels. The investigation is not without risk (dye sensitivity, renal impairment and vessel injury) and is indicated when percutaneous vascular intervention or vascular reconstructive surgery is necessary for arterial disease. Noninvasive tests with Doppler segmental pressures and toe pressures are safe and give dynamic assessment but they do not give anatomical structure information. A decrease in adjacent Doppler segmental pressures of 40 mmHg or more suggests a stenotic segment or occlusion between the segments. This result, together with distal pressure levels within the critical range, requires urgent arteriographic evaluation.

For lesions above the femoral artery, transbrachial or translumbar arteriography is performed, and below this level a transfemoral technique is used. The radio-opaque dye, with serial radiographs or image intensifier recordings, can demonstrate occlusions, stenoses, aneurysm or dilatations and atheromatous areas in all the major arteries from the pelvis to the foot.

Digital subtraction angiography (DSA) with computerized imaging subtraction and dynamic range enhancement has become useful in a wide variety of vascular assessment applications. Visualization of all the lower leg and foot vessels is obtained with intra-arterial DSA, requiring only small amounts of contrast material.

Neuropathy evaluation

Clinical assessment

Standard clinical sensory examination of the diabetic foot provides a general assessment of the degree of impairment and distribution of touch sensation (cotton wool, brush or bristle) and pain sensation (pin prick). These are recorded as normal, reduced or absent and the extent of involvement as none, patchy or diffuse. Vibration (tuning fork) and position sensibility (toe movements) can be recorded as present or absent.

Sensibility threshold tests

Although there are no really objective test methods for assessing the critical sensory neuropathic threshold below which breakdown is likely to occur, there are three sensory modalities that are crudely quantifiable.

Tactile pressure measurement is provided by use of the Semmes–Weinstein monofilament bristle, which, when applied to the skin under bending load, produces a standard pressure dependent upon the thickness. A set of three monofilaments of logarithmic pressure scales giving 1, 10 and 75 g force are in common clinical use. The 10 g (5.07 scale) has been considered the threshold level for neuropathic breakdown (Birke & Sims 1986, Sosenko et al 1987).

Temperature sensibility testing at various levels is difficult to achieve, but specific heat and cold extremes of 45°C and 0°C (with warm water and ice in test tubes) provide a positive or negative response,

Vibration sensibility threshold gives a more accurate and repeatable comparable testing when measured using a mains driven vibrometer (BioThesiometer) (Hockaday et al 1982, Bloom et al 1984). Age and sex charts of normal values have been calculated for different sites, including the feet. However, serial changes over a period in each patient would be more practical in monitoring the neuropathic progress.

Sensory nerve impairment by electroconduction testing and autonomic neuropathy assessment with galvanic skin stimulation provide qualitative indications of the neuropathies but they are not of quantitative clinical value. Similarly, electrodiagnostic motor nerve conduction and electromyography tests are also of a qualitative and diagnostic value only.

Plantar pressure assessment

Corns, calluses, previous scars and ulcerations with bony underlying prominences are clinical indicators of high pressure areas in many diabetic neuropathic feet. Higher pressure sites, particularly in the metatarsal regions, are associated with claw toes, hallux valgus and pes cavus. Restricted movement, as with hallux rigidus, midfoot plantaris, hindfoot varus and ankle stiffness are all associated with increased abnormal loading and clinical pressure problems. A whole range of residual foot deformities from the Charcot osteoarthropathy also produce abnormal bone and joint displacement with further high pressure loading in the often severely insensitive neuropathic foot.

Recently, improved pedobarometric devices have become available for evaluation of the plantar pressure profiles in the at-risk neuropathic foot. Application of the modern electronics and computerized data collection and recording systems has provided such devices for use in clinical settings. These plantar pressure monitoring systems were at first limited to a dynamic bare foot platform, or two plates, for analysis of the pressure recorded from a single foot contact. The high pressure areas are then defined with potential for breakdown and a decision on further management (Stokes et al 1975, Betts et al 1980, Veves et al 1992). More recently still, insole transducers have been developed for in-shoe pressure monitoring. These are still under development but will provide essential feedback on the pressure-relieving characteristics of various insole materials for protective neuropathic footwear (Cavanagh et al 1992). Breakdown threshold pressure levels, or more practically, risk levels at various pressures have not so far been defined, but the values seem to be very device-specific. Other factors, particularly the time-load, are important for ulceration and would be very dependent upon the walking and standing activity of the individual patient. Thus, the currently available plantar pressure monitors are able to define the elevated plantar pressures with plantar ulceration association, but further advances are required for these platform and in-shoe devices to be used for prediction and site of foot ulceration and its subsequent safe footwear treatment (Cavanagh & Ulbrecht 1994).

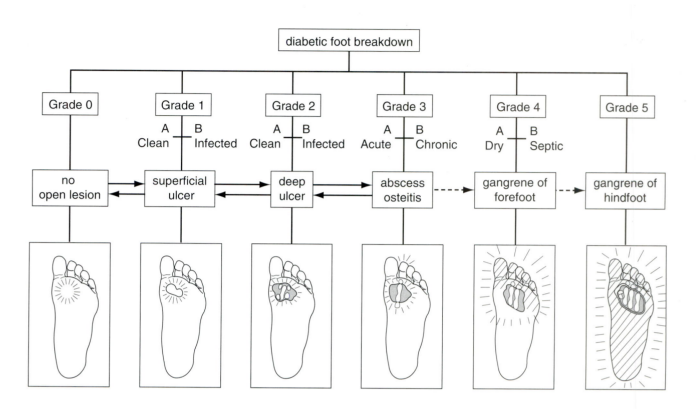

Figure 6

Meggitt–Wagner clinical classification of diabetic foot lesions

Natural history and classification of diabetic foot lesions

The classification of diabetic foot complications, based essentially on the underlying pathology as septic, neuropathic, ischaemic and mixed groups, has improved the understanding of the aetiology of the lesions (Oakley 1954). A clinical classification, developed from a study of the natural history of the progressive diabetic foot breakdown (Fig. 6), has been presented (Meggitt 1972, 1973, 1976, 1988). It has six grades in order to provide a basis for a treatment flow chart. Use of this clinical classification and further development of the flow charts, with application to other dysvascular feet, has also been reported (Wagner 1979, 1981). The six classification grades show progressive severity from the early at risk potential lesions to progressive deeper ulceration, abscess formation with or without bone and joint involvement. Occasionally, closed deep lesions occur; these are secondary to penetrating injuries, infections with small skin defects, and previously healed lesions.

With recent diabetic computer audit records this classification has been improved by separating the acute septic lesions from the cleaner ones at each level. This grading system is as follows:

Grade 0   No open lesions but potential breakdown with sensory neuropathy and high pressure deformities – the at risk foot.

Grade 1   The lesion is superficial through the skin only, usually with prominent underlying bone; 1A – clean ulcer, 1B – infected ulcer

Grade 2   The ulcer is deep, penetrating to bone, tendon or joint; 2A – clean ulcer; 2B – infected sloughy ulcer

Grade 3   Deep abscess formation involving plantar spaces, tendon sheath, osteomyelitis or septic arthritis; 3A – acute abscess; 3B – chronic deep infection

Grade 4   Gangrene present locally in the toes and diffusely over the forefoot; 4A – dry gangrene; 4B – wet infected gangrene

Grade 5   Gangrene involving whole foot requiring higher amputation

The progress from Grade 0 to Grade 3 was a common observation with the original study (Meggitt 1972), with the patient walking on an insensitive foot, causing initial tissue breakdown followed by secondary infection being pumped into the foot or, in some situations, already present from a previously apparent healed lesion. These processes are technically reversible with appropriate treatment. Progress from the deep abscess to forefoot

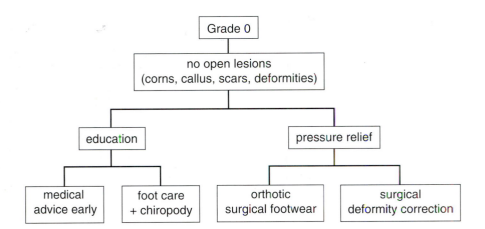

Figure 7

Grade 0: at risk foot treatment flow chart

gangrene, commonly involving one or more toes, can follow increasing tissue pressure with arterial or venous thrombosis, particularly to segments of the anterior pedal arch vessels. However, this may well be associated with a high incidence of peripheral angiopathy with or without calcification and end-artery disease in the diabetic foot. Finally, progress from Grade 4 to Grade 5 is usually associated with major vessel disease in the leg, with critical ankle inflow being unable to meet the demands of the other foot lesions.

Treatment programmes

The working hypothesis that the main cause of diabetic foot breakdown is high local pressure or trauma in the presence of impaired sensibility, foot deformities, or lowered resistance to an infection, with most likely tissue nutritional deficiencies from a basic microvascular disease, can provide a rationale for treatment. The clinical classification (Fig. 6) provides the basis for a comprehensive management framework with the development of a treatment flow chart. This allows recognition of the lesions, comparison of different treatments and their outcome. These flow charts form a sequence of treatment steps for each grade, obtained by matching the requirements for healing against the optimum available materials and techniques.

The patient who is referred with a diabetic foot problem requires full general assessment and specific lower limb and foot evaluation as described above. The essential clinical information required for a full foot evaluation involves the vascularity level in the hindfoot from the ankle and the forefoot from the toes, the neuropathic severity and localization, and the high-pressure sites associated with deformity, which are all recorded before the lesion itself is considered. With signs of clinically reduced arterial flow and ischaemia and with vascularity measurements at a critical or severe ischaemic level

(Doppler ankle index < 40% or toe pressure < 30 mmHg), urgent referral to a vascular reconstruction service is essential. With higher pressure indices and clinically adequate circulation, grading of the lesion and its appropriate treatment plan then follows.

Treatment of Grade 0 disease

This is essentially the at risk diabetic foot (Fig. 7) showing various degrees of neuropathy deformities but no open lesions. Treatment is preventative, with full education of the patient and the patient's family, and relief of pressure over dangerous areas.

Education

Advice on daily feet inspection with a bathroom mirror for the sole, washing with soap and water only and drying well, and the application of a lanolin or other aqueous cream to prevent drying, is given. Direct external heat to the insensitive feet should be avoided, especially from hot water bottles, electric pads and blankets, fires and car heaters. This information, together with other help, is given both verbally and in the foot section of a diabetic advisory booklet.

Orthotic footwear

The principle of 'cushioning the foot' on a total-contact moulded resilient insole is used to provide maximum plantar pressure distribution during weight bearing, thus reducing the local high-load areas. A clearance of at least 1 cm depth of insole from the lowest point of the foot is necessary to prevent 'bottoming out' (Fig. 8a). This is provided with the orthotist's prescription as the 'extra depth insole', which usually has a composite lamination with base high density, intermediate medium density plastizotes and a thin cover of soft calf leather or

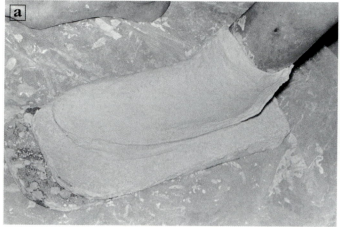

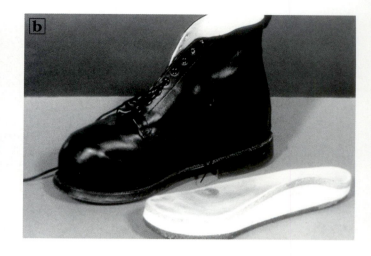

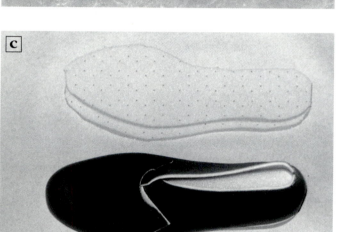

Figure 8

Orthotic extra depth footwear: (a) plaster cast moulding for last; (b) boot with rocker and composite insole leather covered; (c) temporary thermomouldable shoe and insoles

neoprene. Various techniques are available for producing a last of the diabetic feet. One commonly used involves a plaster cast or hard foam last made from plaster of Paris moulding, 50% weight bearing on a thick plaster cast slab (see Fig. 8a). Appropriate rectification of the plaster last is undertaken by the experienced orthotist, with reduction or addition to areas for higher or lower loading. The 'extra depth insole' and custom made 'extra depth shoe or boot', with a firm sole is made from the last (Fig. 8b). Three pairs of insoles are prescribed with each pair of shoes, with variable duration before thinning, and they are replaced when the patient reaches the last pair. A rocker sole is added for foot stiffness, or an ankle orthlene or metal brace is fitted for any ankle weakness. In recent years, thick foam-lined insole trainers with lacing opening to the toe have become available and many patients without severe deformities can be accommodated comfortably and safely with this footwear.

For emergency prescription, or for house use by the elderly, the direct thermomouldable 'extra depth' plastizote insole and lined shoe is fitted using an infrared oven within a few minutes (Fig. 8c). In a patient who has severe neuropathic feet and deformities, which often

follow Charcot's osteoarthropathy in the overweight, the plantar surface is too small to obtain insole pressure relief. The load is then transferred higher with a patellar tendon–tibial condylar bearing brace fitted to the heel of the extra depth shoe. The acute Charcot osteoarthropathy foot is at high risk from breakdown and this requires rested elevation, followed by application of a well-moulded laminate plaster of Paris and synthetic cast to allow mobilization.

Prophylactic surgery

If conservative treatment with the orthotic footwear is not sufficient when breakdown has occurred and healed, and threatens again, then surgical relief of the intrinsic pressure is necessary by correcting the deformities. After adequate assessment and selection, successful treatment with the commoner orthopaedic operations can be obtained. Thus treatment of ingrowing toenails with wedge resections or matrix ablations, hallux valgus with bunionectomy, metatarsal osteotomy or Keller's arthroplasty, claw toes with tendon transfers or arthrodeses, and metatarsal head protrusions with osteotomies or Fowler's procedures have all been undertaken (Fig. 9).

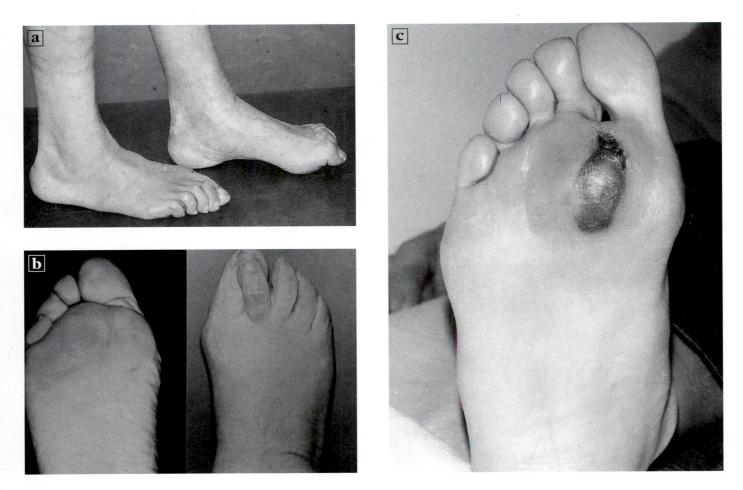

Figure 9

Grade 0 at risk foot – neuropathy and deformities (for prophylactic surgery): (a) pes cavus and claw toes (API = 76%, TP = 43 mmHg); (b) hallux valgus and dislocated second toe with plantar callus (API = 80%, TP = 60); (c) Subcutaneous haematoma with second metatarsal pressure

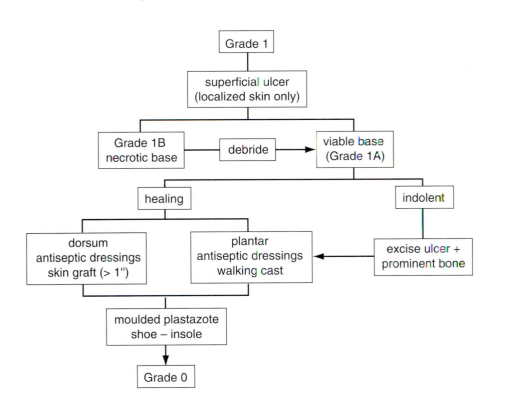

Figure 10

Grade 1: Superficial ulcer treatment flow chart

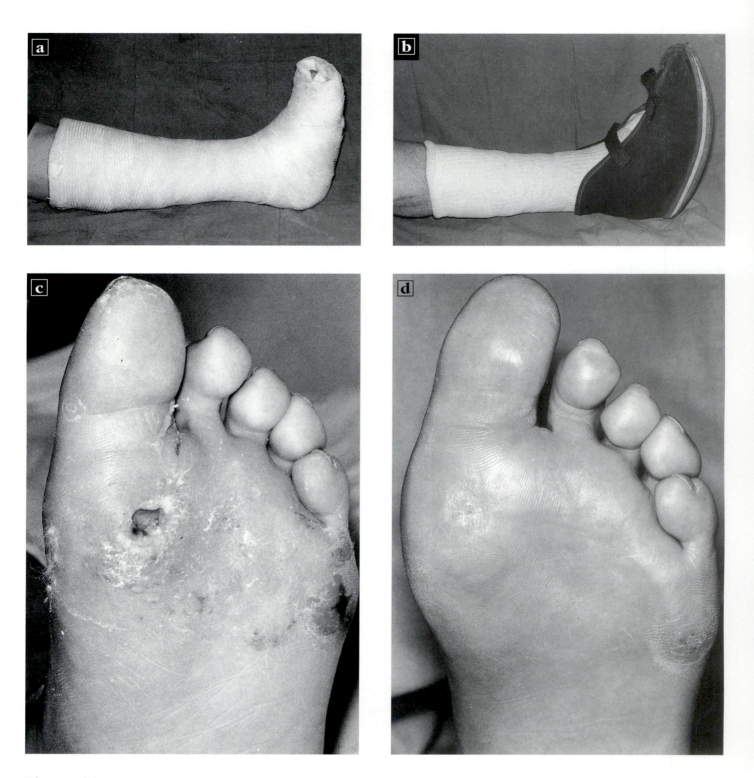

Figure 11

Walking cast treatment of plantar ulcers: (a) total contact cast of plaster – synthetic laminate; (b) rocker cast boot fitted; (c) Grade 1 ulcer lateral and Grade 2 medial anaesthetic foot before cast; (d) lesions healed after 9 weeks' cast treatment

Treatment of Grade 1 disease

Superficial ulcers through the skin only, if infected with a necrotic base (Grade 1B), require bacteriological swab to assess the organisms, a course of systemic antibiotics for the cellulitic infection, and debridement for conversion to a clean ulcer (Grade 1A). The most effective and rapid debridement is mechanical, with forceps, scissors or scalpel, removing the slough from the insensitive ulcer, or with debridement agents, followed by antiseptic cleansing (Fig. 10). The environment for granulation

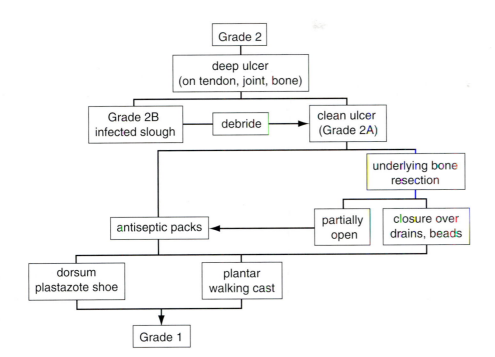

Figure 12

Grade 2: Deep ulcer treatment flow chart

tissue, healing and epithelialization from the edges is maintained with a simple low adherent dressing or paraffin tulle. Ulcers on the dorsum or sides of the foot, usually caused by shoe trauma, will epithelialize satisfactorily if they are small, but larger ulcers (> 0.5 cm diameter), require a skin graft once there is a satisfactory clean granulating base. Support and protection is required with a gauze pad and an elasticated crepe or tubular bandage. Foot protection during this healing phase should be with a thermomoulded plastizoate boot.

On the plantar surface, similar treatment can be undertaken for very small ulcers but for larger ones, once the ulcer is clean, relief of the high local pressure is needed with a below-knee total-contact walking cast. This is a well-moulded plaster of Paris cast with a thin layer of plaster wool over the nonadherent dressing on the ulcer. An improved and lighter design is with a laminate of thin plaster of Paris for total contact and an outer synthetic cast for strength (Fig. 11a). A rocker roll-off cast or overboot is also provided for a more even gait; this allows the patient to remain safely walking out of hospital during the healing phase (Fig. 11b). The cast should mould the toes in a neutral position with either the end open to allow aeration and direct change of

Table 1 Topical agents

Irrigant and antiseptic solutions	
sodium chloride warm solution 0.9%	Clean ulcers (Grades 1A, 2A)
chlorhexidine solution 0.05%	Infected ulcers (Grades 1B, 2B, 3B)
hydrogen peroxide 3% & 6%	
acetic acid 5%	Septic pseudomonas (Grades 1B, 2B, 3B)
potassium permanganate solution 0.01%	Granulating ulcers (Grades 1A, 2A)
Topical antibiotic	
silver sulphadiazine cream 1%	septic sloughy ulcers (Grades 1B, 2B, 3B)
metronidazole geo 0.8%	malodorous septic ulcers (Grades 1B, 2B, 3B, 4B)
antibiotic powders contraindicated	rapid resistance, dermatitis and wound caking
Chemical debridement	
organic acids paste or cream	Aserbine, Variclene
hydrogen peroxide 1.5% cream	Hioxyl
enzymic solution or gel	Varidase
hydrocolloids, hydrogels, xerogels	dressings with debriding action

Table 2   Wound dressing – biological matching

Superficial wound or ulcer (Grades 1 and 2)
(a) Dry	low adherent dressing (e.g. Melonin, Mepore, Release)
	paraffin gauze (e.g. Tulle gras, Bactigras, Inadine)
(b) Low exudate	low adherent dressing (as (a) above)
	semipermeable film (e.g. Opsite, Tegaderm, Bioclusive)
(c) Moderate exudate	viscous monofilament (e.g. Tricotex N-A)
	hydrocolloids e.g. Granuflex, Tegasorb, Vigilon, Biofilm
(d) Heavy exudate	sugar paste
	xerogels beads or paste (e.g. Debrisan, Cadexomer iodine)
	hydrogels granules (e.g. Scherisorb, Geliperm)
	hydrocolloids (as (c) above)
	alginates (e.g. Sorban, Kallostat)
	synthetic foams (e.g. Lyofoam, Allevyn, silastic foam)

Deep ulcers and cavities (Grades 2 and 3)
Variable exudates	gauze ribbon packing with antiseptic (e.g. chlorhexidine, povidone iodine)
	hydrocolloid paste (e.g. Comfeel, Biofilm)
	silastic foam pack

Gangrene (Grade 4)
Antisepsis and odour reduction	Povidone iodine wet pack, Metronidazole gel

dressing, or with the toes completely enclosed. The plaster of Paris allows some absorption of exudate and can be changed every 4 weeks until full healing has occurred (Fig. 11c,d). A temporary plastizoate shoe after removal of the cast protects the foot until a satisfactory extra depth shoe is provided. The rest of the management is then as in Grade 0.

Treatment of Grade 2 disease

In Grade 2 disease, there is deep ulcer penetration through the subcutaneous tissue onto tendon, ligament, bone or joint structures, usually starting with an infected, sloughy lesion of Grade 2B (see Fig. 11c). Treatment again requires culture and sensitivity of the pathogens, a course of antibiotics if associated with cellulitis, and extensive surgical debridement of all the necrotic tissue, often without anaesthetic in the insensitive foot (Fig. 12). Residual necrotic tissue may require further treatment with chemical desloughing agents, with antiseptic if purulent, or with saline cleansing between applications, and appropriate dressings for moderate or heavy exudates. A large number of wound cleansing agents and different dressings have been developed recently but few as yet have received clinical trials. It is now possible to match the healing requirement empirically with the optimum agents and dressings available (Tables 1 and 2). With dorsal foot lesions, the plastizoate moulded boot can be used to maintain safe mobility. On the plantar surface a total contact below-knee walking cast

is used if the ulcer is clean with low exudate. This allows the patient safe walking out of hospital.

A modification of the cast has been used in Cambridge, UK for a number of years for the deeper, larger ulcers with fairly heavy exudate requiring regular cleansing and dressing – a small window exactly over the ulcer, which is usually in the metatarsal or heel region (Fig. 13), is cut out and refashioned with a further segment of cast being attached and overlapping the surrounding cast by 1 cm. This allows regular dressings on removal of the window and reapplication with circumferential elastoplast. The new cast edge prevents sinkage of the window and any increased pressure. A reinforced synthetic cast sole is used, and a rocker plaster overboot (see Fig. 13a,b).

Where there are large bony prominences underlying the ulceration, with slow healing or recurrent breakdown, then relief of this 'intrinsic pressure' is required surgically. Thus Keller's bunionectomy arthroplasty, metatarsal head excisions or elevation osteotomies, claw toe straightening and exostectomies of any prominent underlying bone, may be required. The wounds are kept as small as possible and primary closure undertaken with mini-vacuum drains and intravenous antibiotic cover. In some situations, the ulcer itself may be excised and closed with the same regime. Plantar wound protection may be required with a total contact walking cast for out-patient treatment.

Occasionally, a Grade 2B ulcer may remain indolent with no attempt at healing, in which case further surgical debridement may be necessary to excise the ulcer and the underlying bone to allow the tissues to oppose. This may require partial or complete ray resection in the forefoot,

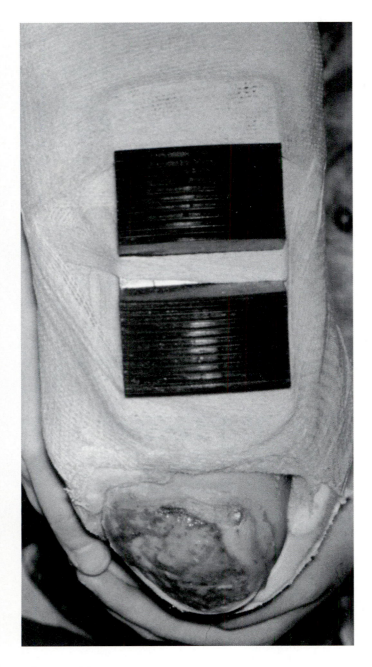

Figure 13

Grade 2 ulcer of the heel – walking synthetic cast with rocker and replaceable window for dressings

large exostectomies, Charcot bone extrusion, or large resection of posterior calcaneum for hindfoot ulceration. Further treatment is then as in Grade 1 and Grade 0.

Treatment of Grade 3 disease

This lesion involves a deep abscess, often with osteomyelitis and joint involvement (Fig. 14), presenting

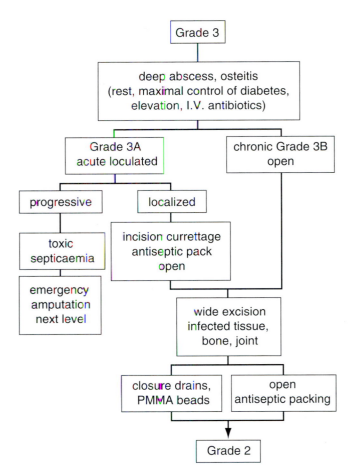

Figure 14

Grade 3: deep abscess – osteitis treatment flow chart.

either as an acute infection (Grade 3A) or a chronic flare with intermittent discharging sinuses or ulceration (Grade 3B). Urgent treatment with limb rest and elevation, intravenous antibiotics and diabetic control is necessary. An acute fluctuant abscess (Fig. 15) is treated primarily with incision, drainage and curettage followed by open antiseptic packing. Once the acute lesion is localized, a second stage is necessary with wide excision of all necrotic tissue, including associated tendons, ligaments, bone or joint structures under appropriate antibiotic cover.

In the diabetic, chronic infections are often very deceptive with a small surface sinus communicating with a deep 'volcano lesion' with infected necrotic tissue. These can prove very difficult to eradicate, since they may extend widely. Surgical debridement procedures often require partial, multiple or complete ray resection and occasionally, with very extensive destruction, partial foot amputation. Similarly the acute plantar space infection can become very destructive and usually enter

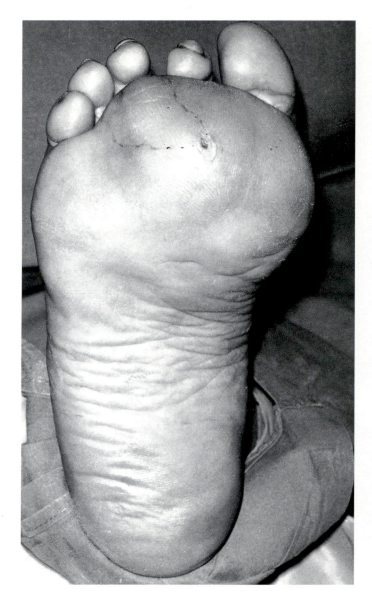

Figure 15

Grade 3 lesion with acute abscess from previous ulcer fluctuant area marked

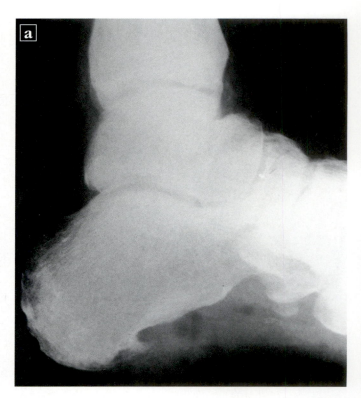

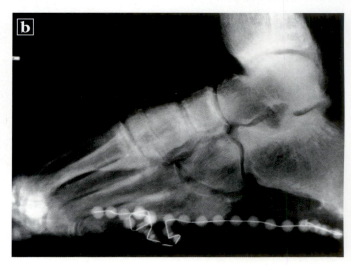

Figure 16

Acute central plantar abscess from a heel ulcer: (a) nonclostridial gas formation; (b) gentamicin bead chain in debrided central space abscess cavity

through penetrating ulcers. Thus the medial and lateral plantar space abscesses commonly occur via pressure ulcers under the first and fifth metatarsals and, the most severe of all, the central plantar abscess through toe infections down the flexor sheaths, and via deep septic metatarsal or heel ulceration (Fig. 16a,b).

Following wide resection or localized amputation, the residual cavity is treated with antibiotic irrigation–drainage system allowing ingress of saline-antibiotic solution through the wound. An alternative and much more nurse-friendly treatment has proved very successful – this is the use of local depot high-level antibiotic by implanting a chain of gentamicin polymethylmethacrylate beads, leaving one protruding through the end of the

sutured incision. A semi-occlusive membrane dressing is applied over the wound and the bead, leaving a small nonvacuum drain in the operation site to prevent haematoma. The chain can be withdrawn after 3 weeks and, usually, there is very little discharge, if any, and the whole operation site becomes quiescent. The slow, high-level antibiotic release has been shown to be far in excess of the mean inhibitory concentrations for all bacteria, providing rapid local control of the infected cavity

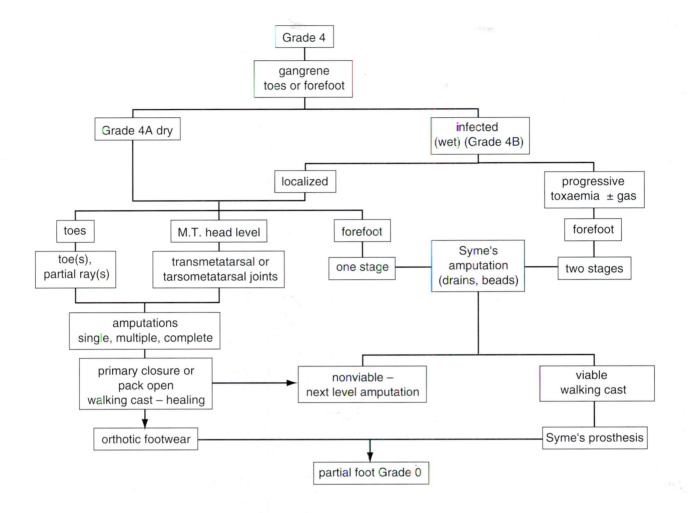

Figure 17

Grade 4: forefoot gangrene treatment flow chart

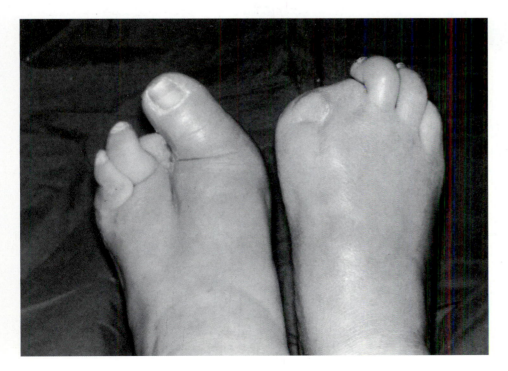

Figure 18

Multiple toectomies and ray resections for forefoot infection and gangrene: five procedures over 12 years with still functional feet (API = 60% left & 52% right, TP = 40 mmHg)

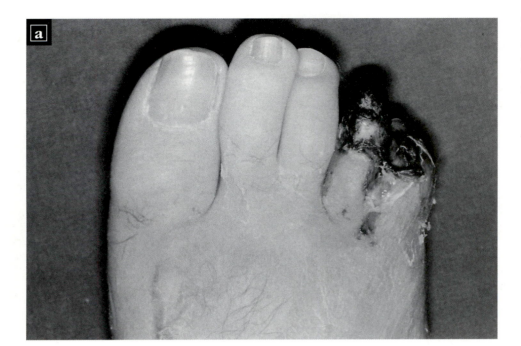

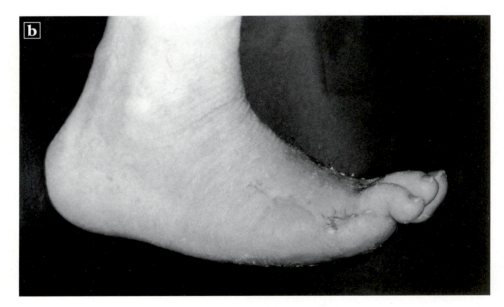

Figure 19

Grade 4A lesion: (a) 'dry' gangrene of fourth and fifth toes (API = 70%, TP = 50 mmHg); (b) After fourth and fifth partial ray resections healed

after adequate surgical debridement (Wahlig et al 1978). The reliability and simplicity of this implant technique has considerable advantages over the more complex nursing required with irrigation–drainage systems.

With the debrided cavities left open, appropriate packing type dressing with alginate ribbon, hydrocolloid paste or silastic foam is undertaken. Once adequate granulation, epithelialization and healing is under way, further treatment is undertaken as in Grade 2.

Treatment of Grade 4 disease

Grade 4A lesions involve noninfected 'dry' gangrene; Grade 4B involves septic 'wet' gangrene of the toes or forefoot (Fig. 17) where partial foot amputation is mandatory, if vascular assessment is satisfactory at the ankle. General treatment involves leg elevation and rest, diabetic metabolic control and systemic antibiotics. Locally the gangrene is treated with regular antiseptic soaks; dressing with povidone solution is very effective in controlling the surface infection and odour. Any combination of resections of the foot may be undertaken to provide viable flap closure involving toes, rays and metatarsal disarticulation as partial, complete, single or multiple procedures (Figs. 18, 19, 20). In cases of (now rare) infected wet type of gangrene, with progressive severe toxaemia and often septicaemia, amputation of the life-threatening limb is an emergency and should be undertaken at the next safe viable level (Fig. 21).

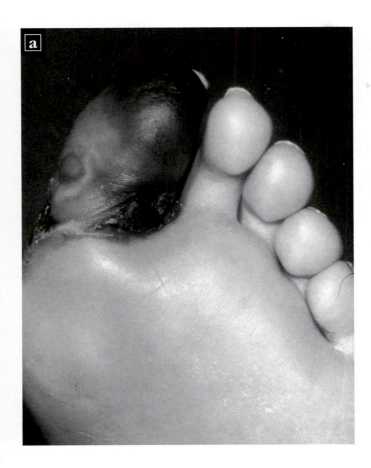

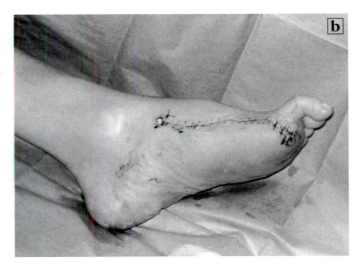

Figure 20

Grade 4B lesion: (a) septic 'wet' gangrene hallux (API = 65%, TP > 42 mmHg); (b) after first ray amputation with small bead gentamicin chain in the cavity

Toe amputation

This is indicated for localized gangrene of the toes as well as for chronic lesions for ulceration, phalangeal osteitis and septic arthritis. The amputation is undertaken through healthy skin with adequate racquet, fishmouth or eccentric flaps. In amputation of the hallux, the base of the proximal phalanx should be preserved if possible to maintain weight bearing push-off tissue over the first metatarsals. In this procedure or, if necessary, with disarticulation through the first metatarsophalangeal joint, the extensor hallucis longus tendon should be sutured to the dorsal capsule under tension, so preserving its dorsiflexion and inversion function in the forefoot. Similarly, the lesser long toe extensors require reattachment to the dorsal capsules and metatarsal heads with metatarsophalangeal joint amputations to rebalance the forefoot and reduce excessive impact pressure in the plantar flexion phase of gait.

Ray resection

When gangrene extends to the base of the toes, or chronic infection involves the metatarsals, then partial or complete ray resection is necessary. All necrotic tissue is excised with, ideally, a racquet incision bringing the long 'handle' proximally over the dorsum of the foot to avoid plantar surface scarring. When there is an associated metatarsal ulcer, this can be included in a plantar skin wedge excision. The metatarsal bone is excised cleanly with a small air saw or, if necessary, disarticulated at the metatarsotarsal joint. Wound closure is partial with low adherent dressing, or complete over a nonvacuum drain or small size gentamicin bead chain with semiocclusive membrane film for 3 weeks. Once the wound is healing satisfactorily, the patient is mobilized in a total contact walking cast, with appropriate window as necessary, as in Grade 3 late management. If reinfection or further breakdown occurs and there is adequate tissue vascularity, then either more extensive local resection is undertaken or, if necessary, a more proximal amputation at the transmetatarsal, tarsometatarsal or Syme ankle level (see Fig. 21).

Transmetatarsal amputation

Transmetatarsal amputation through the metatarsal shafts is indicated when the gangrene or extensive chronic infection extends to the base of multiple toes and into the distal forefoot, or with healing failure of toectomies or partial ray resections. Transmetatarsal amputation for diabetic gangrene and infection has been reported in large series as providing a functional and durable foot (McKittrick et al 1949, Wheelock 1961, Baddeley & Fulford 1965) (Fig. 22).

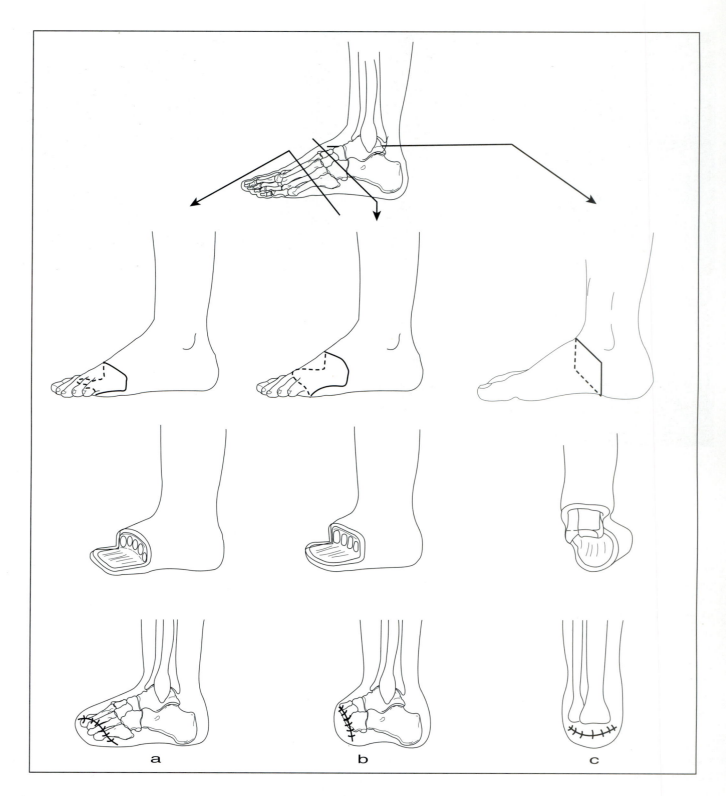

Figure 21

Partial foot amputations: functional levels. (a) Transmetatarsal, (b) Lisfranc, (c) Syme

The transmetatarsal amputation technique (see Fig. 21) involves a curved incision across the dorsum of the foot through all tissues at the level of the metatarsal bone resection. At the sides, the incision is taken vertically and then distally to approximately 1 cm from the base of the toes to give a long plantar flap, slightly longer on the medial side, to allow for greater foot depth there.

The metatarsal shafts are divided from the dorsum with an oblique plantar undercut and, with retraction, dissection is carried forward along the metatarsal plantar

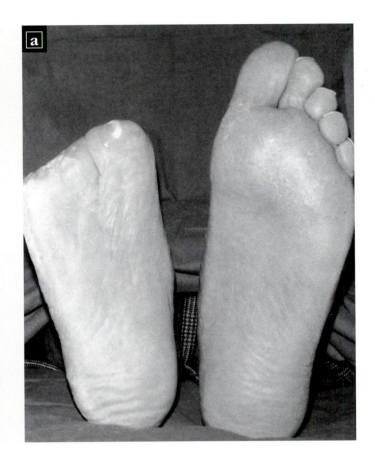

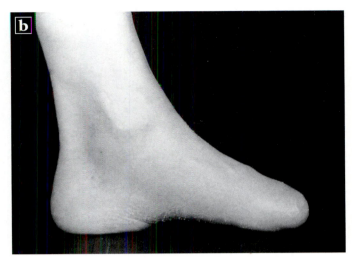

Figure 22

Transmetatarsal amputation: (a) durable amputation after 10 years (API = 65%); (b) functional foot length for normal shoe

surfaces to complete the amputation. With some recent longer-term pressure studies, a plantar–valgus deformity occurs from tendon imbalance, giving high impact in the flat foot gait phase with high medial stump loading on push-off. To provide a long term durable transmetatarsal stump, rebalance of the tendons is required with extensor hallucis longus being sutured to the periosteum via a drill hole through the dorsum of the first resected metatarsal end. The lesser extensor tendons may be similarly sutured to their appropriate metatarsal, with moderate tension, having the foot in slight dorsiflexion. The procedure is completed by closure in two layers, without tension, with a nonvacuum drain or, in cases of infection, with a chain of small gentamicin beads.

Further support with wound detensioning using a semipermeable adhesive dressing can be provided to the suture line, followed by a well-padded posterior cast splint. The drain is removed at 48 hours and the beads are withdrawn at 2 weeks. Once the incision is healed, a total contact laminate walking cast is applied until the scar and end-amputation tissues have matured. An extra depth moulded plastizote shoe with insole and end filler can then be fitted, followed by a similar permanent protective orthotic footwear.

Lisfranc amputation

Disarticulation amputation through the tarsometatarsal (Lisfranc) joints is indicated when gangrene or chronic infection extends proximally to the metatarsal head level and there is insufficient skin for a transmetatarsal amputation (Fig. 23a).

A problem with the Lisfranc amputation, which caused it to fall into disrepute, has been the development of an equinovarus deformity giving problems with walking function, prosthesis and footwear. This deformity results from imbalance loss of the long toe extensors and peroneal brevis and overpull of the Achilles tendon, tibialis posterior and tibialis anterior. This can be overcome with rebalance of the foot by suturing the toe extensors and peroneus brevis laterally. An Achilles tendon lengthening can be undertaken if there is a later tendency for an equinbus deformity to develop, in order to weaken the plantarflexion of the ankle and balance the less powerful dorsiflexors. However, this has not been necessary in a fairly large series of Lisfranc amputations undertaken in Cambridge, UK. A further advantage of the Lisfranc amputation is that the patient is able to wear a normal boot or shoe of a slightly larger size using a soft calf leather lightweight zip closure bootee with a moulded polypropylene sole plate and toe filler (Fig. 24a,b). The 'Cambridge Lisfranc ZIP Appliance' (Meggitt 1980) is lighter and more functional than the older 'Chopart Appliance' with block leather lace-up boot and steel sole plate. Recent development of the 'silicone slipper partial foot prosthesis' is under trial at present (Fig. 24c). The alternative is a Syme's amputation, which requires full prosthesis in the long term and leaves a less functional foot.

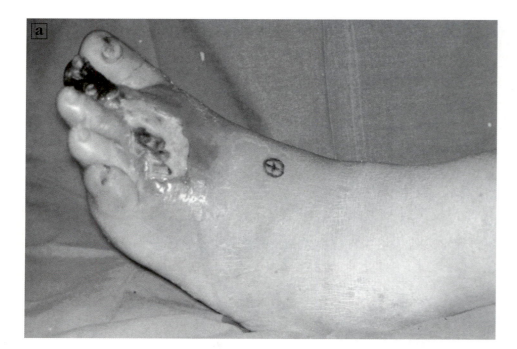

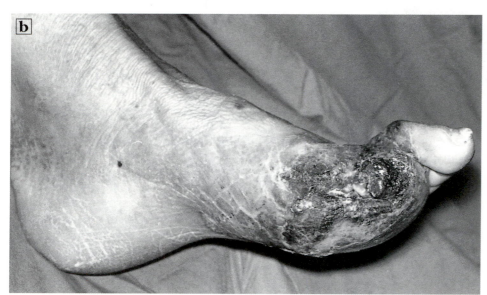

Figure 23

Indications for partial foot amputations: (a) septic forefoot gangrene: Lisfranc salvage (API = 72%); (b) dry gangrene after first ray resection: Syme salvage (API = 52%)

The technique of the Lisfranc amputation (see Fig. 21) involves a transverse dorsal incision over the tarsometatarsal joints level, extending approximately two-thirds down each side vertically and then longitudinally distal, to finish transversely across the metatarsal neck level. The tendons of the extensor hallucis, the lesser toes and the peroneus brevis are divided a little distally to the incision. The tarsometatarsal joints are disarticulated and dissection carried forward beneath them and along the metatarsal plantar surfaces to complete the amputation at the distal transverse incision. The peroneus brevis tendon is then sutured to the remaining capsule from the fifth metatarsal–cuboid joint with the foot in eversion and slight dorsiflexion. The long toe extensors are sutured to the remaining dorsal capsules of the cuboid–metatarsal joints if these are adequate; if not, then fixation is through drill holes in the cuboid–cuneiform bones, beginning with the extensor hallucis longus in the middle and the lesser tendons laterally under moderate tension, as with the peroneus brevis. Thus a dorsiflexion–valgus rebalance is provided. Postoperatively the management is similar to the trans-metatarsal amputation but, once healed, a Lisfranc appliance or the newer silicone slipper partial foot prosthesis is provided by the prosthetic service.

Syme's amputation

A Syme's amputation is indicated if gangrene or deep infection extends proximally past the forefoot, if partial

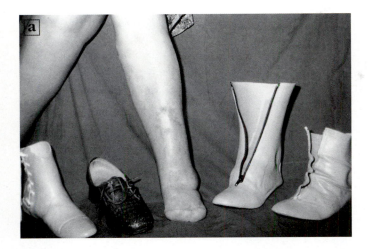

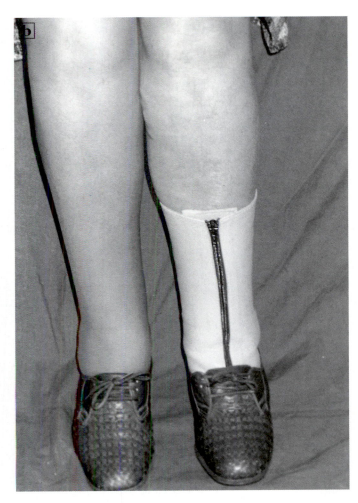

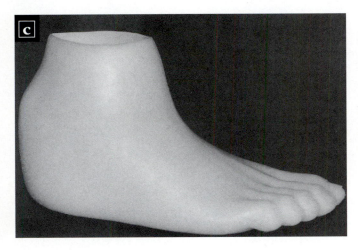

Figure 24

Lisfranc amputation and prosthesis: (a) tendon balanced stump, older heavy Chopart type prosthesis (left) and new lighter Lisfranc ZIP appliances (right); (b) Lisfranc appliance fitted with a larger normal shoe; (c) new silicone slipper foot prosthesis

foot amputations are not possible or if they have failed to heal (see Fig. 23b). Contraindications are necrosis that extends to the heel flap level, chronic oedema of the foot, or ulceration or infection of the heel itself. Adequate vascularity of the hindfoot is essential, with the Doppler ankle pressure index > 40%. The presence of a sensory neuropathy in the heel is not in itself a contraindication if the skin and heel pad are healthy (Harris 1956, Baker & Stableforth 1969).

Although the ankle disarticulation amputation was described over 150 years ago (Syme 1843) it did not become widely accepted until the last 50 years (Alldredge & Thompson 1946, Harris 1961). Reports have indicated the successful use of the Syme's amputation in peripheral vascular disease (Warren et al 1955, Dale 1961, Mazet 1968). A modified Syme amputation has been developed as a two-stage procedure involving primary disarticulation and then later, when healed, a secondary stump formation, for the salvage of failed forefoot reconstructive surgery (Hulnick et al 1949) and

after infected war wounds (Spittler et al 1954). The procedure has been successfully applied to the diabetic foot with gangrene, using the same rationale. Then, with the development of the Doppler ankle pressure index (Carter 1973), improved selection of this two-stage Syme procedure in the diabetic was reported to have an over 90% success rate (Wagner et al 1980).

The original reasoning for the two-stage procedure in the diabetic in the early 1970s was difficulty in controlling the infection and the often doubtful vascularity. This became much less valid with the introduction of wide spectrum antibiotics, improved surgical techniques and better evaluation of tissue vascularity. The modified Syme's amputation requires two operations, a prolonged hospitalization period and difficulty in mobilizing between the procedures. The one-stage Syme involves one operation and a shorter hospitalization.

This has been confirmed in a series in Cambridge, UK with over 20 years' experience of the one-stage Syme's amputation for diabetic midfoot gangrene or chronic

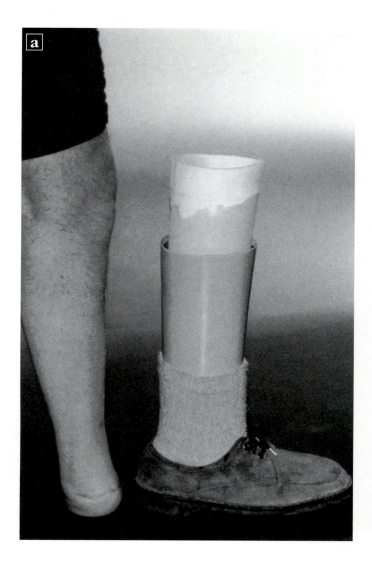
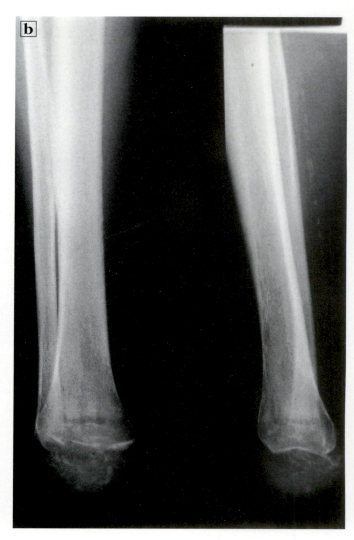

Figure 25

Syme amputation and prosthesis: (a) stable end-bearing stump and temporary prosthesis; (b) radiographs showing ankle disarticulation and malleoli resection

infection, with no failures from secondary infection with adequate vascularity indicated by an API > 40% (Meggitt 1996). A Syme's amputation in one stage is now considered indicated for most unsalvagable foot breakdown lesions extending to the midfoot level, and the two-stage Syme procedure reserved only for the severe acutely infected forefoot. The Syme amputation stump is very functional, with end-bearing (Fig. 25) and allows an easily donned and doffed prosthesis. The energy requirements are much less in a Syme's amputation walker than in higher level amputees, this being significant in the many diabetics who have cardiovascular complications (Waters et al 1976).

The operative technique (see Fig. 21) involves an incision from the tip of the lateral malleolus, extending transversely across the ankle from just below the distal tibia to a point opposite, usually 1 cm below the

tip of the medial malleolus. The incision continues vertically down the sides to the sole, and transversely across at right angles to the foot. The tendons are divided under tension to retract proximally in order to avoid scar adherence, and the vessels are ligated. The ankle joint capsule is opened anteriorly with dissection down the sides of the talus to divide the collateral ligaments from the inside. With the aid of a bone hook, in the talus first and then the calcaneum, dissection is carried out posteriorly taking care to protect the neurovascular bundle posteriomedially. The Achilles tendon and posterior attachment of the long plantar ligament are divided by sharp dissection, but the rest of the os calcis is delivered subperiosteally, working from side to side to preserve the pressure-tolerant fibrofatty heel pad compartments intact. On reaching the plantar incision level, the amputation is completed transversely with the traditional Syme's knife. After plantar vessel ligation and nerve division away from the suture line, the malleoli are dissected and excised level with the abraded tibial articular surface. The remaining sharp corners are rounded off with vertical bone resection by approximately 1 cm. Closure in two layers of the periosteum to deep plantar fascia, and of the skin with absorbable sutures, follows over either an irrigation–drainage tube or antibiotic beads with a nonvacuum overflow drain laterally. An adhesive semipermeable film dressing is used to reduce tension in the Syme wound; this is applied first distally and then, with a little tension, over the wound proximally. With removal of the drain (2 days) or beads (14 days) a well-moulded synthetic below-knee walking cast is applied and the patient mobilized with elbow crutches or frame support. Once the stump is mature, a provisional and then definitive Syme's prosthesis is fitted by the prosthetic service.

With the two-stage procedure, the wound is closed immediately after disarticulation with application of a protective well-moulded below-knee plaster cast. When fully healed, 6–8 weeks later, the malleoli are resected through lateral incisions and the sharp corners are trimmed. A further period of healing is required before application of a walking cast.

Treatment of Grade 5 disease

Once gangrene or severe infection has extended into the hindfoot, a higher amputation is mandatory. Reassessment of the segmental vascular pressure index will determine whether the next best level at the below-knee site is possible, or whether a higher through-knee or above-knee amputation is necessary.

Prognosis

The ultimate management of the at risk foot in the diabetic population depends on the elucidation of the basic pathology of diabetes mellitus and its complications with the finding of a treatable cause. Until then, treatment remains essentially empirical and depends upon an efficient health care system involving:

- early diagnosis and treatment of diabetes mellitus, and evaluation and prophylactic screening for the diabetic foot at risk factors;
- improved assessment and treatment of foot breakdown lesions;
- effective rehabilitation after surgical and medical treatment to return patients to optimal functional level, and then continued education and prophylaxis for the remaining lower limbs.

The most effective prophylactic management of the diabetic foot breakdown is to reduce the incidence of vascular and neuropathic disease. Two recent large studies of insulin-dependent diabetics have reported that intensive glycaemic control significantly reduces the progress of microvascular disease and the development of neuropathy (Riechard et al 1993, Diabetes Control and Complications Trial 1993). Thus the prognosis for the diabetic foot complications currently depends upon providing the best possible glycaemic control long term.

The prognosis for the untreated intact sensory neuropathic foot for primary and secondary threatened ulceration is poor, but it can be significantly improved with patient education (Maloney et al 1989, Fletcher et al 1992), custom extra-depth footwear (Edmonds et al 1986) and corrective orthopaedic surgery for deformities and intrinsic pressure areas (Niklas 1991). When normovascular neuropathic ulceration is present, the prognosis for healing is good, with over 90% success (Meggitt 1976, Wagner 1979) using the Meggitt–Wagner clinical ulcer classification and treatment flow charts for each grade.

Foot breakdown in the neuroischaemic diabetic limb depends for the outcome on whether vascular reconstructive surgery is possible. The prognosis with diabetic iliac and femoropopliteal angioplasty is as successful at 5 years in the diabetic as in the nondiabetic (Stokes et al 1990), and for distal vein bypass to the dorsalis pedis, high foot salvage rates have been reported (Pomposelli et al 1990). Major vessel disease in critical chronic ischaemic lower limbs treated in specialist centres with modern vascular surgery shows considerable improvement in limb survival, with only 20% requiring primary amputation (Second European Consensus Document on Chronic Critical Leg Ischaemia 1991).

The diabetic vasculopathy is a progressive disease and the prognosis for further breakdown shows ipsilateral revision amputation rates of up to 10% between 1–10 years (Larsson & Anderssen 1978) and contralateral primary amputation rates of 30–50% (Mazet 1967, DHSS Amputation Statistics 1989). The life expectancy prognosis in diabetic patients with partial foot amputation has been little reported, but in patients with higher amputation levels, the mortality after 4 years is recorded at 25–50% (Ebskov & Josephsen 1980, DHSS Amputation Statistics 1989), perhaps indicating more generalized vascular disease. Thus it would appear now that the diabetic patients have equal risk for loss of their life as for loss of their limbs, making rapid rehabilitation essential for artificial limb function and contralateral limb preservation. Overall the current prognosis for the patient with the diabetic foot syndrome depends upon an efficient health care system with specialized diabetic foot clinics and multidisciplinary services available for prevention and research to provide the patient with optimal life and limb function.

References

Alldredge R H, Thompson T C 1946 The technique of the Syme amputation. J Bone Joint Surg 28: 415–436

Asbury A K, Johnson P C, Bennington J L (eds) 1978 Diabetic neuropathies. In: Pathology of Peripheral Nerves Vol 9: Major Problems in Pathology. W B Saunders Co, Philadelphia

Axtine S G 1982 Infection and diabetes mellitus. In: Bressler R, Johnson D J (eds) Management of Diabetes Mellitus. Wright, Bristol, Ch 9, p. 175

Baddeley R M, Fulford J C 1965 A trial of conservative amputations for lesions of the feet in diabetes mellitus. Br J Surg 52: 38

Baker G C W, Stableforth P G 1969 Syme's amputation. A review of sixty seven cases. J Bone Joint Surg 518: 482–487

Barnes R W, Thornhill B, Nix L, Rittgers S E, Turley G 1981 Prediction of amputation wound healing. Roles of Doppler ultrasound and digit photoplethysmography. Arch Surg 116: 80

Berquist T H, Brown M L, Fitzgerald R H et al 1985 Magnetic resonance imaging: application in musculo-skeletal infection. Magn Reson Imaging 3: 219–230

Bessman A N, Wagner F W 1975 Non-clostridial gas gangrene: report of 48 cases and review of the literature. JAMA 23: 958

Betts R P, Franks C I, Duckworth T, Burke J 1980 Static and dynamic foot pressure measurement in clinical orthopaedics. Med Biol Eng Comput 18(5): 674

Birke J A, Sims D S 1986 Plantar sensory threshold in the ulcerative foot. Lepr Rev 57: 261–267

Bloom S, Till S, Sönksen P, Smith S 1984 Use of biothesiometer to measure individual vibration thresholds and their variation in 519 non-diabetic subjects. BMJ 288: 1793

Boehm J J 1962 Diabetic Charcot's joint. N Engl J Med 267: 185

Bone G E, Pomajzl M J 1981 Toe blood pressure by photoplethysmography: an index of healing in forefoot amputations. Surgery 89: 569

Borssen B, Bergenheim T, Lithner F 1990 The epidemiology of foot lesions in diabetic patients aged 15–50 years. Diabetic Med 7: 43–44

Bose K 1979 A surgical approach for the infected diabetic foot. Int Orthop 3: 177

Brand P W 1978 Pathomechanics of diabetic neuropathic ulcer and its conservative management. In Bergan J J, Yoa J S T (eds) Gangrene and Severe Ischaemia of the Lower Extremities. Grune & Stratton, New York

Brodsky J W, Wagner F W, Kwong P K et al 1987 Patterns of breakdown in the Charcot tarsus of diabetes and relation to treatment. Orthop Trans 2: 484

Carter S A 1973 The relationship of distal systolic pressures to healing of skin lesions in limbs with arterial occlusive disease with special reference to diabetes mellitus. Scand J Chir Lab Invest 31 Suppl 128: 239

Cavanagh P R, Hewitt F G, Perry J E 1992 In-shoe plantar pressure measurements. A review. The Foot 2: 185–194

Cavanagh P R, Ulbrecht J S 1994 Clinical plantar pressure measurement in diabetes: rationale and methodology. The Foot 4: 123–135

Charcot J M 1868 Sur quelques arthropathies qui paraissent d'une lesion du cerveau ou de la moelle épinière. Archives de Physiologie Normale et Pathologique 1: 161

Cofield R H, Morrison M J, Beabout J W 1983 Diabetic neuropathy in the foot: patient characteristics and patterns of radiographic change. Foot Ankle 4: 15

Cowell J A, Lopes-Vivella M, Halushka P V 1981 Pathogenesis of atherosclerosis in diabetes mellitus. Diabetes Care 4: 121

Dale G M 1961 Syme's amputation for gangrene for peripheral vascular disease. Artif Limbs 6: 44

Dearfield J E, Daggett P R, Harrison M J G 1980 The role of autonomic neuropathy in diabetic foot ulceration. J Neurol Sci 47: 203

DHSS Amputation Statistics for England, Wales and N Ireland 1974–1983

DHSS Amputation Statistics for England, Wales and N Ireland 1989

Diabetes Control and Complications Trial Research Group 1993 The effect of intensive treatment of diabetes on the development and progression of long term complications in insulin dependent diabetes. N Eng J Med 329: 986–997

Dolkart R E, Halpern B, Perlman J 1971 Comparison of antibody responses in normal and alloxan diabetic mice. Diabetes 20: 162

Durham J R, Lukens M L, Campanini D S et al 1991 Impact of magnetic resonance imaging on the management of diabetic foot infections. Am J Surg 162: 150–153

Ebskov B, Josephsen P 1980 Incidence of reamputation and death after gangrene of the lower extremity. Prosthet Orthot Int 4: 77

Edmonds M E, Blundell M P, Morris H E et al 1986 Improved survival of the diabetic foot: the role of a specialised foot clinic. Q J Med 60: 763–771

Eichenholz S N 1966 Charcot Joints. Charles C Thomas, Springfield, Illinois

Eisenberg B, Wrege S S, Morton I A, Moore J W 1989 Bone scan: Indium-WBC correlation in the diagnosis of osteomyelitis of the foot. J Foot Surg 28: 532–536

Eliasson S G 1983 Neuropathy and the diabetic foot. In: Levin M A, O'Neal L W (eds) The Diabetic Foot, 3rd edn. Mosby, St. Louis, Ch 2, p 76

Eymontt M J, Alavi A, Dalinka M K 1991 Bone scintigraphy in diabetic osteoarthropathy. Radiology 140: 475–477

Fagerberg S E 1959 Diabetic neuropathy, a clinical and histological study on the significance of vascular affectations. Acta Med Scand 164: Supp 345

Ferrier T M 1965 Vascular lesions in diabetes. BMJ 2: 819

Fierer J, Daniel D, Davis C 1979 The fetid foot: lower extremity infections in patients with diabetes mellitus. Rev Infect Dis 1: 210

Fletcher E M 1990 Foot care education in the community for people with diabetes. Practical Diabetes 7: 171–172

Galle J, Bessenge S, Busse R 1990 Oxidized low density lipoproteins potentiate vasoconstrictions to various antagonists by direct interaction with vascular smooth muscle. Circ Res 66: 1287–1290

Ganda O P 1980 Pathogenesis of neuromuscular disease in the human diabetic. Diabetes 29: 931

Goldstein J L, Brown M S 1982 Lipoprotein receptors: genetic defence against atherosclerosis. Clin Res 30: 417

Gough S C L, Grant P J 1991 The fibrinolytic system in diabetes mellitus. Diabetic Med 8: 898–905

Gregersen G 1967 Diabetic neuropathy: influence of age, sex, metabolic control and duration of diabetes on motor conduction velocity. Neurology 17: 972

Haimovici H, Shapiro J H, Jacobson H G 1960 Serial femoral arteriography in occlusive disease. Am J Roentgenol Radium Ther Nucl Med 83: 1042

Harris J R & Brand P W 1966 Patterns of disintegration of the tarsus in the anaesthetic foot. J Bone Joint Surg 48B: 4–16

Harris R I 1956 Syme's amputation. The technical details essential for success. J Bone Joint Surg 38B: 614–632

Harris R I 1961 The history and development of Syme's amputation. Artif Limbs 6: 4

Heiple K G, Cammarn M R 1966 Diabetic neuropathy with spontaneous peritalar fracture dislocation. J Bone Joint Surg 48A: 1177–1181

Hockaday T D R, Hilson R M, Smith B 1982 Correlates of deterioration in pedal vibration sensory threshold over 5 years from diagnosis of maturity onset diabetic patients. Diabetologica 23: 174

Hodgson J R, Pugh D G, Young H H 1948 Roentgenologic aspects of certain lesions of bone: neuropathic or infections? Radiology 50: 65

Holstein P, Naer I, Tonnesen K H, Sager P 1978 Distal blood pressure in severe arterial insufficiency. In: Bergan J J, Yao J S T (eds) Gangrene and Severe Ischaemia of the Lower Extremities. Grune & Stratton, New York, Ch5

Hulnick A, Highsmith C, Boutin F J 1949 Amputations for failure in reconstructive surgery. J Bone Joint Surg 31A: 639

Intern Diabetes Fed Congress Proceedings 1991. Washington D C

Janlea H V, Standl E, Mehnert H 1980 Peripheral vascular disease in diabetes mellitus and its relation to cardiovascular role factors. Diabetes Care 3: 207

Johnson J T H 1967 Neuropathic fractures and joint injuries: pathogenesis and rationale of prevention and treatment. J Bone Joint Surg 49A: 1

Jordan W R 1936 Neuritic manifestations in diabetes mellitus. Arch Intern Med 57: 307–366

Karanfilian R G, Lynch T S, Zupal V T et al 1986 The value of laser Doppler velocimetry and transcutaneous oxygen tension determination in predicting healing of ischaemic forefoot ulceration and amputation in diabetics. J Vasc Surg 4: 511

Keenan A M, Tindel N L, Alavi A 1989 Diagnosis of pedal osteomyelitis in diabetic patients using current scintigraphic techniques. Arch Intern Med 149: 2262–2266

Kelly P J, Coventry M B 1958 Neurotrophic ulcers of the feet: review of 47 cases. JAMA 168: 388

Kilo C, Vogler N J, Williamson J R 1972 Muscle capillary basement membrane changes related to ageing and to diabetes mellitus. Diabetes 21: 881

Kozak G P, Rowbotham J L 1984 Diabetic foot disease: a major problem. In: Kozak G P et al (eds) Management of Diabetic Foot Problems. W B Saunders Co, Philadelphia. Ch 1, p 3

Larsson U, Andesson G 1978 Partial amputation of the foot for diabetic or arteriosclerotic gangrene. J Bone Joint Surg 60B: 125

Lee B Y, Trainer F S, Kavner D et al 1979 Assessment of healing potential of ulcers of the skin by photoplethysmography. Surg Gynecol Obstet 147: 232–239

Leslie C A, Supico F L, Bessman A N 1989 Infections in the diabetic host. Compr Ther 15: 23–32

Lipcomb H, Dobson H L, Greene J A 1959 Infection in the diabetic. South Med J 52: 16–23

Lopes-Vivella M F, Sherer G K, Lees A M et al 1982 Surface binding, internalisation and degradation by cultured human fibroblasts of low density lipoprotein isolated from type 1 (insulin dependent) diabetic patients: changes with metabolic control. Diabetologica 22: 430

Louie T J, Bartlet J G, Tally F P, Gorbach S L 1976 Aerobic and anaerobic bacteria in diabetic foot ulcers. Ann Intern Med 85: 461

Maloney J M, Snyder M, Aderson G et al 1989 Prevention of amputation by diabetic education. Am J Surg 158: 520–524

Margo M K 1967 Surgical treatment of conditions of the forepart of the foot. J Bone Joint Surg 49A: 1665

Mazet R 1967 The geriatric amputee. Artif Limbs 11: 33

Mazet R 1968 Syme's amputation. J Bone Joint Surg 50A: 1549

McKittrick L S, McKittrick J B, Risley J S 1949 Transmetatarsal amputation for infection or gangrene in patients with diabetes mellitus. Ann Surg 130: 826–842

Meade J W, Mueller C B 1968 Major infections of the foot. Med Times 96: 154

Meggitt B F 1972 Orthopaedic management of diabetic foot breakdown: classification and local treatment framework for preventative leg amputations, Orthop Seminars – Los Angeles County University, S California 5: 311

Meggitt B F 1973 Orthopaedic management of foot breakdown in the diabetic patient. J Bone Joint Surg 55B: 882

Meggitt B F 1976 Surgical management of the diabetic foot. Brit J Hosp Med 16: 227

Meggitt B F 1980 The Lisfranc partial foot appliance. DHSS–UK Prosthetic Contract Registration, Blackpool, UK

Meggitt B F 1988 Diabetes. In Helal, B, Wilson D W (eds) The Foot. Churchill Livingstone, Edinburgh. pp. 724–736

Meggitt B F 1996 Partial foot amputation in the diabetic: selection, surgery and survival. 5th Malvern Diabetic Foot Conference, 1994 in press

Mehta K, Hobson R W, Jamil Z et al 1980 Fallibility of Doppler ankle pressures in predicting healing of transmetatarsal amputations. J Surg Res 28: 466

Moss S E, Klein R, Klein B 1992 The prevalence and incidence of lower limb extremity amputation in a diabetic population. Arch Intern Med 152: 610–615

Most R S, Sinnock P 1983 The epidemiology of lower extremity amputations in diabetic individuals. Diabetes Care 6: 87–91

Mulder D W, Lambert E H, Bastron J A 1961 The neuropathies associated with diabetes mellitus. A clinical and electromyographic study of 103 unselected diabetic patients. Neurology 11: 275

Neil H A W, Thompson A V, Thorogood M et al 1989 Diabetes in the elderly: the Oxford Community Diabetic Study. Diabetic Med 6: 608–613

Newman J H 1979 Spontaneous dislocation in diabetic neuropathy. J Bone Joint Surg 61B: 484

Newman L G, Waller J, Palestro C G et al 1991 Unsuspected osteomyelitis in diabetic foot ulcers. JAMA 226: 1246–1251

Niklas B J 1991 Prophylactic surgery in the diabetic foot. In Frykberg R G (ed) The High Risk Foot in Diabetes Mellitus, 2nd Edn. Churchill Livingstone, Edinburgh. pp. 513–541

Oakley W 1954 Diabetes in surgery. Ann Royal Coll Surgeons 15: 108

Palumbo P J, Melton L J 1985 Peripheral vascular disease and diabetes. In Harris M I, Haniman R F (eds) Diabetes in America. N I H Pub No 85, 1468 Bethesda

Peterson C N, Jones R O, Koenig R J et al 1987 Reversible haematological sequelae of diabetes mellitus. Ann Int Med 6: 425–429

Pomposelli F B, Jepson S J, Gibbons G W et al 1990 Efficacy of the dorsal pedal bypass forelimb salvage in diabetic patients. J Vasc Surg 11: 745–752

Pratt T C 1965 Gangrene and infection in the diabetic. Med Clin N Amer 49: 987

Quin R O, Evans D H, Fyfe T 1977 Evaluation of indirect blood pressure measurement as a method of assessment of peripheral vascular disease. J Cardiovasc Surg 18: 109

Radcliffe D A, Clyne C A C, Chant A D B, Webster J H H 1984 Prediction of amputation wound healing: the role of transcutaneous pO_2 assessment. Br J Surg 71: 219–222

Raff M C, Asbury A K 1970 Ischaemic mononeuropathy and mononeuropathy multiplex in diabetic mellitus. N Engl J Med 279: 17

Raff M C, Sangalong V, Asbury A K 1968 Ischaemic mononeuropathy multiplex associated with diabetes mellitus. Arch Neurol 18: 487

Rayfield I J, Ault M J, Keush G T et al 1985 Infection and diabetes: the case for glucose control. Am J Med 72: 439–450

Reckless J P, Betteridge D J, Wu P 1978 High density and low density lipoproteins and prevalence of vascular disease in diabetes mellitus. BMJ I: 883

Riechard P, Nilsson B Y, Rosenquist U 1993 The effects of long term insulin treatment on the development of microvascular complications of diabetes mellitus. N Eng J Med 329: 304–309

Ross R 1981 Atherosclerosis: a problem of the biology of the arterial wall cells and their interaction with blood components. Atherosclerosis 1: 293

Sanders L J, Frykberg R G 1991 Diabetic neuropathic osteoarthropathy: the Charcot foot. In Frykberg R G (ed) The High Risk Foot in Diabetes Mellitus, 2nd edn. Churchill Livingstone, New York

Schwartz G S, Berenyi M R, Siegel M W 1969 Atrophic arthropathy and diabetic neuritis. Am J Roentgenol 106: 523–529

Second European Consensus Document on Chronic Critical Leg Ischaemia 1991 Circulation 84 (suppl IV): 1–26

Sibley W A 1982 The neuropathies of diabetes mellitus. In: Bressler R, Johnson D G (eds) Management of diabetes mellitus. Wright, Bristol. Ch 12, p 251

Singer A, Rossi G 1968 Radical local surgery in diabetic gangrene. J Mt Sinai Hosp N Y 35: 390

Siperstein M D, Unger R H, Madison L L 1968 Studies of muscle capillary basement membranes in normal subjects, diabetic and prediabetic patients. J Clin Invest 47: 1973

Smith D, Weinberger M, Katz B 1987 A controlled trial to increase office visits and reduce hospitalization of diabetic patients. J Gen Intern Med 2: 232–238

Sosenko J M, Sadia M T, Natori N et al 1987 Neurofunctional testing for the detection of diabetic peripheral neuropathy. Arch Intern Med 147: 1741–1744

Spittler A W, Brennan J J, Payne J W 1954 Syme amputation performed in two stages. J Bone Joint Surg 36A: 37

Stokes I A F, Faris I B, Hutton W C 1975 The neuropathic ulcer and loads on the foot in diabetic patients. Acta Orthop Scand 46: 839

Stokes K R, Strunk H M Campbell D R et al 1990 Five year results of iliac and femoropopliteal angioplasty in diabetic patients. Radiology 174: 977–982

Strandness D E, Priest R E, Gibbons G E 1964 Combined clinical and pathologic study of diabetic and non diabetic peripheral arterial disease. Diabetes 13: 366

Syme J 1843 Amputation at the ankle joint. Lond Edinb Monthly J Med Sci 3: 93

Thomas P K, Lascelles R C 1966 The pathology of diabetic neuropathy. Q J Med 35: 489

Trap-Jensen J 1971 Permeability of small vessels in diabetes. In: Lundback K, Keen H (eds) Blood vessel disease in diabetes. The Publishing House 'Il Ponte', Milano. Acta Diabetol Cat 8 Suppl I: 192

Veves A, Murray J H, Young M J, Boulton A J M 1992 The risk of foot ulceration in diabetic patients with high foot pressure: a prospective study. Diabetologia 35: 660–663

Wagner F W 1979 A classification and treatment program for diabetic, neuropathic and dysvascular foot problems. In: The American Academy of Orthopaedic Surgeons Instructional Course Lectures 28, C V Mosby Co, St Louis. p. 143

Wagner F W 1981 The dysvascular foot: a system for diagnosis and treatment. Foot Ankle 2: 64

Wagner F W, Buggs H 1978 Use of Doppler ultrasound in determining healing levels in diabetic dysvascular lower extremity problems. In: Bergan J J, Yao J S T (eds) Gangrene and Severe Ischaemia of the Lower Extremities. Grune and Stratton, New York p. 131

Wagner F W, Russ J, Webb J, Buggs H 1980 Syme's amputation of the diabetic foot: results utilising preoperative Doppler evaluation. In: Bateman J E, Trott A W (eds) The Foot and Ankle. Brian C Decker, New York. Ch 15, p 127–130

Wahlig H, Dingelden E, Bergmann R, Reuss K 1978 The release of gentamicin from polymethylmethacrylate beads. J Bone Joint Surg 60B: 270

Waldvogel F A, Medoff G, Swartz M N 1970 Osteomyelitis: a review of clinical features, therapeutic considerations and unusual aspects. N Engl J Med 282: 198

Warren R, Thayer T R, Achenbach H, Kendall L G 1955 The Syme amputation in peripheral vascular arterial disease. Surgery 37: 156

Warren S, Le Compte P M, Legg M A (eds) 1966 The Pathology of Diabetes Mellitus, 4th edn. Lea and Febiger, Philadelphia, Ch 4

Waters R L, Perry J, Antonelli D, Hislop H 1976 Energy cost of walking of amputees. The influence of level of amputation. J Bone Joint Surg 58A: 42

Wheelock F C 1961 Transmetatarsal amputations and arterial surgery on diabetic patients. N Engl J Med 264: 316–320

Whitehouse F W 1978 On diabetic osteopathy: a radiographic study of 21 patients. Diabetes Care I (5): 303

Wilens S L 1951 The nature of diffuse intimal thickening of arteries. Am J Pathol 27: 825

Williamson B R J, Treates C D, Phillips C et al 1989 Computed tomography as a diagnostic aid in diabetic and other problem feet. Clin Imaging 13: 159–163

Wilson R M 1986 Neutrophil function in diabetes. Diabetic Med 3: 509–512

Wyss C R, Matsen F A, Simmonds C W et al 1984 Transcutaneous oxygen tension measurements on limbs of diabetic and non-diabetic patients with PVD. Surgery 95: 339–346

Yamagata S, Yamauchi Y 1969 Diabetic neuropathy and triopathy. In: Diabetes: Proceeding of the Sixth Congress of the International Diabetes Federation, Stockholm. Excerpta Medica Foundation, Amsterdam

Yao J S T 1970 Haemodynamic studies in peripheral vascular disease. Br J Surg 57: 761

Yao J S T, Hobbs J T, Irvine W J 1969 Ankle systolic pressure measurements in arterial disease affecting the lower limbs. Br J Surg 56: 676–679

Young M J, Boulton A J M, Williams D R R et al 1993 A multicentre study of the prevalence of diabetic neuropathy in patients attending UK Diabetic Clinics. Diabetologica 36: 150–154

Yuh W J C, Corson J D, Baraniewski M H et al 1989 Osteomyelitis of the foot in diabetic patients: evaluation with plain films, 99m-Tc-MDP bone scintigraphy, and MRI imaging. AJR 152: 795–800

VI.5 Salvage of Diabetic Neuropathic Arthropathy with Arthrodesis

Mark S Myerson

General concepts of treatment

Neuroarthropathy of the foot and ankle in the diabetic patient is a common orthopaedic problem and the outcome depends on proper management. The incidence of neuroarthropathy and diabetes ranges from 1 to 2.5% (Kristiansen 1980, Griffiths 1985). The most common areas of neuroarthropathy are the midfoot and hindfoot (Sinha et al 1972, Brodsky et al 1987). Owing to the increasing longevity of patients with diabetes, it is anticipated that many orthopaedic surgeons will have an opportunity to manage this problem.

The Charcot joint in the diabetic patient (neuroarthropathy) is a common event, which may lead to ultimate amputation of the limb. Although other elements of neuropathy and ischemia are often present, they may be, to some extent, addressed through revascularization without resorting to amputation. Structural breakdown of the foot, which leads to wound problems, and osteomyelitis are far more difficult to treat.

The treatment of the Charcot foot and ankle is influenced by the stage of arthropathy. Eichenholtz (1966) described three stages of development of the Charcot joint that are fairly typical of the course of events from the initial phase of the arthropathy through healing. In stage I, characterized by acute inflammation associated with hyperemia and erythema, the bone dissolves and fragments, and dislocations are common. In the second stage, characterized by bony coalescence and decreasing swelling, radiographic evidence of periosteal new bone formation is present, even when the initial injury was a joint dislocation rather than fracture. During stage III, bony consolidation and healing occurs. The initial diagnosis of acute neuroarthropathy is relatively straightforward, based on painless swelling associated with warmth of the affected area. Although radiographs are helpful, the typical changes of neuroarthropathy, such as fragmentation and periosteal new bone formation, are not often present during this acute stage.

Treatment concepts of neuroarthropathy have changed significantly over the past decade (Papa et al 1993, Myerson et al 1994). The goal of any treatment program for the Charcot foot is to achieve a plantigrade weight bearing surface that is free of infection. In addition to these parameters, the foot and ankle must be stable and braceable. Whether the phase is acute or chronic and involves the midfoot, hindfoot or ankle, most forms of Charcot breakdown are treated conservatively. The accepted treatment for neuropathic arthropathy of the foot and ankle has been prolonged immobilization in a brace or plaster cast until consolidation and healing are radiographically evident and clinical stability of the foot and ankle have been restored (Harris & Brand 1966, Johnson 1967, Newman 1979, Clohisy & Thompson 1988, Lesko & Maurer 1989, Stuart & Morrey 1990, Papa et al 1993, Myerson et al 1994). These methods of treatment are effective in most patients, particularly when promptly instituted. However, severe deformity may develop despite appropriate immobilization and protected weight bearing, and immobilization of the limb does not guarantee that additional deformity will not occur.

Although some reports indicate that deformity may progress in the immobilized limb even if it is not subjected to weight bearing, my experience has been otherwise (Myerson et al 1993). Deformity may indeed worsen in a cast, but I have observed, without exception, that patients with these conditions do bear weight on the extremity, owing to a combination of neuropathy, noncompliance, and inability to use crutches or a walker because of problems with proprioception and balance. One wonders whether a long leg cast with the knee flexed would achieve a more reliable end result under these circumstances.

The mainstay of treatment for neuropathic arthropathy, once diagnosed, continues to be prolonged external immobilization in a plaster cast or brace. A brace is the traditional method of managing chronic deformity of the hindfoot and ankle. This brace may be a vertical double upright type, a molded polypropylene ankle foot orthosis, a posterior AFO type, or a clam shell type. The patellar-tendon-bearing (PTB) brace has recently been recommended by Saltzman et al (1992), who assessed the effect of shoe wear, custom-made inserts, PTB braces, and extra-padded PTB braces on load transmission to neuroarthropathic feet. They found that a properly fitted PTB brace can reduce load transmission to the Charcot foot, but in a reliable manner only to the hindfoot. Adding extra padding to the brace decreased the mean peak force further by 32%. They recommended that a PTB brace not be used to reduce vertical load transmission to the midfoot or forefoot. For long-term use, the PTB brace should be used for treatment of hindfoot disorders only, and adjusted regularly to ensure adequate fit. However, deformity of the hindfoot and ankle may not be amenable to bracing, since these

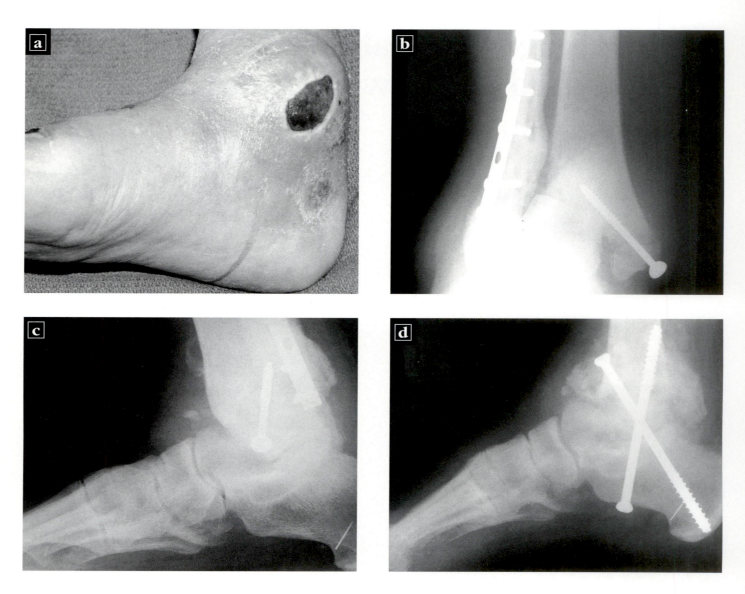

Figure 1

Acute neuropathic dislocation of the ankle after open reduction and internal fixation for an ankle fracture associated with an ulcer (a). Dislocation was present on the anteroposterior and lateral radiographs (b, c). This was treated with a tibiotalocalcaneal arthrodesis which was quite stable 5 years later (d)

structures are far too unstable to be maintained in adequate alignment by either a brace or a cast. The stresses of weight bearing in these patients may preclude the possibility of bracing. To avoid the complications of unstable neuroarthropathy, operative treatment is occasionally warranted, particularly when consolidation and healing of the neuropathic fracture and dislocation has not taken place. This is well exemplified in a patient (Fig. 1) who was treated with a double upright brace for neuropathic deformity of the ankle. Recurrent ulceration over the fibula developed secondary to ankle instability while in the brace. The problem was not appreciated until weight bearing radiographs of the foot inside the brace were obtained.

With either a varus or valgus deformity of the hindfoot or ankle, it is particularly difficult to keep the foot in a plantargrade position centered under the leg. Although a Syme or below-the-knee amputation eliminates the immediate problem, many amputees experience limitations in day-to-day functional activities, necessitating a significant modification in their lifestyle. Amputees have an increased energy requirement, frequently have limited cardiac reserve, are often overweight, and have a marked risk for future contralateral amputation. For these reasons, limb salvage should be attempted wherever possible.

Although operative treatment for neuropathic arthropathy of the foot and ankle is an option, under most circumstances, this should not be the initial treatment of choice. We have reported previously on salvage of intractable diabetic neuropathic arthropathy of the hindfoot and ankle treated with open reduction and arthrodesis (Papa et al 1993). At an average of approximately 4 years after arthrodesis, salvage proved to be successful in 93% of these patients. Certainly, operative treatment must be considered part of one's armamentarium for managing the deformed diabetic foot. This treatment program was, however, complex: 20 complications were encountered in 19 of the 29 patients. Enthusiasm for operative treatment therefore has to be tempered by the potential for complications during a difficult salvage procedure.

Other authors have reported on the results of operative treatment of neuropathic arthropathy (Cohn & Brahms 1987, Lesko & Maurer 1989, Shibata et al 1990, Stuart & Morrey 1990, Cleveland 1993). Shibata et al (1990) reported on results of extended hindfoot fusions in patients with leprotic neuropathic deformity. They used an intramedullary nail for fixation and an arthrodesis occurred in 19 of the 26 patients. Stuart & Morrey (1990) have reported on the results of ankle and hindfoot arthrodesis in 13 patients with insulin-dependent diabetes. Their results were satisfactory in only five of the 13 patients, and complications developed in seven of the nine patients who showed radiographic signs of new neuroarthropathy. One of the problems that may have led to the high rate of failure in their patients was that external fixation was used in nine of the 13 patients. As discussed below, I do not believe that external fixation is the ideal form of stabilization for these deformities.

Healing from the acute inflammatory phase through coalescence and ultimate consolidation takes a long time. Healing of the tarsometatarsal joint and midfoot takes approximately 6–12 months, and that of the hindfoot and ankle takes 12–24 months. The mainstay of treatment for most feet is adequate stabilization during this period to allow the tissues to heal and ultimately consolidate. Although deformity leading to recurrent ulceration may require surgery for claw toes, metatarsal head resections, and exostectomy, intervention with open reduction and arthrodesis is less commonly required. It is important to recognize that open reduction on its own is not sufficient to stabilize these joints.

Ideally, surgery should not be performed in the presence of an open wound. Therefore, if feasible, wounds are first healed with either a total contact cast (Myerson & Wilson 1991, Myerson et al 1992) or a split thickness skin graft. If surgery is performed in the presence of an open wound, the infection rate is increased. Therefore, in the presence of an open wound with or without osteomyelitis, reconstruction and salvage has to be staged. This problem exists, for example, over the malleoli where ulceration associated with deeper infection may be present. In these instances, I prefer to debride the wound and bone, and initiate treatment for osteomyelitis.

The midfoot

The treatment goal for patients with neuroarthropathy of the midfoot is to obtain a durable plantigrade foot for ambulation. Amputation, however, remains a necessary management option in patients with severe infection with or without ischemia. However, by controlling the rate and severity of ulceration, a carefully designed treatment program can decrease the frequency with which amputations are required. It is important to identify the stage of neuroarthropathy to initiate treatment. Once immobilization and rest brings active neuroarthropathy under control, a total contact cast becomes the mainstay of treatment. Nonoperative treatment measures are usually more successful for deformities of the midfoot than for deformities of the hindfoot and ankle.

Acute midfoot neuroarthropathy

For acute neuroarthropathy, the mainstay of treatment is rest of the limb, restricted ambulation and activities, and total contact cast immobilization. The indication for surgery in this acute setting is very specific, and should be performed only for a severe dislocation which is unstable and manually reducible. Invariably, however, a fracture is present, and dislocation without bone fragmentation is not common. Any bone fragmentation or periosteal new bone formation is a contraindication to surgery, and the mainstay of treatment for acute neuroarthropathy remains nonoperative. Open reduction and arthrodesis is indicated in these patients to prevent skin necrosis and acute ulceration after reduction of edema. Since the disease process is acute, the bone density is usually adequate for fixation. Surgery should not be attempted if preoperative radiographs show evidence of bone absorption and fragmentation, since profound osteopenia may be present, precluding stable reduction and fixation.

Surgery should be performed once swelling has resolved, since operating on a swollen foot increases problems with wound closure and the likelihood of infection. This has to be monitored very closely, since the displaced tarsal and metatarsal bones will often cause skin necrosis (Fig. 2). I use the A-V Impulse system foot pump (Kendall, Mansfield, Massachusetts, USA) to reduce edema of the foot (Myerson & Henderson 1993), and this is successful in the presence of neuropathic swelling of the foot. This has to be monitored closely to prevent pressure and ischemic necrosis of prominent parts of the foot. Between 4 and 6 hours of intermittent compression are often sufficient to decrease all edema in the foot and prepare the foot for surgery. Prophylactic cephalosporin antibiotics are used routinely. I do not use a tourniquet, and surgery is performed under regional ankle block anesthetic. Bone graft is occasionally

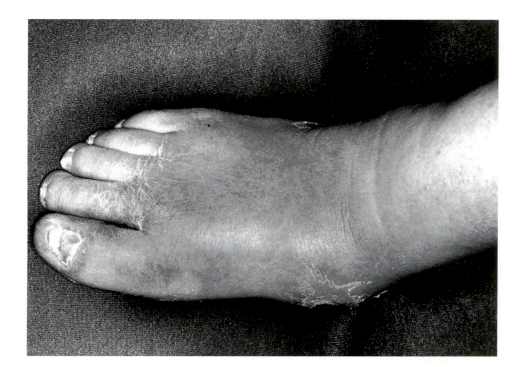

Figure 2

Acute neuropathic dislocation of the tarsometatarsal joint associated with swelling of the foot

required for arthrodesis of acute neuroarthropathy, and depends on the magnitude of the deformity. In the event of significant bone loss, iliac crest bone should be used, but smaller quantities of graft from the calcaneus can be harvested. This is usually unnecessary in the setting of acute fracture dislocation, since minimal bone resorption and destruction has occurred. For reconstruction of chronic neuroarthropathy, bone graft is invariably required.

The incisions are planned according to the pattern of dislocation, the most common of which is disruption of the medial column involving the first metatarsal and medial cuneiform. Here, a single dorsal incision is made medial to the extensor hallucis longus tendon. In patients with middle column disruption involving the second and third metatarsocuneiform joints, a long incision is made centered over the space between the second and third metatarsals, and a second smaller incision is made medially over the first metatarsal and medial cuneiform. Thick skin flaps are raised without much attention paid to superficial nerves. The bones are handled cautiously since they are fragile and, with too much periosteal dissection, a bone may fall out of the wound. Fibrous scar and granulation tissue has to be removed from the joint spaces, and thin, flexible chisels or fine, sharp osteotomes are used to denude the articular surfaces.

Manual reduction is now performed and temporary internal fixation obtained using 0.062-inch Kirschner wires or the guide pins for cannulated screws. It is important to obtain intraoperative anteroposterior and lateral radiographs to assess the reduction. Although fluoroscopic imaging is useful to guide the insertion of

the pins, it is not sufficient to determine alignment. The reduction of the dislocation is usually accomplished by a maneuver that involves grasping the hallux and pulling it into varus while simultaneously pushing with the thumb against the base of the first metatarsal and medial cuneiform. This is the same maneuver used for reduction of a chronically dislocated midfoot following a Lisfranc type injury. If this is not sufficient to reduce the medial cuneiform, a small periosteal elevator can be used. The base of the second metatarsal is the key to an anatomic reduction. Although achieving a precise reduction and alignment of the midfoot is not as important as for the patient without neuropathy, it is still preferable to restore a medial longitudinal arch and prevent recurrent pressure on the medial foot. I therefore prefer to use compression screws for fixation to reduce the medial cuneiform directly into the second metatarsal and *vice versa*. The first screw is introduced medially from the medial cuneiform into the middle and lateral cuneiforms or the second metatarsal, depending on the pattern of dislocation. If the second metatarsal is laterally displaced, I direct the screw obliquely and distally from the medial cuneiform into the second metatarsal base.

Subacute midfoot neuroarthropathy

It is important to distinguish between subacute and chronic neuroarthropathy of the midfoot. Although many feet end up deformed, the chronic stage produces a foot that is stiff as well as deformed. These feet are generally easy to protect in an extra-depth shoe with a molded orthosis and it is unlikely that patients with true chronic neuroarthropathy will require an arthrodesis. Some feet remain permanently in a subacute phase, the midfoot is deformed and unstable, and a 'spongy' fibrous arthrosis is present at the apex of the deformity. A rocker-bottom deformity is present, with an apex medial or lateral, depending on which bones are prominent on the plantar surface of the foot. In these feet, sagittal plane motion occurs through this pseudoarthrosis and the hindfoot remains fixed in equinus. The rocker-bottom deformity is always associated with a fixed hindfoot equinus. The posterior soft tissues, including the Achilles and the flexor tendons, are contracted. An Achilles tendon lengthening is integral to the success of this procedure. The remaining long flexor tendons rarely require lengthening. The magnitude of this equinus contracture is best evaluated on a weight bearing lateral radiograph of the foot. It is then appreciated that the forefoot must be redirected (plantarflexed) in line with the hindfoot, which must be corrected through posterior soft tissue releases.

Prior to the midfoot approach, soft tissue lengthening is performed posteriorly with a percutaneous triple hemisection technique for the Achilles tendon. A stab incision is made centrally in the posterior aspect of the Achilles tendon and then directed subcutaneously. The incisions on the tendon are spaced approximately 20 mm apart. The Achilles tendon should be lengthened before working on the midfoot, as no effective dorsiflexion lever on the foot is present once the midfoot is open. If the hindfoot is still in equinus after Achilles tendon lengthening, the other long flexor tendons may require lengthening. In severe rocker-bottom deformity, this would have to be approached through a lateral incision over the peroneal tendons and a posteromedial incision posterior to the medial malleolus.

I use three incisions to reconstruct these feet: dorso-medial, central, and lateral. Sammarco has recommended a transverse incision across the midfoot with the advantage of improved exposure (GJ Sammarco, personal communication). Transection of superficial nerves is not important; however, I have some concerns about this incision since it disrupts the superficial veins and potentially could cause problems with wound healing, which have not as yet been reported by Sammarco. Thick skin flaps are raised regardless of the method of these incisions. The dislocated joints are approached by resection of the fibrous scar. Although an osteotome may be used here, I find that a small microsagittal saw blade is preferable to perform these planar cuts. The extruded bone fragments on the plantar surfaces must be removed and are usually accessible through the dorsal incisions. A laminar spreader is placed into the wound between the tarsal and metatarsal bones and placed on distraction, and the bone fragments on the plantar surface are removed with a rongeur.

Once the bone fragments, debris, and fibrous tissue have been removed, the forefoot is reduced to the midfoot by adduction and plantarflexion. Large gaps are usually present between the tarsal and metatarsal bones, and approximation of the bone ends should not be attempted at this time. Temporary internal fixation with Kirschner wires is used and anteroposterior and lateral radiographs are obtained. Once the intraoperative radiographs are obtained, permanent fixation and final correction is planned.

Bone graft is usually necessary, and although I prefer to use iliac crest autograft, allograft bone has been recommended in the diabetic patient (Myerson et al 1993). The bone graft is morsellized and only cancellous bone fragments (2 × 3 mm) are used. Permanent fixation of the midfoot is not easy because of osteopenia and the irregular size and shapes of the remaining bones and joints. Although the insertion of crossed pins from the first and fifth metatarsals is relatively easy, this fixation construct is not very stable, and I use compression lag screws. One screw that is always helpful in these chronic midfoot reconstructions is a 6.5 mm lag screw introduced from the medial cuneiform transversely across the foot into the cuboid. The other screws are introduced from the medial and lateral aspects of the foot obliquely. Cannulated screws are much easier to insert, since the guide pins can be introduced and radiographs obtained before inserting the screws. Occasionally threaded Steinmann pins are needed because of the orientation and quality of the bones. Threaded pins are preferable since they cause less motion at the skin interface and are therefore less likely to be associated with pin-tract infections. The pins are left in place for approximately 3 months and should be used cautiously because they are left protruding from the skin.

Chronic midfoot neuroarthropathy

The need for arthrodesis of the midfoot in the setting of chronic neuroarthropathy is less common. Most feet can be successfully treated with accommodative orthoses in a wide, extra-depth shoe with a rocker-bottom sole. If this type of shoe is unsatisfactory, a custom molded shoe with a steel shank or a molded ankle foot orthosis can be used. Unlike the unstable foot seen in subacute neuroarthropathy, these feet are stiff and generally stable, so that the deformity can usually be protected with the appropriate shoe. If recurrent ulceration occurs, tarsal ostectomy is an alternative form of treatment. Unlike the hindfoot and ankle, ostectomy of the midfoot is a good option and should be considered when recurrent ulceration occurs. However, ostectomy only works where the arthropathy is truly chronic, the deformity is rigid and stable, and there is no pseudoarthrosis or false motion across the site of the original fracture dislocation process. Therefore, this is generally easier to treat since

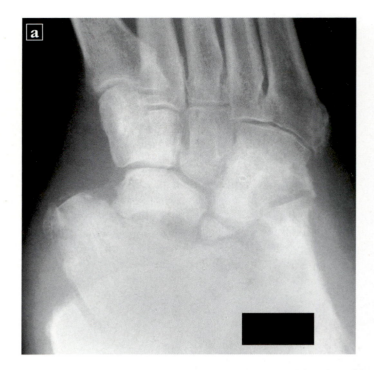

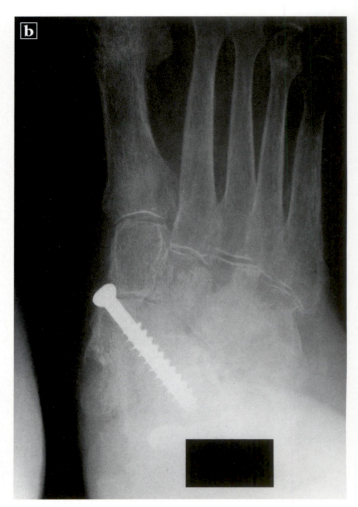

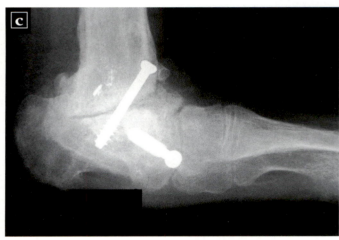

Figure 3

Chronic dislocation of the transverse tarsal joint is demonstrated. This dislocation was grossly unstable, and not braceable (a). This was treated with a modified pantalar arthrodesis by resecting a portion of the talus (b, c)

the foot can be fitted with an appropriate accommodative shoe and orthosis. If recurrent ulceration occurs despite this treatment program, then ostectomy is indicated and the offending bone is shaved down or removed. This may involve the cuneiform, cuboid, navicular, or a combination of these bones.

Rarely, patients with stable chronic neuroarthropathy have pain. Although pain is not associated with neuroarthropathy, this may occur when severe forefoot abduction and midfoot pronation is present. The forefoot is usually abducted, the midfoot pronated, and the hindfoot in equinus. All of these should be corrected as described above for subacute deformity. In most of these feet, the medial soft tissue structures of the hindfoot, including the posterior tibial tendon, spring ligament,

talonavicular capsule and deep deltoid ligament, are stretched out. I have seen perfect correction of the midfoot with a reconstructive arthrodesis only to find that the hindfoot later collapses into severe planovalgus. This is not necessarily a reactivation of the neuroarthropathy, but more likely represents partial treatment of the initial deformity.

Following correction of the midfoot, attention should be directed to the medial hindfoot. If from the preoperative planning, these structures were noted to be attenuated, then soft tissues are corrected as one would do with a posterior tibial tendon reconstruction. In these patients, I perform an osteotomy of the calcaneus and translate it medially. This is performed in conjunction with a flexor digitorum longus tendon transfer to the navicular or cuneiform. An alternative would be to perform a simultaneous subtalar or transverse tarsal arthrodesis. The combination of hindfoot and midfoot arthrodesis is, however, required infrequently.

Hindfoot and ankle deformity

Regardless of the magnitude of the varus or valgus deformity, if the ankle is stable, then bracing usually succeeds. If the foot can be maintained under the axis of the leg during the acute or subacute phases of neuroarthropathy, despite bone dissolution or destruction, the foot will usually be stable. Such a foot, of course, requires prolonged immobilization until the consolidation phase has been reached. This contrasts with the foot where gross dislocation of the tarsus or ankle is present, which may occur during either the acute or chronic phases of neuroarthropathy. Operative treatment should, as a rule, be performed only once a chronic phase is reached. During the acute hyperemic stage, fragmentation of bone occurs and adequate rigid internal fixation is not usually possible. However, some feet do not reach a chronic phase of bony consolidation. Dislocation or subluxation persists, and in these feet reconstruction is performed during the subacute stage of arthropathy.

A decision has to be made with the patient whether amputation or arthrodesis is to be attempted. The efforts to achieve a stable foot and ankle may take a prolonged amount of time, and require immobilization, restricted weight bearing and curtailed activities. If the patient is totally unable to comply with these activity restrictions, then amputation may be an efficient and perhaps even a more cost effective method of dealing with severe neuropathic deformity. In my experience, the success rate of salvage of severe deformity with arthrodesis is approximately 90%, and the failures are treated by amputation (Papa et al 1993).

The indications for arthrodesis in the hindfoot and ankle are limited to the severely unstable joint that is not amenable to bracing. In this group of patients are also those for whom bracing has been attempted but in whom repeated ulceration occurs (Fig. 3).

Surgery is also occasionally indicated during the acute phase of hindfoot neuroarthropathy associated with an acute fracture or dislocation followed by disorderly fragmentation and loss of alignment. In a patient with diabetes, an acute fracture dislocation of the ankle that is amenable to open reduction and internal fixation should be treated in the same manner as that in a patient without neuropathy. Diabetes is not a contraindication to internal fixation of acute fractures of the ankle. In fact, I would exercise even more caution to ensure that the fracture heals uneventfully. Unless these fractures are immobilized postoperatively for a long period of time, malunion and fragmentation of the talus may occur. I prefer to sacrifice full range of motion in these patients

by immobilizing them until complete healing with no signs of any warmth or swelling is evident. The patient is not allowed to bear weight for 3 months, and for a further 3–4 months cast immobilization is continued until warmth and swelling have dissipated.

Despite this caution, deformity may occur very rapidly in patients with neuropathy, and an early arthrodesis should be considered before inevitable ulceration and infection occurs, as in the patient shown in Fig. 1, whose displaced bimalleolar fracture of the ankle was successfully treated with open reduction and internal fixation. Weight bearing on the ankle was begun at 2 months when healing was thought to be present. The patient presented for treatment with significant deformity and a superficial ulcer over the medial malleolus.

The same principles apply to an acute dislocation of the hindfoot and tarsal joints where anticipated deformity is ultimately going to be difficult to brace. An example of this situation is presented in a patient with acute neuropathic dislocation of the naviculum with considerable deformity (Fig. 4). The alternatives for treatment in this patient would be to follow the course of neuroarthropathy with limb elevation, immobilization, and bracing in the hope of avoiding eventual ulceration. With this deformity, however, it is highly likely that ulceration will occur, owing to the prominence of the navicular on the plantar medial aspect of the foot. Salvage could be performed later with excision of the navicular or a later arthrodesis. However, it is likely that, with time, the deformity will increase, which may subsequently be difficult to salvage. Early surgery may therefore be indicated.

As is the case for the midfoot, it is preferable not to operate on the hindfoot and ankle in the presence of an open wound. This is not always easy, since the nature of the instability causing and also perpetuating the wound may preclude the possibility of adequate skin coverage. In these patients, strict bed rest and a split thickness skin graft may be used to obtain coverage followed by reconstructive surgery as soon as is feasible before breakdown occurs again. If the hindfoot is grossly unstable, or if osteomyelitis is present, an external fixator is used to achieve temporary stability. Once the wound has settled down, coverage is obtained, followed by arthrodesis. Osteomyelitis is treated aggressively with debridement and appropriate antibiotics; definitive surgery is delayed until the osteomyelitis is completely resolved. External fixation, however, should not be used routinely to secure fixation, since the risk of infection is markedly increased. Therefore, the only time that I use external fixation is in the presence of severe focal sepsis that cannot be managed by other means. I prefer to use rigid internal fixation for the hindfoot and ankle with large cannulated 6.5 mm or 7.0 mm cancellous screws (Fig. 5).

Prophylactic intravenous antibiotics and a pneumatic tourniquet should be used for the hindfoot and ankle. A standard approach for a triple arthrodesis is used with a lateral incision dorsal to the peroneal tendons and a

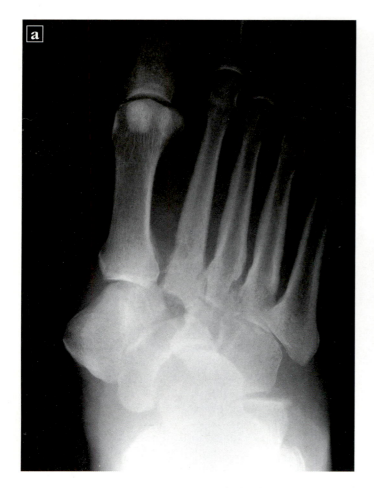

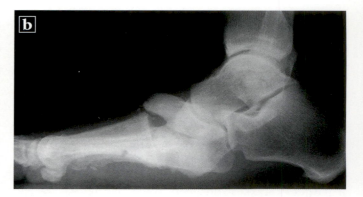

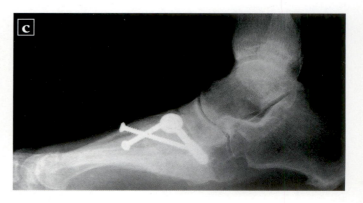

Figure 4

This patient (also presented in Fig. 2) sustained an acute dislocation of the tarsometatarsal joints. On the anteroposterior (a) and lateral (b) radiographs, medial and dorsal dislocation of the medial cuneiform was present which could cause skin necrosis. This was treated with open reduction and primary arthrodesis of the tarsometatarsal and midtarsal joints (c, d)

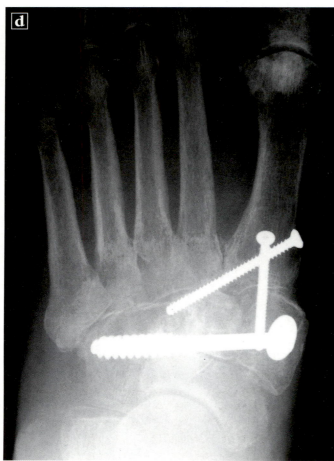

second dorsomedial incision medial to the anterior tibial tendon. A transfibular lateral approach is used for all tibiotalar fusions, and is extended distally toward the sinus tarsi if a tibiotalocalcaneal or pantalar fusion is performed. A small medial incision is used to explore the medial ankle, resect the medial malleolus and debride the talonavicular joint when it is included in the fusion. Full thickness skin flaps should be preserved wherever possible. Congruent surfaces are fashioned in the ankle and hindfoot to allow good bony contact and maximum inherent stability.

If the talus is fragmented and avascular, then a talectomy and tibiocalcaneal fusion is performed (see Fig. 5). If talectomy is to be performed, then supplemental bone graft should be used. This has been successfully used with a femoral head allograft (Myerson et al 1993). Owing to the plantar inclination of the posterior facet, the calcaneus cannot be apposed directly to the tibial plafond. If this is attempted, the hindfoot and calcaneus dorsiflex into a calcaneus position. Instead, a triangular-shaped bone graft needs to be inserted into the space

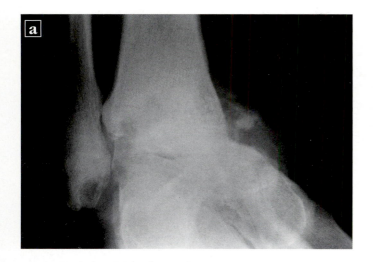

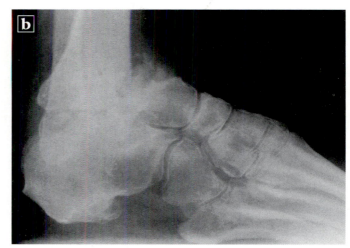

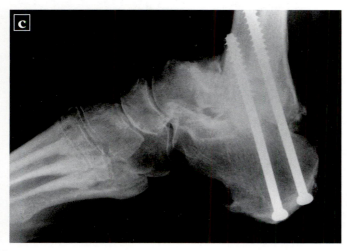

Figure 5

A brace was used unsuccessfully in this patient to control the deformity of the hindfoot. Anteroposterior and lateral radiographs demonstrate the fragmentation of the talus and varus dislocation of the ankle (a, b). This was treated by resecting the body of the talus and a tibiocalcaneal arthrodesis (c)

created by resection of the joint surfaces. This can be fashioned using a strut of the fibula, with a femoral head allograft, or with trapezoidal pieces of tricortical bone from the iliac crest. This is augmented with copious cancellous bone chips. One way to obtain copious cancellous bone is to use a morsellized fibula graft by grinding down the fibula using a small acetabular reamer.

One of the more difficult problems arises when determining the final position in which the foot is to be fused. This is particularly a problem following talectomy. The height of the foot is shortened, and the soft tissue bulk on the medial and lateral ankle obscures and distorts the alignment. For this reason, the limb should be draped proximal to the knee joint to allow full visualization of the foot and knee prior to definitive fixation. The foot is positioned plantigrade with the ankle in neutral dorsiflexion, 5° of hindfoot valgus, and slight external rotation. While slight malunion is tolerated by the patient with neuropathy, varus deformity, no matter how mild, will lead to ulceration along the lateral border of the

foot. Temporary fixation is obtained using cannulated pins, and the position of the foot is checked with anteroposterior and lateral radiographs before definitive fixation with long, partially threaded cancellous screws. The wound is closed in layers and a large bulky dressing is applied, with a plaster splint incorporated into the bandage.

Postoperative management

Prophylactic intravenous antibiotics are utilized for 48 hours, the limb is elevated, and strict bed rest is enforced for 2–3 days. Oral antibiotics are used until the wound is clean or the sutures are removed. Patients commence protected ambulation on the second or third postoperative day. No weight is allowed on the affected extremity for 3 months, and the foot is immobilized in a short leg cast. If patients are not able to comply with these restrictions, a rubber heel can be attached posteriorly on the cast to minimize pressure under the midfoot.

Weight bearing is allowed when the warmth and swelling in the foot decreases, usually by 3 months. A reliable method of determining reduction of warmth is to use a skin thermistor and chart the changes in temperature every 2–3 weeks with the cast changes. The cast should be changed every 2 weeks during the first 6 weeks after surgery and then at 3-week intervals. At approximately 3 months, weight bearing is commenced in a short leg cast for a further 3 months for the midfoot, and for 6–12 additional months for the hindfoot and ankle.

Once weight bearing has commenced, the foot should be inspected more regularly. After midfoot procedures, patients should ambulate in a shoe with a rocker-bottom sole and a protective molded orthosis that should be provided and ready for the patient once casting is discontinued. I usually take the mold for the orthosis 4 weeks prior to the anticipated time for discontinuing the cast. A brace is not usually necessary for the midfoot, but is preferable for the hindfoot and ankle, where it is continued indefinitely.

References

Brodsky J W, Wagner F W, Kwong P K et al 1987 Patterns of breakdown in the Charcot tarsus of diabetes and relation to treatment (abstr). Orthop Trans 2: 484

Cleveland M 1939 Surgical fusion of unstable joints due to neuropathic disturbance. Am J Surg 43: 580–584

Clohisy D R, Thompson R C Jr 1988 Fractures associated with neuropathic arthropathy in adults who have juvenile-onset diabetes. J Bone Joint Surg 70A: 1192–1200

Cohn B T, Brahms M A 1987 Diabetic arthropathy of the first metatarsal cuneiform joint. Introduction of a new surgical fusion technique. Orthop Rev 16: 465–470

Eichenholtz S N 1966 Charcot Joints. Charles C Thomas, Springfield, Illinois, USA

Griffiths H J 1985 Diabetic osteopathy. Orthopedics 8: 401–406

Harris J R, Brand P W 1966 Patterns of disintegration of the tarsus in the anaesthetic foot. J Bone Joint Surg 48B: 4–16

Johnson J T H 1967 Neuropathic fractures and joint injuries. Pathogenesis and rationale of prevention and treatment. J Bone Joint Surg 49A: 1–30

Kristiansen B 1980 Ankle and foot fractures in diabetics provoking neuropathic joint changes. Acta Orthop Scand 51: 975–979

Lesko P, Maurer R C 1989 Talonavicular dislocations and midfoot arthropathy in neuropathic diabetic feet. Natural course and principles of treatment. Clin Orthop 240: 226–231

Myerson M S, Henderson M R 1993 Clinical applications of a pneumatic intermittent impulse compression device after trauma and major surgery to the foot and ankle. Foot Ankle 14: 198–203

Myerson M, Wilson K 1991 Management of neuropathic ulceration with the total contact cast. In: Sammarco G J (ed) The Foot in Diabetes. Lea & Febiger, Philadelphia. pp 145–152

Myerson M, Papa J, Eaton K et al 1992 The total-contact cast for management of neuropathic plantar ulceration of the foot. J Bone Joint Surg 74A: 261–269

Myerson M S, Alvarez R G, Brodsky J W et al 1993 Symposium: neuroarthropathy of the foot. Contemp Orthop 26: 43–64

Myerson M S, Henderson M R, Short K 1994 Management of midfoot diabetic neuropathy. Foot Ankle 15: 233–241

Newman J H 1979 Spontaneous dislocation in diabetic neuropathy. A report of six cases. J Bone Joint Surg 61B: 484–488

Papa J, Myerson M, Girard P 1993 Salvage with arthrodesis in intractable diabetic neuropathic arthropathy of the foot and ankle. J Bone Joint Surg 75A: 1056–1066

Saltzman C L, Johnson K A, Goldstein R H, et al 1992 The patellar tendon-bearing brace as treatment for neurotrophic arthropathy. A dynamic force monitoring study. Foot Ankle 13: 14–21

Shibata T, Tada K, Hashizume C 1990 The results of arthrodesis of the ankle for leprotic neuroarthropathy. J Bone Joint Surg 72A: 749–756

Sinha S, Munichoodappa C S, Kozak G P 1972 Neuro-arthropathy (Charcot joints) in diabetes mellitus. Medicine 51: 191–210

Stuart M J, Morrey B F 1990 Arthrodesis of the diabetic neuropathic ankle joint. Clin Orthop 253: 209–211

VI.6 Amputation

John Angel

Introduction

Controversy surrounds amputations of the foot. When they work well they enable a high level of activity and require a minimum of prosthetic attention. Unfortunately, they are also prone to failure (Irwin 1919), which sometimes does not become apparent for many wearisome months of frustration for both the patient and the rehabilitation team.

There are two guiding principles to be observed. Firstly, the foot must be capable of coming to the plantigrade position, preferably with mobile joints under normal muscular control. Secondly, the weight-bearing area of the sole should be covered with sound, innervated skin (McCowan et al 1987).

The factors that lead to foot amputations and the amputations themselves have a tendency to produce equinus deformities, which often lead to weight-bearing on the scarred ends of the stumps that are unable to tolerate the shear forces and pressure of even the most gentle walking (Fig. 1). This manifests itself as pain or, in the insensate foot, ulceration. The answer is to guard against the development of equinus deformity by using physiotherapy, plaster casts, tenotomy, tendon transfer or even an external fixator (Burgess 1966).

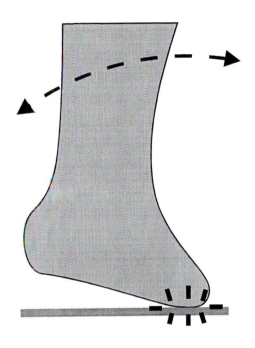

Figure 1

Rocking motion challenges the plantar skin of the partially amputated foot, especially in the presence of fixed equinus

Causes

Trauma and the complications of diabetes mellitus are together responsible for most foot amputations. Lawn mowers and trains account for a significant proportion of the cases of mechanical trauma, and thermal damage occurs in the form of burns, frostbite, trench foot and cold exposure resulting from drug or alcohol abuse.

Arteriosclerosis usually involves the proximal vascular tree (down to the level of the popliteal arteries), and when gangrene occurs with this condition, it usually represents the tip of a large iceberg of disordered tissue for which a foot amputation is inadequate, unless the situation can be improved with reconstructive vascular surgery. In diabetes, arterial blockage tends to occur proximally and also distally in vessels the size of the metatarsal arteries and smaller. Thus, when gangrene occurs in the diabetic it does so at a stage of relatively mild involvement of the proximal vessels, which means that well-perfused tissue can be found quite close to the gangrene. This makes distal amputation possible.

Sometimes diabetic neuropathy leads to severe infection in the foot. Usually this can be cleared by debridement rather than amputation.

Congenital problems requiring amputation include polydactyly, macrodactyly, failed clubfoot and longitudinal deficiency in which either leg length discrepancy or deformity cannot be overcome. Tumours are a less common cause of foot amputations. They include malignant primary tumours, haemangiomata and the occasional recurrent cases of pigmented villonodular synovitis and plantar fibromatosis. Sometimes partial toe amputations are a good solution for overriding second toe, long mallet toes and persistent ingrowing toenail.

Level selection and predictive factors

In general, it is better to sacrifice some of the length of the residual foot rather than violate the principles set out

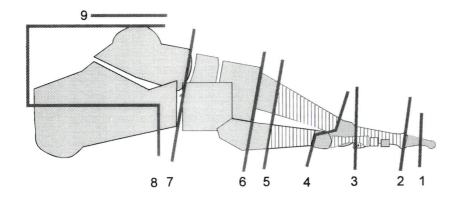

Figure 2

Recommended levels for foot amputations:
(1) through terminal phalanx of big toe; (2)
through interphalangeal joint of big toe
(distal interphalangeal joint for lesser toes);
(3) through metatarsophalangeal joint(s); (4)
through distal transmetatarsals; (5) proximal
transmetatarsals; (6) through tarsometatarsal
joints (Lisfranc); (7) mid-tarsal level
(Chopart); (8) Boyd amputation; (9) ankle
disarticulation (Syme amputation).
Amputations through the shaded areas are
not usually recommended

at the beginning of this chapter. Bearing this in mind, there are certain amputation levels to be avoided and others to be aimed at (Fig. 2).

Partial amputations of the lesser toes have a tendency to develop extension contractures, so much so that Baumgartner (1988) recommended disarticulation at the metatarsophalangeal joint as the only acceptable level. However, the lesser toes do have value as spacers, preventing the remaining toes from bunching together; amputation of the second toe in particular is commonly followed by the development of hallux valgus. To retain its value as a spacer Chapman (1973) recommended partial amputation of the second toe, though not of the lesser three toes. Farquharson (1966) endorsed this policy and recommended an extensor tenotomy and postoperative physiotherapy to prevent deformity. Most authors agree that no toe should be left with less than one complete phalanx. Where this is not possible amputation should be either through the base of the proximal phalanx or through the metatarsophalangeal joint.

In the case of the hallux, good results can be achieved by amputating through the terminal phalanx or at the interphalangeal joint. If this is not possible then an amputation through the base of the proximal phalanx or the metatarsophalangeal joint should be selected. Baumgartner (1988) recommends shaping the head and removing the sesamoid bones in preference to a metatarsophalangeal disarticulation. Disarticulation of all the toes in cases of severe clawing with subluxed tarsometatarsal joints was recommended by Flint and Sweetnam (1960). First and fifth ray resections are occasionally indicated in order to achieve closure or to remove dead infected bone. Occasionally ray resections are carried out on the second, third or fourth rays although the result is rarely satisfactory.

With regard to the transmetatarsal level, most authors are united in their preference for amputating through the metatarsal necks. Chapman (1973) believes in the preservation of metatarsal length as far as possible but Baumgartner (1988) avoids amputation through the cortical bone of the metatarsal shafts because of the

increased risk of infection; he recommends section through their necks or bases instead.

Amputation through the tarsometatarsal joint (Lisfranc amputation – Lisfranc, 1815) produces an irregular bony surface, and it is better to leave the bases of the second and fifth metatarsals. This level of amputation has the advantage of preserving the invertors and evertors of the foot but the disadvantage of removing the insertion of the tibialis anterior tendon, so making the remaining foot vulnerable to developing an equinus deformity in the early postoperative stage. This can be guarded against either by keeping the foot in a cast in slight dorsiflexion in the first six weeks while the cut end of the tendon forms a new insertion into the tarsal bones or by performing a formal tendon transfer.

The classical Chopart disarticulation was performed through the talonavicular and the calcaneocuboid joints (Kirkup 1994). But wherever feasible as much bone as possible should be conserved between the tarsometatarsal and mid-tarsal joints so that the operation usually becomes an *ad hoc* amputation in the mid-foot area. The principal disadvantage of this amputation level is the tendency for the stump to tilt into equinus, owing to the unopposed action of the calf muscles. For the stump to be successful, the tendon of tibialis anterior must be transferred to the neck of the talus or allowed to insert naturally into the remaining tarsal bones while the foot is prevented from tilting into equinus. It should be noted that amputations in this area, at one time condemned, have become acceptable in recent years because of improved postoperative techniques and more advanced prosthetic fitting.

The Boyd amputation (Boyd 1939), in which the distal half of the os calcis is fused to the distal tibia, produces a particularly robust stump and it is appropriate where there is diminished sensation, leg length discrepancy and healthy periarticular bone. The Syme amputation is one that has stood the test of time and it produces marginally better functional results than the trans-tibial level (Harris 1956). However, it is not so much better that it outweighs the cosmetic disadvantage of a bulky stump and so this level cannot normally be recommended for women (Fig. 3).

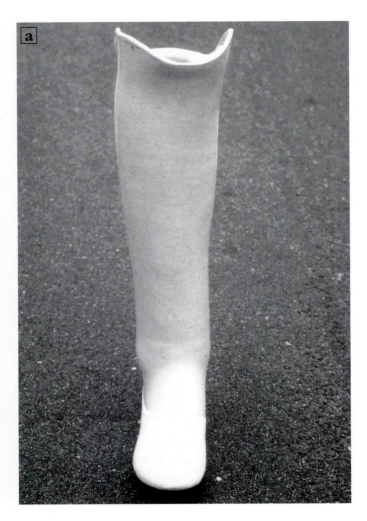 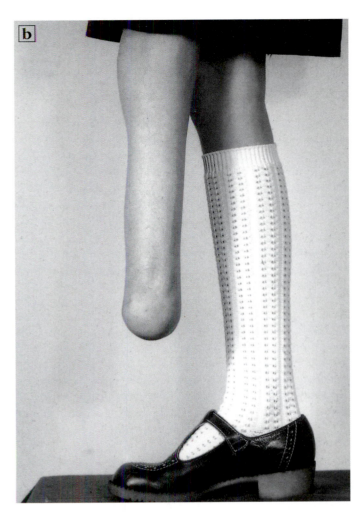

Figure 3

A Syme prosthesis tends to produce a fat ankle (a) unless it is done where there is a marked limb length discrepancy (b), allowing the 'bulb' to be concealed in the shape of the prosthetic calf

With regard to the preoperative assessment of patients with vascular disease, Larssen & Anderson (1978) found significantly worse results in older patients. Other researchers (Schwartz et al 1982, Hodge et al 1989, Rosendahl 1992) looked specifically for this effect but found that their older patients did no worse than the younger. Schwartz et al (1982) and Hodge et al (1989) found that diabetics did better than nondiabetics and assumed that this was due to the different pattern of vascular involvement. But more frequently it has been reported that the results were the same in the two groups of patients.

Hunter (1975) warned that the results of partial foot amputations were worse where a previous amputation had already been undertaken. For this reason he advised against toe amputations on the grounds that this might well mitigate against the success of a trans-metatarsal amputation, which was often required later. Subsequent authors had no worse results following previous amputation.

Many authors (McKittrick et al 1949, Warren et al 1952, Larssen & Anderson 1978) found that better results were

obtained if there was a long interval between the onset of the gangrene and the amputation, and advised two or three weeks of preoperative hospitalization and conservative treatment. However, the beneficial effects may have simply been due to the selecting out of cases with rapidly advancing arterial obstruction.

Special investigations to assess blood supply have not proved as useful for foot amputations as they have at other levels (e.g. the transtibial level). A number of researchers (Barnes et al 1981, Holstein 1984) found that the systolic blood pressure at the ankle gave an indication of the likely success of forefoot amputation, but this has been denied by others (Mehta et al 1980, Bone & Pomajzl 1981, Schwartz et al 1982, Pinzur et al 1986, Doucette et al 1989). Skin perfusion measured by isotope clearance was thought (Holstein 1984, Welch et al 1985) to give a good indication of local viability, with several workers believing it to be the 'gold standard' of predictive factors. However, Boeckstyns & Jensen (1984) found no correlation. Recent papers (Barnes et al 1981, Bone

& Pomejzl 1981, Schwartz et al 1982, Holstein 1984) have pointed to photoplethysmography as an equally valuable method of assessment, especially as it is simpler and more rapidly performed. It has been noted as providing good results in the toes themselves where other methods are less practicable (Doucette et al 1989).

Where tissue damage has been at least in part due to ischaemia and this factor has subsequently subsided (as in frostbite, resolving cellulitis, crush injury or a foot that has been improved by successful vascular surgery), one should be cautious in deciding amputation level. It is worth waiting until incontrovertible demarcation has displayed the most distal limits at which the amputation can be performed.

Pinzur et al (1986) found that amputations in the middle level of the foot were less likely to succeed if the serum albumin was below 3.0 g/dl or the lymphocyte count was below 1500 per ml³. Bailey et al (1979) showed a remarkably high negative correlation between the preoperative haemoglobin level and the success of the amputation, anaemic patients doing far better than those with a normal haemoglobin. This pointed to the possible importance of blood viscosity in amputation surgery. Turnbull & Chester (1988) produced convincing figures to show that the results of forefoot amputations in diabetic patients were dependent on the experience of the operator.

Handling of tissues

Skin covering the parts of the stump that carry weight, not only in the stance phase but at heel strike and toe off, must be healthy, free from scars and have unimpaired sensitivity to pinprick (McKittrick et al 1949, Wagner 1977). The only exception to this rule is the Syme and Boyd amputation stumps where the prosthetic fitting can be used to protect anaesthetic skin (Fig. 4). If dorsal skin or skin grafts are used to make up for inadequate plantar skin the result is rarely satisfactory. To allow the long plantar flap to be sutured to the short or nonexistent dorsal flap, the points from which the two flaps are marked need to be relatively near the plantar surface of the foot.

The cut through the deep tissue is usually tapered to a point just proximal to the bone section. The subcutaneous loculi are damaged as little as possible, those tendons not required for tenodesis are normally cut well back, and the bones are cut usually with an oscillating saw and well rounded with a rasp. Most vessels are coagulated to secure haemostasis but the plantar and dorsalis pedis vessels need to be ligated with an absorbable suture. Named nerves are pulled down and cut high with scissors. Cutting them with a knife allows them to spring proximally leaving the last few fibres to be cut at a much more distal level. These can later form a troublesome neuroma.

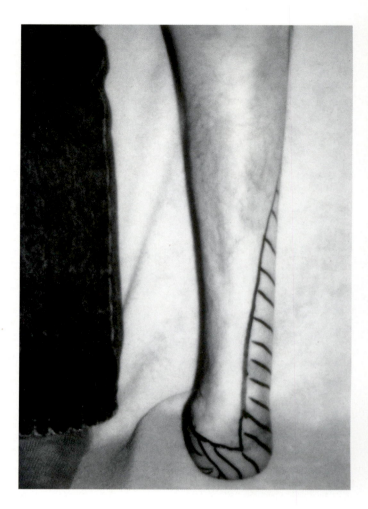

Figure 4
This Boyd amputation stump was totally anaesthetic in the marked area, owing to a complete sciatic nerve palsy. Nevertheless the patient led an almost normal active life wearing an enclosed end-bearing prosthesis

Most wounds are closed using Vicryl for the deep layer and either staples or 3–0 nylon interrupted sutures for the skin. Where there is a tendency for the remaining part of the foot to deviate from the plantigrade position this must be prevented by a cast or even a system of percutaneous pins and distracter.

Operative details

Amputation of the toes

Partial amputation of the distal phalanx of the hallux
A circular incision is made around the nail and taken down to bone (Fig. 5). The disc of tissue so removed must include the nail and the skin enfolding it together

with all the germinal matrix. The distal half of the terminal phalanx is removed. The plantar flap is then approximated to the dorsal. Undue tension may be relieved by excising additional bone.

Disarticulation of the big toe at the phalangeal joint

The skin flaps are marked from two points on either side of the toe, level with the head of the proximal phalanx and slightly more towards the plantar aspect than the dorsal (see Fig. 5). A short dorsal flap and a longer plantar one are required. The incisions are taken down to bone and the distal phalanx is disarticulated after dividing the flexor and extensor tendons. Haemostasis is secured by means of diathermy and the flexor and extensor tendons are sutured to one another over the end of the bone. The flaps are then approximated. It may be necessary to excise extra tissue to ensure that the resulting stump is not bulky and unsightly. These instructions apply equally to a disarticulation at the distal interphalangeal joint of one of the lesser toes as to disarticulation through the interphalangeal joint of the hallux.

Disarticulation of a toe at the metatarsophalangeal joint

A racquet incision is made, with the handle of the racquet lying over the dorsum of the foot to give access to the metatarsophalangeal joint (Fig. 6). The blade part of the raquet is located not at the root of the toe but sufficiently distal to this level to fashion flaps that will easily come together. In the case of the great toe and the little toe the handle of the racquet inclines somewhat to the centre of the foot to avoid pressure on the scar. After the incision has been made, the toe is pulled down and the extensor tendon is divided at its insertion. The capsule of the joint is then divided and the phalanx is stripped away from the plantar structures.

For the first metatarsophalangeal joint, Baumgartner (1988) now recommends excising the sesamoids and trimming the head of the first metatarsal. This can significantly reduce the amount of soft tissue cover required, which can be a considerable advantage in infected dysvascular cases. On the rare occasions when neither blood supply nor contamination is a problem, it may be desirable to suture the tendons over the head of the first metatarsal in order to try to stabilize the sesamoid bones. It may even be possible to leave the base of the proximal phalanx for the same purpose. When removing an infected lesser toe, there may similarly be an advantage in leaving the extreme base of the proximal phalanx in order to avoid opening into the main cavity of the metatarsophalangeal joint. This technique leaves a much smaller wound cavity, so it may be useful in a badly infected case.

Following the removal of the toe or toes, haemostasis is achieved and the wound is either closed loosely with

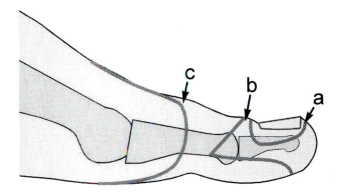

Figure 5

Skin flaps for amputations involving the hallux: (a) partial amputation of the distal phalanx; (b) disarticulation at the interphalangeal joint; (c) disarticulation at the metatarsophalangeal joint

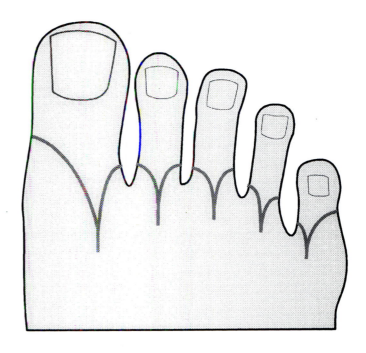

Figure 6

The racquet incisions used for individual toe amputations

a few interrupted sutures or, if infection is present, left open and the flaps are allowed to fall together.

Amputation of all the toes

This can be achieved by means of two single flaps, a dorsal and a plantar. This produces a specimen in which all five toes are linked together by narrow bridges of skin forming the apices of the toe clefts.

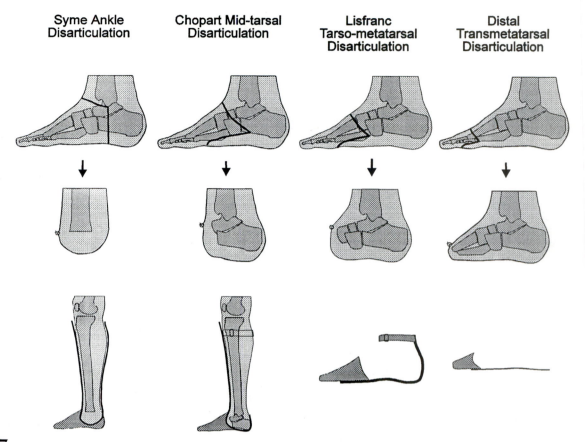

| Syme Ankle Disarticulation | Chopart Mid-tarsal Disarticulation | Lisfranc Tarso-metatarsal Disarticulation | Distal Transmetatarsal Disarticulation |

Figure 7

The Syme and mid-foot amputations, their skin incisions, the resulting shapes and their orthotic or prosthetic requirements

Transmetatarsal amputation

This must be performed through the cancellous bone of either the metatarsal heads or their bases, since the cortical bone of the shafts has a poor resistance to infection. The skin flaps for the more distal procedure are marked from points on either side of the foot level with the metatarsal necks and close to the plantar aspect (Fig. 7). The plantar flap extends virtually to the roots of the toes and the dorsal flap to the metatarsophalangeal joints. The plantar incision is extended through the deeper layers, raking the incision down to the metatarsal necks. For the higher level the flaps are based level with the tarsometatarsal joints. The plantar flap is fashioned longer on the medial side, enabling it to cover the thicker base of the first metatarsal.

The flexor tendons are pulled down and cut as high as possible. The metatarsal nerves are sought and sectioned high. The tourniquet is released and haemostasis secured. The deep tissues are sutured over the ends of the bone with Vicryl 2–0 and the skin with interrupted nylon.

The foot is encased in copious plaster wool and immobilized in a slightly dorsiflexed position in a below-knee plaster cast. The plaster is changed to allow the wound to be inspected at 4–7 days. The plaster is changed again at 2–3 weeks to allow the sutures to be removed, and after this time weight-bearing is allowed. When healing has occurred (Fig. 8), the patient will be able to wear one of his old shoes with a filler occupying the space previously taken up by the toes and a stiff insole to prevent the shoe from deforming because of the more posterior location of the toe-break.

Lisfranc disarticulation

Disarticulation at the tarsometatarsal joint in its pure form is not recommended because of the irregular surface presented by the distal aspect of the tarsal bones. It is better to leave the base of the second and fifth metatarsals in order to fill in the irregularities. A long plantar skin flap is marked out using the same principles as for the transmetatarsal amputation (see Fig. 7). A raking cut is made through the deep tissues of the plantar flap, taking care to avoid damage to the plantar arteries, which are close to the second and third cuneiform bones. The second and fifth metatarsals are divided with an osteotome. The remainder of Lisfranc's joint is then disarticulated. In order to bring the rather stiff plantar flap over the front of the tarsus it may be necessary to reduce its thickness, taking care to avoid

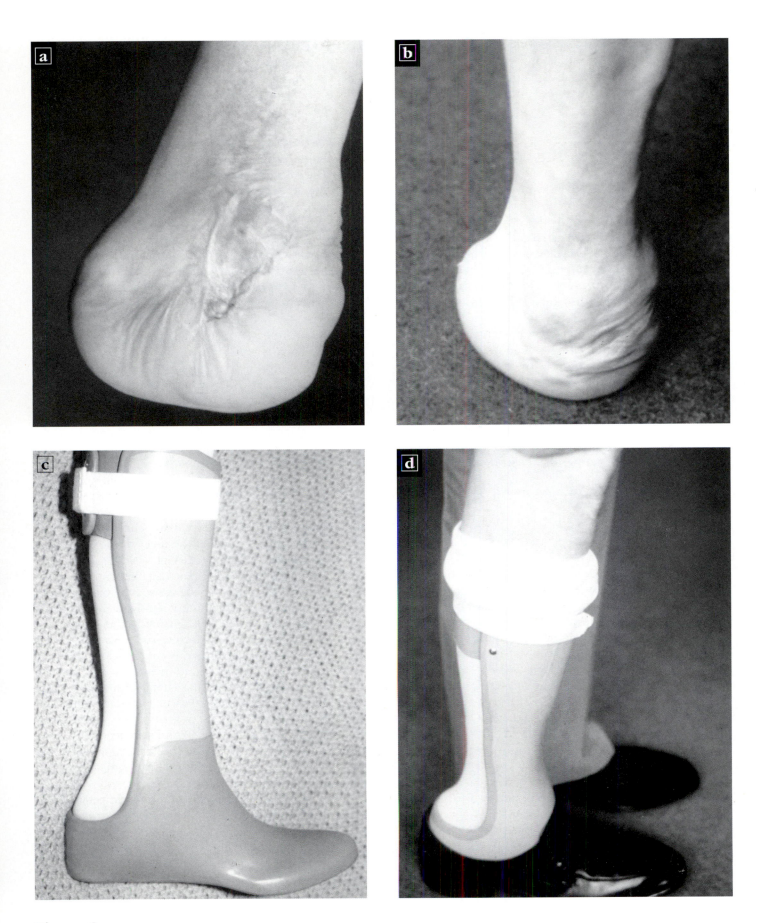

Figure 8

This Chopart stump is capable of strong dorsiflexion (a) and can easily carry the patient's full weight (b). The rigid prosthesis (c) allows ambulation with a normal 'roll-over' and the wearing of a shop-bought shoe (d).

damage to the blood supply and plantar nerves. Before closing the soft tissues, any bony prominences should be rounded. The postoperative care is the same as that described for the transmetatarsal level.

Chopart disarticulation

The skin flaps are fashioned with sufficient length to cover the residual bone or, if it is the skin that is in short supply, the bone is divided to suit the length of the available plantar flap (see Fig. 7). The plantar and dorsalis pedis vessels are ligated and the related nerves are pulled down and cut high. Where the conditions allow and the risk of sepsis is slight, the tibialis anterior tendon is passed through a hole drilled in the neck of the talus and sutured to itself, as described by Christie et al (1980). If the wound is too contaminated for this to be done safely, the Achilles tendon is tenotomized percutaneously and the cut ends of the tendon of tibialis anterior and those of the toe extensors are approximated as far as possible to the dorsum of the foot. The gap is subsequently minimized by immobilizing the foot in plaster in a position of dorsiflexion. The bones are rounded and the wound is closed in layers. The postoperative care is the same as that described for the transmetatarsal level.

Syme amputation

Because of its importance and greater reliability this amputation is described in greater length. The stump is often, though not always, able to take full body weight without a prosthesis, despite the fact that the limb is usually 50 mm (2 inches) shorter than the opposite side. The stump allows the patient to walk short distances and obviates the need to don the prosthesis in the night to go to the toilet, for example. The amputation is suitable when there is complete anaesthesia of the distal end of the stump because the prosthesis largely protects the stump from shear forces. The stump can easily be ruined by failure to attend to points of detail during surgery or in the postoperative phase.

The sides of the posterior flap are marked by lines drawn from the tips of the malleoli perpendicular to the sole of the foot. The distal edge of the flap is produced by joining these two lines across the sole of the foot. It will be noted that this produces a flap that is shorter on the lateral side compared to the medial. The anterior flap is marked by the line taking the shortest route across the front of the ankle from the tips of the malleoli. The anterior incision is deepened down to the flexor retinaculum, which is also incised. The tibialis anterior tendon is grasped with tissue forceps and cut as high as possible. It is cut again distally and the intervening segment

is discarded to prevent it from getting in the way during the rest of the operation. The same procedure is carried out for flexor hallucis longus and flexor digitorum longus. The anterior tibial vessels are identified, divided and ligated with a transfixion ligature using an absorbable material.

The ankle joint is then opened across its full extent from the tip of the medial to the tip of the lateral malleolus. The plantar incision is deepened with a slightly tapering cut that passes through all layers down to bone. The remains of the medial and lateral ligaments of the ankle are divided, allowing the foot to be drawn forwards, giving a view over the back of the talus. A sharp hook introduced in the back of the talus facilitates this. The soft tissues are gradually cleared from the talus, taking care to avoid damage to the flexor hallucis longus tendon, behind which lie the posterior vessels. Working backwards, the soft tissues are cleared from the dorsum and sides of the os calcis. As the dissection proceeds, the sharp hook is transferred to the back of the os calcis. By working steadily from side to side, the surgeon gradually strips the os calcis using sharp dissection with a scalpel. Eventually the os calcis, together with the rest of the amputation specimen, comes free, leaving an empty heel pad. The weight-bearing properties of the tissue are best preserved by leaving the fatty loculi intact and confining the dissection to the subperiosteal plane.

The peroneal, posterior tibial, flexor digitorum longus and flexor hallucis longus tendons are all grasped with tissue forceps and used to help retract the soft tissues as the malleoli are exposed by extraperiosteal dissection. The periosteum is cleared at the level of the ankle joint and the malleoli are removed with a single cut using a tenon saw. It is most important that this cut is perpendicular to the long axis of the tibia and that it is at a level that removes, but only just removes, the subchondral cortical bone of the tibial plafond. After cutting the bone, all the remaining tendons, apart from the Achilles tendon, are pulled down and cut as close to their musculotendinous junctions as possible. The anterior tibial nerve and the medial and lateral plantar nerves are cut high. The three main vascular pedicles are also ligated. The tourniquet is released and haemostasis secured. The wound is tidied and cleared of any poorly vascularized tags. After insertion of a suction drain, the plantar fascia is sutured to the extensor retinaculum and the skin is closed with staples.

The wound is dressed with gauze and the entire stump to the level of the knee is covered with a well-padded plaster cast. Suspension is accomplished by moulding the cast in the coronal plane just above the bulb of the stump. The drain is pulled out from the top of the cast after 2 days and the plaster is changed and the wound inspected after 4–6 days. If wound healing proceeds uneventfully, the patient should be able to walk in the cast by the third or fourth postoperative week. In order to preserve the position of the heel pad, the cast must be maintained until a prosthesis has been supplied.

In the Boyd amputation the bottom half of the os calcis is preserved and secured to the cut distal end of the tibia. It is very similar to the Syme amputation; in fact it may be impossible clinically to distinguish it, since bone is commonly formed by the periosteum contained in the heel pad of a Syme stump. The Boyd amputation may have particular value where the distal tibia has insufficient surface area to provide an adequate platform for the heel pad; its disadvantage is in producing an overlong stump, so it is best used in cases where there has been significant previous shortening.

Prosthetics

When a toe is amputated, the neighbouring digits tend to deviate towards the resulting space. This tendency is minimized by fitting a silastic spacer, supplied by podiatrists or orthotists. The remaining toes are also prone to attract undue pressure from the toe box of the shoe and may need to be fitted with a protective cap. The loss of several toes or of all the toes requires a filler to be located in the end of the shoe. This is usually mounted on a thin insole to maintain its position. A distal transmetatarsal amputation requires, besides a toe filler, a stiffer insole in order to prevent the shoe from deforming.

The proximal transmetatarsal and Lisfranc stumps not only flex the shoe in the wrong place but also tend to cause the heel to come out of the back of the shoe. This can be avoided by means of a strap that passes from the back of the strong insole up around the ankle (see Fig. 7). A similar type of device will work for many Chopart stumps but to achieve a natural gait with 'toe-off' it is necessary to fix a rigid gaiter to a stiff prosthetic foot (see Fig. 8).

A Syme prosthesis comprises a rigid shell, closely fitted around the stump up to the knee, with a prosthetic foot bolted or firmly glued distally. The shock-absorbing and energy-storing capacity that can be built into the foot is largely dependent on the relative shortening of the limb, 50 mm (2 inches) being sufficient to fit a unit adequate for most purposes.

References

Bailey M J, Johnston CL, Yates C J P et al 1979 Preoperative haemoglobin as predictor of outcome of diabetic amputations. Lancet 8135: 168–170

Barnes R W, Thornhill B, Nix L et al 1981 Prediction of amputation wound healing. Arch Surg 116: 80–83

Baumgartner R F 1988 Partial foot amputations: aetiology, principles, operative techniques. In: Murdoch G (ed) Amputation Surgery and Lower Limb Prosthetics. Blackwell Scientific Publications, Oxford. pp 97–104

Boeckstyns M, Jensen C M 1984 Amputation of the forefoot. Acta Orthop Scand 55: 224–226

Bone G E, Pomajzl M J 1981 Toe blood pressure by photoplethysmography: an index of healing in forefoot amputation. Surgery 89: 69–74

Boyd H B 1939 Amputation of the foot with calcaneotibial arthrodesis. J Bone Joint Surg 21: 997–1000

Burgess E 1966 Prevention and correction of fixed equinus deformity in midfoot amputations. Bull Prosthet Res spring volume: 45–48

Chapman M W 1973 Amputations. In: Inman V T (ed) Du Vries' Surgery of the Foot. C V Mosby, St Louis. pp 443–456

Christie J, Cloughs C B, Lamb D W 1980 Amputations through the middle part of the foot. J Bone Joint Surg 62B: 473–474

Doucette M M, Fylling C, Knighton D R 1989 Amputation prevention in a high-risk population through comprehensive wound-healing protocol. Arch Phys Med Rehabil 70: 780–785

Farquharson E L 1966 Textbook of Operative Surgery. Livingstone, Edinburgh, London

Flint M, Sweetnam R 1960 Amputation of all toes. J Bone Joint Surg 42B: 90–96

Harris R I 1956 Syme's amputation: the technical details essential for success. J Bone Joint Surg 38B: 614–632

Hodge M J, Peters T G, Efird W G 1989 Amputation of the distal portion of the foot. South Med J 82: 1138–1142

Holstein P 1984 The distal blood pressure predicts healing on the feet. Acta Orthop Scand 55: 227–233

Hunter G A 1975 Results of minor foot amputations for ischaemia of the lower extremity in diabetics and nondiabetics. Can J Surg 18: 273–276

Irwin S T 1919 The end results of partial amputations of the foot. Br J Surg 7: 327–334

Kirkup J 1994 Foot amputations: (1) Fore- and midfoot. Foot 4: 45–47

Larssen U, Anderson G B J 1978 Partial amputation of the foot for diabetic or arteriosclerotic gangrene: results and factors of prognostic value. J Bone Joint Surg 60B: 126–130

Lisfranc J 1815 Nouvelle méthode opératoire pour l'amputation partielle du pied. Gabon, Paris

McCowan M B, Millstein G A, Hunter M B 1987 Traumatic partial foot amputations: a long-term follow-up study. J Bone Joint Surg 69B: 503

McKittrick L S, McKittrick J B, Risley T S 1949 Transmetatarsal amputation for infection or gangrene in patients with diabetes mellitus. Ann Surg 130: 826–842

Mehta K, Hobson R W, Jamil Z et al 1980 Fallibility of Doppler ankle pressure in predicting healing of transmetatarsal amputation. J Clin Res 28: 466–470

Pinzur M P, Kaminsky M, Sage R et al 1986 Amputations in the middle level of the foot. J Bone Joint Surg 68A: 1061–1064

Rosendahl S 1992 Transmetatarsal amputation in diabetic gangrene. Acta Orthop Scand 42: 78–83

Schwartz J A, Schuler J J, O'Connor R J et al 1982 Predictive value of distal perfusion for the healing of amputation of the digits and the forefoot. Surg Gynecol Obstet 154: 865–869

Turnbull A R, Chester J F 1988 Partial amputations of the foot for diabetic gangrene. Ann R Coll Surg 70: 329–331

Wagner F W 1977 Amputations of the foot and ankle: current status. Clin Orthop 122: 62–69

Warren R, Crawford E S, Hardy I B et al 1952 The transmetatarsal amputation in arterial deficiency of the lower extremity. Surgery 31: 132–140

Welch G H, Lieberman D P, Pollock J G et al 1985 Failure of Doppler ankle pressure to predict healing of conservative forefoot amputations. Br J Surg 72: 888–891

VI.7 Tumours

Brian C Sommerlad and Peter A Revell

In this chapter, tumours, and tumour-like conditions have been divided into those that appear to arise from the skin or immediately subcutaneous tissue, those that arise from soft tissue (excluding synovium), those which may arise from synovial tissue or at least show synovial characteristics, and those which arise from bone. The divisions may not be clear-cut as the tissue of origin of some tumours is uncertain and as tumours may spread to involve adjacent tissue.

Skin

The skin of the foot is prone to most of the tumours and tumour-like conditions occurring elsewhere in the body. However, the skin of the sole is histologically different from that of the dorsum, having profuse eccrine glands, no sebaceous glands, very thick stratum corneum and no hair. This gives a guide as to the sort of tumours which occur at each site. Disorders of the skin of the foot may be part of a generalized disease. Many of these conditions have been dealt with earlier (Chapter VI.2). Only the common and important tumours will be discussed here (Table 1).

Diagnosis

Diagnosis first depends on an adequate history. The duration of the lesion is all-important and change in a previously quiescent lesion should be viewed with suspicion. A history of previous trauma may be important, but may be a 'red herring'. A search should always be made for similar swellings elsewhere, with particular care being taken to examine the other foot. Examination, by demonstrating mobility on deep tissues, should confirm that the tumour arises from the skin. Variation of colour in a pigmented lesion may be important. Ulceration of a skin tumour may indicate malignancy, especially if the margins are raised and indurated. Examination of popliteal and groin lymph nodes should be routine. If doubt about the diagnosis remains, excision biopsy (if the lesion is small) or incision biopsy (if large) is indicated.

General principles of management

Because of the tendency of the sole of the foot to produce hyperkeratotic, fissured scars, and of the dorsum of the foot to produce scars which rub on footwear, unnecessary operations must be avoided on the weight bearing sole. In particular, a benign lesion which will respond to nonsurgical measures such as cryotherapy should not be surgically excised. Where surgical excision is necessary on the weight bearing sole, the aims should be to produce as little scar as possible on and adjacent to the weight bearing area, to preserve as much subcutaneous fat as possible, to leave fibrous attachments to bone as undisturbed as possible and to preserve sensation.

Unfortunately, there is little spare skin on the dorsum of the foot and still less on the sole. Removal of a tumour, therefore, frequently necessitates skin replacement. Split skin grafts may be satisfactory on the dorsum and on non-weight-bearing areas of the sole. Grafts on weight bearing sole tend to be protected by the patient by alteration of gait, if possible (Sommerlad & McGrouther 1978), this being more easily achieved on the heel than on the forefoot (Fig. 1). Random local skin flaps and muscle flaps (Ger 1975) are useful in certain situations. Distant flaps, lacking the specialized skin and subcutaneous tissue of the sole, are best avoided if possible. Neurovascular island flaps from toes which are to be amputated, or from web spaces, may be useful for small defects. The instep flap, based on the medial plantar nerves and vessels (Shanahan & Gingrass 1979, Harrison & Morgan 1981) may be used as an ipsilateral island pedicled flap, a contralateral pedicled flap (requiring subsequent division) or as a free microvascular flap. This may be the most suitable form of reconstruction for a significant area of weight bearing sole.

Table 1 Tumours and tumour-like conditions of skin

Congenital	Haemangioma
	Lymphangioma
	Neurofibromatosis
	Hamartoma
Traumatic	Keratoses – callosities and corns
	Inclusion dermoid cysts
Infective	Pyogenic granuloma
	Warts
	Specific infections (tuberculosis, mycoses, leprosy and yaws)
Degenerative and miscellaneous	Sarcoidosis
	Epidermal cysts
	Granuloma annulare
Neoplastic	Benign fibrous histiocytoma
	Acquired digital fibrokeratoma

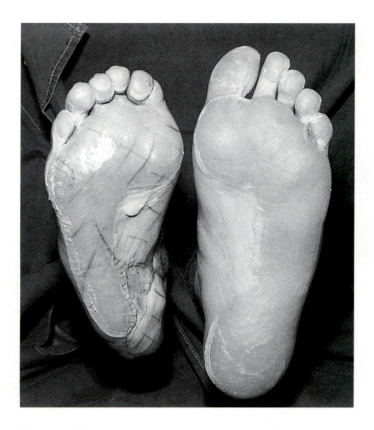

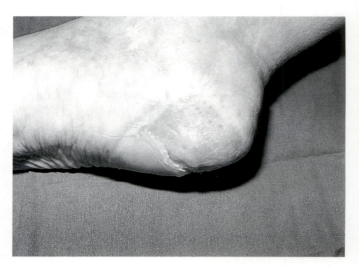

Figure 2

Hyperkeratosis of the sole adjacent to a split skin graft over the heel (with fissuring)

Figure 1

Demonstration of weight bearing patterns (by asking the patient to walk on coloured paint) shows that a skin graft used for heel cover does not actually take weight and is avoided by the patient

Common tumours and tumour-like conditions of skin

Traumatic

Keratoses, callosities and corns
The skin of the sole of the foot responds to abnormality within, or abnormal pressure without, by excessive production of keratin (Jahss 1982) (Fig. 2). In callus, the parakeratin is relatively diffuse; in corns, there is a localized central core of keratin. Pressure of callus may produce underlying necrosis or adjacent fissuring (especially in vulnerable patients such as diabetics). Treatment consists of shaving and paring and subsequent avoidance of pressure by modification of footwear.

Inclusion dermoid cysts
The absence of a relevant history does not exclude penetration by a foreign body and the diagnosis should always be considered when there is an intradermal or subcutaneous swelling (Rowley et al 1978). Soft tissue penetration X-rays may show the offending foreign body. Treatment consists of excision of the entire cyst with its foreign body (if present).

Infective

Pyogenic granuloma
The pyogenic granuloma may follow recognized injury. It is usually red, partly compressible, may or may not be ulcerated or crusted and tends to bleed with minor trauma (Berlin et al 1972). Histologically, the lesion looks like chronic granulation tissue containing many capillaries, simulating a capillary haemangioma. Curettage and diathermy is usually the first line of treatment, although recurrence is not uncommon.

Warts
These are discussed in Chapter VI.2. The surgeon may see them when excessive keratin formation may suggest a neoplasm or underlying foreign body. He must resist all requests to excise them, because the disease is self-limiting, better treated by less radical means and the scar resulting from excision is likely to be a permanent source of trouble from hyperkeratosis and fissuring (Fig. 3).

Specific infection
Infections such as tuberculosis, mycoses, leprosy, sarcoidosis and yaws are discussed elsewhere, but may be mistaken for tumours.

Degenerative and miscellaneous

Epidermoid cysts
These can occur on the dorsum of the foot, where they are not common but may occasionally be large.

Granuloma annulare
This condition may be mistaken for a basal cell carcinoma. It occurs commonly on the dorsum where it usually presents as a raised, reddish lesion, often in the form of

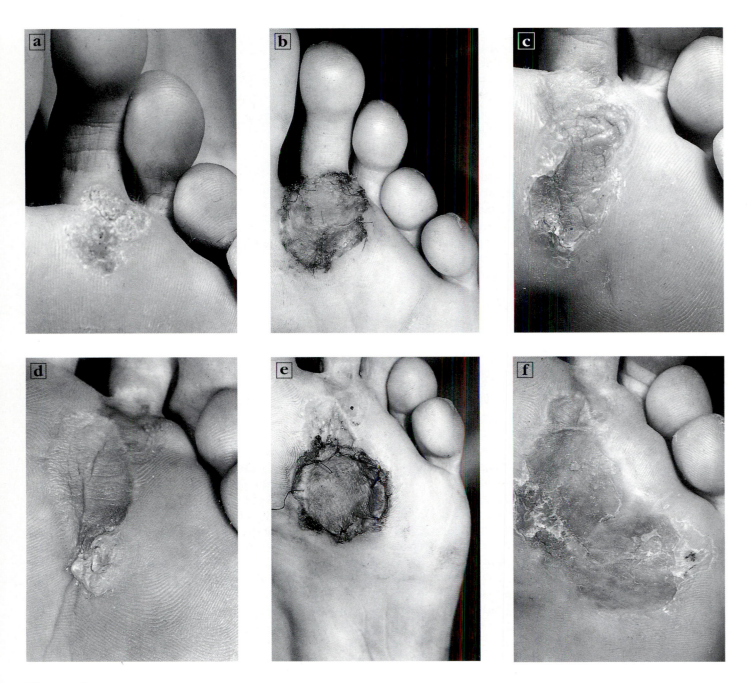

Figure 3

(a) Resistant plantar warts. (b) Treated by excision and graft. (c) Fissuring at the margin of the graft. (d) Increasing hyperkeratosis at the margin of the graft. (e) Wider excision and graft. (f) The most recent appearance following still further excision. This demonstrates that excision of the skin of the sole of the foot must be a last resort. Split skin grafts on the weight bearing sole (particularly the forefoot) are totally unsatisfactory

a doughnut and sometimes composed of discrete papules. No treatment is necessary if the diagnosis is made, as the lesion will almost certainly regress spontaneously.

Neoplastic

Benign fibrous histiocytoma (dermatofibroma or sclerosing haemangioma)
The fibrous histiocytoma or dermatofibroma is a benign tumour, presenting usually as a small, firm reddish-brown and sometimes almost green, painless nodule in the skin. It may be single or multiple and the extremities of adults are most commonly affected. Fibrous histiocytoma is rare on the soles of the feet (Bedi et al 1976) but does occur.

Occasionally these lesions are darker coloured or black, due to heavy deposition of haemosiderin, and under these conditions there may be clinical confusion with malignant melanoma. A firm consistency and the presence of a central dimple on lateral compression are useful clinical signs in making the distinction from melanoma (Fitzpatrick & Gilchrest 1977). The fibrous histiocytoma may occasionally be more deeply situated in the soft tissue of the extremities, again usually in young adults. They are yellow or white, well circumscribed masses on examination.

Histological examination shows that the fibrous histiocytoma is made up of fibroblasts, histiocytes, capillaries and young or mature collagen in varying proportion. The exact name used by the pathologist may vary according to the appearance and sclerosing haemangioma is considered to be the same type of lesion as fibrous histiocytoma (Gross & Wolbach 1943). Many now prefer to use the term 'fibrous histiocytoma' regardless of the particular features present in a given lesion (Enzinger & Weiss 1983). The collagen fibres in these tumours are typically arranged in an intertwined mat-like or 'storiform' pattern, or radiate from a central point in a whorled arrangement. Hyperplasia of the overlying epidermis occurs in over 80% of fibrous histiocytomas (Schoenfeld 1964).

In most cases, a definite clinical diagnosis can be made and no treatment is required unless the lesion is large or causing discomfort. On occasion, a benign fibrous histiocytoma may extend to several centimetres in diameter, arousing suspicion of malignancy which is not confirmed by histological examination.

Acquired digital fibrokeratoma

This is a benign tumour, occurring at any age, but predominantly in middle-aged men. It is a typically solitary sessile or pedunculated lesion, found usually on a toe, though occasionally on the sole of the foot (Verallo 1968) and may be present for months or years before the patient seeks medical advice. Histology reveals hyperkeratosis and acanthosis of the epidermis with thickened branching rete ridges, which cover a vertically arranged core of thick interwoven collagen bundles in which there are variable numbers of elastic fibres (Bart et al 1968, Hare & Smith 1969, Lever & Schaumberg-Lever 1983). The lesion may resemble a rudimentary supernumerary digit clinically, but is readily distinguished on pathological examination. More detailed accounts are available elsewhere (Verallo 1968, Bart et al 1968, Hare & Smith 1969, Hemric & Allen 1979). Treatment is by curettage and cautery or local excision.

Sweat gland tumours

Because of the high density of eccrine glands on the sole of the foot, one might expect a relatively high incidence of sweat gland tumours, but few have been reported (Forman & Streigold 1982). The eccrine poroma is the most common. It presents as a red swelling on the sole (Fig. 4). Histopathological examination shows ducts traversing solid masses of basophilic tumour cells extending into the dermis. Treatment is by local excision.

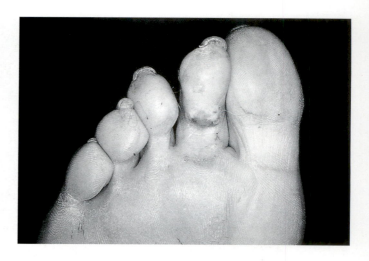

Figure 4

An eccrine poroma of the plantar surface of the second toe, presenting as a red nodule

Malignant sweat gland tumours are extremely rare in the foot.

Melanocytic naevi

These are not uncommon on the foot and there is a tradition that they may be more likely to become malignant than naevi elsewhere, although the evidence for this is thin. There is, however, an argument for removal if this can be done easily. Giant melanocytic naevi pose management problems, especially if situated on the sole of the foot. They can be verrucous and cause problems from friction, and they are also a potential neoplastic risk (Fig. 5). However, in general, the complications produced by excision and grafting would outweigh the risks of treatment by simple observation.

Basal cell carcinoma

The ubiquitous basal cell carcinoma in fact occurs very rarely on the foot (Kurzer & Patel 1979). It occasionally occurs on the dorsum of the foot or ankle, either as a typical raised, pearly 'cystic' lesion or, more commonly, as a crusted and somewhat indurated lesion which may well be disregarded by the patient for some time. Basal cell carcinoma of the sole is rare but not unknown (Robinson 1979). Treatment involves excision, usually with split skin grafting.

Squamous cell carcinoma

The typical, low-grade, actinic squamous cell carcinoma may occur on the dorsum of the foot where treatment consists of excision and grafting. The sole of the foot is one of the more common sites of the verrucous carcinoma or epithelioma cuniculatum (Seehafer et al 1979, Schwartz & Burgess 1980, McCann & Al-Nafussi 1989). These are proliferative lesions, sometimes looking rather

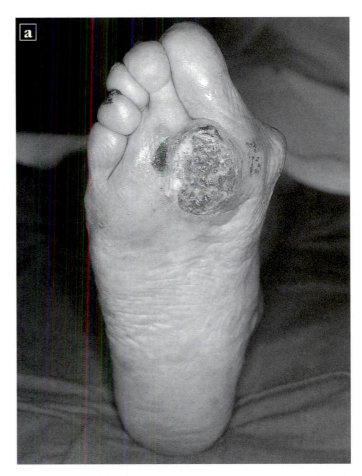

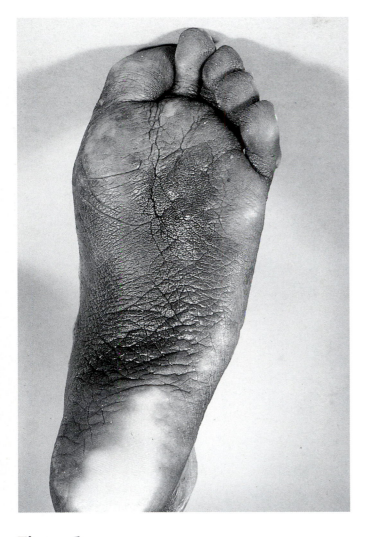

Figure 5

A giant congenital melanocytic naevus, involving the sole of the foot, with verrucous areas. Because of the morbidity from skin grafting, this has been treated conservatively by shaving verrucous areas and observation. Excision and split skin grafting has been avoided because of potential morbidity

warty or friable. They are often foul smelling. Not all squamous cell carcinomas of the sole of the foot are of this histological type (Fig. 6). Wide local excision is indicated (Demuth & Snider 1980) and reconstruction may be difficult, requiring specialized flaps. Lymph node metastases are not uncommon. Subungual squamous cell carcinoma occurs occasionally on the toes and is often diagnosed late. Distal amputation is indicated.

Malignant melanoma
The foot is a relatively common site for this potentially lethal tumour (Sondergaard & Olsen 1980), the incidence on the sole and dorsum being approximately equal. Malignant melanoma of the foot has been well reviewed (Fuselier et al 1985).

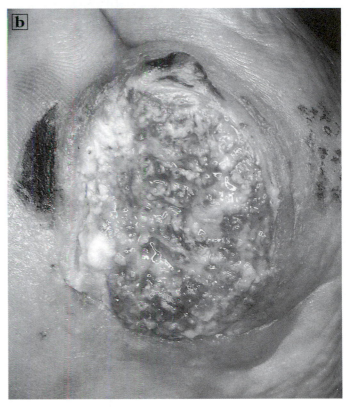

Figure 6

A well differentiated squamous cell carcinoma of the sole of the foot: (a) position; (b) close up

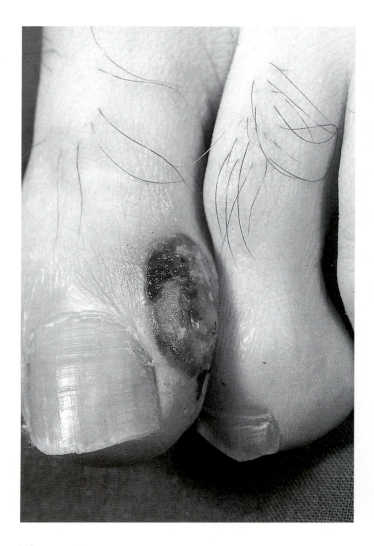

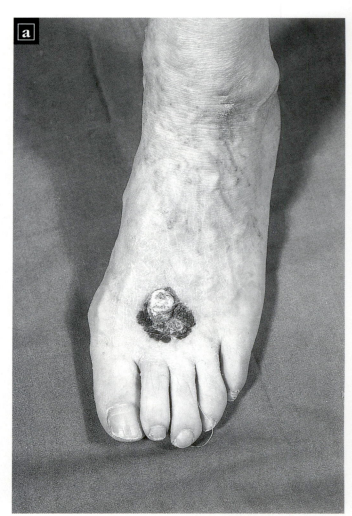

Figure 7

A histologically proven superficial spreading malignant melanoma of the left great toe in a 45-year-old man. Despite a Breslow thickness of 0.9 mm, this patient developed inguinal groin gland metastases. This tends to support the view that malignant melanoma of the foot carries a rather poorer prognosis than elsewhere

Lentigo maligna may occur on the dorsum of the foot, presents as a flat brown to black lesion with irregular margins, and may progress from a superficial noninvasive lesion to invasive nodular melanoma. Histopathological examination reveals intra-epidermal pleomorphic melanocytes, these cells varying from near normality to extreme abnormality.

Superficial spreading malignant melanoma presents as a flat or slightly raised pigmented lesion which may vary in colour from black or brown to tan, red, white or even bluish (Fig. 7). Histopathological examination shows atypical melanocytes arranged singly or in nests within the dermis. There may be lateral extension in the epidermis and dermal invasion in irregular cords and nests. The superficial spreading malignant melanoma may enter an invasive nodular phase (Fig. 8). The level of dermal

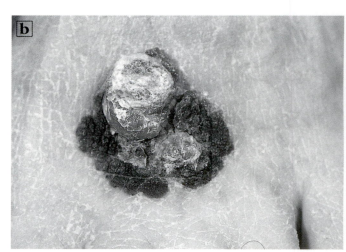

Figure 8

A superficial spreading malignant melanoma of the dorsum of the foot with nodule: (a) position; (b) close up

invasion can be classified according to Clark's level (Clark 1969) and the depth measured in millimetres from the granular cell layer of the epidermis to the depth of the tumour (Breslow 1970).

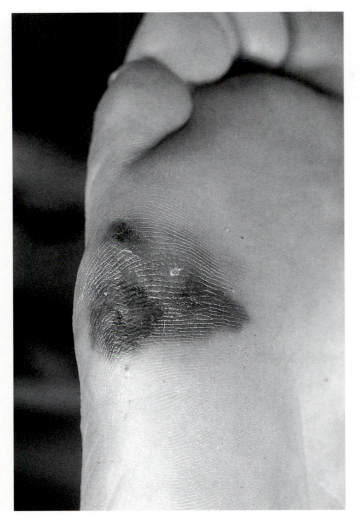

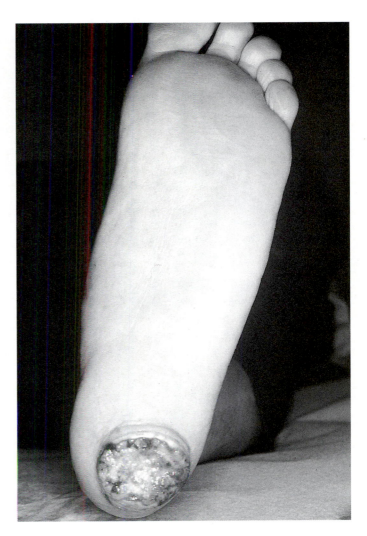

Figure 9

An acral lentiginous melanoma of the sole of the foot

Figure 10

A nodular melanoma of the heel – mainly amelanotic but with small areas of pigment visible

The acral lentiginous melanoma occurs in the foot as a plantar or subungual tumour (occurring also on the hand or on mucosal surfaces). Initially, it presents as a flat, irregular, brown or black lesion. Later it may become more raised and palpable (Fig. 9). Histopathological examination demonstrates large pleomorphic melanocytes in the basal layer. In early lesions, the cells have large nuclei and prominent long dendrites. In later invasive tumours, the cells may be spindle-shaped and non-pigmented. Acral lentiginous melanoma is the most common variety of melanoma in many series (Scrivner et al 1987).

True nodular melanoma occurs as a nodule, usually uniform dark brown or black in colour. However, some may show little pigment although careful examination usually reveals some black areas (Fig. 10). Histologically, it is characterized by direct invasion into the dermis wherever intra-epidermal tumour exists. Subungual melanoma most commonly affects the big toe. Initially,

it presents as a flat brown or black pigmentation of the matrix, nail bed and perhaps eponychium and parony-chium. Later, there may be alteration of the nail bed which may separate.

Surgery remains the mainstay of primary treatment of malignant melanoma. Superficial spreading lesions (less than 0.7 mm in thickness) may be adequately treated by local excision with margins of approximately 1 cm. The greater the nodularity and invasiveness, the wider should be the ideal resection. However, there is a trend in general to narrower excision margins for melanomas and, in the sole of the foot, excision should leave as much weight bearing subcutaneous tissue and skin as is compatible with adequate clearance. Split skin graft is the usual method of reconstruction (Petersen 1968) but primary flap reconstruction, particularly of the weight bearing forefoot, may be indicated to maintain a mobile patient. Amputation of the toe, at least at the interpha-langeal joint, is indicated for proven subungual melanoma. Radical groin lymph node dissection is accepted as the treatment for clinically involved glands. Prophylactic gland dissection is more controversial. The prognosis of acral lentiginous melanoma of the sole and subungual region appears to be poor (Arrington et al 1977, Feibelman et al 1980, Coleman et al 1981). Although lower extremity lesions in general carry a good prognosis, malignant melanoma of the foot seems generally to be an exception (Petersen 1968, Keyhani 1977, Day et al 1981, Scrivner et al 1987).

Kaposi's sarcoma

Kaposi's sarcoma or multiple idiopathic haemorrhagic sarcoma is a condition which has an insidious onset, affects males more often than females and is more common in particular parts of the world such as Eastern Europe and Africa south of the Sahara. There is an association with lymphoma and leukaemia, long-term immunosuppressive treatment and in homosexuals with acquired immunodeficiency syndrome (AIDS) (Cox & Helwig 1959, Reynolds et al 1965, O'Brien & Brasfield 1966, Straehley et al 1975, Harwood et al 1979, Gottlieb et al 1981, Friedman-Kien 1981, Siegal et al 1981).

Lesions most commonly occur first on the legs and feet, commencing on one side, but tending to become bilateral and symmetrical (Fig. 11). Kaposi's sarcoma is characterized by the presence of bluish-red or dark brown plaques or nodules, particularly on the distal parts of the lower limbs and on the arches and soles of the feet where they may become hyperkeratotic. These plaques may undergo ulceration at a later stage, and there is then often lymphoedema of the lower extremity. The clinical course may be indolent, the local disease alone may be progressive or dissemination may occur. Visceral lesions occur in about 10% of cases (Tedeschi 1958) and involve lymph nodes, gastrointestinal tract, liver, lungs and heart. There is a higher incidence of fatal systemic involvement in sub-Saharan Africans and young homosexual men in the USA (Gottlieb et al 1981, Friedman-Kien 1981).

The clinical differential diagnosis of lesions on the foot comprises a long list of conditions, including pyogenic granuloma, neurofibroma, pemphigus vulgaris, verrucae, lichen planus, psoriatic eruption, hyperkeratotic tinea pedis, glomus tumour, haemangioma, angiosarcoma, foreign body reaction, melanoma, sarcomas of various types and infective conditions such as leprosy, filariasis and maduromycosis (Cargialosi & Schmoll 1976).

Histology shows two types of change: vascular malformations with prominent endothelial cells and spindle cell areas containing vascular slits. The presence of inflammatory cells in early lesions gives an appearance resembling granulation tissue (Lever & Schaumberg-Lever 1983). Treatment is largely by medical means using radiotherapy and systemic cytotoxic drug therapy. Surgical excision may be useful for small isolated lesions or as a palliative procedure in fungating lesions not responding to other methods of treatment.

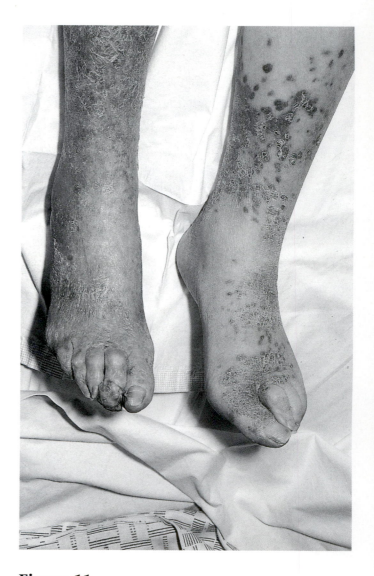

Figure 11

Widespread Kaposi's sarcoma involving both lower legs in a man of Eastern European extraction

Dermatofibrosarcoma protruberans

This tumour may occur in the foot (Sheital et al 1978) where it appears as a raised, firm, irregular, usually dull red swelling within the skin. It may appear to be multi-nodular and inspection and palpation frequently suggest subcutaneous extension. Histology shows whorled fibrous tissue with a degree of pleomorphism. Treatment consists of wide local surgical excision, usually with split skin graft. Local recurrence is frequent but distant metastases are rare.

Deep tumours which may present on the skin

Haemangioma, the fibromatoses, glomus tumour, malignant fibrous histiocytoma, epithelioid sarcoma and fibrosarcoma may all present within the skin. These will be discussed below (pages 546–7).

Tumours and tumour-like conditions of soft tissue (excluding synovium)

Some tumours of the foot arise within subcutaneous fat, from plantar aponeurosis, or from blood vessels, tendons and nerves situated more deeply (Table 2). The origin of some tumours is obscure.

Diagnosis

Once again, the duration of the lesion is of major importance. Examination should reveal the depth of the tumour. In this group of conditions, the skin is mobile over the tumour unless it becomes secondarily involved. X-rays confirm lack of skeletal involvement (unless bone, too, is secondarily involved or eroded) and may show an unsuspected deep foreign body. Exploration and biopsy may be the only way to make a final diagnosis.

General principles of management

Management obviously depends on whether the lesion is benign or malignant. Non-neoplastic swellings (such as haemangiomas and plantar fibromatoses) require surgery only if the diagnosis is uncertain or the condition is causing troublesome symptoms. Benign neoplasms are generally treated by surgical excision. Wherever possible, incision should avoid weight bearing areas and weight bearing plantar subcutaneous fat should be preserved. Malignant soft tissue tumours, unless radiosensitive, require radical surgery which may mean partial or complete amputation of the foot. The various types of incomplete salvage amputations in the foot have been described in Chapter VI.6.

Common conditions

Congenital

Haemangioma

Haemangiomas are vascular tumours produced by the proliferation of vessels and considered by many to be hamartomatous malformations rather than true neoplasms. They may be subdivided into various types, including capillary, cavernous, hypertrophic and cirsoid/racemose (Pack & Miller 1950, Stout 1953).

Haemangiomas are the most common tumours of infancy and childhood. They are relatively rare in the foot, where they may occur in skin, subcutaneous tissues, muscle and other soft tissues or bone. However, 142

Table 2 Tumour and tumour-like conditions of soft tissue (excluding synovium)

Congenital	Haemangioma
	Arteriovenous malformation
	Neurofibromatosis
	Hamartoma
Traumatic	Traumatic neuroma
	Traumatic aneurysm
	Deep retained foreign bodies
Degenerative and miscellaneous	Digital mucous cyst
	Recurrent infantile digital fibroma
	Fibromatoses
	Cicatricial fibromatosis
	Keloid
	Nodular fasciitis
	Plantar fibromatosis
	Aggressive fibromatosis
	Congenital generalized fibromatosis
Neoplastic	Tumours of fat
	Lipoma
	Liposarcoma
	Tumours of nerve
	Neurofibroma
	Neurilemmoma
	Malignant schwannoma
	Tumours of blood vessels
	Capillary haemangioma
	Cavernous haemangioma
	Haemangiopericytoma (benign)
	Glomus tumour
	Angiosarcoma (malignant)
	Haemangiopericytoma (malignant)
	Tumours of fibrous tissue
	Fibroma
	Fibrosarcoma
	Dermatofibrosarcoma protruberans
	Tumours of doubtful origin
	Granular cell myoblastoma
	Malignant fibrous histiocytoma
	Epithelioid sarcoma
	Tumour of muscle
	Leiomyoma
	Leiomyosarcoma
	Rhabdomyosarcoma
	Miscellaneous tumours
	Extra-skeletal chondroma or chondrosarcoma
	Clear cell sarcoma of tendons and aponeuroses

cases of lower extremity haemangioma involved the foot in the early study of Weaver (Someren & Merritt 1978). A capillary haemangioma is seen as a red, slightly raised skin lesion. A cavernous haemangioma in subcutaneous tissue presents as a palpable mass with poorly defined borders, and there may be oedema and pain (Margileth & Museles 1965). The latter may be due to nerve compression. The soft spongy mass has been described as resembling a 'bag of worms' or like 'spaghetti' by an Italian author (Carnevali 1938). If the lesion is close to the epidermis, there may be local red, brown, blue or purple discolouration of the skin. Such discolouration is not seen with all haemangiomas, particularly those occurring more deeply, and the diagnosis should be borne in mind in cases where there is a localized tumour-like swelling. Pulsation of the lesion is not a frequent feature and is indicative of a high arterial input.

The differential diagnosis includes ganglion and other cystic lesions, lipoma, fibroma, neuroma, haematoma, arteriovenous fistula, pigmented villonodular synovitis and malignant soft tissue tumour (Borden & Shea 1976, Cox 1976, Midenberg & Kirschenbaum 1983). Pathological examination usually shows a capillary haemangioma to be situated in the dermis but extending into subcutaneous fat and underlying muscles. Histology shows a network of capillary-like vascular channels of variable calibre which may contain blood. The extent of local involvement by haemangioma can be assessed preoperatively by skin temperature studies, plethysmography, venography and arteriography (Watson & McCarthy 1940).

The typical capillary or cavernous haemangioma is noticed some time after birth, increases in size for months (or occasionally years) and then begins to resolve spontaneously. No treatment is indicated unless growth is rapid. If resolution is slow, and preventing the wearing of footwear, the injection of sclerosant, perhaps combined with compression, may be indicated. This must be performed with care, as considerable necrosis can result. Very rarely, surgical excision may be necessary. Vessel ligation or embolization usually produces only temporary improvement, but may be very useful in reducing flow prior to surgery. Surgical excision should be performed under tourniquet with careful bipolar coagulation of divided vessels. Blood loss may still be considerable when the tourniquet is released. Haemangioma may involve muscles, neurovascular bundles and even bone, and complete removal will probably be impossible. However, persistence of a haemangioma beyond the first two to three years suggests a degree of arteriovenous shunting and if arteriovenous shunts can be embolized and excised, the remaining haemangioma may regress.

The management of persisting high-flow haemangiomas may be a difficult problem. The management of haemangioma of the foot is, generally, complicated by the need for a child to begin walking early (Borden & Shea 1976, Cox 1976, Midenberg & Kirschenbaum 1983, Politz 1976, Bernhard et al 1983).

A relatively uncommon related lesion is the angiokeratoma circumscriptum which may occur on the foot and which frequently recurs following wide excision and skin grafting. The argon laser may be useful in this condition, although results have generally been disappointing.

Arteriovenous malformations

Although many haemangiomas have a degree of arteriovenous shunting, when such shunts are multiple they may cause gigantism of the limb and even high output cardiac failure. There may be capillary haemangiomatous involvement of the skin, dilated veins, obvious temperature increases and possibly thrills or bruits at the site of large shunts. Embolization offers the best chance of control.

Neurofibromatosis (von Recklinghausen's disease)

Neurofibromatosis is inherited as an autosomally dominant trait with an incidence of around 1:3000 live births. Clinically, it is divisible into peripheral and central forms, overlap between which is minimal in any individual kinship. It is the peripheral form of the disease which is important in considerations of foot involvement. The clinical manifestations include the presence of macular pigmented lesions resembling freckles, called 'café au lait' spots which are present early in life and become more numerous with increasing age.

Neurofibromas usually begin to appear in childhood or adolescence and are slowly growing tumours. Pathologically, they may be localized, plexiform or diffuse neurofibromas, the last of these being the rarest (Enzinger & Weiss 1983). Plexiform neurofibroma involves a major nerve which becomes distorted and converted to a 'bag of worms'. The multiple neurofibromas of von Recklinghausen's disease give rise to significant morbidity and mortality and are usually so numerous as to make surgical excision of all tumours impossible. It is not possible to predict which lesions, if any, will undergo malignant transformation, although it is likely that those who have had the disease for many years have the greatest risk of such a development (Guccion & Enzinger 1979).

In the absence of a strong suspicion of malignancy, surgery has to be selective and it has been suggested that it be reserved for lesions which are large, painful or strategically placed so that they impair function significantly (Enzinger & Weiss 1983). The development of a sarcoma typically presents as rapid enlargement or pain in a pre-existing neurofibroma, and either symptom should lead to biopsy followed, on confirmation of malignancy, by radical local excision or amputation.

In the foot, the neurofibroma may present as a deep swelling, tending to be more mobile transversely than longitudinally and associated with a nerve. Unfortunately, in neurofibromatosis, there may be more extensive involvement of skin and subcutaneous tissue in a plexiform neurofibroma (Fig. 12). Finally, there may be gross skeletal deformity with gigantism or dysplasia.

Treatment, if indicated, consists of surgical excision. The isolated small neurofibroma can be excised as it rarely involves a major nerve. The plexiform neurofibroma can be reduced in size if not completely excised,

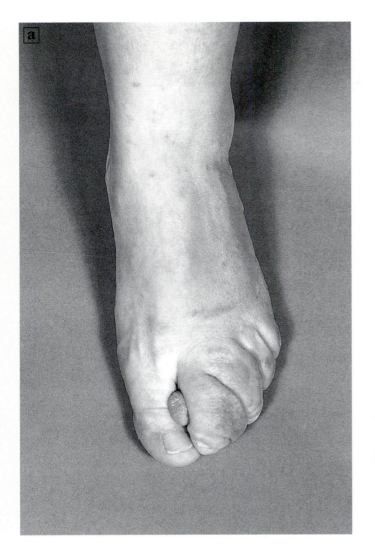

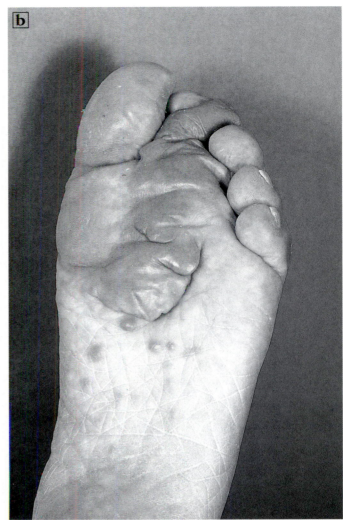

Figure 12

Diffuse plexiform neurofibromatosis of the foot (in a patient with von Recklinghausen's disease): (a) dorsum; (b) sole

as the tumours tend to be particularly lax, although vascular.

Hamartoma

Hamartoma, involving tissues of many origins and producing gross deformity of the foot, may occur (Fig. 13). Histology of tissue removed shows no evidence of neurofibromatosis. Recent examples in the literature are lipofibromatous, eccrine angiomatous, acrosyringeal and vascular hamartoma (Hirakawa et al 1993, Sanmartin et al 1992, Hurt et al 1990, Petrov & Zaremba 1990).

Traumatic

Traumatic neuroma

A traumatic neuroma may present, in the sole of the foot, as a nodule which may be occasionally painful or tender.

It is due to excessive proliferation of the nerve fibre at a site of injury or surgery, occurring, presumably, where regenerative nerve fibres are unable to grow in an orderly fashion into the distal severed end of the nerve sheath. Macroscopically, it is a well circumscribed, whitish-grey nodule in continuity with the affected nerve, and microscopy shows a random overgrowth of nerve fibres, Schwann cells and fibroblasts forming fibrous tissue. Surgical excision is indicated if the diagnosis is in doubt or if the lesion has become symptomatic. Surgery may involve repair of the nerve, dissection of the neuroma if part of the nerve remains in continuity, or excision and burying of the nerve end if pain has been a problem.

Neuroma of the heel affects the medial calcaneal nerve and may be related to direct trauma, the overloading effects of obesity or calcaneal eversion associated with pronation (Altman & Hinkes 1982). Morton's neuroma

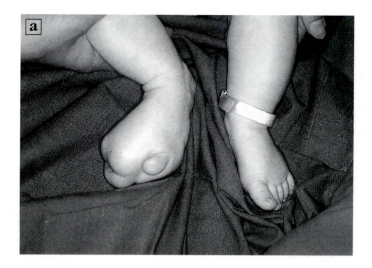

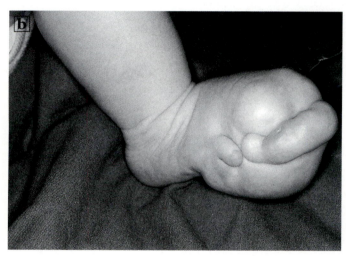

Figure 13

Congenital hamartoma of the foot: (a) comparison with left foot; (b) lateral view

(Morton's metatarsalgia) has been described in Chapter V.4.

Degenerative and miscellaneous

Digital mucous cyst

Digital mucous cysts are benign lesions that occur in the subcutaneous tissues of the toes, particularly on the dorsum near the distal interphalangeal joint and close to the nail bed. They occur at any age and in either sex. Presentation is with a translucent cystic swelling of variable size with little or no tenderness. Occasionally, patients may describe spontaneous rupture with discharge of gelatinous fluid, but the lesion may recur. On other occasions, the lesion spontaneously disappears. Differential diagnosis includes ganglion, lipoma, fibroma, epidermal cyst, nodular pigmented villonodular tenosynovitis and sarcomas of various types. Pathologically,

there is a central myxoid cystic area surrounded by fibrous tissue. Some authorities regard the lesions as ganglia of the distal interphalangeal joint.

Treatment should be directed at complete local excision, usually to the distal interphalangeal joint. This may involve full-thickness skin grafting or local flap cover (if joint or nail bed is exposed) if the overlying skin cannot be peeled off and closed primarily. References to this lesion, sometimes referred to as a myxoma, are available elsewhere (Grosse 1937, Stout 1948, Sugar 1981, Enzinger & Weiss 1983, Lever & Schaumberg-Lever 1983).

Recurrent infantile digital fibroma

Single or multiple nodules are present on the toes (and fingers) in recurrent infantile digital fibroma. More than 50 cases have been reported in the literature, including those occurring in the hand (Shapiro 1969, Santa Cruz & Reiner 1978, Coskey et al 1979). They are usually either present at birth or appear in the first year of life, though development later in childhood sometimes occurs. Recurrent digital fibromas are characteristically circumscribed, reddish-pink nodules which undergo spontaneous involution.

Histopathological examination shows interlacing bundles of collagen fibres with numerous fibroblasts in the dermis and sometimes extension of this process into subcutaneous fat. Characteristic eosinophilic inclusion bodies, 3–10 μm diameter, are present in many of the fibroblasts, and the ultrastructure and significance of these inclusions are discussed elsewhere (Lever & Schaumberg-Lever 1983). Treatment of recurrent digital fibroma should be conservative, with surgical excision reserved for those occasions where there is significant impairment of function because of the lesion. Surgery may well produce even further deformity.

Fibromatoses

Plantar fibromatosis (Fig. 14) may be confused with soft tissue tumours. Its management is discussed in Chapter V.7. The subject has recently been reviewed by Classen & Hurst (1992), Landers et al (1993), and Wu (1994). Nodular fasciitis may occur in the foot and may be difficult to differentiate histologically from fibrosarcoma, especially in children where it may not be suspected (Rao & Luthra 1988).

Neoplastic tumours of fat

Lipoma

This is a benign neoplasm of fat which may contain variable amounts of fibrous and vascular stroma. It presents as a soft swelling which is usually asymptomatic and not tender, although just occasionally it may produce discomfort. Lipomas in the foot are usually situated just beneath the skin (Lisch et al 1982). They may occur within tendon sheaths in the foot or ankle, where they may present with mild discomfort and

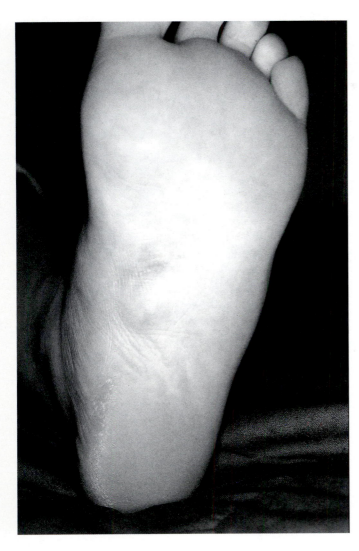

Figure 14

Plantar fibromatosis in a young woman

swelling of the involved tendon sheath (especially peroneal, tibialis anterior and tibialis posterior). Lipomas are the commonest benign soft tissue tumours anywhere in the body and comprise 50% of such lesions in the lower extremity, although occurrence in the foot is relatively infrequent (Booher 1965).

Lipomas may occur at any age and in either sex, but are more common in middle-aged females and rarely affect children. Radiological examination reveals a tumour with a characteristic radiolucency (Cavanagh 1973), while the macroscopic and microscopic appearances are similar to those of normal adipose tissue. Differentiation from low-grade liposarcoma by the histopathologist is on the basis of the presence of pleomorphic lipoblasts. Development of a liposarcoma in a lipoma is uncommon. Liposarcoma of the foot is excessively rare, though single cases have been reported (Sugar & Murphy 1955, Kaufman & Stout 1959, Booher

1965). Treatment of lipoma is by complete surgical excision after which local recurrence is very unusual (Booher 1965).

Neoplastic tumours of nerves

True nerve tumours of the foot are rare; they include neurilemmoma, neurofibroma, neuroblastoma and primary malignant nerve sheath tumours (Berlin et al 1975).

Neurofibroma

This may occur singly or as part of neurofibromatosis (von Recklinghausen's disease). A search should always be made for 'café au lait' spots or other signs of the generalized disease. Solitary neurofibromas are evenly distributed over the body surface and affect the dermoid subcutaneous tissues. They are slowly growing, painless lesions, mostly seen in young adults. Solitary neurofibromas are the commonest nerve tumours in the foot (Berlin et al 1975). Macroscopic examination shows a whitish-grey tumour which may form a fusiform expansion on a larger nerve. Histologically, the appearances are variable but there are interlacing spindle cells, collagen fibres and mucin present and some may be frankly myxoid. Treatment, if indicated, consists of surgical excision.

Neurilemmoma

The neurilemmoma, (or schwannoma) is an encapsulated nerve sheath tumour which may occur at any age but is more common between the ages of 20 and 50 years (Geschickter 1935). It is a relatively rare occurrence on the foot (Luke 1976). It is a slowly growing lesion, usually causing little in the way of pain or neurological problems, and is situated in relation to a nerve. One series included four cases in the foot and there were symptoms of pain, tenderness and paraesthesia (White 1967). A further example was described by Jacobson and Edwards (1993).

On sectioning, the cut surface has a pink, white or yellow appearance, while histological examination reveals characteristic appearances known as Antoni A and B patterns in a tumour made up of spindle cells with variable amounts of collagen fibre deposition (Enzinger & Weiss 1983). The tumour is encapsulated, being surrounded by the epineurium, so that complete removal should be possible without damage to the related nerve. Temporary loss of nerve function may occur but should return (Geschickter 1935). Incomplete excision is needed for cases where attempts at complete removal would give rise to permanent damage to the related nerve (if important).

Malignant schwannoma

This tumour is rare, commonly metastasizes and should be treated by amputation if there is no evidence of distant spread.

Neoplastic tumours of blood vessels

Haemangiomata

These tend to involve multiple tissues and may be situated primarily subcutaneously. They have been discussed previously.

Glomus tumour

Glomus bodies are arteriovenous anastomoses surrounded by a nerve plexus. The glomus tumour is a benign tumour considered to be a hamartoma of the glomus body (Carroll & Berman 1972). They are found particularly in the distal part of the upper and lower extremities and the face. In the foot, the glomus tumour occurs in the papillary dermis of the sole or under the toenails. There may be red or blue discolouration of the skin or nail bed (LaPorta et al 1976, Quigley 1979). The lesion can often be accurately localized by the patient by direct pressure at a specific point. Both cold and pressure produce severe local pain. Glomus tumours may be present at any age, but subungual lesions have been described under the age of 25 years (Vineyard 1975). They are spherical, compressible lesions of small size (often less than 0.5 cm in diameter). Rarely, X-rays show erosion of distal phalanx.

Macroscopically, the lesion is blue, red or violaceous and may resemble a small haemorrhage when located subungually. Histological examination shows blood vessels lined by normal endothelial cells and surrounded by a solid proliferation of round or cuboidal epithelial cells. The differential diagnosis includes haemangioma, neuroma, skin appendage tumour, haemangiopericytoma and Kaposi's sarcoma. Treatment is by surgical excision, which produces immediate relief of symptoms. Subungual glomus tumours require prior removal of the nail, longitudinal incision of the nail bed, and removal of the tumour, which can often be readily enucleated, and the bed curetted. The nail bed should then be repaired under magnification, by fine sutures to minimize subsequent distortion. Recurrence is unusual and metastases are extremely rare (Lumley & Stansfield 1972, Symmers 1973).

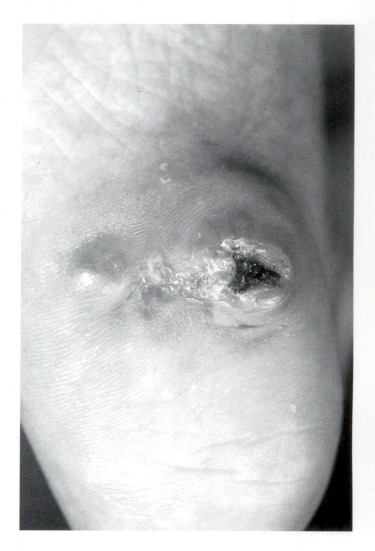

Figure 15

Epithelioid sarcoma of the sole of the foot, which was initially thought to be due to plantar fibromatosis. Following excision (which confirmed the diagnosis), there was early recurrence and the patient had a below-knee amputation. He remains well 12 years later

Neoplastic tumours of fibrous tissues

Fibrosarcoma

This is rare in the foot. It presents as a firm nodule and may be confused with the benign fibromatoses. Histological differentiation may be difficult. The fibrosarcoma is composed of reticulin and collagen, with predominantly spindle-shaped cells. In a well differentiated tumour, the cells may be polarized and mitoses are rare. Biopsy confirms the diagnosis and differentiation. If well differentiated, wide local resection may be resorted to but recurrence may occur. The poorly differentiated, advanced or recurrent tumour should be treated by amputation. Metastases are not uncommon (Campbell 1982).

Neoplastic tumours of doubtful origin

Granular cell tumour (granular cell myoblastoma)

This is rarely diagnosed clinically, usually discovered as an incidental finding on physical examination, and is an unusual tumour in the foot, occurring more frequently in the head, neck and upper limb (Vance & Hudson 1969, Strong et al 1970). It may occur at any age but is more frequent over the age of 40 years. It is a poorly circumscribed lesion and histological examination shows the presence of large uniform cells with eosinophilic cytoplasm and monotonously similar nuclei distributed in bands or nests. Electron microscopical examination shows these cells to have a characteristic appearance and a relationship to Schwann cells is favoured by most pathologists. Treatment is by local excision and recurrence is rare, although metastases occur very occasionally.

Malignant fibrous histiocytoma

This tumour, increasingly recognized elsewhere in the body, is rare in the foot (Smith et al 1976). It may appear as a poorly demarcated nodule or as diffuse thickening beneath and involving the skin. Growth tends to be rapid. It may arise deeply or within subcutaneous tissue. Histologically, it is classically composed of spindle-shaped cells arranged in a 'storiform' pattern and accompanied by pleomorphic giant cells and inflammatory cells. Treatment consists of wide local excision and this may involve amputation in the foot.

Epithelioid sarcoma

This was first clearly described by Enzinger (1970). It is a slowly growing neoplasm occurring mainly in the extremities, including the feet, which were the site of involvement in 9% of cases in one series (Enzinger & Weiss 1983). This tumour occurs mostly in adolescents and young adults (age 15–35 years) though no age group is completely exempt, and men are affected about twice as often as women. The tumour may occur subcutaneously, within plantar aponeurosis or within tendon sheaths. If situated subcutaneously, the tumour may appear as an apparently trivial nodule, sometimes described as 'woody, hard' or it may cause ulceration of the overlying skin. It may be mistaken for a foreign body granuloma. If arising from aponeurosis, it may appear as a poorly defined swelling and may be mistaken for plantar fibromatosis (Fig. 15).

Naked eye examination shows a glistening grey-white or grey-tan mottled surface, with focal areas of necrosis or haemorrhage, while light microscopy shows a distinctive nodular arrangement of tumour cells which may undergo central necrosis. This nodular aggregate of tumour cells may be multiple. Detailed descriptions of the histopathology are available elsewhere (Lever & Schaumberg-Lever 1983, Enzinger & Weiss 1983). Vascular and perineural invasion are seen in surgical excision specimens (Moore et al 1975, Pratt et al 1978) and local recurrence is seen in about 85% of cases, where there has apparently been initial complete excision, because of this diffuse spreading of the lesion (Enzinger & Weiss 1983). The tumour tends to spread locally along nerves, fascial planes and tendons, and these areas should be particularly examined by the histopathologist. Metastases to the lymph nodes and later to the lungs may occur (Pratt et al 1978). The differential diagnosis includes a number of benign conditions in which there are superficial small nodules, such as infective granulomatous lesions, rheumatoid nodules, nodular fasciitis, fibrous histiocytoma, and squamous carcinoma in the case of superficial ulcerated lesions. Larger, deeply situated lesions require differentiation from the fibromatoses, other sarcomas such as synovial sarcoma, fibrosarcoma and angiosarcoma.

Because of the marked tendency for this lesion to recur, adequate treatment requires radical local excision, with amputation if there is involvement of a toe. Amputation should be considered in other sites if there is recurrence. Lymph node metastasis is fairly common and some would argue that lymph node resection should be included in the primary management. Radiotherapy and long-term chemotherapy may be helpful but have not been conclusively shown to improve prognosis.

Neoplastic tumours of muscle

Rhabdomyosarcoma

Although a rare tumour, this is one of the more common soft tissue malignancies of childhood. There are various histological varieties of rhabdomyosarcoma, namely embryonal, botryoid, alveolar and pleomorphic types, and overlapping between these may occur in individual cases (Horn & Enteline 1958). Rhabdomyosarcoma usually occurs in infants and young children, less frequently in older children and adolescents and rarely, if ever, in adults over the age of 45 years (Enzinger & Weiss 1983). Just over 7% of 588 cases occurred in the lower limb in one series and these mainly affected the foot. Clinical presentation is with an enlarging deep-seated mass which may be closely associated with striated muscle. Pain and neurological deficit may occur because of direct nerve invasion and, while erosion of bone is rare with rhabdomyosarcoma, it is in the hands and feet that this feature is sometimes seen. Distal tumours in one series were mostly interosseous in location, although one involved the arch of the foot (Ransom et al 1977).

Macroscopic examination reveals an ill defined rubbery-grey to pinkish-tan coloured tumour, invading into surrounding soft tissues and sometimes showing areas of haemorrhage and necrosis. The histological type of tumour in the foot is variable, although mixed and alveolar types were present in one series (Patcher & Alpert 1964). The histological differentiation from poorly differentiated round and spindle-cell sarcomas like neuroblastomas, Ewing's sarcoma, angiosarcoma, synovial sarcoma, malignant melanoma and malignant lymphoma may be difficult. Treatment should be by surgical excision. Except in low-grade, well encapsulated tumours, this will mean amputation. Surgery may be combined with radiotherapy and adjuvant chemotherapy. The presence of disseminated tumour and the location of the primary tumour on the extremity are significant prognostic features (Ransom et al 1977). Inadequately treated rhabdomyosarcomas recur and metastases are mainly to the lungs, lymph nodes and bone marrow, followed by other viscera, namely heart, brain, meninges, pancreas, liver and kidney.

Leiomyosarcoma

This is a rare tumour which has been described in the foot. Gunzy et al (1992) describes one case and reviews

12 others from the literature. The pathological features and clinical behaviour are like those of leiomyosarcoma in other sites.

Miscellaneous tumours

Extraskeletal chondroma

Chondromas sometimes occur in extraskeletal connective tissue and, when they do so, they are found mainly in the soft tissues of the hands and feet, chiefly the former. There is no connection to underlying bone, though association with tendon, tendon sheath or joint capsule may be present (Murphy & Wilson 1958, Someren & Merritt 1978) and the lesion is usually solitary. Multiple chondroid nodules suggest the possibility of synovial chondromatosis (see below, pages 549–50). Clinical presentation is as a slowly growing mass, which is rarely painful or tender, and adults between the ages of 30 and 60 years are mainly affected. X-ray may show calcification.

Pathological examination shows a well demarcated, firm, round or oval lesion which histologically has the features of a benign tumour. There may be fibrosis, ossification or myxoid change. Fibrochondroma, osteochondroma, myxochondroma and focal calcification may be present towards the centre of the lesion, potentially giving problems with differentiation from tumoral calcinosis in a heavily calcified lesion. Differential diagnosis includes chondroma arising from the outside of the bone (periosteal or juxtacortical chondroma), low-grade chondrosarcoma and synovial chondromatosis, though the latter tends to occur in relation to larger joints like the knee, hip and elbow. Treatment is by local excision. Further detailed information is available in the literature (Lichenstein & Goldman 1964, Dahlin & Salvador 1974, Chung & Enzinger 1978).

Clear cell sarcoma of tendons and aponeuroses

Clear cell sarcoma is a deeply located soft tissue tumour which may be related to malignant melanoma in that there are histological resemblances to the latter, including the presence of melanin (Bearman et al 1975, Boudreaux & Waisman 1978, Toe & Saw 1978). A common feature is involvement of tendons and aponeuroses. Clinical presentation is with a slowly growing mass which is tender and painful in about 50% of cases, and the duration of symptoms ranges from a few weeks to several years. Young adults (age 20–40 years) are mainly affected, but occasionally cases in younger and older patients have been described. Most clear cell sarcomas are situated in the lower limb (Enzinger 1965) and 38% occurred in the foot, heel or ankle in one series (Enzinger & Weiss 1983). Other cases have been described more recently (Bridge et al 1990, Prieskorn et al 1992).

Naked eye examination reveals a lobulated or multinodular mass with a grey-white cut surface, frequently attached to a tendon or aponeurosis and with no connection to the overlying skin. Histopathological examination shows nests of clear, round or fusiform cells with vesicular nuclei and prominent nucleoli. Intracellular melanin

Table 3 Tumours and tumour-like conditions of synovium

Degenerative and miscellaneous	Ganglion
	Local pigmented villonodular synovitis (giant cell tumour of tendon)
	Diffuse pigmented villonodular synovitis (giant cell tumour of tendon)
	Synovial chondromatosis
Neoplastic	Synovial sarcoma

is detected with special stains and by electron microscopy (Kauffman & Stout 1959). The differential diagnosis is from other sarcomas, particularly synovial sarcoma, fibrosarcoma and nerve sheath tumours.

Clear cell sarcoma is a highly malignant tumour which metastasizes to the lung, regional lymph nodes and bone. Radical excision is required, with amputation if necessary, together with chemotherapy and radiotherapy. Removal of regional lymph nodes should be considered and performed, particularly if there is lymphadenopathy. Local experience suggests a particularly good response to radiotherapy and chemotherapy with vincristine and bleomycin (Sugar & Murphy 1955, Radstone et al 1979). Late metastases are not uncommon.

Tumours and tumour-like conditions of synovium

Several tumours and tumour-like conditions either arise from the synovium of the joints and tendon sheaths of the foot and ankle, or have appearances suggesting a synovial origin (Table 3).

Diagnosis

A tumour of synovial origin may be suspected because of the apparent site of the swelling within or adjacent to synovial structures. The appearance of the malignant synovial sarcoma may be deceptively benign.

General principles of management

The benign conditions of synovium have a marked tendency to recurrence following excision. This may be

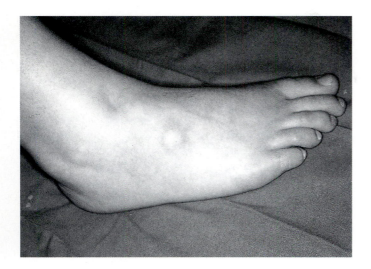

Figure 16

Ganglion of the dorsum of the foot

related to their situation within the fibrous flexor sheath where longitudinal spread and seeding are presumably unobstructed. Perhaps for the same reason, the malignant synovial sarcoma tends to spread readily within the fibrous flexor sheath and the sort of spread suggestive of malignancy may occur late.

Common conditions

Degenerative and miscellaneous

Ganglion
The most common site for a ganglion in the foot is the dorsum over the tarsals (Slavitt et al 1980) (Fig. 16). The swelling may be hard and indistinguishable from an exostosis. An X-ray will confirm the soft tissue nature of the swelling. Microscopic examination shows cellular areas with mucinous degeneration, often in the form of multilocular cysts. Up to 50% of ganglia disappear spontaneously. Some authorities advocate aspiration and instillation of hydrocortisone. However, in general, if treatment is indicated, adequate surgical excision gives the best chance of cure but recurrence is not uncommon.

Local pigmented villonodular synovitis (giant cell tumour of tendon sheath)
Localized (nodular) villonodular tenosynovitis (or giant cell tumour of tendon sheath) can occur at any age, but more commonly occurs between the ages of 30 and 50 years, and in women a little more often than in men. It occurs predominantly in the hand but may also affect the foot and ankle. The tumour is a slowly growing

lesion, occurring in joints or tendon sheaths. Radiological examination shows a soft tissue mass and, in a small number of cases, there may be erosion of bone.

The macroscopic appearance is of a localized nodule, usually mottled yellow or brown, ranging in size between 0.5 cm and 3 cm in diameter, although those occurring in the foot may be larger and more irregularly shaped. Sectioning reveals a pinkish-grey cut surface, which may be flecked with yellow or brown due to lipid or haemosiderin. Histologically there is a discrete nodular proliferation of macrophages and fibroblast cells, forming collagen, with giant cells, foam cells and pigment-laden macrophages also present – features shared with the diffuse form. This raises the possibility that the lesion may be due to reactive hyperplastic inflammatory reaction (Jaffe et al 1941). The exact appearances vary from lesion to lesion, depending on the proportion of macrophages, giant cells, foam cells and collagenization.

Although giant cell tumours are benign, they have a tendency to recur after surgical removal. Recurrence has been quoted at between 10 and 30% (Byers et al 1968, Enzinger & Weiss 1983). Excision involves pursuing the often tortuous route of the tumour to achieve complete removal.

Diffuse pigmented villonodular tenosynovitis (giant cell tumour of tendon sheath)
This mainly affects the large joints such as the knee, though involvement of the ankle and foot occurs in a significant proportion of cases (Enzinger & Weiss 1983). The toe is an uncommon site. Typical symptoms are limitation of movement, pain, tenderness and joint effusion, the latter often due to haemarthrosis. Radiography shows a soft tissue mass and there may be erosion of related bone. At surgery, the synovial membrane is diffusely thickened and brownish-yellow in colour. Microscopy reveals a macrophage and fibroblast proliferation with giant cells, collagen deposition and the presence of pigment-laden macrophages and foam cells.

Treatment is by synovectomy, with curettage of any bony component, but experience shows that there is a high recurrence rate, probably between 40 and 50% (Byers et al 1968, Enzinger & Weiss 1983). The aim should be complete removal of the lesion at first operation, if this is possible without causing severe disability to the patient.

Synovial chondromatosis
This is a term used to describe two quite different conditions, sometimes referred to as primary and secondary chondromatosis. Primary chondromatosis is a condition in which nodules of metaplastic chondroid tissue develop within the synovial soft tissue. Patients may be of any age, and the larger joints are usually those affected, although involvement of toes and ankle has been described (Murphy et al 1962, Jeffreys 1967, Villacin et al 1979). Primary chondromatosis is typically a

monarticular disease, presenting with pain, swelling and limitation of movement. Physical examination shows tenderness, and there may be a mass or effusion. Radiological examination may reveal a soft tissue swelling and there is sometimes erosion of related bone, suggesting the possibility of a malignant tumour.

Pathological study shows chondroid nodules, which may be so numerous as to form an almost continuous mass, and some may break away to become loose bodies in the joint space. Light microscopy shows lobulated collections of chondrocytes, characteristically arranged in small clusters within related matrix. Cellular pleomorphism and the presence of binucleate cartilage cells may at times be alarming, but chondrosarcomatous change is exceedingly rare, if it occurs at all (Murphy et al 1962, Goldman & Lichenstein 1964, King et al 1967, Dunn et al 1974).

One of the chief problems is that the locally erosive character and the histological appearances may lead to the erroneous diagnosis of malignancy. The behaviour of these cartilaginous lesions in the foot is benign (Dahlin 1978). The differential diagnosis is from other loose bodies as formed in secondary chondromatosis, which is perhaps better named synovial osteochondromatosis. Treatment is by local excision of the affected synovial membrane and the removal of loose bodies. Recurrence of the problem after surgery is well known and is not an indication of malignancy.

Secondary synovial chondromatosis is more common than the primary form already described (McIvor & King 1962, Milgram & Addison 1976, Milgram 1977a,b, Villacin et al 1979) and better termed synovial osteochondromatosis, since the loose bodies present in the joint space and incorporated in the synovial membrane comprise both articular cartilage and underlying bone. Large joints are usually those affected, but loose osteochondromatous bodies are sometimes found in the foot and ankle (Villacin et al 1979). In general, they form as a result of processes such as osteochondritis dissecans, osteochondral fractures and traumatic damage and joint disintegration in degenerative, and possible inflammatory, disease (Villacin et al 1979, Milgram 1977a).

Neoplastic

Synovial sarcoma – malignant
Synovial sarcoma accounts for about 8% of soft tissue malignancies. It occurs most frequently in the lower extremities and, in approximately 20% of cases, occurs in the foot or ankle (MacKenzie 1966, Wright et al 1982). It is said to be the commonest sarcoma of the hands and feet. The tumour arises from periarticular structures but not, apparently, directly from synovium (Ryan et al 1982). In fact, many tumours appear to arise when no synovial structures are present (MacKenzie 1966). The tumour presents at any age, but most commonly in young adults, and usually as a painful lump. Microscopically, the tumour consists of two neoplastic cellular elements: the fibrosarcomatous spindle cell and the pseudoepithelial or glandular cell. Fissures, spaces or clefts, suggestive of synovial cavities, are usually found. Cases of synovial sarcoma with extensive osteoid and bone formation have been described, and two of these were in the foot (Milchgrub et al 1993).

Treatment consists of wide resection. The surgeon should not be misled by apparent encapsulation. The general view is that, at least, ray amputation (if involving a digit) or more proximal amputation (if involving major joints) is the correct treatment. Lymph glands are relatively uncommonly involved (Chimenti et al 1982).

Tumour and tumour-like conditions of bone and cartilage

Diagnosis

Tumours, or tumour-like conditions of bone and cartilage (Table 4), usually present as swelling or because of pain. The age of incidence and the rapidity of growth may suggest the diagnosis. X-ray examination may be definitive, but biopsy may be necessary to confirm the diagnosis.

Principles of management

The borderline between benign and malignant tumours is blurred and some bony tumours (for example, giant cell tumour of bone) rarely metastasize. It is therefore essential that an accurate diagnosis is made before definitive treatment is performed. Although the diagnosis may be made on history, X-ray and macroscopic appearance, if there is any doubt biopsy should be taken for paraffin section diagnosis. In general the benign noninvasive tumours are treated by curettage, with or without cancellous bone grafting, while the more aggressive tumours are treated by resection.

Common conditions

Congenital

Bony prominences at the site of previous accessory toes, skeletal anomalies such as accessory navicular bones or skeletal deformity due to hamartoma or neurofibromatosis are unlikely to pose diagnostic problems.

Traumatic

Bony spurs secondary to repeated trauma, and exuberant callosity at a fracture site, may be confused with bony tumours.

Table 4 Tumours and tumour-like lesions of bone and cartilage

Congenital	Abnormal metatarsals or phalanges
	Abnormal tarsals – e.g. accessory navicular
	Neurofibromatosis (with skeletal deformity)
Traumatic	Bony spurs
	Exuberant callus
Miscellaneous	Solitary bone cyst
	Aneurysmal bone cyst
	Fibrous dysplasia
	Eosinophilic granuloma
Neoplastic	Vascular tumours
	Haemangioma
	Lymphangioma
	Haemangioendothelioma
	Haemangiopericytoma
	Angiosarcoma (malignant)
	Chondroid-forming tumours
	Chondroma
	Osteochondroma
	Chondromyxoid fibroma
	Chondroblastoma
	Chondrosarcoma (malignant)
	Osteoid-forming tumours
	Osteoid osteoma
	Subungual exostoses
	Osteoblastoma
	Osteosarcoma (malignant)
	Giant cell Tumour
	Small cell sarcomas
	Ewing's sarcoma
	Neuroectodermal tumour of bone
	Lymphoma
	Myeloma
	Metastatic

Miscellaneous

Solitary bone cyst

This usually appears during childhood or adolescence, most commonly in the os calcis (Campbell 1982). Radiographic examination shows a well demarcated cyst with a sclerotic margin. If seen in the os calcis, it may be safe not to carry out any specific treatment. If the cyst is in another bone, if the diagnosis is in doubt, or if pathological fracture occurs, surgery is indicated. The cyst contains clear fluid and is lined by a thin membrane. At operation, it is curetted and the cavity packed with cancellous bone chips.

Aneurysmal bone cysts

This tumour-like condition is a cystic lesion surrounded by a thin shell of bone. In the past, it was often confused with what is now called giant cell tumour of bone.

Aneurysmal bone cysts occur most commonly in the second and third decades and may be painful. Radiographic examination suggests the condition, but exploration may be necessary. When entered, blood-filled cavities are seen, interspersed with strands of reddish-brown soft tissue. Bleeding may be profuse but is reduced by removal of the abnormal tissue. Histology shows spaces lined by fibrous tissue (with multinucleated giant cells) and occasionally strands of bone. Curettage and bone grafting is the usual treatment and recurrence is rare.

Fibrous dysplasia

This may be monostotic or polyostotic (especially in Albright's syndrome). In the foot, there may be palpable swelling or deformity. Radiographic examination shows lysis which is well demarcated. Treatment, if necessary, consists of biopsy, curettage and packing with bone chips.

Eosinophilic granuloma

This condition affects children and adolescents and presents as pain or swelling. Radiographic examination shows lysis. On exploration, a granulomatous lesion is found. If proven histologically, the treatment is curettage and packing with bone chips. Histology shows granulations with histiocytes, leucocytes and especially eosinophils.

Neoplastic vascular tumours

Haemangioma, lymphangioma, haemangioendothelioma, haemangiopericytoma and angiosarcoma may all rarely involve bone. A review and description of a case of a haemangioendothelioma in the foot was reported by Krajca-Radcliffe et al (1992).

Neoplastic chondroid-forming tumours

Chondroma

The enchondroma is a benign tumour of mature cartilage, usually occurring centrally in the short tubular bones of the hands and feet. Such lesions arising centrally in the bone are referred to as enchondromas. They may occur singly or they may be multiple in enchondromatosis (Ollier's disease). In Maffucci's syndrome, there are multiple enchondromas associated with haemangiomas. They are likely to be asymptomatic, although pathological fractures may occur and cause pain. They are frequently a chance finding on radiological examination, which shows a centrally placed area of radiolucency, most often situated in the diaphyseal region. Macroscopically, the tumour is a lobular bluish-grey mass resembling cartilage, and light microscopy reveals a benign tumour composed of chondrocytes and cartilage matrix. Treatment is by curettage and insertion of cancellous bone chips. It is usually unnecessary to treat the multiple lesions of Ollier's disease.

Osteochondroma and related lesions

Osteochondroma, or cartilage-capped exostosis, is the commonest benign bone tumour but rarely is it found in distal extremities (Dahlin 1978, Fuselier et al 1984). An even rarer lesion has been described and given the name 'bizarre parosteal osteochondromatous proliferation of the hands and feet' (Nona et al 1983). These lesions, too, may occur singly or they may be multiple. They occur at almost any age and, in the foot, present on the proximal phalanges or metatarsals (of which few examples have been described). They are painless, unless involved in pathological fracture or pressure against an adjacent nerve. The cartilage cap contains bizarre binucleate chondrocytes and these appearances mimic chondrosarcoma. Radiographic examination shows the cortex continuous with the cortex at the base of the exostosis and there may be patchy calcification at the margin of the cancellous bone under the cartilage. The lesions can be treated by excision but recurrence may occur in over 50% of cases (Nona et al 1983).

Chondromyxoid fibroma

This is a rare localized tumour affecting males more often than females, presenting at any age in adults, though usually in the second and third decades, and involving the long bones, particularly of the lower limb (Spjut et al 1971, Dahlin 1978). It is not uncommon in the foot (Campbell 1982, Crisafulli et al 1990). Local pain, which may be of some duration, is a common presenting symptom and there may be local tenderness. Radiological examination shows a well circumscribed area of rarefaction and there may be expansion of the outline of the bone. Macroscopically, chondromyxoid fibroma is a grey-white mass with variable amounts of myxoid, cystic or haemorrhagic change. Histology shows myxomatous, fibrous and chondroid areas and oval, round or spindle-shaped cells, resembling the chondroblasts seen in chondroblastoma. Treatment is by local excision. Recurrence may occur after curettage and insertion of bone chips and should be treated by local resection if feasible. Sarcomatous change, if it occurs, is an extreme pathological rarity (Dahlin 1978).

Chondroblastoma

This is a rare tumour occurring in the epiphyseal part of a long bone, usually the femur, tibia or humerus. Occasional cases of involvement at other sites have been described, including the small bones of the hand (Neviaser & Wilson 1972) and foot (Ross & Dawson 1975, Campbell 1982). The majority of patients present in adolescence or adult life. Localized pain is a common clinical feature, although this was absent in a case of chondroblastoma occurring in a toe (Ross & Dawson 1975). There may be considerable swelling. Radiological examination shows a radiolucent area surrounded by a narrow zone of sclerosis, and there may be spotty calcification within the tumour (McLeod & Beabout 1973). Naked eye examination shows a grey or grey-brown tumour with a gritty surface and sometimes cystic or spindle-shaped chondroblasts with chondroid matrix and multinucleated giant cells, showing a lace-like focal calcification (Spjut et al 1971). Treatment should aim at complete local removal by curettage and packing with bone chips, or excision. In the case of a toe,

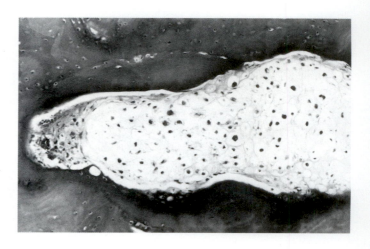

Figure 17

Photomicrograph of chondrosarcoma showing nuclear and cellular pleomorphism. The tumour is invading right up to the adjacent bone

amputation may well be the most suitable choice (Ross & Dawson 1975).

Chondrosarcoma

This is a malignant cartilage-forming tumour of bone which occurs most frequently in the age range 30 to 60 years. Involvement of the small bones of the hand and foot is exceptional and only a small number of cases have been described in the latter, involving either the tubular bones or tarsus (Jakobson & Spjut 1960, Patcher & Alpert 1964, Lewis et al 1975, Dahlin 1978, Miki et al 1978). Local pain and swelling are the usual presenting complaints. Radiological examination shows an expansile destructive mass, often containing mottled radiodensities representing calcification or ossification within the tumour.

The naked eye appearance is that of a bluish-grey lobular mass, while histology shows a tumour in which cartilage matrix is being formed by malignant chondrocytes showing nuclear and cytoplasmic pleomorphism (Fig. 17). Multinucleate tumour cells and mitoses may be present. The question of chondrosarcoma in the hands or feet taking origin from a pre-existing benign enchondroma is not yet resolved, although this would seem unlikely on the basis that enchondromas have a high frequency while chondrosarcomas in this site are rare (Patcher & Alpert 1964). Treatment should aim at complete and wide local excision, with the possibility of prosthetic joint replacement. The involved bone and the soft tissue surrounding it should be excised. In more high-grade chondrosarcomas, amputation is the treatment of choice. Radiotherapy is not indicated, chondrosarcoma being a radio-resistant tumour.

Neoplastic osteoid-forming tumours

Subungual exostosis

This is a benign bone tumour, found adjacent to or beneath the nail on the distal phalanx of a digit. It is a relatively

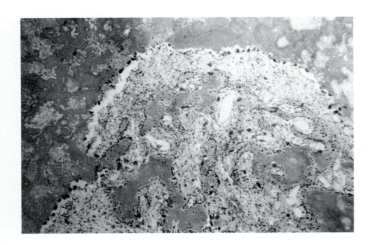

Figure 18

Photomicrograph to show part of an osteoid osteoma, showing nidus of vascular bone-forming tumour (centre and bottom) and sclerotic surrounding bone (top)

uncommon tumour, which comprises trabecular bone with a fibrocartilaginous cap (Evison & Price 1966, Dahlin 1978, Landon et al 1979). These lesions are not related to osteochondromas (exostoses) seen elsewhere in the skeleton and they are not found in patients with multiple hereditary exostoses (Landon et al 1979). Presentation is with a mass in the distal part of the digit, with elevation of the nail bed and often local pain. The vast majority of cases occurring in the foot in one study were present on the great toe (Landon et al 1979). A lateral radiograph shows a dorsal bony outgrowth on the distal part of the phalanx. Surgery involves, first, removal of the nail. As much of the nail bed as possible should be preserved. Through a longitudinal incision, the exostosis is excised with osteotomy at the base and complete removal of the fibrocartilaginous cap. The nail bed should then be repaired.

Osteoid osteoma

Osteoid osteoma is a benign bone-forming tumour, usually affecting the diaphysis or metaphysis of a long bone in the lower limb, particularly the femur and tibia. The great majority of affected patients are aged between 5 and 25 years (Byers 1968, Dahlin 1978). In the foot, the osteoid osteoma is probably the most common osteoid-forming tumour (Jaffe & Lichenstein 1940, Dahlin 1978, Peridue & Olin 1980, Campbell 1982, Kahn et al 1983, Wu 1991). Osteoid osteoma and osteoblastoma are histologically similar lesions. There are no criteria for their separation apart from size, in that osteoid osteomas are less than 1 cm in diameter and typically surrounded by sclerotic bone (Byers 1968, McLeod et al 1976). An osteoid osteoma causes progressively more severe pain and relief from this is obtained with salicylates. Night pain is almost always present and is commonly severe enough to disturb sleep (Dahlin 1978).

Radiological examination typically shows a small area of radiolucency, with a surrounding area of sclerotic bone (Swee et al 1979); tomography and scintigraphy may be valuable in localizing the lesion where typical radiological features are absent yet the diagnosis is suspected (Winter et al 1977). If situated subperiosteally, there may be some new bone formation adjacent to the tumour. Macroscopic examination may reveal a friable red-grey 'nidus' of tumour in the centre of sclerotic bone, though finding this nidus may prove difficult and radiology of excised bone should be considered as an aid to its detection. Histologically, the nidus is composed of cellular, highly vascular tissue with benign osteoblasts lining the surface of osteoid trabeculae, which themselves show a totally random arrangement, while the surrounding bone shows sclerosis (Dahlin 1978) (Fig. 18). The differential diagnosis includes chronic abscess, other benign or malignant tumours, fibrous dysplasia, bone cysts and healing fractures, particularly stress fractures (Freiburger et al 1959).

Treatment is by complete excision en bloc and the nidus can be identified on an X-ray of the biopsy specimen. In the phalanges and metatarsals, curettage is carried out and the nidus looked for histologically. The prognosis is excellent. Unfortunately, cases occur in which there is return of pain and local recurrence, most likely due to inadequacy of primary excision.

Osteoblastoma

This is a benign bone-forming tumour with histological similarity to osteoid osteoma, but differentiated from the latter on the basis of size. Osteoblastomas are more than 1.5 cm in diameter (McLeod et al 1976). Although there is a marked tendency for osteoblastomas to occur in the vertebrae, other sites include the ilium, ribs and long bones. The short tubular bones of the hand and foot are sometimes affected (Spjut et al 1971, Dahlin 1978), and the talus and os calcis (Giannestras & Diamond 1958, Khermosh & Schujman 1977). Pain may be present but is not a marked feature, in contrast to osteoid osteoma. Radiological appearances are nonspecific, the lesion sometimes being radiolucent, sometimes more dense, with a variable amount of sclerosis demarcating the margin. These appearances may be mistaken for osteosarcoma, chondrosarcoma, aneurysmal bone cyst or even osteoid osteoma (Khermosh & Schujman 1977).

The diagnosis is confirmed by biopsy. Naked eye appearance is of a vascular and haemorrhagic dark purple lesion, with a gritty surface, lacking a dense reactive margin but often with a surrounding thin shell of new bone. Histology shows a connective tissue stroma containing osteoid and bone trabeculae formed by benign osteoblasts. Treatment should be local removal of the lesion by conservative surgery, either by excision or by curettage and packing with bone graft if necessary, to fill any defects. Local recurrence does occur.

Osteosarcoma

Osteosarcomas are, by definition, malignant tumours showing evidence of osteoid or bone formation by the malignant tumour cells (Fig. 19). Most cases occur

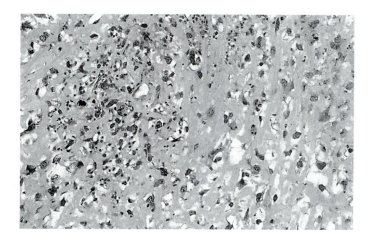

Figure 19

Photomicrograph of osteosarcoma, showing osteoid matrix formation by malignant pleomorphic tumour cells

between the ages of 10 and 20 years, and boys are affected more often than girls. Osteosarcomas may occur in any bone, although the lower femur, upper tibia, upper femur and upper humerus are most frequently involved. The sites of involvement have been summarized elsewhere for five series of cases (Revell 1981). This shows that between 1 and 2% of osteosarcomas occur in the ankle or foot and this is confirmed by other sources (Dahlin 1978, Dahlin & Unni 1977). Matsumoto and colleagues (1993) described involvement of the talus of a 20-year-old male.

Pain and local swelling are the most common modes of presentation and a long history is unusual. The radiological appearances are variable, but there is usually evidence of bone destruction and the tumour mass, which often shows evidence of ossification or calcification in the radiograph, may extend into the surrounding soft tissue. Skeletal surveys, computerized tomography and radioisotope scanning may all be valuable in assessing the clinical extent of the disease.

Naked eye appearances vary according to the composition of the tumour, which may be osteoblastic, chondroblastic, fibroblastic or telangiectatic. Histological features are similarly extremely variable. Classically, a malignant proliferation of spindle-shaped or oval cells, with variable numbers of mitoses, shows evidence of bone or osteoid formation. Haematogenous metastasis to the lungs and other bones is the usual form of spread. Differential diagnosis is between osteosarcoma and the other destructive malignant tumours, and it is essential that an adequate biopsy is available in order that an accurate diagnosis can be made in view of the close similarities there might be to other sarcomas, for example chondrosarcoma or fibrosarcoma, in large parts of any individual lesion.

Surgical treatment should be directed at complete removal with a wide margin of normal tissue. In the foot, this is likely to involve amputation, although limb preser-

vation is being used with prosthetic replacement for osteosarcoma at other sites. Radiotherapy and chemotherapy are important adjuvant features in the modern management of osteosarcoma.

Neoplastic giant cell tumour (osteoclastoma)
Giant cell tumours (osteoclastomas) occur mostly in the age range 20 to 55 years and affect women more often than men (Schajowicz 1961, Hutter et al 1962, Goldenberg et al 1970, Dahlin 1978). Giant cells are often present in other bone lesions in considerable numbers, particularly nonosteogenic fibroma, chondroblastoma, chondromyxoid fibroma, aneurysmal bone cyst and the so-called 'brown' tumour of hyperparathyroidism, and these are a potential source of confusion in biopsy interpretation, together with nodular villonodular tenosynovitis.

Giant cell tumours are situated more often in the epiphyseal region of long bones, frequently around the knee, but may be present almost anywhere, including the hands and feet where they are most commonly located in the tarsal or metatarsal bones. A giant cell lesion affecting the small bones of the foot is more likely to be due to hyperparathyroidism or bone involvement with localized nodular tenosynovitis (Murphy & Ackerman 1956). The clinical presentation of a giant cell tumour of bone is with pain and swelling, and a mass palpable on physical examination may crepitate. Particularly if there is extensive soft tissue involvement, the overlying skin may be red. There are no specific radiological features, the observed eccentric position of a lytic lesion as being an osteoclastoma (Jaffe et al 1940) is considered to be nonspecific. (Spjut et al 1971, Dahlin 1978).

Macroscopic examination shows a heterogeneous cut surface showing solid, pale yellow fibrous areas alternating with cysts, grey-red vascular tissue, necrosis and haemorrhage. The bone is expanded and the overlying cortex thinned. Light microscopy shows multinucleate giant cells, intermixed with numerous oval or spindle-shaped cells. Systems of grading have been devised in the past (Jaffe et al 1940, Hutter et al 1962), but have unfortunately proved of no value in predicting the way in which an individual lesion will behave (Spjut et al 1971, Dahlin 1978), since some tumours with apparently benign histological appearance may unexpectedly assume a malignant course.

Although treatment by curettage has been practised in the past, it is increasingly realized that total excision of the tumour and its surrounding shell of bone (and, if involved, soft tissue) is the treatment of choice, especially in a small bone. This may be difficult in some sites in the foot. Following curettage, the recurrence rate is approximately 50% and, of these, 10% metastasize (Goldenberg et al 1970). More radical excision and amputation should be reserved for cases of multiple recurrent tumour. Radiotherapy should not normally be used because of the possible risk of inducing malignant change, and because giant cell tumours are anyway relatively radio-resistant.

Neoplastic small cell sarcomas

Ewing's sarcoma

This is a primary bone neoplasm, made up of small, round, relatively uniform cells. Although previously considered to be a bone marrow derivation, it is now generally thought to be part of a spectrum of tumours of neuro-ectodermal origin. Patterns of proto-oncogene expression include c-myc, N-myc, c-myb and c-mil/raf-1, which are similar to those seen in peripheral neuro-ectodermal tumour (PNET) (McKeon et al 1988). Ewing's sarcoma is an uncommon malignant tumour, the usual sites being the femur, tibia, humerus, ilium and ribs, and occurs mostly before the age of 20 years. Small numbers of cases in the ankle, tarsals, metatarsals and phalanges have been described (Bhansali & Desai 1963, Marcove & Charosky 1972, Dunn et al 1976, Dahlin 1978, Campbell 1982).

The most common symptoms are swelling and pain; the latter may be intermittent initially. Physical examination shows a palpable tender mass, and the body temperature and erythrocyte sedimentation rate may both be raised, sometimes together with aleucocytosis (Bhansali & Desai 1963, Dahlin 1978). These features may lead to an erroneous diagnosis of osteomyelitis, and this was certainly the case in one specific report relating to Ewing's sarcoma in a great toe (Dunn et al 1976). It is frequently stated that Ewing's sarcoma can be distinguished by its radiological appearances alone, the lytic tumour mass being surrounded by multiple layers of subperiosteal reactive new bone to give an 'onion skin' appearance. Ewing's sarcoma may, however, be equally difficult to distinguish from osteosarcoma, eosinophilic granuloma, malignant lymphoma, metastatic disease or osteomyelitis.

Macroscopically, it is a soft, grey-white lesion and light microscopy shows a small, round cell tumour arranged in cords, nests or sheets, sometimes with a rosette pattern (Fig. 20). The demonstration of glycogen granules, at light and electron microscopical level, aids in the differentiation of the small round cell tumours of bone (Dahlin 1978, Revell 1986). Opinions differ as to the best mode of treatment for Ewing's sarcoma, some favouring radiotherapy, others surgical excision. In the foot, the radiotherapy required may produce significant disability to necessitate subsequent amputation. One large study (Bhansali & Desai 1963) concluded that surgery was the superior treatment when feasible, and amputation should be strongly considered in lesions of the foot. Where there is evidence of metastases, radiotherapy and/or chemotherapy is indicated.

Neuro-ectodermal tumour of bone

This tumour is closely similar to Ewing's sarcoma in clinical, radiological and light microscopical appearances. The distinction is on the basis of the demonstration of well defined ultrastructural and immunohistochemical evidence of neuro-ectodermal differentiation.

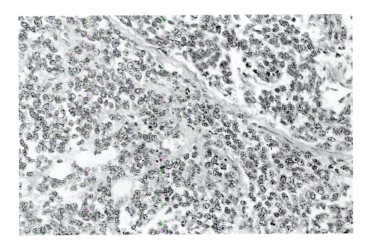

Figure 20

Photomicrograph of Ewing's sarcoma composed of closely packed small round cells

Neoplastic metastatic tumours

Much the most common malignancy affecting bone is metastatic carcinoma, with the likeliest primary sites being lung, breast, prostate, thyroid and kidney. Metastatic carcinoma usually involves the more centrally placed bone marrow-containing parts of the skeleton, namely the spine, ribs, pelvis, proximal femur and skull. Spread to the distal parts of the limbs is decidedly uncommon, there being just over 50 documented cases of such an occurrence in the foot and ankle (Gall et al 1976, Sundberg et al 1982, Zindrick et al 1982). Lung, colon and urogenital carcinomas are reported to be the most frequent source of metastases to the foot and ankle, followed by breast, cervix, uterus, ovary, prostate and submandibular gland (Gelberman et al 1975, Gall et al 1976, Kumar & Kovi 1978, Harkohen & Olin 1980, Sundberg et al 1982, Dripchack & Robertson 1990, Troncoso et al 1991, Bloom et al 1992, Cooper et al 1994). The metastatic lesions have no particular predilection for a specific part of the foot and involve multiple sites: the os calcis, the talus, a phalanx, metatarsal or other tarsal bone. The differential diagnosis includes osteomyelitis, gout, and the peripheral arthropathy of Reiter's syndrome or rheumatoid arthritis. Radiology, tomography and radio-isotope scanning methods are all useful in making the diagnosis and technetium scanning is a particularly effective way of detecting metastatic disease (Revell 1986).

Treatment should be aimed at maintaining maximum function and mobility, with short hospitalization in these patients who are likely to be terminally ill. Radiotherapy and external splinting may prove sufficient to control pain and limit local growth, although amputation may sometimes be required if these less invasive procedures are ineffective.

References

Altman M I, Hinkes M P 1982 Heel neuroma. A case history. J Am Podiatry Assoc 72: 517–519

Arrington J H III, Reed R J, Ichinose H, Krementz E T 1977 Plantar lentiginous melanoma: a distinctive variant of human cutaneous melanoma. Am J Surg Pathol 1: 131

Bart R S, Andrade R, Kopf A W et al 1968 Acquired digital fibrokeratomas. Arch Dermatol 97: 120–129

Bearman R, Noe J, Kempson R 1975 Clear cell sarcoma with melanin pigment. Cancer 36: 977–984

Bedi T R, Pandhi R K, Bhutania L K 1976 Multiple palmoplantar histiocytomas. Arch Dermatol 112: 1001–1003

Berlin S J, Block L D, Donick I I 1972 Pyogenic granuloma of the foot. A review of the English literature and report of four cases. J Am Podiatry Assoc 62: 94–99

Berlin S J, Donick I I, Block L D, Costa A J 1975 Nerve tumours of the foot: diagnosis and treatment. J Am Podiatry Assoc 65: 157–166

Bernhard L M, Brant R G, Bakst M J, Coleman W B, Nickamin A 1983 Hypertrophic haemangioma vs haemangiopericytoma. J Foot Surg 22: 308–313

Bhansali S K, Desai P B 1963 Ewing's sarcoma. Observations of 107 cases. J Bone Joint Surg 45A: 541–553

Bloom R A, Sulkes A, Freilick G, Libson E 1992 Breast metastases to bones of the extremities: simultaneous involvement of all four limbs. Clinical Oncol 4: 58–59

Booher R J 1965 Lipoblastic tumours of the hands and feet: review of literature and report of 33 cases. J Bone Joint Surg 47A: 727–740

Borden J I, Shea T P 1976 Cavernous haemangioma of the foot. A case report and review. J Am Podiatry Assoc 66: 484–490

Boudreaux D, Waisman J 1978 Clear cell sarcoma with melanogenesis. Cancer 41: 1387–1394

Breslow A 1970 Thickness, cross-sectional areas and depth of invasion in the prognosis of cutaneous melanoma. J Am Surg 172: 902–915

Bridge J A, Borek D A, Neff J R, Huntrakoon M 1990 Chromosomal abnormalities in clear cell sarcoma. Am J Clin Pathol 93: 26–31

Byers P D 1968 Solitary benign osteoblastic lesions of bone: osteoid osteoma and benign osteoblastoma. Cancer 22: 43–47

Byers P D, Cotton R E, Deacon O D, Lowy M, Newman P H, Sissons H A, Thomson A D 1968 The diagnosis and treatment of pigmented villonodular synovitis. J Bone Joint Surg 50B: 290–305

Campbell C J 1982 Tumours of the Foot In: Jahss M H (ed) Disorders of the Foot, 1st edn. W B Saunders, Philadelphia. Ch 34 pp 986–988

Cargialosi C P, Schmoll S J 1976 Kaposi's sarcoma of the foot. J Am Podiatry Assoc 66: 523–527

Carnevali S L 1938 Sugli angioma dei muscoli striati. Arch Orthop 54: 476–507

Carroll R E, Berman A T 1972 Glomus tumours of the hand. Review of the literature on twenty-eight cases. J Bone Joint Surg 54A: 691–703

Cavanagh R C 1973 Tumours of the soft tissues of the extremities. Semin Roentgenol 8: 73–89

Chang J L, Ireland M L 1993 Osteoid osteoma of the os calcis in a teenage athlete. Med Sci Sports Exercise 25: 2–8

Chimenti S, Calvieri S, Ribuffo M 1982 Synovial sarcoma of the foot. J Dermatol Surg Oncol 8: 882–886

Chung E B, Enzinger F M 1978 Benign chondromas of soft parts. Cancer 41: 1414–1424

Clark W H Jnr 1969 In: From L, Bernardina E A, Mihm M C The histogenesis and biologic behaviour of primary human malignant melanomas of the skin. Cancer 29: 705–727

Classen D A, Hurst L N 1992 Plantar fibromatosis and bilateral flexion contractures: a review of the literature. Ann Plastic Surg 28: 475–478

Coleman W P, Loria P R, Reed R J, Krementz E T 1981 Acral lentiginous melanoma. Arch Dermatol 116: 773

Cooper J K, Wong F L, Swenerton K D 1994 Endometrial adenocarcinoma presenting as an isolated calcaneal metastasis. A rare entity with good prognosis. Cancer 73: 2779–2781

Coskey R J, Nabbai H, Rahbari H 1979 Recurring digital fibrous tumour of childhood. Cutis 23: 359–362

Cox F H, Helwig E B 1959 Kaposi's sarcoma. Cancer 12: 289–298

Cox K L 1976 Subcutaneous haemangioma of the foot – a case report. J Am Podiatry Assoc 66: 519–521

Crisafulli J A, Adams D, Sakhuja R 1990 Chondromyxoid fibroma of a metatarsal. J Foot Surg 29: 164–168

Dahlin D C 1978 Bone Tumours. General Aspects and Data on 6221 Cases. 3rd edn. Thomas, Springfield. p 111

Dahlin D C, Salvador H 1974 Cartilaginous tumours of the soft tissues of the hands and feet. Mayo Clin Proc 49: 721–726

Dahlin D C, Unni K K 1977 Osteosarcoma of bone and its important recognizable varieties. Am J Surg Pathol 1: 61–72

Day C L, Sober A J, Kopf A W 1981 A prognostic model for clinical stage I melanoma of the lower extremity. Am Surg 193: 599

Demuth R J, Snider B L 1980 Primary squamous cell carcinoma of the plantar surface of the foot. Am Plast Surg 4: 310–314

Dripchack P O, Robertson J R 1990 Breast cancer metastatic to the foot with massive bone loss. Orthop Rev 19: 877–879

Dunn E J, McGavran M H, Nelson P, Greer R B 1974 Synovial chondrosarcoma. J Bone Joint Surg 56A: 811–813

Dunn E J, Yuska K H, Judd D M, Garner F L, Varano L A 1976 Ewing's sarcoma of the great toe. Clin Orthop 83: 224–231

Enzinger F M 1965 Clear cell sarcoma of tendons and aponeuroses. An analysis of 21 cases. Cancer 18: 1163–1674

Enzinger F M 1970 Epithelioid sarcoma. A sarcoma simulating a granuloma or a carcinoma. Cancer 26: 1029–1040

Enzinger F M, Weiss S W 1983 Soft Tissue Tumours. C V Mosby, St Louis

Evison G, Price C H G 1966 Subungual exostosis. Br J Radiol 39: 451–455

Fechner R E, Mills S E 1993 Tumours of bones and joints. Atlas of Tumor Pathology. 3rd Series. Fascicle 8. AFIP, Washington. pp 195–199

Feibelman C E, Stoll H, Maize J C 1980 Melanomas of the palm, sole and nailbed: a clinicopathological study. Cancer 46: 2492–2504

Fitzpatrick T B, Gilchrest B A 1977 Dimple sign to differentiate benign from malignant pigmented cutaneous lesions. New England J Med 296: 1518

Forman W R, Streigold H 1982 Eccrine poroma: review of literature and case reports. J Foot Surg 21: 330–334

Freiburger R H, Loitman B S, Helpern M, Thompson T C 1959 Osteoid osteoma: a report of 80 cases. Am J Roentgenol 82: 194–199

Friedman-Kien A E 1981 Disseminated Kaposi's sarcoma syndrome in young homosexual men. J Am Acad Dermatol 5: 468–471

Fuselier C O, Binning T, Kushner D et al 1984 Solitary osteochondroma of the foot: an in-depth study with case reports. J Foot Surg 23: 3–24

Fuselier C O, Cachia V V, Wong C et al 1985 Selected soft tissue malignancies of the foot: an in-depth study with case reports. J Foot Surg 24: 162–204

Gall R J, Sim F H, Pritchard D J 1976 Metastatic tumours to the bones of the foot. Cancer 37: 1492–1495

Gelberman R H, Salamon P B, Huffer J M 1975 Bone metastasis from carcinoma of the uterus. Clin Orthop 106: 148–150

Ger R 1975 The surgical management of ulcers of the heel. Surg Gynecol Obstet 140: 909–911

Geschickter C F 1935 Tumours of the peripheral nerves. Am J Cancer 25: 377–410

Giannestras N J, Diamond J R 1958 Benign osteoblastoma of the talus. J Bone Joint Surg 40A: 469–478

Goldenberg R R, Campbell C J, Bonfiglio M 1970 Giant cell tumour of bone. An analysis of two hundred and eighteen cases. J Bone Joint Surg 52A: 619–664

Goldman R L, Lichenstein L 1964 Synovial chondrosarcoma. Cancer 17: 1233–1240

Gottlieb G J, Raggaz A, Vogel J V, Friedman-Kien A, Rylin A M, Wiener E A, Ackerman A B 1981 A preliminary communication on extensively disseminated Kaposi's sarcoma in young homosexual men. Am J Dermatopathol 3: 111–114

Grosse R E 1937 Recurring myxomatous, cutaneous cysts of the fingers and toes. Surg Gynecol Obstet 65: 289–302

Gross R E, Wolbach S D 1943 Sclerosing haemangiomas: Their relationship to dermatofibroma, histiocytoma, xanthoma and to certain pigmented lesions of the skin. Am J Pathol 19: 533–551

Guccion J G, Enzinger F M 1979 Malignant schwannoma associated with von Recklinghausen's neurofibromatosis. Virch Arch (Pathol Anat) 383: 43–57

Gunzy T R, Quintavalle P R, Tursi F J 1992 Leiomyosarcoma: a rare pedal finding. J Foot Surg 31: 88–92

Hare P J, Smith P A 1969 Acquired (digital) fibrokeratomas. Br J Dermatol 81: 667–670

Harkohen M, Olin P E 1980 Rectal carcinoma metastasizing to a toe. Acta Med Scand 207: 235–236

Harrison D H, Morgan B D G 1981 The instep island flap to resurface plantar defects. 34: 315–318

Harwood A R, Osuba D, Hofstader S L, Goldstein M B, Cardella C J et al 1979 Kaposi's sarcoma in recipients of renal transplants. Am J Med 67: 759–765

Hemric J R, Allen H B 1979 Acquired digital fibrokeratoma. Cutis 23: 304–306

Hirakawa E, Miki H, Kobayashi S, Ohmori M, Arima N 1993 Lipofibromatous hamartoma of nerve in the foot. Acta Pathol Japan 43: 265–267

Horn R C, Enteline H T 1958 Rhabdomyosarcoma: A clinicopathological study and classification of 39 cases. Cancer 11: 181–199

Hurt M A, Igra-Serfaty H, Stevens C S 1990 Eccrine syringofibroadenoma (Mascaro) An acrosyringeal hamartoma. Archiv Dermat 126: 945–949

Hutter R V P, Worces J N, Francis K C, Forte F W, Stewart F W 1962 Benign and malignant giant cell tumours of bone. A clinicopathological analysis of the natural history of the disease. Cancer 25: 1377–1383

Jacobson G F, Edwards M C Jr 1993 Neurilemmoma presenting as a painless mass on the dorsum of the foot. J Am Podiatry Med Assoc 83: 228–230

Jaffe H L, Lichenstein L 1940 Osteoid osteoma: further experience with this benign tumour of bone. J Bone Joint Surg 22: 645–682

Jaffe H L, Lichenstein L, Portis R B 1940 Giant cell tumour of bone. Its pathologic appearance, grading, supposed variants and treatment. Arch Pathol 30: 993–1031

Jaffe H L, Lichenstein L, Sutro C J 1941 Pigmented villonodular synovitis. Arch Pathol 31: 731–765

Jahss M H 1982 Examination. In: Jahss M H (ed) Disorders of the Foot, 1st edn. W B Saunders Company, Philadelphia

Jakobson E, Spjut H J 1960 Chondrosarcoma of the bones of the hand. Report of three cases. Acta Radiol 54: 426–432

Jeffreys T E 1967 Synovial chondromatosis. J Bone Joint Surg 49B: 530–534

Kahn M D, Tiano F J, Little R C 1983 Osteoid osteoma of the great toe. J Foot Surg 22: 325–348

Kauffman S L, Stout A P 1959 Lipoblastic tumours of children. Cancer 12: 912–925

Keyhani A 1977 Comparison of clinical behaviour of melanoma of the hands and feet: a study of 283 patients. Cancer 40: 3168–3173

Khermosh D, Schujman E 1977 Benign osteoblastoma of the calcaneus. Clin Orthop 127: 197–199

King J W, Spjut H J, Fechner R E, Vanderpool D W 1967 Synovial chondrosarcoma of the knee joint. J Bone Joint Surg 49A: 1389–1396

Krajca-Radcliffe J B, Nicholas R W, Lewis J M 1992 Multifocal epithelioid haemangioendothelioma in bone. Orthop Rev 21: 973–975, 978–980

Kumar P P, Kovi J 1978 Metastases to bones of the hands and feet. J Natl Med Assoc 70: 837–840

Kurzer A, Patel M 1979 Basal cell carcinoma of the foot. Br J Plast Surg 32: 300–301

Landers P A, Yu G U, White J M, Farrer A K 1993 Recurrent plantar fibromatosis. J Foot Ankle Surg 32: 85–93

Landon G C, Johnson K A, Dahlin D C 1979 Subungual exostoses. J Bone Joint Surg 61A: 256–259

LaPorta G A, Davis W S, Scarlet J 1976 Glomus tumour of the foot. Discussion and case report. J Am Podiatry Assoc 66: 528–533

Lever W F, Schaumberg-Lever G 1983 Histopathology of the Skin. 6th edn. Lippincott, Philadelphia

Lewis M M, Marcove R C, Bullough P G 1975 Chondrosarcoma of the foot. A case report and review of the literature. Cancer 36: 586–589

Lichenstein L, Goldman R L 1964 Cartilage tumours in soft tissues, particularly in the hand and foot. Cancer 17: 1203–1209

Lisch M, Mittleman M, Albin R 1982 Digital lipoma of the foot: an extraordinary case. J Foot Surg 21: 330–334

Luke R D 1976 Neurilemmomas of the foot. J Am Podiatry Assoc 66: 547–549

Lumley J S P, Stansfeld A G 1972 Infiltrating glomus tumour of lower limb. Br Med J 1: 484–485

McCann J J, Al-Nafussi A I 1989 Epithelioma cuniculatum plantare. Br J Plast Surg 42: 79–82

McIvor R R, King D 1962 Osteochondromatosis of the hip joint. J Bone Joint Surg 44A: 87–97

MacKenzie D H 1966 Synovial sarcoma: a review of 58 cases. Cancer 19: 169–180

McKeon C, Thiele C J, Ross R A et al 1988 Indistinguishable patterns of protooncogene expression in two distinct but closely related tumors: Ewing's sarcoma and neuroepithelioma. Cancer Res 48: 4307–4311

McLeod R A, Beabout J W 1973 The roentgenographic features of chondroblastoma. Am J Roentgenol Radium Ther Nucl Med 118: 464–471

McLeod R A, Dahlin D C, Beabout J W 1976 The spectrum of osteoblastoma. Am J Roentgenol Radium Ther Nucl Med 126: 321–335

Marcove R L, Charosky C B 1972 Phalangeal sarcomas simulating infection of the digits. Clin Orthop 83: 224–231

Margileth A M, Museles M 1965 Current concepts in diagnosis and management of congenital haemangiomas. Paediatrics 3: 410–416

Matsumoto K, Hukuda S, Ishikawa M, Fujita M, Egawa M, Okabe H 1993 Osteosarcoma of the talus. A case report. Clin Orthop 296: 225–228

Midenberg M, Kirschenbaum S E 1983 benign cavernous haemangioma of the ankle. J Foot Surg 22: 294–297

Miki T, Yamamuro T, Oka M, Urushidani H, Itokazu M 1978 Chondrosarcoma developed in the distal phalangeal bone of the third toe. Clin Orthop 136: 241–243

Milchgrub S, Ghandur-Mnaymneh L, Dorfman H D, Albores-Saavedra J 1993 Synovial sarcoma with extensive osteoid and bone formation. Amer J Surg Pathol 17: 357–363

Milgram J W 1977a The classification of loose bodies in human joints. Clin Orthop 124: 282–291

Milgram J W 1977b The development of loose bodies in human joints. Clin Orthop 124: 292–303

Milgram J W, Addison R G 1976 Synovial osteochondromatosis of the knee. J Bone Joint Surg 58A: 264–266

Moore S W, Wheeler J E, Hefter L G 1975 Epithelioid sarcoma masquerading as Peyronie's disease. Cancer 35: 1706–1710

Murphy A F, Wilson J N 1958 Tenosynovial osteochondroma in the hand. J Bone Joint Surg 40A: 1236–1240

Murphy F P, Dahlin D C, Sullivan C R 1962 Articular synovial chondromatosis. J Bone Joint Surg 44A: 77–86

Murphy W R, Ackerman L V 1956 Benign and malignant giant cell tumours of bone. A clinical evaluation of thirty one cases. Cancer 9: 317–339

Neviaser R J, Wilson J N 1972 Benign chondroblastoma in the finger. J Bone Joint Surg 54A: 389–392

Nona F E, Dahlin D C, Beabout J W 1983 Bizarre parosteal osteo-chondromatous proliferations of the hands and feet. Am J Surg Pathol 7: 245–250

O'Brien P H, Brasfield R D 1966 Kaposi's sarcoma. Cancer 19: 1497–1502

Pack G J, Miller T R 1950 Haemangiomas: Classification and treatment. Angiology 1: 405–426

Patcher M R, Alpert M 1964 Chondrosarcoma of the foot skeleton. J Bone Joint Surg 46A: 601–607

Peridue R L, Olin F H 1980 Osteoid osteoma of the talus, a case study. J Am Podiatry Assoc 70: 353–355

Petersen N C 1968 Malignant melanoma of the foot. Scan J Plast Reconst Surg 2: 144–153

Petrov O, Zaremba J S 1990 Vascular hamartoma. A case report. J Am Podiatry Assoc 80: 377–380

Politz M J 1976 Haemangioma of the digits. Two cases. J Am Podiatry Assoc 66: 515–518

Pratt J, Woodruff J M, Marcove R C 1978 Epithelioid sarcoma. Cancer 41: 1472–1487

Prieskorn D W, Irwin R B, Hankin R 1992 Clear cell sarcoma presenting as an interdigital neuroma. Orthop Rev 21: 963–970

Quigley J T 1979 A glomus tumor of the heel pad. J Bone Joint Surg 61A: 443–444

Radstone D J, Revell P A, Mantell B S 1979 Clear cell sarcoma of tendons and aponeuroses treated with bleomycin and vincristine. Br J Radiol 52: 238–241

Ransom J L, Pratt C B, Shanks E 1977 Childhood rhabdomyosarcoma of the extremity. Results of combined modality therapy. Cancer 40: 280–281

Rao G S, Luthra P K 1988 Dupuyter's disease of the foot in children: a report of three cases. Br J Plast Surg 41: 313–315

Revell P A 1981 Diseases of bones and joints. In: Berry C L (ed) Paediatric Pathology. Springer, Berlin. pp. 451–485

Revell P A 1986 The Pathology of Bone. Springer, Berlin

Reynolds W A, Winkelmann R K, Soule E H 1965 Kaposi's sarcoma. Medicine (Baltimore) 44: 419–443

Robinson J K 1979 A gigantic basal cell carcinoma on the plantar arch of a foot: report of a case. J Dermatol Surg Oncol 5: 958–960

Ross J A, Dawson E K 1975 Benign chondroblastoma of bone. J Bone Joint Surg 57B: 78–81

Rowley L C., Winston L, Hovernale T, Ruskin J 1978 Epithelioid inclusion cyst of the foot: a literature review and case report. J Am Podiatry Assoc 68: 829–833

Ryan J R, Baker L H, Benjamin R S 1982 The natural history of metatarsal synovial sarcoma: experience of the Southwest Oncology Group. Clin Orthop 164: 257–260

Sanmartin O, Botella R, Alegre V, Martinez A, Aliaga A 1992 Congenital eccrine angiomatous hamartoma Am J Dermatol 14: 161–164

Santa Cruz D J, Reiner C B 1978 Recurrent digital fibroma of childhood. J Cutan Pathol 6: 339–346

Schajowicz F 1961 Giant cell tumours of bone (osteoclastoma): a pathological and histochemical study. J Bone Joint Surg 43A: 1–29

Schoenfeld R J 1964 Epidermal proliferations overlying histiocytomas. Arch Dermatol 90: 266–270

Schwartz R A, Burgess G H 1980 Verrucous carcinoma of the foot. J Surg Oncol 14: 333–339

Scrivner D, Oxenhandler R W, Lopez M, Perez-Mesa C 1987 Plantar lentiginous melanoma. Cancer 60: 2502–2509

Seehafer J R, Rahman D, Soderstrom C W 1979 Epithelioma cuniculatum: verrucous carcinoma of the foot. Cutis 23: 287–290

Shanahan R E, Gingrass R P 1979 Medial plantar sensory flap for coverage of heel defects. Plast Reconstr Surg 64: 295–298

Shapiro L 1969 Infantile digital fibromatosis and aponeurotic fibroma. Arch Dermatol 99: 37–42

Sheitel P L, Scheffer N M, Hawthorne F A 1978 Dermatofibrosarcoma protruberans. J Foot Surg 17: 174–176

Siegal F P et al 1981 Severe acquired immunodeficiency in male homosexuals, manifested by chronic perianal ulcerative herpes simplex lesions. N Engl J Med 305: 1439–1444

Slavitt J A, Behesht F, Lenet M, Sherman M 1980 Ganglions of the foot: a six year retrospective study and a review of the literature. J Am Podiatry Assoc 70: 459–465

Smith L S, Lenet M, Sherman M 1976 Malignant fibrous histiocytoma. A rare soft tissue tumour of the foot. J Am Podiatry Assoc 66: 459–464

Someren A, Merritt W H 1978 Tenosynovial chondroma of the hand: a case report with a brief review of the literature. Human Pathol 9: 476–479

Sommerlad B C, McGrouther D A 1978 Resurfacing the sole. Br J Plast Surg 31: 107–116

Sondergaard K, Olsen G 1980 Malignant melanoma of the foot. A clinicopathological study of 125 primary cutaneous malignant melanomas. Acta Pathol Microbiol Scand 88: 275–283

Spjut H J, Dorfman H D, Flechner R E, Ackerman L V 1971 Tumours of bone and cartilage. In: Atlas of Tumour Pathology (fascicle 5). Armed Forces Institute of Pathology, Washington DC

Stout A P 1948 Myxoma, the tumour of primitive mesenchyme. J Surg 127: 706–719

Stout A P 1953 Tumours of the soft tissues. In: Atlas of Tumour Pathology, Section II, Fascicle 5, Armed Forces Institute of Pathology, Washington DC

Straehley C J, Santos J I, Downey D M, Lewin K J 1975 Kaposi's sarcoma in a renal transplant recipient. Arch Pathol 99: 611–613

Strong E W, McDivitt R W, Brasfield R D 1970 Granular cell myoblastoma. Cancer 25: 415–422

Sugar M H 1981 Benign myxomas of the digits: a surgically resistant neoplasm. J Foot Surg 20: 67–69

Sugar S, Murphy B M 1955 Liposarcoma of the foot. Case Report. J. Michigan State Med Soc 54: 468–469

Sundberg S B, Carlson W O, Johnson K A 1982 Metastatic lesions of the foot and ankle. Foot Ankle 3: 167–169

Swee R G, McLeod R A, Beabout J W 1979 Osteoid osteoma. Radiology 130: 117–123

Symmers W St C 1973 Glomus tumours. Br Med J 2: 50–51

Tedeschi C G 1958 Some considerations concerning the nature of the so-called sarcoma of Kaposi. Arch Pathol 66: 656–684

Toe T K, Saw D 1978 Clear cell sarcoma with melanin. Report of two cases. Cancer 41: 235–238

Troncoso A, Ro J Y, Grignon D J, Hans W S, Wexler H, von Eschenbach A, Ayala A 1991 Renal cell carcinoma with acrometastases: report of two cases and review of the literature. Mod Pathol 4: 66–69

Vance S, Hudson R 1969 Granular cell myoblastoma. Am J Clin Pathol 52: 208–211

Verallo V V 1968 Acquired digital fibrokeratomas. Br J Dermatol 80: 730–736

Villacin A B, Brigham L N, Bullough P G 1979 Primary and secondary synovial chondrometaplasia. Histopathologic and clinico-radiologic differences. Human Pathology 10: 439–451

Vineyard W 1975 Glomus tumour. Clin Dermatol 2: 1–10

Watson W L, McCarthy W D 1940 Blood and lymph vessel tumours. Surg Gynecol Obstet 71: 569–588

White N 1967 Neurilemmomas of the extremities. J Bone Joint Surg 49A: 1605–1610

Winter P F, Johnson P M, Hilal S K, Feldman F 1977 Scintigraphic detection of osteoid osteoma. Radiology 122: 177–178

Wright P H, Sim F H, Soule E H, Taylor W F 1982 Synovial sarcoma. J Bone Joint Surg 64A: 112–122

Wu K K 1991 Osteoid osteoma of the foot. J Foot Surg 30: 190–194

Wu K K 1994 Plantar fibromatosis of the foot. J Foot Ankle Surg 33: 98–101

Zindrick M R, Young M P, Daley R J, Light T R 1982 Metastatic tumours of the foot: case report and literature review. Clin Orthop 170: 219–225

VI.8 Crystal Arthropathies

H L F Currey

Introduction

This chapter covers a group of joint disorders that result from the deposition in articular tissues of a variety of metabolic products ('metabolic deposition diseases'). The clinical manifestations of these disorders depend not so much on the chemical composition of the substance deposited as on the physical presence of the crystalline material within the joint tissues. The crystal arthropathies (Table 1) include two common diseases: gout and pyrophosphate arthropathy. Ochronosis (alkaptonuria) is a rare inborn error of metabolism, mentioned only to complete the classification. Finally, crystals of hydroxy-apatite (the mineral component of bone) have been identified in synovial fluids in a number of circumstances. However, their possible role in the pathogenesis of joint disease and in the production of symptoms remains a matter for speculation at present. Each of these four conditions is discussed below.

In addition to these naturally occurring diseases, a wide range of crystalline materials produces inflammation when injected into the joints of experimental animals. The occasional acute flare-up that follows a therapeutic injection of (crystalline) corticosteroid into a joint probably represents a similar reaction.

in the tissues. In the joints this causes recurrent episodes of acute inflammatory arthritis. Untreated, this may later progress to local accumulations of urate as 'tophi' and to chronic destructive joint changes. Fortunately, for most patients, the drug allopurinol provides effective control of both the underlying metabolic defect and the clinical features.

The disease is known to be of great antiquity. It remains a common disorder, and affects predominantly adult males, often with familial clustering. As described below, plasma levels of uric acid depend on the interplay between many influences. However, gout is described as 'primary' when the hyperuricaemia is due mainly to an inborn metabolic fault, and 'secondary' when it results mainly from an environmental factor or acquired disease state.

The clinician dealing with disorders of the foot needs to be familiar with gout. Apart from the characteristic acute podagra of the first metatarsophalangeal joint, other joints in the foot and the ankle joint are commonly affected. Diagnosis can be difficult; gout may closely mimic a local infective lesion, and vice versa. Further, while modern drug therapy should be highly effective in the management of gout, there continues to be widespread misunderstanding of how these drugs should be deployed.

Gout

Gout is a disorder in which an excess of uric acid in the plasma (hyperuricaemia) leads to precipitation of urate

Clinical features

Primary gout is predominantly a disease of men, and the first attack usually occurs between the ages of 20 and

Table 1 Metabolic and crystal-induced arthropathies			
Disorder	Material deposited	Distribution of arthritis	Clinical features
Gout	Urate	Peripheral small joints	Initially acute and episodic; later chronic deforming arthritis
Pyrophosphate arthropathy (Pseudogout)	Calcium pyrophosphate dihydrate	Larger limb joints	Acute episodic and/or chronic 'degenerative' arthritis
Apatite associated arthritis	Hydroxyapatite	?	Inflammatory episodes in OA? Chronic destructive arthritis?
Alkaptonuria (Ochronosis)	Homogentisic acid metabolites	Central joints (mainly spine)	Chronic 'degenerative' arthritis

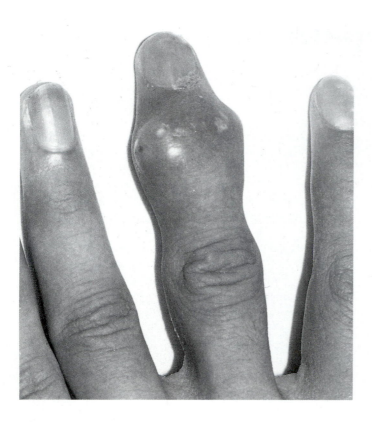

Figure 1

Gouty tophus in a finger (reproduced by permission from Scott 1986)

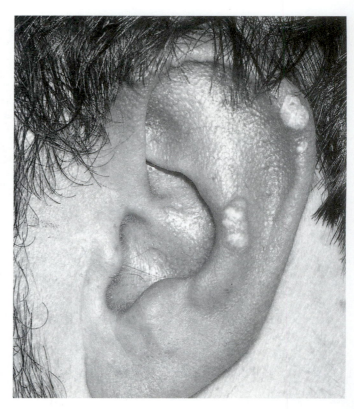

Figure 2

Gouty tophus in the ear (reproduced by permission from Scott 1986)

50. A tendency to gout – like frontal baldness – appears to be inherited as an autosomal dominant trait, with male sex hormone status exerting a 'permissive' effect on its expression (Hippocrates noted that eunuchs were spared both conditions). Complications include urate stone formation in the urinary tract (urate urolithiasis) and a metabolic nephropathy ('gouty kidney').

The acute attack

The initial attack characteristically involves one or other first metatarsophalangeal joint ('podagra'). The patient may be awoken with a dull ache in this joint which, over the next few hours builds up to an almost intolerably acute pain. The joint becomes swollen and red. Walking may become impossible. Untreated the joint reverts to complete normality over the following week to 10 days. There follows a symptom-free ('intercritical') period, lasting weeks, months or even years, before the next attack occurs. This then follows a similar pattern, returning perhaps to the same or the opposite first metatarsophalangeal joint, or some other peripheral joint. Proximal limb joints (shoulder and hip) are seldom involved. Acute attacks may be triggered by trauma, surgical operations, or a sudden lowering of the plasma urate level (as occurs for example when allopurinol therapy is introduced). The mechanism of this is not understood.

Chronic tophaceous gout

Untreated, this sequence of acute episodic attacks may continue for years. However, there is usually a gradual change in the pattern, with the individual attacks becoming less acute, lasting longer, and the joints failing to return completely to normal between attacks. With the passage of time this can evolve into a picture of widespread peripheral polyarthritis and gross, crippling joint deformities with occasional superadded subacute flares in individual joints.

The deformities are due to solid deposits of monosodium urate or 'tophi'. These usually originate in the cartilage of joints and enlarge to produce irregular lumps related to peripheral joints (Fig. 1). Similar masses arising from the cartilage of the pinna of the ear appear as cream-coloured nodules on the helix (Fig. 2), a site where they should always be sought as an important diagnostic lead. Tophi also penetrate into subchondral bone to produce large radiological 'erosions' (Fig. 3)

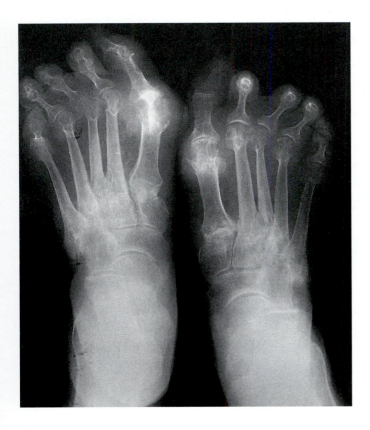

Figure 3
Radiological erosions in gout

Many cases of gout do not progress to a chronic tophaceous stage. Pointers to a severe outcome are a first attack at a young age, e.g. below 25 years, and a short interval between the first attack and the appearance of tophi, e.g. within four years. Fortunately modern methods of management have made it possible in most cases to prevent or even reverse chronic tophaceous lesions.

Urinary tract complications

Gout may be complicated by urinary tract stone formation or by an interstitial metabolic nephropathy. The liability to stone formation is due to the fact that many gouty patients excrete an abnormally high daily load of uric acid in the urine. Uric acid is relatively insoluble, particularly in an acid environment. Hence the two renal processes of concentration and acidification both predispose to the crystallization of uric acid out of solution to form stones (urate urolithiasis) or 'gravel'. A hot, dry environment predisposes to stone formation, and ill-understood, genetically determined aspects of renal tubular function are probably also involved.

The stones are usually small and easily passed and, unless secondarily calcified, are radiolucent. Their chemi-cal nature can be established by polarized light microscopy. In subjects liable to uric acid stone formation, this can usually be prevented by maintaining a dilute urine (through adequate hydration) and reducing urinary acidity by oral sodium bicarbonate. Failing this, administration of allopurinol (see below) is highly effective.

The process of urinary concentration in the renal medulla also predisposes to the precipitation of urate crystals in the interstitial tissues. This can lead eventually to chronic renal failure. Many patients with severe chronic tophaceous gout show some evidence of 'gouty kidney' in the form of proteinuria, impaired tubular functions of concentration or acidification, hypertension or renal failure. Occasionally this is the direct cause of death. All patients with gout require renal evaluation. Fortunately, allopurinol provides not only an effective means of preventing renal damage in those at risk, but will also often improve function in the damaged kidney.

Gout, diabetes, hypertension and vascular disease

Apart from nephropathy attributable to gout, there is also a greater than expected association between gout, hypertension, ischaemic heart disease, diabetes and plasma lipoprotein abnormalities. There is a variety of reasons for this. Genetic association is one. Common aetiological factors such as diet and obesity may play a role. Also, drugs used in the treatment of hypertension may contribute to hyperuricaemia. The important practical point is that there is no evidence that hyperuricaemia itself contributes directly to hypertension, vascular disease or diabetes. This has to be remembered when considering whether asymptomatic hyperuricaemia requires treatment.

Pathology

Acute gouty arthritis (crystal synovitis)

The central event in an acute attack of gout is the interaction between microcrystals of urate and the polymorphonuclear leucocyte. This has been established beyond all reasonable doubt in experimental animals (Phelps & McCarty 1966). However, the factors which initiate and terminate the attack remain unclear (Dieppe 1984). The solubility of urate in physiological saline at body temperature is about 530 μmol/l (8.8 mg/100 ml). Protein and other components of the plasma allow it to hold a higher concentration of urate than this, but at some point this is exceeded and precipitation of urate crystals occurs into the tissues. The predilection for deposition into joint cartilage may depend on differing rates of diffusion into this avascular structure by urate and other components of the synovial fluid. Possibly also cartilage provides the nucleating factor essential to set off crystal-lization. Evidence from 'secondary gout' (see below) suggests that hyperuricaemia has to be present for some years before the first attack of gout occurs. This seems to point to a requirement for a critical load of urate in the tissues.

How trauma or fluctuations in urate levels trigger the attack is unknown. Coating of urate crystals with IgG is probably an essential prerequisite for phagocytosis. Once synovial fluid polymorphs start phagocytosing micro-crystals of urate, lysosomal and cytoplasmic enzymes, cytokines, prostaglandins, toxic oxygen-derived free radicals, and other mediators of inflammation are released by these cells (Platt & Dick 1984, Bhoola et al 1992). In addition, activation of the complement cascade of enzymes, as well as contributing to the inflammation, provides a chemotactic stimulus drawing more neutrophils from the circulation into the synovial fluid (Russell et al 1982). Because of their surface properties, urate crystals have a destructive effect on cell membranes. Thus the phagosomes that ingest them rupture and the cell is killed, adding to the release of inflammatory mediators. This amplification scheme accounts for the rapid build-up of the acute attack. It is not clear what causes an attack to end, unless through intervention: aspiration of the fluid removes crystals, while administration of colchicine (a drug without effect on uric acid metabolism) interferes with neutrophil function (Fordham et al 1981).

Predictably, the characteristic finding in the synovial fluid during an acute attack is numerous neutrophils, many containing ingested microcrystals of urate (see below). However, it is notable that a few crystals may occasionally be identified in fluid from apparently unaffected joints of gouty patients, while a dusting of urate may be seen on the surface of cartilage from uninflamed joints.

Chronic gouty arthritis

The characteristic lesion is the tophus. Multicentric deposits of monosodium urate crystals grow by further deposition of crystals until each deposit consists of a nidus of radially arranged crystals with an interstitial matrix, and is surrounded by a foreign body giant cell reaction. With continued growth, these deposits coalesce to form increasingly large chalky concretions which may eventually become secondarily calcified. Starting as a nidus in the joint cartilage, such tophi will expand to destroy the cartilage locally, and also grow inwards to invade subchondral bone (producing radiological erosions) as well as growing outwards to appear clini-cally as periarticular masses (see Fig. 1). Necrosis of the overlying skin may then result in the discharge of chalky material. Other periarticular tissues, the helix of the ear (see Fig. 2), bursae, tendons, the kidneys and (rarely) almost any other tissue may be the site of tophus forma-tion.

Diagnosis

'When in doubt, think of gout' remains a useful maxim. However, the ready availability of plasma uric acid deter-minations as part of autoanalyser printouts has now made overdiagnosis of gout an equal hazard. The follow-ing points require consideration:

The clinical presentation

While the classical picture of acute podagra in a young or middle-aged man with a positive family history is unmistakable, milder attacks involving other joints or multiple joints may cause confusion. Local infections in the foot, particularly cellulitis, may mimic acute gout. Careful examination will usually give the correct answer. With acute crystal synovitis any passive movement of the joint is very painful. In the case of periarticular cellulitis, while extremes of passive movement will cause pain (by distorting the soft tissues), careful testing should reveal some range of painless movement. Other clues may come from the presence of a site of entry of infection such as a skin crack between the toes or lymphangitis.

Plasma uric acid levels

Unless the patient is taking a urate-lowering drug, a persistently normal plasma level of urate almost completely excludes a diagnosis of gout. By contrast an elevated plasma level, especially a single reading, certainly does not establish a diagnosis of gout. As explained below, a single tablet of aspirin may produce hyperuricaemia. Also, many subjects with persistently elevated levels of plasma urate never develop gout. Failure to appreciate this is the cause of much inappro-priate prescription of allopurinol.

Crystals in joint fluid (Chayen 1983)

Identification of crystals of urate within synovial fluid is the 'gold standard' for the diagnosis of gout. While sparse extracellular crystals may occasionally be found in nongouty fluids, the typical appearance of numerous intracellular crystals establishes the diagnosis beyond doubt. Fluid for this examination should not have anti-coagulant added. Aspiration of even a drop or two from a small joint may be sufficient to establish the diagno-sis. A drop of fluid, either the centrifuged deposit or a fragment of clot, is examined under a coverslip by polar-ized light microscopy. Viewed with 'crossed polars' the birefringent urate crystals stand out brightly against the dark background. These are generally needle-shaped, about 2–12 μm in length, and many lie within polymorphs.

More precise identification of the crystals (and differ-entiation from pyrophosphate crystals) is obtained by rotating the microscope stage with polars crossed. This shows that the bright birefringence of the crystals 'extin-guishes' when parallel with the polars. Next, a 'first order red' quartz compensator is introduced into the optical axis of the microscope. Rotation of the stage now shows the urate crystals taking on a yellow colour (against the red background) when the crystal is parallel with the 'slow component' of the compensator, and a blue colour when at right angles to it. By convention this colour pattern indicates 'negative birefringence'. Further details of the technique of examining synovial fluids for crystals will be found in standard texts (Hartshorne & Stuart 1970).

Examination of tophi and synovial tissue
Solid matter scraped from a tophus with a needle is readily examined by polarized light microscopy. The clusters of needle-shaped crystals are unmistakable (Fig. 4). Similarly synovial or any other biopsy material can be examined in this way. However, if such material is to be fixed before examination, it is important to use a nonaqueous fixative (such as absolute alcohol) to avoid dissolving the crystals.

Radiology
Acute gouty arthritis shows no change on X-ray apart from soft tissue swelling. Once tophaceous deposits extend into bone these appear as bony erosions (see Fig. 3). There may also be loss of joint space and changes of secondary osteoarthritis. Pure urate tophi are radiolucent, but secondary calcification may occur in advanced cases.

While these radiological changes indicate the severity of joint damage, they are rarely of any value in establishing the diagnosis. This is because the gouty erosions, in contrast to the situation in rheumatoid arthritis, are a late feature. By the time they appear, clinically apparent tophi will almost invariably have made the diagnosis obvious.

Plasma levels of uric acid

Epidemiological surveys show that there is broad correlation between plasma levels of urate and the prevalence of gout. However, as has been pointed out above, the duration of hyperuricaemia is an important determining factor. Short term increases in urate levels in the plasma, even if extreme, seldom lead to clinical gout.

In children, plasma urate levels are low, but rise at puberty, particularly in boys, so that young adult males in general have levels 60 μmol/l (1 mg/100 ml) higher than females. At the menopause levels in women rise, possibly because of an adrenal androgenic effect, to approach those for men.

Plasma uric acid levels for gouty and nongouty subjects form two separate distribution curves. In an English study (Snaith & Scott 1971) the mean level for normal men was 306 μmol/l (±60) (5.1 mg/100 ml), that for gouty men 474 μmol/l (±54) (7.9 mg/100 ml). The two distribution curves overlap between 360 and 450 μmol/l. For practical

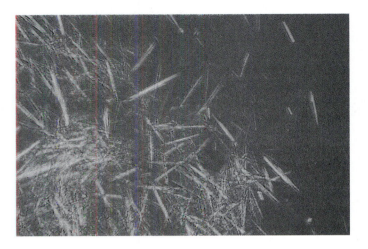

Figure 4
Scrapings from a tophus viewed by polarized light microscopy. Numerous needle-shaped birefringent crystals

purposes the 'upper limit of normal' for men may be taken as 420 μmol/l (7.0 mg/100 ml), and for women 360 μmol/l (6.0 mg/100 ml). There are racial differences. For example, New Zealand Maoris have higher urate levels as well as a greater prevalence of gout.

Uric acid metabolism

Uric acid is a weak dibasic organic acid. At the near neutral pH of the plasma and the body tissues generally it is in the form of the monosodium salt. At the lower pH of the urine much is converted to free uric acid.

Uric acid formation
Uric acid is produced as the end product in the degradation of the purine bases adenine and guanine (constituents of nucleic acids and nucleotides) according to the following (much simplified) scheme:

$$\text{ADENINE} \longrightarrow \text{GUANINE}$$
$$\downarrow \qquad\qquad \downarrow$$
$$\text{HYPOXANTHINE} \rightarrow \text{XANTHINE} \rightarrow \text{URIC ACID}$$

In this respect the purines differ from most other nitrogen-containing body constituents, in that they are not degraded to urea. In lower mammals this degradation is taken one stage further by the enzyme uricase, which converts uric acid to the readily soluble and easily eliminated substance allantoin. Humans, however, have suffered an apparently deleterious mutation and no longer code for uricase. This leaves the relatively insoluble uric acid as the end product to be eliminated.

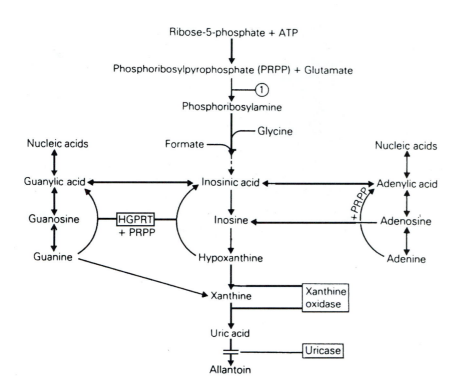

Figure 5

Purine metabolism pathways. Reaction (1) is brought about by the enzyme amidophosphoribosyltransferase, and is the site of feedback inhibition by purines. HGPRT = hypoxanthine guanine phosphoribosyl-transferase, the enzyme missing in the Lesch-Nyhan syndrome. Man lacks uricase. (By permission from Currey 1984)

A complex system of enzymatic reactions controls the synthesis, interconversions and catabolism of purines. Some of these pathways are illustrated in Fig. 5. Factors which add purines to the pool (and hence contribute to uric acid formation) are synthesis of new purines (as in cell replication), breakdown of tissue nucleic acids (as in cell death) and dietary intake of purines.

Uric acid elimination

In the mammalian kidney, urate, being a relatively small molecule and bound, if at all, only very lightly to plasma proteins, is filtered freely through the glomerulus. It is then completely, or almost completely, reabsorbed in the proximal tubule by an active transport process. This is a bidirectional tubular transport system, and most of the urate eliminated in the urine comes from secretion back into the tubule. Some more distal reabsorption also occurs.

The bidirectional active tubular transport system is relatively nonspecific, being shared by many other weak organic acids. Thus competition at this level by other weak organic acids (e.g. ketoacids or aspirin) may markedly influence the renal handling of urate and hence account for fluctuations in plasma and urinary levels of urate. On a purine-free diet the mean normal 24-hour urinary uric acid is about 2.4 mmol (400 mg) with an upper limit of normal of 3.6 mmol (600 mg).

About 30% of urate excretion takes place into the gut. Within the lumen this urate encounters uricase synthesized by the gut flora.

Hyperuricaemia

The factors determining the level of urate in the plasma are illustrated in Fig. 6. Clinical gout is represented as a spill-over of urate from the plasma into the tissues by crystallization (and effective treatment with allopurinol as this process in reverse). Plasma levels of urate depend mainly on the balance between synthesis and renal elimination. Gouty patients in whom hyperuricaemia is due to increased synthesis are referred to as 'overproducers', while those in whom renal elimination is defective are 'underexcretors'. Similarly, when hyperuricaemia is clearly due to some environmental factor or other disease process (e.g. overproduction of purines in leukaemia or renal retention due to a drug) it is called 'secondary', while 'primary' gout results from hyper-uricaemia attributable mainly to an inherited abnormality in the control of purine metabolism. In practice many cases of gout are multifactorial. The mechanism of the association of other factors with hyperuricaemia remains uncertain.

Increased formation of uric acid

Specific enzyme abnormalities (Nuki 1983)
A group of rare inherited enzyme defects has thrown important light on purine intermediate metabolism. Most interest has centered on the Lesch-Nyhan syndrome (Kelly et al 1969). This is an X-linked disorder of boys who develop spasticity, choreoathetosis, mental

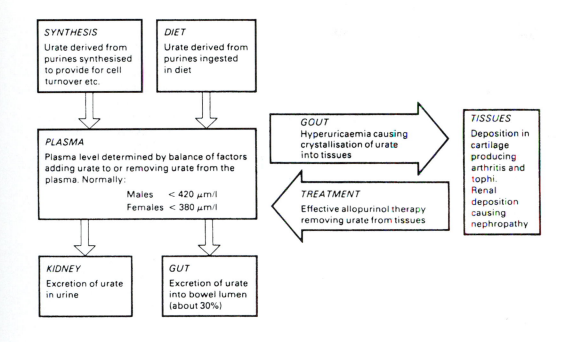

Figure 6

Factors determining the level of urate in plasma and deposition into the tissues. (By permission from Currey 1983)

deficiency and striking compulsive self-mutilation with biting of fingers and lips. Plasma and urinary urate levels are very high, and may result in gout, urolithiasis and renal failure. The massive overproduction of urate is due to lack of the enzyme hypoxanthine guanine phospho-ribosyltransferase (HGPRT) (see Fig. 5).

Increased nucleoprotein turnover
Any proliferative disorder of the haemopoietic system is likely to produce hyperuricaemia. In practice the myelo-proliferative diseases (chronic myeloid leukaemia, polycythaemia rubra vera, myelofibrosis, etc.) are the disorders most associated with gout.

High purine diet
The difference between a high and a low purine diet can account for a difference of about 50 µmol/l in plasma urate levels.

Decreased excretion of uric acid
Altered renal function
Severe renal failure results in progressive hyperuricaemia. In practice, gout secondary to renal disease is rare, perhaps largely because such patients do not survive long enough for the critical load of urate to be deposited.

Drugs
The bidirectional renal tubular transport mechanism accounts for the paradoxical biphasic action of drugs such as aspirin. Plasma salicylate levels of 10 mg/100 ml or more produce uricosuria, while lower levels cause urate retention. Attention has already been drawn to how easily this can lead to misinterpretation of laboratory results: one or two aspirin tablets can readily account for a considerable elevation of urate level in the plasma. Other drugs lack this biphasic action. Thiazide and other diuretics cause urate retention and are an important cause both of hyperuricaemia and (secondary) gout. Probenecid and similar drugs are potent uricosurics and are used for this purpose therapeutically (see below).

Lactic acidaemia
Lactic acid competes with urate for renal tubular transport. This contributes to the hyperuricaemia which may accompany physical exercise, type 1 glycogen storage disease and alcoholic intoxication.

Ketoacidosis
Ketoacids such as aceto-acetic acid act like lactic acid at the level of the renal tubule. Thus both starvation and diabetic ketoacidosis cause hyperuricaemia.

Hypertension
The well known association between hypertension and gout is accounted for by various factors, including treatment of hypertension with diuretics, 'gouty kidney', and a genetic linkage between predispositions to both conditions. There is no evidence that correcting hyper-uricaemia influences essential hypertension.

Lead poisoning
'Saturnine gout' results from renal urate retention secondary to tubular damage by lead.

Hypercalcaemia

The hyperuricaemia (and occasionally gout) which sometimes accompanies hypercalcaemic conditions such as hyperparathyroidism may result from altered renal handling of urate secondary to calcium deposition in the renal tubules.

Hypothyroidism

Urate retention has been reported in myxoedema. The mechanism is unknown.

Other factors associated with hyperuricaemia and gout

Genetics

A positive family history is obtained in about 40% of cases of primary gout. Inherited variations in the renal handling of urate and in the 'setting' of feedback controls in the intermediate metabolism of purines probably account for this. Single biochemical defects underlie the inheritance of conditions such as HGPRT deficiency.

Body weight

Obesity is associated with both hyperuricaemia and gout. Correction of obesity results in a fall in plasma urate, a point of obvious therapeutic importance.

Affluence and intelligence

There is some evidence of a positive correlation between gout and affluence, intellectual capacity and 'drive'.

Alcohol

A relatively high proportion of gout patients indulge in alcohol, and a reduction in alcohol intake will predictably reduce plasma urate levels.

Plasma lipids

There is a well established association between hyperlipoproteinaemia and hyperuricaemia (and gout). Again, the metabolic explanation is unclear.

Ischaemic heart disease and diabetes

Attention has already been drawn to the association between coronary artery disease, diabetes and gout. The association is probably a genetic one. Correction of hyperuricaemia does not influence heart disease or glucose metabolism.

Management of gout

Once a diagnosis of gout is established the patient requires investigation to exclude causes of secondary gout, including questioning about alcohol and drugs, particularly diuretics (Gibson 1988, Dieppe 1991). Splenomegaly may provide the clue to a myeloproliferative disorder. A full blood count, renal function tests, fasting plasma urate determinations, and urinary 24 hour urate (on a low urate diet) should be obtained.

Urate overproducers (over 3.6 mmol (600 mg) urinary urate per 24 hours) should have red cell lysates examined to exclude a deficiency of HGPRT (see page 565).

In planning drug management it is essential to appreciate that terminating an acute attack is an entirely separate issue from introducing long-term (urate-lowering) therapy. The latter must never be started during an acute attack. Lowering urate levels at this stage may both worsen and prolong the attack.

The acute attack

The affected joint will need rest and protection. Most of the nonsteroidal anti-inflammatory drugs are effective in aborting the attack if given early and in large doses. Indomethacin 50 mg four times daily or naproxen 250 mg three times daily are examples of drug regimens which are usually satisfactory. As the attack subsides over the next few days, the dose is tapered down. Once an effective regimen is established, the patient should always carry the drug with him to start at the first warning of an attack.

Colchicine, the time-honoured (and specific) remedy for acute gout (1 mg immediately, followed by 0.5 mg 2-hourly until the attack subsides) tends to produce diarrhoea as the effective total dose is reached. For this reason it has largely given way to the newer drugs.

If a gouty joint is aspirated for diagnostic purposes, the opportunity can be taken to inject corticosteroid locally.

Patients on established allopurinol therapy should continue the drug during the acute attack. However, as mentioned above, such therapy should on no account be started during an acute attack.

Long-term management

After the acute attack has subsided a decision will need to be taken about whether urate-lowering treatment should be started. Once started, such therapy should normally be continued indefinitely. Indications for starting this treatment include:

Frequent acute attacks
Tophi
Urate nephropathy
Severe hyperuricaemia (above about 500 µmol/l,
   8.3 mg/100 ml))

In the absence of one of these indications it is usually advisable to await events. Sometimes the experience of an acute attack and having faced up to the implications of the diagnosis may produce changes in the patient's lifestyle such that he has few or no further attacks.

Allopurinol

If urate lowering treatment is considered necessary, allopurinol is the drug of choice. By competitive inhibition of the enzyme xanthine oxidase (see Fig. 5), it reduces urate production and it also has a second action in inhibiting purine synthesis. The result is a predictable reduction in plasma urate levels, which can usually be brought within the normal range. A single tablet of 300 mg daily is normally sufficient. Occasionally larger doses are needed. For patients in renal failure the dose should be reduced. The final dose should be that which will just maintain a normal plasma urate level. Acute attacks are particularly liable to occur during the period of introducing allopurinol. The chance of this happening is reduced by 'covering' the patient with a small daily dose of colchicine (0.5–1 mg) or a nonsteroidal anti-inflammatory drug during the period of urate lowering, and possibly by starting with a small dose of allopurinol. Apart from occasional skin rashes (which unfortunately require the drug to be stopped) side-effects are uncommon. Once steady-state metabolic control is achieved, attacks of acute gout cease, and tophi begin to get smaller.

Uricosuric drugs

Uricosuric drugs specifically block renal tubular transport of urate, resulting in a net increase in urinary urate. The choice lies between probenecid or ethebenecid (both 0.5–1.0 g twice daily) and sulphinopyrazone (100 mg three or four times daily). These drugs are less effective than allopurinol, particularly in patients with renal failure, and they may actually increase the risk of stone formation. They are used when allopurinol is not tolerated, or in order to get an added effect.

Diet

Strict dietary limitations are not necessary if allopurinol is given, but moderation in the intake of high-purine foods and alcohol are normally advised. Similarly, any obesity should be corrected.

Pyrophosphate arthropathy (pseudogout: chondrocalcinosis)

In a manner similar to gout, pyrophosphate arthropathy results from the deposition in joints of a crystalline metabolite. The metabolite in this case is calcium pyrophosphate dihydrate (CPPD) (McCarty et al 1965). Being opaque, this material produces a characteristic appearance on X-ray: 'chondrocalcinosis'. Attacks of acute arthritis due to CPPD are referred to as 'pseudogout'. The cause of pyrophosphate deposition is unknown, but it probably differs from urate deposition in that the pyrophosphate is generated locally in the cartilage by the chondrocytes.

Clinical features

Pyrophosphate arthropathy is most common in the middle-aged and elderly. The two sexes are equally affected. A positive family history is uncommon, except in certain geographical localities such as former Czechoslovakia (Zitnan & Sit'aj 1963) where familial clustering of severely affected patients at an earlier age represents a more severe form of the disease. A few examples of familial chondrocalcinosis have been described in English families (Doherty et al 1991).

Chondrocalcinosis is a relatively common radiological finding in the elderly, and this is often not associated with evidence of arthritis. When chondrocalcinosis (or CPPD crystals) and arthritis occur together there may – as discussed below – be a 'chicken-and-egg' problem of whether the CPPD deposition is the cause or the result of the arthritis. The present evidence suggests that CPPD deposition can be the cause of:

Episodic attacks of acute arthritis
Chronic 'degenerative' joint damage
Progressive chronic changes punctuated by acute episodes
Subacute polyarthritis mimicking rheumatoid arthritis

The acute attack

The pseudogout attack may mimic acute gout, but is usually somewhat less severe. It generally affects one or a few joints at a time. An important difference is that pyrophosphate arthropathy tends to affect large, rather than small, limb joints. Podagra has been described, but much the most common site is the knee joint, and the hips and shoulder joints are often affected. Acute attacks may be precipitated by trauma, surgical operations, or the taking of a diuretic. Untreated, the acute attack lasts about 10 days, but may grumble on in a subacute form for some weeks. At the height of the acute attack there may be a systemic disturbance, with malaise, fever, leucocytosis and elevated erythrocyte sedimentation rate. The association of these features with an acutely inflamed joint can easily lead to an erroneous diagnosis of septic arthritis, if the tell-take sign of chondrocalcinosis is overlooked on the knee X-ray, and if the synovial fluid is not examined for crystals (Hamblen et al 1966).

Chronic arthritis

The clinical features of chronic pyrophosphate arthropathy do not differ significantly from those of 'primary' osteoarthritis. This diagnosis is made when a patient with what appears to be degenerative joint disease of a knee or shoulder joint is found to have in addition radiological chondrocalcinosis and/or CPPD crystals in the synovial fluid. In some cases this picture is punctuated by episodes of acute crystal synovitis (see above). In others there may be no such attacks.

Usually only a few joints are involved but, particularly in the younger-onset familial cases, there may be widespread polyarthritis, including involvement of finger and spinal joints. Elderly patients with severe destructive changes in one or both shoulder joints are sometimes found to have pyrophosphate deposits in the affected joint(s), and severe destructive lesions are sometimes seen with CPPD deposition in other joints (Richards & Hamilton 1974). However, in general the prognosis is usually good and the condition is not necessarily progressive (Doherty et al 1993). It is not known to what extent these are associated specifically with pyrophosphate deposition. Another association with pyrophosphate deposition is carpal tunnel syndrome. Routine examination of material removed at the time of median nerve decompression sometimes reveals unsuspected pyrophosphate deposits. A case has been described of wrist extensor tendon rupture due to pyrophosphate deposition (Jones et al 1992).

Subacute polyarthritis

An uncommon presentation of pyrophosphate arthropathy is as subacute polyarthritis affecting many joints. There may be an associated systemic disturbance, with elevation of the sedimentation rate, so that the condition may closely mimic rheumatoid arthritis.

Associated conditions

In most patients with pyrophosphate arthropathy, there is no identifiable predisposing cause, except perhaps for advancing years. In a minority, however, there is a general or local associated condition which appears to play a role in determining either the appearance or the distribution of the pyrophosphate deposition. The general conditions include hyperparathyroidism and other causes of hypercalcaemia, hypophosphatasia, haemochromatosis, and Wilson's disease. There may also be a slight association with acromegaly and diabetes. Local predisposing causes include neuropathic (Charcot) arthropathy, previous meniscectomy in a knee joint, and urate gouty arthritis. There may be a tendency for pyrophosphate to be deposited in any badly damaged joint.

Radiology

Chondrocalcinosis is the characteristic radiological sign (Fig. 7). In hyaline articular cartilage this shows as a fine stippled line of opacification running parallel to the subarticular bone cortex and narrowly separated from it. In fibrocartilage the calcification shows as coarser opacities in the knee menisci, labrum acetabulare, triangular ligament of the wrist, etc. When degenerative changes result in destruction of cartilage the chondrocalcinosis predictably may disappear. Much the most common site in which to identify chondrocalcinosis is the knee, and

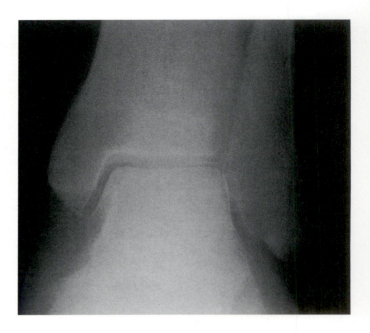

Figure 7

Chondrocalcinosis. The best site to screen for chondrocalcinosis is the knee joint. Only in gross cases can it be identified (as in this illustration) as a thin line of opacification between the ankle and tarsal bones

this is the joint which should be X-rayed when screening for the condition. The next most common sites are the wrist, shoulder, symphysis pubis, hip, elbow and metacarpophalangeal joints. The last are involved particularly in patients with haemochromatosis. It needs to be emphasized that chondrocalcinosis is an increasingly common finding with advancing years. Amongst the very elderly, something like 10% have at least some cartilage calcification. This is often asymptomatic, or associated with no more than the degenerative changes to be expected at that age.

Investigations

In a patient with arthritis, the association of chondrocalcinosis and crystals of CPPD in the synovial fluid (or in the synovial membrane) is generally accepted as evidence of pyrophosphate arthropathy. Rarely the chondrocalcinosis is lacking, sometimes because of cartilage destruction (see above). The technique of identifying CPPD crystals by polarized light microscopy is similar to that described above for urate crystals. CPPD crystals exhibit weak positive birefringence and oblique extinction (Fig. 8). A diagnosis of pyrophosphate arthropathy, or the presence of radiological chondrocalcinosis, demands investigations to exclude hyperparathyroidism, haemochromatosis and the other conditions listed above.

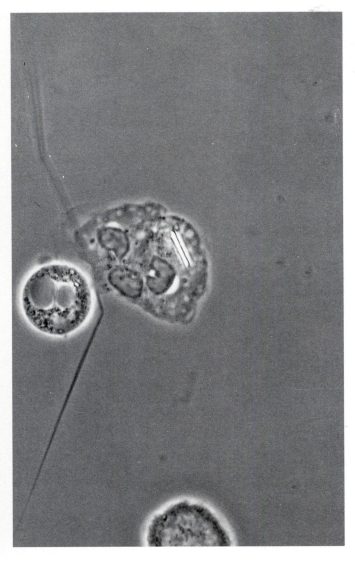

Figure 8

A crystal of calcium pyrophosphate dihydrate lying within a polymorph in synovial fluid from a patient suffering from pyrophosphate arthropathy (phase contrast and partially crossed polars). (Photomicrograph kindly provided by Professor B Vernon-Roberts, reproduced by permission from Currey 1975)

Pathogenesis and aetiology

Acute pyrophosphate arthropathy (pseudogout) seems to be an example of crystal synovitis in which the inflammatory mechanism is similar to that described for urate gout (Casewell et al 1983). There is some evidence that acute attacks can be precipitated by factors which increase crystal solubility, leading to crystal shrinkage and shedding from the cartilage surface into the synovial fluid (McCarty 1993). It appears likely that the pyrophos-

phate originates in the chondrocytes, where it is generated as an intermediate metabolite in the synthesis of macromolecules such as proteoglycan and collagen. What upsets the balance so that it is released in excess to accumulate in crystalline form in the cartilage is unknown. Age-related changes are probably important, but how conditions such as hyperparathyroidism operate is unknown. Some evidence points to cartilage damage from any cause stimulating chondrocytes to overproduce pyrophosphate. From this stems the chicken-and-egg problem of whether, in the case of chronic pyrophosphate arthropathy, cartilage damage causes the deposition of CPPD, or vice versa (Doherty 1983). Familial cases probably have a primary biochemical defect.

Management

An acute attack of pyrophosphate arthropathy is treated in exactly the same way as an attack of urate gout (see page 566) by the immediate administration of relatively large doses of a nonsteroidal anti-inflammatory drug. The dose is then tailed off as the attack settles. In addition, because pseudogout so often affects larger joints, particularly the knee, it is often easy to drain off the effusion and inject a corticosteroid preparation locally. This usually produces dramatic relief. No effective interval treatment is known (although colchicine has been tried). Treatment of underlying conditions such as hyperparathyroidism does not influence the arthritis.

Apatite-associated arthritis

The description by Dieppe et al (1976) and Schumacher et al (1977) of hydroxyapatite crystals within synovial fluids from osteoarthritic joints raised the possibility that a further type of crystal arthropathy has been identified. This question has not yet been settled (Hamilton et al 1990, Reginato 1990). Crystals of hydroxyapatite (the mineral component of bone) are too small to identify by the simple optical microscopy methods which can be used in the case of urate or pyrophosphate crystals. Their identification requires electron microscopy and other elaborate techniques (Paul et al 1983, Crocker et al 1976). Examination of synovial fluid from osteoarthritic joints has shown something like one-quarter of them to contain apatite crystals (Dieppe et al 1979, Giblisco et al 1982). Some fluids contained also crystals of other basic calcium phosphates. The presence of apatite crystals correlated with the severity of the joint damage, but the physical form of the crystals makes it unlikely that they arrived in the synovial fluid through simple grinding away of exposed bone ends. Like urate and pyrophosphate, such crystals are phlogistic in experimental animal models (Glatt et al 1979).

Views about the possible role of apatite crystals in osteoarthritis have varied widely. At one extreme was the suggestion that they might play a central role in the pathogenesis of the disorder. A more popular view has been that hydroxyapatite crystal synovitis might account for some of the more 'inflammatory' features of osteoarthritis. They might, however, represent no more than an unimportant epiphenomenon. By and large the present evidence seems to point to the presence of apatite crystals being a consequence rather than a cause of osteoarthritis (Nuki 1984).

It is notable that intra-articular apatite crystals are often associated with perivascular calcification in tendons and elsewhere. These calcific deposits also consist of hydroxyapatite, and they may certainly induce soft tissue inflammation (Pinals & Short 1966).

Dieppe and his colleagues (1984) described a group of 12 elderly patients with a distinctive type of destructive arthritis affecting predominantly their shoulders and knees. These painful joints progressed rapidly to instability, with very large, cool effusions and noninflammatory characteristics in the synovial fluids. All contained large numbers of ovoid bodies ranging from 0.5 to 5 µm in diameter and consisting of aggregates of apatite crystals. Many of the fluids also contained some crystals of pyrophosphate. The clinical description of these patients is reminiscent of similar case reports from France (de Seze et al 1968) and from North America (McCarty et al 1981). Here again, a pathogenic role for the apatite crystals remains to be proven. At present it appears best to classify these various conditions as 'crystal associated diseases' (Nuki 1984).

Ochronosis (alkaptonuria)

This extremely rare congenital metabolic disorder is mentioned here only to complete the classification of metabolic deposition arthropathies. It is an autosomal recessive defect in which the absence of the enzyme homogentisic acid oxidase blocks the degradation of tyrosine, so that homogentisic acid accumulates. The urine darkens on standing and pigmented metabolites accumulate in cartilage. Arthritis develops in a centripetal distribution and may lead to gross spinal rigidity (O'Brien et al 1963).

References

Bhoola K D, Elson C J, Dieppe P A 1992 Kinins – key mediators in inflammatory arthritis? Br J Rheum 31: 509–518

Casewell A, Guilland-Cumming D F, Hearn P R, McGuire M K B, Russell R G G 1983 Pathogenesis of chondrocalcinosis and pseudogout. Metabolism of inorganic pyrophosphate and production of calcium pyrophosphate dihydrate crystals. Ann Rheum Dis 42 (Suppl): 27–37

Chayen J 1983 Polarised light microscopy: principles and practice for rheumatologists. Ann Rheum Dis 42 (Suppl): 64–67

Crocker P R, Dieppe P A, Tyler T, Chapman S K, Willoughby D A 1976 The identification of particulate matter in biological tissues and fluids. J Pathol 121: 37–40

Currey H L F 1975 In: Mason R M, Currey H L F (eds) An Introduction to Clinical Rheumatology. Pitman, London

Currey H L F 1983 Essentials of Rheumatology. Pitman, London

Currey H L F 1984 Crystal deposition diseases. In: Dickson A, Wright V (eds) Integrated Clinical Science. Musculoskeletal Disease. V. Heinemann. London

de Seze S, Babaut A, Ramdon S 1968 L'épaule senile hemorrhagique. In: L'Actualité Rheumatologique Vol 1 Expansion Scientific Française, Paris, pp 107–115

Dieppe P A 1984 Crystal deposition and inflammation. Quart J Med 53: 309–316

Dieppe P A 1991 Investigation and management of gout in the young and the elderly. Ann Rheum Dis 50: 263–266

Dieppe P A, Crocker P, Huskisson E C, Willoughby D A 1976 Apatite deposition disease: a new arthropathy. Lancet i: 266–268

Dieppe P A, Crocker P R, Corke C F, Doyle D V, Huskisson E C, Willoughby D A 1979 Q J Med 48: 533–553

Dieppe P A, Doherty M, Macfarlane D G, Hutton C W, Bradfield J and Watt I 1984 Apatite associated destructive arthritis. Br J Rheum 23: 84–91

Doherty M 1983 Pyrophosphate arthropathy – recent clinical advances. Ann Rheum Dis 42 (Suppl): 38–44

Doherty M, Dieppe P, Watt I 1993 Pyrophosphate arthropathy: a prospective study. Br J Rheum 32: 189–196

Doherty M, Hamilton E, Henderson J, Misra H, Dixey J 1991 Familial chondrocalcinosis due to calcium pyrophosphate dihydrate crystal deposition in English families. Br J Rheum 30: 10–15

Fordham J N, Kirwan J R, Cason J, Currey H L F 1981 Prolonged reduction in polymorphonuclear adhesion following oral colchicine. Ann Rheum Dis 40: 605–608

Giblisco P A, Schumacher H R, Sieck M 1982 Studies on the role of synovial fluid apatite and calcium pyrophosphate crystals in osteoarthritis (abstract). Arthritis Rheum 25 (Suppl): S43

Gibson T 1988 The treatment of gout: a personal view. Reports on Rheumatic Diseases (Series 2 No 8). Arthritis and Rheumatism Council, Chesterfield.

Glatt M, Dieppe P A, Willoughby D A 1979 Crystal-induced inflammation, enzyme release and the effect of drugs in the rat pleural space. J Rheum 6: 251–258

Hamblen D L, Currey H L F, Key J J 1966 Pseudogout simulating acute suppurative arthritis. J Bone Joint Surg 48B: 51–55

Hamilton E, Pattrick M, Hornby J, Derrick D, Doherty M 1990 Synovial fluid calcium pyrophosphate dihydrate crystals and alizarin red positivity: analysis of 3000 samples. Br J Rheum 29: 101–104

Hartshorne N H, Stuart A 1970 Crystals and the Polarising Microscope. Edward Arnold, London

Jones A, Barton N, Pattrick M, Doherty M 1992 Tophaceous pyrophosphate deposition with extensor tendon rupture. Br J Rheum 31: 421–423

Kelly W N, Greene M L, Rosenbloom F M, Henderson J F, Seegmiller J E 1969 Hypoxanthine-guanine phosphoribosyltransferase deficiency in gout. Ann Int Med 70: 155–206

McCarty D J 1993 Calcium pyrophosphate dihydrate crystal deposition disease. Br J Rheum 32: 177–179

McCarty D J, Kohn N N, Faires J S 1965 The significance of phosphate crystals in the synovial fluid of arthritis patients: the pseudogout syndrome. Ann Intern Med 56: 711–737

McCarty D J, Halverson P B, Carrera G F, Brewer B J, Kozin F 1981 'Milwaukee shoulder' – association of microspheroids containing hydroxyapatite crystals, active collagenase and neutral protease with rotator cuff defects 24: 474–483

Nuki G 1983 Human purine metabolism: some recent advances and relationships with immunodeficiency. Ann Rheum Dis 42: (Suppl): 8–11

Nuki G 1984 Apatite associated arthritis (editorial). Br J Rheum 23: 81–82

O'Brien W M, La Du B N, Bunim J J 1963 Biochemical, pathological and clinical aspects of alkaptonuria, ochronosis and ochronotic arthropathy. Review of the world literature (1584–1962). Am J Med 34: 813–838

Paul H, Reginato A J, Schumacher H R, 1983 Alizarin Red S staining as a screening test to detect calcium compounds in synovial fluid. Arthritis Rheum 26: 191–200

Phelps P, McCarty D J 1966 Crystal-induced inflammation in canine joints II Importance of polymorphonuclear leucocytes. J Exp Med 124: 115–126

Pinals R S, Short C L 1966 Calcific periarthritis involving many sites. Arthritis Rheum 9: 566–574

Platt P, Dick W C 1984 Crystals and inflammation. Ann Rheum Dis (Suppl) 42: 4–7

Reginato A J 1990 Clinical significance of calcium salts in synovial fluid. Br J Rheum 29: 82–83

Richards A J, Hamilton E B D 1974 Destructive arthropathy in chondrocalcinosis articularis. Ann Rheum Dis 33: 196–203

Russell I J, Mansen C, Kolb L M, Kolb W P 1982 Activation of the fifth component of human complement (C5) induced by monosodium urate crystals; C5 convertase assembly on the crystal surface. Clin Immunol Immunopathol 24: 239–250

Scott J T 1986 In: Currey H L F (ed) Clinical Rheumatology. Churchill Livingstone, London

Schumacher H R, Somlyo A P, Tse R L, Maurer K 1977 Arthritis associated with apatite crystals. Ann Intern Med 87: 411–416

Snaith M L, Scott J T 1971 Uric acid clearance in patients with gout and normal subjects. Ann Rheum Dis 30: 285–289

Zitnan D, Sit'aj S 1963 Chondrocalcinosis articularis I. Clinical and radiological study. Ann Rheum Dis 22: 142–152

VII.1   Surgical Approaches

Piet de Boer

Every surgeon has his or her individual surgical technique. Certain principles, however, apply regardless of individual variations. Of these principles perhaps the most important one is that of pre-operative planning. Planning should cover not only the actual surgery that is to be performed but should also concentrate on the surgical approach that is to be used. The surgical approach is as precise a procedure as the insertion of a pre-planned screw or the creation of the triplanar osteotomy. Planning for a surgical approach must include consideration of the position of the patient on the operating table, the exact landmarks that are to be used for the incision, the precise location and length of the incision, the superficial and deep structures that are to be encountered and, above all, consideration must be given to the potential dangers of any approach.

It is always worth taking time to ensure that the patient is in the best position. Operating tables are well padded, but certain bony prominences, notably the head of the fibula, are not. These prominences must always be padded adequately to prevent skin breakdown and nerve entrapment during surgery.

Tourniquets are frequently used to create a bloodless field in surgery of the foot and ankle. The use of a tourniquet makes identification of vital structures easier but, by definition, the use of a tourniquet involves ischaemia to the limb. Tourniquets should be applied to the thigh and should always be padded with a soft dressing to prevent wrinkles and blisters that inevitably occur when the skin is pinched. A tourniquet around the calf should never be allowed. The inflated pressure of the tourniquet should be approximately 400 mmHg in the lower limb, depending on the circumference of the limb. A tourniquet should not be left inflated for more than 1.5 hours in the lower limb, so as to minimize ischaemic damage. Do not use tourniquets when the peripheral circulation is suspect or in the presence of sickle cell disease. Partial exsanguination of the limb, achieved by elevating the limb for 2 minutes, leaves blood in the venous structures. This makes for a bloodier field during surgery but it does make it easier to identify neurovascular bundles.

The landmarks are critical to the planning of any incision. All skin incisions must be accurately related to the landmarks. Skin incisions heal with the formation of scar tissue, which contracts with time. For this reason, skin incisions should not cross flexion creases at 90°. Incisions that must cross major flexion creases are sited to traverse the crease at about 60°.

Approaches to the structures of the foot and ankle are usually straightforward. The bones and joints that are explored are usually superficial, and many are subcutaneous. The most common problem in foot and ankle surgery is poor wound healing. That is why it is very important to evaluate both the circulation and the sensation of the foot. Wound healing is also affected by the thickness of the skin flaps you cut; it is important to cut skin flaps as thickly as possible and to avoid forceful retraction. Remember that skin incisions heal from side to side and not end to end. Longer incisions heal in the same time as shorter ones. Longer incisions require less retraction force to achieve the same exposure as deep structures.

Approaches to the ankle

Anterior approach

The anterior approach to the ankle provides an excellent exposure of the ankle joint. Its major use is in arthrodesis of the joint. It may also be used for drainage of infection and removal of loose bodies, although these two latter uses have been largely superseded by the development of arthroscopic techniques.

With the patient in the supine position, apply a tourniquet and make a 15 cm longitudinal incision on the anterior aspect of the ankle. The centre of the incision should be midway between the malleoli. Incise the deep fascia of the leg in line with the skin incision, taking care to avoid branches of the superficial peroneal nerve. Identify and develop the plane between extensor and digitorum longus and extensor hallucis longus. You will find the neurovascular bundle (anterior tibial artery and deep peroneal nerve) just medial to the tendon of the extensor hallucis longus. Retract the neurovascular bundle medially with the tendon of the extensor hallucis longus.

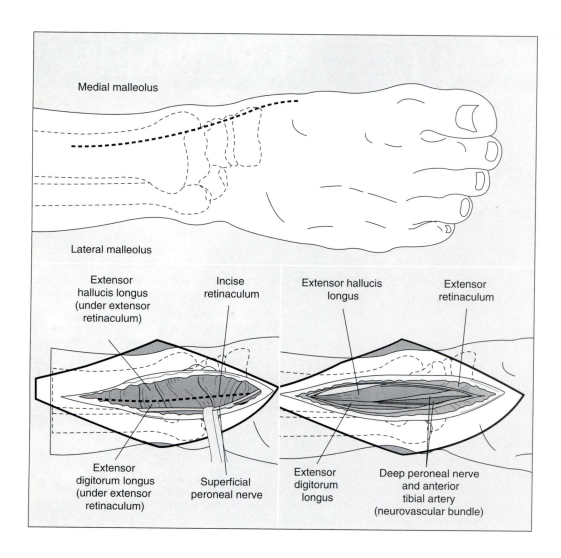

Figure 1

You will need to divide branches of the artery on its lateral aspect to allow its mobilization. Next divide the remaining soft tissues down to the anterior surface of the distal tibia, staying in the line of the skin incision. Incise the ankle capsule and the soft tissue overlying the anterior aspect of the dome of the talus in this line. Expose the full width of the ankle joint by detaching the anterior ankle capsule from the tibia and talus by sharp dissection (Figs 1,2).

Approaches to the medial malleolus

This approach is used mainly for open reduction and internal fixation of fractures of the medial malleolus. The malleolus may be approached either anteromedially or posteromedially. The choice of approach depends on the anatomy of the fracture and the presence of any associated posteromedial tibial fragments. The anterior approach will usually suffice for simple medial malleolar fractures. It is inadequate if you need visualization of the posterior margin of the tibia.

With the patient supine on the operating table apply a tourniquet and make an incision over the medial malleolus. For an anterior exposure make a 10 cm longitudinal curved incision on the medial aspect of the ankle. Begin 5 cm above the malleolus over the middle of the subcutaneous surface of the tibia. Cross the anterior third of the medial malleolus and curve the incision forward to end some 5 cm anterior and distal to the malleolus.

For a posterior exposure make a 10 cm incision on the medial aspect of the ankle. Begin 5 cm above the ankle on the posterior border of the tibia and curve the incision downwards following the posterior border of the medial malleolus (Figs 3,4).

Mobilize the skin flaps as little as you need to ensure good visualization of the fracture site. Take care not to damage the saphenous vein, which runs anterior to the medial malleolus. Running with the vein is the saphenous nerve, division of which often leads to troublesome neuroma formation.

In cases of fracture, the remaining dissection is often already done for you. It is important to preserve as many of the soft tissue attachments as possible to avoid

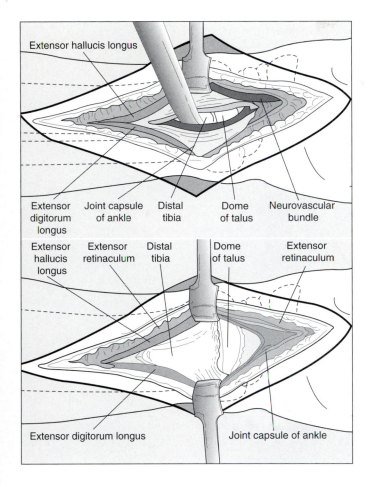

Figure 2

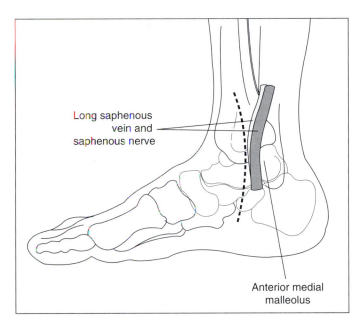

Figure 3

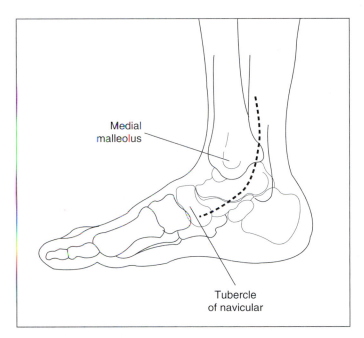

Figure 4

increasing the damage to the blood supply at the fracture site. Anteriorly make a small incision in the anterior capsule of the ankle joint so that the joint surface can be seen after the fracture is reduced (Fig. 5). Posteriorly incise the retinaculum behind the medial malleolus. Mobilize the tendon of tibialis posterior and retract it anteriorly. Staying in a periosteal plane, continue the dissection posteriorly to expose the posterior malleolus of the tibia (Fig. 6).

It is important to note that, although this approach will give good visualization of posteromedial fractures and allow their anatomical reduction, it is often not possible to insert lag screws through this approach. In these cases, you will need to use this approach to reduce the fracture and then insert appropriate lag screws from anterior to posterior using separate stab incisions on the anterior aspect of the ankle.

Medial approach to the ankle

The medial approach to the ankle involves an osteotomy of the medial malleolus. It permits excellent visualization of the dome of the talus and is useful for removal of loose bodies and excision of osteochondral fragments from the medial side of the talus. Arthroscopic surgery has made the use of this approach less important.

With the patient in the supine position apply a tourniquet and make a 10 cm longitudinal incision on the medial aspect of the ankle joint, centring it on the tip of the medial malleolus (Fig. 7). Mobilize the skin flaps

Figure 5

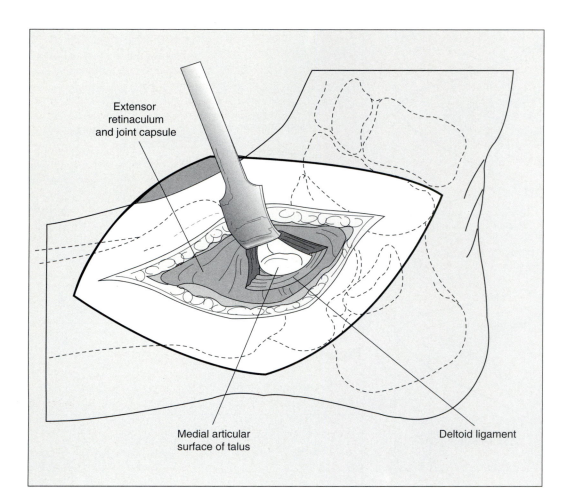

Extensor
retinaculum
and joint capsule

Medial articular
surface of talus

Deltoid ligament

Figure 6

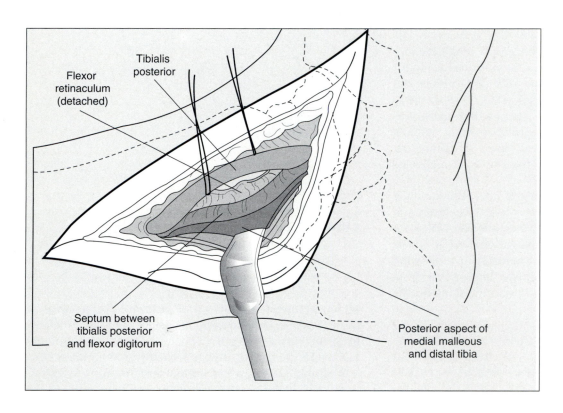

Tibialis
posterior

Flexor
retinaculum
(detached)

Septum between
tibialis posterior
and flexor digitorum

Posterior aspect of
medial malleous
and distal tibia

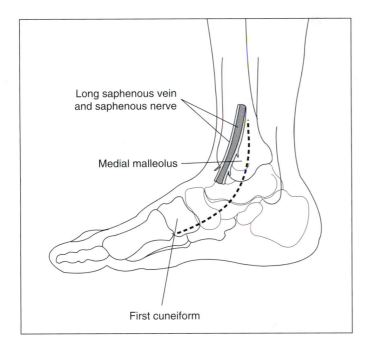

Long saphenous vein
and saphenous nerve

Medial malleolus

First cuneiform

Figure 7

carefully to expose the medial malleolus covered by soft tissue. Make a small longitudinal incision in the anterior aspect of the joint capsule to identify the point at which the medial malleolus joins the shaft of the tibia. Incise

the flexor retinaculum to expose the tendon of tibialis posterior and retract the tendon posteriorly. Score the bone longitudinally to ensure correct rotational alignment of the malleolus during its reattachment. Drill and tap the medial malleolus before osteotomizing it (Fig. 8). Using an oscillating saw, cut through the medial malleolus obliquely from top to bottom until you are almost at the joint surface. Complete the osteotomy by gently using an osteotome. Retract the medial malleolus downwards and evert the foot to bring the dome of the talus into view (Fig. 9).

The bone surfaces of the naturally occurring fracture interdigitate with each other, and this interdigitation prevents rotation between the two fragments when a screw is inserted and tightened. All bone osteotomies are however smooth. Therefore, the use of the single screw is inadequate to stabilize an osteotomy since when you tighten it up the fragments will rotate. Two screws, or a screw and a K wire, should be used to prevent this. Alternatively, tension band fixation may be used.

Posteromedial approach to the ankle

Although this approach can be used for access to the posterior malleolus of the joint in cases of fracture, it is most commonly used for exploring the soft tissues in

Figure 8

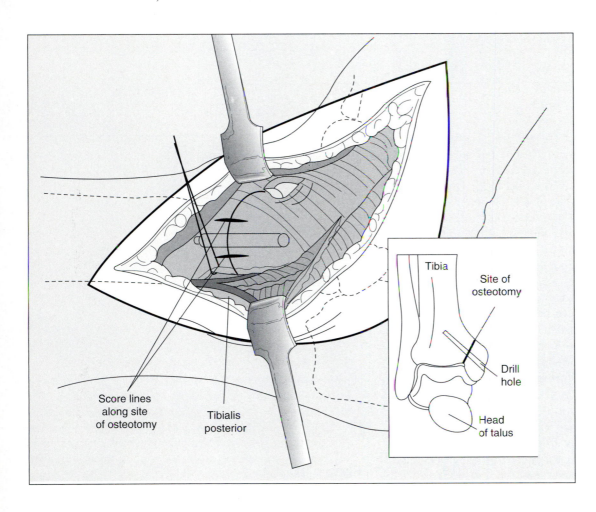

Score lines
along site
of osteotomy

Tibialis
posterior

Tibia

Site of
osteotomy

Drill
hole

Head
of talus

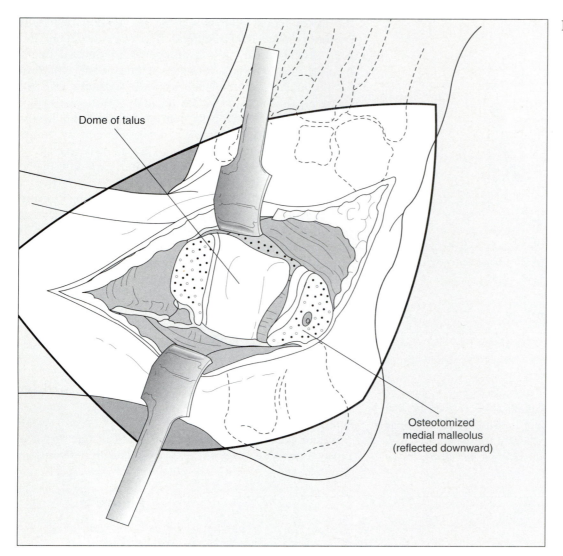

Figure 9

Dome of talus

Osteotomized
medial malleolus
(reflected downward)

this area. It is often used in soft tissue correction of clubfoot, and it can be extended onto the medial aspect of the hind foot for soft tissue correction of joints.

With the patient supine on the operating table, flex the hip and knee and place the lateral side of the affected ankle on the anterior surface of the opposite knee. Apply a tourniquet and make a 10 cm longitudinal incision midway between the medial malleolus and the Achilles tendon (Fig. 10). Make the incision deeper through subcutaneous fat, entering a plane between the Achilles tendon posteriorly and the flexor hallucis longus anteriorly.

Next identify the tendon of flexor hallucis longus. This is easily recognized because it is the only tendon with muscle fibres inserting into it at this level. Continue the dissection anteriorly towards the back of the medial malleolus identifying and preserving the neurovascular bundles and identifying the tendon of flexor digitorum longus and tibialis posterior (Fig. 11). Note that in infants the tibial nerve is the same size as, if not larger than, the tendons of tibialis posterior and flexor digitorum longus. It can be mistaken for these structures because it looks so surprisingly large.

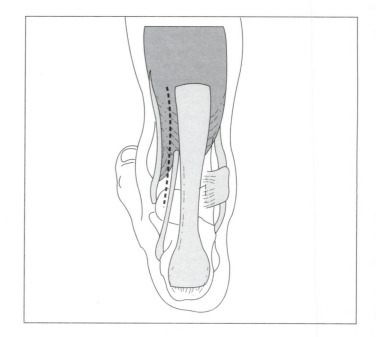

Figure 10

Figure 11

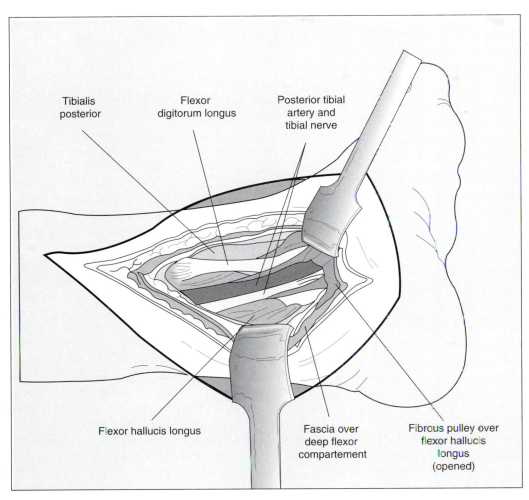

Tibialis posterior

Flexor digitorum longus

Posterior tibial artery and tibial nerve

Flexor hallucis longus

Fascia over deep flexor compartement

Fibrous pulley over flexor hallucis longus (opened)

Figure 12

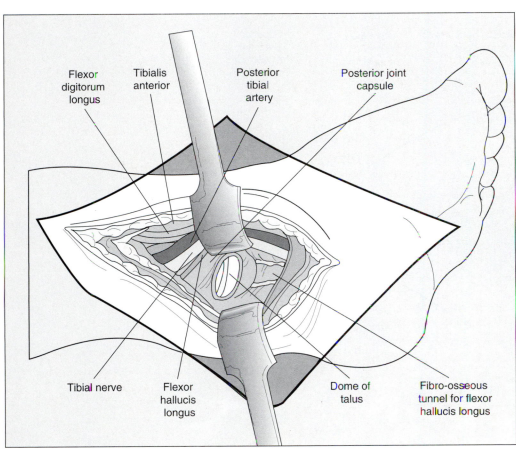

Flexor digitorum longus

Tibialis anterior

Posterior tibial artery

Posterior joint capsule

Tibial nerve

Flexor hallucis longus

Dome of talus

Fibro-osseous tunnel for flexor hallucis longus

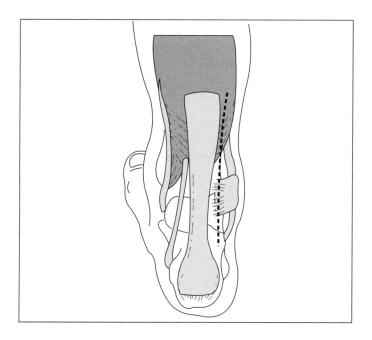

Figure 13

To enter the ankle joint in fracture surgery, develop a plane between the lateral border of the flexor hallucis longus and the peroneal tendons, which lie just lateral to flexor hallucis longus. By retracting the tendon of flexor hallucis longus medially you will expose the posterior capsule of the ankle joint (Fig. 12).

Posterolateral approach to the ankle

This approach gives unrivalled exposure to the posterolateral aspect of the tibia as well as the posterior aspect of the fibula. It allows accurate reduction of fractures in this area and also permits internal fixation. The major drawback of this approach is however that, because the patient is prone, approaches to the medial malleolus cannot be carried out without changing the position of the patient on the table during the operation.

With the patient prone on the operating table apply a tourniquet and make a 10 cm longitudinal incision halfway between the posterior border of the lateral malleolus and the lateral border of the Achilles tendon (Fig. 13). Identify the short saphenous vein on the posterior aspect of the lateral malleolus. Preserve the vein and its associated sural nerve. Incise the deep fascia of the leg in line with the skin incision. Incise the peroneal retinaculum to expose the tendons of peroneus brevis and peroneus longus, and retract the muscles laterally and anteriorly to expose the tendon of flexor hallucis longus (Fig. 14). Next, retract the flexor hallucis longus

Figure 14

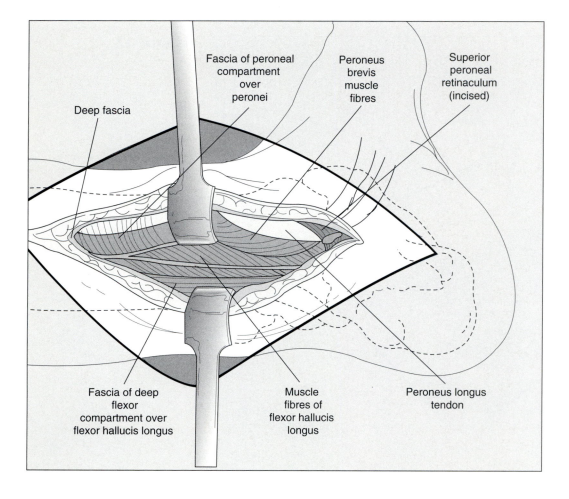

Deep fascia

Fascia of peroneal compartment over peronei

Peroneus brevis muscle fibres

Superior peroneal retinaculum (incised)

Fascia of deep flexor compartment over flexor hallucis longus

Muscle fibres of flexor hallucis longus

Peroneus longus tendon

tendon medially, incising some of the lateral muscular fibres arising from the tendon to allow you to mobilize the tendon more easily. The periosteum over the posterior aspect of the tibia is now exposed (Fig. 15). In cases of fracture, the remaining dissection will have already been done for you. In cases without a fracture, follow the posterior aspect of the tibia inferiorly and incise the posterior ankle joint capsule transversely (Fig. 16).

Approaches to the hindpart of the foot

Anterolateral approach to the ankle and hindpart of the foot

This is the 'workhorse' approach to the hindpart of the foot. It allows exposure of the ankle joint, talonavicular, calcaneocuboid and talocalcaneal joint. The approach is most commonly used for triple arthrodesis and it is also invaluable in the treatment of talar dislocation by open reduction.

Place the patient supine on the operating table. Place a large sandbag underneath the affected buttock to rotate the leg internally. Place a rest against the opposite iliac crest and tilt the table away from you to increase further the internal rotation of the leg.

Apply a tourniquet and make a 15 cm curved incision on the anterolateral aspect of the ankle. Begin some 5 cm proximal to the ankle joint, just in front of the anterior border of the fibula. Curve the incision downwards, staying just anterior to the border of the fibula, and continue on to the lateral aspect of the foot, ending over the base of the fourth metatarsal. Incise the fascia in line with the skin incision, taking care to preserve any dorsal cutaneous branches of the superficial peroneal nerve you may come across. Divide the superior and inferior extensor retinacula to expose the tendons of the extensor digitorum longus and peroneus tertius (Fig. 17).

Identify the extensor digitorum brevis muscle and detach it at its origin from the calcaneus by sharp dissection. Reflect the extensor digitorum brevis distally

Figure 15

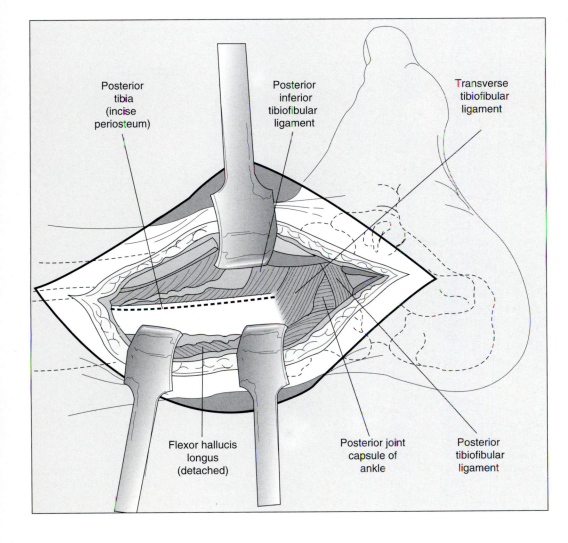

Figure 16

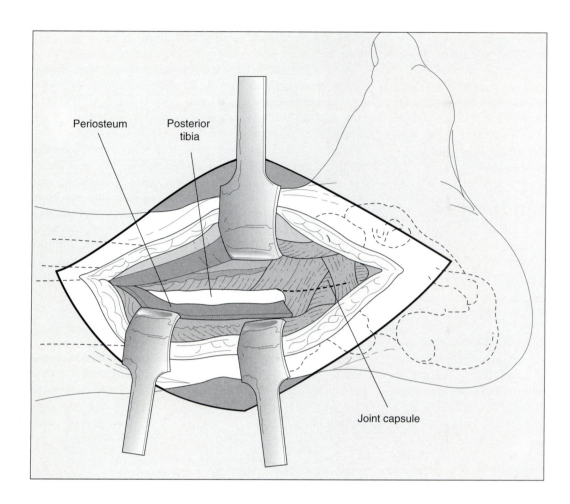

Periosteum   Posterior
               tibia

Joint capsule

Figure 17

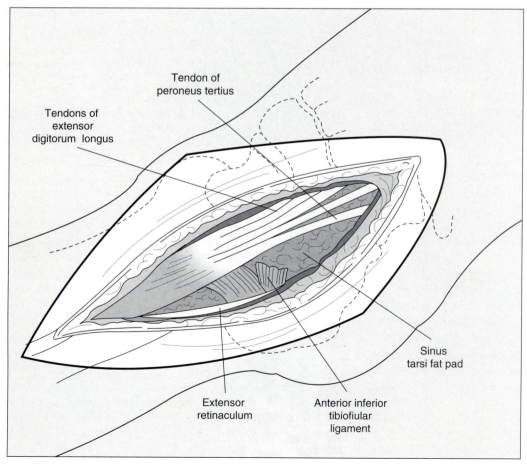

Tendon of
peroneus tertius

Tendons of
extensor
digitorum longus

Sinus
tarsi fat pad

Extensor
retinaculum

Anterior inferior
tibiofiular
ligament

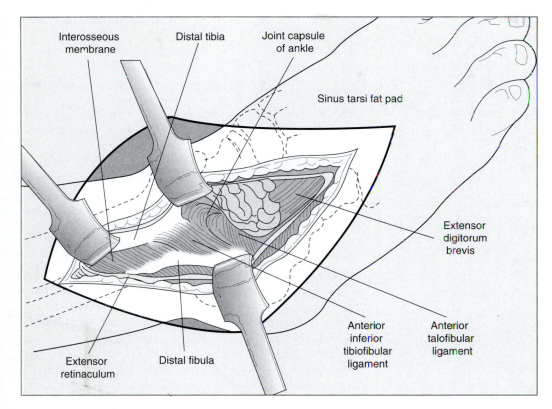

Figure 18

Interosseous membrane

Distal tibia

Joint capsule of ankle

Sinus tarsi fat pad

Extensor digitorum brevis

Anterior inferior tibiofibular ligament

Anterior talofibular ligament

Distal fibula

Extensor retinaculum

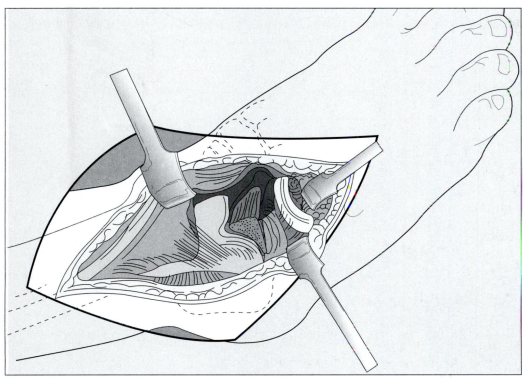

Figure 19

and medially. Try to lift the single flap that consists of extensor digitorum brevis, fascia, fat and skin. Trying to dissect out these layers separately leads to haematoma formation and also devitalizes the overlying skin. You should now be able to see the dorsal capsules of the calcaneocuboid and talonavicular joints (Fig. 18).

Mobilize the fat pad in the sinus tarsi, turning it downwards. Try to preserve this fat pad if possible to aid wound healing and reduce cosmetic deformity. Incise the dorsal capsules of the exposed joints and, by forcibly flexing and inverting the foot, open these joints up (Fig. 19).

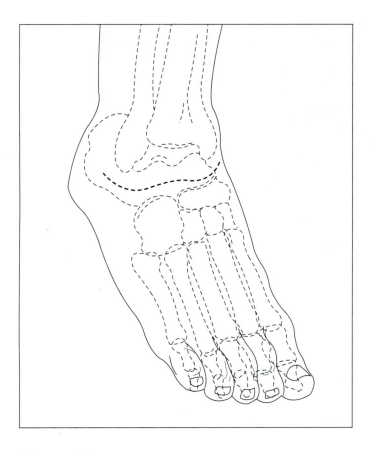

Figure 20

Lateral approach to the hindpart of the foot

The lateral approach provides exposure of the talo-calcaneonavicular, posterior talocalcaneal and calcaneo-cuboid joints. It does not allow access to the ankle joint, unlike the anterolateral approach. Its most common use is in triple arthrodesis.

With the patient in the supine position and a sandbag placed under the affected buttock, place a rest against the opposite iliac crest and tilt the table away from you. Apply a tourniquet and make a curved incision, starting distal to the distal end of the lateral malleolus, and curve it gently along the lateral side of the hind part of the foot to end over the talocalcaneonavicular joint (Fig. 20). Deepen the dissection in the line of the skin incision, ligating any veins that cross the operative field. Open the deep fascia and retract the tendons of peroneus tertius and extensor digitorum longus medially.

Next identify the fat pad lying in the sinus tarsi and partially detach it, leaving it attached to the skin flap. This will expose the origin of the extensor digitorum brevis muscle, which is next detached from its underlying bone using sharp dissection. The dorsal capsule of the talocalcaneonavicular and the dorsal capsule of the calcaneocuboid joint are now exposed (Fig. 21). Incise these capsules and forcibly invert the foot to expose the joints (Fig. 22).

Figure 21

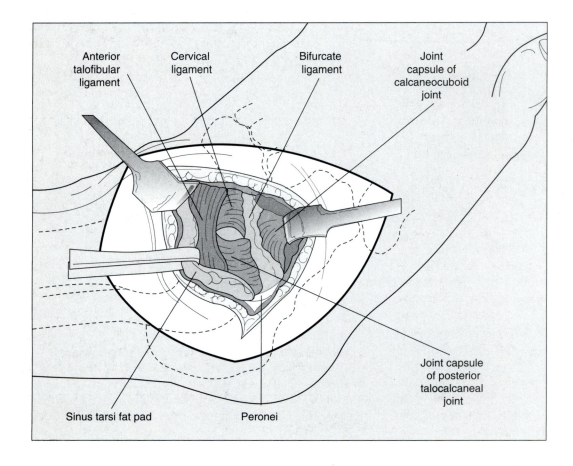

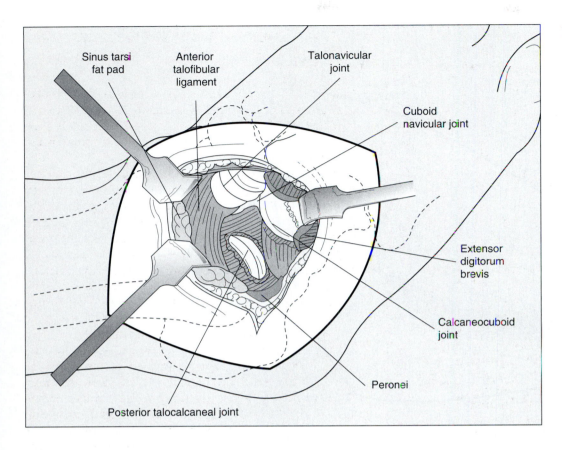

Figure 22

Lateral approach to the posterior talocalcaneal joint

This approach was classically used for the isolated fusion of the talocalcaneal joint. It is now most commonly used for the surgical approach to the calcaneus in cases of fracture where treatment by open reduction and internal fixation is becoming more accepted and widely practised.

With the patient in the supine position on the operating table, place a sandbag under the buttock of the affected side to internally rotate the limb. Then further internally rotate the limb by tilting the table away from you. Place a rest against the opposite iliac crest. Apply a tourniquet and make a curved incision some 15 cm long on the lateral aspect of the ankle. Begin 5 cm above the tip of the lateral malleolus overlying the posterior border of the fibula. Follow the posterior border of the fibula down to the tip of the lateral malleolus and then curve the incision forward to cross the peroneal tubercle. Deepen the approach in the line of the skin incision and incise the deep fascia to uncover the peroneal tendons. Take care not to damage the sural nerve, which runs with the short saphenous vein just behind the lateral malleolus. Incise the peroneal retinacula to mobilize the peroneal tendons and then retract these tendons anteriorly over the distal end of the fibula. It is important for peroneal function that the tendons be replaced in their grooves and that the retinacula be repaired during closure.

The lateral aspect of the calcaneus is now exposed. The joint is difficult to identify. Incise the periosteum overlying the os calcis and by subperiosteal dissection identify and then open the lateral aspect of the joint. In cases of fracture, this dissection will have already been done for you (Figs 23,24,25).

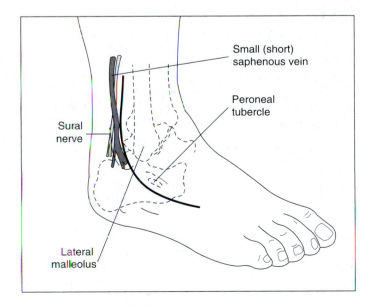

Figure 23

Figure 24

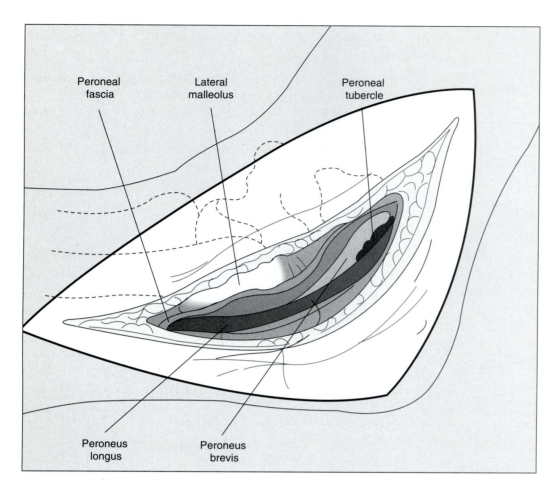

Peroneal
fascia

Lateral
malleolus

Peroneal
tubercle

Peroneus
longus

Peroneus
brevis

Figure 25

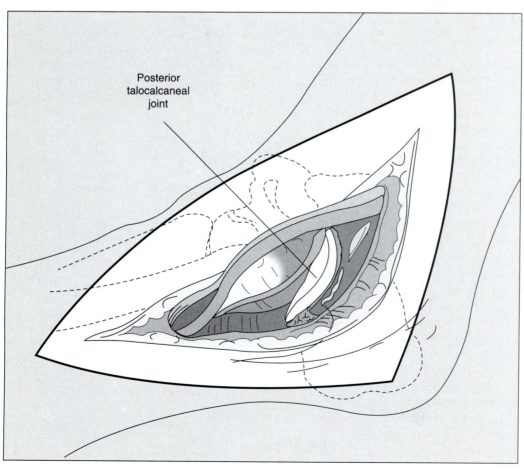

Posterior
talocalcaneal
joint

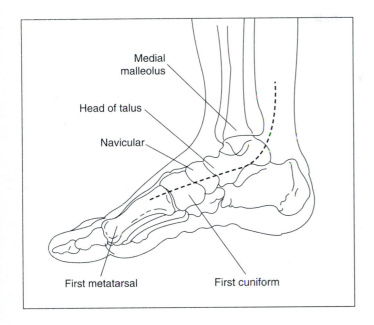

Medial
malleolus

Head of talus

Navicular

First metatarsal

First cuniform

Figure 26

Medial approach to the hindpart of the foot

The medial approach is commonly used for soft tissue release, either of joint capsules or of the tendons of

tibialis anterior and peroneus longus. The approach is also useful for open reduction and internal fixation of os calcis fractures, and it can also be used for subtalar arthrodesis where skin conditions or previous sepsis make a lateral approach undesirable.

With the patient supine on the operating table, apply a tourniquet and make a longitudinal incision extending from just behind the medial malleolus to cross the head of the talus, the navicular, the first cuneiform and the base of first metatarsal (Fig. 26). Deepen the skin incision and incise the deep fascia in its line. Do not mobilize skin flaps widely and take care to preserve as many branches of the cutaneous nerves as possible. The insertion of tibialis anterior, the joint capsules of the talonavicular, the navicular medial cuneiform and the first metatarsocuneiform joint are not exposed and can be excised to suit the surgery (Fig. 27).

Surgical exposure of the toes

Dorsal and dorsomedial approaches to the metatarsophalangeal joint of the great toe

This approach is probably the commonest approach used in foot surgery. The approach is suitable for first

Figure 27

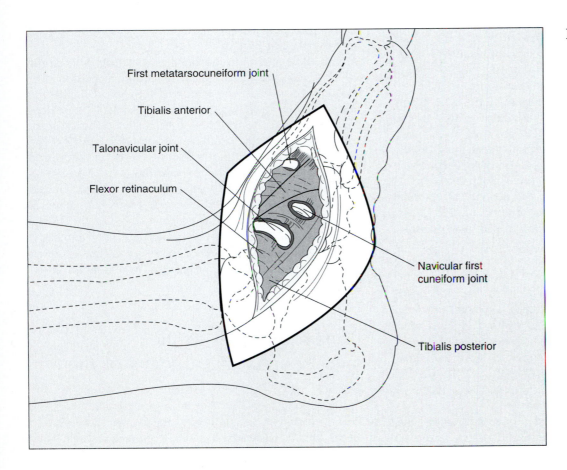

First metatarsocuneiform joint

Tibialis anterior

Talonavicular joint

Flexor retinaculum

Navicular first cuneiform joint

Tibialis posterior

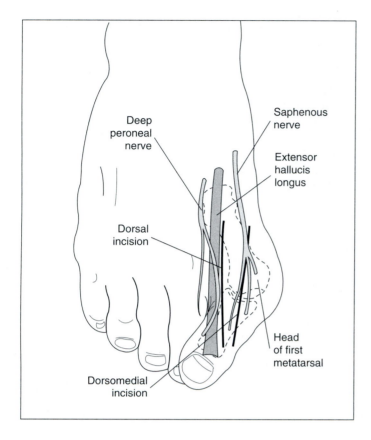

Deep
peroneal
nerve

Saphenous
nerve

Extensor
hallucis
longus

Dorsal
incision

Head
of first
metatarsal

Dorsomedial
incision

Figure 28

performed on the proximal phalanx, it should be noted that the tendon of flexor hallucis longus is bound in a fibro-osseous tunnel on the plantar surface of the proximal phalanx. If that bone is to be divided, care must be taken that the underlying tendon is not damaged.

Although subperiosteal dissection protects soft tissue from damage, it must be noted that this dissection interferes with the blood supply to the bone. Extensive soft tissue stripping of the first metatarsal combined with a first metatarsal osteotomy can render the metatarsal head avascular, and subperiosteal stripping of that bone should be limited to what is required for adequate safe exposure.

Dorsal approach to the metatarsophalangeal and proximal interphalangeal joints of the second, third, fourth and fifth toes

This commonly used approach exposes the metatarsophalangeal and proximal interphalangeal joints whilst avoiding the creation of a scar in the weight bearing area. It is of use in the correction of fixed flexion deformities of the proximal interphalangeal joint and is also useful in excisional surgery of the proximal end of the proximal phalanx. If the metatarsophalangeal joint of the affected toe is dislocated dorsally then the proximal phalanx will be easily accessible. The metatarsal head will not, however, be accessible unless the proximal end of the proximal phalanx is excised, because it is lying underneath that part of the bone.

With the patient supine on the operating table apply a tourniquet and make a 2 cm longitudinal incision over the dorsal aspect of the joint to be exposed. Incise the deep fascia in the line of the skin incision. If the extensor tendon is to be lengthened then divide the extensor tendon to allow this – otherwise retract it laterally. The dorsal aspect of the joint capsule is now exposed and is incised longitudinally to expose the joint (Figs 29,30).

For isolated exposure to the proximal interphalangeal joints in cases of fixed flexion, a transverse elliptical incision excising the pathological skin over the dorsal aspect of the joint is to be preferred. This transverse ellipse will still give excellent exposure of the interphalangeal joint but cannot of course be extended either proximally or distally.

metatarsal osteotomy, soft tissue correction of hallux valgus, arthrodesis of the metatarsophalangeal joint, insertion of joint implants, dorsal wedge osteotomy of the proximal phalanx and resectional arthroplasties.

With the patient supine on the operating table, apply a tourniquet and make a dorsomedial skin incision overlying the metatarsophalangeal joint of the hallux. Begin just proximal to the interphalangeal joint on the dorsomedial aspect of the great toe and curve the incision over the dorsomedial aspect of the metatarsophalangeal joint, remaining well medial to the tendon of extensor hallus longus. The dorsal digital branch of the medial cutaneous nerve should lie lateral to this skin incision, but it may appear on the lateral edge of the wound. Take care to look for this nerve and if seen to preserve it. More dorsally based incisions endanger the nerve.

Incise the deep fascia in the line of the incision down to the bone of the first metatarsal and the proximal phalanx. Retract the tendon of extensor hallucis longus laterally. The type of incision into the joint capsule will depend on the surgical procedure to be undertaken. Longitudinal incision will usually suffice, but distally based flaps have been described for certain soft tissue corrections (Fig. 28).

The most important superficial structure in this approach is the cutaneous nerve. If surgery is to be

Plantar approach to the metatarsophalangeal joints of the toes

This approach is only indicated for excisional surgery to all the metatarsal heads. Its use is confined to those cases

Figure 29

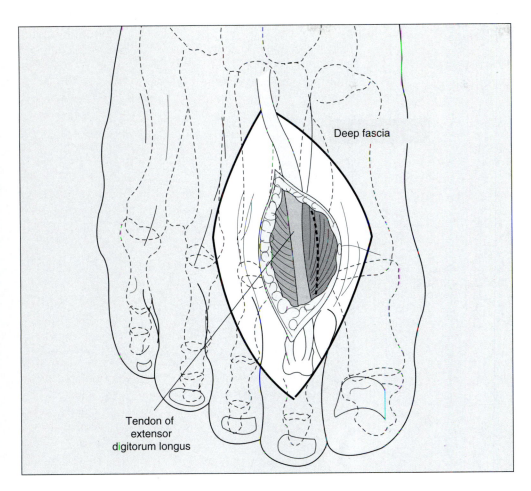

Deep fascia

Tendon of
extensor
digitorum longus

Figure 30

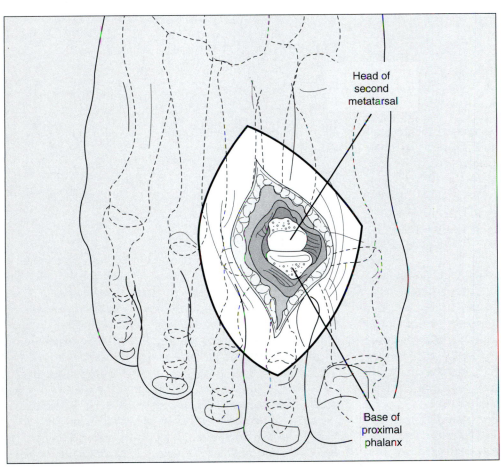

Head of
second
metatarsal

Base of
proximal
phalanx

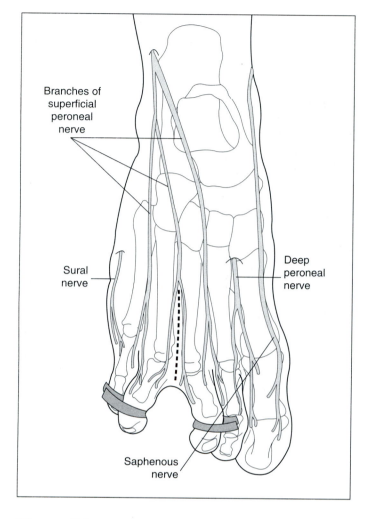

Figure 31

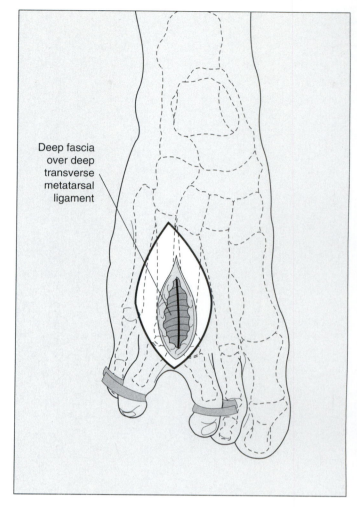

Figure 32

where there is dislocation of the metatarsophalangeal joints of the second, third, fourth and fifth toes such that the metatarsal heads lie underneath the proximal phalanges of these toes. In these cases, the plantar skin overlying the metatarsal heads is pathological, usually with callosities, and the excision of this skin, which is allowed in this approach, is desirable for surgical correction of the forefoot deformity. This condition is seen most commonly in rheumatoid arthritis.

With the patient lying supine, identify the prominent metatarsal heads by palpation. Apply a tourniquet and excise a transverse ellipse of skin overlying the metatarsal heads. Excision of this ellipse of skin usually reveals the prominent metatarsal heads. In these cases, the neurovascular bundles lie more dorsally than in the nondislocated state. Approach each metatarsal head individually by incising directly onto the neck of the bone and placing bone levers around it. Next, excise each metatarsal head so as to produce a smooth arch of remaining metatarsals. Take care to keep the dissection that involves excision of the metatarsal heads in a strictly

subperiosteal plane in order to avoid damage to the neurovascular bundles.

Approaches to the dorsal web spaces

This approach is most commonly used for exploration of the dorsal web spaces. Commonly used for the excision of an interdigital neuroma in Morton's metatarsalgia, the approach can also be used for drainage of sepsis. Dissection of the first web space can be used for division of the adductor hallucis tendon and also the exposure of the sesamoid bones at the base of the hallux.

With the patient supine on the operating table, apply a tourniquet and move separately the two toes of the affected web space. This can easily be done by wrapping a swab around the toes or using a wide band (Fig. 31). Make a dorsal longitudinal incision over the centre of the web space extending some 3 cm onto the dorsum of the foot. Deepen the approach in the line of the skin incision to divide the deep transverse metatarsal ligament. This ligament may be an important factor in the genesis of the pathology of Morton's metatarsalgia (Fig. 32). Division of the deep transverse metatarsal ligament will allow exposure of the neurovascular bundle. Digital pressure on the plantar surface of the affected interspace usually moves the neuroma into the operative field.

Plantar approach for excision of digital neuroma

The plantar approach for a digital neuroma gives excellent exposure of the common plantar digital nerve. The approach can be extended proximally to expose more of the nerve. Its major disadvantages are that it creates a plantar scar, and that healing times are often longer than for dorsal approaches.

Place the patient supine on the operating table. Exsanguinate the limb and apply a tourniquet. Make a 4–5 cm longitudinal incision on the plantar aspect of the sole of the foot overlying the interspace that is to be explored. Deepen the approach in the line of the skin incision and identify the flexor tendons running to the two affected toes. Between the flexor tendons you should find the common plantar digital nerve running with its artery. Trace the nerve from proximal to distal identifying its bifurcation. Proximal section of the nerve should be proximal to the metatarsal heads. Excision of a neuroma should always be confirmed histologically.

This approach is a local approach to the digital nerves and should not be extended proximally or distally.

VII.2 Principles of Patient Care
Basil Helal

The importance of general patient care and management is not always sufficiently appreciated. Often too much emphasis is laid on the surgery, which is but an incident in the overall management. A holistic approach is important. There are stages in such an approach to foot surgery which make general medical training mandatory. The overall care is divided into four stages: pre-operative management, intra-operative management, post-operative management and rehabilitation.

Pre-operative management

History
Careful history taking cannot be over-emphasized. Allow patients to tell you in their own words the complaints and the sequence of events that have led them to you. Only then should you probe with leading questions on the sequence of events that have produced symptoms. In soccer, American football and rugby players, footedness may be important.

You should enquire into the patient's general health and ask about the presence of allergies (especially to anaesthetic drugs, analgesics and antibiotics). A drug history must be taken – this is especially important in the case of patients on steroids, which may be taken for a large variety of reasons and which will need to be boosted to protect against the stress of surgical trauma; similarly, non-steroidal antiinflammatory drugs and their effects should be determined.

A past history is taken of serious illness or operations or accidents, and a family history must be recorded. An enquiry should be made for diabetes and bleeding diatheses. A social history is taken, this should include the patient's work circumstances, sports and hobbies.

See also Chapter II.1.

General examination
This should include a thorough systemic examination and an assessment of the more proximal portions of the limb.

Local examination
Examine the local state of the circulation and the skin and its appendages, including skin elasticity, scars, and callosities. The absence of hair may indicate a poor circulation. Note deformities, alignment and then the active and passive mobility of joints. The patient should be seen walking or running if necessary. The state of the footwear, especially the pattern of wear on the sole of the shoe and warping of the uppers will provide clues to clinical stresses.

Special investigations
Urine analysis, routine chest X-ray and ECG are done when necessary, and they are done routinely in the elderly. Blood screening – including screening for those conditions that put the surgeon and the ward and theatre staff at risk, such as hepatitis and HIV states – is mandatory. In certain ethnic groups, conditions such as sickle cell disease should be tested for. X-ray, CT screening, MRI, technetium and gallium scans, gait analysis, and pedobarography all have their indications.

Admission to a peri-operative ward is advantageous, as nursing care is more concentrated than in a large ward, though less so than in an intensive care ward.

A final assessment is made before surgery and before the patient has any premedication. Here the part to be operated is marked and symbols are used to describe what is to be done; these are written on the limb with marker ink, away from incision site to avoid tattooing in the incision.

In theatre

The patient's identity and the site of surgery is checked. When necessary, a prophylactic antibiotic is given with the premedication and before a tourniquet is applied. Care is taken in exsanguinating the limb before the pneumatic tourniquet is inflated. The author's preference is to use a torus exsanguinator, as it is kind to even the most fragile rheumatoid skin (Fig. 1).

The position of the foot is important for comfortable access – the position depends on the surgical approach. It is sometimes useful to have the foot plantargrade and to be able to load the limb in ankle and hindfoot surgery (Fig. 2). Occlusive adhesive dressings must be used with care, especially on rheumatoid skin, which can be avulsed with removal of the dressing.

Incisions should generally follow Lange's lines and allow for extensile exposure. They should be either straight or zig-zagged to avoid crossing flexion creases. Undermining should be avoided. During closure, any dead space should be obliterated.

Intraoperative wound lavage removes debris and bacteria and reduces infection. Keep the tissues from

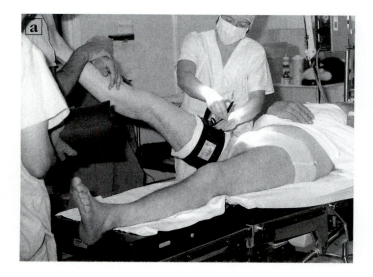

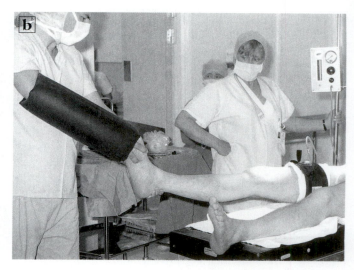

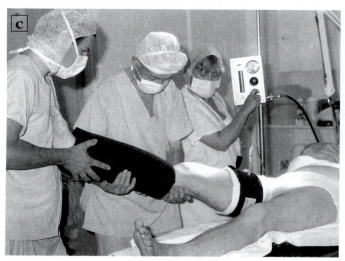

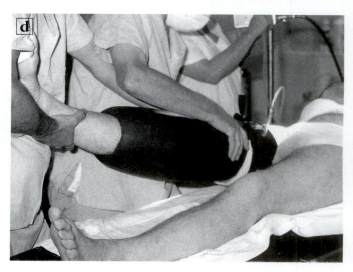

Figure 1

(a–d) Method of application of the torus exsanguinator

overdrying using normal saline. Find the correct tissue planes and stay in them, avoiding damage to vessels and nerves. Always handle tissues delicately and take the pressure off self-retaining or hand held retractors from time to time to avoid compression and tissue damage.

Close the fascial layers over drainage first, ensuring meticulous haemostasis. Suture the skin with minimum trauma and without tension. Elevate and apply compression bandaging to reduce venous congestion and to stop postoperative ooze, oedema, and swelling.

Check that the tourniquets have been removed, especially ring tourniquets applied for toe surgery. Around the nail bed take care to avoid any damage. Reapply an avulsed nail as a template or use an artificial nail to guide nail growth and prevent deformity to the new nail.

During surgery, precautions aimed at avoiding venous stasis, such as elasticated stocking or a calf or foot pump, are useful. Always avoid undue pressure on the skin as

this can cause postoperative subcutaneous fat and skin necrosis.

Bandaging
Even pressure is very important. Bandaging should be started distally and move proximally. Alignment of toes by crepe bandaging can be well tolerated. Even pressure should be applied and the bandaging correcting any malalignment. A useful device for keeping the bandage neatly in place is an elasticated netting support (Fig. 3).

Postoperative management

Check the state of the circulation and assess sensation. Postoperative instructions to the ward staff and physiotherapists should be recorded in the patient's notes. The

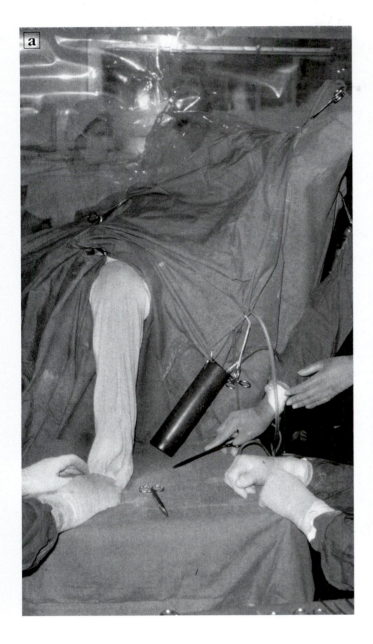

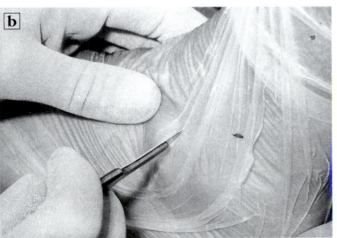

Figure 2

(a,b) The plantargrade position for foot surgery can be helpful in alignment of ankle and subtalar joints

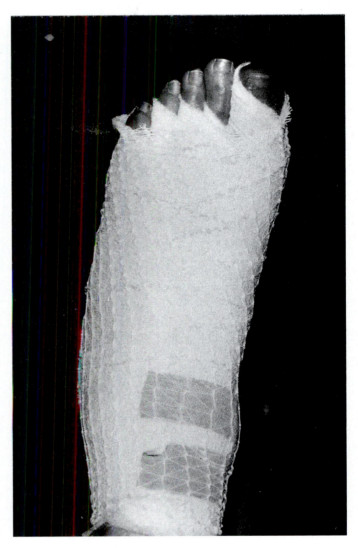

Figure 3

Careful bandaging will encourage correct alignment and an elasticated netting support will prevent displacement and rucking of the bandage.

operator should dictate or write an account of the procedure himself, and sign it. Dressings should not be allowed to become moist through to the surface, as this would allow easy passage of bacterial infection.

Plaster casts – half casts or split plasters – should be the rule until postoperative oedema subsides, when a definitive cast can be applied.

Rehabilitation

Joint mobility should be maintained if possible, as long as there is no risk of displacement or dehiscence of any repair, and no risk of malalignment of bone or dislocation of joint.

Dependency of a limb for long periods, such as occurs when sitting in a chair, should be avoided. Muscle wasting can be prevented by isometric, isotonoic exercise or by electrical stimulation. As soon as feasible, the joints should be moved and muscles exercised.

After removal of casts, the part should be protected from swelling by elasticated bandages or supports, and elevation and exercise should be encouraged. Shoes that can be adjusted to accommodate dressings and swelling are worn.

Shoes will help to remould the foot. Women's feet can be weaned into shape by the usual elegant, narrow women's footwear, and female patients can be encouraged to start wearing them for short periods when they get up in the morning, as the foot is least swollen then. The time periods that these shoes are worn can be gradually extended. If high heels are worn, the heel platform within the shoe should be horizontal to the ground to prevent the foot sliding forwards in the shoe and so displacing weight onto the toes and metatarsals.

VII.3 Casting and Splintage

Jeffrey Hallett

Two important principles of casting and splintage must be stressed:

- The surgeon is as responsible for the cast or bandage as he or she is for the rest of the surgical procedure
- Do not allow good surgery to be spoilt by poor bandaging and casting technique

The lesson that as much or even more care is needed in application of bandages and casts at the end of an operation as in the more obviously surgical parts of the procedure comes as a surprise to many trainees. The lesson usually has to be re-emphasized during a surgical career as the opportunity to delegate grows with experience and authority. Theatre staff must also understand this and be encouraged to provide the exact materials required and to maintain the plaster trolley with the same care as other theatre equipment. The understandable temptation to rush the application of bandages and casts to make time for the coffee break or the next case must also be resisted, especially when trainees feel sensitive about the time they take for operations. Even our anaesthetic colleagues may appreciate an explanation that the patient should stay asleep and relaxed until the plaster has set and will not be damaged by any postoperative restlessness.

The small size of many of the structures involved in foot surgery means that the fixation that can be achieved by sutures or internal fixation is relatively weak. In some circumstances (e.g. Wilson's metatarsal osteotomy) there is no attempt at internal fixation. This is why external support from bandages and casts is so important in protecting and maintaining the surgical correction until healing has taken place.

Before starting to apply a cast several questions will have had to be considered and decided.

Will the cast be applied before or after release of the tourniquet, if one has been used?

If the tourniquet is released well before wound closure and good surgical haemostasis is obtained there is usually no problem. If release is after closure but before plastering there is often messy bleeding from the unsupported wound through the dressings during application. The blood-soaked padding may become stiff and adherent as well as smelly. When the cast is applied before release of the tourniquet some extra allowance must be made to accommodate swelling from bleeding by using extra padding, a backslab principle or a split cast.

Will the cast be expected to support weight-bearing, or only rested on the ground (when not elevated as it should be most of the time)?

Not only will a weight-bearing cast need to be much stronger but its shape and edges will need close attention to avoid pressure problems and chaffing. Synthetic materials may be needed which are lighter and stronger but are less forgiving in application and for adjustment.

Will the patient be likely to go out of doors in the cast or is he or she likely to stay inside?

Even a non-weight-bearing cast may need to be water resistant if it will be rested on wet ground, grass etc. A weatherproof overshoe instead of a synthetic cast may provide a relatively easy solution.

Does the patient have a dog at home?

Many patients report that their pet dogs take a great interest in foot wounds, so it may be prudent to ensure that the cast can protect against the occasional lick or even some chewing!

Who is going to need to remove the cast?

The tools needed to remove a fibreglass-based cast are usually available only in hospitals and a few private consulting rooms. It is therefore not sensible to apply a synthetic cast or even a strong unsplit plaster of Paris cast if the general practitioner will be removing sutures. A backslab or a fully split cast may be the most suitable.

Is it certain that adhesive strapping has not been used to hold a dressing on the wound pending application of the final cast?

Even so-called hypoallergenic adhesive tapes can cause very unpleasant maceration of the skin when covered by full casts, and they should be avoided. Dressings can be held in place by non-elasticated stockinette rolled carefully over the foot, or by a short burst of plastic dressing spray under the corners of the dressing. The author has not encountered any skin problems using this method.

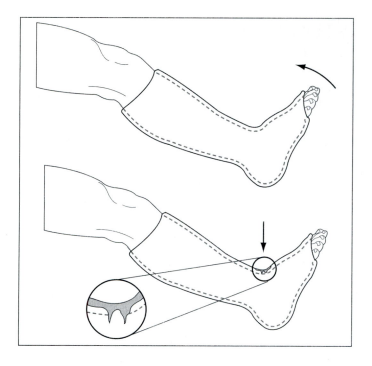

Figure 1

Internal ridges in the cast caused by late correction of incorrect equinus position of the foot

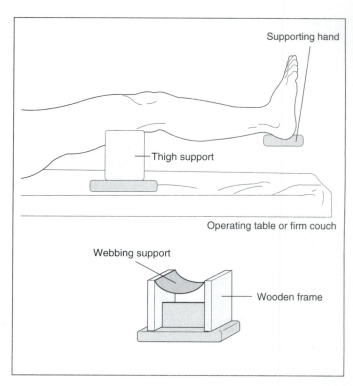

Figure 2

Position for casting with thigh or knee properly supported

Have the ends of the toes been left unobscured by dressings so that circulation can be assessed in the recovery period?

If the toes are stained with a coloured skin disinfectant it may be best to clean it off with spirit before applying the cast so that the circulation checks that are needed following both tourniquet use and application of a cast are made as easy as possible.

What position does the surgeon want the cast to maintain?

It is important that the foot is placed in the desired position and held steady before bandages and any cast are applied. If the position is allowed to alter during the casting process and then corrected once the bandage, padding and cast are in place, there is likely to be creasing of the casting material (Fig. 1) which will cause internal ridges and subsequent pressure sores. Some trainees are disconcerted when the author looks as closely at the image of the plaster cast on post operative radiographs as he does at the operative bony correction!

What position of the patient will make the application of the cast easiest?

In most cases the supine position is suitable but there must be a support to place under the knee or lower thigh (Fig. 2). This will take most of the weight of the leg and enable the surgeon to concentrate on supporting the foot

and ankle in the desired position. There are suitable supports of wood and webbing, or of shaped semi-rigid plastic foam. These supports must be available in the emergency theatres as well as for routine cases.

Where surgery has been carried out at the back of the foot and ankle it may be best to lie the patient prone (with the agreement of the anaesthetist) and cast the foot and ankle with the knee flexed to a comfortable position. Dressings can be applied more easily and the position carefully checked.

What is the preferred material for the cast?

The choice between plaster of Paris and a synthetic cast has been mentioned in terms of strength and water resistance. Fibreglass-based casts tend to have much rougher and sharper edges and this is made worse by trimming, because it exposes more glass fibres. Plaster of Paris can be made very smooth and is also easier to bend and trim at the edges, especially around toes.

Non-glass-based synthetic casts are now available, often using polypropylene for the strong flexible bandage that is coated with water-activated polyurethane resin. These produce a cast that is not quite so strong as fibreglass but that is less harsh at the edges. Thermoplastics in sheet or mesh form are usually too fiddly to be used for immediate postoperative casts.

An important property of plaster of Paris is its extreme mouldability and lack of any tendency to spring back to a cylindrical or flat shape when setting. A combination

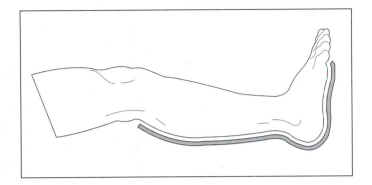

Figure 3

Unsatisfactory 'single strip' backslab

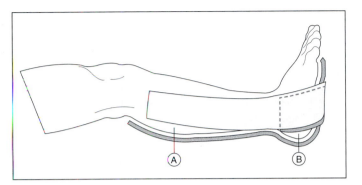

Figure 4

Backslab with side reinforcing slabs (note that gaps at A and B have been left for clarity of illustration; in practice the slabs overlap to give even support)

of materials is sometimes sensible so that accurate moulding and support is provided by the plaster of Paris, and once set this can be covered by tough, rapidly hardening fibreglass to form a weather- and patient-proof cast.

Is everything ready to hand that will be needed for the cast?

This is a basic principle of good casting technique but it can be easily overlooked. A glance at the plaster trolley will reassure the surgeon about most items but he or she will also need to ensure that the assistant will not be called away half way through. The presence of a bucket of water is equally obvious but it is the author's practice always to check the water temperature as this can have such a great effect on the way that casting materials handle and set. Theatre staff will have ensured that proper protection has been provided for the theatre floor, the patient, and perhaps the surgeon, if messy casting materials are being used.

Casts and accessories most commonly used after foot surgery

Below-knee backslab

This is one of the most important casts in orthopaedic and trauma surgery but it is often one of the worst applied. Too many people simply apply a strip of plaster down the back of the leg, ankle and foot as suggested by the name (Fig. 3). This type of backslab is a very weak structure and often fails in plantar flexion before the patient reaches the recovery room. A much stronger cast with ample provision for swelling is formed using reinforcing side strips as well as the original back strip (Fig. 4). If applied rapidly and then bandaged neatly, considerable moulding is possible while final setting

occurs. The cast resembles a shaped trough and is much more resistant to drooping into plantar flexion even before final setting.

Full below-knee cast

This will be used where the surgeon requires all-encompassing support for the foot and ankle, maintaining them in specific positions. It should not be used where considerable swelling is anticipated. Consideration should be given to the choice between stopping the cast at the bases of the toes, providing a toe platform, or even enclosing all but the tips of the toes. If the cast is to be weight bearing, a walking surface will be needed. A toe platform may be indicated if toe protection is needed or if it is not desirable for the toes to be flexed (e.g. after repair of extensor tendons). Rockers fixed to the bottom of the cast are now used less often as they are difficult to apply well, easily cause bad twisting gait patterns and are so high that the other shoe may have to be raised. They also have to go to bed with the patient, causing soiling or even tearing of bedclothes! A well-designed overshoe, strapped firmly to a strong level cast, is usually the most convenient and socially acceptable for the patient.

Split below-knee cast

A full cast, split immediately after application, is used when a combination of good support and an accommodation to swelling is needed. It is important to ensure that all potentially constricting materials are divided right down to skin level along the full length of the cast. Any deviation from this principle must be clearly recorded, preferably on the cast itself. This should prevent an incompletely split cast giving a false sense of safety. It is usually better to cut out a narrow strip of casting material completely rather than simply making a single incision in the cast. Whether this is done by plaster knife, saw or shears must depend on the skill of the operator and the equipment available.

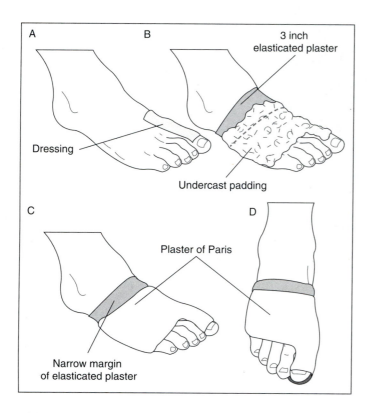

Figure 5

Application of a forefoot cast

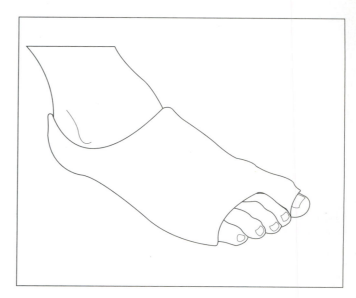

Figure 6

Slipper cast

This type of cast is not suitable for weight bearing and should be repaired or overbandaged as soon as the risk of swelling has passed.

Forefoot cast

This is a cast that is very useful for all first metatarsal osteotomies and metatarsophalangeal fusions. It extends only from toes to midfoot (Fig. 5). It provides adequate stabilization while causing very little constriction and allowing the patient to heel-walk, perhaps with a felt pad under the heel to compensate for the thickness of cast under the forefoot. It is prevented from falling off partly by the widening shape of the forefoot, partly by careful dorsal–plantar moulding of the cast, and partly by a layer of adhesive strapping under its proximal quarter. For a first metatarsal osteotomy, where some abduction is wanted, the cast can encircle the big toe. For a first metatarsophalangeal fusion there is no abduction so there is insufficient room to encircle the toe, and a side trough must be used instead. Plaster of Paris is used for the first cast but a synthetic material is used for the new cast at 2 weeks when sutures are removed. It is important that a thick layer of wide adhesive strapping is used and the casting material is well rubbed into it. If applied in strong ankle dorsiflexion there will not be chaffing from the edge of the cast at the front of the ankle (which is not included in the cast) when the ankle is subsequently in resting or functional positions. (The

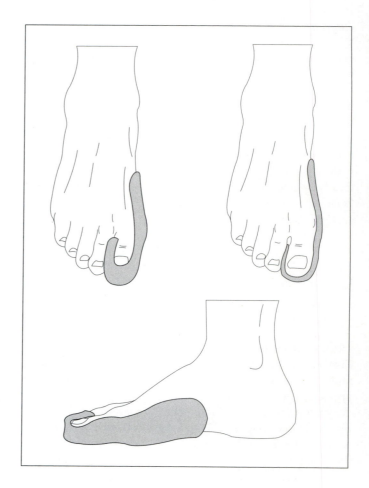

Figure 7

'J' slab for big toe

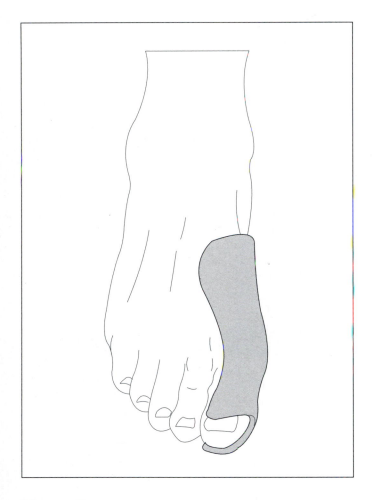

Figure 8

Side gutter toe slab

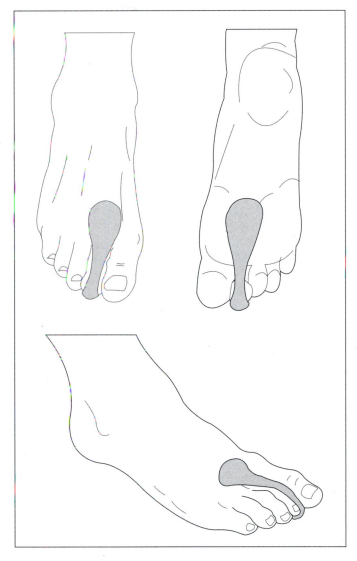

Figure 9

Protective toe loop

edge of the cast will have been pushed away from the front of the ankle while the cast is setting.)

Slipper cast

This cast is popular with many surgeons but it is difficult to apply well. Most of the difficulties arise at the heel and Achilles tendon. Good padding is needed, as is care to trim it below the tendon so that it cannot cause blisters or even tendinitis (Fig. 6). As with other casts where exact shaping of edges is needed, the surgeon will have to choose between trying to apply the material exactly in the hoped-for final position, or plastering beyond the level and then trimming back with a plaster knife as it sets. The latter probably gives better results but needs a good knife and a practised hand.

Bootee cast

This is really a cut-down below-knee cast giving less ankle stabilization. The benefits are doubtful as the upper edge is prone to dig in when the patient moves. A longer cast needs less edge pressure on the skin to resist a given angular deformity.

'J' slabs and gutter slabs

When relatively light support of the big toe is needed, a simple plaster slab along the medial border of the foot may be appropriate. This can be applied as a J-shaped slab (Fig. 7) applied medially and going around the end of the toe, or as a gutter (Fig. 8) applied to cover the plantar, medial and dorsal surfaces of the first ray. The latter leaves the tip of big toe open for regular inspection of circulation and sensation. These slabs are held in place by bandages.

Protective toe loops

It may be appropriate to protect one or more of the lesser toes from direct knocks or twists. Sometimes a K wire has been left protruding from the end of the toe and this needs to be protected. A loop of plaster of Paris can be fashioned in such a way that it is attached to the plantar and dorsal surfaces of the bandage or cast over a fairly wide base, and pinched in to make a narrow loop that stands away from the end of the toe and protects it (Fig. 9). A pencil or small finger held inside the loop as it sets is one way to form the shape of the loop without resting on the end of the toe or wire.

Equinus casts

These may be needed to protect repairs of Achilles tendon. Too much padding may make them liable to fall off, and much more stress than usual may be placed on the forefoot part of the cast if any weight bearing occurs, or even if the cast is rested down. If appreciable weight bearing is to be allowed it will be necessary to attach a Bohler iron to the cast so that weight is transmitted down the normal centre of gravity axis just in front of the ankle. Bohler irons are no longer readily available and may have to be made in a hospital workshop. The shoe for the opposite foot will need to be raised so that the patient walks level. Equinus casts can be applied with the patient in either supine or prone positions.

Cast brace for ankle surgery

Where controlled flexion and extension is desired while providing firm valgus–varus support, a cast brace with heel cup and ankle hinges can be used. A well-shaped and closely fitting gaiter cast is applied to the leg, and a plastic heel cup with hinges at ankle level is attached once the gaiter cast has set. Modern hinges allow the heel cup to be removed or bent back to allow cleaning of the foot. The hinges can also be set to permit specified ranges of movement which can be changed as recovery progresses.

Casting children's feet

Young children's feet pose special problems because they are small, because they have a relatively large amount of soft mobile soft tissue, and because the children may not have the ability or inclination to cooperate with instructions, both when casting and when the cast is in use. Thought also needs to be given to their tendency to poke things down inside the cast and to get them wet.

Most surgeons will have had the embarrassing experience of a mother returning with a child who has wriggled out of a cast very soon after application. Sufficient padding must be applied to protect the skin but too much will make the cast very likely to slip off the foot. If great care is taken, hypoallergenic adhesive felt may be used to protect bony prominences and the tibial crest. This will also help the cast stay in place. Tincture of benzoin has been recommended to hold padding on the skin but the possibility of an allergic skin reaction must be considered. It may be advisable

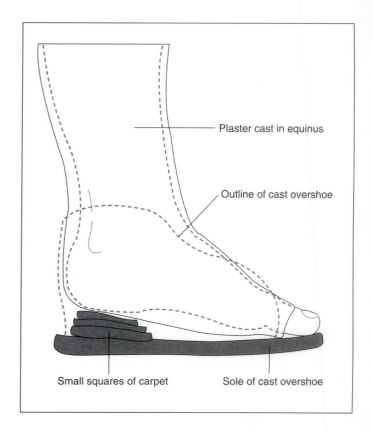

Figure 10

Small squares of carpet placed inside a cast overshoe to compensate for a small amount of equinus of the cast position

to extend the cast above the moderately flexed knee simply to stop it being kicked off. The choice of materials is especially important for children. Plaster of Paris remains unsurpassed as the best material for close and comfortable moulding onto the foot and ankle. The addition of covering layers of fibreglass or other synthetic casting materials gives both rapid and lasting strength as well as a reasonable degree of water resistance.

Cast overshoes

The design and the fitting of overshoes are both of equal importance. It is essential that the overshoe attaches in a stable manner to the cast. The types resembling sandals seem to work best. They should have a firm sole with a good non-slip tread, enough side canvas or rubber moulding to locate around the edges of the cast, and a system of easily adjustable straps to fasten the whole structure in such a way that it does not slip about on the cast. The straps work best if they loop through a 'D' ring before fastening back on themselves with Velcro fabric. This gives a 2:1 purchase and enables the strap to be fastened tightly even with one hand. The shape of the sole is a matter of personal preference but a plain flat shape seems the most adaptable and natural. If the actual cast has been applied with a little equinus at the ankle, as is sometimes inevitable, the effect of a raised heel can be produced by inserting layers of carpet or felt below the heel of the cast inside the overshoe (Fig 10). This allows a normal walking pattern rather than tiptoe to be used, and it is both more stable and more comfortable.

It should be remembered that cast overshoes are often excellent for covering bulky foot bandages so that the patient can walk and be protected from wet and muddy conditions. They are much safer and more comfortable than using plastic bags or disposable theatre shoe covers.

Gait training

Patients who are allowed to take partial or full weight on their foot after surgery sometimes adopt the most bizarre gait patterns because of the awkwardness of dressings and casts. The advantages of proper cast shoes have been mentioned but many patients will also benefit from instruction by a physiotherapist in how to achieve correct gait and how to use properly adjusted sticks or crutches.

Care of the cast and observation of the foot after application of a cast

After operating on the foot, the surgeon will nearly always specify elevation of the foot to minimize swelling and pain. This is even more important when a cast has been applied. Elevation may be achieved by the use of pillows, a frame with slings, and elevation of the foot of the bed.

A newly applied cast must be allowed to dry thoroughly and as evenly as possible. Bedclothes should usually be drawn back to allow free circulation of air. Direct heat should be avoided. Although a waterproof sheet may be needed to protect underlying pillows from moisture, an absorbent layer such as a towel which can be changed frequently, should be placed between the cast and the waterproof sheet. This will avoid the cast resting in a puddle of condensed water from the cast. Nursing staff and the patient should be given the usual warnings to report pain and to observe for signs of constriction and circulatory or other problems.

The duration for which the cast is needed will depend on the type of surgery performed but many casts will be needed for 6 weeks and some for 3 months. The patient will have plenty of time to discover whether this important aspect of patient care has been given the care it warrants and will have formed an early impression of the overall management of his or her condition and the prospects of a good result.

VII.4   Plastic Surgery

Douglas H Harrison and Nicholas Parkhouse

Principles of skin replacement and soft tissue reconstruction of the foot

The principle aim of reconstruction of the foot is to provide stable skin and soft tissue which is capable of bearing weight and withstanding shear stresses. Sommerlad & McGrowther (1978) showed that patients who had had plantar reconstruction tended to avoid bearing weight on the reconstructed residual areas and took pressure instead through areas of undamaged plantar skin where sensation was intact.

Recent endeavour in the field of plastic surgery of the foot has been directed at replacing damaged weight bearing sole skin with skin from non-weight-bearing areas and preserving the cutaneous sensation. The primary area of concern is the heel, where 80% of the body weight is borne on standing, the remaining 20% being taken along the lateral side of the foot and across the metatarsal heads.

An advantage of replacing 'like with like' relates to the subcutaneous structure of sole skin. Fibrous septa attaching the skin to the deep longitudinal ligament break up the intervening fat into compartments; this arrangement prevents shear and provides the feeling of stability. Where the subcutaneous architecture is lost, as occurs in extensive abdominal flap replacements, the patient will comment on the 'feeling of walking on a bar of soap'.

Sole skin naturally forms a thick layer of keratin to protect the basement cells from damage. In people accustomed to not wearing shoes this layer is thicker than in the habitually shod. The keratin layer may become pathologically exuberant where an incision is made into the sole skin or at the interface between a flap or skin graft. Unfortunately, this hyperkeratosis does not improve with time and requires repeated paring to control discomfort.

Clearly, the sole skin is of primary significance in respect of the fact that unsatisfactory replacement can precipitate amputation but the skin of the dorsum of the foot and over the Achilles tendon are also important. The skin over the dorsum is thin and freely mobile but when the toes are plantarflexed the skin becomes taut, so that functionally there is little to spare. In major skin loss of the dorsum, particularly in burns or abrasion injuries, inadequate skin replacement and secondary scar contracture causes hyperextension of the toes at the metatarsophalangeal joints and dorsal subluxation of the phalanges. Providing that the paratenon is intact, skin grafts may prove sufficient to resurface the dorsum. Skin grafts, however, do tend to contract and, although they are an easily available source of skin in quantity, they do not always provide good quality cover. The skin grafts tend to adhere to underlying structures and are therefore liable to break down. Stabilization and mobility do occur with time, but dermal overgrafting, as recommended by Hynes (1957), may prove necessary.

The Achilles tendon area is liable to skin loss by serious abrasion injury or pressure, or iatrogenically as a result of surgical repair of a ruptured Achilles tendon. Skin grafts do not take well over the Achilles tendon, particularly if this structure has been damaged. Flap cover is not easily available locally and may indeed be rendered impossible by previous incisions in the area. Distant flaps may be essential, particularly when the Achilles tendon requires lengthening, as in equinus deformities. The disadvantage of most distant flaps in this site is their bulk, which makes the wearing of shoes difficult.

Causes of skin loss

The causes of skin loss are protean, but they do fall into several recognizable categories. The main congenital cause of skin loss is epidermolysis bullosa. Types of injuries that cause skin loss include lacerations and abrasions, burns, injuries in which the foot is run over, and undue pressure secondary to sensory loss. Iatrogenic procedures can also lead to skin loss: these causes include harvesting and microvascular flaps.

Vascular pathology can cause skin loss. These conditions can be divided into arterial disease, deep vein thrombosis, and emboli (meningococcal, septicaemic, or secondary to subacute bacterial endocarditis).

Conditions that require surgical excision will naturally cause skin loss. These include benign verruca and Dupuytren's disease, as well as the various malignant conditions that can affect the skin of the sole of the foot (e.g. melanoma and squamous cell carcinoma, as well as other rare tumours).

Standard methods of replacement

When the surgeon is faced with a problem of skin loss on the foot he must have in mind a number of methods available whereby the skin loss may be replaced. It may be that the first method chosen will fail and a secondary means will then prove necessary. In any method of

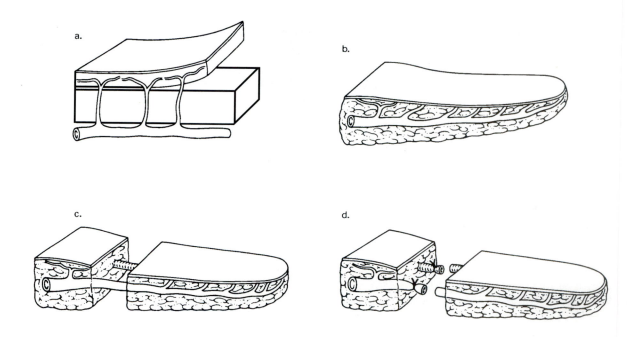

Figure 1

Vascular patterns of flaps in descending order, a = random, b = axial, c = island and d = free flaps

reconstruction, a period of at least 10 days is generally required before the patient is permitted dependency of the limb. This is to prevent disruption of new vascular connections by premature venous engorgement.

Sole of foot

Full-thickness skin grafts

Injuries in which skin has been clearly excised or in degloving injuries, where the proximal part of a distally based flap is not going to survive as determined either clinically or by fluorescein injection studies, there is a place for replacing the skin as a full-thickness graft. In order to achieve a successful outcome to this manoeuvre meticulous defatting of the skin must be carried out. The recipient bed on to which the graft is to be applied should be carefully cleaned and necrotic tissue removed, since survival of the graft will be hampered by infection or tissue breakdown beneath it. Examples of excellent takes of these full-thickness grafts have been reported and may be well worth the attempt. It must be accepted, however, that full-thickness grafts are prone to failure, particularly in circumstances in which the skin itself is damaged, as in degloving injury. The recipient area is usually the rather avascular longitudinal ligament, which forms the plane of shear and provides a poor bed for graft.

Split-thickness skin grafts

Providing that there is a vascularized bed, split-thickness skin grafts (SSG) should take without difficulty. They enable rapid re-epithelialization of the area of skin loss and protect underlying structures from further damage. Long-term cover by SSG is acceptable in non-weight-bearing areas such as the medial area of the sole, but is unlikely to withstand heavy duty wear on a weight bearing area. SSG, if used in such areas, should be considered as interim cover before proceeding to a more durable replacement. SSG do not have sufficient dermis to provide movement over the immobile recipient site. The dermis can be augmented by dermal overgrafting (Hynes 1957), which constitutes removal of the epidermal layer from the SSG and placement of a thick SSG on top; this process can be repeated. By this means, mobility of the epidermal layer can be achieved and the skin made more resilient to ulceration. If skin grafts are to be used on the sole, suitably adapted footwear will be required to protect the grafts from injury. Split thickness skin grafts are commonly used in conjunction with pedicled muscle flaps in foot reconstruction.

Flaps

Flaps constitute an area of skin and underlying fat with an intact vascular network sufficient to maintain their viability.

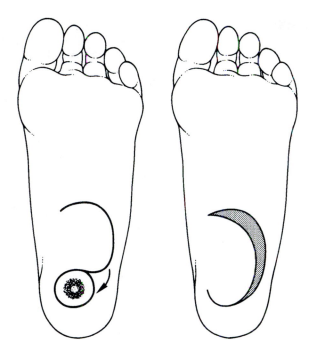

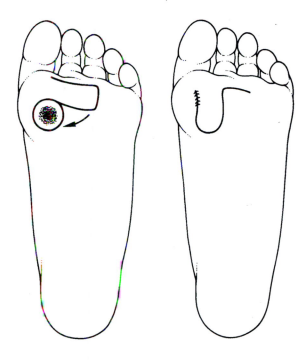

Figure 2

Medially based transposition flap to resurface a heel defect. Cross-hatched donor site is skin grafted

Figure 3

Transposition flap from distal sole to resurface an excised defect over the first metatarsal head

They may be divided into random and axial pattern types. Random pattern flaps have no specific vascular pedicle enclosed within them and are supplied by perforating vessels; in consequence they have constraints regarding length-to-breadth ratios. Axial pattern flaps are created around known vascular pedicles and, providing the pedicle is not damaged, their length may be unrelated to the breadth of the skin base. Free flaps are extensions of the axial pattern flaps whereby the whole flap may be disconnected from the donor site and placed into a recipient site with viability restored by microvascular anastomotic techniques (Fig. 1).

Flaps may be distant or local depending on the proximity of the donor site to the recipient site. They may be sensory or insensitive depending on the inclusion of a cutaneous nerve.

Local random pattern flaps

These flaps have been the mainstay of treatment for major skin loss in the weight bearing sole in past times and do have occasional application, but they have been largely superseded by one-stage reliable axial pattern flaps.

The most commonly employed are transposition flaps (Fig. 2), which require a skin graft to close the donor site and are usually medially based (Maisels 1961). Laterally based flaps do have the benefit of a donor site which can be placed in the non-weight-bearing medial

sole (Curtin 1977). For larger transposition flaps, a delay procedure is advisable to ensure survival of the terminal part of the flap, but this does make the flap more rigid.

Transposition flaps from the distal sole area (Fig. 3) are ideal for resurfacing excised plantar warts or callosities over the metatarsal heads. There is a relative redundancy of skin between the metatarsal heads and the proximal phalangeal crease; therefore a transversely orientated flap may be raised and transposed longitudinally into the defect over the head. The flap is reliable and may be carried out in one stage. Rotation flaps are relatively uncommon as it is unusual to close the donor site of the flap because of the inelastic quality of sole skin.

All transposition flaps of the foot are insensitive.

Axial pattern local flaps

These flaps are based on a known vascular pedicle. They are therefore more flexible than the previously described transposition flaps and are generally more reliable. They also have the advantage of incorporating a cutaneous sensation.

Filleted toes

The big toe (Kaplan 1969) or the second and third toes (Snyder & Edgerton 1965) may be filleted by removing the skeletal support, and the skin transferred to resurface

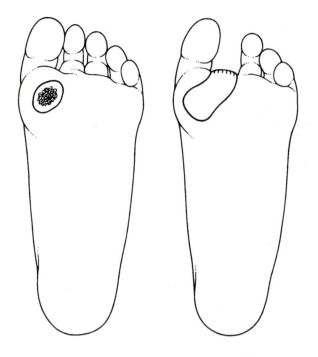

Figure 4
To resurface a more extensive defect over the first metatarsal head the second toe may be filleted to provide sensory skin cover

defects in the distal weight bearing sole or the heel area if required. The digital nerves to the toes are preserved and therefore perfect sensation is retained.

Filleted toes are safe and are used to resurface areas over the metatarsal heads. Here, it is unnecessary to divide the dorsal skin and the veins are therefore left intact. If a single toe, such as the second, is employed, a minimal cosmetic deformity is apparent (Fig. 4).

Filleted toes can be used to resurface the heel area; these are neurovascular island flaps, and detailed knowledge of the vascular pattern of the individual foot is required before proceeding.

The arterial supply to the toes on their plantar aspect is derived from three main sources: 81% of 361 feet dissected by Vann (1943) were found to have the deep plantar branch of the dorsalis pedis artery playing the major role in the formation of the plantar arterial arch. Except for the deep plantar branch of the dorsalis pedis, the plantar arterial circulation is formed by the lateral plantar branch of the posterior tibial artery. The medial plantar artery plays only a minor role. The deep arteries of the foot do have accompanying venae comitantes; thus, the medial and lateral plantar veins drain into the posterior tibial vein and so into the deep venous system.

Whereas there is no superficial arterial arch as in the hand, there is a superficial venous arch at the level of the metatarsal heads, which drains into the long saphenous vein.

The foot is extremely variable in its blood supply and this may be intensified by pre-existing vascular impairment. Arteriography is therefore virtually mandatory if a toe fillet is to be used to resurface a heel. Variations such as no medial plantar or dorsalis pedis artery, may occur, or alternatively the dorsalis pedis artery may be the only source of the plantar metatarsal arch. Both of these anatomical situations may render toe fillets difficult. Generally the lateral plantar artery (or medial plantar) is the desirable vessel on which to base the toe.

The surgery is carried out under tourniquet. The whole toe may be filleted or alternatively just the plantar aspects of the toes may be used, preserving the dorsal skin. The neurovascular pedicle is then dissected out as far as the proximal sole.

The area of skin available from one or more toes is not great and therefore the procedure has limitations in proximal sole resurfacing. It is probably the method of choice, however, in distal sole resurfacing where loss of a toe is of minimal functional importance. This method provides rapidly available sensory flap tissue.

Medial plantar island flap (instep island flap)
Shanahan & Gingras (1979) transposed a medial plantar sensory flap for coverage of heel defects. This flap was based on the medial plantar artery and the cutaneous nerves, but retained a skin bridge and because of a delay took two stages to reach the recipient site. As the flap was an axial pattern flap, based on the medial plantar artery, there was no advantage in the skin bridge and therefore the medial plantar island flap (Harrison & Morgan 1981) was described shortly afterwards. A flap measuring 10 cm by 7 cm may be taken from the medial plantar area of the foot without invading the weight bearing area (Fig. 5). A larger flap can be taken and will be supplied by the medial plantar artery but will then pass on to the weight bearing area. The flap is based on the medial plantar artery and the cutaneous nerves, and it may be raised as an island flap without a delay. This provides a large area of sole skin that is freely mobile on a neurovascular pedicle, retains normal sensation and is ideally suited for resurfacing the vital area of the heel.

Surgical anatomy
The nerve supply to the medial two-thirds of the sole of the foot comes from the cutaneous branches of the medial plantar nerve. The lateral one-third of the sole is supplied by the cutaneous branches from the lateral plantar nerve. These cutaneous branches emanate from the common digital branches of the plantar nerves, usually in fine fascicles piercing the plantar fascia. The neurovascular bundles pass along the intermuscular septum between the abductor hallucis and the flexor digitorum brevis on the medial side and between the flexor digitorum brevis and the abductor digiti minimi on the lateral side. It is thus unnecessary to raise the

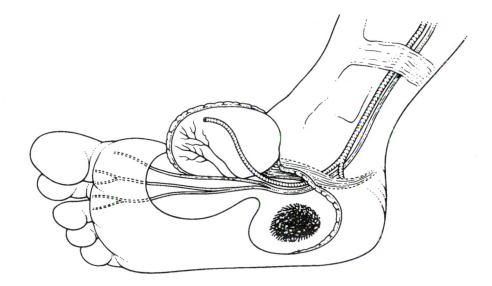

Figure 5

The medial plantar island flap elevated, based on the medial plantar artery and vena comitans and the cutaneous branches of the medial plantar nerves, prior to transfer

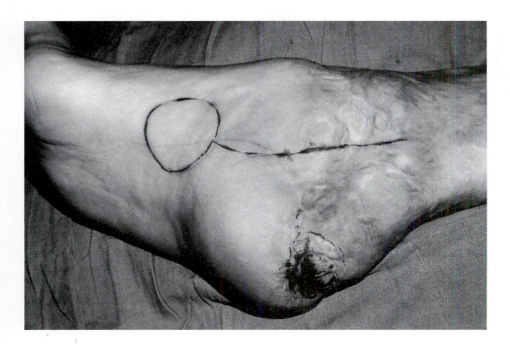

Figure 6

Medial plantar flap designed to reconstruct an area of unstable scarring on the heel. The proximal extension marks the line of the vascular pedicle

medial plantar flap with included muscle, as it is not myocutaneous but dependent on perforating vessels passing through the intermuscular septum. It is possible to raise the medial plantar flap either on the medial plantar neurovascular bundle or on the lateral plantar neurovascular bundle, but the former is easier, quicker and does not invade a weight-bearing surface (Fig. 6).

The flap is raised distally by marking out the area of skin required and then deepening the distal incision in the cleft between the abductor hallucis and the flexor digitorum brevis, where the medial plantar neurovascular bundle is easily found.

The vessels are divided – the plane of dissection is between the medial plantar vessels and the medial

plantar nerve. As the dissection proceeds proximally, great care must be taken to avoid damaging the cutaneous nerves which emanate from the medial plantar nerve. Magnification is certainly desirable for this procedure. As the cutaneous fascicles are defined they can be split off the medial plantar nerve by intraneural dissection to provide increased mobility of the flap. The medial plantar neurovascular bundle is traced as far as the lateral border of the abductor hallucis beneath which it passes. It is usually unnecessary to dissect proximal to the abductor hallucis as the pedicle thus formed is usually sufficient for transposition to the heel area.

Normal two-point discrimination of the heel skin is about 20 mm and therefore the sensitivity required for this area is not high. In the early postoperative period following transfer of the medial plantar flap, sensation is often quite poor and may well reflect neuropraxia of the fine cutaneous fascicles. Over the course of the succeeding few weeks the sensation recovers. In a series of 10 flaps, none has proceeded to ulceration and all have withstood normal weight bearing.

Morrison et al (1983) suggested that it would be desirable to resurface the whole calcaneal area as a unit rather than resurfacing only the ulcerated area, in order to avoid scars passing across the weight bearing sole. Hyperkeratosis along the suture lines can occur and is not easily treated. Unfortunately, this can occur in scars even along the lateral border of the foot, which is apparently non weight bearing, but may bear weight in certain phases of gait. The medial plantar flap may be used as a free vascularized transfer and the cutaneous nerves may also be repaired, providing a sensory free flap.

Innervated skin grafts to provide sensation to the reconstructed heel

In circumstances in which the calcaneal area has been resurfaced with a distant flap, sensation may remain poor over the weight bearing area, which therefore becomes susceptible to recurrent ulceration. Lister (1978) described a case in which a crossed thigh flap had been used to resurface skin loss over the calcaneum. Five months later the sural nerve on the same foot was blocked with local anaesthetic just above the ankle, delineating an area of sensory loss over the lateral aspect of the dorsum of the foot. At surgery the sural nerve was then dissected behind the lateral malleolus and traced along the lateral aspect of the foot. A full-thickness innervated skin graft was then raised from the lateral aspect of the dorsum of the foot. This skin graft based on the sural nerve was transposed to the central area of the flap overlying the calcaneum, and the donor site was skin grafted using a split-thickness graft. The innervated skin graft then took and provided sensation to this previously insensitive area.

Providing the surgical technique is meticulously carried out and a good take of the graft achieved, this is a useful method of introducing sensory tissue into the weight bearing area of an insensitive flap.

Distant flaps

Distant flaps are introduced into the recipient foot from an unconnected donor site. Again they may be divided into random pattern flaps or axial pattern flaps. Random pattern flaps as previously described are not based on a known vascular pedicle and depend for their blood supply on perforating vessels. They are in general less reliable than axial pattern flaps and, since the pedicle of such flaps is relatively short, the positioning and fixation between the recipient and donor sites are much more critical.

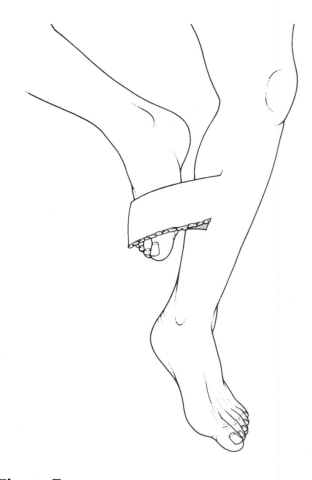

Figure 7

Medial calf cross leg flap inset into the dorsum of the foot

The art of raising these flaps, insetting them and achieving a satisfactory outcome requires a high degree of skill. They are mentioned here for two reasons – first historical and, second, because modern and sophisticated methods occasionally do go wrong and a secondary method may prove necessary.

Cross leg flaps

This group of flaps may be divided into three: the medial calf cross leg flap, the cross thigh flap, and the cross foot flap.

The medial calf cross leg flap

This flap was possibly the most commonly used flap for resurfacing the anterior part of the lower tibia before the advent of the axial pattern flap. It can be used for the heel area, but it is not ideally suited for this and is better used for resurfacing the dorsum of the foot when this is necessary (Fig. 7). The flap is based on the cutaneous markings of the long saphenous vein. The length-to-breadth ratio is important and the flap should not be raised longer than its width. The plane of elevation of the

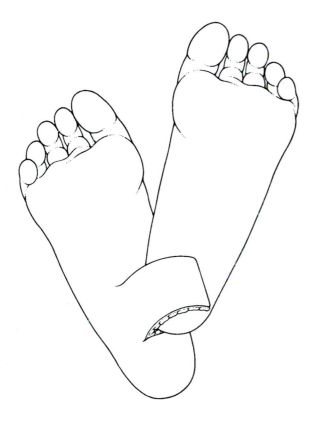

Figure 8

Cross foot flap inset into the heel of the recipient foot. The donor site is the medial plantar area which is non-weight-bearing

flap is immediately above the fascia. The flap can be raised deep to the fascia on the premise that this increases the viability, though it is doubtful that this is true, since the fascial vessels run longitudinally down the limb. If the fascia is included with the flap it is stiffer and less easy to inset; furthermore, skin grafts, which are required for the donor site of the flap, will then be placed directly on to the muscle, causing discomfort particularly in the early postoperative period.

Once the flap is raised, it is inset into the recipient area and must be retained in this position for some 3 weeks before division. Maintaining this often uncomfortable position for three weeks can be achieved in a number of different ways but perhaps the commonest are the use of heavily padded plaster of Paris or an adapted orthopaedic external fixation device. Whatever the method, considerable care has to be taken to avoid pressure sores on exposed bony points.

Cross thigh flap

The principle is similar to the previously described medial calf cross leg flap, but the cross thigh flap is more suitable for resurfacing the heel area because of the

direction of its raw surface. It is, however, acceptable only in patients with very flexible knees that can hold the position of 90° of knee flexion for three weeks, which is likely to be extremely uncomfortable, particularly in a rather stiff-jointed Caucasian. The more flexibly jointed Eastern races are at a distinct advantage if this flap is to be used. The flap is raised on a superiorly orientated base and again its length-to-breadth ratio should not exceed 1:1.

Preoperative planning is of considerable importance in the siting of the flap. The donor site is skin grafted and the recipient foot placed into association with the flap. Following insetting the flap, it is important to avoid pressure between the recipient foot and the underlying quadriceps muscle, otherwise the pressure of the foot itself can cause necrosis of the underlying muscle. The flap is divided at 3 weeks and then inset.

Cross foot flap

Mir y Mir (1954) described the transfer of a laterally based flap from the sole of the opposite foot. Its principle was to provide skin from the medial plantar area of the opposite foot to resurface the heel area of the recipient foot. A double pedicle flap was prepared from the non-weight-bearing part of the sole of the donor foot and a thick graft was applied immediately to the raw surface beneath it.

In the second stage, 2 weeks after the delay, the bridge flap on the medial side was detached and then inset into the recipient heel. The standard procedure was to place the sole of the donor foot against the inner side of the recipient foot and then place the flap into position (Fig. 8). A single plaster bandage is usually sufficient to secure absolute immobilization of the operative site. The flap was divided at 3 weeks.

The advantage of this flap was that it provided specially adapted sole skin to resurface the important heel area. The skin used from the medial plantar area does not interfere with the physiology of the donor foot. A modern adaptation of this flap is to carry out the surgery in one stage, dissecting out the cutaneous nerve supply to the medial plantar skin. The flap is then transferred to the recipient foot and the cutaneous nerves are sutured to suitable nerves in the recipient foot, thus restoring sensation to the flap in its new site.

Abdominal tube pedicles

The abdominal tube pedicle described by Gillies (1920) had been the mainstay of major reconstruction on the sole of the foot before the advent of the axial pattern flaps. It constitutes the use of two conjoined random pattern flaps of abdominal skin. The flap is usually designed 18 cm long and 9 cm in breadth. It is based over the groin area and the lateral flank. It has been appreciated in recent years that the survival of these flaps probably depends on incorporating the epigastric artery and vein inferiorly and the lateral branches of the intercostal vessels laterally. The flap requires delays and has to be taken down to the foot on a wrist carrier. On average the surgery takes some 5.8 months to achieve its termination and some five operations (Stranc et al 1975). The position required of the patient where the hand has to be in close association with the foot is again highly uncomfortable and usually is only tolerated by young people.

Axial pattern flaps

The distant axial pattern flaps which may be of value in resurfacing the foot form three categories: musculo-cutaneous, fascial, and free flaps (see Fig. 1).

Musculocutaneous flaps

The two musculocutaneous flaps that may be of partic-ular use in resurfacing parts of the foot are the medial gastrocnemius musculocutaneous flap (McCraw 1977) and the tensor fasciae latae flap (Nahai 1980). There are a number of areas on the body surface where the blood supply to the skin is largely from the perforating vessels from the underlying muscle. It is therefore possible to elevate skin and the underlying muscle as a unit and, providing the hilar vessels of the muscle are not divided, this unit may be transferred to another area and the skin expected to survive.

The medial gastrocnemius flap constitutes a musculo-cutaneous unit 10 cm broad and 23 cm long based on the medial gastrocnemius muscle of the contralateral calf. The muscle itself is 8 cm by 15 cm in size, so clearly the distal part of the cutaneous blood supply relies on a fascial plexus. The hilar vasculature to the muscle origi-nates close to its origin and therefore the flap is freely mobile. The distal end of the flap can be taken to within 8 cm of the medial malleolus. After inset of the flap to the recipient area on the damaged foot, it is left connected to the recipient area for 3 weeks before division. It is a highly reliable flap but because it contains muscle it is rather thick. Its further disadvan-tage is that it does cause an unsightly defect on the donor leg, and oedema of the ankle may be slow to settle. It is insensitive.

The dominant vascular pedicle of the tensor fasciae latae flap is the terminal branch of the lateral circumflex femoral artery and its vena comitans. The skin territory supplied by the tensor fasciae latae muscle is the skin overlying it and most of its tendon. The skin of the lateral thigh can therefore be raised with the tensor fasciae latae and its muscle included, and this provides a very safe flap for covering defects. To use the flap, much as with the random cross thigh flap, does require the patient to have flexible knees. The lateral cutaneous nerve of the thigh may be incorporated with the tensor fasciae latae flap and at the time of division of the pedicle the nerve may be further dissected proximally and then taken with the flap across to the recipient foot. If there is a suitable cutaneous nerve into which to inset

the divided distal part of the lateral cutaneous nerve, the flap may be rendered sensory.

Fasciocutaneous flaps

The fasciocutaneous flap includes skin, the subcutaneous fat and the deep fascia but not the muscle. The most useful of these flaps was described by Ponten in 1981 using skin on the medial side of the calf measuring some 18 cm in length by 8 cm broad. The vascular anatomy of the flap has been well described by Haertsch (1981a, b), who showed that there are axial vessels running just superficial to the deep fascia, forming a network to supply the overlying skin. The axial feeding vessel is the saphenous artery, which arises as a common trunk with the descending genicular vessel running deep to sarto-rius and entering the leg between the tendons of the sartorious and the gracilis muscle.

The flap is planned with the base sited proximally. The incision is carried through the skin, subcutaneous tissue and fascia, but the underlying muscle is left intact. Inclusion of the saphenous vein is important in order to provide good venous drainage. Although the free flap transfers are probably the treatment of choice for distant flap cover, the fasciocutaneous flap does have special advantages. The flap itself is easy to raise and it is safe (Barclay et al 1982). The pedicle may be long, and there-fore rigid plaster of Paris fixation between the donor and recipient site is probably not necessary. The flap is thin, which may not be so in free flap transfers. The time in hospital required for a fasciocutaneous flap differs only moderately from that for free flap transfer (Barclay et al 1983). The operating time is considerably shorter and the expertise required to raise the flap and inset it is much less than for a free flap transfer. These flaps are suitable for covering dorsal or plantar surfaces of the foot.

Free flap transfers

Free flaps constitute a flap of skin with fat and sometimes muscle based on a known artery, which is transferred from one part of the body to another and whose circulation re-established by the use of micro-vascular anastomotic techniques. A considerable number of these flaps have been described; perhaps the best known are the groin flap and the latissimus dorsi flap (O'Brien & Shanmugan 1973, Taylor & Daniel 1975, Serafin et al 1980). It would be a needless waste of space to describe every microvascular free flap that would be suitable for resurfacing the sole, heel, or dorsum of the foot. The surgeon has merely to consider the clinical problem and choose a suitable transfer. These techniques have revolutionized the ability with which flaps may be transferred to the foot. The surgery is time consuming but essentially the flap reaches its recipient area in one operation, dispensing with the previous 5–8 months (Stranc et al 1975) required by the tube pedicle. It is also more comfortable for the patient, since it avoids a lengthy period in a fixed position. Before a free flap transfer to the foot is done, an arteriogram is often valuable. As previously mentioned, the variation in anatomy of the foot can be marked and, although assessment with a Doppler ultrasound may well provide most of the information, errors can be made.

Every flap has advantages and disadvantages and these must be understood by the surgeon before embarking on the technique. When importing a flap to the foot it is desirable to have it fairly thin. This is particularly relevant on the dorsum and in the area over the Achilles tendon. If the flap introduced is too thick then thinning procedures may have to be carried out in order to enable the patient to wear shoes satisfactorily. On the sole of the foot the thickness is possibly of not quite so much importance. Conflicting arguments exist as to the importance of a thick flap on the sole. Excessive bulk may aggravate the effects of shear stress and be subjectively unstable. If, however, the flap is thin then it is possibly more vulnerable to ulceration, since pressure is not distributed evenly. A thick flap, such as the latissimus dorsi musculocutaneous free flap, certainly undergoes considerable muscular degeneration, but nevertheless does remain thick as a result of the subcutaneous bulk. Satisfactory cutaneous stability can be achieved with less bulk by applying split skin grafts to the muscle alone.

It is possible now to introduce sensation into the recipient area on the sole of the foot. The tensor fasciae latae flap previously described is suitable, since it has a reliable vascular pedicle and the lateral cutaneous nerve of the thigh supplies sensation to the cutaneous area. It is therefore possible to take the flap down to the sole of the foot and provide sensation to the skin by neurorrhaphy to either a divided cutaneous nerve present in the recipient area or to the medial or lateral plantar nerve according to availability. Morrison et al (1983) have extended the value of the medial plantar flap by elevating this flap from the contralateral foot on the medial plantar artery and its cutaneous nerves and transferring it to the heel area on the injured side. In some respects it has similarities to the crossed foot flap described by Mir y Mir (1954), but the procedure is carried out in one stage and restoring the continuity of the cutaneous nerve pathways should be of real benefit to the patient.

An additional possibility is the introduction of vascularized bone grafts (Fig. 9). In some severe injuries to the foot, continuity of the bony skeleton may be lost and the stability of the foot may be improved by restoring the lost bone. A deep circumflex iliac artery osteocutaneous flap is of particular value in this reconstruction (Taylor 1983). The bone is viable and will therefore withstand infection without being sequestrated, and because of its vascularization it does not have to be reconstituted by 'creeping substitution', since the osteocytes remain viable within the Haversian systems.

In circumstances in which there has been complete loss of tendon continuity on the dorsum of the foot, both of the long and short extensors, and there is foot drop,

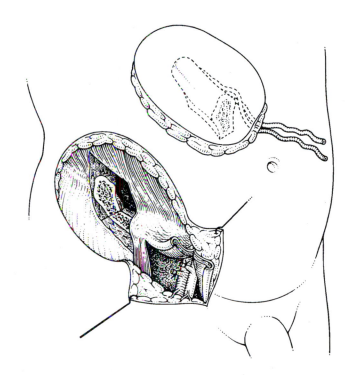

Figure 9
The deep circumflex iliac artery supplies the iliac crest and an area of overlying groin skin. An osteocutaneous flap based on this vessel may therefore be elevated

vascularized tendon grafts can be used. The simplest method of achieving this is the use of a radial artery free flap (Song et al 1982). Thin skin from the volar aspect of the forearm is provided, incorporating within the flap the flexor carpi radialis and also the palmaris longus. These tendons can be used to restore the continuity of the lost tendons. The surgery can then be carried out in one stage rather than two.

Plan of reconstruction for specific areas apart from the sole

Dorsum of the foot

The dorsum of the foot is not exposed to the same vertical loads and shear forces as the sole. In consequence, skin grafts are usually sufficiently stable. For the first 6 months after the skin has been applied, minor ulcerations will occur and require treatment, but after this time the skin graft becomes more mobile on the underlying structures and ulceration becomes less frequent. The area over the base of the first and second metatarsals receives most wear and is therefore more liable to ulceration. A dermal overgraft may be sufficient to correct this and avoid the need to proceed to flap cover. If the area suffers recurrent ulceration, flap cover may be required; this can be either a free microvascular transfer or a cross leg fasciocutaneous flap. The choice between these two will depend on the requirements of the recipient area, the desire of the patient and the technical skill of the surgeon. The decision to introduce a vascularized bone graft with the free flap or vascularized tendon grafts is more relevant in resurfacing the dorsum of the foot.

The Achilles tendon area

The skin overlying the Achilles tendon can be damaged directly by trauma; it can be necrosed by pressure exposing the Achilles tendon in the base of an ulcer; and it can be damaged iatrogenically in an attempt to repair the Achilles tendon surgically. Skin replacement may also be required when the Achilles tendon is lengthened in equinus deformity. The overriding problem in reconstruction is to provide stable re-epithelialization without excessive soft tissue bulk.

Skin grafts

Shaving of the exposed Achilles tendon and splitting of the tendinous fibres longitudinally commonly permits granulation tissue to penetrate through tendon fibres. If this can be achieved, a skin graft can be expected to take on the tendon itself. The Achilles tendon is thick just above its insertion into the calcaneum and therefore considerable shaving of its fibres can be carried out without disrupting its continuity. If this fails, flap cover must be considered.

Transposition flaps

The most useful of these flaps is a proximally based flap that extends between the lateral malleolus and the defect almost to the sole skin. The axial vessel that is incorporated within the flap is the terminal branches of the peroneal artery, which emanates from beneath the flexor hallucis longus muscle. The donor site will require a skin graft (Fig. 10).

The turn over flap

A flap may be raised based on the edge of the ulcerated area, de-epithelialized and then turned over to resurface the Achilles tendon. The raw surface that then presents externally may be skin grafted (Thake 1981).

Axial pattern flap

The dorsalis pedis artery flap to be described below will reach the heel, but the transfer is tight. Considerable dissection needs to be carried out to achieve this trans-

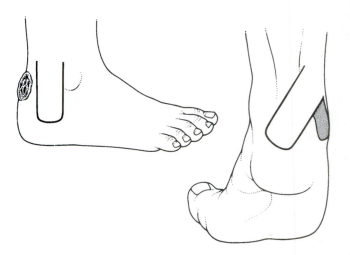

Figure 10

Transposition flap for resurfacing the Achilles tendon area. It is designed to include the terminal branches of the peroneal artery and the sural nerve. The donor site is skin grafted

fer. The medial plantar flap may also be used but the abductor hallucis muscle has to be divided to achieve sufficient freedom for the vascular pedicle.

Muscle flaps

The abductor hallucis muscle originates from the medial part of the calcaneum and inserts into the base of the proximal phalanx of the first toe. Its innervation and blood supply emanate from the medial plantar neurovascular bundle. In order to elevate the flap an incision is made along the non-weight-bearing surface and the tendon divided distally. The muscle is then separated from the fibres of the flexor hallucis brevis. The muscle is turned over on itself and elevated up to its pedicle. In order to resurface defects on the posterior heel, however, it will be necessary to divide the medial plantar artery distally and elevate the artery with the flap up to its bifurcation with the posterior tibial artery. The muscle may then be transposed to the area of the Achilles tendon and skin grafted. The procedure is satisfactory but depends on the size of the abductor hallucis muscle. In general it is probably easier to take a medial plantar flap, since the dissection is similar.

Free flap transfers

When circumstances demand, a free flap transfer may be used to resurface the area over the Achilles tendon. In particular, this may be necessary when the Achilles tendon is to be lengthened in equinus deformities. A thin flap is desirable, and therefore flaps such as the radial

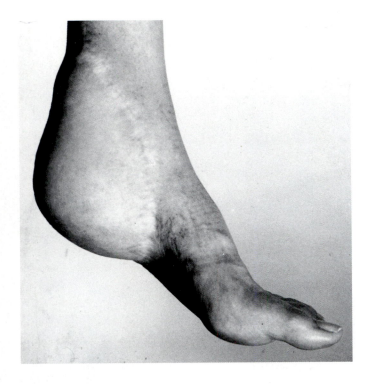

Figure 11

A 15 × 22 cm groin flap transferred as a microvascular free flap to the heel and posterior ankle over the Achilles tendon

artery forearm flap may be particularly useful. If the area to be resurfaced is extensive, as may occur in injury, then a groin flap or a tensor fasciae latae flap may be more suitable (Fig. 11).

In an effort to try and produce the thinnest possible re-epithelialization of this area, a recent innovation is the use of vascularized fascial grafts.

Vascularized fascial grafts
The most commonly used donor sites for vascularized fascia is the radial artery fascial flap, which comprises the radial artery and an expanse of the deep fascia on the forearm but not the overlying skin. The radial artery and the fascia may be then transferred to the lower leg where the radial artery is anastomosed to the posterior tibial artery and vein, and the fascia is used to cover the area over the exposed Achilles tendon. The vascularized fascia may then be skin grafted and in consequence the area re-epithelialized. A further suitable donor site for vascularized fascia is the galeal flap. The hair-bearing scalp may be elevated over an extensive area of the lateral side of the scalp and the galea beneath raised on the superficial temporal artery and vein. Following removal of the galea, the scalp may be closed directly. The galea may then be transferred to the ankle region, revascularized by microvascular anastomosis, and skin grafted.

In conclusion, there are many methods of resurfacing the sole of the foot, the dorsum of the foot and Achilles tendon. It is highly desirable, if possible, to try and provide sensory flap tissue to resurface the sole, and the medial plantar flap and filleted toes are particularly useful in achieving this aim. When a distant flap has to be introduced (the most useful of which are innervated free flap transfers) a period of at least 9 months of non-weight-bearing on the flap is probably essential to avoid pressure ulceration due to insensitivity.

Congenital deformities of the foot

The surgery of congenital deformities of the foot should be designed to correct functional deficits simply and quickly. Functional deficits in the foot generally relate to the wearing of shoes and this may be prevented by such conditions as polydactyly, gross clinodactyly of the pre- or postaxial digits or macrodactyly.

Complex multiple stage operations are generally less successful than simple procedures. The earlier the surgery is carried out, the more easily the child adapts to the change and makes use of it.

The classification of congenital deformities of the hand prepared by the American Society for Surgery of the Hand is equally applicable to the foot:

1. Failure of formation of parts (developmental arrest)
2. Failure of differentiation or separation of parts
3. Duplication
4. Overgrowth (gigantism)
5. Undergrowth (hypoplasia)
6. Congenital constriction bands
7. Generalized skeletal abnormalities

Failure of formation of parts
Arrest of development may be transverse or longitudinal. Transverse arrest produces congenital amputations and can occur at any level. Congenital ring constriction can also produce amputation of the terminal digits and should be differentiated from a true arrest. Longitudinal arrest includes central or preaxial and postaxial failures of development.

There is little that need or indeed that can be done for most of these conditions but a central deficit may produce spreading of the lateral segments, as in lobster claw deformities. In this condition, wearing shoes may prove difficult because of the width of the foot.

Correction is directed at trying to narrow the foot and may necessitate osteotomies of the lateral metatarsals to permit them to fall into the central defects, suitable excisions of central skin, and usually the maintenance of the position by a wire or fascial loop around the necks of the metatarsals.

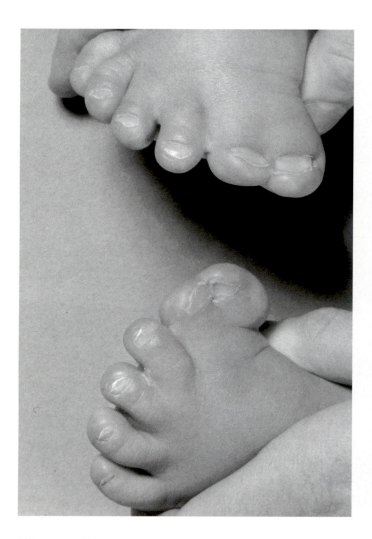

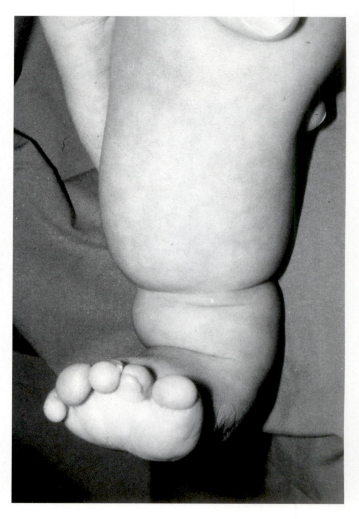

Figure 12

Preaxial polydactyly and associated syndactyly

Figure 13

Congenital constriction ring of the lower leg

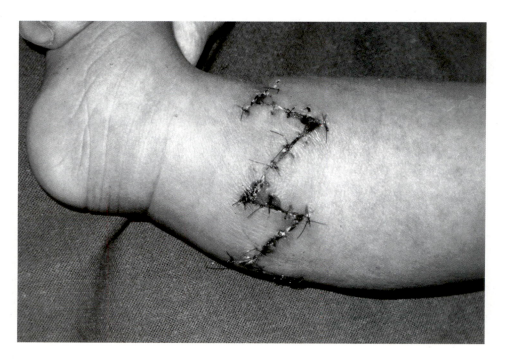

Figure 14

Congenital constriction ring closed with the incorporation of a series of Z-plasties

Failure of differentiation (or separation) of parts

Syndactyly of the toes is one of the most common congenital deformities. Functionally it produces no deficit and its correction is a purely cosmetic exercise; advice should therefore be given against separation.

Modern techniques of desyndactylization emphasize a long dorsal flap into the base of the cleft to prevent distal creep, zigzag design of interdigitating skin flaps along the adjacent sides of the cleft and full-thickness grafts in areas where the skin flaps do not meet. Scarring on the dorsum of the foot is therefore inevitable and draws attention to a deformity which, prior to surgery, would probably not have been apparent to any but the most careful observers. Scarring along the sides of the cleft from incisions and skin grafts will lead to clinodactyly towards the cleft. Finally, scars on the plantar surface of the foot are undesirable as they may become hyperkeratotic and therefore painful.

Exceptions to this rule are 'fenestrated syndactyly' (acrosyndactyly), often associated with the ring constriction syndrome, in which cleaning the cleft between the toes may be troublesome and separation of the toes is particularly easy as the base of the cleft is well formed. The other indication for surgical correction is the syndactylized nail, where difficulty may be experienced in trimming. Separation of the distal phalangeal segment only is recommended and is usually achieved by turning a flap from the pulp of one of the toes into the cleft and placing a full-thickness graft onto the donor site of the other toe.

Polydactyly

This is probably the most common congenital deformity of the foot. It is commoner in black races and is more frequently seen in females. It is often associated with polydactyly of the fingers.

An extra digit is normally seen on the postaxial side of the foot and may be connected with the foot by a narrow stalk; alternatively a fully formed toe may be attached to the foot at metatarsophalangeal or interphalangeal joint level.

Correction is directed to narrowing the foot to enable the wearing of shoes, and this is usually simply achieved.

Preaxial polydactyly can be associated with medial deviation of the big toe (Fig. 12). The accessory digit can be removed, but the deviation is caused by an inclination of the metatarsal head, and in order to straighten the toe to permit the wearing of shoes a lateral wedge osteotomy at the metatarsal neck may be required.

Macrodactyly

This is a congenital pathological enlargement of soft tissue and associated skeletal enlargement. Fortunately it is rare and usually affects one digit, but if more than one is involved they are adjacent. The digital nerves in macrodactyly are commonly enlarged with fatty tissue, and the condition may be associated with neurofibromatosis.

The enlargement may be stable, in that the size of the digit remains in proportion, or progressive, in that the digit increases out of proportion to the rest of the foot. The surgical treatment is either conservative or ablative. Conservative methods constitute reducing the bulk of the digit by thinning soft tissue and controlling excessive growth by shortening bone and preventing epiphyseal growth.

Thinning of soft tissue has to be carried out with care in order to avoid skin necrosis. The results of conservative surgery are usually poor, with a stiff, enlarged digit commonly the outcome. Amputation of the digit is usually the best method of treatment and permits the wearing of shoes.

Congenital constriction rings

Ring constrictions consist of deep grooves in the lower leg running transversely to the long axis. The depth varies and may be sufficient to cause autoamputations.

Commonly, the groove passes down to the deep fascia and deep structures are unaffected. The constriction rings produce obstructions to the superficial lymphatics and therefore distal lymphoedema.

Constriction rings are often multiple and autoamputation of digits or fenestrated syndactyly may be found in association.

The aetiology is debatable: the condition may be caused by the fetus pushing its foot into the amniotic sac with subsequent development of a tight band around it, by filamentous strands from the amnion wrapping around the limb, or by a local dysplasia of the mesoderm.

Treatment is undertaken early in order to prevent the distal lymphoedema becoming chronic with irreversible skin changes. Excision of the constriction ring is carried out to its full depth, if necessary including the deep fascia, and is repaired with multiple Z-plasties. In view of the fact that a circumferential excision will be necessary, there is a risk to the distal viability of the limb and it may be advisable, particularly where there is suspected deep involvement, to carry out the correction in two stages, doing half the circumference of the limb at a time (Figs. 13, 14).

Following surgery the distal lymphoedema usually disperses completely.

References

Barclay T L, Cordoso E, Sharpe D T, Crockett D J 1982 Repair of lower leg injuries with fasciocutaneous flap. Br J Plast Surg 35: 127–132

Barclay T L, Sharpe D T, Chisholm E M 1983 Cross-leg fasciocutaneous flaps. Plast Reconstr Surg 72: 843–846

Curtin J W 1977 Functional surgery for intractable conditions of the sole of the foot. Plast Reconstr Surg 59: 806–811

Gillies H D 1920 The tubed pedicle in plastic surgery. N Y Med J III:1

Haertsch P A 1981a The surgical plane in the leg. Br J Plast Surg 34: 464–469

Haertsch P A 1981b The blood supply to the skin of the leg: a post mortem investigation. Br J Plast Surg 34: 470–477

Harrison D H, Morgan B D G 1981 The instep island flap to resurface plantar defects. Br J Plast Surg 34: 315–318

Hynes W 1957 The treatment of scars by shaving and skin graft. Br J Plast Surg 10:1

Kaplan I 1969 Neurovascular island flap in the treatment of trophic ulceration of the heel. Br J Plast Surg 22: 143–148

Lister G D 1978 Use of an innervated skin graft to provide sensation to the reconstructed heel. Plast Reconstr Surg 62: 151–161

McCraw J B 1977 In Converse J M (ed) Reconstructive Plastic Surgery, Vol. 7, Saunders, Philadelphia, p 3563

Maisels D O 1961 Repairs of the heel. Br J Plast Surg 14: 117–125

Mir y Mir L 1954 Functional graft of the heel. Plast Reconstr Surg 14: 444–450

Morrison W A, Crabb D McK, O'Brien B McC, Jenkins A 1983 The instep of the foot as a fasciocutaneous island and as a free flap for heel defects. Plast Reconstr Surg 72: 56–63

Nahai F 1980 The tensor fasciae latae flap. Clin Plast Surg 7: 51

O'Brien B McC, Shanmugan M 1973 Experimental transfer of composite free flaps with microvascular anastomosis. Aust NZ J Surg 43: 285–288

Ponten B 1981 The fasciocutaneous flap: its use in soft tissue defects of the lower leg. Br J Plast Surg 34: 215–220

Serafin D, Sabatier R F, Morris R L, Gengicide N G 1980 Reconstruction of the extremity with vascularised composite tissue: Improved tissue survival and specific indications. Plast Reconstr Surg 66: 230–241

Shanahan R E, Gingras R P 1979 Medial plantar sensory flap for coverage of heel defects. Plast Reconstr Surg 64: 295–298

Snyder G B, Edgerton M T 1965 The principle of the neurovascular flap in the management of ulcerated anaesthetic weight-bearing areas of the lower extremity. Plast Reconstr Surg 36: 518–528

Sommerlad B C, McGrowther D A 1978 Resurfacing the sole: long term follow-up and comparison of techniques. Br J Plast Surg 31: 107–116

Song R, Gao Y, Song Y, Yu Y, Song Y 1982 The forearm flap. Chir Plast Surg 9: 21–26

Stranc M F, Labandter H, Roy A 1975 A review of 196 tubed pedicles. Br J Plast Surg 28: 54–58

Taylor G I 1983 Current status of free vascularised bone grafts. Clin Plast Surg 10: 185–209

Taylor G I, Daniel R K 1975 Anatomy of several free flap donor sites. Plast Reconstr Surg 56: 243

Thake R L 1981 Random pattern de-epithelialised 'turn-over' flaps to replace skin loss in the upper third of the leg. Br J Plast Surg 34: 312–314

Vann H M 1943 A note on the formation of the plantar arterial arch of the human foot. Anat Rec 85: 269

VIII   INFECTIONS

VIII.1   Infections and Infestations

Both acute and chronic infections are discussed in the following section. Although not common in the West in world terms, some of the exotic infections are extremely common and there are no apologies for including them.

Other sections may deal with specific aspects of infection and in particular the reader is referred to Chapter VI.4 on diabetes.

Pyogenic infections
David Stuart

Introduction

Surgical experience with major foot infection mirrors general medical experience over the years. In most developed countries the incidence has lessened with improved standards of living, improved nutrition, hygiene and cleanliness, better shoe wear and protective shoe wear in industry and agriculture. The more effective management of injuries, improved worldwide communications, appropriate preoperative preparation, and the availability of adequate chiropody have all played a part in reducing the incidence of foot infection. The introduction of antibiotics has revolutionized the treatment and outcome. Even so, management can still prove difficult.

In the more developed parts of the world a large part of experience is concerned with the increasing age of the population, and patients with diabetes, secondary infection in rheumatoid arthritis, neuropathic disorders and circulatory problems of the lower limbs, both arterial and venous. Added to these are patients with secondary sepsis from ingrowing toe nails and ill-fitting fashionable shoes. Any general or orthopaedic ward will also have its share of patients with secondary sepsis following operative surgery or chiropody.

In the less developed world, experience is probably the same as in the past in western Europe, with secondary sepsis following trauma by far the most common. Interestingly, with increasing urbanization and industrialization, the large cities of the developing world are faced with ancient problems as well as those presently occurring in the richer countries.

The importance of major foot infections lies not only with the fact that a great reduction in this incidence is

possible, but also, that should infection occur, it is often necessary for these patients to be admitted to hospital. This carries important economic implications both to the individual and the society in which they live.

Aetiology

Being the distal end of the longest extremity, and having a ready exposure to trauma, the foot has a naturally lower vitality due to relatively poor circulation compared with elsewhere. There is a reduced potential for healing. As sensation lessens with age, the foot demonstrates the effect of diminished resistance to infection, no matter what the virulence of the organism. Rheumatoid patients, the elderly, those with malnutrition, patients with diabetes and nephritis, alcoholics and the debilitated constitute the 'at risk' patient. These now include immunosuppressed patients, those on steroids and patients with local circulatory problems such as varicose veins and ulcers, arterial insufficiency related to smoking, neuropathies and gout. Other predisposing local factors include rigid deformity (with corns) and the use of physical agents causing trauma.

Primary acute infections of the foot

Primary acute haematogenous osteomyelitis of the foot is rare compared to elsewhere. The incidence is higher in the poorer communities, but it can attack the fittest and the best fed quite unexpectedly. Local trauma usually determines the localization. Acute septic arthritis in neonates is known as Tom Smith's arthritis. In the neonate there is probably an immature defence mechanism. However, persisting reduction in host defences after acute haematogenous osteomyelitis in childhood was not found by Gillespie et al (1983). In adults the condition occurs in patients with lowered resistance and there is reason to believe that in some there is a transient or continued immune deficiency as in acquired immune deficiency syndrome (AIDS). Thus any of the 'at risk' patients may suffer the same infection (see the section by John Jellis below, pages 625–9).

Subacute and chronic primary infections of the foot

Such diseases as brucellosis, actinomycosis and other fungal infections are often associated with local trauma as well as generally poor nutrition and are common in less developed countries in the malnourished. Tuberculosis is dealt with below.

Chronic primary osteomyelitis seems to affect the calcaneus more frequently than other bones. Osteomyelitis of the metatarsals and other tarsal bones is more frequently secondary to crushing injuries or compound fractures.

Secondary major infections of the foot

Secondary infection is far more widespread. In the less developed parts of the world (as in earlier times elsewhere) the major cause is trauma. The type of case is determined by the environment, whether urban or rural, coastal, forest or desert. In more developed countries similar examples would include industrial, farming or gardening injuries. Major infections following compound fractures of the foot from industrial or road traffic accidents, and especially from blast or explosive injuries such as land mines, are a difficult group of cases. They are frequently associated with multiple injuries.

Many have iatrogenic causes such as skeletal pin track infection of the calcaneus, forefoot operations with or without prosthetic implants and poor chiropody. Recent infection of a bunion or ingrowing toenail increases the likelihood of secondary infection if definitive surgery on the same foot is undertaken too early. Moreover the use of local anaesthetic or the use of a tourniquet is unwise in the presence of infection for fear of spread.

Secondary infections from puncture wounds form an interesting group. They may be from thorns, needles, pins, rusty nails or splinters of wood. They may result in gram-negative osteomyelitis which is relatively rare, as described by Gordon et al (1974), Miller & Semian (1975) and Nuber & Anderson (1982). Such puncture wounds can affect all ages. The organism found is not from the usual flora or commensals, but is probably opportunistic from the environment carried in with the foreign body which may be retained (Cracchiolo & Goldberg 1977). Pseudomonas aeruginosa osteomyelitis after puncture wounds has been described by MacKinnon (1975).

Clinical presentation and diagnosis

Acute osteomyelitis

Acute haematogenous osteomyelitis may affect any bone of the foot or ankle region but is less common than elsewhere in the limbs; one or more bones may be involved. Typically it follows relatively minor local recent trauma such as a bruise, although there may be no known incident. There is also frequently a history of infection such as a boil or furunculosis elsewhere and it usually occurs in the ill nourished, puny child. In the infant the condition may be difficult to diagnose with poor localizing signs initially and hence the presentation as a pseudoparalysis.

The os calcis and talus are the most frequently affected bones in the foot. The patient arrives with local pain, ill with fever and unable to walk on the painful foot. The general toxaemia may seem out of proportion to the local signs in some cases. Later, oedema and even blistering of the skin occur. Spreading proximal lymphangitis and then adenitis follow. Rigors may develop, the child becoming rapidly ill and requiring admission to hospital.

Patients with reduced resistance may present late, with severe, spreading, local changes, but often with relatively little pain and toxaemia. Neonates may be brought in extremis, with the whole limb or foot full of pus.

In acute haematogenous osteomyelitis the brief history is typical. Initially there will be no X-ray changes. In this phase a blood culture is necessary and, if positive, the antibiotic sensitivity. The erythrocyte sedimentation rate (ESR) is almost invariably raised. Above 20 mm/h is significant, even in children and in subacute infections. A normal blood count is possible and unhelpful in making a diagnosis. Changes in the blood counts and sedimentation rates are important in the assessment of progress and response to treatment.

Recording the clinical progress is all important. This includes not only the local signs but also the systemic effects and observations of the temperature, the extent of the pain, especially in acute haematogenous osteomyelitis, the spread of the swelling, inflammation, lymphangitis, adenitis and oedema.

Differential diagnosis

Foot sepsis must be distinguished clinically from soft tissue trauma, fractures, stress fractures, Still's disease and perhaps any form of paralysis in children. Additionally, consideration has to be given to gouty conditions, rheumatoid arthritis, arterio-venous malformation, metastatic aneurysm in association with bacterial endocarditis and other forms of polyarthritis, including seronegative forms as described by Capen & Sheck (1981).

Ultimately surgery may be necessary for drainage or biopsy. This carries the advantage of definitive diagnosis by enabling the actual organism and its antibiotic sensitivity to be characterized, although this may not be possible if antibiotics have already been commenced.

Sickle-cell osteomyelitis

Tests for sickle-cell disease are important, particularly where there are multiple sites of osteomyelitis. Both sickle-cell trait (AS) and sickle-cell disease (SS or SC) show a tendency for osteomyelitis whether in acute or less acute forms. Sickle-cell disease itself is characterized by osteomyelitis at various sites and is of a recurrent nature, associated with crises.

Complications

These include proximal spread, ultimately causing an inguinal abscess, direct spread and necrosis of adjacent structures in the foot – metatarsals and joints. Involved tendons rapidly necrose, especially if exposed. Joint destruction and sequestration, with chronic sinus formation, are features of chronic infection of the foot.

Increasing skin necrosis occurs with chronic ulceration and secondary infection, aided and abetted by powerful topical applications and careless surgery. Such chronic infection leads to destruction of the tissues, causing contractures and deformities of the foot and ankle. This inevitably implies chronic pain, instability and permanent lameness.

With very prolonged chronic osteomyelitis and chronic discharge from a sinus, a Marjolin's ulcer with neoplastic change is a possibility.

Anatomical spread of infections

Infection adjacent to the toenail may spread to the dorsal fascial space. Infections of the toe itself, particularly on the plantar surface, may cause a secondary infection of the superficial plantar fascial space. This is the same as the first plantar fascial space of the central compartment (as described in Gray's Textbook of Anatomy). Interdigital infection, if it spreads to a fascial space, will follow the lumbrical muscles to involve the second and third fascial spaces of the central compartment. An infection of the dorsal subcutaneous space likewise will follow the course of the lumbrical muscles to infect the second and third spaces of the central compartment.

Since the dorsal subcutaneous space and the middle two spaces of the central compartment are connected, an infection of the second and third fascial spaces may result in swelling on the dorsum of the foot. In cases of a penetrating wound, the infection may be carried directly to the central compartment.

Cellulitis presenting with swelling, redness and induration may be associated with a localization of the infection in the deep fascial space and the formation of pus. Deep pus is often present when there is pitting oedema.

Clinical bacteriology

In osteomyelitis of the feet the range of possible organisms responsible is wide. However, by far the most common is *Staphylococcus aureus*. Whitehouse & Smith (1970) listed other possible organisms affecting the feet. Acute infection from *Streptococcus haemolyticus* should be considered in the presence of cellulitis, especially in the 'at risk' patient. Uncommon forms of osteomyelitis due to *Salmonella*, *Brucella*, coccidiomycosis, blastomycosis, actinomycosis, Madura foot, lues, leprosy and *Bacteroides* were described by Curtis (1973). Typhoid osteomyelitis of the calcaneus due to direct inoculation was reported by Monsoor (1967). Clostridial myonecrosis (gas gangrene) may follow severe trauma and neglect. It is frequently seen when tissues are devitalized and usually necessitates urgent amputation.

Most diabetic foot infections are polymicrobial. The most common pathogens seem to be a *Staphylococcal* species, and *Bacteroides*, followed closely by one of the *Streptococcal* species (particularly Group D streptococci, and enterococci). The most commonly encountered gram-positive aerobe in foot infections is still *Staphylococcus aureus*, and the most common gram-negative organism is *Pseudomonas aeruginosa*. *Bacteroides* species are the most common anaerobes isolated, followed closely by *Peptococci* (Johnson & Hall 1994).

In debilitated patients, *Staphylococcus aureus* is the most commonly identified organism, and the most commonly identified gram-negative bacteria are *Escherichia coli*, *Pseudomonas*, *Klebsiella* spp and *Aerobacter* spp. Puncture wounds of the foot are usually colonized with *Pseudomonas*.

X-ray diagnosis

X-rays are important not only to demonstrate late destruction and reactive changes of the bones and joints, but also to localize foreign bodies, e.g. metal and glass. Sinography should be considered in the presence of a chronic sinus; non-opaque foreign bodies as well as sequestra and the presence of bone cavities may be detected in the chronic phase. More sophisticated soft tissue X-rays are useful, including tomography on occasions. MRI, if available, is a very powerful tool in localizing infective foci.

Imaging

Plain radiographs do not generally show bone infection until about 10 to 20 days after the onset of symptoms (Capitanio & Kirkpatrick 1970), and at this stage, further imaging studies may not be needed. Radiographic signs of osteomyelitis are osteopenia, small ill-defined lucencies in the medullary bone and cortex and cortical breakthrough. Periostitis of a metatarsal should not be considered a sign of infection since it can be due to either a stress fracture or a neuropathic joint.

After the plain radiograph the most frequently used study to evaluate osteomyelitis is the three-phase 99m technetium-labelled diphosphonate bone scan. The first phase of the scan is a radionuclide angiogram to assess relative blood flow to the area. The second phase is a blood pool image obtained immediately following the angiogram. This shows soft tissue activity due to hyperemia. The third phase is obtained after 3 to 4 hours, and reflects bone uptake of radionuclide due to osteoblastic activity. In osteomyelitis there is both increased blood flow and increased osteoblastic activity. There are numerous causes of positive three-phase bone scans, and thus the test is not specific for sepsis. Such a false-positive bone scan might be due to a neuropathic joint. Cellulitis can also cause false-positive bone scans (Unger et al 1988), and may be due to inflammation of the periosteum from overlying cellulitis and ulcers.

Bone scanning with indium-111-labelled white blood cells may increase the specificity of using technetium bone scans. Indium scanning has been reported to be positive at an earlier stage of osteomyelitis than the bone scan (Raptopoulos et al 1982). However, false positives occur in cases of a fracture, and the indium scanning has poor spatial resolution, which can make it difficult to determine whether the activity is in bone or soft tissue. These scans are reported to be positive in as many as 31% of non-infected neuropathic joints (Seabold et al 1990).

CT scanning is a useful method to diagnose osteomyelitis. CT will demonstrate increased density of bone marrow in cases of osteomyelitis because the marrow is infiltrated with inflammatory cells and pus. It will also show areas of cortical destruction, periostitis, and sequestra (Kuhn & Berger 1979, Ram et al 1981). Intraosseous gas has been reported as a sign of osteomyelitis visible on CT (Ram et al 1981).

MRI has been found to have a very high sensitivity (92–100%) for osteomyelitis (Tang et al 1988). A focus of osteomyelitis will demonstrate low signal intensity on T1-weighted images, and high signal intensity on T2-weighted and STIR sequences. Potential causes of false-positive scans include occult fracture and bone infarction, postoperative changes and neuropathic joints.

Crim et al. (1996) recommend using the following procedure based on cost and accuracy in order to optimize radiographic diagnosis of osteomyelitis. Plain radiographs are used as a screening examination. If the radiograph is positive and there are other signs of an infection, then no further investigation is necessary. If a radiograph is negative, a three-phase bone scan is the next logical choice for diagnostic imaging because of its low cost. If a three-phase bone scan is negative, osteomyelitis cannot be completely excluded early in the course of disease. Thus, if clinical suspicion is high an MRI, which has virtually 100% sensitivity, can be performed. An MRI is also the procedure of choice when a three-phase bone scan is equivocal. CT scanning is more sensitive to outline a sequestra than our plain radiographs, and therefore it can be most useful in planning treatment (Seltzer 1984). MRI can also be used to detect sequestra.

Ultrasonography has been useful in detecting foreign bodies in the soft tissues, such as wooden splinters.

Treatment

Antibiotics

The use of antibiotics is crucial in limb- or life-threatening conditions particularly in established acute major infections of the foot. Appropriate antibiotics are chosen from the blood or local culture and tested for antibiotic sensitivity. Where possible antibiotic blood levels should be monitored.

Until the laboratory results are available broad spectrum antibiotics or combinations of these are favoured, especially to cover mixed infection. They should be bactericidal. Depending upon the environment, in acute major infections high doses of intravenous systemic crystalline penicillin still play a part. In patients who have been in hospital for any length of time, cloxacillin, flucloxacillin or ampicillin may be necessary.

Specific antibiotic drugs will vary widely depending on where treatment is being performed. Generally a broad spectrum antibiotic is best. When the organism is unknown one must treat for gram-positive and gram-negative organisms.

Intravenous antibiotic therapy is the quickest and best way to provide the necessary blood concentration in serious major foot infections. The regime described by O'Brien et al (1982) is preferred: 100 mg/kg per day of cloxacillin in four divided doses and 30 mg/kg per day of fusidic acid in three divided doses are given in a bolus injection. These achieve serum levels exceeding the usual inhibitory concentrations for staphylococcal strains as reported by Garrod et al (1973). The additional use of metronidazole is advisable where anaerobic infection is suspected.

When employed, antibiotics are usually necessary for at least six weeks for major bone or joint infections, but for purely soft tissue infections the period may be less. Antibiotic use is guided by the local and general signs, the level of pain and the blood sedimentation rate during the course of management. Oral use of antibiotics after the initial phase, particularly after discharge from hospital and management as an outpatient, should be considered depending upon compliance of the patient and relatives, and the costs.

In the acute infection in particular, the response must be monitored closely and the regime changed if necessary. What would be applicable today may well change in the course of time, especially as hospital pathogenic organisms have a habit of changing their resistance to antibiotics. Combinations of antibiotics may not be the answer indefinitely. The choice of antibiotics must necessarily take into consideration the relative cost, avoiding the habit of using the most costly when there is a genuine choice.

Other systemic measures

In addition to appropriate prophylactic antibiotics, the use of antisera should be considered to prevent tetanus and gas gangrene. The use of antiserum in the presence of gas gangrene is generally agreed. It should also be considered prophylactically in severe wounds where there is delay in treatment and especially those occurring in wartime injuries, in patients involved in agricultural work and in patients with serious devitalizing injuries with much muscle damage and with compound fractures of the foot and lower limb. However, antiserum in tetanus has largely fallen into disuse, certainly as a prophylactic measure, because of the incidence of allergic reactions (including anaphylaxis) to the horse serum from which it is prepared. In the presence of clinical tetanus, special preparations are necessary, including those prepared from human sera.

Antitetanus toxoid immunization is obligatory in soiled wounds, especially in agricultural workers, those with foot injuries in the under developed world and in children running about barefoot. Even minor foot injuries, such as a small puncture wound, in those keen on gardening should be considered for immunization against tetanus.

Other systemic measures include the need for analgesics, sedatives and fluid replacement as well as the treatment of accompanying disorders such as diabetes.

Hyperbaric oxygen therapy has been used in the treatment of chronic osteomyelitis (Morrey et al 1980), and in gas gangrene (Maudsley & Colwill 1966, Colwill & Maudsley 1968). With reasonably economic means (100% oxygen in two atmospheres of pressure undertaken for two hours twice daily, in a small one-man chamber) it was possible to reduce the mortality. Hyperbaric oxygen is only an adjunct to surgery and antibiotics, and these two sets of workers related their failures to inadequate surgery.

Local measures

To prevent infection, old injuries, severe injuries with compound fractures and crush injuries should not be closed primarily. This does not mean there should be no surgery. Debridement is necessary, excising severely damaged and devitalized tissues and muscles after the usual wound toilet. Indeed the surgery itself is important, with careful handling of tissues at all times to prevent further devitalization and damage. When left open, the wound is gently packed with gauze and kept moist with saline. The foot should be supported with a well padded plaster of Paris slab in the anatomical position with the ankle at 90° to avoid permanent contractures and deformity. The limb is elevated. After about five days most cases are suitable for secondary suturing to reduce the possibility of gross scarring. However, some may be left open to granulate and epithelialize. Occasionally split skin grafting is necessary. Some of the more chronic cases or those with considerable skin loss require cross-leg pedicle or myocutaneous grafting as described by Ger (1983) to provide a more supple foot, and the latter also provides a better circulation to combat infection.

A free tissue transfer can also be performed. The added bulk of the muscle flap provides a weight bearing surface and adheres to the calcaneus, preventing heel pad migration (Anderson et al 1990).

It is emphasized that in all severe, contaminated and crushing injuries, as well as old injuries, primary closure should be avoided. The urge to stitch all lacerations indiscriminately frequently results in secondary infection and necrosis in foot and lower limb injuries.

An indication for surgery is a localized abscess in the bone, with inadequate drainage, or the presence of a sequestrum. Drainage of the abscess is obtained by opening the cavity with minimum trauma to the surrounding tissue. The local management includes packing of the wound gently with Vaseline gauze, and supporting the limb in a plaster of Paris cast with a window cut out for sterile dressings. Hauser elevated the limb to about the height of an ordinary pillow to facilitate circulation and to prevent oedema and swelling. The general management has not altered much; he advised rest, fluids (to produce 1500 ml of urine daily), analgesics and sedatives. In those days sulphanilamide was the only antibiotic available and was used for surgical sepsis, especially that due to *S. haemolyticus*.

In summary, the principle in the treatment of established severe infection of the foot involves eradication by antibiotics, surgical drainage if necessary, general systemic treatment, local rest and assisting the circulation, usually by elevating the limb. Admission to hospital is generally necessary. With any life-threatening stage, amputation should be considered although this is now less often indicated.

Chronic infections and salvage procedures

In the aftermath of acute osteomyelitis, the presence of necrosed cortical bone will be seen at the base of the wound, or on X-ray, or presumed to be there. If still attached to healthy bone there is no urgency to remove it provided there is no gross sepsis. It should be left as long as possible to preserve the architecture of the foot, particularly in children. With sequestrated or loose bone, the bone with gross sepsis and chronic sinuses, surgery is necessary; the infection will not clear until the necrotic material is removed. This includes foreign bodies or implants used in surgery.

Any resulting pain or deformity may necessitate secondary surgery: the excision of bony prominences and the need for limited or extensive arthrodesis where there has been destruction of weight bearing joints. Radical measures may be necessary to eliminate chronic infection, from partial to total removal of the affected bone. This is possible even after many years of chronic infection with sinuses.

Ultimately, with any spreading infections or with gross destruction which is disabling and deemed to be incurable, some form of amputation may be necessary and indeed beneficial. The likelihood of spread, septicaemia, malignancy, chronic pain and disability can be prevented or overcome.

Chronic infection of a weight-bearing joint which has lost its articular cartilage is best treated by means of a formal surgical fusion, especially where the condition remains painful. Spontaneous fusion characteristically may occur, but the foot requires adequate and prolonged support in plaster or in surgical boots while this process is continuing.

Infections at special sites

Sesamoids

Although unusual, infection of the metatarsal sesamoid under the great toe is important in that the diagnosis is frequently late. Infection will not clear until the sesamoid is removed.

Acute osteomyelitis of the metatarsal sesamoid is rare. The responsible organism is usually *S. aureus*, as reported by Colwill (1969), who described three patients and indicated that five previous cases had been reported. Rome (1963) reported a patient with acute haematogenous osteomyelitis of the sesamoid. Torgerson & Hammon (1969) reported two other cases, one of which was in an adult with diabetes and the other an acute case due to *S. aureus* in a 12-year-old.

Talus

According to Antoniou & Conner (1974) the diagnosis of osteomyelitis of the talus is often made late and the condition is usually subacute. If due to *S. aureus*, it tends to be the coagulase negative organism. The most common incorrect diagnosis was a ligamentous injury. Most developed an abscess in the bone. Primary haematogenous osteomyelitis was also reported by Skevis (1984) in four children. These had proved difficult to diagnose and again presented late.

Chronic infection of the talus usually responds to local curettage and antibiotics. The antibiotics should be continued for six months. Similarly, plaster fixation may be necessary for six months. Transfixing Steinmann pins or Schantz screws with some form of external skeletal fixation is a useful method, particularly if chronic wounds and sinuses have to be dressed and inspected regularly.

Os calcis

Where there are persistent large ulcers of the heel, satisfactory results can be obtained by partial resection of the calcaneus, tailoring the skin incision around the ulcer and carrying out a primary closure as described by Horwirz (1972), who detailed four cases. Martini et al (1974) advocated partial or total resection and obtained satisfactory results in 20 cases. A shoe insert for the heel produced a reasonable gait. The split heel technique of Gaenslen was reported by Broudy et al (1976), who described three children with refractory osteomyelitis and a central sinus. They considered excision unnecessary.

Winkelmann & Schulitz (1977) reported the difficulties experienced in managing 59 cases with chronic infection affecting the calcaneum. Various operations were discussed. Only 10 out of 29 cases followed up had good results. There were frequent deformities, skin trophic changes, scars and ulcers. Amputation was necessary in some. Infection was usually due to *S. aureus*, but next in frequency were those due to gram-negative organisms. Mueller & Biebrach (1978) discussed their experience with 46 cases over 10 years, emphasizing the need for correct early diagnosis and treatment. Only six were eventually symptom-free.

These examples from recent literature illustrate the tendency to chronicity in osteomyelitis of the calcaneus and serve to demonstrate the difficulties in management. The choice of surgery depends upon the site and extent of involvement. Although conservative surgery is preferable, subtotal or total resection may be necessary. The results overall may not be satisfactory without proper planning and thorough investigation of the extent of involvement.

Tuberculosis
John E Jellis

Introduction

Disease of the ankle and foot accounts for less than 10% of osteoarticular tuberculosis. Although in the northern hemisphere examples are rarely seen, bone and joint tuberculosis is becoming more common (Scott & Taor 1982, Sammon 1983) and has a great propensity to mimic other lesions in bone (Standish et al 1977). Thus the diagnosis and treatment of tuberculosis of the foot and ankle have retained their importance in orthopaedic practice. Even in temperate climes such lesions are more common than primary bone tumours.

Pathology

Incidence

The incidence of tuberculosis is rising in most areas of the world, including Britain and the United States (Centers for Disease Control 1988). An estimated 1.7 billion people are infected with *Mycobacterium tuberculosis* (Kochi 1991) and 8 million new cases are reported each year (WHO 1991). Urban overcrowding, immigration, wars and attendant poverty are contributing to this, but the human immunodeficiency virus (HIV) epidemic is the most significant factor. In several African countries, 30% of the adult population are infected with the virus (Kehoe & Jellis 1994) and a similar pattern is developing in Asia.

HIV specifically attacks and depletes the lymphocytes, bone marrow mononuclear phagocytes and tissue macrophages that are the main components of the body's defence against tuberculosis (Chretian 1990). This synergism has produced a dual epidemic of tuberculosis and HIV (Elliott et al 1990) and, in Zambia for example, 62% of adults with bone and joint tuberculosis are HIV positive (Jellis et al 1995a).

Classically, orthopaedic tuberculosis was predominantly a disease of childhood and adolescence, but in many areas of the world fewer children now develop the disease, possibly because of BCG vaccination in infancy. Where HIV disease is common tuberculosis is a disease of young adults (Jellis et al 1995a). In temperate regions, the high risk groups are the indigenous elderly and the young adults among immigrant populations (Medical Research Council 1980, Davies et al 1984, Janssens & Haller 1990).

Anatomical distribution

Disseminated cystic tuberculous osteitis (multiple pseudocystic tuberculosis of bone) is a rare disease of infants and young children (O'Connor et al 1970, Shannon et al 1990) and polyarticular tuberculosis may affect the ankle and foot (Garrido et al 1988, Hameed et al 1993), but generally osteoarticular tuberculosis is a centripetal disease.

The spine is involved in between 30% and 60% of cases, while the hip and knee are the next most common sites of disease (Jellis 1979, Sammon 1983, Davies et al 1984, Jellis et al 1995a). In the series quoted above, tuberculosis of the ankle, tarsus and forefoot was present in between 2% and 12% of patients.

Types of lesions

Periarticular granuloma of bone

A granuloma in the distal metaphysis of the tibia or in the subchondral bone of the talus or other tarsal bone is the usual lesion in the ankle or foot. Infection spreads to the neighbouring joint and in children the physeal plate does not act as a barrier. A secondary synovitis occurs with erosion of bone at the synovial attachments and beneath the articular cartilage, but lysis of the articular cartilage is slow. Eventually, cold abscesses and sinuses appear which drain the joint debris. Secondary infection may subsequently complicate the picture. Cultures for tuberculosis should be set up for all biopsies taken for bone infections because mixed infections do occur and underlying tuberculosis may be masked by the more obvious staphylococcal infection (Sinnott et al 1990). Under favourable conditions or chemotherapy, the infection may resolve and a fibrous ankylosis develops.

Osteitis of a single bone

Rarely, a central granuloma of the calcaneum may occur (Manzella et al 1979) and occasionally tuberculous osteitis of a metatarsal base or phalanx without spread to adjacent joints has been seen. In childhood tuberculous dactylitis, a phalanx or phalanges may be expanded as if distended by air (Chapman et al 1979), giving the appearance known as spina ventosa.

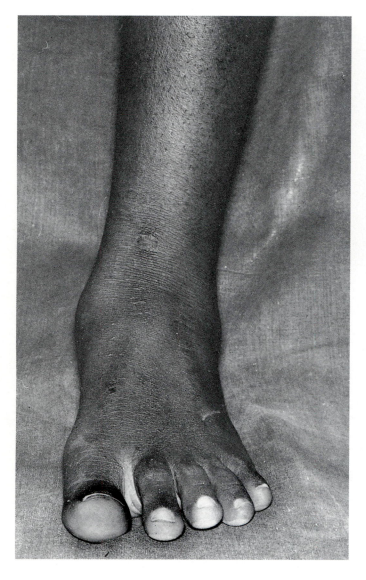

Figure 1a

Tuberculosis of the talonavicular joint. This 20-year-old woman had complained of pain and swelling over the dorsum of the foot for 6 months. She had received repeated courses of simple analgesics. There was moderate swelling and tenderness over the talonavicular joint. The overlying skin showed slight hyperpigmentation and the transverse scars of traditional treatment. Dorsiflexion of the foot was limited and weight bearing painful. A Heaf test was strongly positive and the ESR 33 mm/h. Debridement was performed and histology showed typical tuberculous granulation tissue and synovitis. The patient was treated with streptomycin and Thiazina and the foot was rested in a walking cast. Painless resolution occurred

Synovitis

Primary haematogenous synovitis probably occurs, but in the foot and ankle it is usually possible to demonstrate an adjacent bony lesion from which the infection has spread.

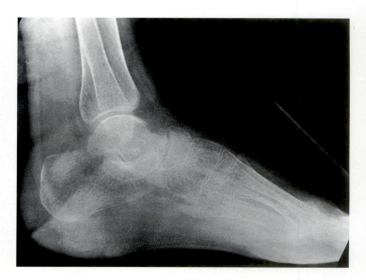

Figure 1b

Lateral radiograph

Tenosynovitis

Tenosynovitis and bursitis are usually the late sequelae of established infection of the underlying bones.

Clinical presentation

Patients may be of any age and either sex. The onset of disease is insidious, with a history of aching pain in a bone or joint increasing over weeks or months. Swelling of the surrounding tissue is at first soft and decreases overnight, but later hardens to a brawny oedema. Hyperpigmentation of the overlying skin occurs in black patients and, in Africa, generations of scarification from traditional treatment may substantiate the length of history (Fig. 1).

Delay in diagnosis is common. Tuberculosis should be considered in the differential diagnosis of any subacute or chronic bone or joint lesion that is not responding to treatment. The warm swollen foot of Kaposi's sarcoma and mycoses may produce a similar appearance in the tropics and in immunocompromised patients.

Investigations

Radiology

In the typical radiological pattern, an area of bone lysis develops in the metaphyseal, subepiphyseal or subchondral bone with surrounding osteoporosis and soft tissue swelling. There is usually little or no periosteal reaction

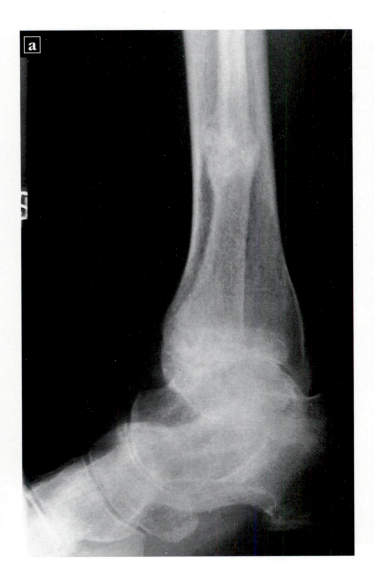

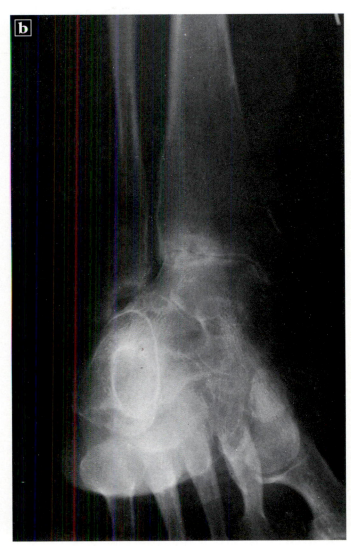

Figure 2

(a) Lateral and (b) anteroposterior radiographs of tuberculous arthritis of the ankle

and sclerosis around the lesion is uncommon except in the healing phase. The margins of the articular bone surface are hazy and ill defined, but the joint space is preserved (Fig. 2) longer than in pyogenic arthritis because lysis of the sequestrated cartilage is slower.

In predominantly synovial disease, there is erosion of bone at the synovial attachments. Because much of the synovial inflammation may be non-specific, it is important to locate any granuloma in the adjacent bone for biopsy. Computerized tomography is particularly helpful in this respect, while magnetic resonance imaging better delineates the extent of soft tissue extensions of the disease.

Apart from pseudocystic expansile lesions of the phalanges, metatarsals and os calcis in infants and young children and tuberculous osteitis of the calcaneum in adults (Manzella et al 1979), a wide range of uncommon

appearances occur. Osteoarticular tuberculosis is the great mimic of other pathologies (Standish et al 1977, Naidoo 1980). When tuberculosis is suspected, or indeed proven, a search for lesions elsewhere in the patient should include radiography of the chest, spine and renal tract.

Other investigations

A raised sedimentation rate (ESR), which is usually in the range of 29 mm to 100 mm/60 min (Westergren), and a relative lymphocytosis, are fairly constant features of established disease. In HIV infections, however, the ESR is always high while there will be a progressive lymphopoenia, depending on the stage of disease, thus

Table 1 Chemotherapeutic agents in current use

Drug	Dose	Administration	Length of treatment
Streptomycin	Adult	0.75–1.0 g/d	Intramuscular	60–90 days
	Child	15–25 mg/kg/d		
Isoniazid	Adult	300 mg/d	Oral single dose	Usually for 18 months but may be continued for several years if doubt of cure exists
	Child	10 mg/kg/d		
Rifampicin	Adult	600 mg	Oral single dose	90–180 days
	Child	10 mg/kg/d		
Ethambutol	Adult	25 mg/kg/d reducing to 15 mg/kg/d after 60 d	Oral single dose	60 days at full dose then continued at reduced dose for 18 months with isoniazid

making these tests poor indicators for tuberculosis.

Tuberculin skin tests (Haef or Mantoux) now have less significance. Because of the almost universal use of BCG vaccination in infancy and childhood and irregular suppression of the immune response in HIV disease, little reliance can be put on such tests.

As evidence of tuberculosis of other systems is sought, bacteriological examination of urine and sputa should be included.

Definitive diagnosis

A definitive diagnosis can only be made by the isolation and culture of *Mycobacterium tuberculosis* from the lesion, but bacteria are comparatively scanty in osteoarticular disease. Atypical mycobacterial infections are becoming more common in immunocompromised patients in Europe and America.

Histology

The typical appearance of the tuberculous granuloma stained by the Ziehl-Neelson technique is almost diagnostic, especially if acid-fast bacilli are demonstrated. There are possibilities of confusion with sarcoid disease and other granulomatous lesions, however, and a synovial biopsy may show only non-specific changes of chronic inflammation if the granulomatous area is missed.

Management

Treatment of orthopaedic tuberculosis consists of rest, chemotherapy and a variety of surgical interventions, and considerable judgement is needed to match therapy with demands of individual patients.

Chemotherapy

Modern chemotherapy (Table 1), especially when combined with surgical clearance of the lesion, is effective in eliminating tuberculous infection. The eventual prognosis and the place of surgery in those patients with both HIV disease and tuberculosis has yet to be evaluated. In such patients, severe drug reactions are common, especially to thiacetazone which is no longer used.

Surgery

The role of surgery is five-fold:

(1) To obtain material for diagnosis.
(2) To assess the damage to the bone or joint. However, the joint can also be assessed by performing an MRI or an arthroscopic evaluation of the joint.
(3) Debridement, which in this context is taken to mean the removal of sequestra, granulomata and any fibrotic barrier to the blood supply of the area.
(4) Synovectomy if the synovium is excessively thickened.
(5) Arthrodesis of an irretrievably destroyed joint.

In early lesions a single exploration, biopsy and curettage may suffice and healing is achieved by chemotherapy and rest. It may be impossible, however, to predict whether a damaged joint will heal well enough to bear weight without pain.

When severe destruction has occurred, especially in the presence of sinuses and secondary infection, initial biopsy and debridement may usefully be followed by several months of chemotherapy before arthrodesis is performed.

In HIV positive or other immunocompromised patients it is important to assess the degree of immune competence remaining before any surgery is contemplated. This can be done by physical examination and estimation of the CD4 helper/inducer T-lymphocyte subsets (WHO 1990). While the magnitude of ankle or foot surgery is unlikely to overstress the patient's remaining immune competence, complications of surgery, especially infections and poor wound healing, are likely to increase in advanced stages of HIV disease (Jellis et al 1995b).

Biopsy

A drill biopsy may be carefully guided into an identified area of eroded bone by radiological screening, but open biopsy can usefully be combined with assessment of the joint and debridement.

The approach should be the most direct available, excising any sinuses or draining abscesses if these exist. A representative specimen of tuberculous granulation should be sought for histological and bacteriological investigation.

Debridement should include the removal of sequestra, pus or caseous material, loose or damaged cartilage and any synovium or capsule that is excessively thickened. The bone lesion should be curetted or cut back to normal bone and any thick fibrous encapsulation excised.

Future prospects

Since the first edition of this chapter in Helal & Wilson (1988) the incidence of osteoarticular tuberculosis has risen in many parts of the world. Tuberculosis should be considered within the differential diagnosis of any chronic erosive condition of the foot and ankle and a high index of suspicion maintained. With surgery combined with modern chemotherapy, bone and joint tuberculosis is eminently treatable unless complicated by HIV infection. In these cases the initial response to chemotherapy seems promising, but whether a cure can be effected remains to be seen.

Tropical infections and infestations
Sureshwar Pandey

Leprosy

Synonyms: Hansen's infection, Hansen's disease, Elephantiasis graecorum, Leontiasis or Satyriasis, Kusth (India).

Leprosy, a chronic, complex infectious granulomatous condition – erroneously associated with 'Biblical leprosy' – is caused by *Mycobacterium leprae* (discovered by the Norwegian scientist Dr Gerhard Armauer Hansen at Bergen in 1873). Although a multisystem disease, it essentially affects the nerves to the skin in susceptible human hosts. Specific cell-mediated immunity, through thymus-sensitized lymphocytes, determines its wide range of clinical manifestations. Leprosy remained endemic all over the globe until the end of the Middle Ages. However, today it is most prevalent in tropical countries (Fig. 3).

Aetiology

M. leprae is an obligate, intracellular, acid-fast bacillus, multiplying mainly inside the macrophages of the skin and the Schwann cells of the nerves. The organism has not yet been cultured *in vitro*. Leprosy bacilli are found in nasal secretions, nasal mucosa, erosions, ulcers and blisters of lepromatous and borderline patients and patients in reactional states. They are also excreted in sputum, semen, sweat, sebum, tears and breast milk of lepromatous patients (Thangaraj & Yawalker 1986).

Epidemiology

Untreated multibacillary leprosy cases are the main reservoir of the bacilli. The infective capacity of these cases is 4 to 11 fold greater than those of paucibacillary leprosy. Although the role of insect vectors of bacilli is still not established, mosquitos (Narayanan et al 1978) and flies (Geater 1975) may be effective carriers. However, by and large the infected human being is considered to be the only source. *M. leprae* can remain viable outside the human body in dried nasal discharge for seven days (Daney & Rees 1974) or even more.

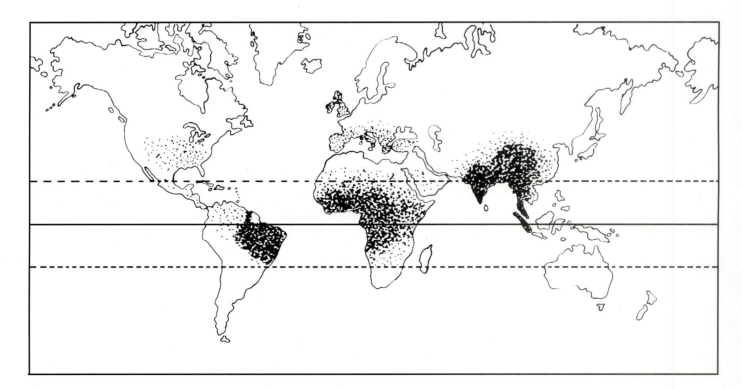

Figure 3

Geographical distribution of leprosy

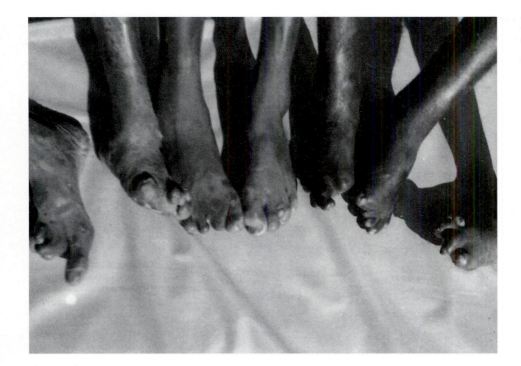

Figure 4
The forefoot is more commonly affected in leprosy than the hindfoot

Pathogenesis

Entering through the skin, bacilli enter the nerve endings and endoneural fine blood vessels and migrate upwards through the Schwann cells and the axons to localize at the site of predilection in the nerve trunk. There they excite a delayed type of hypersensitivity reaction with aggregation of macrophages, epitheloid and lymphoid cells and with a minimal bacterial population. The lepromatous granuloma leads to intraneural compression, ischaemia and axonal degeneration.

Bacilli entering through respiratory or gastrointestinal tracts circulate and excite antibody formation to form immune complexes with suppression of cellular immunity. Bacilli multiply unbridled within the macrophages. Well recognized 'globi', foam cells and macrophage-granulomata dominate the picture.

Classification

Leprosy has been classified mainly in relation to host immune response. With the introduction of the infection the bacilli may or may not be completely phagocytosed and quickly destroyed. The defence mechanisms produce a reaction which is usually transient and may produce spontaneous healing in up to 75% of cases.

Based upon the immunological spectrum, Ridley & Jopling (1966) have proposed a five-group system of classification of leprosy, which is useful in assessing the disease and its prognosis. The groups, according to severity and infectivity across the spectrum are tuberculoid (TT), borderline tuberculoid (BT), borderline (BB), borderline lepromatous (BL) and lepromatous (LL). With proper chemotherapy, the borderline type shows an upgrade towards the TT end of the specrum, and without treatment a downgrade to a subtype of LL subpolar lepromatous leprosy (known as LLs to differentiate it from the polar type LLp). Group LLp is immunologically stable, LLs is not.

Clinical features

Due to a variable incubation period (2 to 30 years) and bizarre manifestations, one must be vigilant in suspecting and diagnosing leprosy (Fig. 4). The clinical features of only the polarized cases are more or less clear. The onset of the disease is mostly gradual and insidious, however it may appear suddenly and even with malaise, fever and pain.

Intermediate type

Typically, a child with prolonged contact develops one or two hypopigmented weals, papules or pale macules with decreased sweating in an area of normal or slightly depressed sensation. These lesions may persist for months to a year and in 50 to 75% of cases there is spontaneous recovery. In others, depending upon the cell-mediated immune response and proper treatment,

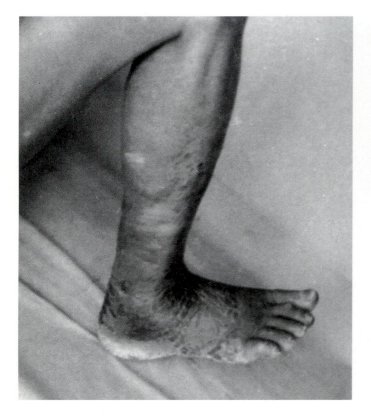

Figure 5
Tuberculoid lesions of the foot – infiltration on the periphery and scaling in the central area, with atrophy

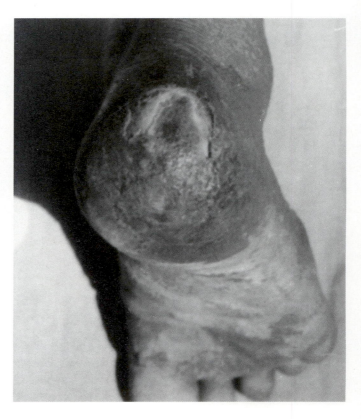

Figure 6
Friction ulcers due to a tight closed boot

there may be either upgrading towards the tuberculoid pole or downgrading towards the lepromatous pole, or persistence as borderline unstable leprosy.

Tuberculoid type

Jadassohn used the term 'tuberculoid' leprosy to describe a type in which the histopathological features resemble non-caseous tuberculosis. The main clinical manifestation in this type of leprosy is the peripheral nerve involvement with or without dermal lesions (Fig. 5). Motor loss is mainly manifest in involvement of the ulnar (ulnar claw hand) or ulnar and median (main en griffe), common peroneal (footdrop) and, rarely, radial (wrist drop) nerves. Other nerves affected are greater auricular, superficial peroneal, antebrachial cutaneous, posterior tibial and lateral cutaneous nerve of thigh. Very rarely there may be trigeminal, olfactory and facial nerve involvement.

The nerves are thickened and there may be cold abscesses in their course. Anaesthetic skin of the foot and hand can be subjected to repeated and prolonged trauma, leading to trophic ulceration. Anaesthesia, disuse, repeated trauma and trophic ulceration lead to osseous atrophy with shortening and absorption of the digits of the toes and fingers.

Lepromatous type

Most cases of this type develop from borderline leprosy. The main clinical manifestations in this form are the dermal and mucosal lesions. The neural affections are comparatively late. The peripheral nerves at the sites of predilection laden with leprosy bacilli (even in early stage) may be enlarged, soft and tender. Later the nerve trunks are liable to become fibrosed and paralysed, leading to a glove and stocking anaesthesia, claw hand and foot-drop. Icthyosis and chronic oedema of legs and feet (more in the evening) are common in this type of leprosy, and they may even be the early manifestations.

The long bones of the foot and hand usually undergo osteoporosis, atrophy and destruction. Trophic changes are mostly seen in the feet. In the phalanges atrophic changes start from the periphery and ultimately the whole diaphysis may look like a stick of bone before dissolution (concentric bone atrophy). In the metatarsals the trophic and absorptive changes usually start in the heads and proceed proximally, leading to gradual thinning of the bone which looks like a pencil tip. Ultimately the stumpy end of the toes may remain loosely connected to the foot without any bony continuity.

The joints of the feet may undergo subluxation, deformity and ankylosis due to muscular paralysis, disuse, infiltrative lesions in the overlying skin, trophic ulceration and secondary infection through ulcers. Secondary neuropathic joints may also develop due to continued sensory loss which also predisposes to friction lesions (Fig. 6).

Borderline or dimorphous type

This type usually occurs in individuals with limited cell-mediated immunity. Here dermal lesions present the mixed picture of tuberculoid and lepromatous types, but there is always marked neural involvement. These cases remain unstable until they polarize to either side depending upon the treatment given and the level of immunity. Usually there is downgrading to a lepromatous type.

Diagnosis

Subjects presenting with hypopigmented or discoloured skin patches, vague sensory complaints like hyperaesthesia, tingling or unnoticed burning of the hands and feet, non-healing ulcers on the sole, non-traumatic foot-drop or persistent blood-tinged nasal discharge must be investigated for leprosy.

Investigations

Leprosy, being a chronic disease, has no reactive haematological changes. However more than 50% of patients (whether treated LL type or BL type and occasionally even untreated ones) suffer from the antigen-induced reactive phenomenon of erythema nodosum leprosum (probably derived from dead lepra bacilli). At this time abnormal laboratory tests may show a polymorphonuclear leucocytosis and raised sedimentation rate. Otherwise, there may be comparative lymphocytosis, a low haemoglobin and little elevation of the sedimentation rate.

Nasal scrape

Nasal blowings or nasal scrapings taken from the anterior part of the septum always show enough organisms in the untreated LL type, but are always negative in BB, BT and TT types. In BL types they are usually negative.

Skin smear

Skin smears can be taken from active leprosy ulcers or, better, from an active lesion on the ear lobules and dorsum of the fingers. The smear, collected by the slit and scrape method, is stained by the Ziehl–Neelsen technique. Plenty of acid fast bacilli are always demonstrable in LL, BL and BB lesions and scanty in BT, but none show in the TT (except during reactions) and intermediate groups.

Skin biopsy

This is essential to classify the type of lesion accurately, by properly analysing the histological changes and cell infiltrates. The biopsy material should be taken from the most active part of the lesions (e.g. the edge in tuberculoid (TT) and centre in the lepromatous (LL)) and must include the subcutaneous fat. To show the bacilli in sections Fite–Faraco's method of staining is used.

Foot in leprosy

The affections of the foot are caused both directly by the disease process and secondarily due to nerve involvement, deformity and secondary infection. True leprosy infection manifests on the dorsum of the foot, mainly in the lepromatous variety and during lepra reactions, as a swollen foot with nodularity and painful joints. In secondary affections the dominant role is played by nerve damage, mainly of the lateral popliteal, posterior tibial and the calcaneal branch of the posterior tibial nerves.

Trophic ulcers

Synonyms: plantar ulcer, perforating ulcer, neuropathic ulcer, foot pressure ulcer.

Plantar ulcer is a chronic resistant recurrent ulcer of an anaesthetic foot, where walking is still possible. Of all the complications of leprosy, it is the most unpleasant and annoying. It occurs in about 12% of leprosy patients (Languillon 1964, Srinivasan 1976). Males are affected about two or three times as often as females. Patients with ulcers are very rare below the age of 20, and usually have tuberculoid or indeterminate leprosy (paucibacillary type). Price (1964a,b) has classified these ulcers into:

(1) Infected wounds (caused by thorns or sharp nails and burns).
(2) Friction ulcers usually develop on the dorsum of the foot, due to sandal straps and unsuitable footwear, and on the sole on the projecting part of the deformed foot.
(3) Plantar ulcers occur on any insensitive sole, where the patient still walks. The precipitating factor in producing the ulcer is pressure, unbalanced in both amount and time. Trauma due to stones, nails and pointed objects may also lead to some changes.

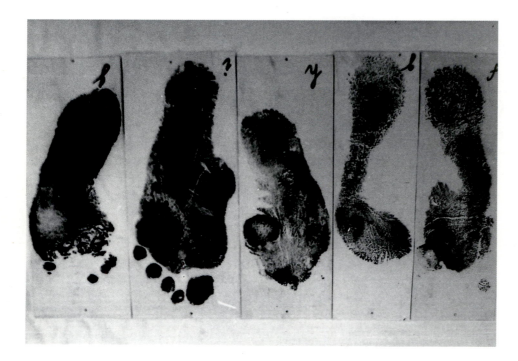

Figure 7

(a) Footprint in leprosy: absorbed and distorted great toe; fallen second, third and fifth toes; ulcer beneath the anterior end of the tarsal border of the foot. (b) Absorbed and fallen toes; healed ulcer beneath base of fifth toe. (c) Fallen toes; secondary punched-out healing ulcer on the collapsed anterior end of the medial arch; partially healed ulcer on the lateral border of the foot.
(d) Collapse of both longitudinal and transverse arches of the foot; partially healed ulcer beneath the base of the great toe and a healed ulcer on the anterior end of the collapsed medial arch. (e) Extensive active deep ulcer beneath the bases of first, second, third, fourth and fifth toes with varying absorption of all the toes; secondary varus and adduction deformities of the forefoot

Table 2 Primary deformities (Lennox 1964)	
Muscle imbalance	*Site of ulcer*
Foot drop (with loss of peroneal)	Anterolateral border
Foot drop (peronei intact)	Anteromedial border
Claw toes	Dorsum and pulp of toes, Metatarsal heads

Healing, if it happens at all, occurs at cessation of exudate, epithelial cover and consolidation (Price 1964a,b); the ultimate result is scarring. Further progress involves the cycle of scar–ulcer–scar (Anderson 1964). Due to various factors (intrinsic paralysis, ligamentous avulsion and damage and destruction of bones and joints) collapse of the foot (lateral, medial and total) develop (Fig. 7). These, together with fixed deformities, favour the development of secondary ulcerations (Table 2).

Management

General

A good rapport between doctor and patient, proper education about disease and morale boosting of the patient are essential in order to gain confidence and co-operation of the latter, in order that the disease may be finally arrested by therapy without any major deformity or disability of the foot, except for some sensory loss (unavoidable) and motor palsy (which can be compensated for). Admission to a hospital for a few days proves useful for establishing the rapport and educating the patient.

Segregation

This used to be indicated at the start of treatment but now, except for the initial few weeks in an open LL type, it is unnecessary and avoids putting stigma upon the patient. However, close contact with others (especially infants and children) should be avoided.

General health care

The patient must be properly educated and shown how to take care of his hands, feet and eyes, as preventative and therapeutic measures.

Specific chemotherapy

Chaulmoogra oil is now superseded. Dapsone, 4:4″-diaminodiphenylsulphone (DDS) is the drug of choice and is essentially bacteristatic in action. The dose (in adults) is 1–2 mg per kg body weight (WHO 1982), given regularly as a component of a combination regime. Rifampicin is the most potent bactericidal antileprosy drug today.

Multidrug therapy (MDT)

In 1982 the WHO Study Group recommended multidrug regimens for treating the paucibacillary and multibacillary leprosy patients. The aims were to prevent and/or overcome the emergence of drug resistance, to help reduce bacterial persistence and to rapidly arrest the transmission of the disease.

Surgery

The role of decompressing the posterior tibial nerve and vessels in the fibro-osseous tunnel behind the medial malleolus in accelerating the healing process and retarding the rate of recurrence of the ulcers is being increasingly recognized (Carayon 1971, Panande & Azhaguraj 1975, Rao & Panda 1985, Patond & Srivastava 1991). If the posterior tibial nerve conduction velocity is found to be decreased, its decompression may help in prevention of plantar ulceration.

Tio et al (1986) have reported more than 75% success with ambulatory treatment of plantar leprosy ulcers in rural areas. The ulcers were plugged with Zincoil (75% zinc oxide and 25% cod liver oil) and the patients were instructed to modify their walk, according to the site of the ulcer. Topical application of zinc sulphate (40% emulsion as a tape applied to trophic plantar ulcers) induces a local hyperaemic state, which reduces the healing time.

Foot deformities should be adequately corrected to prevent recurrent ulceration problems. For foot-drop, a splint should be tried initially for at least six months. Thereafter, the deformity can be corrected by tendon transfer (tibialis posterior or peronei to the dorsum of the foot with or without extensor hallucis longus plication) or by a stabilization procedure (Lambrinudi's) or modified (Pandey 1990) triple arthrodesis. Fixed deformities like equinovarus will require an 'oblique sliding osteotomy' of foot or wedge resection. Persistent ulcers and unstable adherent scars at the metatarsal heads should be resected. Excessive scarring in the forefoot is better managed by forefoot amputation followed by the use of well moulded special footwear. Equinus deformities usually yield to Achilles tendon lengthening and posterior capsulotomy, but for resistant cases dorsal wedge resection or oblique sliding osteotomy of the foot (Pandey 1986) may be required.

For mobile claw toe, transposition of the flexor digitorum longus to the dorsum of the proximal phalanx can be performed, but in the big toe interphalangeal joint fusion is better (Rose 1962). Rigid claw toes, where the forefoot is relatively intact, should be treated by fusing the interphalangeal joints of the toes. Where there is superficial forefoot scarring, fusion of the interphalangeal joints should be followed by use of well soled footwear, but where there is loss of subcutaneous tissue and metatarsal heads, it is better to amputate the forefoot proximal to the metatarsal heads. Claw toes, with the proximal phalanges grossly hyperextended and a relatively intact forefoot, should be managed by excision of the proximal phalanges of the second to fifth toes through a plantar incision.

Leprotic neuroarthropathic ankle should be arthrodesed, since it not only clears the local symptoms and improves the alignment and stability of the affected ankle, but also helps in halting the neuropathic destruction of mid tarsal joints (Shibata et al 1990).

Footwear in leprosy foot

The purposes of footwear (Girling 1966, Brand 1977) are

(1)   to take care of anaesthetic skin,
(2)   to prevent undue pressure on the vulnerable sites for trophic ulcers and on scarred areas,
(3)   to protect from thorns or nails and
(4)   to substitute for the deficiencies.

It is difficult to get an 'all-in-one' design. Usually special footwear is not cosmetically acceptable. Open slippers have been more beneficial and acceptable, and simple strap microcellular rubber chappals have proved quite useful (Karat 1969).

Rehabilitation

Properly cared for, no leprosy foot should become a problem in rehabilitation of the patient back to his original or a modified occupation. A word of caution: 'patients must not walk on wounded feet' (Rose 1962) is mandatory. The sole aim of physical therapy for Hansen's foot should be prevention and management of neuropathic foot lesions

Treponematosis

Endemic treponematosis continues to be a health problem in some tropical countries. Treponematosis includes

(1)   yaws due to *Treponema pertenue*,
(2)   pinta due to *T. carateum* and *T. herrejoni*,
(3)   syphilis:
         (a) non-venereal, and
         (b) venereal,
         both due to *T. pallidum*.

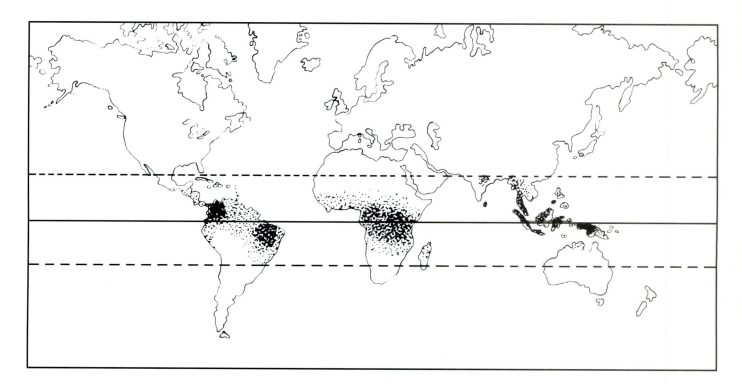

Figure 8

Geographical distribution of yaws

Although the epidemiological behaviour and the clinical features of the different treponematoses could be adequately differentiated, the impossibility of cultivating these spirochaetes on artificial media, the common serological reactions and the details of the pathological changes have led to the concept of a unitary theory of the aetiology of these forms of treponematosis.

The foot is not affected in the early stage of pinta, but plantar manifestations are seen in even the early stages of yaws and non-venereal syphilis and infrequently in the secondary stage of venereal syphilis. In tertiary stages, gummetous and destructive lesions can be seen in all these forms, but mostly in yaws.

Yaws

Yaws is a contagious granulomatous disease caused by a non-venereally transmitted spirochaete, *Treponeme pertenue*; it mainly involves the skin and bones, and is usually crippling but not fatal. Yaws is mostly confined to the hot and humid forest regions of the tropics, although it is prevalent in the Far East and China, where it extends into temperate zones (Fig. 8).

With the eradication programme against yaws (WHO) it has ceased to be a public health problem. However, the problem of residual yaws or recrudescence of yaws will persist for some time; in fact there was a resurgence in the 1980s in West and Central Africa and the South Pacific.

It is a disease of childhood (after 1 year of age) (it is not congenital) and adolescence. In hyperendemic areas the peak incidence is in the 2 to 5 year age group, whereas in the low endemic areas the highest seroprevalence is in the older age group. However, 70% of infections occur before the age of 15. Males are more frequently affected than females. The causative organism is *T. pertenue* (tightly coiled, rigid and motile spirochaetes measuring 16 μm × 0.2 μm), which exists in the epidermis of the lesions, the lymph nodes, spleen and bones. They cannot be cultured *in vitro*. Baboons may act as a reservoir for yaws.

The disease is transmitted by direct contact: organisms from the discharge of an infectious lesion enter through a breach in the epidermis. Transmission from an infected mother to her infant and vice versa is often possible. Vectors (Hippelates, flies, cockroaches) may spread the infection.

Pathology

Animal experiments show that immediately after entering through the breached or intact skin the treponemes are carried to the lymph nodes and also circulate in the body. Lesions are localized, either in the skin or the bone, or both, in all three stages of the disease. The basic pathology is the development, at the site of

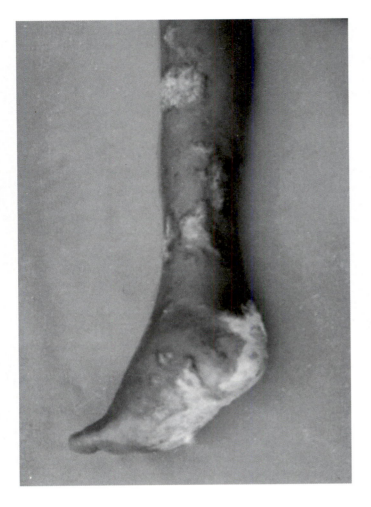

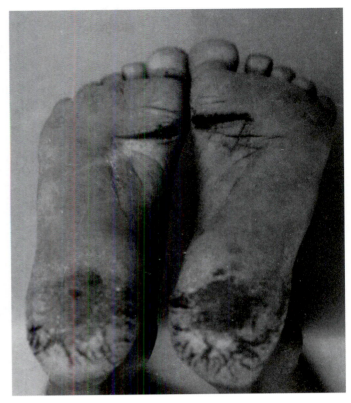

Figure 10

Almost symmetrical 'crab yaws' – late hyperkeratotic lesions with cracks and fissures, partly due to prolonged barefoot walking

Figure 9

Early framboesiform lesion (the patient had adherent skin at sole and heel following burn in early childhood)

cutaneous invasion, of a proliferative granuloma containing numerous treponemes in the epidermis.

Clinical features

The incubation period varies between 10 days and 6 months (average 3 to 5 weeks). As in other trepanosomal infections the clinical manifestations of yaws can be divided into three distinguishable stages: primary, secondary and tertiary (Hacket 1957), separated by latent periods. The early lesions are multiple, non-destructive and contagious, whereas the late lesions are destructive and non-contagious.

Primary stage

Synonyms: mamanpion, mother yaws, protopianoma, buba madra.

Lesions usually develop at the site of inoculation of infection in an exposed part of the body, three-quarters being on the lower part of the leg and foot (Fig. 9).

They start with erythematous infiltrated papules, then nodules form which gradually enlarge into papillomatous, broad-based granuloma exuding whitish-yellow, serous discharge, swarming with treponemes. This later forms a yellow scab. Ultimately, typical raspberry lesions are produced, which are painless but bleed easily. Mother yaws heal spontaneously without much scarring. Soles of feet are not common sites, but margins and the clefts are affected. There may be mild constitutional features.

Secondary stage

The secondary lesions usually appear 8 to 16 weeks after the onset of the disease, after the primary lesions have healed, but overlap is not infrequent and the period of appearance may also vary widely. The lesions are basically similar to the primary ones, but are multiple and of various sizes. Lesions erupting in successive crops spread widely, but gradually tend to localize around the body orifices (mouth, nose and urogenital regions), the periaxillary regions and the soles and palms. General symptoms such as headache, irregular fever, loss of appetite and weight, pains in the bones and joints and generalized lymphadenopathy may precede the eruptions.

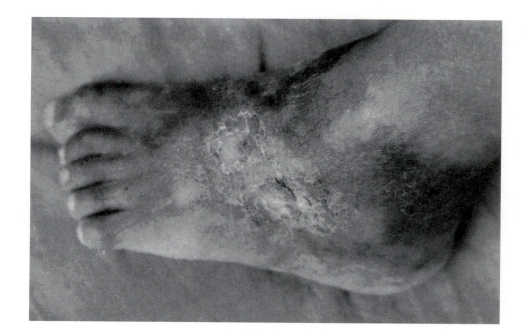

Figure 11
Late yaws – infiltrative lesion
mimicking lupus vulgaris

Skin lesions The exudative papillomatous eruptions covered with yellowish or brownish crusts resemble mother yaws. They are known as 'daughter yaws', pianomas or framboesiomas. Smaller lesions are miniature yaws, and peripheral extension of daughter yaws may produce circinate yaws (tineal yaws). Cutaneous yaws are painless but may itch.

Plantar lesions Those on the sole and palm, where the epithelium is thick and firm, appear late and are painful. The plantar skin becomes dry and peels and is irregularly thickened by hyperkeratotic plaques, cracks and fissures. A cherry-like granuloma appears in the well of the fissured horny layers. The granulomatous tissue is commonly present on the outer and inner borders of the sole, and in the clefts of the toes. The yaws on the soles produce painful disability and the patient tries to walk on the margin of the foot, giving rise to the term crab yaws (Fig. 10) (Basset et al 1972). The scattered areas of hyperkeratotic plaque on the sole may fall out, leaving behind punched out excavations, known as clavus. The bones (leg, forearm, hand, foot, skull) are commonly involved; the basic lesions are periostitis and gummatous osteitis. In the foot basic osseous lesions are thickening, cortical expansion and/or destructive focal rarefaction occurs in the metatarsals and phalanges. Late secondary lesions of skull and facial bones may lead to gangosa (collapse of nose with perforation of palate) and goundou (periosteal deposit across the face on the sides of the nasal bridge). In joints, hydrarthrosis and rheumatic manifestations (rheumatic yaws) may occur.

Latent yaws After spontaneous resolution of 'early yaws' serological changes may persist to manifest later as early yaws, late yaws or tertiary lesions.

Tertiary stage
In this stage also the main affections are of skin, subcutaneous tissue and bones. The basic reactions are those of active and destructive granulomata, in which the gummatous lesions are at first hard, mobile and painless. Gradually lesions undergo central necrosis with cold abscess formation. The abscess bursts, forming a chronic, indolent, slowly progressive ulcer with yellowish slough and deep connections (Fig. 11). They ultimately heal with severe scarring, which may lead to disfigurement and deformity. Keloid formation and secondary elephantiasis may occur. Very rarely the chronic ulcers may end in epithelioma. The most common legacies are keratoderma and diffuse or localized hyperkeratosis of the sole and palm. Such painful lesions on one side of the sole lead to crab yaws. Osseous lesions in this stage are limited, but of a serious nature (osteoperiostitis, oval cortical rarefaction, necrosis, sequestrum formation, pathological fracture).

Investigation

Isolation of *T. pertenue* from the exudate of the suspected primary and secondary lesions by dark ground examination or with silver stains is confirmatory. Inoculations of treponema have been possible in monkeys, rabbits and hamsters. Serological tests carried out for syphilis (e.g. Wassermann, Kahn etc) are positive in increasing titre from four weeks after the appearance of the primary lesions, with possible cross-immunity. Differential diagnosis:

- Framboesiomas from framboesoid leishmaniasis, framboesiform syphilides, paracoccidioidomycosis.
- Bubides or piamides in yaws from pityriasis versicolor, psoriasis, pityriasis rosea.

- Hyperkeratotic lesion of sole from keratoma plantare sulcatum, plantar warts.
- Late yaws from leprosy and tuberculosis.

Treatment

Penicillin G has dramatically revolutionized the treatment and control of yaws (also bejel, pinta and syphilis). The early lesions become dark field negative within 48 hours and disappear within two weeks, even with the single dose treatment. (Age below 5 years: 0.3 Mu as single dose; 5 to 15 years: 1.2 Mu in divided doses, at 4 to 5 days; adults: 2.4 Mu in divided doses at 4 to 5 days). Ulcerated yaws lesions should be adequately dressed and supported.

Pinta

Synonyms: carate (among Carib and Aztec Indians), mal del pinto (Cuba).

Pinta, essentially a disease of childhood and affecting only the skin, is the weakest of the human treponematoses, caused by *T. carateum*, which is morphologically indistinguishable from *T. pertenue* and *T. pallidum*. The disease is now restricted to the Philippines and some areas of the Pacific.

Aetiology and pathology

T. carateum gains access mostly through abraded skin. The incubation period is 2 to 3 weeks. There is a weaker cross-immunity with syphilis than in yaws, and pinta may co-exist with syphilis.

The essential granuloma develops slowly in the subcutaneous layer along with hypertrophy of the overlying skin, which later undergoes atrophy or depigmentation. Local and regional lymphadenitis may develop.

Clinical features

Progress is through three overlapping stages. In the primary stage, itchy erythematous papules, gradually changing into elevated erythematous patches, develop on the exposed parts of the body (dorsum of the foot and leg, the forearm and/or dorsum of the hand, elbows, neck, face, buttocks and thigh). After about a year the secondary stage creeps in, characterized by generalized cutaneous rashes or papules known as pintides; these multiply and may coalesce, and may be hypopigmented, pigmentary or erythematosquamous. The tertiary stage is manifest 2 to 5 years later and lesions consist of irregular pigmented spots in different shades of grey, steel, ash or blue (Lawton-Smith 1971). Eventually depigmented areas appear, especially near bony prominences. In the later stages there may be overlap lesions of dyschromia, hypochromia and achromia in the same patient (Fig. 12).

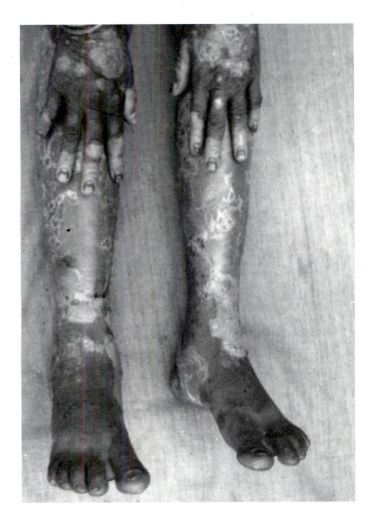

Figure 12

Late pinta with mixed overlapping lesions of dyschromia, hypochromia and achromia. Areas with complete loss of melanin mimic vitiligo

Treatment

Repository long-acting penicillin (procaine penicillin G in oil with 2% aluminium monostearate) or benzathine penicillin G in a total dosage of 2.4 Mu is the drug of choice (Marquez et al 1955). Except for the prolonged depigmented and atrophic lesions of the tertiary stage, other manifestations can be cured with proper treatment.

Filariasis

Synonyms: tropical elephantiasis, lymphatic filariasis, Malabar legs.

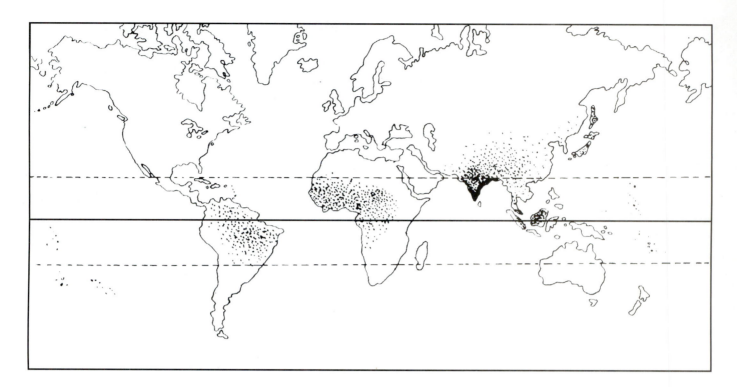

Figure 13

Geographical distribution of filariasis

Filariasis is distributed worldwide (between the latitudes 45° north to 25° south), and is found mainly in Asia (Fig. 13). Globally, filariasis appears to be on the increase (WHO 1967). Of the various filariodea nematodes, *W. bancrofti* and *B. timori* are responsible for producing lymphatic filariasis. Numerically, the public health problem of lymphatic filariasis is greatest in China, India and Indonesia – accounting for two-thirds of the estimated World problem. WHO (1992) reported that 3287 million people live in countries where this disease is endemic; 751 million are at risk of infection and 78.6 million are actually infected (72.8 million by *W. bancrofti* and 5.8 million by *B. malayi* or *B. timori*).

Life cycle of W. bancrofti

Man is the only known definitive host. Infective larvae pass from the peripheral blood to the lymphatics, where they mature. Mature worms copulate and the viviparous female gives off microfilaria (about 50 000 per day) which appear in the peripheral blood one year after infection. Mosquitoes are the intermediate host.

Pathogenesis

The pathogenesis of lymphatic filariasis falls into three stages: inflammatory, obstructive and definitive elephantiasis.

Inflammatory stage

Prolonged repeated infection with the adult worm and later with microfilaria is an essential factor, but the individual's acquired immunosensitivity also plays an important role (Edeson et al 1960, Schacher & Sahyoun 1967, Dandero et al 1975, Denham & Rogers 1975). There is a temporary lymphatic obstruction leading to lymphoedema, which improves with subsidence of inflammation, leaving the lymphatic wall weaker. With repeated intermittent rise in lymph pressure, afferent lymphatics become dilated and tortuous, resulting in permanent lymph varices.

Occlusive stages (lymphoedema and elephantiasis)

Maturing worms induce endothelial thickening, obliterature endolymphangitis and fibrin deposition. The death of worms locally produces an epitheloid granuloma and a foreign body giant-cell reaction and even calcification, which press upon the lymphatics leading to occlusion. The inflammatory processes gradually lead to permanent fibrotic obliteration of the lymphatic channels, especially those lying in the compact connective tissue of the leg. The regional lymph glands lose their filtering capacity due to fibrosis, which further augments the back pressure producing lymphoedema. Secondary infection (β haemolytic streptococci leading to local abscess formation, which may rupture and/or fibrose) also adds to the lymphatic obstruction. Gradually those parts of the limb below the obstruction become enlarged with fibrotic infiltration and thickening of the tissues leading to irreversible elephantiasis.

Histology

The fibro-fatty tissues are oedematous and irregularly infiltrated with mature fibrous tissue, round cells and eosinophils. The lymphatic system in the affected region becomes hypertrophic and dilated with lobulations. It is rare to find the filarial worm in the elephantoid tissue, however a dead or calcified worm (usually detected by X-ray) may be detected in the lymphatic channels and glands.

Clinical features

The incubation period (interval between invasion by infective larvae and clinical manifestations) is about 8 to 16 months whereas the prepatent period (interval between inoculation of infective larvae and the first appearance of detectable microfilaria) is not exactly known. Although there can be an overlap, the clinical presentation may be considered in relation to the stages of the disease.

Early filariasis or invasion stage
During invasion stage lymphatic filariasis may pass through the following stages (WHO 1984):

(1) Asymptomatic amicrofilaraemia: it is not possible to detect the disease at this stage by available diagnostic procedures.
(2) Asymptomatic microfilaraemia: in this group individuals do not manifest clinically, but they show microfilaria in blood. They are the carriers of the disease in the community.

Acute inflammatory stage
This stage is clinically manifest by filarial fever, retrograde and centrifugal lymphangitis lasting for a few days, lymphadenitis, and lymphoedema. These are most probably produced by the toxins liberated while the dead worms undergo absorption, disintegration or calcification. These features usually come in recurrent episodes. It usually affects the legs in the malleolar region, the testes, spermatic cord and breasts in bancroftial filariasis and the legs or arms in *B. malayi* infection. The affected lymph vessels feel like cords and are acutely tender. The overlying skin is oedematous and itchy and presents congested red streaks running along the course of the affected vessels. Local or regional lymphadenitis and local abscess may develop.

Chronic obstructive manifestation
Repeated inflammatory reactions over 10 to 15 years end in progressive obstruction of the lymph vessels, resulting in various pathologies. There may be no history of an earlier episode, yet chronic filarial manifestations (e.g.

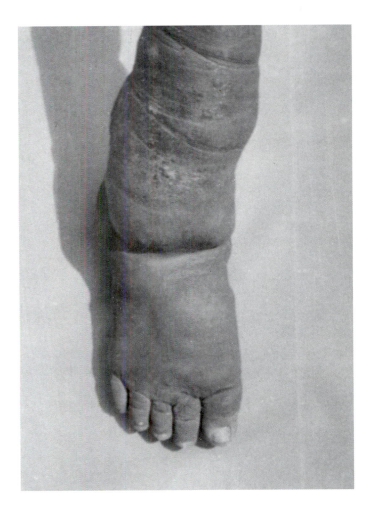

Figure 14

Elephantiasis of the foot and leg with deep transverse grooves, ulcers and pachydermia

hydrocele, lymph varices, filarial arthropathy, filarial osteomyelitis) may be found.

Elephantiasis

Lymphoedema and elephantiasis are the result of anatomical and/or functional blockage of the lymphatics and are usually seen in individuals with recurrent infections over prolonged periods who reside in endemic areas for 15 to 20 years (Figs 14 and 15).

Treatment

During the inflammatory stages treatment consists of rest with the affected part supported, antipyretics, anti-allergics and corticoids during reactions, and laxatives or purgatives for constipation.

Specific chemotherapy
Microfilaricidal drugs (antimony, Antrypol and arsenicals) kill adult filarae, but are too toxic for general human use.

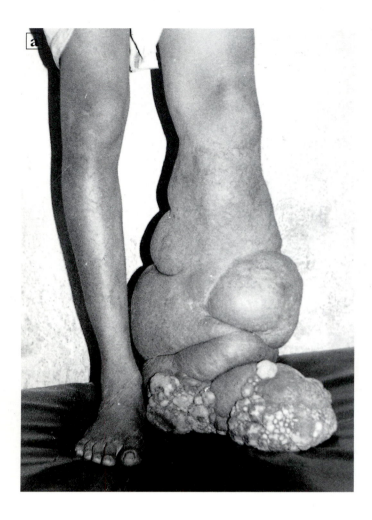

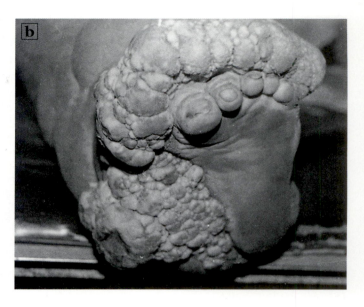

Figure 15

(a, b) Elephantiasis, with enormous swelling of the foot and ankle, furrows, lobulations, nodules and warty projects. The toes and soles are not affected (by courtesy of Dr K D Sharan)

On the other hand, microfilaricidal drugs (diethylcarbamazine citrate) are quite effective in controlling the disease.

Physical measures
Reducing the likelihood of developing chronic obstructive lesions, by repeated DEC therapy, can prevent lymphoedema. Measures such as elevation of the limb, prolonged firm sponge-elastic bandaging, spiral elastic stockings, pneumatic stockings, pulsatile air pressure devices, intermittent positive pressure apparatus and the avoidance of prolonged standing or sitting with the leg dependent are effective in the early stages.

Dracuncalosis

Synonyms: dracontiasis, guinea worm, serpent worm, medina worm, dragon worm, naru.

Dracunculosis is a chronic parasitic infection of human connective and subcutaneous tissues caused by the nematode worm, *Dracunculus medinensis*, the females being solely responsible for clinical manifestations. Infection is more or less limited to tropical and subtropical regions since the larvae thrive best at temperatures

between 25° and 30° C. They cannot develop below 19° (Muller 1979). Out of an estimated 48 million cases in the world, the majority are in Africa and Asia (Harman 1979) and also in the Caribbean islands, Brazil, Guyana, southern Russia and North and South America) (Fig. 16). *D. definensis* has two hosts: the definitive host is man (but it has been found in dogs and cats), and the intermediate host is the crustacean Cyclops. Cyclops thrive in dirty, stagnant and shallow water (e.g. ponds and step-wells in India, rural pods in Ghana, desert cipterus in Iran). Natives use such water for drinking.

Clinical features

Clinical manifestations are due to toxins liberated from the anterior end of the worm, the presence of a gravid female worm superficially just prior to discharge of the larvae, or to the resultant ulcers due to rupture of the vesicles. General features may appear as anaphylactic reactions due to the absorption of toxins liberated by the worm, and these are generalized urticaria, pruritus, giddiness, nausea, vomiting, asthma, rigors or diarrhoea. With the subsidence of the general features local reactions appear, usually at night. The patient feels a sharp pain at the site of the worm piercing the cuticle, where a

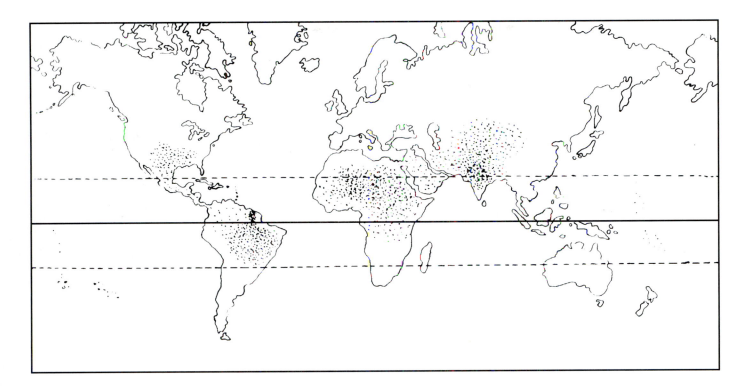

Figure 16

Geographical distribution of guinea worm

papule develops. For a couple of days, the site remains erythematous, indurated, raised and tender, followed by the appearance of a vesicle in the centre, due to raising of the epidermis over the head of the piercing worm. The patient feels a marked burning sensation and likes to immerse the part in cold water. The vesicle ruptures, resulting in a superficial ulcer of about 1.5 cm diameter with copious discharge of serosanguinous fluid. The periphery of the ulcer shows spontaneous healing, but at the centre a minute hole is left, through which the head of the worm can be seen protruding. With superimposed staphylococcal or streptococcal or other infections, the features may be complicated and become chronic.

Investigation

The differential white cell count shows a high eosinophilia during the appearance of active general and early local symptoms. The milky fluid ejected after cold douching around the vesicular area, if examined under the microscope, shows myriads of coiled up larvae.

Complications

Allergic reactions may be very serious. The victims are usually poor farmers and labourers, who suffer economically due to prolonged incapacitation. Arthritis and contractures may disable the patient.

Management

Prodromal symptoms (of urticaria, pruritis, fever, vomiting, etc) being allergic in origin are controlled by antihistaminics. Chemotherapy employs several drugs (niridazole, thiabendazole, metronidazole, diethylcarbamazine), which have been found effective in the early stages (Hawking 1956). If chemotherapy is effective, manual removal of the worm may not be required. However, the worm should usually be removed with care. The ruptured vesicle should be cleaned and dressed. Cold compressing and douching of the region for two or three days usually stops the larval discharge. The head of the worm should be identified in the centre of the ulcer, and is caught with forceps and cautiously pulled, while the other hand is used to massage the worm towards the wound to expel it. Gaining a sufficient length, the head end of the worm is tied on a sterile stick and the worm is gradually wound over it (Fig. 17). Each day, 5 to 10 cm or even more of the worm can be extracted and should the worm break, it should be left in situ without any surgical attempt at removal (Fig. 18).

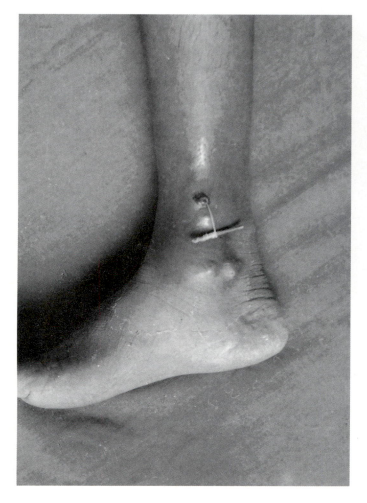

Figure 17
The traditional method of removing the worm by coiling on a match stick. At a distal level two fresh vesicles are appearing

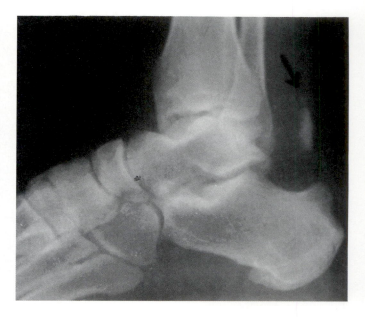

Figure 18
Radiograph showing a late calcified worm (arrowed) around the Achilles tendon

Tungiasis

Synonyms: Jiggers, chigoe, chique.

This condition, caused by a small parasite, *Tunga penetrans* (chigoe flea), is mainly seen in South America, the West Indies, tropical Africa, Madagascar and the Indian subcontinent. In spite of being formerly restricted to the equatorial zones, the disease is being reported in Europe.

The parasites mainly thrive in dry sandy soil. When gravid, the female flea usually tries to enter the sole crevices and fissures, the toe webs or around the toenails. The flea immediately starts burrowing through the skin deep into the dermis, and will reach the stratum granulosum in as short a time as ten minutes. Except for the narrow posterior part, the whole of the flea becomes enveloped in the host skin. A horny mass develops around the burrow which appears as a pit with a black dot in its centre. In one to two weeks, the gravid female distends to the size of a pea as the eggs mature and this causes inflammation and irritation. Itching causes the subject to scratch and the eggs are gradually discharged and, more rarely, the whole flea. A localized abscess and later an ulcer may form. Secondary infection may develop with sheddings of ulcerated skin. The remnants of the parasite are expelled with the necrotic tissue, leaving behind a pitted sole (Fig 19). Regional lymphangitis, lymphadenitis or more severe complications may occur, such as thrombophlebitis, secondary pyogenic infection, tetanus or even gangrene (Harman 1979, White 1982), which may even prove fatal.

Usually one or two jiggers are seen at a time, but there may be numerous lesions, producing a honeycomb of solid patches. With lesions beneath the nail, an irregular pocket of pus may form. However, there may be spontaneous recovery.

Treatment

When detected at an early stage, a thin sterilized needle should be used to enucleate the parasite from the penetrated skin. Care of the ulcer and inflamed area by regular antiseptic dressings should be undertaken. At a later stage it is very difficult to remove the flea, and then they are best killed by turpentine, chloroform or parasiticidal drugs.

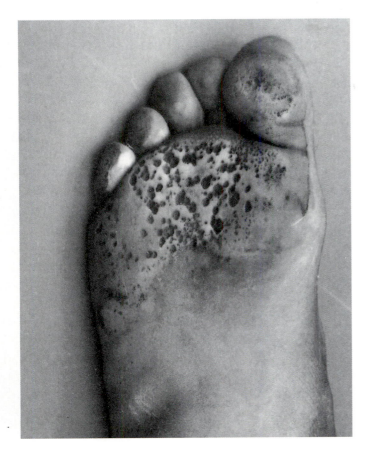

Figure 19

Old unusual jiggers in the sole of the foot

Mycetoma

Synonyms: Madura foot, Maduramycosis, Vincent's white mycetoma, actinomycosis madurae, pseudo-actino-mycosis.

Madura foot is chronic granulomatous systemic fungal disease caused by several species of 'true' fungi, mainly actinomycetes, affecting any part of the body exposed to trauma and resulting in severe damage to skin, sub-cutaneous tissues and bones. It is typically characterized by a painless nodular indurated swelling, suppuration and multiple sinuses discharging coloured granules. Mycetoma is known to occur all over the world, but is most common in tropical and subtropical areas (Africa, India, Mexico, Central America, South Vietnam, Senegal, South America and Italy) (Fig. 20). Abbott (1956) has confirmed its high incidence in the Sudan.

Aetiology

Mycetoma, literally meaning 'fungal tumour', is caused by two main groups of organisms:

(1) the 'true' fungi causing eumycetoma, and
(2) the aerobic actinomycetes causing actinomycetoma.

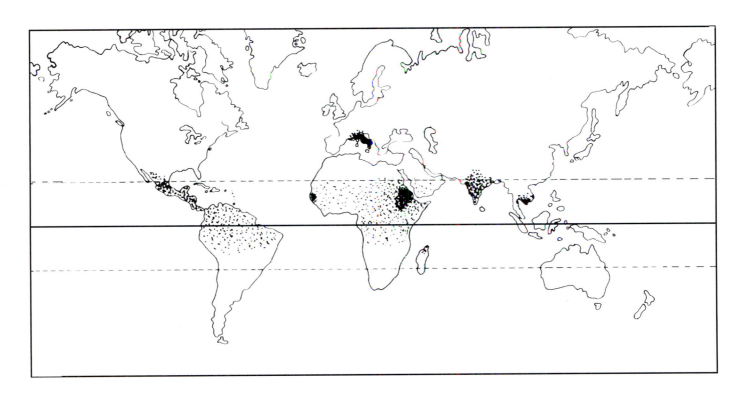

Figure 20

Geographical distribution of mycetoma

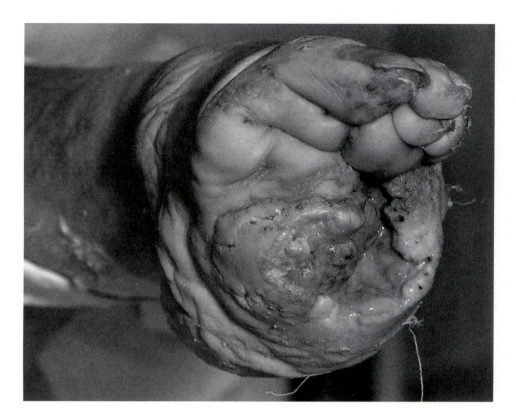

Figure 21
Mycetoma affecting the forefoot

Both groups are characterized by the formation of typical coloured granules ranging from 60 µm to 3 mm in diameter. They occur as saprophytes in soil and on plants or rotting vegetable matter, usually during the hot and rainy seasons. The main victims are poor rural labourers, working bare-footed in the fields, farms or forests. The infection usually gains entry to the subcutaneous tissues through a penetrating injury, caused by a thorn or splinter.

Pathology

The painless swollen foot riddled with numerous nodules and dry or discharging sinuses spreading all over the foot, once seen cannot be mistaken. Nodules develop under the epidermis and rupture into sinuses comminuting with abscesses at various depths and having fibrous or epithelial collars around the opening.

On section it is difficult to identify different tissues except for tendons and fascia. Even bony tissue can disappear in the fungal mass. The whole surface presents a pale greyish-yellow, oily and greasy look, an amalgam of the different tissues. The overall look presents a network of cystic spaces containing friable material of different colours, depending upon the variety of mycetoma.

Histology

The chronic granulomatous reaction results in dense scar formation. In the cystic spaces, characteristically coloured granules are seen and are discharged in pus through multiple sinuses. Epitheloid, plasma and giant cells in the areas of fibrosis may dominate the picture. Actinomycetoma can be recognized by the positive reaction to gram, haematoxylin and eosin or periodic acid-Schiff stains, whereas the fungi are identified by their broad ramifying and often irregular mycelium.

The pathology spreads locally, but lymphatic spread is rare. Systemic spread may occur in actinomycetoma, but never in eumycetoma.

Mycetoma is not a contagious disease. Madura foot patients are deficient in cell-mediated immunity. Precipitating and complement-fixing antibodies develop in mycetomal infection and their level varies in direct proportion to the activity of infection.

Clinical features

Irrespective of the causative fungus of actinomycete, the clinical features are essentially the same: the triad of

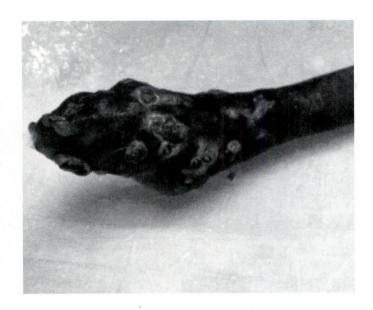

Figure 22

Advanced mycetoma of the foot and lower leg with ulcers and sinuses. Marked equinus deformity

tumefaction, sinus tracts and grains representing micro-colonies of the aetiological agent. The foot is the commonest site (Figs 21 and 22), however, hand, face, leg and shoulder may be affected.

The first manifestation is the appearance of one or more irregular and lumpy, subcutaneous, indurated, pale and painless nodules (Fig. 23). Growing slowly, these nodules rupture producing ulcers or sinuses, through which foul-smelling purulent or seropurulent fluid, containing coloured grains of the fungus, is discharged. The foot gradually enlarges in size, presenting an ugly look with deformed toes and plantarflexed ankle. The leg muscles atrophy. Pain and systemic symptoms are conspicuously absent until there is advanced secondary bacterial infection. Usually pyogenic infection does not penetrate the depths until very late, probably because of antibody activity by the fungi. However, secondary infections and long-standing disabilities may incapacitate the patient, resulting in debility, anaemia and toxaemia. The regional lymph nodes are not affected, and neurological complications and trophic ulceration do not occur in Madura foot. The lesions should be differentiated from chronic infections (tuberculosis, leprosy, pyogenic), botromycosis, mossy foot, neoplasms, etc.

Investigations

Radiographs reveal soft tissue swelling with irregular margins and textures with destructive and proliferative reactions in the underlying bones. Cystic appearances may be seen in the bones. The demonstration of the characteristic granules (grains of mycetoplates) in the discharge from a sinus is essential to clinch the diagnosis. Direct microscopy of the pus is made by placing the granule in a drop of 10% sodium hydroxide and crushing it under a cover slip to examine it for hyphae. Saline-washed granules must be cultured to demonstrate the responsible fungi. Serological studies by immunodiffusion and counterimmunoelectrophoresis with the appropriate antigens can be helpful in studying the responsible organisms with accuracy.

Management

Although the clinical manifestations are almost indistinguishable, the differentiation between Eumycates and actinomycetes is crucial, since the former have resisted the development of any effective chemotherapy while the medical treatment of actinomycetoma is more helpful.

Various drug combinations have been found useful: Dapsone (1.5 mg/kg twice daily with streptomycin (14 mg/kg daily intramuscularly) or co-trimoxazole with streptomycin or oral rifampicin (4 mg/kg daily) have been used successfully. The efficiency of the treatment can be checked by assessing the precipitating antibodies, which disappear with successful treatment. In eumycetoma, although certain fungi have been found relatively sensitive to amphotericin B and griseofulvin *in vitro*, their clinical efficiency has yet to be proved. However, penicillin and griseofulvin should be used postoperatively to check recurrence.

Localized lesions can be best treated by thorough surgical excision. In the case of eumycetoma, due to its resistance in chemotherapy and the inexorability of the disease, complete surgical excision is the only effective management. In most of the advanced cases, planned amputation is the answer. In cases where amputation is not desirable, surgical excision followed by local infiltration of 1–2 ml of tincture of iodine into the suspicious areas every tenth day for 2 months or more should be tried.

In neglected cases the destruction is progressive and often necessitates amputation. In the long-lasting secondary infection, depression and prolonged disabilities incapacitate the patient and may end in death. It is very seldom self-limiting.

Tropical ulcer

Synonyms: tropical sloughing, phagedena, tropical phagedene, tropical phagedenic ulcer, naga ulcer (India).

Tropical ulcer is a clinical syndrome of no definite known aetiology characterized by an initial acute or

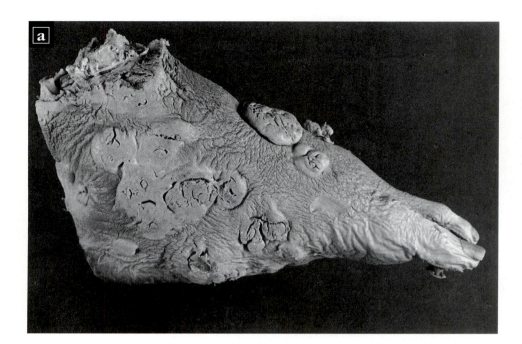

Figure 23

(a) Specimen of Madura foot showing varying swelling of the foot with multiple fungus-like nodules of various sizes spreading up to the ankle. The skin over the nodules is depigmented; the centre of the nodules shows sinuses. (b) The cut surface of Madura foot shows many yellowish granules invading the soft tissues and bones (by courtesy of Professor A V Dhaded, Belgaum)

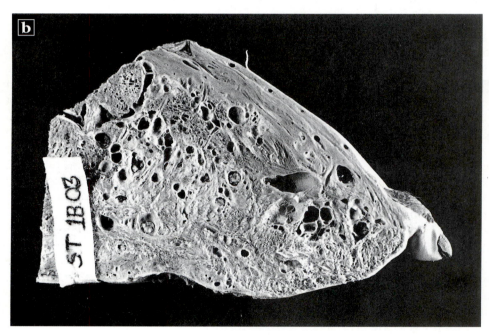

subacute dermal necrosis followed by a chronic non-specific persistent ulcer, usually seen in poor patients inhabiting hot and humid areas.

Geographical distribution

It is commonly found in Africa (commonest in northern Nigeria), South and Central America and India, but can be seen in other parts of the world. No definite cause is known (Simons 1952, Basset 1969, Canizares 1975), but minor trauma has been blamed for the initial tissue necrosis. Children, labourers and farmers working barefoot in crowded, unhygienic surroundings are the usual victims. Anaemia, hypoproteinaemia, malnutrition and chronic morbidity predispose to the condition by devitalizing the tissues. Tropical ulcer may be endemic, eg after famine and flood, or in refugee and prison camps. Although no specific causative organisms have been proved, in acute lesions (not in closed blebs) *Borrelia Vincentii* and *Bacillus fusiformis* are commonly found. Secondary invaders are seen in advanced lesions.

Clinical features

There is usually a history of minor trauma, a scratch or an insect or mosquito bite, a burn or even an antecedent

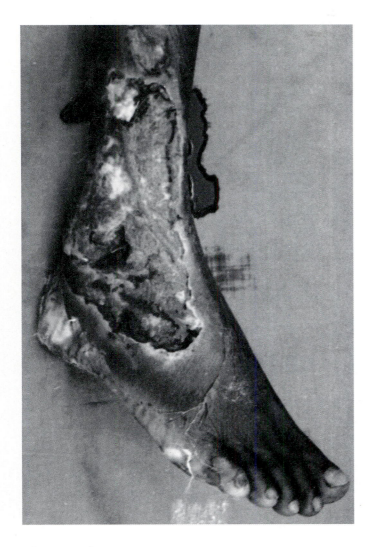

Figure 24
This extensive ulcer developed in 14 days following an insignificant injury caused by the leg of a cot

local bacterial infection (eg impetigo or furunculosis). Soon after the area becomes slightly erythematous and vesicles or bullae containing serous or serosanguinous fluid appear. The surrounding area may be slightly indurated. There may be mild constitutional features with pyrexia. Within 24 to 48 hours the bullae rupture leaving behind a dirty, painful, foul-smelling, superficial ulcer. The margin of the ulcer is indurated, and may be undermined or raised. The floor is covered by dirty, purulent, friable green-grey slough (Fig. 24).

The ulcer spreads rapidly in all directions. The underlying muscles, fascia and tendons die and dissolve and the ulcer encroaches upon bone, where periostitis or osteomyelitis develops. The regional lymph nodes are usually not enlarged, except when there is superimposed infection. The surrounding tissues remain indurated, the skin becomes atrophic, adherent and depigmented. In favourable circumstances the ulcer may heal with an atrophic, tissue paper like scar with a hyperpigmented margin. This scar breaks down easily.

The margins of long-standing ulcers become hyperplastic and squamous cell carcinoma may develop. Variable contractures, deformities or ankylosing occur and contracting cicatrices may strangulate the circulation, necessitating amputation (McLaren 1979). In severe types, the rapid extension of the ulcer debilitates the patient, occasionally resulting in death.

Investigation and differential diagnosis

In acute stage demonstration of *B. fusiformis* or *B. Vincentii* spirochaetes may be taken as diagnostic, but in the chronic stage no specific investigation is helpful. The chronic tropical ulcer should be differentiated from ulcers in yaws, syphilis, tuberculosis, cutaneous diphtheria, varicose, Buruli ulcers, cutaneous leishmaniasis, epithelioma, burns and malignant melanoma.

Management

In the acute stage, rest, nutritious diet and hospital supervision are helpful. The limb should be kept elevated and the wound dressed three times daily with some bland application after thorough irrigation with hydrogen peroxide and normal saline, hypertonic saline or magnesium sulphate. As the ulcer becomes healthy, the number of dressings is reduced to once daily. It is better to carry out a split skin graft on the healthy granulating surface.

If the ulcer is deep, and affecting the underlying bone, excision of the ulcer with curettage or limited excision of the underlying affected bone and skin grafting speeds the recovery. For chronic indolent and incapacitating ulcer, amputation may be considered on the patient's request.

Chemotherapy

1 Mu of penicillin in divided dosage should be started. Other antibiotics should be given according to the chemosensitivity of the secondary invaders. Metronidazole (600 to 1200 mg daily) may assist recovery.

There is no specific preventative measure, but improved nutrition and living standards, and the care of injuries will decrease the likelihood of developing the tropical ulcer.

Chromomycosis

Synonyms: chromoblastomycosis, verrucous dermatitis.

This is a chronic systemic fungal disease caused by

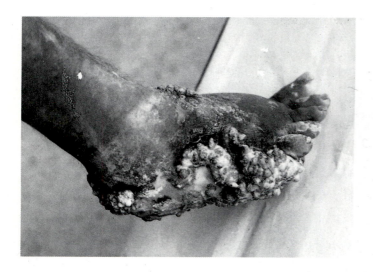

Figure 25

Papulonodular lesions with ulcerations spread over the foot, mainly on the dorsolateral aspects (by courtesy of Dr A S Prasad)

species of *Phialophora*, *Cladosporium* or *Fonsecaea* acquired through the skin by traumatic implantation and characterized by slowly growing, verrucous, ulcerated and crusted or wart-like lesions affecting the skin and subcutaneous tissues.

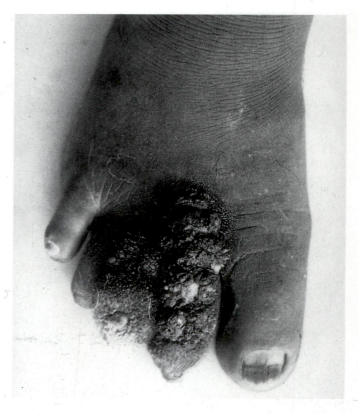

Figure 26

Tuberculous verruca cutis may present with similar features to those of chromomycosis: nodules are normally absent (by courtesy of Dr A S Prasad)

Aetiology

Adult male labourers of low living standards (especially timber and soil workers) working barefoot in rural areas of the tropics and having indifference to minor injuries of the extremities, are most susceptible. Numerous fungi have been blamed, but the most common are *P. verrucosa* (named by Thaxter), *P. pedrocoi*, *P. compacta*, and *P. dermatitides*. Remaining single, or grouped in the tissues, each appears as round, thick walled, 6–12 μm budding cells of the brown colour from which the disease derives its name. These fungi can be cultured, and mycelia vary according to genus and species.

Pathology

Histopathologically the infection appears as a foreign body granuloma with isolated microabscesses. Six or seven fungal bodies may be seen crowded in a giant cell, looking like peas in a pod. Fungal cells are readily discernible with haematoxylin and resin stains.

Clinical features

Though the lesion in the first reported patient was on the buttock, they are usually seen on exposed sites,

especially the feet, legs, hands, forearm, arm, face, neck and shoulders. Initially a small papule, nodule or pustule develops, which persists for months. Finally it ulcerates, spreads laterally, becomes dry and crusted and may assume a papular or even wart-like appearance (Fig. 25). It may remain flat or grow papillomatous, with masses of elevated hard brownish or reddish nodules surmounting the plaques, with a stalk as long as 3 cm, resembling a cauliflower. The lesion may heal centrally, but spontaneous cure does not occur. The lesion spreads marginally and by lymphatic channels and may affect the function of the leg or arm in 4 to 15 years, although muscles and bones are hardly affected. There may be satellite lesions due to autoinoculation while scratching. Haematogenous spread may lead to brain abscesses or other cerebral lesions.

The patient complains of considerable itching, but hardly any pain, unless ulcers develop due to secondary infection. Extensive fibrosis may lead to lymphoedema or even lymphoedematous elephantiasis.

Investigations

In examination of the superficial crusts removed from the lesions, dark brown spheroid mycelia spores 4–8 μm

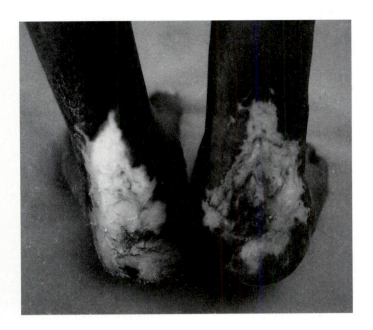

Figure 27

Typical burn ulcer on the back of the heel from a rural area where people warm their feet over a fire in winter

in diameter can be recognized and cultured on media containing chloramphenicol or other antibiotics and incubated at 30°C.

Diagnosis

This is based on a very chronic history, a typical lesion, the demonstration of the spores of the causative organism microscopically from the biopsy specimen and by culture. Lesions should be differentiated from blasto-

mycosis, tuberculosis, leprosy, yaws, leishmaniasis, syphilis and neoplasms (Fig. 26).

Management

There is no certain chemotherapy for these fungi, but oral 5-fluorocytosine, 30–50 mg per kg body weight, six hourly for several months, may be effective. However, blood levels should be monitored regularly, especially in renal risk cases. In resistant cases amphotericin B may be added (0.5 mg to 1.0 mg per kg body weight, for a month or longer). For early lesions complete surgical resection is the most effective treatment. When diagnosed, early small localized lesions can also be destroyed, by thermal cautery or diathermy.

Local infiltration with amphotericin B and excision with or without skin grafting has been recommended by Whiting & Cloete (1968). However, relapses have been frequent. For stubborn and extensive lesions, amputation may be required to eliminate the disease.

Cold-fired feet

The labourers, farm and field workers, working barefooted develop thick soles and often have increased threshold for pain. In winter they usually warm their feet over a fire or charcoal burning in earthenware. It is not unusual to see a burn ulcer on the heels of such persons, which may even penetrate to the underlying bone (Fig. 27).

Initially, they are treated by dressings, avoidance of pressure and suitable antibiotics. In severe cases, surgical excision of the ulcer with infected bone may be required.

Ainum in Africa
Godwin Iwegbu

Ainhum is an acquired and progressive constrictive disease, affecting mainly the little toe, characterized by a circumferentially spreading and deepening fissure or groove in the plantodigital fold which eventually undergoes autoamputation. The word ainhum is derived from a Yoruba word.

Aetiology

The cause is essentially unknown. It is predominantly a disease of blacks over the age of 30 years. It may be no coincidence that most of the victims walk barefoot most of their lives, and minor trauma cannot be discounted. There is no evidence that any particular infective organism is associated with the disease.

Pathogenesis

The little toe is the predominant site (Browne 1965). Two-thirds of cases are bilateral. It starts as a groove which may go right round the circumference of the toe and it inevitably becomes secondarily infected from time to time, which adds to progressive scarring. Browne (1961) describes four stages from the start of the sulcus to eventual autoamputation. The bone progresses from periostitis, through resorption to pathological fracture at the site of the constriction inevitably leading to autoamputation.

Diagnosis

Pain and fissure are followed by oedema, scarring and deformity. The toe is classically bulbous and eventually dangles as a useless appendage.

Management

If treated early, secondary infections may be controlled, and once infection has cleared the decision is whether to conserve the toe or electively amputate. Generally, amputation is simple and effective, although some advocate excision of the fissure followed by Z-plasty (Brown 1959).

References

Abbott P 1956 Mycetoma in Sudan. Trans R Soc Trop Med Hyg 50:11

Anderson J G 1964 Treatment and prevention of plantar ulcers. A practical approach. Lepr Rev 35, 4a: 251–258

Anderson R, Foster M, Gourd J, Hanel D 1990 Free tissue transfer and calcanectomy as treatment of chronic osteomyelitis of the calcaneus: a case report. Foot Ankle 11: 168–171

Antonious D, Conner A M 1974 Osteomyelitis of the calcaneus and talus. J Bone Joint Surg 56A: 338–345

Bassett A 1969 In: Simons R D G P, Marshall J (eds) Essays on Tropical Dermatology. Excerpta Medica, Amsterdam. p25

Bassett I, Faye I, Maleville J, Malgras J 1972 Yaws and endemic syphilis. In: Marshall J (ed) Tropical Dermatitis, 2nd edn. Excerpta Medica, Amsterdam. p 304

Brand P W 1977 Leprosy today. Insensitive feet. A practical handbook on foot problems in leprosy. The Leprosy Mission, London. pp 1–77

Broudy A S, Scott R D, Watts H G 1976 The split heel technique in the management of calcaneal osteomyelitis. Clin Orthop 119: 202–205

Brown E C 1959 Bilateral ainhum treated by multiple Z-plasties. Plast Reconstr Surg 23: 550

Browne S G 1961 Ainhum: a clinical and aetiological study of 83 cases. Ann Trop Med Parasitol 55: 314–320

Browne S G 1965 True ainhum: its distinctive and differentiating features in a clinical study based on 100 patients. J Bone Joint Surg 47B: 52–55

Canizares O 1975 Clinical Tropical Dermatology. Blackwell Scientific Publications, Oxford. p96

Capen D, Scheck M 1981 Seronegative inflammation of the ankle and foot. Clin Orthop 155: 147–155

Capitanio M A, Kirkpatrick J A 1970 Early roentgen observations in acute osteomyelitis. Am J Roentgen 130: 488–496.

Carayon A 1971 Investigations on the physiopathology of the nerve in leprosy. Int J Lepr 39: 278–294

Centers for Disease Control 1988 Tuberculosis: final data in the United States (1986). Morbidity and Mortality Weekly Report 36: 817

Chapman M, Murray R O, Stoker D J 1979 Tuberculosis of bones and joints. Semin Roentgenol XIV: 266–282

Chretian J 1990 Tuberculosis and HIV: the cursed duet. Bulletin of the International Union against Tuberculosis and Lung Diseases 65: 25–32

Colwill M 1969 Osteomyelitis of the metatarsal sesamoids. J Bone Joint Surg 51B: 464–468

Colwill M R, Maudsley R H 1968 The management of gas gangrene with hyperbaric oxygen therapy. J Bone Joint Surg 50B: 732–742

Cracchiolo A, Goldberg LS 1977 Local and systemic reactions to puncture wounds by the sea urchin spine and date palm thorn. Arthritis and Rheumatism 20: 1206–1212

Crim J R, Cracchiolo A III, Hall R L 1996 Imaging of the Foot and Ankle. Martin Dunitz, London. p. 144

Curtis P H J 1973 Uncommon forms of osteomyelitis. Clin Orthop 96: 84–87

Davey T F, Rees R J W 1974 Lepr Rev 45: 121. In: Manson-Bahr P E C, Apted F I C (eds) 1982 Manson's Tropical Diseases, 18th edn. Ballière Tindall, London. p 300

Davies P D O, Humphries M J, Byfield S P et al 1984 Bone and joint tuberculosis. A survey of notification in England and Wales. J Bone Joint Surg 66B: 326–330

Denham D A, Rodgers R 1975 Structural and functional studies on the lymphatics of cats infected with Brugia pahangi. Trans R Soc Trop Med Hyg 69: 173–176

Deysine M, Rafkin H, Teicher I et al 1975 Diagnosis of chronic and postoperative osteomyelitis with gallium 67 citrate scans. Am J Surg 129/6: 632–635

Dondero T T, Mullin S W, Balasingham S 1975 In: Manson-Bahr P E C, Apted F I C (eds) 1982 Manson's Tropical Diseases, 18th edn. Ballière Tindall, London. p 179

Edeson D F B, Wilson T, Wharton R H, Laing A B G 1960 Experimental transmission of Brugia malayi and Brugia pahangi to man. Trans R Soc Trop Med Hyg 54: 229–234

Elliott A M, Luo N, Tembo G et al 1990 Impact of HIV on tuberculosis in Zambia: a cross sectional study. Br Med J 301: 412–415

Garrido G, Gomez-Reino J, Fernandez-Dapica P et al 1988 A review of peripheral tuberculous arthritis. Semin Arthr Rheum 18: 142–149

Garrod L P, Lambert H P, O'Grady F 1973 Antibiotic and Chemotherapy. Churchill Livingstone, Edinburgh

Geater J C 1975 Lepr Rev 46: 279

Gelfand M J, Silberstein E B 1977 Radionuclide imaging: use in the diagnosis of osteomyelitis in children. JAMA 237: 245-247

Ger R 1983 Muscle transposition in the management of perforating ulcers in the forefoot. Clin Orthop 175: 186–189

Gilday D L, Paul D J, Paterson J 1975 Diagnosis of osteomyelitis in children by combined blood pool and bone imaging. Radiology 117: 331–335

Gillespie W J, Farmer M H, Fong R, Harding S M 1983 The result of a case study of host defences in haematogenous osteomyelitis of childhood. J Bone Joint Surg 65B: 520

Girling J, Hameed M A, Selvapanadian A J 1966 Experimental moulded soles and shoe lasts. Lepr Rev 37, 2: 103–107

Gordon S L, Evans C, Greer R B 1974 Pseudomonas osteomyelitis of the metatarsal sesamoid of the great toe. Clin Orthop 99: 188–189

Hackett C J 1957 An International Nomenclature of Yaws Lesions. WHO Monograph Series 45, Geneva. p 88

Hameed K, Karim M, Islam M, Gibson T 1993 The diagnosis of Ponset's disease. Br J Rheumatol 32: 824–826

Harman R R M 1979 Parasitic worms and protozes dracunculosis. In: Rook A, Wilkinson D S, Ebling F J G (eds) Textbook of Dermatology, 3rd edn. Blackwell Scientific Publications, Oxford. p 876

Hawking F 1956 Treatment of filariasis. Trop Dis Bull 53: 829

Helal B, Wilson D 1988 The Foot. Churchill Livingstone, Edinburgh

Horwitz T 1972 Partial resection of the os calcis and primary closure in the treatment of resistant large ulcers of the heel with and without osteomyelitis of the os calcis. Clin Orthop 84: 149–153

Hughes S 1980 Radionuclides in orthopaedic surgery. J Bone Joint Surg 62B: 141–150

Janssens J-P, de Haller R 1990 Spinal tuberculosis in a developed country. Clin Orthop 257: 67–75

Jellis J E 1979 Tuberculous arthritis and osteitis in Zambia. Proc Assoc Surg East Afr 2: 56–59

Jellis J E, Mulla Y, Youbo C, McSweeney L, Forester A, Mouritzen L 1995a Bone and joint tuberculosis and HIV. East Central Afr J Surg 1(2): in press

Jellis J E, Mulla Y, McSweeney L, Forester A, Youbo C, Mouritzen L 1995b Orthopaedic surgery in HIV-positive patients: a preliminary report. East Central Afr J Surg 1(2): in press

Johnson J E, Hall R L 1994 Management of foot infections. In: Gould J (ed) Operative Foot Surgery. W B Saunders, Philadelphia pp. 263–291

Karat S 1969 The role of microcellular rubber in the prevention of anaesthetic feet in leprosy. Lepr Rev 40: 165–170

Kehoe N S, Jellis J E 1994 The incidence of human immunodeficiency virus in injured patients in Lusaka. Injury 25: 375–378

Kochi A 1991 The global tuberculosis situation and the new control strategy of the WHO. Tubercle 72: 1–6.

Kuhn J P, Berger P E 1979 Computed tomographic diagnosis of osteomyelitis. Radiology 130: 503–506

Languillon J, Yawalkar S J, McDougall A C 1979 Therapeutic effect of adding Rimactane 450 mgm daily or 1200 mg once monthly in a single dose to dapsone 50 mg daily in patients with lepromatous leprosy. Int J Leprosy 47: 37

Languillon M C J 1964 Translated by Ross J. Frequency of localization of plantar perforating ulcers of leprosy patients. Lepr Rev 35, 4A: 239–244

Lawton-Smith J et al 1971 Neuro ophthalmological study of late yaws and pinta. II The Caracas project. Br J Vener Dis 47: 226

Lennox W M 1964 A classification of leprosy foot deformities. Lepr Rev 35, 4A: 239–44

MacKinnon A E 1975 Pseudomonas osteomyelitis following puncture wounds. Postgrad Med J 51: 33–34

McLaren D S 1979 Cutaneous changes in nutrition sciences. In: Fitzpatrick et al (eds) Dermatology and General Medicine. McGraw-Hill Books Co, New York. p 1024

Manzella J P, Vanvoris L P, Hruska J F 1979 Isolated calcaneal tuberculous osteomyelitis. J Bone Joint Surg 61A: 946–947

Marquez F et al 1955 WHO Bulletin 13: 229

Martini M, Benkeddache Y, Bekhechi T, Daoud A 1974 Treatment of chronic osteomyelitis of the calcaneus by resection of the calcaneus. J Bone Joint Surg 56A: 542–548

Maudsley R H, Colwill M R 1966 Hyperbaric oxygen in the management of gas gangrene. J Bone Joint Surg 48B: 584

Medical Research Council 1980 National survey of tuberculosis notifications in England and Wales 1978/79: report from the Medical Research Council Tuberculosis and Chest Diseases Unit. Br Med J 281: 985–898

Miller E H, Semian D W 1975 Gram negative osteomyelitis following puncture wounds of the feet. J Bone Joint Surg 56A: 535–537

Monsoor I A 1967 Typhoid osteomyelitis of the calcaneus due to direct inoculation. J Bone Joint Surg 49A: 732–734

Morrey D F, Dunn J M, Heimbach R D, Davis J, Petersen L F A 1980 Hyperbaric oxygen as an adjunct in the treatment of chronic osteomyelitis. J Bone Joint Surg 62B: 132

Mueller K H, Bierbrach M 1978 Calcaneal osteomyelitis: Biomechanics, clinical features, treatment and results. Unfallheilkunde 81: 585–592

Muller R 1979 Guinea worm disease, epidemiology, control and treatment. Bull World Health Org 57: 683

Naidoo K S 1980 The great imitator. J Bone Joint Surg 62B: 279

Narayanan E, Sreevatsa Raj A D, Kircheimer W F, Bedi B M S 1978 Persistence and distribution of *Mycobacterium leprae* in Aedes aegypti and Culex fatigans experimentally fed on leprosy patients. Lepr India 50: 26–37

Nuber D W, Anderson P R 1982 Acute osteomyelitis of the metatarsal sesamoid. Clin Orthop 167: 212–213

O'Brien T, McManus F, MacCauley P H, Ennis J T 1982 Acute haematogenous osteomyelitis. J Bone Joint Surg 64B: 450–453

O'Connor B T, Steel W M, Sanders R 1970 Disseminated bone tuberculosis. J Bone Joint Surg 52A: 537

Panande D D, Azhaguraj M 1975 Surgical decompression of posterior tibial neurovascular complex in chr. plantar ulcers and posterior tibial neuritis. Int J Lepr 43: 36–40

Pandey S 1986 Oblique sliding osteotomy. Proceedings of the CIP World Congress, Lausanne, 1984. pp 51–54

Pandey S 1990 Modified triple arthrodesis. Presented at the CIP World Congress, Bologna

Patond K R, Srivastava S K 1991 Surgical decompression of posterior tibial neurovascular bundle in plantar ulcers of leprosy. J Foot Surg 6: 39–43

Price E W 1964a The etiology and natural history of plantar ulcers. Lepr Rev 35, 4A: 259–266

Price E W 1964b The problem of plantar ulcers. Lepr Rev 35, 4A: 267–272

Ram P C, Martinez S, Korobkin M, Beriman R S et al 1981 CT detection of intraosseous gas: a new sign of osteomyelitis. Am J Roentgenol 137: 721–723

Rao P T, Panda D 1985 Posterior tibial neurovascular decompression in plantar ulcer in leprosy. J Bone Joint Surg 67B: 497

Raptopoulos V, Doherty P W, Goss T P, King M A, Johnson K, Gantz N M 1982 Acute osteomyelitis: advantage of white cell scans in early detection. Am J Roentgenol 139: 1077–1082

Ridley D S, Jopling W H 1966 Classification of leprosy according to immunity. A five group system. Int J Lepr 34: 255–275

Rome M 1963 Osteomyelitis of the metatarsal sesamoid. Br Med J 1: 1071

Rose W F 1962 Etiology and treatment of plantar ulcers. Lepr Rev 33, 1: 25–40.

Sammon D J 1983 Bone and joint tuberculosis in Glasgow: the present situation. Scott Med J 28: 48–56

Schacher J F, Sahyoun P F 1967 A chronological study of the histopathology of filarial diseases in cats and dogs caused by *Brugia pahangi* (Buckley and Edeson 1956). Trans R Soc Trop Med Hyg 61: 234

Scott J E, Taor W A 1992 The changing patterns of bone and joint tuberculosis. J Bone Joint Surg 64B: 250

Seabold J E, Flickinger F W, Kao S C S et al 1990 Indium-111-leukocyte/technetium-99m-MDP bone and magnetic resonance imaging: difficulty of diagnosing osteomyelitis in patients with neuropathic osteoarthropathy. J Nucl Med 31: 549–556

Seltzer S E 1984 Value of computed tomography in planning medical and surgical treatment of chronic osteomyelitis. J Comput Assist Tomogr 8: 482–487

Shannon F B, Moore M, Houkom J A, Waecker N J Jr 1990 Multifocal cystic tuberculosis of bone. J Bone Joint Surg 72A: 1089–1092

Shibata T, Tada KL, Hashizume C 1990 The results of arthrodesis of the ankle for leprotic neuroarthropathy. J Bone Joint Surg 72A: 749–756

Sinnott J T, Cancio M R, Frankle M A, Gustke K, Spiegel P G 1990 Tuberculous osteomyelitis masked by concomitant staphylococcal infection. Arch Intern Med 150: 1865–1868

Skevis X A 1984 Primary subacute osteomyelitis of the talus. J Bone Joint Surg 66B: 101–103

Srinivasan H 1976 Heel ulcers in leprosy patients. Lepr India 48: 355–361

Standish W, Hyndma J, Forsythe M 1977 Skeletal tuberculosis the great imitator. J Bone Joint Surg 59B: 511

Tang J S H, Gold R H, Bassett L W, Seeger L L 1988 Musculoskeletal infection of the extremities: evaluation with MR imaging. Radiology 166: 205–209

Thangaraj R H, Yawalkar S J 1986 Historical background. In: Leprosy, 1st edn. CIBA-Geigy Ltd, Basle

Togerson W R, Hammond G 1969 Osteomyelitis of the sesamoid bones of the first metatarsophalangeal joint. J Bone Joint Surg 51A: 1420–1422

Unger E, Moldofsky P, Gatenby R, Hartz W, Broder G 1988 Diagnosis of osteomyelitis by MR Imaging. Am J Roentgenol 150: 605–610

White G B 1982 Fleas. In: Manson-Bahr P E C, Apted F I C (eds) Manson's Tropical Diseases, 18th edn. Ballière Tindall, London. p 820

Whitehouse W M, Smith W S 1970 Osteomyelitis of the feet. Semin Roentgenol 5: 367–377

Whiting D A, Cloete G N 1968 Chemotherapy and conservative surgery in the treatment of Chromoblastomycosis. S Afr Med J 42: 885–886

WHO 1967 Technical Report Series (on Filariasis) no. 359. World Health Organization, Geneva

WHO 1982 Chemotherapy of leprosy for control programmes. Tech Rep Ser 675. World Health Organization, Geneva

WHO 1984 Lymphatic filariasis. Fourth report of the WHO expert committee on filiarsis. Technical Report series no 702. WHO, Geneva

WHO 1990 AIDS: Interim proposal for a WHO staging system for HIV infection and disease. Weekly Epidemiological Record 65: 221–228

WHO 1991 Guidelines for tuberculosis treatment in adults and children in national tuberculosis programmes (WHO/TB/91.161). Tuberculosis Unit, Division of Communicable Diseases, WHO, Geneva

WHO 1992 WHO Technical Report Series (821) Lymphatic filariasis: the disease and its control. Fifth report of the WHO Expert committee on filariasis. WHO, Geneva

Winkelmann W, Schulitz K P 1977 Chronic osteomyelitis in the subtalar tarsus. Orthop Prax 13: 848–851

VIII.2 Poliomyelitis

P K Sethi

Although poliomyelitis has almost been controlled in most countries in the Western hemisphere ever since a successful polio vaccination programme was launched and surgeons in these countries are unlikely to encounter fresh cases of paralytic foot disorders resulting from this disease, vast territories in Asia and Africa are still awaiting the benefits of an effective vaccination programme. Poliomyelitis, as a consequence, still continues to be the leading cause of physical disability in these continents. Of more than 2000 nations in the world, 108 have reported no fresh cases of polio for three consecutive years (Adamson 1994). It should be understood, however, that not every case of polio is reported. For every confirmed case of polio there are an estimated fourteen unreported ones (WHO 1994).

Surveys have computed that between 200 000 to 300 000 children are affected by polio every year in India alone (LSSH Newsletter 1988). Huckstep (1975) had reported a very similar situation in many African countries. It has to be realized that only 30 per cent of the world's population lives in areas that are probably free from polio and that at present 10 million people are lame from poliomyelitis (WHO 1989).

Special problems in developing countries

The hospital based services, where adequate evaluation and management of postpolio paralytic patients could be carried out, are located in developing countries only in large metropolitan towns. It is inevitable, therefore, that the bulk of patients from rural areas suffer neglect, with gross deformities and contractures, the like of which would seldom be encountered in the West. Some of the illustrations from Jones and Lovett's (1929) classical text on orthopaedics are as pertinent in Afro-Asian countries today as they were over six decades ago in the west. The surgical management of such gross deformities demands interventions with which an average surgeon in the West would hardly be familiar these days.

Even if such patients are spotted in rural areas, it is difficult to prevail on them to travel long distances to hospitals where such specialized surgery could be carried out. Alternative strategies, designed both for prevention of avoidable deformities and for simplifying orthotic appliances and surgical procedures (Huckstep 1975, Werner 1987, Sethi 1989a,b) in such situations to 'reach the unreached' are clearly called for.

For climatic, economic and cultural reasons, the majority of patients in developing countries move around barefoot or else use open, well ventilated footwear. Orthoses mounted on closed laced up shoes are often rejected and thus there is an understandable tendency to operate on young feet merely to be able to dispense with the need for orthoses. On the other hand, operations primarily designed to avoid pressure or friction caused by closed shoes on deformed feet are often not performed – hallux valgus, a cocked-up great toe, or claw toes usually remain asymptomatic in a barefoot population.

Clinical features

In all but a few patients, polio is a minor illness with sore throat, gastrointestinal upset or transient fever. In susceptible patients, probably no more than 1 in 500, the central nervous system is invaded with production of an acute and widespread central nervous infection. The polio virus almost selectively affects the motor neurone cells of the anterior horns of the spinal cord and brain stem, which are either destroyed or rendered temporarily functionless with the production of flaccid paralysis of muscles supplied by affected cells. The sensory components are spared, though during the acute stage the affected limbs may reveal widespread muscle tenderness or hyperaesthesia with signs of meningism. There is never any sensory loss.

Neuronal lesions

Those motor nerve cells that are totally destroyed are never replaced. Other cells show histological changes short of complete chromatolysis in which a ring of Niesl substance forms at the periphery of the cell. Such a cell may recover during subsequent weeks. In yet further cells, no histological changes may be seen though function in them is temporarily lost because of surrounding inflammatory oedema and vascular change. Function can recover in these cells within a few days of the subsidence of the acute illness.

Several factors have been shown to increase the severity of the paralysis. Peripheral trauma during the 2 weeks preceding the onset of the paralysis can affect the localization of paralysis in anatomically related segments of the cord. Such trauma can include intramuscular injection, injury, excessive physical activity or an operation performed during the two weeks preceding the onset of the major illness (Russel 1956). In developing countries it is a common practice to give drugs by injection for any febrile illness in infants and children and it is often stated by parents that the paralysis in a particular limb was a result of an injection given in that limb. The practice of administering drugs through injections in a vulnerable population can be strongly criticized (Werner 1987). Possibly excessive sensory stimulation of half-dead cells may tip the scales against them.

By the end of 3–4 months, the damage caused by the infection has largely been cleared. Areas of gliosis with lymphocytic cell collections occupy the site of destroyed motor nerve cells. Any remaining nerve cells show little or no histological abnormality (Sharrard 1971).

Muscle paralysis in poliomyelitis

Initial paralysis

The most important and the most interesting feature of the disease is the muscle paralysis and its sequelae. The paralysis usually reaches its maximum severity within 48 hours, though it sometimes continues to increase or involves other limbs during the course of several days. Occasionally a second wave of paralysis may follow a week or more after the complete subsidence of the initial bout of paralysis, especially if the patient has been allowed to become ambulant too soon.

At the end of the paralytic stage, a patient may have any combination of paralysis from weakness of one or two muscles in a limb to complete quadriplegia. Fortunately for those who are extensively affected, the level of paralysis at this time is not directly related to the degree of recovery that may ultimately occur. For instance, one limb, all of whose muscles are paralysed at the height of acute illness, may show a return of activity in almost every muscle after 2 or 3 weeks, while the equally affected opposite limb may remain permanently paralysed.

Muscle recovery

A convenient time to make a detailed assessment of the residual paralysis and paresis that bears some relation to the future state of the limb is at the end of the fourth week when the patient has recovered from the effects of acute illness as such, and much or all of the pain and tenderness in the muscles has subsided.

In routine clinical work, no better method has been devised to record the residual power than that devised by Lovett and described by his assistant, Wright (Wright 1912). Muscle power was graded on its ability to move the appropriate segment of a limb against gravity, with a force greater than gravity or with gravity eliminated. Almost all systems of clinical testing of muscle power

Table 1 Grades of muscle power used in manual testing (modified MRC scale)
Grade 0 - No contraction
Grade 1 - Flicker or trace of contraction
Grade 2 - Active movement with gravity eliminated
Grade 3 - Active movement against gravity
Grade 4 - Active movement against gravity and some resistance
Grade 5 - Active movement against gravity and considerable resistance
Grade 6 - Normal power

invented since have used this principle (Medical Research Council, 1943). Between MRC scale 4 and 5, many insert an additional grade because so often there is a need to record the power of a muscle that will contract against considerable resistance, but that is still not strong enough to be considered as normal (Table 1).

Recovery of paretic muscles
Sharrard (1955b) studied 149 patients whose muscles were tested every 2 months for the first year and at 6-monthly intervals for the following 2 years. He described a unit of recovery as a move up from one grade to the next; for instance, a muscle which was grade 2 at one muscle examination but became grade 3 at the next examination had made one unit recovery. Histograms were thus charted showing unit increase in power for each affected muscle. It was seen that the recovery is rapid between the end of the first month and the end of the second but after this the rate steadily diminished until, at the twelfth month, for practical purposes recovery ceased.

If the recovery of individual muscles is analysed separately, all muscles, whatever their function, size and position in the limb, are found to recover at the same rate and to the same extent. This is quite different from the recovery in peripheral nerve injuries in which proximal muscles recover before distal muscles as axons grow down the axon sheaths. The point of practical importance is that if one muscle is stronger than the other in the early months of the disease, it will remain stronger throughout the period of recovery and will still be the stronger one at the end.

The other point is that electrical stimulation of the paralysed muscles does not have any rational place in the management of polio, unlike its role in recovery during peripheral nerve injuries (Seddon 1954).

Recovery in paralysed muscles
Unlike the paretic muscles (i.e. muscles that are active however weak they may be), the prognosis for recovery

in completely paralysed muscles is quite different. Among muscles that are paralysed at the end of the first month, 68% never recover while the remainder will begin to function again with time. Among muscles that are still paralysed at the end of the fourth month, 90% remain paralysed permanently and at the end of the sixth month the figure is 95%. After the fourth month, it is unlikely that a completely paralysed muscle will recover any useful function.

Distribution of permanent paralysis

At first sight the pattern of distribution of paralysis in polio seems to be different in every case and to be quite haphazard in its distribution but as Lovett (1915, 1917) and Legg (1929, 1937) point out, it is not quite as disorderly as it would seem to be. Sharrard (1957) carried out a very laborious but elegant analysis of this problem. In addition to studying the distribution of paralysis in over 2000 lower limb muscles in 149 patients, he also studied seven spinal cords from patients who had died more than 3 months after the onset of the acute disease, five of them after the end of the first year. All of them had been examined before death and records made of the power of individual muscles in their limbs. Serial sections of the whole length of the lumbosacral cords to show the number and position of residual nerve cells in the grey matter were made and three-dimensional reconstructions worked out. The main findings can be summarized as follows:

1. Amongst those muscles that were paretic, quadriceps, hip abductors and inner hamstrings were often affected, leg muscles less often and intrinsic muscles of foot the least.
2. In the same group of patients, the situation of muscles that remained permanently paralysed was almost reversed. The highest incidence of permanent paralysis was in tibialis anterior, tibialis posterior and long flexors and extensors of toes. Hip and thigh muscles were much less often paralysed. The rate of paralysis to paresis represents the susceptibility of each muscle to permanent paralysis. For instance, tibialis anterior is seven times as likely to be paralysed as hip adductors or flexors and twice as likely as peronei.
3. There is a tendency of certain muscle groups to be paralysed or spared together. Gluteus minimus, medius and maximus behave often as one group. Likewise, tibialis anterior and tibialis posterior, both invertors, often go together, even though one is a dorsiflexor and the other a plantarflexor.
4. One of the most surprising findings was the frequency with which gastrosoleus and biceps femoris are involved together. If one of them is paralysed, in nine out of 10 cases the other one is also paralysed.
5. Equally surprising, some muscles one would have expected to be functionally associated together are not affected together. For example, inner and outer hamstrings are not involved simultaneously, nor are the long flexors and intrinsic flexors of toes.
6. The explanation of some of these bizarre findings lies in the disposition of motor-cell columns, or longitudinal cell representation in the cord. The motor-cell columns of some muscles are short and of other muscles are long. Tibialis anterior and posterior possess short columns and are surrounded by longer columns belonging to the quadriceps, hamstring muscles and adductors. A small focus of poliomyelitic destruction affecting mainly the 4th lumbar segment severely damages the nuclei of the two tibialis muscles. But muscles with long motor-cell columns are more likely to remain unaffected or suffer a paresis.
7. It has been possible to correlate the proportion of functioning motor-cells that remain and the clinical grading of power. A muscle graded 0 is always associated with total loss of all supplying nerve cells. A clinical grade of 3 corresponds to a residue of 5–10% motor cells and grade 4 to 10–20% of residual cells. Clinically detectable weakness is only present when more than 60% of the motor cells have been destroyed (Sharrard 1955a) and similar findings have been recorded in experimental poliomyelitis in monkeys (Bodian 1949).

Many features remain unexplained, however. Why the virus should select the cervical and lumbar enlargements of the cord in preference to other spinal segments or why the lower limbs should be involved twice as frequently as upper limbs remains inexplicable.

The acute phase of polio

The acute stage of the disease and the first 2 or 3 weeks following it has a curious feature, relevant to treating the foot, which has defied a convincing explanation. There is a tendency to rapid development of an excessive fibrosis of fascial planes between muscles, particularly around the tensor fascia latae, gluteus medius, iliotibial tract, the fascia in the popliteal region and the calf, the pectoral fascia and in the flexor crease of the elbow. It is associated with the laying down of considerable quantities of collagen in the affected tissues, and if not treated adequately during this stage, marked fixed deformities may result. For a detailed discussion of this puzzling feature, the monograph by Clark (1976) makes for thought-provoking reading.

Position of the lower limbs in the acute phase
To prevent early contractures from occurring, the lower limbs should be maintained parallel to each other and

cradled on two pillows to maintain the hips and knees in slight flexion, just enough to provide comfort. The limbs should not be allowed to roll out with the hips flexed, abducted and externally rotated and the knees flexed. This is the commonest cause of an abduction–flexion deformity at the hip and a flexion contracture at the knee. A splint or a board to maintain the ankles dorsiflexed at a right angle would prevent an equinus deformity. Ready-made below knee splints or plaster of Paris shells with a cross-bar connecting the two limbs are effective in preventing these avoidable contractures. Canvas shoes, nailed to a wooden box at a distance so that the lower limbs remain parallel, have been found to be a simple and effective measure to achieve this objective.

The maintenance of passive movements at all joints twice daily and the relief of painful spasm is important. These exercises can be taught to the mother of a child and it is unnecessary to employ a physiotherapist for such measures. It is a wrong notion that uneducated parents are incapable of understanding and implementing these essentially simple principles. In the third world, a village health worker can, if available, be a useful agent to ensure that this positioning and passive movements are being properly implemented.

Where there is a marked spasm and discomfort on movement, the time-honoured use of hot moist packs is probably still the best means of relieving pain and allowing passive movements.

During the acute stage, it is generally not possible or necessary to draw out a detailed muscle rating chart; the irritable infant would not allow it. Merely handling the limb, lifting it up at the hips and allowing the leg to drop, stroking the sole of the foot and gently moving the joints provides a fair estimate of the extent and severity of paralysis.

Phase of recovery – the convalescent phase

The convalescent stage is characterized by progressive recovery of the paralysis. If the patient is seen for the first time during this phase, the scattered nature of the paralysis, which is practically never symmetrical, the absence of sensory loss, and the history of feverish illness is usually diagnostic. Recovery after the first month usually shows steady progress.

Muscle power increases very rapidly from the first to the fourth month following the onset of the disease and then more gradually until, at the end of the first year, $\frac{14}{15}$ of the total amount of recovery has occurred (Sharrard 1955b). In the lower limbs the ultimate grade of power of a partially paralysed muscle at the end of treatment may be estimated by adding 2 to its grade at 1 month, 1.5 to its grade at 2 months, 1 to its grade at

4 months and 0.75 to its grade at 6 months. At the end of the first month, a completely paralysed muscle may possess no residual anterior horn motor nerve cells or there may be viable cells that have not yet recovered from neuronal injury. Any muscle that is still paralysed after 6 months is almost certain to remain paralysed permanently.

Deformity in poliomyelitis

Fixed deformity at a joint, if still present at the end of the fourth month, is usually due to the true fibrous contracture that had developed during the acute stage. The development of secondary deformity due to the absence of the protection by active muscles can develop in joints that are not properly splinted. Deformities secondary to muscle imbalance do not usually develop until the end of the first year.

Primary or early contractures

In the foot and ankle the deep transverse fascia of the leg and the plantar aponeurosis are the main sites of these early contractures. The deep fascia of the leg is thickened in two areas, the popliteal and the deep transverse fascia of the leg which forms a broad intermuscular septum between the calf muscles superficially and the muscles of the posterior compartment of the leg underneath. The deposition of collagen in this area provides a braking action on muscle leading to a contracture of the calcaneal tendon.

This shortening of the calcaneal tendon will induce an equinus deformity at the ankle. Attempts to stand or walk on such a foot will either modify the foot deformity or cause a compensatory knee deformity or possibly do both. If the hamstrings are paralysed, the heel can reach the ground only at the expense of a genu recurvatum. When, however, the hamstrings are intact, or at least so long as the semimembranosus is active, 'back knee' will not occur. Standing or walking will modify any pure equinus deformity provided the subtalar joint is mobile. The modification of the foot deformity consists of the addition of valgus or varus to the basic equinus. With the commoner coincidental knee flexion deformity, inversion of the foot is the more likely deformity, but with a straight knee the foot may move into valgus through the agency of the body weight. In some severe cases, an equinovarus may be seen in one foot and an equinovalgus in the other, according to whether there is a knee flexion deformity in one and a genu recurvatum in the other.

Plantar aponeurosis

In peripheral paralysis the plantar aponeurosis is one of the prime repositories for the deposition of collagen.

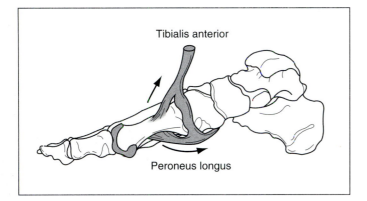

Figure 1

Tibialis anterior is an elevator of first metatarsal; peroneus longus is a depressor, causing the first metatarsal head to dig on to the floor and anchor it during 'take-off'. Isolated paralysis of tibialis anterior leads to a drop of first metatarsal; the forefoot is pronated and so the heel has to invert to provide a plantargrade foot (medial cavovarus). Contrariwise, a loss of action of peroneus longus causes the forefoot to supinate helplessly during push-off because the 'bite' is lost. The use of peroneus longus for tendon transfers can be questioned

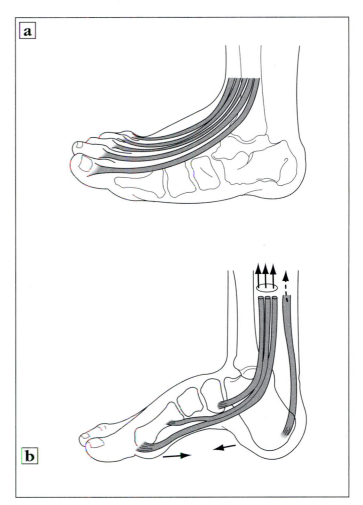

Figure 2

Examples of secondary contractures in muscle imbalance. (a) A valgus foot with a combined paralysis of tibialis anterior and tibialis posterior induces a medial bow of the foot. The active long extensors of toes and peroneus tertius bowstring across the dorsum of foot actively abduct the forefoot. (b) Weak gastrosoleus allows the calcaneum to be drawn towards the forefoot, which in turn is pulled backwards by active long flexors and intrinsics of the foot. The active tibialis posterior pulls up the keystone of the arch. A calcaneocavus foot results

Hicks (1955) has shown the action of plantar aponeurosis as a tie beam connecting the anterior and posterior pillar of the longitudinal arch of the foot and its arch raising action as the 'windlass' mechanism. As the toes are dorsiflexed at the metatarsophalangeal joints, such as when rising on toes or during the push-off stage in walking, the plantar aponeurosis raises the arch and because its proximal attachment is anchored to the undersurface of the calcaneum, medial to the oblique subtalar axis, the heel also inverts. Inversion at the subtalar joint locks the transverse tarsal joint, stiffening up the foot to support the body weight at push-off (Mann 1985).

The retrogression of the metatarsal heads during passive extension of the toes is greatest in the first ray and least in the fifth. The effect of this inequality of movement is to impose a pronation twist on the forefoot. This always shows up on weight bearing as a compensatory inversion of the hindfoot. The use of such feet for walking will result in painful callosities under the metatarsal heads, and in the shod foot, on the dorsum of the proximal interphalangeal joints.

In the child, further bone growth will accentuate the height of the arch and cause the individual bones to grow eccentrically. Such structural changes in the bones are irreversible and a small, rigid painful foot will be the inevitable legacy of failure to deal with the contracture of the plantar aponeurosis at an early stage in the disease. Inman & Mann (1973) have shown how a Steindler's plantar fasciotomy prevents a rise in the height of the arch on passive dorsiflexion of the toes.

This simple operation needs to be utilized fairly early in the recovery phase if a normal foot growth is to be allowed.

Muscle imbalance as a cause of deformity

Gross disparity in the power of agonist muscles over that of their antagonists is bound to cause progressive deformity. The influence of muscle imbalance will be aggravated by weight bearing and gravity. Gross valgus deformity of the foot is a common result of weakness or paralysis of tibialis anterior and tibialis posterior muscles. Isolated paralysis of tibialis anterior, curiously, seldom leads to a valgus foot. Tibialis anterior is primarily an elevator of the first metatarsal, and in its absence, and with an unopposed action of peroneus longus, whose main action is to act as a depressor of the first metatarsal, there is a drop of the first metatarsal. This pronates the forefoot (Figure 1). A medial cavus results and the heel gets inverted as a compensatory mechanism. A cavovarus deformity is often an aftermath of an isolated tibialis anterior paralysis.

A valgus foot with a combined paralysis of tibialis anterior and posterior induces a medial bow of the foot with bowstringing of the long extensors of the toes and that of the peroneus tertius muscle. The pull of these tendons across the concavity of the deformity will actively increase the abduction of the forefoot (Fig. 2a).

The persistent action of normal or predominant muscles in the posterior compartment of the leg (tibialis posterior, long flexors of toes and peroneus longus), while the calf muscles are weak, may actively maintain or augment any existing calcaneus deformity. The attachment of the tibialis posterior muscle to the navicular bone and the anterior portion of the calcaneus will permit traction on the keystone of the medial longitudinal arch and so further elevate it. The anterior and posterior pillars of the arch are thus drawn together and so will tilt the calcaneus into an almost vertical position and a calcaneo-cavus results (Figure 2b).

An entirely flail foot cannot develop any intrinsic deformity because muscle forces are absent. However, a collapse of the flail foot such as this would lead to a stretching of ligaments and eventually to a passive deformation of immature bones. Yet the presence of even a minor degree of muscle power in a portion of a flail part, although incapable of effective action in normal circumstances, can induce a deformity because it alone is active. For instance, toe flexor action, especially that of flexor hallucis longus, in an otherwise flail foot, will cause the forefoot to supinate and adduct. This forces the patient to walk on the lateral border of the foot and leads to a secondary inversion of the heel.

Deformities of the foot can also be caused by the presence of deformity at a more proximal level. Contracture of the iliotibial band often leads to a flexion deformity at the knee, genu valgum and external rotation of the tibia. This induces an equinovarus deformity of the foot to compensate for the proximally located deformity.

A mild degree of tibial torsion is often brought to light by the fitting of a walking calliper. It is common to see an apparent varus deformity of the foot in a child wearing a calliper because the tibial torsion has not been noted. The varus deformity appears because the axes of the knee and ankle joints in the patient do not occupy the same coronal planes whereas the calliper joints do. Material improvement in the foot can be obtained by setting the thigh stem of the calliper in lateral rotation or by altering the socket alignment in the shoe. A

Lehneis tibial torsion measuring device can be very useful in this respect (Lehneis 1972).

Clinical examination

An accurate chart should be drawn up during the recovery phase because this is the only means of noting progress by a serial examination of muscle power and thereby forming an estimate of the prognosis.

The testing of the muscle power should not be left entirely to the physiotherapists even though they are a great help in relieving the surgeon from a time consuming activity and the child often gets to be more familiar and therefore co-operative with them. But any clinician who lacks the ability or the patience needed for complete muscle assessment should not undertake the care of poliomyelitis (Seddon 1954). This is particularly important when a tendon transfer is being contemplated.

In the presence of a fixed deformity, it is often very difficult to make an accurate assessment of muscle power and this may again have to be deferred to a later time after the deformity is corrected.

Muscle tests should be made monthly for the first 6 months, second-monthly for the second 6 months, and finally at 18 months and 2 years following the onset of the disease.

Useful deformities

The lower limbs are linked structures and the foot cannot be viewed in isolation from the suprapedal segments. In this context it is important to visualize the ground reaction force (GRF) which can be conceptually drawn by connecting the centre of gravity of the body and the point of contact of foot with the ground. In an equinus deformity the initial contact during gait cycle is at the forefoot, which causes the GRF to pass in front of the knee axis and the same body weight now locks the knee in extension (Fig. 3). In a polio patient with quadriceps paralysis, a fixed equinus thus becomes a useful deformity by providing alignment stability to the knee. An ill-judged correction of this equinus deformity can destabilize such a knee. Use is made of this observation while designing a floor-reaction orthosis (Fig. 4) for stabilizing an unstable knee following quadriceps paralysis.

Likewise, a mild genu recurvatum moves the knee axis behind the line of weight and provides alignment stability. Excessive or progressive genu recurvatum is obviously undesirable because it interferes with initiation of knee flexion and leads to a halting gait. Mild, nonprogressive genu recurvatum is a useful deformity.

If the patient is ambulatory, considerable information can be gleaned by observing the gait. Not only does one

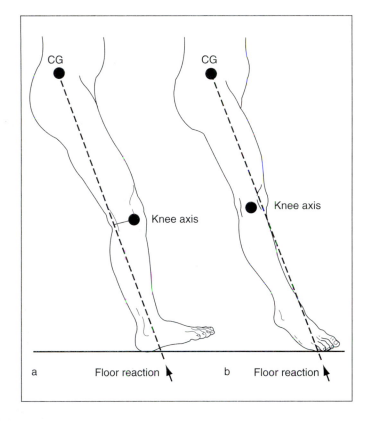

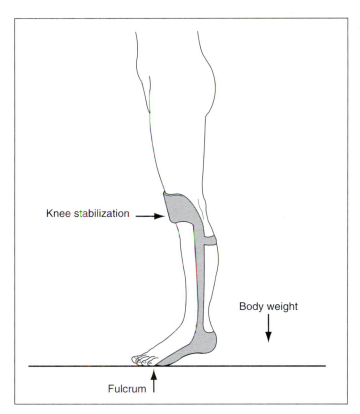

Figure 3

(a) A mild equinus is a useful deformity when the knee is unstable because of quadriceps paralysis. It is important to visualize the relation of the knee to the weightline extending from the centre of gravity to the point of contact of foot on floor. In normal individuals, a heel-strike provides initial contact; the quadriceps is needed to prevent the knee from buckling. A fixed equinus shifts the initial contact to forefoot. The weightline now passes in front of the knee axis. The body weight locks the knee by providing alignment stability. (b) A mild, non-progressive genu recurvatum likewise provides alignment stability and is a useful deformity

Figure 4

Floor reaction orthosis – this not only provides alignment stability but, acting like a cranked lever, with the fulcrum at the forefoot, it causes the descending body weight on the heel to push the knee back via the lateral uprights and a cross-piece in front of the knee

gather information about the limbs in their entirety but the relation of the foot and ankle can be viewed in relation to the suprapedal segments. For example, a paralytic drop foot is usually allowed to clear the ground in the classical steppage gate by raising the knee higher. This, however, depends on an adequate power in the hip flexors. If the hip flexors are weak, the foot would scrape the floor. On the other hand, if the limb length has been affected, a short limb would allow an easy clearance. This may have an implication in the management of the drop foot. In a pure drop foot, with a short limb, often the case could be left alone and an appliance or surgery avoided. Likewise, a fixed equinus may be helping an individual with zero quadriceps in stabilizing the knee.

In weakness of plantarflexors, the calcaneus gait is characterized not only by a lack of push-off but also an excessive knee flexion during midstance; the controlled forward movement of the tibia exercised by an eccentric contraction of gastrosoleus is missing. Westin (1985) has drawn attention to the fact that instead of heel rise, in such cases, the ankle actually rotates into dorsiflexion and ultimately into a posterior subluxation at the ankle and a simultaneous toe-rise (Fig. 5).

Passive movement and the effects of weight bearing should be examined. It is important always to examine each patient in three different positions – lying supine, prone and standing. Examination in the prone position is often overlooked despite being the most informative (Fitton 1988). It is the best position to test for hindfoot equinus and to assess varus or valgus deformity of the calcaneus. Equinus is tested with the knee straight and then bent. This makes it possible to tell if and by how much elongation of the Achilles tendon will correct the

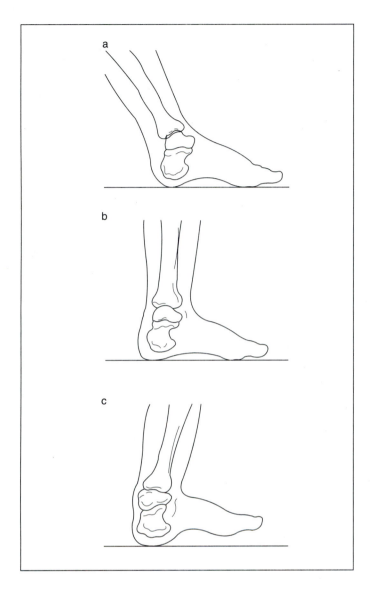

Figure 5

Westin (1985) pointed out how the talus subluxates backwards at the ankle at push-off in a paralytic calcaneus foot, causing the forefoot to rise up (c)

heel. The contribution of equinus to valgus is ascertained by holding the knee erect and the foot in the plantar-grade position when the knee is straight. This is also a good position in which to test the ankle joint for instability.

The size of the feet can be compared and the location and severity of any callosities marked out. These provide as much information as any pressure studies in a more sophisticated setting.

Wasting of the calf and thigh should be recorded, and this would be a good time to inform the parents that surgery for polio would not result in the girth of the limb improving. This is a very common assumption of parents.

Management

Management during the convalescent phase

Treatment during the convalescent stage is directed towards the correction of any deformity that may be left over from the acute stage, the avoidance of any new or progressive deformity, the enhancement of recovery or paretic muscles by graduated exercises, and the resumption of as normal a function as possible.

The management of early deformity

The splintage that was required during the acute stage should be removed by the end of the third or fourth week. If all the joints have full passive movements, putting each joint through a full passive range each day is usually sufficient to prevent deformity. Only when serial records of movements show that a range is becoming progressively more limited should splintage at night be used to supplement passive movements.

While stretching an equinus deformity at the ankle, the heel should be pulled down rather than pushing the forefoot up, as this latter manoeuvre can overstretch the plantar ligaments and also damage the ankle joint. For stretching out a contracture of the plantar fascia, one hand should stabilize the heel while the forefoot is straightened out using a three-point principle by pressing down the middle of the dorsum of the foot as the forefoot is pushed up. In severe calcaneus deformities the dorsiflexors of the ankle and the anterior capsule of the ankle joint can suffer a contracture and the ankle should be stretched into plantarflexion.

If full movement has not been achieved by the sixth month, simple operative division of tight fasciae and elongation of the short tendons should be carried out.

Measures to aid muscle recovery

Spontaneous recovery can be accelerated by measures to encourage hypertrophy of surviving muscles and by functional activity to aid the reorganization of connections to surviving motor cells (Eccles 1953, quoted by Sharrard 1971). The basis of treatment is encouragement of activity in individual muscle groups and later of functional activity of the limb as a whole. Two types of exercise treatment can be employed.

Specific exercises
Individual muscles or groups of muscles are made to act to the maximum of their capability for up to 10

contractions per day. This will achieve as much improvement as any activity greater than this. Fatigue should be avoided as it may lead to a temporary diminution of performance similar to that encountered by athletes who have overtrained. The load on the muscles should initially be minimal and, as the power returns, the load is increased. This type of exercise predominates between the sixth week and sixth month.

General exercise

After the fourth month, more general activities such as rolling and crawling, sitting up and lying down, sling suspension, pool activities and later cycling, walking and climbing can be gradually added.

Walking

The recommencement of walking needs to be adapted carefully to each individual patient and the degree of paralysis in the lower limbs and trunk as a whole. Premature unsupported walking in severely paralysed cases may be frustrating as well as harmful, and parents need to be warned about this. However, early walking when the paralysis has been mild is beneficial. Appropriate supports must be applied when needed to prevent further deformities from developing as a result of weight bearing.

Walking with appliances and crutches can usually begin in the third or fourth month. Too much delay, as was customary in the past, is demoralizing and the general benefits, psychological as well as physical, should not be underrated.

Management of permanent paralysis

Once permanent paralysis is established, no further improvement can be expected by natural means. Treatment is directed towards the prevention and, if necessary, the correction of deformity, and the use of reconstructive surgical procedures that may enhance residual function. These two aims are to some degree interdependent.

The management of progressive paralytic deformity

It is unwise to wait for fixed deformity to be allowed to develop and lull oneself into a sense of complacency just because an orthosis has been prescribed. Orthoses can, within their own limitations, minimize the occurrence of gross deformity if there is a minor imbalance of muscle power, but no splint can contain or minimize deformity if there is marked dominance of one group of muscles over its antagonist group. As Clark (1976) remarked, 'it is no more reasonable to expect external equipment to be strong enough to withstand the combined deforming force of muscle power and growth than it should continue to be a source of wonder that a small growing plant can split a rock... Once deforming forces have been brought under proper control, splintage may then have a place in sustaining body weight during walking and standing. A calliper is a mere crutch.'

It is often possible to anticipate the type of deformity that is likely to arise in any given pattern of residual paralysis. If there is a marked predominance of evertor power over invertor power, for instance, the development of a fixed valgus deformity can be anticipated. The rapidity with which such deformity can develop is less easy to predict. Each case must therefore be assessed individually at 3- to 6-monthly intervals as to the range of movement at each joint, gait, shoe wear, callosities on the skin even when orthoses are worn, and general functional ability.

The only measure that can be relied upon to halt the progress of such a deformity is to somehow balance the muscle action by tendon transfer.

The chief protagonists of tendon transfers were Sir Robert Jones (1908) and Naughton Dunn (1920) but, being also the sternest critics of the method and being aware of an increasing number of indifferent functional results, they laid down an elaborate code of rules for the indications of such transfers. Much of what has been subsequently written on this matter has confirmed their conclusions, and more recently the introduction of electromyography has given scientific support to their clinical impressions.

After a long experience of transfer operations, Dunn (1928) concluded that:

1. Transfers must be made only in their own muscle grouping.
2. A transfer from a foreign muscle grouping will require prolonged education.
3. The anterior tibial group of muscles are all suitable as dorsiflexors.
4. The peroneal muscles and the posterior tibial group of muscles are all suitable for plantar flexion.

In general, the phasic activity of muscles in the lower limbs reflects their effectiveness when they are transplanted (Close & Todd 1959). In normal gait, muscles in the lower limbs can be defined as swing-phase muscles (such as hamstrings and foot dorsiflexor muscles) and stance-phase muscles (quadriceps and calf muscles). A euphasic transfer regains activity more constantly and rapidly. Nonphasic transfers can modify their activity (Blodgett & Houtz 1960) as for instance when the peroneal tendons are transplanted anteriorly or the tibialis anterior muscle is transplanted to the heel, but if a mixed transfer of phasic and nonphasic muscles is done, it is often very difficult to train the nonphasic muscle.

Mortens & Pilcher (1956) advised that it is better to delay operation until a child is more than 5 years old because of the difficulty in accurate assessment of muscle power below this age. Injudicious or incorrect tendon transfer can lead to overcorrection of deformity, production of a new deformity, or instability at joints from which tendons have been removed. All these considerations show that, whilst tendon transfers can be an extremely important and useful measure in poliomyelitis, the judgement regarding the results is difficult.

Principles of tendon transfers

The requirements to be met in order to ensure success were laid out by Barr (1949) and his list of instructions continues to be a table of law:

1. There must be a free range of movement and no deformity in the joints to be moved by the transposed tendon.
2. Apart from the removal of a deforming force, the power so set free should be strong enough to reinforce the weaker muscles.
3. The line of pull of the transposed tendon must be direct and preferably as near as possible to the course of the one to be replaced.
4. The transposed tendon must be inserted into bone wherever possible, best through a drill hole or else into a subperiosteal groove. A transposed tendon fixed into that of the paralysed muscle will cause the recipient tendon to stretch and the functional benefit of the operation will progressively decrease.
5. Normal blood and nerve supply to the transposed muscle must be preserved.
6. Muscles that have similar or related actions are greatly to be preferred to antagonists except when an antagonist in movement becomes a synergist in stabilization.
7. The amplitude of pull of the transferred tendon ought to be equal to that of the tendon replaced.
8. A suitable bed ought to be provided for the transposed tendon to enable it to form a gliding mechanism.
9. Although it is preferable for a transposed tendon to run in a muscular or subfascial compartment, it will perform very well when placed subcutaneously and this situation may afford an additional mechanical advantage. Deliberate bowstringing of a tendon on the dorsum of the foot will allow the distal attachment of the transfer to be brought further forward than it would otherwise reach, and the leverage can thus be increased.
10. The transferred tendon must be under the right amount of tension.
11. Immobilization of the part is needed until the tendon attachments are secure. This is about 6 weeks in the lower limb.
12. Functional education of the transfer is the main object of rehabilitation.

Orthoses for the paralysed ankle and foot in poliomyelitis

During the convalescent phase when ambulation is permitted and sometimes in permanent paralysis while awaiting a definitive surgical solution, the use of orthoses is most useful in order to facilitate walking or prevent the occurrence of deformities caused by weight bearing. It is essential that fixed deformities are corrected before an orthosis can be tolerated.

The traditional metal–leather callipers are gradually giving way to polypropylene orthoses (Fig. 6). By suitably altering the trimlines, flexibility, stiffness, and control of the heel inclination can be arranged. In hot climates, some patients do find excessive sweating intolerable and allergic reactions have been encountered. Large windows, however, can be opened up in such polypropylene orthoses and necessary stiffness restored by providing corrugations, as designed by Engen in his TIRR AFO (Fig. 7).

In the developing countries, such appliances are available only in large metropolitan centres and skilled manpower is not available. Huckstep (1975), working in Uganda, worked out cheaper analogues and worked out a logistics of supply that eliminated any waiting lists. His wooden clog, used in lieu of a shoe, however, was oversimplistic and its rocker, with its see-saw action, led to a very abrupt heel rise. Work done at Jaipur (Sethi 1974) allowed a much smoother roll-characteristic during the stance-phase (Fig. 8). A hybrid design, mounting a polypropylene AFO (ankle–foot orthosis) on a Jaipur clog, can overcome the footwear costs and permit a better ventilation in hot tropical climates (Fig. 9).

There is no suitable orthosis for a calcaneus foot which could provide a proper take-off. However, a rigid sole with a rocker can permit the heel to rise when the forefoot is pressed down (Sethi 1977).

The floor-reaction principle can be utilized, not only to control the unstable foot and ankle but also to stabilize a knee with quadriceps paralysis by keeping the ankle in just enough equinus as to prevent the heel from touching the ground at the time of the initial contact during gait cycle. Connected via two lateral uprights and a cross-piece in front of the knee, this floor-reaction orthosis (FRO) functions like a cranked lever (Saltiel 1969). As the body weight descends down to the heel, the forefoot acts as the fulcrum, the lateral uprights together with the cross-piece tilt backwards to press the front of the knee and thus prevent the knee from

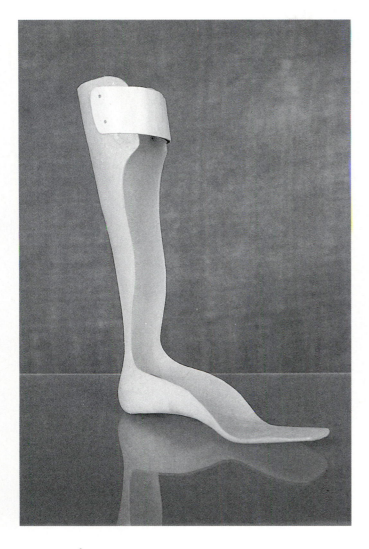

Figure 6

Polypropylene AFO – biomechanically more efficient, lightweight, cosmetically preferred, and permitting interchangeability of shoes, these are increasingly finding greater patient acceptance. By suitably arranging the trimlines, flexibility can be modified and three-point application of force-systems can be effectively used. Skin–orthosis interface problems demand care and expertise: if these cover large areas of skin, sweating poses problems in hot climates

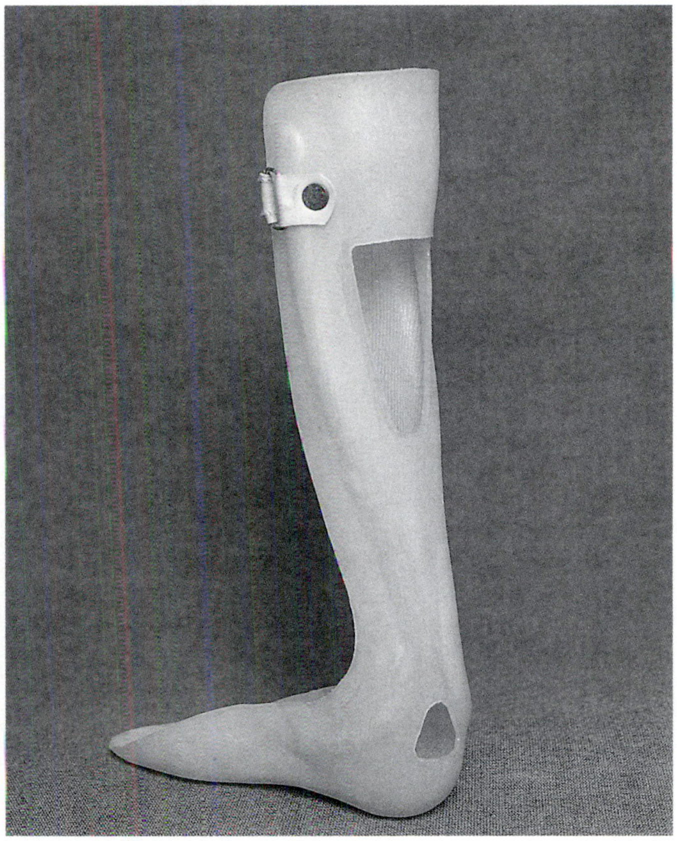

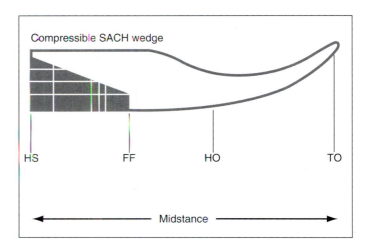

Figure 7

ITRR AFO – opening windows allows skin to breathe, and corrugations add to strength and stiffness

buckling (Fig. 10). What a hand-on-thigh gait can achieve in such cases by using the body weight from above via the hand to press the thigh back is achieved by harnessing the ground reaction from below.

In well over 1250 cases this device has been found acceptable in 90% of patients, as opposed to an almost 80% rejection rate of conventional above-knee callipers (Sethi 1989). The prerequisite, however, is adequate rotational control at the hip to ensure an initial forefoot contact. Callosities under metatarsal heads are avoided by moulding the footplate accurately to the sole for dispersal of the pressure over a wide area.

Compressible SACH wedge

HS   FF   HO   TO

Midstance

Figure 8

A Huckstep wooden sandal is inexpensive and easy to construct. A rocker bar, essential for heel rise, has a sharp leading edge and provides an abrupt, see-saw action that makes it difficult to control, especially when walking down a slope. The Jaipur wooden clog illustrated here has better 'roll-characteristic'. By providing a compressible SACH wedge, the side bars can be attached without the need of an ankle joint. HS, heel-strike; FF, foot-flat; HO, heel-off; TO, toe-off

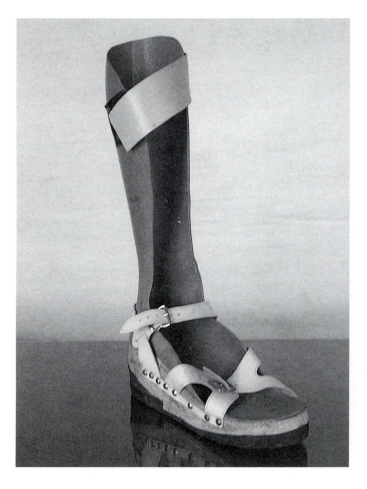

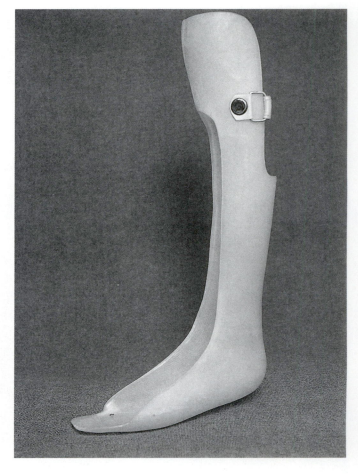

Figure 9

Polypropylene AFO mounted on a Jaipur clog. An open, well-ventilated footwear is often preferred in villages in developing countries

Figure 10

Floor-reaction orthosis – while conventional above-knee calipers have an 80% rejection rate in developing countries, such FROs have a 90% acceptance rate. A prerequisite is to posses enough rotational control at the hip to ensure a forefoot initial contact

For controlling a valgus inclination of the heel, the principles used in UCBL (University of California Biomechanics Laboratory) foot support can be used while preparing a negative wrap cast for an AFO.

Surgery of the paralysed ankle and foot in poliomyelitis

Once the final phase of permanent residual paralysis is reached, a long-term plan for any surgical intervention should be worked out and this programme should be clearly spelt out to the parents. This preliminary discussion is often omitted and this continues to remain the commonest reason for frustration for the family. Each operation then arouses an expectation that after this surgery everything would be all right when in fact this is often not possible. In growing children it is extraordinarily difficult to predict accurately the future, and periodic check-ups are needed. The requirements of satisfactory function of the foot are stability, plantigrade weight bearing, absence of significant deformity, and power sufficient to allow toes to clear the ground.

The operations can be grouped under the following headings:

- For correction of deformities.
- For restoration of muscle balance.
- For stabilization of flail joints.

Many of these operations have to be staged procedures to avoid an excessive surgical assault which may sometimes have disastrous consequences.

There are some important points to realize in this context.

1. If there are proximally located deformities at the hip or knee, these should be corrected first before tackling the ankle and foot. For example, in a patient with flexion deformity at the knee and an equinus deformity at the ankle, the knee should be straightened before correcting the equinus deformity. If a plantigrade foot is aimed at as a first stage and then the flexed knee is corrected later, the foot can end up with a calcaneus deformity.

2. In an equinovarus foot where a Steindler's release and an Achilles tendon lengthening are required, it is always wiser to tackle the cavus element first. This permits the forefoot to be pushed up effectively against a fixed hindfoot anchored by the tight heel cord which can be released at a second stage. An initial heel cord release allows the hindfoot to become mobile, and when the forefoot is later pushed up after a Steindler release, the force is lost in pushing up the ankle into calcaneus (Steindler 1920).

3. A varus hindfoot is a much worse deformity than a valgus deformity. The weight is borne on the thin skin of the outer border of the foot, which rapidly develops painful callosities. The ankle also becomes vulnerable to recurrent inversion sprains. In a valgus foot, there is a much larger area of thick plantar skin for weight bearing and painful callosities are not seen except when wearing a polypropylene orthosis which may lead to callosities over the medial malleolus or a prominent navicular tuberosity. If this precaution of avoiding a varus deformity is not guarded against when performing a triple fusion, the patient may suffer a disability that demands revision surgery. The commandment laid down by Perkins (1954), 'Thou shalt not be varus' must be written in bold letters on the surgeon's desk.

4. If there is a gross muscle imbalance, the operation for correction of deformity should be followed by a suitable tendon transfer to prevent a recurrence.

Operations on soft tissues

In children, before asymmetric bone growth has had time to develop, soft tissue release alone may be needed to get rid of the deformity followed by the use of an appropriate orthosis. With a superadded bony component, and before skeletal maturity is reached, in order to permit operations for joint stabilization, some selected osteotomies may be combined, in the same sitting or as a two stage procedure to bring the foot into a plantigrade position.

There are three soft tissue operations which are often needed in a post-polio foot:

- Steindler's release for contracture of plantar fascia;
- posterior release for a fixed equinus; and
- posteromedial release for an equino-varus foot.

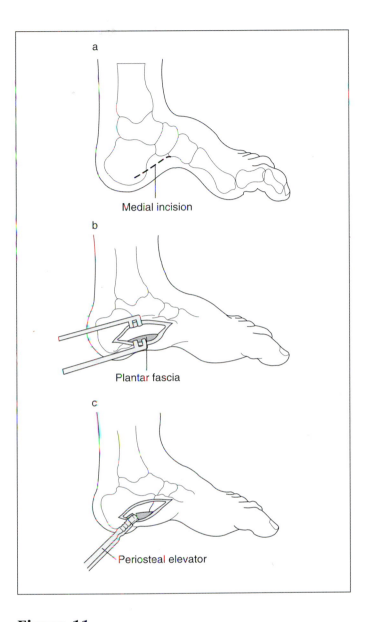

Figure 11

Steindler's plantar release. (a) Skin incision; (b) exposure of plantar fascia along its width; (c) elevating tissues from under the calcaneum

Steindler's plantar fasciotomy

There are many variants of this operation, depending on the severity of the deformity. A mild deformity may require a mere subcutaneous fasciotomy. This is often used as a preliminary to a Dwyer's calcaneal osteotomy in a cavovarus deformity.

Full plantar release is usually performed through a medial incision (Figs. 11 and 12). It is important to preserve the specialized plantar subcutaneous fat and its septa, and retraction to retain this plane is the key to successful surgery. If the medial border of the foot is concave, and the abductor hallucis is found to be tight, its attachment to calcaneus is erased from the medial

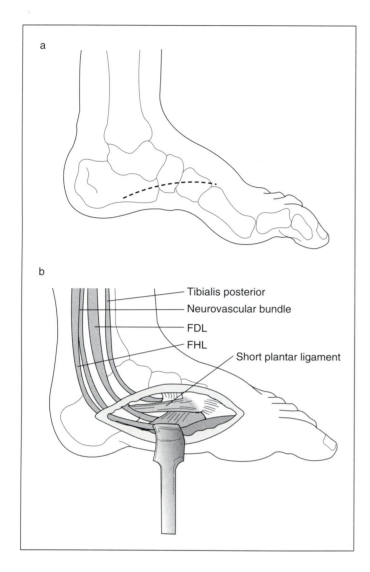

Tibialis posterior
Neurovascular bundle
FDL
FHL
Short plantar ligament

Figure 12

Extended plantar release. (a) Incision; (b) exposure

surface as well as the flexor retinaculum. The entire plantar surface of plantar aponeurosis is exposed to its lateral border. Then the undersurface of the calcaneum is exposed, gradually working distally, lifting the short muscles of the foot forwards till the long plantar ligament is exposed. After carefully sectioning it, the short plantar ligament is also severed, making sure that peroneus longus is not injured. Then the forefoot is pushed up against a fixed hindfoot (a heel cord lengthening should not be attempted before or during this operation, as already mentioned). Skin alone is sutured, taking care that subcutaneous fat does not keep protruding out as it often does.

This is not an easy operation to perform meticulously. The space is cramped and an injudicious use of periosteal elevators can break through the rather thin-walled calcaneus of these paralysed limbs.

A Steindler procedure may have to be added to a wedge tarsectomy or a triple fusion where the cavus element is excessive. It is always included as a part of the two-stage Elmslie procedure for a calcaneocavus foot.

Posterior release at ankle for equinus deformity

Having made sure that the quadriceps muscle has adequate power to stabilize the knee, an equinus deformity usually can be corrected by a lengthening of the Achilles tendon. With a paralysed quadriceps and a severe equinus deformity, an Achilles tendon lengthening may still be carried out, but just enough to leave behind a mild equinus that could be utilized to stabilize the knee.

In skeletally mature feet, a very severe equinus may demand an excessive resection of a wedge from the talus in a Lambrinudi triple fusion, with a subsequent risk of inviting its avascular necrosis. A preliminary lengthening of the heel cord may reduce the size of this wedge.

A pure equinus deformity is rarely encountered; it is commonly combined with a varus or a valgus element. A coronal section of Achilles tendon, erasing the distal attachment to calcaneum medially in an equinovarus or laterally in an equinovalgus, can cause the gastrosoleus to exercise a corrective pull to minimize such deformities.

Unlike the equinus deformity of a congenital clubfoot, it is seldom necessary to perform a posterior capsulotomy at the ankle or the subtalar joints. In fact, if a future Lambrinudi fusion is contemplated, it is wiser to leave the posterior capsule intact; this permits the posterior margin of the talus to remain hitched against the posterior lip of the ankle mortice and permits the forefoot to be brought up firmly while closing the wedge in a Lambrinudi triple fusion.

An extra-articular subtalar fusion for a valgus foot should be done after preliminary correction of any equinus deformity at the ankle. This can usually be carried out by a sliding lengthening sutureless operation of the Achilles tendon (Fig. 13). Any of the standard methods can be used (White 1944).

Posteromedial soft tissue release

An equinovarus foot is occasionally encountered in polio children before bony changes have occurred and it is difficult to fit an orthosis because of the deformity. In such cases a posteromedial release, much as is done for a congenital clubfoot, is needed. It is a much easier proposition because the foot is larger and does not have the same degree of stiffness as in a congenital deformity. Almost always, an orthosis fitted after such surgery would serve as a holding device before a triple fusion is done at the age of 12 years.

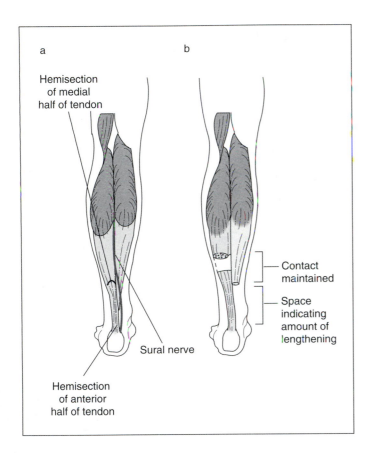

a b

Hemisection of medial half of tendon

Contact maintained

Space indicating amount of lengthening

Sural nerve

Hemisection of anterior half of tendon

Figure 13

Sliding-lengthening of Achilles tendon

Osteotomies in the foot

Except for an extra-articular Grice subtalar fusion, most surgery on the bones in the surgically immature foot is in the form of joint-sparing osteotomies. These may also be a prelude to a subsequent tendon transfer operation to forestall a recurrence of the deformity. The advantages of osteotomy over arthrodesis are that the length of the foot is not reduced to a significant extent nor mobility lost. Because growing cartilage is not disturbed, growth of the foot is unaffected and surgery can be done at an earlier age.

The usual sites for such osteotomies are in the calcaneum, the base of the first metatarsal and rarely the lower end of the shaft of the tibia. A wedge tarsectomy, even though it transgresses some of the intertarsal or tarsometatarsal joints, does not significantly diminish the mobility of the foot and could be classified in the group of osteotomies.

Calcaneal osteotomy

The best-known example of this group was popularized by Dwyer (1959) who advocated a wedge osteotomy of a closed wedge or open wedge variety. Lately, however, displacement osteotomies are becoming popular though the long term results of their many variants are still awaited. While Dwyer initially described his oblique osteotomy with removal of wedge from the lateral side (closed wedge) or from the medial side with insertion of a bone graft (open wedge) for a varus heel in congenital clubfoot or idiopathic cavovarus foot, the basic principle can also be utilized in paralytic post-polio feet. By restoring the posterior end of a varus heel to a vertical or even a valgus position, the deforming force of weight bearing as well as the pull of Achilles tendon is converted into a correcting force. A closed wedge osteotomy from the lateral side is a simple operation and is preceded by a subcutaneous plantar fasciotomy. By shifting the weight line towards the inner border of the foot, a progressive correction of the deformity takes place. The skin at the site of incision is not under tension and its healing poses no problem. It, of course, shortens the size of the heel.

An open wedge osteotomy from the medial side is a more complicated procedure and closure of the skin becomes difficult because the size of the heel is elongated. Wound breakdowns are often encountered and this has never really become popular. In polio, the deformity so corrected would recur unless controlled by an orthosis or followed by a suitable tendon transfer.

Posterior displacement osteotomy of calcaneum

In paralytic calcaneus feet, the heel becomes vertical, bringing it closer to the axis of rotation at the ankle joint. Any tendon transfer into the heel therefore has to function with a short lever arm and suffers a mechanical disadvantage. An operation to make the calcaneum horizontal is a desirable prelude to tendon transfers. Dwyer (1964) had described a closed wedge osteotomy based superiorly to alter this heel inclination but this actually shortens the calcaneum. Mitchell (1977) attempted to increase the length of the calcaneum by performing a posterior displacement osteotomy (Fig. 14). To be able to shift the osteotomized body of the calcaneum backwards, soft tissue plantar release is essential. Two incisions are needed, a medial incision to perform a Steindler plantar release (including division of the long and short plantar ligaments), and a curved lateral incision, dividing the bone obliquely below the peroneal tendons. The posterior fragment is displaced backwards and upwards to restore the normal arch of the foot. A Steinmann pin is driven across the site of osteotomy.

An open wedge osteotomy of the anterior part of the calcaneum was described by Evans (1975) for correction of a calcaneovalgus deformity for patients between the ages of 8 and 12 years. A cortical tibial graft is used as a strut to hold the fragments apart. Evans reported good results from this operation in 25 patients with calcaneovalgus deformity due to poliomyelitis.

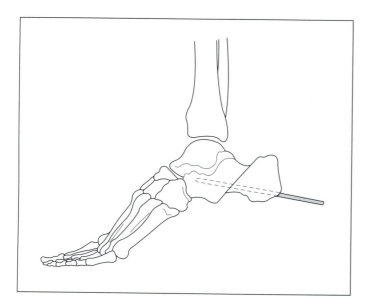

Figure 14
Posterior displacement calcaneal osteotomy of Mitchell. This increases the length of the posterior lever arm and adds to the mechanical advantage of any subsequent tendon transfer. A Steindler's release is mandatory before calcaneum can be displaced posteriorly. Temporary fixation with a pin is necessary

Osteotomy of the base of the first metatarsal
In paralysis of tibialis anterior, with an active peroneus longus, the first metatarsal gets plantar flexed and gradually, with age, a fixed deformity develops leading to a pronated forefoot with a medial cavus deformity. A dorsal based osteotomy centred on the base of the first metatarsal allows the first metatarsal to be pushed up till the forefoot is no longer pronated (McElvenny & Caldwell 1958). The osteotomy is best fixed with a Kirschner-wire or a screw.

Supramalleolar osteotomy of the tibia
Though rarely necessary, osteotomy of the lower end of tibia is a valuable adjunct to render the foot plantargrade in cases of severe equinus deformity where even after a Lambrinudi triple fusion, a residual equinus persists. A residual valgus or varus deformity following a triple fusion can also be corrected at this level without the necessity of revising the triple fusion.

Operations to restore muscle balance

The aim of muscle balancing operations is to achieve a balanced power of dorsiflexion and plantarflexion against each other and of inversion and eversion of the hindfoot and forefoot. To do this it may sometimes be appropriate to sacrifice control of stability in inversion and eversion in order to obtain active dorsiflexion or plantarflexion so that progressive deformity may be avoided. Inversion and eversion can always be controlled by stabilizing operations.

The general principles governing tendon transfer operations have already been discussed. Of the nine tendons available for transfer, only a few transfers have been shown to function effectively. A lot of improvement could be attributed to removal of the deforming influence of an overactive muscle or often to a mere tenodesing effect, which, however, tends to stretch out with time. The gastrosoleus muscle has a very large cross-section and there is no muscle that can ever equal its power. Several tendons are used to jointly work together to restore some effective power of plantar flexion. Restoration of dorsiflexion function is easier, partly because the functional demand is merely to be able for the foot to clear the ground during the swing phase and partly because of a much longer lever arm being available with the longer length of the forefoot available for insertion of the transferred tendon.

An important issue is the use of peroneus longus for tendon transfers. Peroneus longus is primarily a depressor of the first metatarsal leading to pronation of the forefoot, which is so necessary for an effective push-off. If peroneus longus is used for some other purpose, the effectiveness of the first metatarsal during take-off is lost and this adversely affects the gait (see Fig. 1). As far as possible, peroneus longus is best left alone. If tibialis anterior is strong, removal of peroneus longus results in an elevated first metatarsal and a hallux flexus develops. This is a very awkward deformity to treat.

While the literature is full of a very large variety of tendon transfers, the following selection of transfers takes care of most situations in poliomyelitis.

Transfer of peroneus brevis to the dorsum of the foot
Where there has been severe paralysis of tibialis anterior and posterior with preservation of activity to grade 4 or greater in peroneus longus and brevis, some weakness of the remaining dorsiflexors of the toes, and an overall predominance of plantarflexors over dorsiflexors, a fixed valgus deformity may need to be corrected by concomitant lateral soft tissue release of the subtalar joint and any fixed equinus by lengthening of the Achilles tendon. In such cases, the peroneus brevis is transferred into the base of the second metatarsal or, if the tendon is too short to reach it, the intermediate cuneiform bone. Even though this is not a euphasic transfer, the peroneus brevis seems to learn its new action fairly quickly (Fig. 15).

Transfer of tibialis anterior laterally
A paralysis of the peroneus muscles with retention of activity in the tibialis muscles occurs relatively rarely in

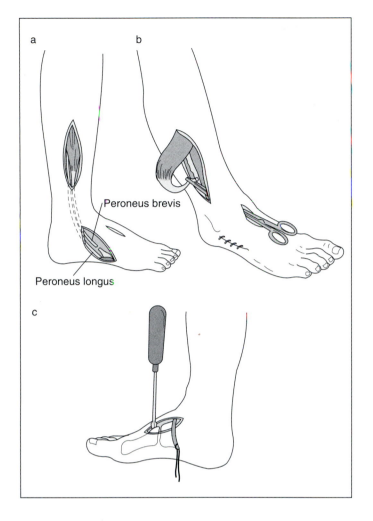

Figure 15

Transfer of peroneus brevis to dorsum of foot. This illustrates some of the dictums laid down by Barr (1949) – subcutaneous tunnel; direct line of pull; bony attachment. Even though this is not a euphasic transfer it seems to function well.

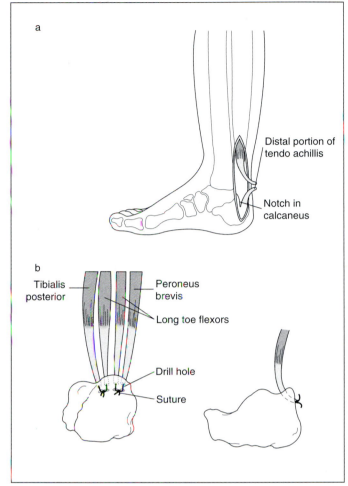

Figure 16

Somerville's (1979) technique of cutting a notch into the calcaneum and drilling holes from the calcaneal tuberosity into the notch to secure a sound bony attachment to transferred tendons

poliomyelitis but is commoner in meningomyelocele with paralysis below L4. The tibialis anterior is detached from the medial cuneiform and the first metatarsal bones, pulled up into the leg and inserted through a tunnel in the base of the fourth or fifth metatarsal or the cuboid.

Transfer of tibialis posterior to dorsum of foot

Paralysis of all the dorsiflexors of the foot and toes is seen more commonly in a lesion of the common peroneal nerve or in leprosy but it sometimes occurs in poliomyelitis. Equinus deformity may require concomitant elongation of the Achilles tendon and medial release of the hindfoot. The power of the tibialis posterior must be normal or at least grade 4. This transfer is done through the intraosseous membrane just above the ankle. It acts mostly as a tenodesis.

While some authorities prefer the interosseous route to bring the tibialis posterior through a window in the interosseous membrane, most leprosy groups have preferred a circumtibial route subcutaneously (Selvapandian 1974). Again, Sherrard (1993) prefers to insert the tendon into the cuboid, while Selvapandian feels that this may lead to excessive eversion and the intermediate cuneiform is to be preferred as the site of distal attachment.

Transfer of posterior tendons to the calcaneus

Paralysis of the gastrosoleus leads to a calcaneus foot. If, as frequently occurs, there is strong or normal activity in the dorsiflexors and the long flexors of toes are active, a calcaneocavus deformity always develops. If there is a cavus deformity it should be corrected as a separate procedure. Lengthening of the dorsiflexors tendons – tibialis anterior and toes extensors – may need to be done as a preliminary to transfer the posterior tendons. These could all be done at the same operation.

Before operation, the presence of activity in the tibialis posterior, peroneus brevis and long toe flexors should be confirmed clinically. To replace the strength of the triceps surae, the tendons of at least three and preferably four other strongly acting muscles must be transferred – tibialis posterior, peroneus brevis and both long toes flexors. The peroneus longus, as a plantarflexor of the forefoot should, as already mentioned, be left to counteract the action of the tibialis anterior. Somerville's technique (1979) of cutting a notch on the upper surface of the posterior part of the calcaneus to place the tendons in this notch is recommended (Fig. 16).

Transfer of dorsiflexor tendons to the Achilles tendon

Where the ankle plantarflexors are weak and the dorsiflexors strong, tibialis anterior can be passed through the interosseous membrane (Peabody 1949). If there is no side-to-side imbalance of dorsiflexor action, the peroneus tertius can be transferred together. Because these tendons are generally short, insertion into the calcaneus is not possible and attachment must be made to the Achilles tendon by interlacing the tendons through it with the foot pulled into plantarflexion.

It is difficult to demonstrate this out-of-phase transfer to function during actual walking; even if this acts as a tenodesis, the foot grows straight and the patients seem to be happy with the result.

The Robert Jones tendon transfer

With an isolated paralysis of tibialis anterior, two consequences follow. The peroneus longus, now unopposed, pulls the first metatarsal down, pronating the forefoot. The extensor hallucis longus (EHL) tries to prevent a foot drop during swing phase by overaction, thus pulling the proximal phalanx into excessive dorsiflexion, riding up on to the dorsum of the first metatarsophalangeal joint and further depressing the head of the first metatarsal down. This 'cocked-up-great toe' tightens up the flexor hallucis longus to flex the terminal phalanx.

In shoe-wearing people this causes a callosity on the dorsal skin and the Robert Jones tendon transfer of extensor hallucis longus to the first metatarsal with fusion or tenodesis of the joint of the big toe (Jones 1916) gets rid of this problem effectively (Fig. 17). In a barefoot population this is seldom symptomatic. The increase in dorsiflexor power does not seem to be very convincing.

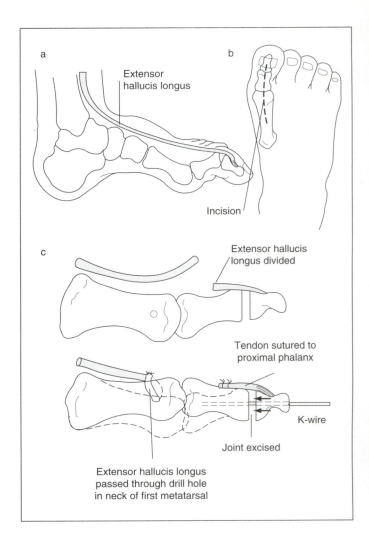

Figure 17

Robert Jones operation for cocked-up great toe when tibialis anterior is paralysed. This is seldom needed in a barefoot population

Stabilizing operations on bones and joints – arthrodeses

Some degree of stability at the ankle and foot is essential for an individual to be able to walk confidently. A wobbly foot, supporting the overlying body weight, forces an individual to walk very carefully, slows walking speed, and increases the energy consumption. A stable foundation should not be viewed as a stiffening up situation; it is in real terms a liberating procedure.

To be able to provide enough stability to allow orthotic devices to be discarded, one has to wait till the tarsal bones have skeletally matured. This, in general, means a waiting period till the patient is about 12 years of age. Trying to perform these operations at an earlier age, when the tarsal bones are still largely cartilaginous, can lead not only to failure of fusion but also to a stunting of the growth of the foot. The only arthrodesis which is permitted in a younger foot is an extra-articular subtalar fusion of the Grice variety.

The basic design of these arthrodeses is a triple fusion (i.e. a fusion of the posterior subtalar joint, the talocalcaneonavicular joint, and the calcaneocuboid joint). By planning to resect appropriate wedges, any residual deformity of the hindfoot and midfoot can be corrected.

If there is a muscle imbalance, sometimes it becomes necessary to also perform a tendon transfer to prevent a recurrence of a deformity. Such tendon transfers can be done prior to the bony stabilization, or the two procedures could be done together in one sitting or the tendon transfer could be done at a second stage after the fusion.

The correct amount of tension in a tendon transfer is the key to its success and, if the transfer is carried out before the correction of a deformity, this tension is likely to be disturbed when the deformity is corrected later. If done at the same time as the fusion, early movements after 6 weeks cannot be commenced to mobilize the transfer in its new bed, so the chances of the transferred tendon getting frozen by adhesions are likely. Ideally, therefore, it seems rational to carry the transfer as a second stage procedure after the fusion is complete and the foot mobilized. This does mean two operations and more time but the results seem to justify this policy.

Triple arthrodesis

This is the basic operation for providing subtalar stability and correcting a deformity by removal of suitable wedges. An equinovarus foot is easier to operate upon. The bases of the wedges are located dorsolaterally and the foot is easy to dislocate to ensure that all the articular cartilage at the subtalar joint, especially the posterior tubercle of the talus and covering the sustentaculum tali are removed. If left behind, a proper opposition of the subtalar joint is difficult to achieve.

Triple fusion in a valgus foot is always more difficult. The peroneal tendons are tight and may on occasion be even required to be divided before an adequate exposure of the medial side is made possible. The talonavicular component is rather inaccessible from a single lateral incision and it is wiser to make an additional incision on the medial side to properly section the talonavicular joint.

There are two variations of triple arthrodesis which have a special place: the Lambrinudi fusion and the Elsmlie operation.

Lambrinudi triple arthrodesis (Lambrinudi 1927)
This has two different indications:

* for correction of a fixed equinus deformity; and
* for a paralytic foot drop without a fixed equinus deformity.

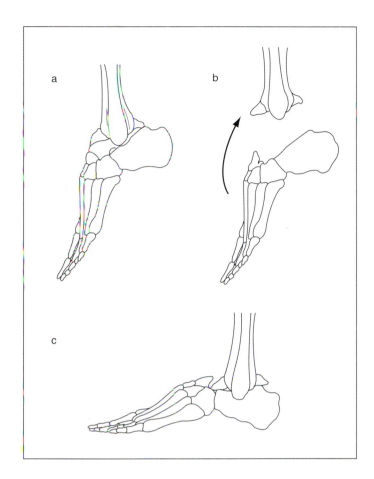

Figure 18

Lambrinudi triple fusion is excellent for a fixed equinus deformity. Against a fully plantarflexed talus, the calcaneum is dorsiflexed to cancel out the deformity.

Lambrinudi conceived of the idea that if a deformity cannot be corrected at one level, its effects can be cancelled out by creating an opposite deformity at a more distal level. For instance, a fixed equinus deformity at the ankle can be corrected by removal of a wedge at the ankle joint itself and fusing the joint. But this would not control the subtalar joint if there is an invertor–evertor weakness. Lambrinudi did not touch the ankle joint at all; instead he created an opposite deformity to the plantarflexed talus by dorsiflexing the calcaneum, which is possible by removing a wedge from talus based anteriorly. The head of the talus thus gets transformed into a beak which is fitted into a slot made along the inferior position of the navicular. The navicular thus rides on top of the talar beak in front of the ankle joint. The size of the wedge removed depends on the severity of the equinus. Since the subtalar joint is also fused, any invertor–evertor imbalance is automatically taken care of (Fig. 18).

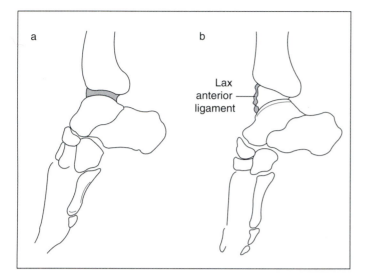

Figure 19

For a paralytic drop foot that is otherwise plantargrade, Lambrinudi fusion is somewhat unpredictable. If the anterior ligament of ankle is lax, the joint hinges open anteriorly. Pre-operative stress skiagram with ankle in full plantarflexion may reveal an anterior ligament laxity

A Lambrinundi fusion can also control a paralytic foot drop where the foot otherwise is plantigrade on weight bearing (Fig. 19). The principle depends on the fact that the talus can be plantarflexed at the ankle till its posterior margin moves up to hitch against the posterior articular margin of the lower end of tibia. Then it cannot be plantarflexed further.

Reviews by Fitzgerald & Seddon (1937), Patterson et al (1950) and MacKenzie (1959) show that about 80% of results are good and fair, but there is a failure rate of about 20%. In order of frequency, the complications include varus deformity, callosities, pain, recurrent equinus, instability, and delayed wound healing with infection.

Elmslie's operation (Elmslie 1934, Cholmeley 1953)
In the UK, many authorities prefer an Elmslie operation, especially when the cavus element is rather marked. This operation is done in two stages. In the first stage the cavus deformity is corrected, followed 6 weeks later by correction of the calcaneus deformity combined with tendon transfer (Fig. 20).

In his original description, Elmslie (1934) used part of the Achilles tendon and sutured it under tension to itself by passing it through drill holes located on the posterior surface of the tibia. This practice is not generally followed now.

Cholmeley (1953) reviewed five patients and found that the power in the calf muscle had increased by three to four grades and there was no recurrence of deformity. This is popular with us for what is otherwise a difficult problem to treat in a calcaneocavus foot.

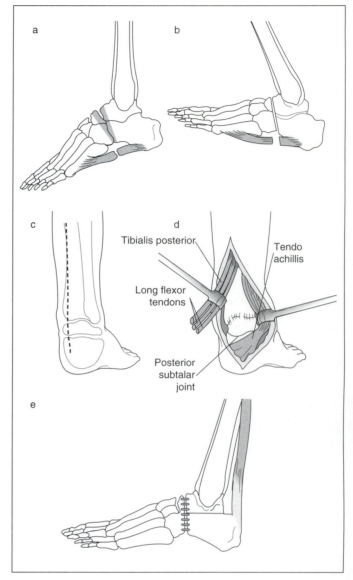

Figure 20

Elmslie's operation for calcaneocavus foot. Even though this requires two stages, the results have been better than when performing a one-stage triple fusion.

Pan-talar arthrodesis

In a completely flail ankle and foot, it is not uncommon to find that a pantalar arthrodesis has been performed. One must be careful before embarking on this kind of surgery, in which mobility is totally sacrificed for the sake of stability.

It may, on the whole, be preferable to perform a triple fusion and let the patient accept a steppage gait. A shoe designed for a calcaneus foot (SACH heel, stiff shank and a rockered sole) would allow for a comfortable stance phase. All that the patient has to learn is to adjust to the idea of a steppage gait during the swing phase. Some of the poor results of surgery have been when a

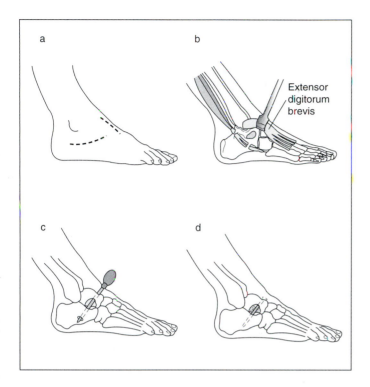

a

b

Extensor
digitorum
brevis

c

d

Figure 21

Dennyson & Fulford (1976) technique of fixing a paralytic valgus foot with a strong screw and cancellous bone filling the sinus tarsi. It is a particularly effective procedure in skeletally mature feet where wedges have to be removed to correct fixed deformities. The strong fixation and the adequate supply of cancellous bone leaves one satisfied at the end of the operation

pan-talar fusion has been performed and the foot is not perfectly plantargrade.

Extraarticular subtalar arthrodesis

Instability of the subtaloid joint is often due to paralysis or weakness of inversion or dorsiflexion and inversion. This leads to a paralytic valgus or an equinovalgus foot. In skeletally immature feet, it is possible to stabilize such valgus feet with an extra-articular subtalar fusion, an idea first suggested by Green to Grice (Grice 1952). Several modifications of this concept have since been devised.

This operation should not be performed in very young feet where the talus and calcaneum are still largely cartilaginous. It is wise to wait till the child is about 5 years old. Too premature a fusion can also force compensatory changes at the ankle leading to a ball and socket joint (Mann 1985). It is essential to correct any equinus before operation by wedging casts or by lengthening the Achilles tendon because equinus deformity of more than 15° prevents the calcaneum from being brought far enough distally beneath the talus to allow the correction

of the valgus deformity. Six weeks after this procedure, the peroneus brevis tendon can be transferred to the dorsum to prevent a recurrence.

It is always wise to get an anteroposterior radiograph of the ankle to make sure that there is no valgus tilt at the tibiotalar level. Often the distal tibial epiphysis is wedge-shaped, with the lateral malleolus at a higher level. If overlooked it is embarrassing to find a persistent valgus at ankle level (Smith & Westin 1968, Paluska & Blount 1968). A temporary stapling of the medial aspect of the distal epiphyseal plate has been suggested in such situations.

Grice used two trapezoidal tibial bone grafts fixed in the sinus tarsi and this still remains the most satisfactory method in young feet.

Both undercorrection and overcorrection are undesirable. When the deformity is undercorrected, a residual fixed valgus remains and the situation become analogous to the fixed valgus of congenital talocalcaneal coalition; such patients are liable to develop peroneal muscle spasm and pain. However, it is better to fuse the heel in slight valgus position than overcorrect the deformity, for even a slight varus deformity seems to increase with growth.

Several studies of the results of Grice fusion have been published; in more than 600 patients the results were found to be satisfactory in 60–70% (Ingram 1985).

Dennyson & Fulford (1976) described a modification of the Batchelor procedure where, instead of a fibular graft, a strong cancellous screw was used to transfix the talus to the calcaneus. The sinus tarsi is exposed, the undersurface of neck and talus and superior surface of calcaneus is decorticated and, with the heel held in a neutral position, the track for the screw is made by an awl, inserted through a small incision overlying the talar neck and directed downwards, posteriorly and laterally to emerge at the posterolateral corner of the calcaneum. A screw then firmly holds this position and the sinus tarsi is packed with cancellous bone (Fig. 21).

This is a satisfying procedure but probably more suitable for slightly older children in whom there is an easier supply of cancellous bone. After a triple fusion for a valgus deformity in mature feet, this method of internal fixation ensures that there is no loss of correction while applying or changing a cast.

Wedge tarsectomy for cavus deformity

Pure cavus deformity of the foot is not commonly encountered in poliomyelitis, but it is a very common accompaniment to a calcaneus or an equinus foot in skeletally mature feet. In younger patients, a soft tissue plantar release gets rids of the deformity. In calcaneocavus, the two-stage Elmslie procedure takes care of this deformity.

In severe neglected equinus, however, a marked cavus element is superadded. This equinocavus deformity is

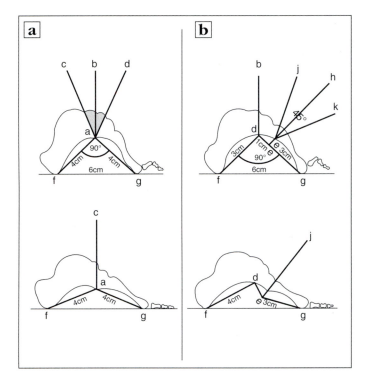

Figure 22

The apex of the deformity in a severe cavus foot is located at the mid-tarsal level. If a wedge tarsectomy is performed at this level (a) the dorsal hump disappears and a greater foot length is obtained. A subsequent Lambrinudi fusion, however, may be rendered more difficult. A more distally located Cole's anterior wedge tarsectomy (b) leaves behind a bump on the dorsum but permits an easier triple fusion. The apex line of the cavus deformity is usually located at the talonavicular articulation (a–b in Fig. 22): the two sides of this cavus triangle correspond to the lines from apex a to the point of the os calcis and head of the first metatarsal (a–f and a–g). The base of the triangle (f–g) is the length of the foot from the heel to the head of the first metatarsal. Lines d–a and c–a bisected by b–a form the angle of osteotomy which is 45° in a cavus of 90°. By removing a bone wedge of 45° and closing the gap, c–a and d–a will overlap, the length of the arch will increase from 6 cm to 8 cm, and the foot will have a more normal shape. If, however, with the same degree of cavus a dorsal osteotomy of 45° is performed 1 cm forward at the tarsometatarsal level, the lines j–e and k–e will overlap and the foot will acquire an odd shape and increase only 1.5 cm in length. This is why the foot acquires an odd shape and less length when tarsal osteotomies, such as Cole's anterior tarsal wedge osteotomy, are performed beyond the apex angle of osteotomy (c–a–d).

very frequently encountered in developing countries. The dorsal surfaces of the tarsal bones overgrow and without a wedge restriction the deformity cannot be corrected.

Sotelo-Oritz (1982) has discussed in detail the disadvantages of an anterior tarsal wedge osteotomy of Cole

(1940). This is performed anterior to the apex of the deformity, which is located at the talonavicular junction. Since Cole's wedge tarsectomy is performed at the tarsometatarsal level, a dorsal hump at the Chopart level remains uncorrected and may be uncomfortable in a closed shoe (Fig. 22).

If the predominant fixed deformity is a drop of the first metatarsal, while the other metatarsals have a mobile deformity (medial cavus), McElvenny & Caldwell's (1958) technique of a first metatarsal–medial cuneiform resection–arthrodesis is a suitable procedure.

Arthrodesis of ankle

A paralytic foot drop at the ankle can be controlled effectively by fusing the ankle joint. This works well if the invertor–evertor balance is satisfactory so that subtalar instability does not pose a problem. However, such a situation is seldom encountered in poliomyelitis. The actual indications for an ankle fusion are few indeed.

Conclusions

Surgery of the foot in poliomyelitis cannot be viewed in isolation from the rest of the lower limb. If the limb is flail and would require an orthosis to control the hip or knee, there seems to be little point in operating on the foot unless there is a deformity that does not allow a comfortable containment within such an orthosis; in such situations the role of surgery is merely to allow the orthosis to be worn comfortably. It is always desirable to aim at discarding an orthosis if the proximal segments (hip and knee) are stable and this really becomes the major role of surgery.

It should be realized that poliomyelitis offers a very different outlook compared to spina bifida or cerebral palsy. Almost always, the afflicted individual aims at becoming a community walker. Speed and walking distance become important objectives and a stable base for the lower limb makes for a confident gait. So some form of stabilizing operation, supplemented, if feasible, with an appropriate euphasic tendon transfer, can achieve this objective in many patients.

References

Adamson P 1994 The Progress of Nations. UNICEF, New York. p. 17

Barr J S 1949 The management of poliomyelitis; the late stage. In: Poliomyelitis: Papers and discussions presented at the first International Conference. J B Lippincott Co, Philadelphia. p. 201

Blodgett W H, Houtz S J 1960 Clinical and electromyographic evaluation of patients with anterior transposition of peroneal tendons. J Bone Joint Surg 42A: 59

Bodian D 1949 Poliomyelitis: pathological anatomy. In: Poliomyelitis: Papers and Discussions Presented at the First International Conference. J B Lippincott Co, Philadelphia. p. 62

Brown A 1968 A simple method of fusion of the subtalar joint in children. J Bone Joint Surg 50B: 369–71

Cholmeley J A 1953 Elmslie's operation for the calcaneus foot. J Bone Joint Surg 35B: 46–49

Clark J M P 1976 Tether, Contracture and Deformity. William Heinemann, London. pp. 26–48

Close J R, Todd F N 1959 Phasic activity of muscles of the lower extremity and the effect of tendon-transfer. J Bone Joint Surg 41A: 189

Cole W H 1940 The treatment of claw foot. J Bone Joint Surg 22: 895

Dennyson W G, Fulford G E 1976 Subtalar arthrodesis by cancellous grafts and metallic screw fixation. J Bone Joint Surg 58B: 507

Dunn N 1920 The causes of success and failure in tendon transplantation. J Orthop Surg 2: 554

Dunn N 1928 Surgery of muscle and tendon in relation to infantile paralysis. Proc R Soc Med 22: 243

Dwyer F C 1959 Osteotomy of the calcaneum for pes cavus. J Bone Joint Surg 41B: 80–86

Dwyer F C 1964 Relationship of variations in the size and inclination of the calcaneum to the shape and function of the whole foot. Ann R Coll Surg Eng 34: 120

Eccles J C 1953 The Neurophysiological Basis of Mind, Waynflete Lectures 1952. Oxford University Press, London

Elmslie R C 1934 In: Grey Turner G (ed.) Modern Operative Surgery, 4th edn, vol. 1, pp. 67–68

Evans D 1975 Calcaneo-valgus deformity. J Bone Joint Surg 57B: 270–278

Fitton J 1988 Other neurological disorders: poliomyelitis. In: Helal B, Wilson D (eds). The Foot. Churchill Livingstone, London. pp. 347–77

Fitzgerald F P, Seddon J H 1937 Lambrinudi's operation for dropfoot. J Bone Joint Surg 25: 283

Grice D S 1952 An extra-articular arthrodesis of the subastragalar joint for correction of paralytic feet in children. J Bone Joint Surg 34A: 927–940

Hicks J H 1955 The foot as a support. Acta Anat 25: 34

Hoffmann D 1950 Local innervation in partially denervated muscles. Austr J Exper Biol Med Sci 28: 38B

Huckstep R L 1975 Poliomyelitis – A Guide for Developing Countries. Churchill Livingstone, Edinburgh. p. 6

Ingram A J 1985 Paralytic Disorders. In: Cranshaw A H (ed.) Campbell's Operative Orthopaedics, 7th edn, Vol. 4. C V Mosby Co, St. Louis. p. 2963

Inman V T, Mann R 1973 Biomechanics of the Foot and Ankle. In: Inman V T (ed.). Duvries Surgery of the Foot. CV Mosby Co, St. Louis. pp. 3–22

Japas L M 1968 Surgical treatment of pes cavus by tarsal V-osteotomy; preliminary report. J Bone Joint Surg 50A: 927–944

Jones R 1908 Arthrodesis and tendon transplantation. BMJ 1: 728

Jones R 1916 The soldier's foot and the treatment of common deformities of the foot, claw foot. BMJ 1: 749

Jones R, Lovett R W 1929 Orthopaedic Surgery. Oxford University Press, London. pp. 426–491

Lambrinudi C 1927 New operation on drop-foot. Br J Surg 15: 193–200

Legg A T 1929 An analysis of the 1927 epidemic of infantile paralysis in Massachusetts. JAMA 92: 31

Legg A T 1937 An analysis of the 1935 epidemic of infantile paralysis in Massachusetts. JAMA 217: 507

Lehneis H R 1972 New developments in lower limb orthotics through bioengineering. Arch Phys Med Rehabil 53: 303–310

Lovett R W 1915 The treatment of infantile paralysis. JAMA 64: 2118

Lovett R W 1917 Fatigue and exercise in the treatment of infantile paralysis. JAMA 69: 168

LSSH Newsletter 1988 Cited in State of India's Health (1992). Voluntary Health Association of India, New Delhi. p. 381

MacKenzie I G 1959 Lambrinudi's arthrodesis. J Bone Joint Surg 41B: 738–748

Mann R 1985 Biomechanics of the Foot. In: Atlas of Orthotics, American Academy of Orthopaedic Surgeons, 2nd edn. CV Mosby Co, St. Louis. pp. 112–125

McElvenny R T, Caldwell G D 1958 A new operation for correction of cavus foot. Clin Orthop 11: 85

Medical Research Council 1943 War Memorandum No. 7. Aids to the Investigation of Peripheral Nerve Injuries. HMSO, London

Mitchell G P 1977 Posterior displacement osteotomy of the calcaneus. J Bone Joint Surg 59B: 233–235

Morris D D B 1953 Recovery in partially paralysed musles. J Bone Joint Surg 35B: 650

Mortens J, Pilcher M F 1956 Tendon transplantation in the prevention of foot deformities after poliomyelitis in children. J Bone Joint Surg 38B: 633

Paluska D J, Blount W P 1968 Ankle valgus after the Grice subtalar stabilization: the late evaluation of a personal series with a modified technique. Clin Orthop 59: 137

Patterson R L Jr, Parrish F F, Hatheway E N 1950 Stabilizing operations on the foot: a study of the indications, techniques used, and end results. J Bone Joint Surg 32A: 1

Peabody C W 1949 Tendon transposition in the paralytic foot. In: American Academy of Orthopaedic Surgeons. Instructional Course Lectures, Vol. 6. J W Edwards, Ann Arbor, Michigan, USA

Perkins G 1954 The Foundations of Surgery. E & S Livingstone Ltd, Edinburgh. p. 229

Perkins G 1970 The work of Lambrinudi. In: Ruminations of an Orthopaedic Surgeon. Butterworths, London. pp. 139–142

Russel W R 1956 Poliomyelitis, 2nd edn. Arnold, London

Saltiel J 1969 A one piece laminated knee locking short leg brace. Orthop Prosth 23: 68–75

Seddon H J 1954 Poliomyelitis part II. Treatment of poliomyelitis. In: Carling E R, Ross J P, British Surgical Practice. Surgical Progress 1954. Butterworths, London. p. 162

Selvapandian A J 1974 Surgical correction of foot drop. In: McDowell F, Enna CD (ed.) Surgical Rehabilitation in Leprosy. William & Wilkins Co, Baltimore. pp. 330–341

Sethi P K 1977 The foot and footwear. Prosth Orthot Int 1: 173–182

Sethi P K 1989a Designing aids for physically handicapped in developing countries. Proc Indian Natn Sci Acad B55: 7–14

Sethi P K 1989b Technological choices in prosthetics and orthotics for developing countries. Knud Jansen Lecture. Prosth Orthot Int 13: 112–124

Sharrard W J W 1955a The distribution of permanent paralysis in the lower limb in poliomyelitis. A clinical and pathological study. J Bone Joint Surg 37B: 540–557

Sharrard W J W 1955b Muscle recovery in poliomyelitis. J Bone Joint Surg 37B: 63

Sharrard W J W 1957 Muscle paralysis in poliomyelitis. Br J Surg 44: 471

Sharrard W J W 1971 Paediatric Orthopaedics and Fractures. Blackwell Scientific Publications, Oxford and Edinburgh. p. 470

Sharrard W J W 1993 Operations for paralysis. In: Evans D (ed.) Techniques in Orthopaedic Surgery. Blackwell Scientific Publications, London. pp. 335–416

Smith J B, Westin G W 1968 Subtalar extra-articular arthrodesis. J Bone Joint Surg 50A: 1027

Somerville E W 1979 Multiple tendon transfers into the heel. In: Robb C, Smith R, Bentley G (eds) Operative Surgery. Orthopaedics Part II. Butterworth, London. pp. 872–875

Sotelo-Oritz F 1982 Poliomyelitis and the foot. In: Jahss M H (ed.) Disorders of the Foot, vol 2. W B Saunders Co, Philadelphia. pp. 1123–1168

State of India's Health 1992 Radhika Mullick Alkazi: Disability. Voluntary Health Association of India, New Delhi. pp. 377–400

Steindler A 1920 Stripping of the os calcis. J Orth Surg 2: 8

Werner D 1987 Disabled Village Children. The Hesparian Foundation, Palo Alto, California, USA. pp. 59–76

Westin W G 1985 Cited in: Crenshaw A H (ed.) Campbell's Operative Orthopaedics, 7th edn, vol. 4. CV Mosby Co, St. Louis. p. 2966

White J W 1944 Torsion of the Achilles tendon. Arch Surg 46: 784–787

World Health Organization 1989 Poliomyelitis: global eradication by the year 2000. Expended Programme on Immunization Update. Cited in Status Report on Polio Eradication. World Immunization News 1989

Wright W G 1912 Boston Med Surg J 167: 567

IX TRAUMA

IX.1 Ankle Fractures

Isadore Yablon and Edward S Forman

Ankle trauma is a very common injury. It may involve isolated bony or ligamentous structures, or it can involve both. The severity of the trauma can range from a stable ankle sprain to an unstable bi- or trimalleolar fracture dislocation. Anatomically, the ankle joint is composed of the distal tibia with its medial malleolus; the distal fibula terminating in the lateral malleolus; the talus, which is positioned between the two malleoli; and three distinct groups of ligamentous structures.

The stability of the ankle joint is provided by the configuration of the mortise and by its ligamentous structures. The syndesmotic ligaments, which include the anterior and the posterior tibiofibular ligaments, the inferior transverse ligament, and the interosseous ligament, resist the axial, translational, and rotational forces between the tibia and the fibula which attempt to separate these two bones (Rice 1968). The fibular collateral ligaments prevent inversion of the talus, whereas the deltoid ligament by itself offers very little stability.

Biomechanics

The ankle joint bears up to five times the body weight and it is the most congruent joint in the lower extremity (Seireg & Arvikar 1975). The stability of the ankle is provided by the bony and ligamentous structures described. It is important to note that an intact syndesmosis is critical in maintaining the normal relationship of the distal tibia and the fibula during ankle function (Amendola 1992).

The talus articulates within the ankle mortise throughout the ranges of motion (Close 1956, Inman 1976). Recent studies demonstrate that the amount of separation of the malleoli during dorsiflexion and plantar flexion ranges from 0.2 to 1.8 mm with weight bearing and from 0.0 to 1.6 mm during non-weight bearing (Grath 1960, Inman 1976). Motion analysis studies demonstrate that a minimum of 10° of dorsiflexion and 20° of plantar flexion are required for ankle function during walking (Inman 1976). Many studies (Barnett & Napier 1952, Cailliet 1968, Rice 1968, American Academy of Orthopaedic Surgeons 1972, Cunningham 1972, Gray

1973, D'Ambrosia 1977) have shown a wide variation in the amount of dorsiflexion and plantar flexion, with 'normal' values ranging from 15°–32.5° for dorsiflexion and from 15°–50° for plantar flexion.

The method used at our institution has been previously described (Segal 1979). The patient bears weight while standing and the angle of dorsiflexion is measured between the tibia and the lateral border of the foot. By measuring the angle with the patient bearing weight, motion is restricted in the foot and only takes place in the ankle joint. To measure plantar flexion, the angle between the tibia and the lateral border of the hindfoot is measured. The mean dorsiflexion was 29.13° and the mean plantar flexion was 34.51° (Inman 1976).

The fibula is thought to bear up to one-sixth of the patient's weight while the tibia carries the rest (Lambert 1971, Takebe et al 1984). Because the talus is securely attached to the fibula and has been shown to follow the displacement of the lateral malleolus in ankle injuries (Yablon et al 1977, Harper 1987b) the slightest widening of the syndesmotic interval may result in a talar shift and joint incongruence.

In order to investigate the role of ankle instability further, cadaveric studies have been performed. The studies assessed the effects of ankle stability after isolated division of the deltoid ligament, isolated division of the fibular collateral ligaments, transverse osteotomy of the medial malleolus at the level of the joint with all ligaments intact, and short oblique osteotomy of the lateral malleolus with all ligaments intact (Yablon 1977, Harper 1987a,b).

Results of these cadaveric studies have demonstrated that no lateral displacement or valgus tilting of the talus was possible in any intact specimen (Harper 1987a,b). When the deltoid ligament alone was divided, no instability resulted. When the medial malleolus was osteotomized at the level of the joint line, 10–15° of rotatory displacement occurred, but very little valgus instability resulted. When only the lateral malleolus was osteotomized with all other ligaments intact, no talar instability resulted. However, when the anterior tibiofibular ligament was divided after osteotomizing the lateral malleolus, a talar tilt was present. When the ligament was repaired or the lateral malleolus was fixed with a plate, stability of the ankle was restored. These studies demonstrated that the lateral structures (i.e. the fibular collateral ligaments and the lateral malleolus) are the prime stabilizers of the ankle.

When evaluating the significance or amount of lateral talar shift, it is important to note that Ramsey & Hamilton (1976) demonstrated that 1 mm of lateral displacement of the talus caused a 42% decrease in tibiotalar articulation; with 3 mm of lateral shift, the articular contact area decreased by over 60%. Because the pressure is inversely proportional to the area (according to the formula $P = F/A$) a decrease in the contact area causes an increase in the pressure the talus must bear. Many clinical studies of ankle fractures have confirmed that good results depend upon an anatomic reduction of the fracture, and there is a direct correlation between the amount of residual talar displacement and the occurrence of degenerative arthritis (Lewis & Graham 1940, Burwell & Charnley 1965, Brodie & Denham 1974, Mitchell et al 1979, Wheelhouse & Rosenthal 1980).

Classification

There are many classification systems for describing ankle fractures. The two most often used are the Lauge-Hansen and the AO Danis–Weber systems.

Lauge-Hansen system

Based on experimental, clinical, and radiographic work, Lauge-Hansen (1950) demonstrated that the type of fracture a patient sustained depended on the position of the forefoot, the direction of the force, and the direction of the ankle on the foot. He observed five different fracture patterns, each of which was subclassified into stages. As the force continued to act, the severity of the injury was increased.

Supination–eversion injury

A supination–eversion injury occurs when the forefoot is placed in supination and an external rotatory force is applied to the foot on the ankle. The first structure to fail is the anterior tibiofibular ligament followed by an oblique or short spiral fracture of the lateral malleolus. As the force continues, the posterior lip of the tibia is fractured, and finally a fracture of the medial malleolus occurs or the deltoid ligament may be torn.

Supination–adduction injury

A supination–adduction injury occurs with the foot in supination and with a medially directed force. A transverse fracture of the lateral malleolus or a tear of the fibular collateral ligaments is observed, followed by a vertical fracture of the medial malleolus at the level of the joint.

Pronation–eversion injury

When the forefoot is held in pronation and an external rotatory force is applied, a pronation–eversion injury occurs. The first structure to fail is either the medial malleolus or the deltoid ligament. As the injury progresses, there is a disruption of the anterior tibiofibular ligament and the interosseous membrane. A short oblique fracture of the fibula 8 cm or more proximal to the lateral malleolus results, a disruption of the posterior tibiofibular ligament follows, and a fracture of the posterior lip of the tibia eventually occurs. These injuries are characterized by a diastasis of the tibiofibular joint.

Pronation–abduction injury

A pronation–abduction injury occurs when the forefoot is in pronation and a force is directed laterally on the foot. The medial malleolus is fractured or the deltoid ligament is torn. This is followed by development of an oblique fracture of the lateral malleolus in which there is usually comminution of the lateral cortex. This fracture is horizontal when viewed on the lateral radiograph.

Pronation–dorsiflexion injury

A pronation–dorsiflexion injury occurs when the forefoot is in pronation and the ankle is forcibly dorsiflexed, as in axial loading of the tibia. The medial malleolus is fractured, and a fracture of the tibial plafond follows. The amount of comminution is determined by the magnitude of the force. With further progression a fracture of the posterior lip of the tibia may be noted, followed by a high transverse or oblique fracture of the fibula.

Danis–Weber system

The Danis–Weber system (Müller et al 1988a) is based on the level of the fracture of the fibula and the level of the syndesmotic disruption (Table 1). There are three types of fractures in this system, each with three subgroups (Müller et al 1988b).

A Type A fracture is characterized by a transverse fibular fracture at or below the joint line with no involvement of the syndesmosis. The Weber A fracture corresponds to the Lauge-Hansen supination–adduction injury.

A Type B fracture involves a fracture beginning at the level of the joint and a partial syndesmotic injury. The Weber B fracture corresponds to the Lauge-Hansen supination–eversion type injury.

In a Type C fracture, the fibular fracture is proximal to the joint line and there is an associated disruption of the syndesmosis. Type C fractures are divided into diaphyseal fractures (Dupuytren) and proximal fractures (Maisonneuve). The Weber C fracture corresponds to the Lauge-Hansen pronation–eversion or pronation–abduction injury.

Reduction

The ultimate goal in treating ankle fractures is to achieve an anatomical reduction of the articulating surfaces so that normal function may be restored. The literature confirms that excellent long-term results are obtained only when an anatomical reduction is achieved, and this is more predictably done by open reduction and internal fixation than by closed means. Any residual talar displacement or instability will predispose the patient to late degenerative changes (Lee & Horan 1943, Denham 1964, Burwell & Charnley 1965, Cedell 1967).

Radiographic evaluation of the ankle joint should include at least three views: an anteroposterior view, a lateral view, and a mortise or internal oblique view. One method commonly used to evaluate the reduction is measurement of the joint space. The importance of this has been demonstrated in the literature (Bonnin 1970, Burns 1943, Denham 1964). The joint space measurement can be assessed by the distance between the inner surface of the lateral and the medial malleoli and the opposing articulating surface of the talus. The joint space may also be measured between the talus and the tibial plafond. Less than 2 mm of difference in the measurements should be considered normal; residual talar displacement should be suspected if any of these measurements is over 2 mm.

The problem with this method is that all three measurements cannot be obtained in a single view. A routine anteroposterior projection of the ankle in which the X-ray beam is parallel to the inner surface of the medial malleolus cannot show the space between the talus and the lateral malleolus. Similarly in the mortise view, with the leg internally rotated 15–20° so that the X-ray beam will be nearly perpendicular to the intermalleolar line and parallel to the inner surface of the lateral malleolus, the space between the talus and the medial malleolus cannot be appreciated. It is strongly recommended that if radiographic evaluation is to be used to access the reduction, all three views named above should be obtained.

From these views, the following data may be observed: the clear space between the talus and the medial and lateral malleoli and the tibial plafond, the fibular length, talar tilt, talar shift, talocalcaneal angle, and the interosseous clear space.

Probably the most accurate radiological description of the ankle joint was given by Joy et al (1974), who found that the amount of talar displacement and the width of the medial clear space influenced the final clinical result. With a standard anteroposterior X-ray, a vertical line is drawn down the center of the tibial shaft passing through the talus. The line should pass through the center of the talus. If it does not, then the talus has shifted either laterally or medially depending on which way the line was displaced. The amount of displacement represented by the distance between the midline of the tibia and the midline of the talus should not exceed 0.5 mm. Anterior or posterior displacement of the talus may be evaluated on the lateral projection by drawing a vertical line along the middle of the tibia through the talus. This line should pass through the most superior part of the dome of the talus.

Talar tilt may be evaluated on either the anteroposterior or the mortise X-rays. In the anteroposterior view, the distances between the articular surfaces of the tibia and the talus in the lateral and medial aspects of the joint are measured. In the mortise view, lines drawn parallel to the articular surface of the distal tibia and the articular surface of the talus should be parallel to each other. Another method of measuring talar tilt on the mortise view, described by Tile (1987) is to draw an intermalleolar line and measure the angles between the intermalleolar line and each of the articular surface lines. The difference between the two angles is the talar tilt. The normal talar tilt angle is 0°, with a range of −1.5–1.5°.

The talocrural angle is the superior medial angle of a line perpendicular to the distal tibial articular surface and the intermalleolar line. The normal adult talocrural angle is 83 ± 4° (Sarkisian & Cody 1979). The medial clear space is the distance between the lateral border of the medial malleolus and the medial border of the talus at the level of the talar dome in the mortise view. A space of greater than 4 mm is abnormal (Joy et al 1974).

The syndesmotic integrity is determined in two ways: first, the tibiofibular clear space is measured from the lateral border of the posterior tibial malleolus to the medial border of the fibula on the anteroposterior X-ray. The normal value for this is 5 mm. Another method of evaluating the syndesmotic integrity is to measure the overlap of the tibia and fibula from the medial border of the fibula to the lateral border of the anterior tibial prominence on the anteroposterior X-ray. This is abnormal if less than 10 mm.

From a practical point of view, it may be difficult to obtain precise X-rays, especially if the ankle is immobilized in either a cast or a splint. Therefore, it has been our policy to accept a reduction in which the lateral or medial malleolus may have a residual displacement of less than or equal to 2 mm from the anatomical position.

Treatment options

Ankle fractures may be treated by either closed reduction and cast immobilization or by open reduction with internal fixation. The main goal of treatment, whether operative or nonoperative, is to obtain an anatomic reduction and to maintain it. Multiple studies have been done to compare operative and nonoperative treatment (Charnley 1961, Klossner 1962, Wilson & Skillbred 1966, Philips et al 1969, Eventov et al 1978, Wheelhouse & Rosenthal 1980, Yde & Kristensen 1980a, Yde & Kristensen 1980b, Pettrone et al 1983, Tunturi et al 1983, Leeds & Ehrlich 1984, Kristensen & Hansen 1985, Phillips et al 1985, Rowley et al 1986).

These studies strongly suggest that closed reduction with cast immobilization should be reserved for nondisplaced stable fractures, for displaced fractures which are reduced anatomically and maintained without multiple manipulations, or for patients who are not operative candidates because of underlying medical conditions. Unstable fractures, however, should be treated with open reduction and internal fixation.

Stable injuries include isolated fractures of the lateral and medial malleolus when no ligaments are torn, avulsion fractures, and fractures of the anterior or posterior tibial lips that involve less than 25% of the articular surface.

Unstable injuries are those in which there is 2 mm or more displacement of the talus or lateral malleolus or those in which a talar tilt exists as determined radiographically. These fractures are characterized by injury to both the medial and lateral structures.

Closed reduction

To obtain a successful closed reduction, the surgeon should have an understanding of the mechanism of injury and realize that a good reduction is obtained by reversing the mechanism of injury (Rockwood et al 1991). Closed reductions should be performed under general or spinal anesthesia. It is helpful to flex the knee over the end of the operating table to assist in the reduction. Manual traction is applied along the longitudinal axis of the leg to bring the fragments out to length. Following this, a corrective force is used to reduce the fracture.

The Lauge-Hansen classification is useful in this regard because, if the surgeon is aware of the forces that caused the injury, he is better able to reduce the fracture by reversing the forces. For example, a supination–eversion injury is denoted radiologically by an oblique or short spiral fracture of the lateral malleolus just above the joint and a transverse fracture of the medial malleolus at or below the level of the joint. Reduction is achieved by pronating the forefoot and forcibly internally rotating the foot on the ankle. The same reasoning applies to fractures caused by other forces.

If the ankle has a considerably increased amount of swelling at the time of reduction, a bulky Jones dressing with plaster reinforcements or a splint may be applied after reduction to maintain immobilization and also to allow for the swelling to decrease. When the swelling has subsided, and if the reduction has been maintained, a short leg cast is applied with three-point fixation and molded to maintain the corrective force. If post-reduction radiographs show that the position has been maintained, then the knee is brought out to 15° of flexion and the cast is extended to the groin. Radiographs are obtained after the cast has been applied, at 48 hours, 7 days, 2 weeks, and then at 2-week intervals until 4–6 weeks have passed, to detect any loss of reduction. The patient is allowed to ambulate during this time with crutches but is not permitted to bear weight on the affected extremity. Immobilization of the foot in equinus should be avoided.

If the position of the fracture is satisfactory, a short leg cast is applied at 6 weeks and the patient is allowed to start ambulating with touch-down weight bearing and crutches. The patient's weight bearing status is advanced as evidence of healing is seen on X-rays. The cast must be changed if it becomes too loose or is excessively constricting.

These fractures generally show evidence of union at 12–16 weeks, at which time the cast is removed, an elastic bandage or an air cast stirrup is applied, and physical therapy is started for range-of-motion activities.

If intraoperative radiographs after the first manipulation show that the fracture has not been adequately reduced, a further attempt may be made. If one elects to treat ankle fractures by closed reduction and cast immobilization, post reduction X-rays must be of good quality and close attention must be paid to the position of the fragments, since some detail may be obscured by the cast. If this fails to achieve a satisfactory result, the surgeon must decide whether to continue with repeated closed reductions or to proceed with an open reduction and internal fixation.

In the presence of marked swelling, it may not be possible to achieve an anatomical reduction and the surgeon may prefer to accept an incomplete reduction and immobilize the extremity in a short leg cast or splint with elevation and ice for 48 hours until the swelling subsides. A repeat closed reduction at this time has a better change of succeeding. The same principle of ice and elevation to reduce swelling prevails if any open reduction is contemplated. Edema is the enemy of wound healing and should be treated before the ankle is opened.

The condition of the skin must also be evaluated prior to considering an open reduction. Surgery should not be performed on any patient with blisters or open contaminated wounds that have been present for more than 12 hours. In such instances it is advisable to treat the soft tissues and do an open reduction when the skin has healed, even if the surgery is performed as late as 3 weeks after the injury. This is preferable to operating in the presence of suboptimal conditions and risking infection. Surgery is not recommended in the presence of established infection. In these cases it is better to treat the infection by debridement and appropriate antibiotic therapy and to fix the fracture when the acute phase of the infection has been brought under control.

Rarely, the skin is so damaged that neither cast immobilization nor open reduction is possible. In such instances, the displaced ankle may be reduced by manipulation and the position of the talus secured with a Steinmann pin, which is drilled through the plantar aspect of the calcaneum, traverses the talus, and enters the tibial shift. Alternatively, an external fixator may be used. Although these methods may not afford a complete repositioning of the bones, this may be achieved at a later date.

The only advantages that a closed reduction offers are the avoidance of a scar and the possible avoidance of infection. The disadvantages are related to several features: the difficulty in obtaining an anatomical reduction and maintaining that reduction, repeated attempts at closed reduction and cast changes, prolonged immobilization, non-weight-bearing, post-reduction edema, and post-reduction stiffness, which may often prevent the ankle from regaining a full range of motion (Braunstein & Wade 1959, Denham 1964, Philips et al 1969). Unless an anatomical reduction is achieved there will be a significant incidence of late post-traumatic degenerative arthritis (Magnusson 1944, Iselin & De Vellis 1962, Cedell 1967, Solonen & Lauttamus 1968).

Open reduction

With appropriate open reduction and internal fixation of ankle fractures, early range-of-motion exercises and weight bearing may be instituted and cast immobilization may be avoided. Thus the advantages of achieving predictable results by open reduction and internal fixation, which permit early range of motion and weight bearing, far outweigh the apparent advantages of closed reductions.

Open reduction with internal fixation is recommended for failure of closed reductions, when closed reduction requires forced abnormal positioning of the foot, for displaced or unstable fractures of either or both malleoli that result in displacement of the talus or widening of the mortise greater than 1–2 mm, and in many open fractures (Yablon & Wasilewski 1980, Tile 1987, Müller et al 1988a).

Operative techniques
The goal of operative treatment is to establish an anatomical reduction with secure fixation and to allow early postoperative range of motion.

Bimalleolar fractures
The incision is placed midway between the anterior and posterior borders of the fibula, extending 5 cm proximal to the fracture and to the tip of the lateral malleolus. By sharp dissection, the incision is carried down through the tissues until the periosteum is identified. At the proximal aspect of the incision, care should be taken to avoid the cutaneous branch of the lateral peroneal nerve. The periosteum is incised at the fracture site only. The distal fragment is pulled distally and internally rotated. To insure an anatomical reduction, the fracture should be visualized in two planes, that is in the lateral plane and the posterior plane. The reduced fragments are held in position with a small self-locking bone clamp. A five- or six-hole semitubular plate is used to secure the fracture. The screws should avoid purchasing on small fragments and should be engaged in the intact portion of the proximal and distal fibula (Fig. 1). The distal fibula differs significantly among individuals, therefore the plate may require bending to conform to the shape of the bone.

Interfragmentary screws without the use of a plate may afford anatomical reduction of the fractured lateral malleolus but the fixation is not strong enough to allow for early motion and weight bearing. The one exception in which interfragmentary screws may be used is a long noncomminuted fracture of the lateral malleolus in which the length of the fracture is equal to or greater than twice the width of the fibula.

The use of circlage wires or intramedullary rods to stabilize the lateral malleolus is contraindicated if early motion and weight bearing are to be instituted. These devices do not prevent shortening or rotation of the fragment and may lead to malunion. In the presence of marked comminution they provide insufficient fixation. A tapered, triflanged, V-shaped malleable intramedullary nail has been described to fix the lateral malleolus (McLennan & Ungersma 1986). This yielded good results in the hands of these authors, but to date we have had no experience with this method. Occasionally the lateral malleolar fracture is extremely unstable because of comminution so that it is difficult to hold the reduction with a clamp while the plate is being applied. An interfragmentary screw placed across the fracture is a useful adjunct to maintain the position in such instances.

During surgery, the distal part of the peroneus tertius muscle originating from the anterior edge of the distal fibula should be gently elevated and the anterior tibiofibular ligament visualized throughout its length. A torn anterior tibiofibular ligament should always alert the surgeon to the possibility of other torn syndesmotic ligaments. This ligament represents the first line of defense, and it is the only ligament that can be visualized adequately at surgery. Manually pulling the distal fibula laterally in the presence of intact syndesmotic ligaments is impossible. However, if the fibula can be pulled laterally, it is an indication of a diastasis and the fibula should be stabilized with a syndesmotic screw as described below. On rare occasions when there is marked comminution of the fibula, rather than using

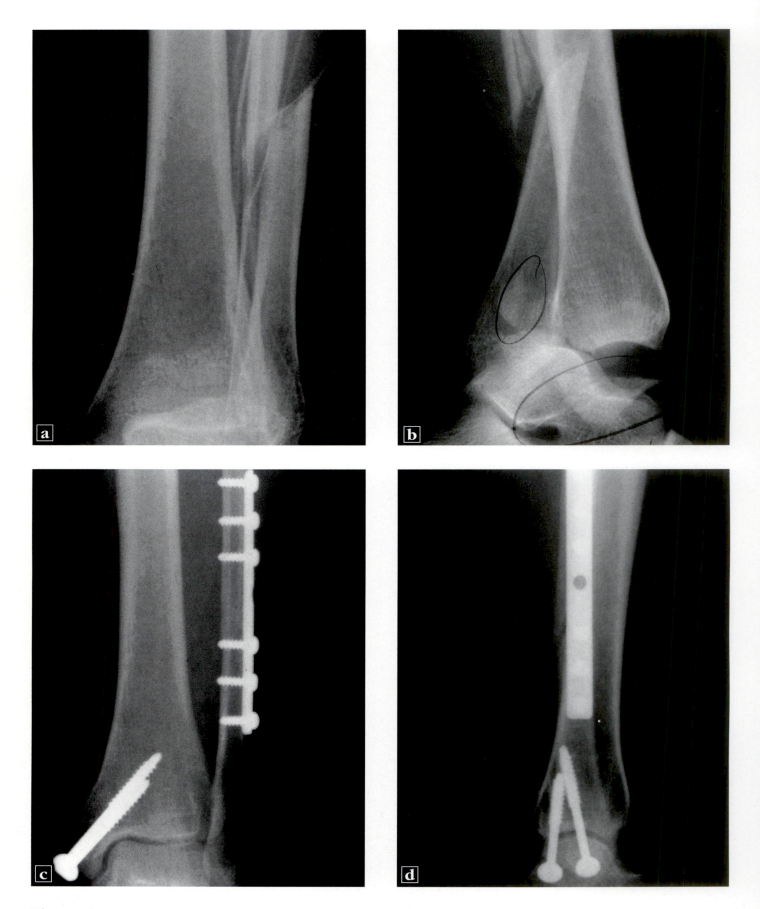

Figure 1
This bimalleolar fracture was associated with posterior dislocation of the ankle, but an intact distal tibiofibular syndesmosis (a,b). This was treated with open reduction and internal fixation of the malleoli (c,d)

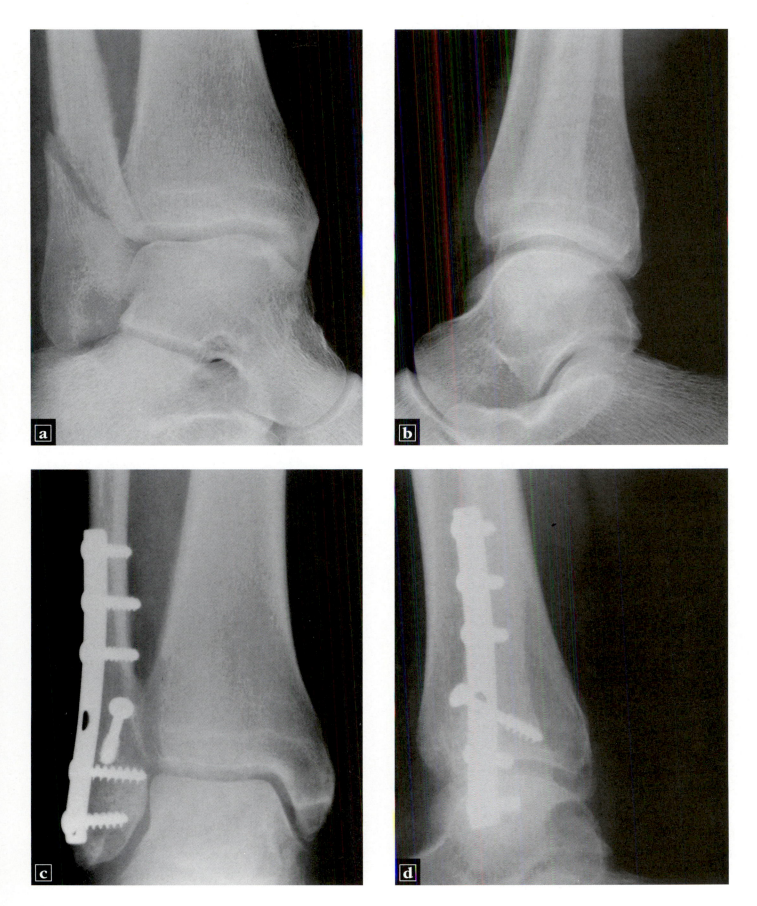

Figure 2

Isolated Weber B distal fibula fracture (a,b) treated with open reduction and internal fixation (c,d)

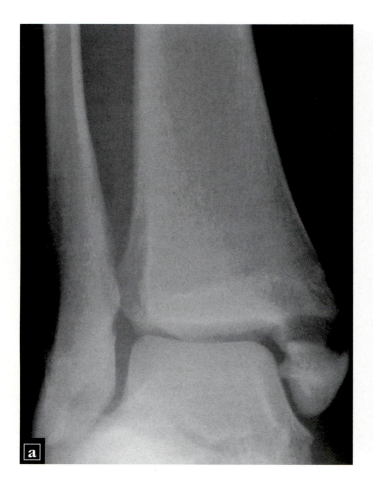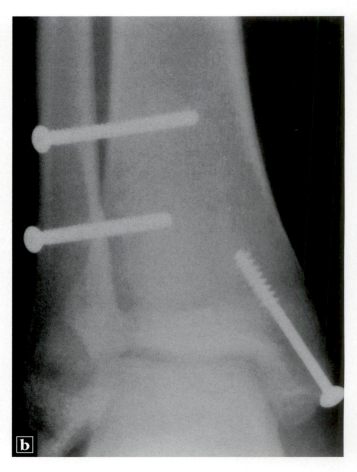

Figure 3

This isolated fracture of the medial malleolus was associated with disruption of the distal syndesmosis (a) and treated with open reduction and internal fixation of the medial malleolus, and fixation of the syndesmosis (b)

longer plates and more extensive surgery, the proximal and distal fibular fragments may be secured by screws into the lateral cortex of the tibia. In this way the lateral cortex of the tibia is used as a stabilizing structure. This method is also helpful in the presence of severe osteoporosis, when the purchase of the screws in the fibula is not firm.

Fibular shaft fractures

Fractures of the fibular shaft that occur in the lower diaphyseal region are called Dupuytren's fracture (Fig. 2), those in the middle third of the shaft are called Hugier or high Dupuytren's fractures, and those at the neck of the fibula are called Maisonneuve fractures. These injuries may be misleading and are often overlooked. When examining patients with fibular fractures, whether proximal, midshaft or distal, the surgeon should palpate the entire shaft. Tenderness anywhere along the shaft of the fibula should warrant additional radiographs, since the initial ones may miss the fracture if only the ankle region has been examined.

Tenderness along the medial aspect of the ankle or over the anterolateral area should alert the examining physician to a tear of the deltoid ligament or anterior tibiofibular ligament. If a disruption of the syndesmosis is suspected, it may be necessary to obtain inversion stress X-rays under local anesthesia. This will demonstrate a diastasis and talar displacement. These have been described by Lauge-Hansen (1950) as pronation–eversion injuries.

In pronation–eversion injuries, the pronated foot has a laterally directed force applied to it, which first causes either a tear of the deltoid ligament or a fracture of the medial malleolus. This is followed by a rupture of the anterior tibiofibular ligament and a tear of the interosseous membrane, resulting in a diastasis. With the continued lateral forces acting proximally through the interosseus membrane, the fibula eventually fractures. It should be borne in mind that, although isolated fibular shaft fractures may occur, quite often shaft fractures are associated with severe ligamentous disruption. This results in a diastasis between the tibia and the fibula, leading to marked instability.

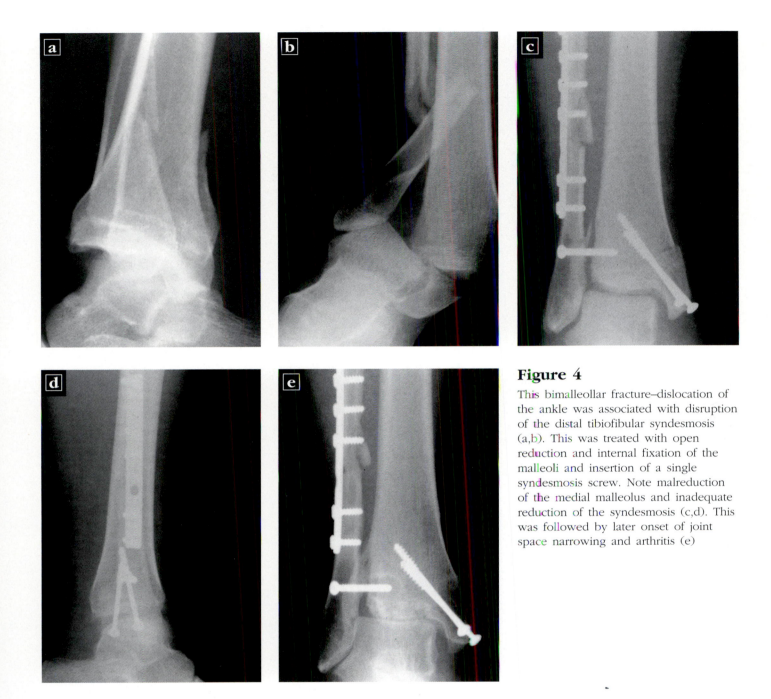

Figure 4

This bimalleollar fracture–dislocation of the ankle was associated with disruption of the distal tibiofibular syndesmosis (a,b). This was treated with open reduction and internal fixation of the malleoli and insertion of a single syndesmosis screw. Note malreduction of the medial malleolus and inadequate reduction of the syndesmosis (c,d). This was followed by later onset of joint space narrowing and arthritis (e)

If a syndesmotic disruption has occurred, a syndesmotic screw is required to maintain the fibular and talar reduction. Prior to placing the syndesmotic screw, all bony structures must be stabilized and the ankle joint must be reduced (Fig. 3). The syndesmotic screw is then inserted through one of the holes in the plate approximately 2 cm proximal and parallel to the joint. When inserting the syndesmotic screw, the ankle should be fully dorsiflexed to maintain the ankle mortise in its widest position and to preserve its full range of dorsiflexion. Olerud (1971) demonstrated that the dorsiflexion of the ankle joint decreased by an average of 0.1° for every degree of decrease in plantar flexion when the screw was being inserted. The cortices of both the fibula and the tibia should be drilled anteriorly at approximately 30° in order to center the screw in the tibia. The AO manual states that a 4.5 mm cortical screw, through three cortices (two fibular and the lateral tibial), should be used (Ramsey & Hamilton 1976, Müller et al 1988a). We and others (Stiehl 1990), however, prefer to engage four cortices with either a 3.5 mm or a 4.5 mm screw to prevent painful screw micromotion or screw failure (Fig. 4).

Although some authors (Phillips & Spiegel 1979, Phillips et al 1985, Müller et al 1988a, Orthopaedic

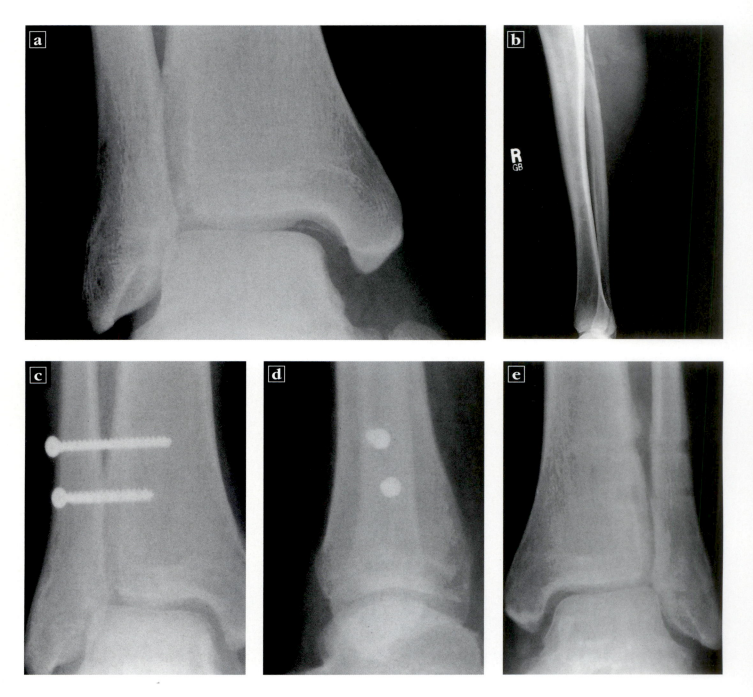

Figure 5

Anteroposterior and lateral radiographs of a Maisonneuve type fracture of the fibula (a,b) treated with tricortical syndesmosis screw reduction (c,d). The appearance of the ankle following screw removal (e)

Knowledge Update 1990) believe that syndesmotic screws should be removed prior to full weight bearing, we have permitted patients to bear weight as tolerated. Complications involving screw breakage or loosening may be avoided if the screw is placed close to and parallel to the ankle joint. We recommend the use of a 4.5 mm screw, securing four cortices. The screw should be removed under a local anesthetic at 10–12 weeks

(Roberts 1983, Phillips et al 1985, Orthopaedic Knowledge Update 1990).

For fractures of the proximal fibular shaft, open reduction and internal fixation with a small fragment plate may be used. Care should be taken not to damage the common peroneal nerve, which crosses over the neck of the fibula. Many surgeons prefer one or two syndesmotic screws inserted from the fibula into the tibia for Dupuytren's and Maisonneuve fractures. This will be effective only if the fibular fracture is reduced (Fig. 5). If the fibular fracture is not reduced, a residual increase in the medial joint space between the talus and the medial malleolus will remain. This will not be corrected by increasing the compression between the fibula and tibia because this deformity is due to a residual externally rotated position of the talus rather than to an incompletely reduced diastasis. The reason for this is the trapezoidal shape of the talus, which is wider anteriorly and narrower posteriorly. Therefore if the talus is externally rotated the narrower posterior border is brought into view and on the radiograph, this is observed as an increase in the medial joint space. If the fracture is fresh, the syndesmotic screws should be removed and the fibular fracture anatomically reduced. This will correct the talar rotation. If the fibular fracture has united, then a fibular osteotomy just proximal to the joint should be performed. The distal fragment is pulled distally and internally rotated.

Tears of the deltoid ligament

Isolated tears of the deltoid ligament are extremely rare. They may occur in lateral dislocations of the talus not associated with fractures of the malleoli. The majority of deltoid tears occur in conjunction with ankle fractures in which the lateral malleolus or the distal fibula is fractured. Controversy still exists as to the indications for opening the medial side in an injury with ankle diastasis and as to whether it is necessary to repair the deltoid ligament. We do not believe that an isolated tear of the deltoid ligament causes ankle instability.

Fractures of the medial malleolus

A 10 cm incision is placed midway between the anterior and posterior borders of the medial malleolus and is carried down to the periosteum, and full-thickness subcutaneous flaps are developed. Often, the displaced fragment will have some periosteum or fibrous tissue interposed. The interposed tissue and clots are removed, but stripping of the periosteum is limited to that affording visualization of the fracture site.

The next step is to identify the anterior inferior part of the medial malleolus. Occasionally, this will require dissecting the capsule from the distal tibia as it inserts into the medial malleolus. The joint is irrigated and inspected, and bone or cartilaginous fragments are removed. It is essential that the medial malleolus should be visualized in two planes. This will ensure accurate repositioning and has proven very reliable. The medial malleolus is secured either with one or two screws. The screw has the advantage of adding compression to the fixation, thus reducing the incidence of nonunion. Small fragments that cannot be fixed can be safely excised, especially if they are distal to the tibial plafond. Figure-of-eight tension band wiring principles do not apply to either the medial malleolus or the lateral malleolus since joint motion occurs in a plane parallel to the malleoli

rather than perpendicular to them, which is a prerequisite whenever tension band fixation is utilized.

On the rare occasions when the fracture of the medial malleolus extends proximally and posteriorly to include a significant portion of the tibial plafond, the surgical incision is extended more proximally. Occasionally such large fragments must be fixed with a buttress plate because of comminution at the junction of the fragment and the distal tibia to avoid collapse and varus deformity of the ankle.

Posterior tibial lip fractures

Isolated fractures of the posterior tibial lip, also referred to as the posterior malleolus, are rare. Most posterior tibial lip fractures are associated with malleolar and ligamentous injuries. An isolated posterior tibial lip fracture may be caused by an avulsion of the posterior inferior transverse ligament or by direct impingement of the talus when the talus is forcibly displaced posteriorly (Bonnin 1970, Wilson 1975). Posterior lip fractures may be subdivided into avulsion fractures of the posterior tuberosity, fractures of the posterior margins involving less than 25% of the articular surface, and those that involve greater than 25% of the articular surface. Avulsion fractures and fractures of less than 25% of the articular surface do not require fixation, whereas fractures involving more than 25% of the articular surface require open reduction and internal fixation because the injury involves a significant portion of the tibial plafond. With displaced posterior tibial lip fractures, the peroneal and Achilles tendons are retracted to allow for identification of the fracture site. The fracture may then be manipulated under direct visualization with the foot in plantar flexion in order to obtain an anatomic reduction (Fig. 6). If it is diffuclt to obtain good exposure of the fracture site the distal fibula should be osteotomized and turned down on itself (Gateleier 1931).

After obtaining a reduction, a K-wire is inserted from anterior to posterior to engage the fragment and the reduction is verified radiographically. If this is satisfactory, a lag screw is inserted to lag the fragment and maintain the reduction. When doing this, it is important to keep the K-wire in place so that the fragment does not rotate. The use of cannulated screws has made internal fixation easier, and has almost eliminated the potential for a rotational deformity to occur during fixation.

Anterior tibial lip fractures

Fractures of the anterior tibial lip are less common than fractures of the posterior tibial lip. These fractures may present in three forms. The first type is an avulsion of the anterior margin of the tibia by the capsule usually caused by forceful plantar flexion. The other two types are those that involve less than 25% of the articular surface, and those that involve more than 25%. As with posterior tibial lip fractures, fractures of the anterior tibial lip which involve more than 25% of the articular surface

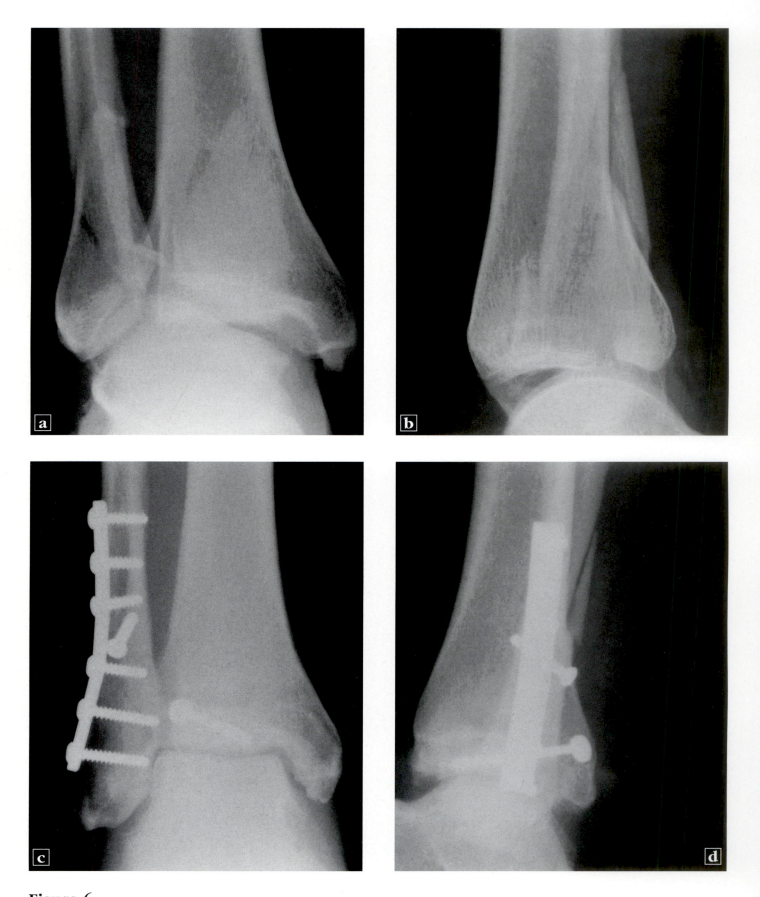

Figure 6

This comminuted fracture of the distal fibula was associated with a fracture of 30% of the posterior tibial plafond with posterior subluxation of the ankle joint (a,b). This was treated with open reduction and internal fixation of the fibula and the posterior malleolus (c,d)

require open reduction and internal fixation. The extensor tendons are retracted laterally, exposing the anterior tibia and allowing for manipulation of the fragment into position under direct visualization. By using an anterolateral exposure, the fracture may be visualized in two planes, thus allowing the surgeon to be more certain of the reduction. The fracture fragment is fixed in the same manner as the posterior tibial lip fracture.

Open fractures

Management of open fractures should be based on the principles that have been described by Gustillo & Anderson (1976). Open fractures may be classified into three types. Type I is an open fracture with a clean wound less than 1 cm long and with minimal soft tissue injury. Type II is an open fracture over 1 cm long with moderate contamination and soft tissue damage. A type III open fracture may also be further broken down into three sub-types. Type IIIA usually has a wound greater than 10 cm long with a high level of contamination and severe soft tissue damage. Type IIIB has a wound greater than 10 cm long with a high level of contamination and loss of soft tissue coverage. Type IIIC involves a wound greater than 10 cm long with a high level of contamination and loss of soft tissue plus a vascular injury.

On initial presentation with an open ankle fracture, the patient should be thoroughly evaluated for any other injuries. Swabs from the wound should then be cultured, and the injury should be assessed for the grade of the fracture and then covered with a sterile dressing not to be removed until the patient is brought to the operating room. This attempts to limit the potential for iatrogenic infection.

The fracture is splinted and radiographs should be obtained in the emergency room in as many views as possible to assist with preoperative planning. Tetanus prophylaxis should then be administered. In types II and III wounds, broad spectrum perioperative antibiotics are started after initial cultures have been obtained and before the patient goes to the operating room. In type III wounds, an aminoglycoside should be added to a cephalosporin. Recent increased experience with internal fixation in open fractures has led to successful application of these techniques in open fractures (Chapman 1986, Wiss et al 1989).

Following the initial evaluation and immobilization of the fracture, the patient should be brought to the operating room expeditiously. A tourniquet is applied but is not used unless absolutely necessary. If needed, the tourniquet is inflated without exsanguinating the limb to prevent the potential hematogenous spread of infection.

The operative procedure may be broken down into three stages:

1. Irrigation and Debridement.
2. Open Reduction and Internal Fixation.
3. Soft Tissue Evaluation and Wound Closure.

The wound must be copiously irrigated and debrided of all foreign material and dead necrotic tissues. This requires careful inspection of the joint and removal of any loose or foreign material from within the joint. Following a thorough irrigation and debridement, open reduction internal fixation is performed using methods previously described. After stable fixation has been secured, the wounds are packed open and scheduled for repeat irrigation and debridement in 48–72 hours in the operating room.

It cannot be overemphasized that type II and III wounds should never be closed primarily regardless of how benign they may appear. Failure to recognize this principle has led to disastrous consequences culminating in septicemia, chronic osteomyelitis, and even the need for amputation. Wound care should be performed as many times as needed prior to final closure or possible soft tissue coverage procedure.

Postoperatively, the patient should remain on broad spectrum intravenous antibiotic coverage for 72 hours or until cultures are negative. Antibiotics are not advised past this time period because of the potential for the development of superinfection.

For the more severely comminuted fractures where internal fixation may not be applicable, external fixation or skeletal traction may be acceptable treatment modalities provided the soft tissue protocols outlined above for open reduction internal fixation are followed in order to preserve soft tissues and prevent infection.

Postoperative management

Postoperative management of ankle fractures has traditionally consisted of immobilization of the extremity with the patient ambulating with crutches for 6 weeks. Then, as fracture healing continued, weight bearing was gradually permitted until complete union occurred. Following radiographic evidence of union, the cast was removed and physical therapy was started to assist the patient in regaining range of motion and muscle strength.

With the rigid internal fixation method as described above, early mobilization of the involved joint in order to restore function and prevent fracture disease should now be the primary goal of postoperative management (Danis 1979, Lund-Kristensen et al 1981, Müller et al 1988a). This applies to most ankle fractures with the exception of those involving the tibial plafond and the anterior and posterior tibial lip fractures with more than 25% articular surface involvement.

Our preferred method of treatment is to place the patient in a derotation AO splint postoperatively for 48 hours and to elevate the extremity to decrease postoperative swelling while in bed. During this immediate postoperative period, the patient is ambulating non-weight-bearing with crutches on the affected side. After 48 hours the patient is permitted graduated weight bearing in the ankle orthosis as tolerated. The orthosis is worn 24 hours a day for the first 4 weeks. Following this, the patient may discard the orthosis at night but should wear the brace when ambulating until union occurs at approximately 12 weeks. In patients who have had syndesmotic screws placed, the screws are removed under local anesthesia between 10 and 12 weeks postoperatively. Owing to the nature of anterior and posterior tibial lip fractures involving more than 25% of the articular surface, weight bearing is avoided until radiographic union occurs. These patients wear a short leg cast for 2 weeks, and then an air cast boot for 4 weeks to allow them to actively dorsiflex and plantarflex the ankle to maintain range of motion and strength.

Tibial plafond fractures

Tibial plafond fractures, also commonly referred to as pilon fractures (from the French, meaning crutch), are fractures of the distal tibia that extend into the distal articular surface of the tibia and potentially disrupt the tibiotalar joint and its respective articular surfaces. These injuries are usually the result of an axial compression force applied through the foot, which drives the talus into the distal tibia or through a torsional loading force, which may extend a tibial fracture into the distal tibia. Rüedi & Allgöwer (1973) have classified plafond fractures on the basis of the severity of the comminution and the displacement of the articular surfaces. Type I is an articular fracture without significant displacement; type II involves an articular fracture with significant incongruity but minimal comminution; and type III involves a severely comminuted and impacted articular fracture. Evaluation of tibial plafond fractures should include standard anteroposterior, lateral, and mortise X-rays, and either a CT scan, anteroposterior and lateral tomograms, or a CT scan with three-dimensional reconstructions.

Fractures of the tibial plafond that involve less than 20% of the articulating surface or in which the fractures are displaced less than 2 mm may be treated nonoperatively. There are circumstances in which the surgeon may decide not to intervene surgically and to treat the patient with early range of motion and delayed weight bearing. One such occasion is a markedly comminuted plafond injury considered by the surgeon to be beyond reconstruction, which appears on X-ray as a 'bag of bones'. Other structures include peripheral vascular disease, diabetes, and a plafond fracture associated with paralysis.

The patient should be hospitalized and the affected extremity should be elevated. Ice and a compression dressing are applied to decrease edema. Close observation of the neurovascular status is essential. Occasionally, swelling may be associated with a compartment syndrome or ischemic changes of the skin, necessitating fasciotomies. Usually evaluation and immobilization in a well-padded cast or posterior splint with ice packs will reduce the swelling within a period of 5–7 days. At this stage, active dorsiflexion and plantar flexion is encouraged. An ankle brace with rigid hinges, which permits motion in the sagittal plane, is prescribed, but weight bearing is delayed for 3 months or until bony union occurs.

In the past, we have followed the general trend of treating the type II and III Ruedi fractures by meticulous open reduction and internal fixation. After reviewing these results, we were less than satisfied. There was a high incidence of postoperative infection (approaching 8%), anatomical reduction was almost never obtained, and the patients ultimately required an arthrodesis. Because of this we now recommend a more restricted surgical approach. If there is comminution to the point where the tibial articular surface cannot be anatomically restored we feel that it is better to do a limited internal fixation, encourage early motion, and retain as much bone stock as possible so that an ankle arthrodesis can be done at the appropriate time. This generally requires reduction of the fibula by direct exposure and the application of a five- or 6-hole plate followed by early range-of-motion exercises. There are occasions when the fracture is composed of two or three large fragments that can be fixed securely. In such instances it is obviously advisable to attempt an anatomical reduction. However, if an anatomical reduction cannot be achieved it is better for the patient to have less surgery and for an ankle fusion to be planned in the future.

Postoperative care of tibial plafond fractures

The patient's neurovascular status should be monitored closely and frequently in the first 24 hours after surgery. If any concerns arise about possible loss of either circulation or sensation, the cast or the splint should be bivalved immediately down to the skin. Within 5–7 days, as the swelling subsides, the patient is instructed in active dorsiflexion and plantar flexion exercises. Reliable patients may be discharged in an air cast boot and instructed in range-of-motion exercises while non-weight-bearing. One of the criteria for discharge is that the patient can actively dorsiflex the ankle to at least neutral and preferably achieve a few degrees of dorsiflexion. Patients who cannot dorsiflex their ankle to at least neutral should preferably be discharged in a short leg cast, which is applied under minimal sedation to position the ankle in slight dorsiflexion. Unreliable patients should be discharged in a short leg cast. No weight bearing is allowed for at least 3 months in patients with tibial plafond fractures or until bony union can be confirmed radiographically.

Complications

Malunion

Malunion may occur in any fracture. In ankle fractures, malunions are more common than nonunions because most ankle fractures occur in metaphyseal bone and therefore usually heal (Rockwood et al 1991). The major symptoms of malunion secondary to malleolar displacement are pain, which is usually localized over the lateral aspect of the ankle and swelling. The most common cause for a malunion of the lateral malleolus is a failed closed reduction. The lateral malleolus is usually shortened and externally rotated. As described above in unstable fractures of the lateral malleolus, the talus follows the displacement of the fibula. When the ankle is reduced by closed reduction, the talus is often forced into what appears to be an acceptable position. This forced reduction of the talus occurs at the expense of the fibular collateral ligaments, which are stretched. Post-reduction X-rays usually demonstrate satisfactory talar alignment but the lateral malleolus is incompletely reduced.

When the external immobilization is discontinued the residual talar instability causes pain and ultimately arthrosis. If the patient's symptoms persist and interfere with activities of daily living, surgery may be necessary. This is done by exposing the fibula through a lateral approach as described above and performing a transverse osteotomy above the joint. After the osteotomy is complete, the anterior tibiofibular joint should be exposed and cleaned of scar and fibrous tissue. A unicortical hole is then drilled in the posterior aspect of the distal portion of the lateral malleolus, into which a bone hook is inserted. The lateral malleolus is then distracted distally and is internally rotated to restore the integrity of the anterior tibiofibular notch on the tibia. The lateral malleolus is held in a corrected position with a five-hold plate. A slight gap may be present at the osteotomy site and this should be packed with autogenous bone graft obtained locally from the tibia.

Malunion of the medial malleolus can also occur. This is usually due to an incomplete closed reduction or to failure to observe the fracture in two planes during open reduction. Patients with malunion of the medial malleolus will usually complain of increased pain when the ankle is dorsiflexed. This is because the talus is wider anteriorly, and as patients dorsiflex their ankle, impingement of the medial malleolus will occur. This results in pain and degenerative changes in the area. Treatment consists of osteotomizing the medial malleolus through the original fracture and obtaining an anatomical reduction. The fragment should then be repositioned anatomically and fixed with a malleolar screw. Recently, the use of cannulated screws has decreased the potential for loss of reduction. If the fragment has united and is in an unacceptable position where it impinges on the medial aspect of the talus and causes symptoms, it may be best to excise it.

Posterior malleolar malunions are significant only when there is involvement of more than 25% of the articular surface. Preoperative X-rays and CT scans with three dimensional reconstructions are helpful in assessing the extent of the articular surface involvement. The malunited fragment must be approached under direct visualization to be osteotomized and then reduced anatomically. This is best performed by using the Gatelier approach (Gatelier 1931). The skin incision is identical to that described for the treatment of the lateral malleolus. The distal fibula is identified and osteotomized about 6 cm

proximal to the tip of the lateral malleolus. With sharp dissection the lateral malleolus is freed from the interosseous membrane and ligament, and from the anterior and posterior tibiofibular ligaments, and turned distally on itself; the calcaneofibular ligament is left intact. This will now bring the whole of the lateral aspect of the tibia into view. The malunited fragment is osteotomized and pulled into its anatomical position with a bone hook. A K-wire is inserted from an anterior to posterior direction to transfix the fragment, and intraoperative radiographs are obtained. If these are satisfactory, fixation is augmented with a compression screw inserted through the anterior fragment into the posterior aspect of the tibia. The K-wire is cut and bent on itself to prevent migration. The fibula is then fixed with a plate.

Nonunion

Most nonunions in ankle fractures involve the medial malleolus. They are more common after a closed reduction (Mendelsohn 1965). Because ankle fractures commonly occur in metaphyseal bone, healing generally occurs, so that if there are complications, these manifest themselves as a malunion rather than a nonunion. Treatment of nonunions should be by direct visualization using the usual exposures. The fracture needs to be completely exposed and any soft tissue interposition needs to be cleared. The ends of the fracture should be curetted and freshened up so that rigid internal fixation can be achieved. Fixation of the medial malleolus should be with a screw. Fixation for the lateral malleolus should be with a plate. The fracture site should be bone grafted with autologous bone obtained locally to assist in healing.

Distal tibiofibular synostosis

In some ankle fractures associated with significant soft tissue injury, a bony synostosis may develop at the distal tibiofibular joint. Ossification usually occurs at the level of the fibular fracture site. It is unclear whether the synostosis is caused by the fracture healing, the use of a syndesmotic screw, or both (Kaye 1989). Although some patients have increased pain with fibular motion and these may benefit from excision of the heterotopic bone (McMaster & Scranton 1975) a synostosis usually does not require treatment, especially if there is a good range of motion at the ankle (Grath 1960).

Infection

The infection rate in patients undergoing open reduction and internal fixation of closed ankle fractures has been shown to be approximately 1% (Mitchell et al 1979, Mast & Teipner 1980, Meyer & Kumler 1980). Should an infection occur, it is necessary to follow the same principles that one would follow for any other orthopaedic infection.

For superficial infections, local wound care and antibiotics may be all that are required. There are, however, differences of opinion regarding the treatment of deep infections. Some authors have recommended formal debridement with removal of the hardware (Phillips et al 1985), while others have recommended debridement with appropriate antibiotic therapy (Roberts 1983, Rockwood et al 1991). We feel that antibiotics are not indicated if the wound is open and draining exteriorly. If the hardware is securely holding the fracture then it is recommended that it should not be removed and that the wound should receive local care. This is continued until the fracture has healed, which takes approximately 10–12 weeks. At that time, the patient is admitted to hospital, the hardware is removed and a formal debridement is done. Cultures are obtained and the appropriate antibiotic administered intravenously for 4 to 6 weeks. If a deep seated infection is present and the hardware is loose then it should be removed and the infection treated according to accepted principles that is, debridement, packing the wound open, taking appropriate cultures and instituting appropriate intravenous antibiotic therapy.

Wound dehiscence

The application of a plate on a subcutaneous bone such as the fibula should not cause undue complications if care is taken to close the wound carefully and to prevent edema. Special attention must be paid in order to achieve a good subcutaneous closure. The best way of avoiding edema is to elevate the ankle and to apply ice over the dressing immediately in the recovery room. These measures if carefully followed will promote wound healing and will allow for an uneventful post-operative recovery. The limb should be suspended from an overhead frame and the level of the ankle should always be higher than the heart to ensure physiologic drainage. Pillow elevation is inadequate to prevent swelling.

References

Amendola A 1992 Controversies in diagnosis and management of syndesmosis injuries of the ankle. Foot Ankle 13: 44–50
American Academy of Orthopaedic Surgeons 1972 Joint Motion: Method of Measuring and Recording. Churchill Livingstone, New York
Anderson M E 1985 Reconstruction of the lateral ligaments of the ankle using the plantaris tension. J Bone Joint Surg 67A: 930–934

Barnett C H, Napier J R 1952 The axis of rotation at the ankle in man. Influence upon deformity of the talus and mobility of the fibula. J Anat (Lond) 86: 2–9
Bonnin J G 1970 Injuries to the Ankle. Hefner Publishing, Darien, Conn.
Braunstein P W, Wade P A 1959 Treatment of unstable fractures of the ankle. Ann Surg 149: 217
Brodie I A D, Denham R A 1974 The treatment of unstable fractures of the ankle. J Bone Joint Surg 56B: 252–262
Burns B H, 1943 Diastasis of the inferior tibiofibular joint. Proc R Soc Med 36: 330
Burwell N H, Charnley A D 1965 Treatment of displaced fractures at the ankle by rigid internal fixation and early joint movement. J Bone Joint Surg 47B: 634–660
Caifliet R 1968 Foot and Ankle Pain. F A Davis, Philadelphia
Cedell C A 1967 Supination–outward rotation injuries of the ankle. A clinical and roentgenological study with special reference to the operative treatment. Acta Othop Scand (suppl) 110
Chapman M W 1986 Fractures and fracture–dislocation of the ankle. In: Mann R A (ed) Surgery of the Foot, 5th Ed. C V Mosby, St Louis pp. 568–591
Charnley J 1961 The Closed Treatment of Common Fractures, 3rd ed. Livingstone, Edinburgh
Close R B 1956 Some applications of functional anatomy of the ankle joint. J Bone Joint Surg 38A: 761–781
Cunningham's Textbook of Anatomy 1972 11th ed Oxford University Press, London
D'Ambrosia R D 1977 Musculoskeletal Disorders: Regional Examination and Differential Diagnosis. J B Lippincott, Philadelphia
Danis R 1979 The aims of internal fixation. Clin Orthop 138: 23–25
Denham R A 1964 Internal fixation for unstable ankle fractures. J Bone Joint Surg 46B: 206–211
Eventov I, Salema R, Goodwin D R A, Wiessman S L 1978 Evaluation of surgical and conservative treatment of fractures of the ankle in 200 patients. J Trauma 18: 271–275
Fritschy D 1989 An unusual ankle injury in top skiers. Am J Sports Med 17: 282–286
Gatelier J 1931 The juxtaretroperoneal route in the operative treatment of fracture of malleolus with posterior marginal fragment. Surg Gynecol Obstet 52: 67
Grath G B 1960 Widening of the ankle mortise. Acta Chir Scand (suppl): 263
Gray's Anatomy 1973 35th British ed. W B Saunders, Philadelphia
Gustillo R B, Anderson J T 1976 Prevention of infection in the treatment of 1025 open fractures of long bones. J Bone Joint Surg 58A: 453
Harper M C 1987a Deltoid ligament: an anatomical evaluation of function. Foot Ankle 8: 19–22
Harper M C 1987b Posterior malleolar fractures in the ankle: results with and without internal fixation and effect on ankle stability. Orthop Trans 11: 483
Inman V T 1976 The Joint of the Ankle. Williams & Wilkins, Baltimore
Iselin M, De Vellis H 1962 La primaute du perone dans les fractures du cou-du-pied. Mem Acad Chir 87: 399
Joy G, Patzakis M J, Harvey J P 1974 Precise evaluation of the reduction of severe ankle fractures. J Bone Joint Surg 56A: 979–993
Kaye R A 1989 Stabilization of ankle syndesmosis injuries with a syndesmotic screw. Foot Ankle 9: 290–293
Klossner O 1962 Late results of operative and non-operative treatment of severe ankle fractures. Acta Chir Scand (suppl) 293: 1–93
Kristensen K D, Hansen T 1985 Closed treatment of ankle fractures: stage II supination–eversion fractures followed for 20 years. Acta Orthop Scand 56: 107–109
Lambert K L 1971 The weight bearing function of the fibula. A strain gauge study. J Bone Joint Surg 53A: 507–513
Lauge-Hansen N 1950 Fractures of the Ankle II. Combined experimental–surgical and experimental–roentgenologic investigations. Arch Surg 60: 957–985

Lee H G, Horan R B 1993 Internal fixation in injuries of the ankle. Surg Gynecol Obstet 76: 493

Leeds H C, Ehrlich M G 1984 Instability of the distal tibiofibular syndesmosis after bimalleolar and trimalleolar ankle fractures. J Bone Joint Surg 66A: 490–503

Lewis B W, Graham W D 1940 Secondary osteoarthritis following fractures of the ankle. Am J Surg 49: 210–218

Lund-Kristensen J, Greiff J, Riegels-Nielson P 1981 Malleolar fractures treated with rigid internal fixation and immediate mobilization. Injury 13 191–195

Magnusson R 1944 On the late results in non-operated cases of malleolar fractures. Clinical–roentgenological–statistical study. I. Fractures by external rotation. Acta Chir Scand (suppl): 84

Mast J W, Teipner W A 1988 A reproducible approach to the internal fixation of adult ankle fractures: rationale, technique, and early results. Orthop Clin North Am 11: 661–679

McLennan J G, Ungersma J A 1986 A new approach to the treatment of ankle fractures: the inyo nail. Clin Orthop 213: 125

McMaster J H, Scranton P E 1975 Tibiofibular synostosis. Clin Orthop 111: 172–174

Mendelsohn M A 1965 Nonunion of malleolar fractures of the ankle. Clin Orthop 42: 103–118

Meyer T L Jr, Kumler K W 1980 ASIF technique and ankle fractures. Clin Orthop 150: 211–216

Mitchell W G, Shaftan G W, Sclafani S J, 1979 Mandatory open reduction: its role in displaced ankle fractures. J Trauma 19: 602–615

Müller M E, Allgöwer M, Schneider R, Willenegger H 1988a Manual of Internal Fixation Techniques Recommended by the AO Group, 2nd ed. Springer-Verlag, New York

Müller M E, Nazarian S, Kock P 1988b The AO Classification of Fractures. Springer-Verlag, New York

Olerud S 1971 Subluxation of the ankle without fracture of the fibula. J Bone Joint Surg 53A: 594–596

Orthopaedic Knowledge Update III 1990. AAOS, Park Ridge, Illinois. pp. 613–624

Pettrone F A, Mitchell G, Pee D, Fitzpatrick T, Van Herpe L B 1983 Quantitative criteria for prediction of the results after displaced fracture of the ankle. J Bone Joint Surg 65A: 667–677

Philips R S, Balmer G A, Monk C J E 1969 The external rotation fracture of the fibular malleolus. Br J Surg 56: 801

Phillips W A, Spiegel P G 1979 Evaluation of ankle fractures: non-operative vs operative (editorial comment). Clin Orthop 138: 17–20

Phillips W A, Schwartz H S, Keller C S et al 1985 A prospective randomized study of the management of severe ankle fractures. J Bone Joint Surg 67A: 67–78

Ramsey P L, Hamilton W 1976 Changes in tibiotalar area of contact caused by lateral talar shift. J Bone Joint Surg 58A: 356–357

Rice C O 1968 Classification of the Industrial Disabilities of Extremities and the Back, 2nd ed. Charles C Thomas, Springfield, Illinois

Roberts R S 1983 Surgical treatment of displaced ankle fractures. Clin Orthop 172: 164–170

Rockwood C A, Green D P, Bucholz R W 1991 Fractures in adults, volume II, 3rd Ed. J B Lippincott, Philadelphia. p. 201

Rowley D I, Norris S H, Duckworth T 1986 A prospective trial comparing operative and manipulative treatment of ankle fractures. J Bone Joint Surg 68B: 610–613

Rüedi T P, Allgöwer M 1973 Fractures of the lower end of the tibia into the ankle joint: results nine years after open reduction and internal fixation. Injury S130

Sarkisian J S, Cody S W 1979 Closed treatment of ankle fractures: a new criterion for investigation. A review of 250 cases. J Trauma 16: 323–326

Segal D 1979 Unstable ankle injuries. In Instructional Course Lectures, AAOS, Vol 28. C V Mosby, St Louis

Seireg A, Arvikar R J 1975 The prediction of muscular load sharing and joint forces in the lower extremities during walking. J Biomech 8: 89–102

Simon W H, Friedenberg S, Richardson S 1973 Joint incongruence. A correlation of joint congruence and thickness of articular cartilage in cogs. J Bone Joint Surg 55A: 1614

Solonen K A, Lauttamus L 1968 Operative treatment of ankle fractures. Acta Orthop Scand 39: 223

Stiehl J B 1990 Ankle fractures with diastasis. In: AAOS Instructional Course Lectures, Vol. 39. AAOS, Park Ridge, Illinois. pp. 95–103

Takebe K, Nakagawa A, Minami H, Kanazawa H, Hirohata K 1984 Role of the fibula in weight bearing. Clin Orthop 184: 289–292

Tile M 1989 Fractures of the ankle. In Schatzker J, Tile M (eds) The Rationale of Operative Fracture Care. Springer-Verlag, New York, pp. 371–405

Tunturi T, Kemppainen K, Patiala H, Soukas M, Tamminen O, Rokkanen P 1983 Importance of anatomical reduction for subjective recovery after ankle fracture. Acta Orthop Scand 54: 641–647

Wheelhouse W W, Rosenthal R E 1980 Unstable ankle fractures: comparison of closed versus open treatment. South Med J 73: 45–50

Wilson F C 1975 Fractures and Dislocations of the Ankle. J B Lippincott, Philadelphia

Wilson F C, Skillbred L A 1966 Long-term results in the treatment of displaced bimalleolar fractures. J Bone Joint Surg 48A: 1065–1078

Wilson M J, Michele A A, Jacobsen E W 1939 Ankle dislocations without fracture. J Bone Joint Surg 21: 198–204

Wiss D A, Gilbert P, Merritt P O, Sarmiento A 1989 Immediate internal fixation of open ankle fractures. J Orthop Trauma 2: 265–271

Yablon I G, Wasilewski S 1980 Management of unstable ankle fractures. In Bateman J, Trott A (eds) The Foot and Ankle. Thieme-Stratton, New York. pp. 11–19

Yablon I G, Heller F G, Shouse L 1977 The key role of the lateral malleolus in displaced fractures of the ankle. J Bone Joint Surg 59A: 169–173

Yde J, Kristensen K D 1980a Ankle fractures: supination–eversion fractures stage II, primary and late results of operative and non-operative treatment. Acta Orthop Scand 51: 695–702

Yde J, Kirstensen K D 1980b Ankle fractures: supination–eversion fractures stage IV, primary and late results of operative and non-operative treatment. Acta Orthop Scan 51: 981–990

Additional reading

Bauer M, Bergstrom B, Hemborg A, Sandegard J 1985 Malleolar fractures: nonoperative versus operative treatment. Clin Orthop 199: 17–27

Bauer M, Johnson K, Nilsson B 1985 Thirty-year follow-up of ankle fractures. Acta Orthop Scand 56: 103–106

Baxter D E Traumatic injuries to the soft tissue of the foot and ankle. In: Mann R A (ed) Surgery of the Foot, 5th Ed. C V Mosby, St Louis pp. 456–471

Boruta P M, Bishop J O, Braly W G, Tullos H S 1990 Acute lateral ankle ligament injuries: a literature review. Foot Ankle 11: 107–113

Brostrom L, Sundelin P 1966 Sprained ankles: IV. Histologic changes in recent and 'chronic' ligament ruptures. Acta Chir Scand 132: 248–253

Chapman M W, Mahoney M 1979 The role of early internal fixation in the management of open fractures. Clin Orthop 138: 120–127

Cox J S 1985 How to prevent chronic ankle instability. J Musculoskel Med 2: 65–75

De Souza I J, Gustillo R B, Meyer T J Results of operative treatment of displaced external rotation–abduction fractures of the ankle. J Bone Joint Surg 67A: 1066–1073

Freeman M A R 1965 Instability of the foot after injuries to the lateral ligament of the ankle. J Bone Joint Surg 47B: 669–676

Freeman M A R, Dean M R E, Hanham I W F 1985 The aetiology and prevention of functional instability of the foot. J Bone Joint Surg 47B: 678–685

Garrick J G The frequency of injury, mechanism of injury, and epidemiology of ankle sprains. Am J Sports Med 5: 241–242

Harper M C 1986 The deltoid ligament: an evaluation of function and need for surgical repair. Orthop Trans 10: 446

Hopkinson W J, St Pierre P, Ryan J B, Wheeler J H 1990 Syndesmosis sprains of the ankle. Foot Ankle 10: 325–330

Kannus P, Renström P 1991 Treatment of acute tears of the lateral ligaments of the ankle. J Bone Jont Surg 73A: 305–312

Leach R E 1979 Fractures of the tibial plafond. Instructional Course Lectures Volume 28. C V Mosby, St Louis p. 88

Lovell E S 1968 An unusual rotary injury of the ankle. J Bone Joint Surg 50A: 163–165

Marymont J V, Lynch M A, Henning C E 1986 Acute ligamentous diastasis of the ankle without fracture: evaluation by radionuclide imaging. Am J Sports Med 14: 407–409

Needleman R L, Skrade D A, Stiehl J B 1990 Effect of the syndesmotic screw on ankle motion. Foot Ankle 10: 17–24

Pankovich A M 1978 Fractures of the fibula proximal to the distal tibiofibular syndesmosis. J Bone Joint Surg 60A: 221–229

Pankovich A M, Shivaram M D 1979 Anatomical basis of variability in injuries of the medial malleolus and deltoid ligament. Acta Orthop Scand 50: 217–223

Reckling F W, McNamara G R, DeSmet A A 1981 Problems in the diagnosis and treatment of ankle injuries. J Trauma 21: 943–950

Sammarco G J, Di Raimondon C V 1988 Surgical treatment of lateral ankle instability syndrome. Am J Sports Med, 16: 501–511

IX.2 Talar and Peritalar Injuries

David B Thordarson and Andrea Cracchiolo III

Injuries involving the talus can be divided into two categories:

1. Soft tissue injuries: injuries to the lateral ligaments, especially the anterior talofibular ligament, which is very common; the chronic instability that sometimes results could lead to secondary injury to the talar cartilage. (These injuries are described in Chapter IX.1.)
2. Fractures and dislocations of the talus: this chapter will deal with fractures of the talus, but it will omit the osteochondral lesions (see Chapter IX.8). Dislocations of the talus and around the talus are extremely rare unless accompanied by a fracture.

Functional anatomy

The talus has several unique characteristics. It is one of the few moveable bones that has no tendinous attachments, yet it is surrounded by a multitude of tendons. In the lower extremity it represents one of the smaller bones that has a considerable range of motion. Also, despite its small size, it must bear the body weight like the much larger proximal bones. It is surprising that the talus functions so well and that its articular cartilage receives relatively less damage than the larger hip and knee joint.

The connection between the lower leg and the foot is maintained by the talus. It is enclosed between the lateral malleolus, the lower articular surface of the tibia, the medial malleolus, the calcaneus and the navicular bone. It forms the keystone for movements between the foot and the lower leg. It thus has the combined function of stability and mobility in the ankle joint (Goldie 1988). The talus consists of the neck and head articulating against the navicular bone, the trochlea against the tibia and fibula, and the body against the calcaneus (Fig. 1). During the growth period the talus changes its internal direction in two ways. First in infancy the neck is directed about 30° medially. With increasing age this direction diminishes to 15–20°. Secondly, in infancy the neck is longitudinally rotated more laterally than in adulthood, when it straightens up (Goldie 1988).

The neck and head

The neck continues into the head, which articulates against the navicular bone. This joint forms the medial part of Chopart's joint. The head also articulates against an anterior facet of the calcaneus. Further, it articulates against a ligament that joins the sustentaculum tali of the calcaneus with the tuberosity of the navicular bone. This is the spring or calcaneonavicular liagment. Part of pronation–supination or eversion–inversion occurs in this multiaxial joint.

The trochlea

The trochlea is enclosed in the malleolar mortise, giving the lower leg – and consequently the whole body – stability during the stance phase of gait. It is covered

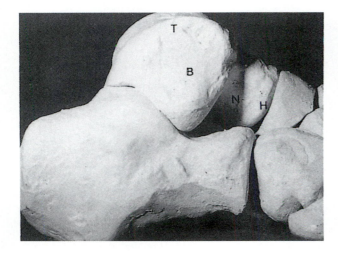
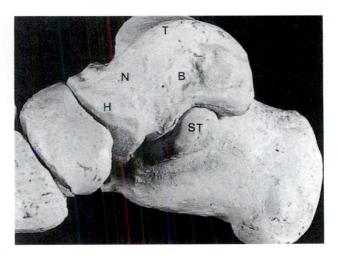

Figure 1

Surface anatomy of the talus. T–trochlea; B–body; N–neck; H–head; ST–sustentaculum tali. (From Goldie 1988)

by cartilage on the superior aspect, which articulates with the tibial plafond and on both sides articulating against the medial and the lateral malleoli.

The axis for the rotation of the trochlea is constantly changing within a narrow limit. In the coronal plane, the axis runs at an inclination downward from the medial malleolar tip to just distal to the lateral malleolar tip, but deviates posteriorly from the coronal plane (Goldie 1988).

The body

By its connection with the navicular bone, the talus has an important influence on the function of the forefoot. The talus represents a substantial component of the hindfoot. It rests on the calcaneus, which supports the talus by its posterior, middle and anterior articular surfaces. Between the posterior and middle articular facets there is a groove, the sulcus calcanei, which together with the sulcus tali forms the sinus tarsi.

The movement of the subtalar joint occurs around an axis inclined in two planes, one running in the sagittal plane at an inclination of 42° and the other in the horizontal plane from posterolateral to anteromedial at an angle of 23° from the midline of the foot. The range of motion varies markedly and values from 10° to 60° have been reported.

Vascular supply

The talus is in the midst of an arterial network, with vascular sources including the artery of the tarsal canal, the anastomosing artery of the sinus tarsi, branches that course along the deltoid ligament, branches from the dorsalis pedis artery, which enter the neck of the talus, and the small arteries in capsules and ligaments which connect the talus with the surrounding bone. Goldie et al (1974) showed that, apart from these arteries, there are rich vascular connections between the tibial and the talar marrow spaces by way of the interconnecting capsules and ligaments. Gelberman & Mortensen (1983) have investigated both the extraosseous and intraosseous vascular supply of the talus (Fig. 2).

Extraosseous blood supply
The talus receives its blood supply from branches of the anterior tibial, posterior tibial, and peroneal arteries. The surface branches of these arteries enter the five nonarticulating surfaces of the talus. The surfaces are: the superior surface of the neck, the inferior surface of the neck (the roof of the tarsal canal), the medial surface of the body, the sinus tarsi, and the posterior tubercle.

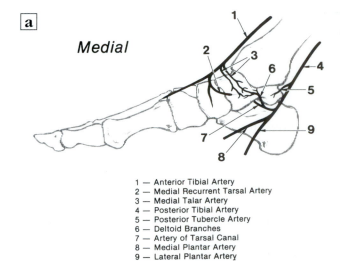

Medial

1 — Anterior Tibial Artery
2 — Medial Recurrent Tarsal Artery
3 — Medial Talar Artery
4 — Posterior Tibial Artery
5 — Posterior Tubercle Artery
6 — Deltoid Branches
7 — Artery of Tarsal Canal
8 — Medial Plantar Artery
9 — Lateral Plantar Artery

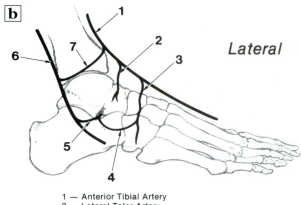

Lateral

1 — Anterior Tibial Artery
2 — Lateral Talar Artery
3 — Lateral Tarsal Artery
4 — Posterior Recurrent Branch of Lateral Tarsal
5 — Artery of Tarsal Sinus
6 — Perforating Peroneal
7 — Anterior Lateral Malleolar Artery

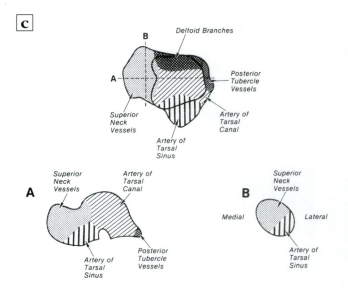

Figure 2

Vascular supply to the talus. (a) Medial side; (b) lateral side; (c) intraosseous blood supply of the talus: (A) Sagittal section through the midtalus; (B) coronal section through the neck of the talus. (From Gelberman & Mortensen 1983)

Anterior tibial artery

The anterior tibial artery provides six branches to the talus. The most frequent branches are the medial talar branches, which are at the level of the talar neck (87%), and the lateral talar branches, which are present in 65% of specimens.

Posterior tibial artery

The posterior tibial artery provides three local branches to the talus.

1. Small branches to the posterior tubercle (78%).
2. The artery of the tarsal canal (91%); this important artery courses between the flexor digitorum longus and flexor hallucis longus to enter the tarsal canal on the medial aspect of the talus.
3. The deltoid branch (91%), which enters the medial surface of the body of the talus.

Peroneal artery

The peroneal artery provides two branches to the talus. The major branch is the perforating peroneal artery, present in 83% of specimens.

Surface arteries

There are five nonarticulating surfaces of the talus through which blood vessels enter the bone.

1. The superior surface of the neck receives its main blood supply from the anterior tibial artery.
2. The medial surface of the body of the talus is supplied by the deltoid branch of the posterior tibial artery.
3. The posterior tubercle is supplied by direct branches from the posterior tibial artery in most specimens.
4. The inferior surface of the neck is supplied by the artery of the tarsal canal which anastomoses with the artery of the sinus tarsi.
5. The sinus tarsi is supplied by the artery of the sinus tarsi.

The intraosseous blood supply (see Fig. 2c)
1) The head of the talus is supplied by vessels entering the superior neck and sinus tarsi.
2) The body of the talus is supplied by the anastomotic artery in the tarsal canal, the deltoid branches and the sinus tarsi branch.

The single major arterial supply to the body of the talus is from the artery of the tarsal canal. It supplies the middle one-half to two-thirds of the body directly and, through internal anastomoses, could supply the remainder.

The blood supply to the head of the talus is from the superior neck vessels from the anterior tibial artery to the superiomedial two-thirds and from branches of the artery of the sinus tarsi to the inferolateral one-third. Thus the blood supply to the talus is much more complex than has been previously noted. These vascu-

lar studies correlate well with the reports of avascular necrosis (AVN) noted after certain injuries. For example: a vertical fracture of the neck of the talus probably interrupts only a portion of the contribution from the artery of the tarsal canal. However, it probably does not damage the minor four sources of arterial supply to the body. Fracture of the talar neck with a subtalar dislocation damages both arterial supplies; thus the greater incidence of AVN. If one adds a dislocation of the ankle joint, then 100% of the blood supply is disrupted, which correlates well with the nearly 100% incidence of AVN.

Fractures of the neck of the talus

Mechanism of injury

Fractures of the neck of the talus account for approximately half of the significant injuries to the talus. Classically, they have been described as Aviator's Astragalus, owing to their frequent occurrence following crash landings of airplanes. Fractures of the talar neck are now more commonly caused by high-velocity trauma, such as motor vehicle accidents and falls from a height (Hawkins 1970, Penny & Davis 1980, DeLee 1983). Many authors have theorized that the fracture is caused by a hyperdorsiflexion injury, the neck of the talus impacting against the anterior lip of the tibia. However, creating this fracture in the laboratory is difficult, and it was found not to be possible by forced dorsiflexion in cadaver feet (Peterson et al 1974). Peterson and Romanus (1976) were only able to fracture the talar neck reproducibly by placing the ankle in a neutral position and compressing the calcaneus against the overlying talus and tibia. Depending on the force, a nondisplaced talar neck fracture may result. However, increased force ruptures the posterior talocalcaneal and the interosseous ligaments, producing a subluxation of that joint. The calcaneus displaces anteriorly with the remainder of the foot and also usually dislocates medially. The talar body tips into equinus and the talar head is displaced dorsally on the neck. With continued force, the posterior ligamentous attachments to the ankle rupture and the body of the talus is dislocated posteromedially from the ankle mortise (Penny & Davis 1980). Sneppen and Buhl (1974) described 26 talar neck fractures in 1806 ankle fractures, and found that a supination force was most commonly associated with these combined injuries. This also correlates with the observation of others (Hawkins 1970, Penny & Davis 1980).

Classification

In 1970, Hawkins described a classification of fractures of the neck of the talus. He based it on the displacement

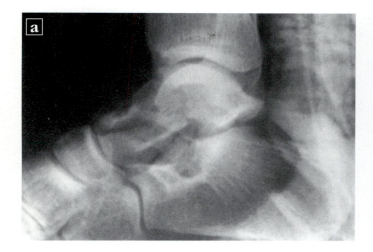
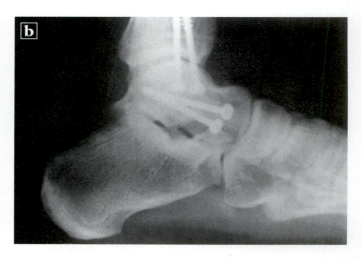

Figure 3

(a) Lateral radiograph of a Hawkins' II fracture following a motor vehicle accident. Note the incongruous subtalar joint with uninvolved ankle joint. There is also a nondisplaced fracture of the talar head and a medial malleolus fracture; (b) postoperative lateral radiograph revealing healed fracture with anatomic reduction of the talar neck and congruent subtalar joint

of the fracture site in the neck of the talus and the congruency of the subtalar joint and ankle joint. The higher grades involve greater trauma, greater displacement, and a poorer long-term prognosis. A Hawkins I fracture occurs vertically in the neck of the talus and is nondisplaced. In theory, this fracture disrupts only the blood vessels entering the dorsolateral aspect of the neck of the talus. Such fractures carry the best prognosis, usually heal, and have an avascular necrosis (AVN) rate ranging from 0–13% (Canale & Kelly 1978).

In a Hawkins II fracture, the neck of the talus is displaced and, as a result, the subtalar joint is subluxated or frankly dislocated (Fig. 3). This fracture pattern disrupts the blood supply both from the dorsolateral aspect of the talar neck and from the vascular sling in the sinus tarsi and tarsal canal. Accordingly, Hawkins II fractures carry a poorer prognosis with AVN rates of 20–50% (Hawkins 1970).

In a Hawkins III fracture, both ankle and subtalar joint incongruities exist and the body of the talus usually extrudes posteromedially between the posterior aspect of the tibia and the Achilles tendon (Figs 4,5). Owing to the severity of the trauma, Hawkins III fractures are frequently open injuries. An associated fracture of the medial malleolus occurs in many cases. The blood supply to the talus is completely disrupted, with the possible exception of that from the deltoid branches, which can be kinked because of the displaced and rotated body of the talus. Avascular necrosis has been reported in 80–100% of these fractures (Coltart 1952, McKeever 1963, Mindell et al 1963, Pennal 1963, Hawkins 1970, Penny & Davis 1980).

Canale & Kelly (1978) expanded Hawkins's original talar fracture classification. They defined a fracture of the

neck of the talus, accompanied by disruption of the ankle, subtalar, and talonavicular joints as a Hawkins IV fracture (Fig. 6). Not only is the blood supply of the body of the talus disrupted, but the head might also suffer impaired vascularity.

Clinical findings

Talar neck fractures generally result from high-velocity trauma and thus frequently occur in young adults. They occur three times more often in males than females and they are most frequent in the third decade of life (Penny & Davis 1980). In addition, associated injuries frequently occur to the musculoskeletal system (64% in Hawkins patients) or to other organ systems (Hawkins 1970). Medial malleolar fractures have been described in 20–30% of reported cases. These fractures occur especially in Hawkins III fractures with an extruded body of the talus (Lorentzen et al 1977, Canale & Kelly 1978) (see Figs 4,5). Calcaneal fractures also occur in 10% of talar neck fractures (Lorentzen et al 1977).

On examination, fracture displacement and possible dislocation of the talus can be masked by the rapid onset of swelling, making palpation of the fracture and dislocation impossible. In patients with a Hawkins III fracture with extrusion of the body of the talus, the skin overlying the talar body is frequently tented and can rapidly become necrotic. The neurovascular structures generally are spared from serious injury. However, soft tissue damage can be extensive, and a compartment syndrome of the foot or the leg may develop.

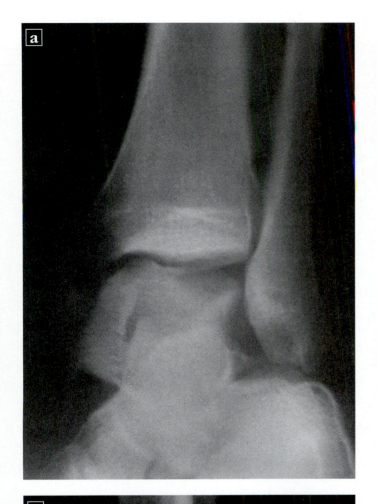

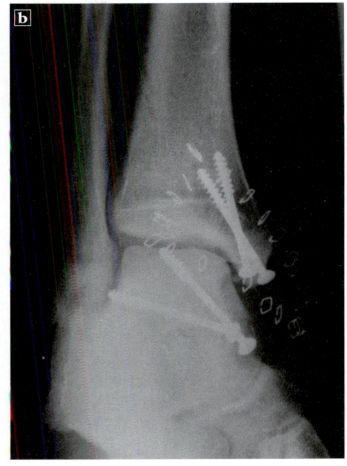

Figure 4

(a) Anteroposterior radiograph of a Hawkins' III fracture following a motorcycle accident. The talar body had extruded from the mortise posteromedially and was tenting the skin upon presentation. The medial malleolus has also been fractured; (b) anteroposterior radiograph following anatomic internal fixation. Note the skin staples medially in the region of skin graft, where the patient developed full thickness skin slough due to pressure from the talar body; (c) lateral radiograph demonstrating anatomic internal fixation with congruent ankle and subtalar joints

Radiographic evaluation

The presence of the talar neck fracture is readily apparent on anteroposterior (AP) and especially lateral radiographs of the talus. The lateral view demonstrates the displacement of the neck fracture, as well as any incongruity of the subtalar, ankle, or talonavicular joints (see Figs 3,6). However, varus or valgus displacement of the talar neck can be difficult to demonstrate on a routine AP radiograph. Since varus displacement occurs frequently, Canale & Kelly (1978) have described a modified AP radiograph that better profiles the alignment of the talar neck in the transverse plane. With a cassette

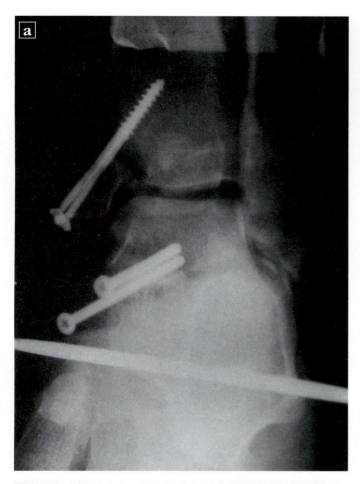

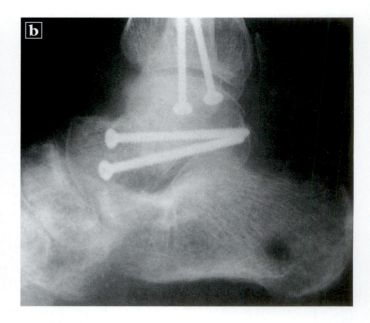

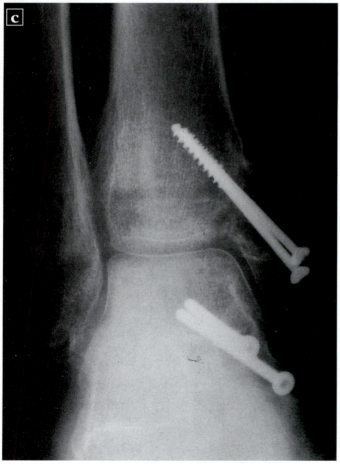

Figure 5

(a) Intraoperative anteroposterior radiograph demonstrating an anatomic reduction of fractures of the medial malleolus and talar neck with placement of a calcaneal pin used for traction to assist in reduction of the talar body into the ankle mortise; (b) lateral radiograph of the same patient following fracture consolidation with evidence of the posteroinferior pin site in the calcaneus; (c) anteroposterior radiograph of the same patient 8 weeks after open reduction and internal fixation, with a subchondral radiolucency (Hawkins' sign) extending across the entire dome of the talus indicating an absence of AVN

placed beneath the foot, the ankle is placed in maximal plantar flexion, the foot is pronated 15° and the X-ray beam is angled cephalad at an angle of 75° relative to the cassette. This view is extremely helpful in assessing alignment following fracture reduction.

Treatment

Although the treatment of these fractures depends upon the classification type, a common treatment goal is urgent anatomic reduction to restore congruency of the ankle and subtalar joints and to reduce the risk of avascular necrosis by preserving any remaining blood supply. However, despite the increased knowledge which we have concerning this fracture, treatment is still difficult. Daniels & Smith (1993), in their excellent review, point out three reasons for this problem:

1. These fractures are infrequent so they are not often seen by any individual orthopaedic surgeon.
2. Exposure, reduction and fixation are difficult, owing to the anatomy of the area.

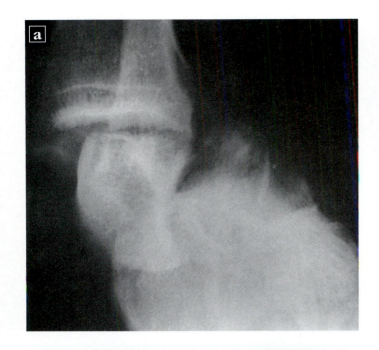

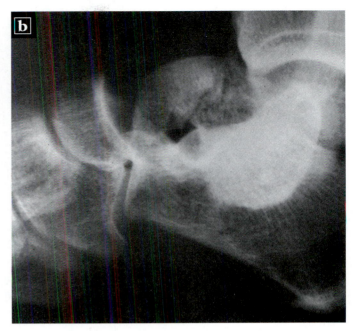

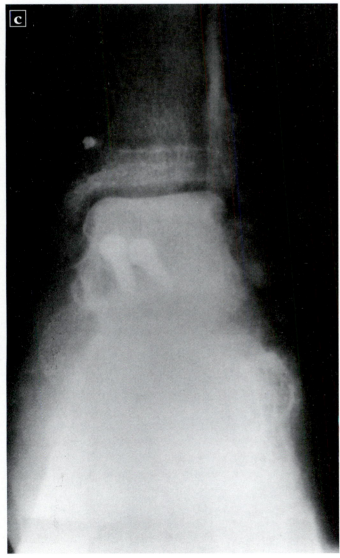

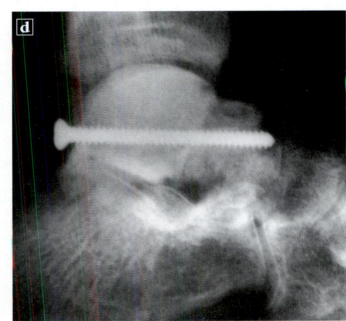

Figure 6

(a) Anteroposterior radiograph of a patient with a Hawkins' IV fracture following a fall from the third floor of a building. Note extrusion of the body of the talus posteromedially; (b) lateral radiograph of a Hawkins' IV fracture demonstrating incongruous ankle, subtalar and talonavicular joints; (c) three months after open reduction and internal fixation with two parallel screws; note the sclerotic body of the talus indicating whole body avascular necrosis; (d) a lateral radiograph at 3 months postoperatively demonstrating placement of screws from posterior to anterior and the sclerotic body of the talus

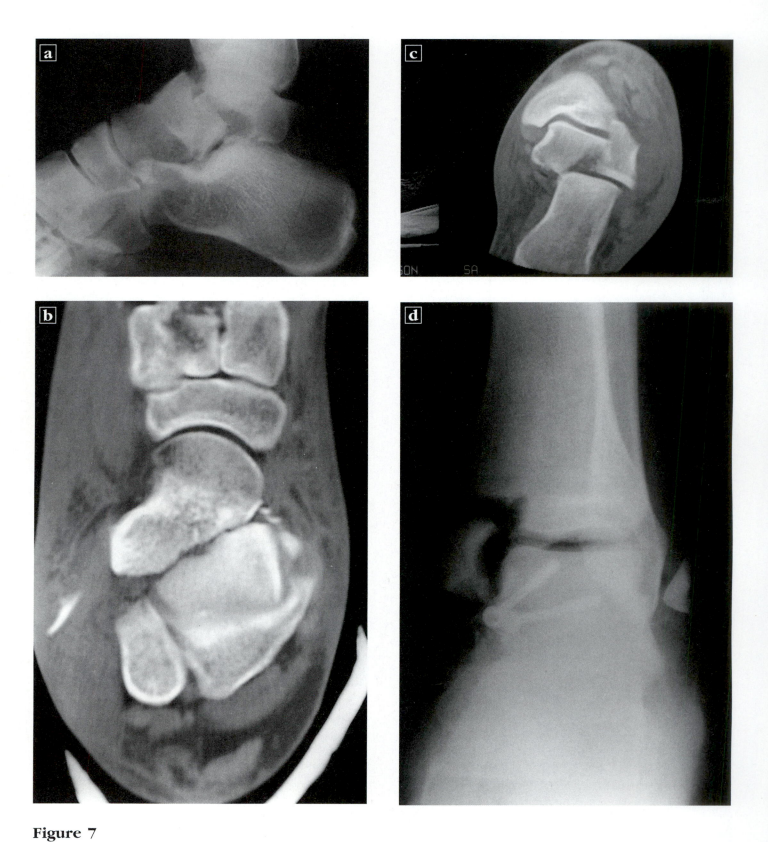

Figure 7

(a) Lateral radiograph of a comminuted talar body fracture following a motorcycle accident; (b) preoperative transverse CT scan and (c) preoperative coronal CT scan demonstrating the complex anatomy of this fracture; (d) an intraoperative radiograph demonstrating a step-cut osteotomy of the medial malleolus which provides excellent exposure and is easily repaired following fixation of the talus fracture; (*contd*)

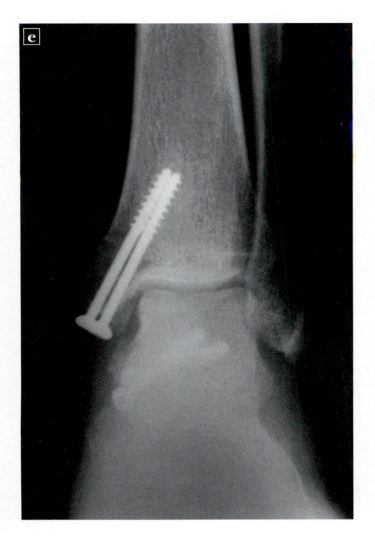

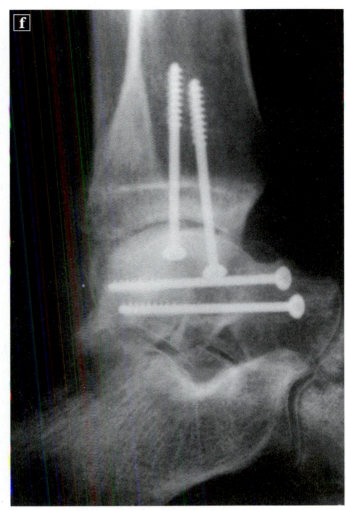

Figure 7 *continued*

(e) anteroposterior and (f) lateral radiographs following fracture consolidation demonstrating anatomic reduction of the talar body fracture with congruent ankle and subtalar joints and bony union of the malleolar osteotomy

3. There is a complex relationship between the ankle, subtalar and midtarsal joints, which is not clearly understood.

Hawkins I fractures

Since this group represents a nondisplaced, stable fracture, the ankle should be casted in a neutral position until radiographic union is achieved. This usually requires 4–6 weeks in a short leg, non-weight-bearing cast. The patient can then be protected an additional 2 weeks in a walking cast.

Hawkins II fractures

Hawkins II fractures represent displacement at the fracture site with subtalar joint incongruity or dislocation. All of these fractures should be managed with an immediate closed reduction. This maneuver requires both maximal plantar flexion of the foot to realign the head with the body fragment, as well as varus or valgus stress to realign the neck in the transverse plane. Some authors recommend casting the patient in plantar flexion until radiographic healing is evident and then gradually bringing the foot into dorsiflexion. The total duration of immobilization should be approximately 10–12 weeks (Pennal 1963, Hawkins 1970, Canale & Kelly 1978, Penny & Davis 1980).

Although all authors recommend open reduction and internal fixation following a failed closed reduction, we also recommend the same strategy when an anatomic closed reduction of a Hawkins II fracture has not been achieved (Lemaire & Bustiri 1980) (see Fig. 4). The benefits of open reduction and internal fixation include the avoidance of an equinus contracture, since plantar flexion casting is unnecessary; immediate mobilization if stable fixation is obtained; and the prevention of any shearing across the fracture site, which can damage capillary ingrowth.

An anteromedial approach is used to expose the neck of the talus (Adelaar 1989). This can be extended over the medial malleolus should a malleolar osteotomy be necessary for exposure (though we generally find this unnecessary) unless the fracture extends into the body of the talus. If we are uncertain as to the adequacy of the reduction of the fracture, or if we want to explore the subtalar joint for articular debris, we make a second anterolateral incision over the sinus tarsi. Following anatomic reduction of the fracture site, 3.5 mm cortical screws or partially threaded 4.0 mm cancellous screws can be used for fixation across the neck of the talus. Screws are definitely superior to Kirschner wires. Fractures occurring in the distal aspect of the talar neck require the screws to be countersunk into the head of the talus in order to obtain adequate fixation. One of us (DT) routinely uses titanium screws to allow for postoperative MR imaging of the talus (Thordarson et al 1994).

When an anatomic reduction has been achieved preoperatively, a posterolateral approach to the talus can be performed with the patient in the prone position, and screws can be inserted from posterior to anterior thus allowing fixation perpendicular to the fracture site. Swanson et al (1992) have recommended using a single 6.5 mm cancellous screw for fixation. Lemaire & Bustiri (1980) reported good results with this technique performing fracture manipulation under fluoroscopic control. We are reluctant to rely solely on fluoroscopy for assessing the reduction of the fracture. Therefore, we insert screws posteriorly only after an open reduction through an anteromedial approach, after which the fracture has been provisionally stabilized with smooth Kirschner wires.

Hawkins III fractures

Hawkins III fractures represent a surgical emergency for two reasons. First, the skin overlying the extruded talar body will quickly become necrotic if the tension is not relieved. Secondly, the body of the talus pivots upon the deltoid ligament, thus kinking the only remaining blood supply from the deltoid branches. Although closed reduction is usually unsuccessful, one can attempt it using a half pin external fixator for temporary distraction followed by closed manipulation. If the reduction is successful, screws can be inserted, as described by Lemaire & Bustiri (1980).

We generally prefer immediate open reduction and internal fixation via an anteromedial approach extending from the talar neck along the posterior aspect of the medial malleolus (see Figs 4,5). In patients with an intact medial malleolus, we perform the step-cut osteotomy described by Alexander & Watson (1991) in order to protect the deltoid ligament with its deltoid blood vessels (Fig. 7). The step-cut osteotomy allows for a large cancellous surface, which can be easily reduced at the conclusion of the case and which rapidly heals.

Despite the excellent exposure of the talar body with this approach, reduction is frequently very difficult and we routinely place a large Steinmann pin through the posteroinferior aspect of the calcaneus to act as a traction device (see Fig. 5). Following fracture reduction, rigid fixation is achieved with screws placed as described previously.

Patients are kept non-weight-bearing in a short leg cast or brace for approximately 3 months until radiographic evidence of fracture union exists. In reliable patients, range of motion exercises of the ankle and subtalar joints can be begun 2 weeks after surgery to minimize post-operative stiffness.

Type IV fractures

The fourth type of talar neck fracture includes a dislocation of the talonavicular joint which accompanies a Type II or III talar neck fracture (see Fig. 6). Fortunately, such injuries are rare. In addition to all the problems associated with treating Type II and III fractures, it is essential to recognize the talonavicular dislocation and to reduce and stabilize the joint.

Complications

Skin necrosis and osteomyelitis

Skin necrosis can occur following Hawkins II and, more frequently, Hawkins III fractures if the body of the talus is displaced posteromedially. These wounds require aggressive debridement and either early skin grafting or free muscular transfer to minimize the risk of osteomyelitis.

Osteomyelitis can occur following open fractures of the talus with contamination, or following wound dehiscence or skin slough. Osteomyelitis of the talus is extremely difficult to eradicate after it has developed and generally requires excision of the body of the talus (Canale & Kelly 1978, Dunn et al 1966).

Nonunion and malunion

Nonunion following talar neck fracture is unusual. Even in patients with avascular necrosis of the body of the talus, the viable neck of the talus can heal to the body. Delayed union is commoner but is still infrequent. Peterson et al (1977) found 13% of Type IV fractures had a delayed union, but none went on to develop a nonunion.

Malunion of a talar neck fracture is much commoner and can result in both incongruity and subsequent degenerative arthritis in the ankle and subtalar joints. The commonest type is a varus malalignment due to medial talar neck comminution which has not been properly realigned with a closed reduction or (less often) an open reduction. The complication has been seen more often in Type II fracture – 27% (Canale & Kelly 1978); 28%

(Lorentzen et al 1977). In Type III fractures, Lorentzen et al (1977) reported 18% varus malunion. The reason for the higher incidence of this malunion in Type II fractures is that they were not always managed by open reduction and rigid internal fixation. These varus malunions are difficult to treat because of the marked biomechanical disruption of the ankle and hindfoot joints. A stiff, supinated forefoot results from this deformity, with subsequent increased weight bearing on the lateral border of the foot. Even resorting to a triple arthrodesis may be an unsatisfactory salvage procedure (Canale & Kelly 1978, Daniels & Smith 1993). Dorsal malunion can also occur with limitation in ankle range of motion. Treatment can consist of excising the dorsal beak of the malunion (Canale & Kelly 1978).

Talar and ankle joint arthritis and arthrofibrosis
All patients who have suffered a talar neck fracture are at risk of developing arthrofibrosis of the ankle and, more commonly, the subtalar joint. Dunn et al (1966) reported that decreased range of motion of the ankle and subtalar joints accounted for poor results in over half their patients. McKeever (1963) also noted that arthrofibrosis of the subtalar joint was a frequent complication, and he recommended early range of motion exercises which we agree should be done whenever possible.

Arthritis of the ankle and subtalar joints also can occur in the absence of avascular necrosis of the talus and joint incongruity. Canale & Kelly (1978) noted subtalar arthritis in approximately half of their patients but only one-third of this group had a malunion of their fracture. Chondral damage from the initial injury or from prolonged immobilization could theoretically account for the cases of arthritis without AVN or joint incongruity.

Fortunately, many patients with radiographic evidence of post-traumatic arthritis are relatively asymptomatic or have symptoms that are not disabling. Arthrodesis of these joints in patients with pain and disability is not uniformly successful, and it has been difficult to select those patients who will benefit most from such operations. Therefore, if possible, nonoperative treatment should be advised, using nonsteroidal anti-inflammatory drugs, orthotic devices, shoe modifications and possibly the other general modalities used to treat chronic pain.

Avascular necrosis
The diagnosis of avascular necrosis has classically been made on plain radiographic evaluation. Hawkins (1970) reported that the presence of subchondral bony atrophy is an active process and, therefore, rules out the possibility of avascular necrosis (AVN). This 'Hawkins' sign is evaluated on an AP view of the ankle, out of plaster, 6–8 weeks after injury (see Fig. 5c). Its absence, however, does not always indicate the presence of AVN. Increased density of the body of the talus relative to the distal tibia is also typically felt to be a reliable sign for AVN (see Fig. 6c).

Owing to the equivocal nature of some of these radiographic findings, other methods for evaluating AVN have been explored. Bone scanning with a pinhole collimator has been reported as successfully detecting AVN (Canale & Kelly 1978, Penny & Davis 1980). We have been evaluating AVN using magnetic resonance images (MRI) performed 6–12 weeks after Hawkins II and III fractures (Thordarson et al 1994). Although stainless steel markedly scatters MRI, titanium screws cause little distortion of the image and allow for high-quality scans to be performed. In a preliminary series of 10 patients, the MRI scans documented AVN in four patients where plain radiographs had shown evidence of AVN, and partial AVN of the talar body in four patients where plain radiographs were equivocal. We hope to be able to identify early those patients who are at risk of talar collapse with this imaging modality.

It is difficult to determine if the present proper care of these patients can prevent the occurrence of AVN. However, the revascularization process can certainly be enhanced by early and prompt recognition, by reduction of the fracture, and by a careful surgical technique that does not further injure the viable blood vessels to the talus.

AVN of the talus is difficult to treat, owing to the uncertain long-term prognosis of these patients and the prolonged period of revascularization. Penny & Davis (1980) reported that a sclerotic talus requires over 2 years to revascularize completely. They stated that the sclerotic body rarely collapses; however, if revascularization occurs quickly and in a patchy distribution, the risk of collapse of the dome of the talus is greater. DeLee (1983) reported that late segmental collapse occurs only in one-third of the patients with whole body AVN and rarely in patients with only partial body AVN. In addition, some authors report that the development of AVN does not guarantee a poor result (Dunn et al 1966). Hawkins (1970) found that AVN did not necessarily lead to a poor result. He also noted that collapse of the dome was well tolerated in many patients and that it occurred despite prolonged non-weight-bearing.

Owing to the uncertainty regarding the prognosis following AVN, some authors allow weight bearing following fracture healing, while others recommend prolonged non-weight-bearing. Hawkins (1970) recommends delaying weight bearing until the fracture has healed. O'Brien et al (1972) also advises against prolonged non-weight-bearing, since it may not prevent late segmental collapse.

In an attempt to prevent collapse of the talar body, Mindell et al (1963) and Pennal (1963) recommend protecting the foot until the talus is fully revascularized. Canale & Kelly (1978) reported that patients who were kept non-weight-bearing for prolonged periods with AVN had a better outcome than did those who were allowed to bear weight. They recommended a patellar tendon bearing brace as an alternative to a non-weight-bearing short leg cast. Unfortunately, the relationship of AVN to the final clinical result is still unresolved.

MRI scans on all of our patients are now being obtained by one of us (DT), 6–12 weeks after injury as a supplement to the radiographic evaluation (Thordarson et al 1994). The current protocol is that, in patients without AVN or with less than one-third involvement of the talar body, weight bearing is allowed following fracture consolidation. Patients with AVN involving more than one-third of the talar body are advised of the risks of late segmental collapse, should it occur, following early weight bearing. They are offered a patellar tendon bearing brace to be used for the 1–2 years of revascularization. Nevertheless, many patients refuse the brace and begin weight bearing after the fracture has healed.

Fractures of the body of the talus

Fractures of the body of the talus are extremely uncommon, being present in about 1% of all talar fractures (Coltart 1952). DeLee (1986) utilizes a classification for these fractures which divides the talar body into five groups: Group I are osteochondral fractures of the talar dome (see Chapter IX.8); Group II are shearing fractures, either in the coronal, sagittal or horizontal plane; Group III are fractures of the posterior process of the talus; Group IV are fractures of the lateral process of the talus; the Group V are comminuted fractures of the body of the talus.

Diagnosis of these injuries is made by analysis of the patient's radiographs and, wherever practical, the use of computerized tomography (CT).

Group II – fractures of the body of the talus

Coronal fractures of the body of the talus may be difficult to distinguish from posterior fractures of the talar neck. Fractures involving the talar body usually exit the talus posteriorly and involve not only the articular space of the talus, but also the posterior facet of the subtalar joint. Perhaps the only importance in making a distinction between the two types of fracture is that the prognosis of talar body fractures is worse than that for talar neck fractures. The major complications are the development of AVN and secondary traumatic arthritis. In coronal fractures, the more posterior the fracture in the body, the higher the risk of disruption of the blood supply from the deltoid ligament branches. A complete separation from the blood supply occurs in horizontal fractures (Sneppen & Buhl 1974, Sneppen et al 1977).

Treatment

Treatment of talar body fractures is based on whether the fracture is displaced or nondisplaced. Usually, CT is essential to make this determination (see Fig. 7).

Shearing fractures of the body in the coronal or sagittal plane, if truly nondisplaced, are treated by immobilizing the ankle in a neutral position and keeping the patient non-weight-bearing until the fracture has healed. DeLee (1986) indicates that if there is minimal displacement (2–3 mm, with no evidence of subtalar dislocation) he prefers closed reduction and then considers percutaneous K wire fixation. Early ankle motion is allowed, and the K wires are usually removed at about 6 weeks. Weight bearing is allowed when the fracture has healed.

Fractures with more than 3 mm of displacement usually involve subluxation of the subtalar joint. Such dislocations are reduced under a general or spinal anesthetic by closed methods. Longitudinal traction on the heel and forefoot, along with plantar flexion, usually reduces the fracture. Once anatomic reduction has been attained, the fracture should be fixed using an A-O compression screw.

Fractures of the talar body with complete dislocation of the body are surgical emergencies, and they are treated by open reduction and internal fixation. A Steinman pin can be placed into the calcaneus for traction during open reduction. An osteotomy of the medial malleolus is performed to preserve whatever blood supply may still be present through the deltoid ligament (see Fig. 7). Internal fixation is used with a screw after reduction.

Group III

The posterior process of the talus is composed of two tubercles, medial and lateral, separated by the groove for the flexor hallucis longus. The lateral tubercle is known as Steida's process and is the larger and more posteriorly placed. Fractures of this tubercle are known as 'posterior process' fractures, but they should be called 'lateral tubercle' fractures. The eponym 'Shepherd's Fracture' is also used for any fractures of the posterior talus. These fractures are often nondisplaced and can be mistaken for ankle sprains. They may also be confused with a large os trigonum. Fractures of the medial process are much less common, and are avulsions by the posterior portion of the deltoid ligament. They respond well to surgical excision.

Fractures of the entire posterior process are rare, and they require anatomical reduction and internal fixation. The mechanism of fracture is probably a forced maximum plantar flexion which compresses the posterior process between the posterior tip of the tibia and the calcaneus. The few fractures of this type that have been reported heal, but there is some loss of ankle and subtalar joint motion (Nasser & Manoli 1990). Hallux dorsiflexion is limited, probably because of scarring around the FHL.

Group IV

Fractures of the lateral process of the talus are more common, accounting for about 24% of all fractures of the body of the talus (DeLee 1986). This fracture is often overlooked. A fracture of the lateral process of the talus usually involves both the talofibular articulation of the ankle joint and the posterior talocalcaneal articulation of the subtalar joint. The lateral process also serves as a point of attachment for several lateral ligaments. Therefore, this process is an important structure in the stability of the ankle and the motion of the ankle and subtalar joint.

Mechanism of injury

There are several mechanisms that can produce this injury. The fracture can be caused by a shearing force, or the lateral process can be avulsed by either the anterior talofibular or talocalcaneal ligaments. A direct blow can also cause this fracture. Most authors agree that the lateral process fractures are the result of acute dorsiflexion and inversion of the foot.

Diagnosis

These fractures may be confused with an inversion sprain of the ankle, and therefore not only clinical evaluation, but also radiographic evaluation, is essential, keeping in mind a high degree of suspicion. Generally, lateral process fractures are easily seen on a standard set of ankle radiographs. Obviously, CT shows the fracture, but more importantly, it indicates the type of fracture. One must be careful not to confuse this fracture with some of the more common accessory bones in this area.

Treatment

Nondisplaced fractures are treated by immobilization, with about 4 weeks of non-weight-bearing followed by 2 weeks of a walking cast. Displaced fractures usually cannot be reduced by closed means. One must choose whether to excise a small fragment, or perform an open reduction and internal fixation of any fracture fragment that is probably large enough to allow some form of stable internal fixation. The surgical approach is usually through an anterolateral incision. If a small fragment has been excised, then the patient can be kept in a short leg cast for about 3 weeks and then started on early motion. A fracture that has been internally fixed should be in a cast for about 2–3 weeks, and then started on early motion with weight bearing being allowed at about 6 weeks.

Group V comminuted fractures

These unusual injuries may have only a minimal displacement of the fracture fragments. Closed treatment is preferable, particularly if it appears that open reduction and internal fixation of these multiple fragments will be hopeless. A short leg non-weight-bearing cast is used until there is evidence of some fracture consolidation. Motion is then started, protecting the foot from weight bearing until it appears that the fragments will not further collapse. An arthrodesis of these ankles may eventually be necessary.

Fractures of the head of the talus

Fractures of the head of the talus are rare injuries, being present in about 5–10% of reported fractures of the talus (Coltart 1952, Pennal 1963). Two types of fractures are usually seen: the first is a compression fracture, which is probably caused by impaction of the talar head. This injury can be associated with a compression fracture of the tarsal navicular. The second type is a longitudinal or oblique fracture through the talar head, which results in two or more major fragments of the head of the talus. Compression mechanisms have been postulated for these types of injuries. Additional injuries can be subluxation of the calcaneocuboid joint, and associated midtarsal joint dislocations (Coltart 1952).

Diagnosis is made by physical examination which usually reveals a swollen, tender area on the dorsal and medial side of the hindfoot, and occasionally some gross deformity. Radiological evaluation usually shows the fracture if one looks carefully at the anteroposterior and oblique views, but particularly if one looks at the lateral radiographs. Since the fractures are often comminuted and seldom displaced (because they are held in place by the strong intertarsal ligaments), radiographs may be insufficient to analyze the fracture completely. In such cases CT is very helpful.

Treatment

Isolated head fractures of the impaction type that are nondisplaced are treated by immobilization using a non-weight-bearing cast for about 3 weeks, and then a walking cast for about 3 weeks. Displaced fractures usually require open reduction and internal fixation of the major fracture fragments or excision of small fragments. At least two-thirds of the head of the talus should be retained, though smaller fragments can be excised. Fixation may be attempted using small screws, Herbert-type screws, or occasionally K wires; though these are certainly not so useful. If internal fixation is used, then the foot must be protected in a cast until there is some evidence of bony union, which is usually at about 6 weeks. If some small fracture fragments have been removed, then the foot can be immobilized in a short leg walking cast for a few weeks and then started on early motion. Patients who develop symptomatic traumatic arthritis will need to undergo a talonavicular arthrodesis. Obviously, other displaced injuries must be treated. For example, if the

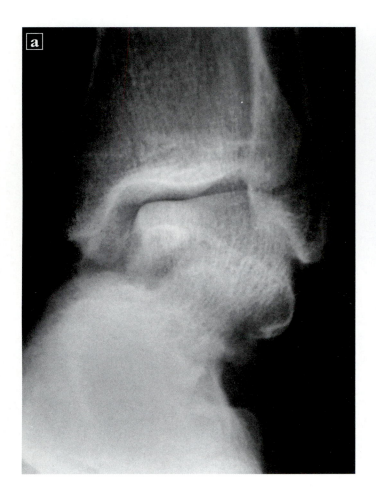

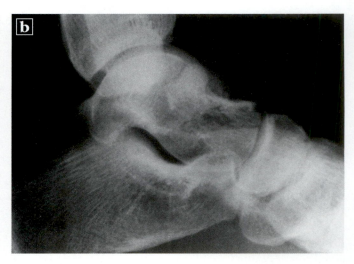

Figure 8

(a) Anteroposterior radiograph of a medial subtalar dislocation; (b) following closed reduction of this subtalar dislocation, note the nondisplaced talar head fracture

calcaneocuboid joint is subluxated, weight bearing should be delayed for about 3 weeks so that the calcaneocuboid joint capsule can heal.

Dislocations about the talus

There are three types of dislocations involving the talus without fracture of the talus.

1. Talocrural dislocation, where the talus is dislocated from the ankle mortise, but the other joints remain intact.
2. Subtalar dislocation, where the talus remains intact in the ankle mortise, but the subtalar and talonavicular joints are simultaneously dislocated.
3. Total dislocation of the talus, where the talus is disrupted from the ankle mortise and the subtalar joint.

Subtalar dislocations

By definition, this injury is not associated with a fracture of the neck of the talus (DeLee & Curtis 1982, DeLee

1986, Dunn et al 1966, Dunn 1974). This is an uncommon injury and Leitner reported this dislocation to make up about 1% of all traumatic dislocations. Pennal (1963) reported that these dislocations occur in only 15% of all injuries to the talus. Most authors prefer to use the classification of Broca & Malgaigne (DeLee 1986). Medial dislocations make up the vast majority of subtalar dislocations followed in frequency of occurrence by lateral, posterior and finally anterior dislocation. Men are affected about three to 10 times more frequently than women (Figs 8, 9).

Anatomy

Several ligaments and capsules must be disrupted for a subtalar dislocation to occur. These are:

1. The strong interosseous talocalcaneal ligament in the sinus tarsi;
2. The fibrous capsule that connects the three talocalcaneal facets;
3. Medially, the superficial portions of the deltoid ligament;
4. Laterally, the calcaneofibular ligament;
5. The weak talonavicular capsule.

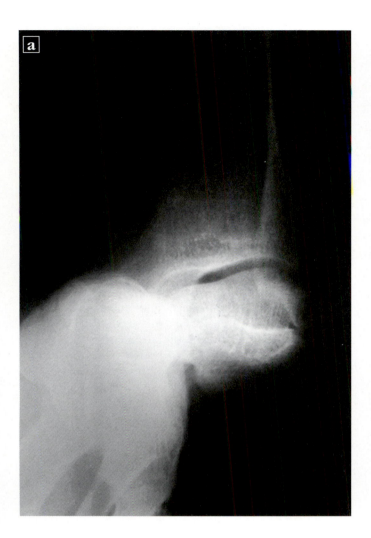

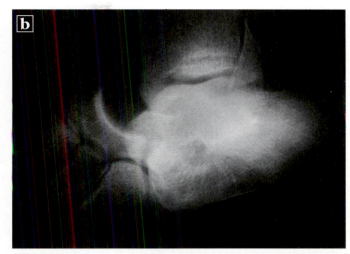

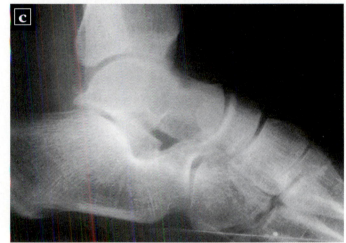

Figure 9

(a) Anteroposterior and (b) lateral radiographs of a medial subtalar dislocation with an associated talonavicular dislocation; (c) lateral radiograph following open reduction, which demonstrates anatomic reduction of the talonavicular and subtalar joints. At operation, reduction was found to be blocked by the talar head protruding through the extensor retinaculum and the extensor digitorum longus which was wrapped around the neck

The surfaces of the subtalar joint also provide some intrinsic stability. Because of this bony stability, a dislocation may cause fractures of the lateral process of the talus, and the posterior tubercles of the talus (DeLee & Curtis 1982, DeLee 1986). In a medial subtalar dislocation, the head of the talus appears on the lateral side of the foot between the extensor hallucis longus and the long toe extensors and can rest on either the navicular or the cuboid bone. In lateral dislocations, the head of the talus can be palpated over the medial aspect of the foot while the heel is displaced laterally. Thus the term 'acquired clubfoot' has been used for a medial dislocation while a lateral dislocation has been called an 'acquired flat foot' (Buckingham 1973).

Mechanism of injury

The medial subtalar dislocation usually occurs secondary to plantar flexion of the foot with forceful inversion of the forefoot (Buckingham 1973). The less common lateral dislocation occurs with plantar flexion of the foot by forceful eversion of the forefoot. Depending upon the injury, there may be only soft tissue damage or bony damage. For example, Grantham (1964) noted medial subtalar dislocation mostly in basketball players. The mechanism of injury may not have been as violent as in other injuries, and may not have produced bony fractures, as he did report a good range of motion and minimal evidence of subtalar arthritis. Alternatively, those injuries produced by motor vehicle accidents or falls are probably associated with more trauma, and have a higher incidence of associated intraarticular fractures. They usually have a poorer clinical result (DeLee & Curtis 1982, DeLee 1986).

Clinical diagnosis

The patient may give a history of an injury secondary to only minor trauma, such as missing a step, or it may be obvious that they have been involved in a major accident. In addition to the deformity as described above, the entire foot is swollen, and movement of the ankle or subtalar joint is either nonexistent or very painful. The foot and ankle appear deformed. Any of the subtalar dislocations may present as an open injury. Additionally, the dislocation may result in compromise of the circulation to the overlying skin, so that an immediate reduction will be necessary to try to prevent skin necrosis.

Radiographic diagnosis

In addition to anteroposterior, lateral and oblique radiographs of the foot, a superior–inferior view of the foot was stressed by Barber et al (1961). This view will clearly demonstrate the absence of the head of the talus in the articulation with the navicular. It is important to analyze carefully the initial films for associated fractures, which may be easily masked by the deformities (DeLee & Curtis 1982, DeLee 1986).

Fahey & Murphy (1965) reported that medial dislocations may produce:

1. Impacted fracture of the medial portion of the head of the talus produced by the navicular;
2. Fracture of the posterior process of the talus;
3. Fracture of the navicular.

Lateral dislocations may be associated with fractures of:

1. The lateral malleolus;
2. The calcaneus; or
3. The cuboid.

DeLee & Curtis (1982) reported that over half of their patients had associated fractures, and that lateral subtalar dislocations had a higher incidence of associated intra-articular fractures than medial dislocations. It is probably a good idea to perform CT after reduction of these dislocations in order to ascertain whether any fractures exist.

Treatment

Following the diagnosis, a closed reduction should be attempted. It may be possible to use intravenous sedation, but cases that have been dislocated for some time usually require a general or spinal anesthetic. Closed reduction is done by flexing the knee to relax the gastrocsoleus muscles and traction is placed on the heel in line with the deformity. Then, in the medial dislocation the heel is everted and the forefoot abducted before attempting dorsiflexion. The reverse is true for a lateral dislocation. Postoperative radiographs are essential, and CT may be indicated if one is suspicious of fractures or if a lateral dislocation has occurred.

Should the closed reduction fail, one should proceed directly to an open reduction. For a medial dislocation, a lateral incision parallel to the long axis of the foot and over the talar head, which is easily palpated, is utilized. This approach allows excellent access to the extensor retinaculum, which frequently blocks reduction in the irreducible medial dislocation. In an irreducible lateral dislocation an oblique anterolateral incision is made over the sinus tarsi, which can expose both the subtalar and midtarsal joints. It also allows access to the posterior tibial tendon, which commonly blocks reduction in a lateral dislocation. In patients with an irreducible anterior or posterior dislocation a lateral longitudinal incision is made parallel to the sole and just below the distal fibula, which allows access to the subtalar joint.

Following reduction of a dislocation, the foot and ankle are immobilized in a non-weight-bearing cast for 3 weeks, and then started with subtalar and ankle joint motion using both active and active-assisted physical therapy. Range of motion exercises of the metatarsophalangeal joints are begun immediately to prevent adhesions to the extensor tendons. If an open operation is required, and if there have been fractures, then the period of protected weight-bearing may need to be longer.

Results

Subtalar dislocations can give good functional results (Buckingham 1973). However, this depends on the nature of the dislocation and the amount of trauma that has occurred. Most authors report poor results if the injuries have been open, and if the reduction has been delayed (Mindell et al 1963, DeLee & Curtis 1982, DeLee 1986). This is also true if intra-articular fractures are associated with the subtalar dislocation. Aseptic necrosis of the talus following uncomplicated dislocation is rare (Pennal 1963, Buckingham 1973, Parkes 1977). Loss of motion of the subtalar joint is common and depends to some degree on the amount of trauma that caused the dislocation and whether the joint was promptly relocated. Later, degenerative joint changes in the subtalar joint are reported, and can be seen in a majority of cases (Pennal 1963). Many of these patients have also had an intra-articular fracture involving the subtalar joint or an open injury. Recurrent dislocation rarely, if ever, occurs following subtalar dislocation (DeLee & Curtis 1982, DeLee 1986).

Total dislocation of the talus

Total dislocation of the talus is a rare injury, being present in less than 5% of all major injuries to the talus (Coltart 1952). Total dislocation of the talus describes a talus which is dislocated both from the ankle joint and from the rest of the foot. Mostly, isolated case reports appear in the literature.

Mechanism of injury

Probably the most common mechanism is the end point of a supination injury to the ankle (Leitner 1954). Thus, a third degree supination injury results in a total lateral dislocation of the talus. Conversely, a third degree pronation injury results in a total medial dislocation of the talus. Leitner reports more supination injuries than pronation injuries, and therefore total lateral dislocations are more common. A posterior dislocation of the talus is also possible, but it is usually accompanied by further injury to the ankle.

Clinical findings

At least 75% of these injuries are open injuries (Coltart 1952). Those that are not closed usually show a foot in marked inversion, and the skin over the prominence of the talus is usually severely compromised. Some evidence of ischemia can also be present. This dislocation is usually easy to recognize and can be seen on standard radiographs. At times only the dislocation of the talus from the ankle mortise is evident. However, when the foot is stressed, even moderately, the instability between the talus and the calcaneus and midtarsal joints can also be seen. Therefore some type of stress radiographs may be important.

Treatment

With such a massive injury there is a very high incidence of the talus becoming completely avascular. In some incomplete dislocations, there may be some ligamentous attachments remaining on the talus, particularly the deltoid ligament, which may retain some blood supply to the talus.

A closed total dislocation of the talus is a surgical emergency. One attempt can be made at closed reduction and this may be facilitated by placing a Steinmann pin in the distal tibia, and a wire in the calcaneus for traction. The displaced talus should be manipulated either in a posteromedial or a posterolateral direction, depending on the direction of the displacement of the talar body. If this is unsuccessful the ankle should be opened directly over the displaced talus and an open reduction performed. Following reduction, the ankle should be protected in a cast for about 6 weeks. Protected weight bearing will be needed until one can determine the consequences of the AVN. If an open reduction is required, it may be best to close the skin at a subsequent procedure about 3–5 days later to determine whether significant soft tissue damage has occurred.

An open total dislocation is also a surgical emergency. The skin edges should be debrided and the bone should also be debrided, if necessary. Obviously, the surgeon needs to use his or her judgement as to whether the talus should be saved or discarded. Certainly, it would be best to save the talus if possible. It may be that this gives some support to the soft tissues, and a talectomy can be done later as a staged procedure.

With open injuries the possibility of an infection exists and appropriate intravenous antibiotics should be given. The length and type of antibiotic will vary according to the clinical condition. The wounds should be cultured prior to performing any surgery. A mixed flora of bacteria will probably be present, so that the antibiotic treatment must be individualized.

References

Adelaar R S 1989 The treatment of complex fractures of the talus. Orthop Clin North Am 20: 691–707

Alexander I J, Watson J T 1991 Step-cut osteotomy of the medial malleolus for exposure of the medial ankle joint space. Foot Ankle 11: 242–243

Barber J R, Bricker J D, Haliburton R A 1961 Peritalar dislocation of the foot. Can J Surg 4: 205–210

Buckingham W W 1973 Subtalar dislocation of the foot. J Trauma 13: 753–765

Canale S T, Kelly F B 1978 Fractures of the neck of the talus. J Bone Joint Surg 60A: 143–156

Coltart W D 1952 Aviator's astragalus. J Bone Joint Surg 34B: 545–566

Daniels T R, Smith J W 1993 Talar neck fractures. Foot Fellows' Review. Foot Ankle 14: 225–234

DeLee J C 1983 Talar Neck Fracture with Total Dislocation of the Body. Report of the Committee on Trauma of the American Orthopaedic Foot Society, Anaheim, California

DeLee J C 1986 Fractures of the head of the talus. In Mann R A (ed) Surgery of the Foot, 5th edition. C V Mosby, St. Louis

DeLee J C, Curtis R 1982 Subtalar dislocation of the foot. J Bone Joint Surg 64A: 433–437

Dunn A R, Jacobs B, Campbell R D 1966 Fractures of the talus. J Trauma 6: 443–468

Dunn A W 1974 Peritalar dislocation. Orthop Clin North Am 5: 7–18

Fahey J J, Murphy J L 1965 Dislocations and fractures of the talus. Surg Clin North Am 45: 79–102

Gelberman R H, Mortensen W W 1983 The arterial anatomy of the talus. Foot Ankle 4: 64–72

Goldie I 1988 Talar and peritalar injuries. In: Helal B, Wilson D W (eds) The Foot. Churchill Livingstone, Edinburgh pp. 916–931

Goldie I, Peterson L, Lindell D 1974 The arterial supply of the talus. Acta Orthop Scand 45: 260

Grantham S A 1964 Medial subtalar dislocation: five cases with a common etiology. J Trauma 4: 845–849

Hawkins L G 1970 Fractures of the neck of the talus. J Bone Joint Surg 52A: 991–1002

Leitner B 1954 Obstacles to reduction in subtalar dislocations. J Bone Joint Surg 36A: 299–306

Lemaire R G, Bustiri W 1980 Screw fixation of fractures of the neck of the talus: using a posterior approach. J Trauma 20: 669–673

Lorentzen J E, Christensen S B, Krogsoe O, et al 1977 Fractures of the neck of the talus. Acta Orthop Scand 48: 115–120

McKeever F M 1963 Treatment of complications of fractures and dislocations of the talus. Clin Orthop 30: 45–52

Mindell E R, Cisek E E, Kartalian G W, Delob JM 1963 Late results of injuries to the talus. J Bone Joint Surg 45A: 221–245

Nasser S, Manoli A 1990 Fracture of the entire posterior process of the talus: a case report. Foot Ankle 10: 235–238

O'Brien E T, Howard J B, Shepard M J 1972 Injuries of the talus. J Bone Joint Surg 54A: 1575–1576

Parkes J C II 1977 Injuries of the hindfoot. Clin Orthop 122: 28–36

Pennal J F 1963 Fractures of the talus. Clin Orthop 30: 53–63

Penny J N, Davis L A 1980 Fractures and fracture–dislocations of the neck of the talus. J Trauma 20: 1029–1037

Peterson L, Romanus B 1976 Fracture of the collum tali – an experimental study. J Biomech 9: 277–279

Peterson L, Goldie I, Irstam L 1974 Fracture of the neck of the talus. An experimental and clinical study. Thesis, Göteborg

Peterson L, Goldie I F, Irstam L 1977 Fracture of the neck of the talus. A clinical study. Acta Orthop Scand 48: 696–706

Sneppen O, Buhl O 1974 Fracture of the talus: a study of its genesis and morphology based upon cases with associated ankle fracture. Acta Orthop Scand 45: 307–320

Sneppen O, Christensen S V, Krosgsoe O, et al 1977 Fractures of the body of the talus. Acta Orthop Scand 48: 317–324

Swanson TV, Bray TJ, Holmes GB 1992 Fractures of the talar neck. J Bone Joint Surg 74A: 544–551

Thordarson D B, Triffon M, Terk M 1994 MRI of AVN of the Talus Following Displaced Talar Neck Fracture. Presented at American Orthopaedic Foot and Ankle Society Meeting, Coeur d'Alene, Idaho

IX.3 Calcaneal Fractures

Mark S Myerson

Introduction

Over the past decade, the philosophy of treatment for fractures of the calcaneus has undergone a marked change, both in the USA and in Europe, and the fact that more intra-articular fractures are now treated surgically is largely attributable to an increased understanding of the three-dimensional nature of the injury, as well as to evolving operative techniques and methods of fixation.

However, the surgical reconstruction of these fractures is difficult – indeed, sometimes impossible – and restoration of the articular surfaces, the maintenance of calcaneal height and width, and the preservation of motion in the subtalar joint is quite a challenge. For these reasons, a sense of nihilism often obtrudes when patients present with these injuries, and the fracture is treated by cast immobilization. Nonoperative treatment, however, is associated with marked complications, which make subsequent efforts at reconstruction most difficult.

These injuries typically occur in young adult males as a result of falls in the work place or motor vehicle accidents. Regardless of the mechanism of injury, however, the personal life and economic productivity of most patients is severely compromised. Many patients, for example, are unable to return to work for up to 2 years, and some are unable to return at all. Therefore, efforts should focus on minimizing the period of disability after injury. Described below is an approach to understanding various methods of evaluating and treating these injuries based on the clinical, radiographic, and anatomical perspectives.

Anatomy and fracture classification

The superior portion of the calcaneus is made up of the articular facets of the subtalar joint and the posterior third of the tuberosity, which is nonarticular. In 1931, on a lateral radiograph, Bohler described the angle formed by the intersection of lines from the posterior tuberosity to the anterior process of the calcaneus. Variations of a normal Bohler's angle have been described by Bohler (1931) (30–35°), Stephenson (1983, 1987) (25–40°), and Palmer (1948) (10–40°). Although some authors have stated that this angle reflects the amount of compression of the posterior facet (Bohler 1931, Stephenson, 1983, 1987), changes in Bohler's angle may not reflect a collapse of the posterior facet, and may be affected by extra-articular fractures. I have not relied on this angle in the evaluation of calcaneal fractures, as it provides little information on the spatial changes affecting outcome. The same can be said for the 'crucial angle' of Gissane, so termed by Gissane in 1947, since the angle varies greatly between individuals and does not have any prognostic value. The floor of Gissane's angle, however, does give some idea of the relationships of the posterior, anterior, and middle facets. The apex of Gissane's angle is of more significance intraoperatively, and may be used to restore alignment of the posterior (tuberosity segment) to the more anterior (neck segment) calcaneus.

The lateral process of the talus fits into the floor of the neck of the calcaneus, or the apex of Gissane's angle, and is driven into the calcaneus with axial loading, causing the primary fracture line. Secondary fracture lines occur, depending on the position of the heel on impact, but typically all arise from the primary fracture line (Stephenson 1987). The most consistent pattern of fracture is depression of the posterior facet combined with various secondary fracture lines, with an intact sustentaculum tali medially. This latter bone is hard and dense, and since it is anchored by the interosseous talocalcaneal ligament, it rarely displaces or fractures. The sustentaculum can therefore be reliably used as an anchor for internal fixation.

Several authors have classified intra-articular fractures according to their appearance on plain radiographs and, more recently, on CT scan (Conn 1926, 1935, Bohler 1931, Essex-Lopresti 1952, Rowe et al 1963, Romash 1988, Crosby & Fitzgibbons 1990). In 1908, Cotton & Wilson stated that it was not possible to classify 'the fracture of a nut subjected to the stresses in a nutcracker'. I agree wholeheartedly with this statement, since I find that it is impossible accurately to describe and categorize so many parts of a bone in so many pieces. From a descriptive standpoint, classification by CT has some merit, but I do not subscribe to the use of CT to predict prognosis and determine treatment as suggested (Crosby & Fitzgibbons 1990). CT scanning, however, has markedly increased our understanding of the three-dimensional nature of these fractures and is essential in preoperative planning.

Diagnosis and management

Diagnosis and initial interventions

The clinical findings of an acute calcaneal fracture include severe swelling, pain, and ecchymosis. Severe burning pain and sensory deficits may also be present if associated with a compartment syndrome. After 1–2 days, fracture blisters may involve the hindfoot and ecchymosis may extend to the knee. These fractures are associated with high-energy etiologies, and the patient's general medical condition, lumbar spine, pelvis and lower extremities must be evaluated carefully. Anteroposterior, lateral, oblique, and axial radiographs of the foot are obtained. If there is uncertainty regarding involvement of the posterior facet (particularly if comminuted), a CT scan is obtained, which is essential for preoperative planning. A CT scan obtained in two planes (coronal and oblique) is essential to determine the need for operative treatment. Other authors have demonstrated that fractures involving the posterior facet with less than 2 mm of displacement of the posterior facet do well with nonoperative treatment (Conn 1926). I routinely obtain a CT scan, although I do not adhere rigidly to a classification system to determine the need for operative treatment. The CT scan is obtained using 2 mm cuts in the coronal and oblique planes at 90° to each other. In this manner, it is possible to examine more accurately the posterior facet, the sustentaculum tali, and the calcaneocuboid joint.

If a compartment syndrome is suspected because of increasing pain, paresthesias, or pain on passive dorsiflexion of the toes, compartment pressures must be measured. In one series of 98 intra-articular fractures, 13% had compartment pressures greater than 30 mmHg (Saxby et al 1992, Myerson & Manoli 1993). I recommend fasciotomy if the pressure is greater than 40 mmHg, if there is associated sensory loss or relentless pain, but only if the patient is evaluated within 24 hours of the injury. Myerson & Henderson (1993) have documented the successful use of an intermittent compression pump device (A-V Impulse System, Kendall, Mansfield, Massachusetts, USA) in acute trauma in the foot and the use of the pump specifically for calcaneal fractures is also under investigation.

Initially, the intermittent compression device was used for selected patients who presented 3–5 days after injury and who had signs and symptoms of a compartment syndrome. Since the lengthy time from injury physiologically precluded fasciotomy in these patients, the intermittent compression device was used and found to reduce not only the swelling, but the compartment pressures as well. Subsequently, this device has been tried in the acute setting, and again it decreased both swelling and elevated compartment pressures. The use of fasciotomy to treat compartment pressure elevation associated with calcaneal fractures is now generally rare.

This intermittent compression device is therefore particularly useful for treating patients who present with significant swelling in the foot, and in whom surgery is to be expedited.

These patients are now routinely evaluated for evidence of myoneural ischemia, admitted, and scheduled for a CT scan. Although elevation, ice, and a bulky compressive dressing may be used immediately after evaluation to control swelling, I routinely use the intermittent compression device to manage the swelling, since it allows surgery on the foot to be performed within 6–12 hours, regardless of the magnitude of the initial swelling. If this device is not available, it is important to evaluate and treat elevated compartment pressures expeditiously with fasciotomy.

Management options

Management options of these fractures include closed treatment, open reduction with internal fixation, and primary subtalar arthrodesis. To a large extent, the choice of operative versus nonoperative methods of treatment is determined by the magnitude of the injury, the degree of comminution, and the experience of the surgeon.

Nonoperative treatment

Most extra-articular fractures and nondisplaced intra-articular fractures may be treated nonoperatively. Although nonoperative methods of treatment have been recommended (Lance et al 1964, Pozo et al 1984), it is quite clear from recent literature that anatomic reduction is most likely to be associated with a good outcome.

Intra-articular calcaneal fractures that are treated conservatively are complicated by loss of calcaneal height, lateral wall extrusion, subtalar arthritis, and hindfoot varus. Anatomic reduction and internal fixation restores the normal alignment, bony architecture, and the joint surfaces. This preserves motion and prevents sequelae such as peroneal impingement and arthritis.

If nonoperative treatments are selected, it is important to commence early range of motion and restricted weight bearing. I am not in favor of closed methods of reduction, which serve only to compress already tenuous skin and soft tissues. Immobilization has a purpose initially in reducing swelling and minimizing pain, but is counterproductive in that it causes severe arthrofibrosis. Other sequelae of cast immobilization may include tarsal tunnel syndrome and, more seriously, reflex sympathetic dystrophy. If nonoperative methods are selected, early range of motion exercises are therefore recommended. No study has documented further collapse of the subtalar joint with early range of motion of the foot and ankle. Early weight bearing is, however, not recommended, since further collapse will occur. I use swimming pool exercises and encourage early and aggressive movement, including swimming, followed by progressively increasing weight bearing initially in the pool.

Operative treatment

Over the past three decades, there have been many conflicting reports in the literature concerning the merits of surgical treatment. Perhaps the major difficulty in evaluating these reports is that, before the use of routine preoperative CT scans, calcaneal fractures were not classified, and one cannot infer anything about the severity of the fracture from these reports. In addition, the methods of evaluating patients after surgery differed in each of these reports, and interpretation of the results is therefore less meaningful than it would otherwise be. More recent literature on calcaneal fractures has emphasized anatomic reduction and has more carefully evaluated the ability of a patient to resume a lifestyle comparable to his or her preinjury one.

The options for operative management of calcaneal fractures include open reduction and internal fixation (Soeur & Remy 1975, Stephenson 1983, 1987, Leung et al 1989, Eastwood 1993, Leung et al 1993, Myerson & Multhopp-Stevens 1993, Paley & Hall 1993), percutaneous fixation (Essex-Lopresti 1952), or primary arthrodesis (Dick 1953, Hall & Pennal 1960, Noble & McQuillan 1979). Of these methods, open reduction is most frequently used, whether by a medial approach (McReynolds 1982, Burdeaux 1983, Paley & Hall 1993) or lateral approach (Stephenson 1983, 1987, Leung et al 1989, Eastwood 1993, Myerson & Multhopp-Stevens 1993).

Open reduction and internal fixation is indicated for management of a displaced intra-articular fracture in a medically fit patient. Although old age is a relative contraindication to operative management, the individual who sustains this fracture is often very active. It does not seem appropriate, therefore, to treat an elderly active individual any differently than someone younger, since the potential complications of nonoperative treatment are similar. One should be cautious when treating these fractures in patients who have attempted suicide by jumping, although the indications for operative treatment are again similar.

Although comminution certainly decreases the likelihood of success regardless of the method of treatment (Paley & Hall 1993), it is my firm belief that the more comminuted the fracture, the greater the need for operative treatment. If these comminuted fractures are treated nonoperatively, it is highly likely that subsequent arthrodesis will be required (Myerson 1992, Myerson & Quill 1993). The reconstruction of the severely deformed foot is difficult, and delayed arthrodesis is made far easier if some semblance of the height and width of the hindfoot is restored acutely. Although severely comminuted fractures seem impossible to fix correctly and secure fixation seems an impossible goal, a subsequent salvage procedure (i.e. arthrodesis), is simplified once alignment is restored.

Timing of surgery

Surgical planning and timing is critical. The skin should regain its normal turgor with fine surface wrinkles before surgical intervention. A useful sign is to pinch the skin on the lateral aspect of the foot, and if wrinkling occurs, the tissues are less likely to be compromised. Swelling is usually resolved within 5–7 days of injury, at which time surgery may be safely performed. Although the fracture is ideally treated 6–8 hours after injury, the necessary imaging studies at this stage are seldom completed. As stated above, these fractures undergo surgery within 12–24 hours of injury because of the rapid reduction in swelling produced by the intermittent pressure device. If an intermittent compression foot pump device is not available, then strict bed rest and limb elevation should be enforced, and surgery performed between 5 and 7 days. The only time that surgery should be performed as an emergency is when the fracture is associated with a compartment syndrome, when the fracture is open, or when a tongue-type fracture is present and is tenting the skin posteriorly over the Achilles tendon. This type of fracture is associated with the most severe swelling, fracture blisters, and skin necrosis if the fracture is not treated operatively and expeditiously.

If an open fracture is present, urgent operative debridement is required, but not necessarily the definitive fracture care. Clinicians differ as to whether fracture blisters should be debrided when they appear or left intact until the time of surgery. Although the fracture blister is an indication of underlying skin and tissue distension, surgery can be safely performed, provided the skin wrinkles. In my experience, using the intermittent pressure device to reduce swelling has not caused any increase in wound complications. Fracture blisters are not debrided, and an incision may be made through the blister, provided swelling has resolved and the skin turgor is normal.

Surgical technique

The patient is positioned on a beanbag and a pneumatic thigh tourniquet is applied. After induction of general anesthesia, the patient is placed in a lateral decubitus position with the involved extremity facing upwards. The foot should lie in a perfectly lateral position to prevent the limb from 'falling away' during surgery. The leg and the ipsilateral anterior iliac crest are prepared and

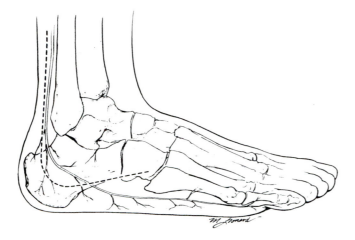

Figure 1

The skin incision is marked. Note its proximity to the sural nerve, which remains in the skin flap with the peroneal tendons. (Reprinted by permission from Myerson & Multhopp-Stevens 1993)

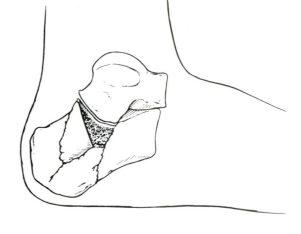

Figure 2

A typical joint depression fracture where the posterior facet is compressed into the substance of the tuberosity. (Reprinted by permission from Myerson & Multhopp-Stevens 1993)

draped. (Although I never use bone graft for routine open reduction and fracture fixation, graft is required if primary arthrodesis is performed.) Other authors have recommended the use of autogenous bone graft, and bone graft substitutes and allograft bone are used by some to fill the defect following open reduction.

Prophylactic antibiotics are administered and surgery is begun with an extensile lateral approach using a long J- or L-shaped incision with the apex inferior and posterior to the peroneal tendons and sural nerve (Fig. 1). More distally, the sural nerve crosses over the peroneal tendons, and it should be visualized during dissection of the calcaneocuboid joint. The apex of the incision is gently curved to prevent necrosis of the tip of the flap. If the incision is made parallel to the plantar surface of the foot, then the dissection should be dorsal to the abductor digiti minimi muscle. Although a medial approach is recommended by some authors, I find that it is necessary only if there is an extruded medial fracture fragment that is not accessible from the lateral approach.

The flap, including the peroneal tendons with their sheath intact, is then elevated directly off the lateral wall of the calcaneus. It is important to dissect the flap sharply. The sural nerve is not visualized in the main part of the flap and should not be looked for except in the most distal part of the incision where the nerve crosses over the peroneal tendons. Subperiosteal dissection is continued along the lateral calcaneus and the calcaneofibular ligament is usually excised. Once the subtalar joint is identified, short 0.45 inch Kirschner wires are inserted into the fibula posteriorly and the talus anteriorly and bent to retract the skin flap without constant manual retraction on the skin. The skin flap is kept moist throughout the procedure.

The dissection is carried anteriorly to the level of the calcaneocuboid joint, which is exposed only if the fracture extends distally. Using this incision, the distal dissection over the peroneal tendons is difficult and one may need to work both dorsal and plantar to the tendons, particularly if the anterior process of the calcaneus requires reduction. The lateral wall is fully exposed and the lateral portion of the tuberosity or posterior facet is retracted away from the body of the calcaneus (Fig. 2). This fragment is often free of soft-tissue attachments and can be exteriorized and placed in saline-soaked gauze on the back table (Fig. 3). Although avascular, this fragment rarely undergoes complete avascular necrosis and late collapse.

Once this fragment is removed, the primary fracture line extending toward the medial aspect of the subtalar joint can be visualized. The rotated posterior facet fragment is identified and gently disimpacted by inserting a large periosteal elevator or osteotome under the anterior aspect of what Souer & Remy (1975) referred to as the thalamic fragment. A Schantz pin is inserted into the posterior inferior and lateral aspect of the calcaneus to aid in the reduction (Fig. 4). The pin should not be inserted percutaneously but through the exposed bone at the apex of the incision. The combined force applied to this pin is distraction and valgus while visualizing the medial subtalar joint and palpating the medial wall of the calcaneus (Fig. 5). The varus deformity of the fracture should be appreciated by palpating the shortened tuberosity fragment while placing an index finger over the fracture line. It is easy to feel the shift in this fracture line, which is actually the most posterior edge of the sustentacular fragment.

Once the primary fracture is reduced and heel height and valgus are restored, 0.062 or 0.045 inch Kirschner

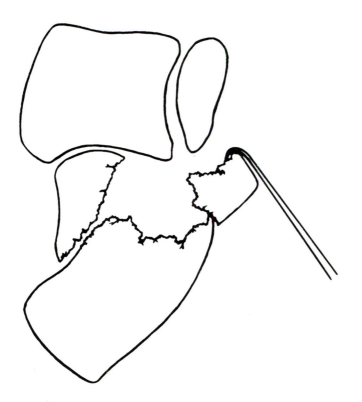

Figure 3

The posterior facet is elevated and it may need to be removed completely from the calcaneus during the reduction maneuver. (Reprinted by permission from Myerson & Multhopp-Stevens 1993)

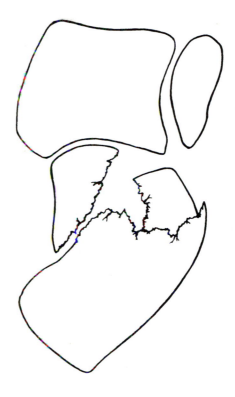

Figure 4

The tuberosity usually tilts into varus and shortens. The heel is now wider, and shorter. (Reprinted by permission from Myerson & Multhopp-Stevens 1993)

wires are inserted from plantar and posterior across the primary fracture into the talus as provisional fixation. These Kirschner wires restore the height and concavity of the medial wall (Fig. 6). One should attempt to avoid placing them into the defect created by the fractured tuberosity, since they will block reduction of the posterior facet if they are not intraosseous. The midportion of the posterior facet is now aligned, and it is held reduced with Kirschner wires introduced from lateral to medial (Fig. 7). Since these wires should be positioned to avoid interfering with the permanent fixation, they should be angled slightly so that the lateral screw fixation does not necessitate their immediate removal (Fig. 8).

Many forms of internal fixation are available to stabilize this fracture, including a 3.5 mm reconstruction plate, a vertical H-plate, and a specially designed calcaneal plate (Synthes, Paoli, Pennsylvania, USA) (Fig. 9). I generally try to restore the height of the tuberosity using a vertically oriented H-plate or a calcaneal plate, which can be planned to include the fixation of the facet through the superior three plate holes. The articular facet is then reduced and fixed provisionally, including the fragment that was removed, and 3.5 mm cortical screws are used to lag the subchondral bone just beneath the articular facet and hold the articular reduction. The correctly sized H-plate is selected, applied to the lateral

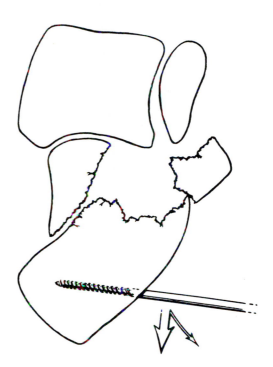

Figure 5

To reduce the tuberosity, it is pulled plantarward and laterally with a Schantz pin. This allows the posterior facet to be elevated out of its impacted position. (Reprinted by permission from Myerson & Multhopp-Stevens 1993)

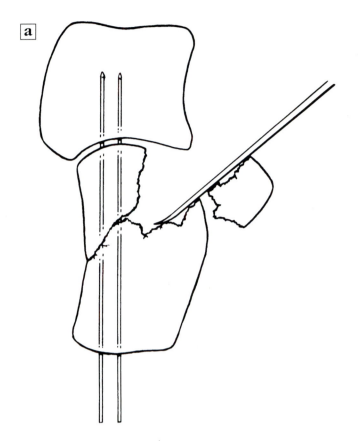

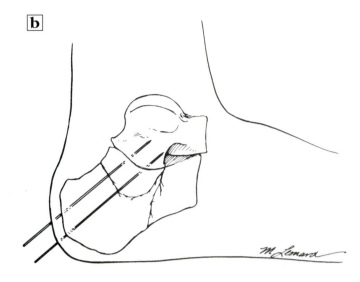

Figure 6

The medial wall is reduced first and held with 0.062 inch Kirschner wires introduced from the inferior, posterior heel. It is not always necessary to pass the pins across the subtalar joint. (a, reprinted by permission from Myerson & Multhopp-Stevens 1993)

wall as a buttress, and secured with 3.5 mm screws. These screws are inserted in a lag fashion for the thalamic fragment, preferably by inserting the three superior screws in a lag fashion through the plate. The rest of the screws are then inserted with a gliding hole (Figs 10 and 11). Any involvement of the calcaneocuboid joint is reduced and fixed temporarily with Kirschner wires and then with 3.5 mm cortical or 4.0 mm cancellous screws.

Bone grafting of the defect, rarely necessary if correct fixation technique is used, may be performed if it is felt it will increase the stability of the reduction. This depends to a large extent on the type of fixation used and the pattern of bone loss under the posterior facet. With the vertical H-plate, the entire lateral wall is supported, and the defect under the plate is irrelevant since the facet is held elevated and reduced. Using a vertically oriented H-plate, there is no fixation between the tuberosity and the neck across the primary fracture line, which has to be supported with additional rigid fixation. If a longitudinal reconstruction plate is used, the primary fracture is held rigidly, but the posterior facet may not be adequately supported. This depends on the size of the thalamic fragment. If the fragment is large, then the inferior edge may be secured by the dorsally curved portion of the plate. Occasionally more than one plate system is necessary for fixation, including the vertical H-plate and a second H-plate or reconstruction plate longitudinally.

The subcutaneous tissue does not require suture and the skin is closed using modified vertical mattress nylon

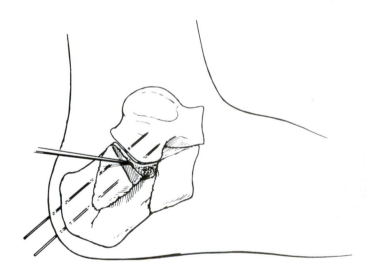

Figure 7

The posterior facet is replaced and, under direct vision, reduced. (Reprinted by permission from Myerson & Multhopp-Stevens 1993)

sutures over a suction drain. A bulky compressive dressing is applied postoperatively and early range of motion is commenced once the sutures are removed. A posterior splint may be used for comfort, but this is removed at regular intervals to perform the range-of-motion

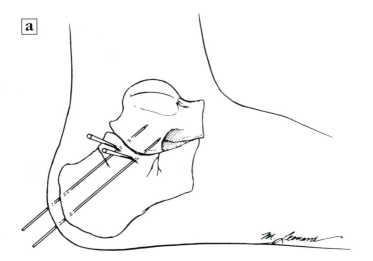

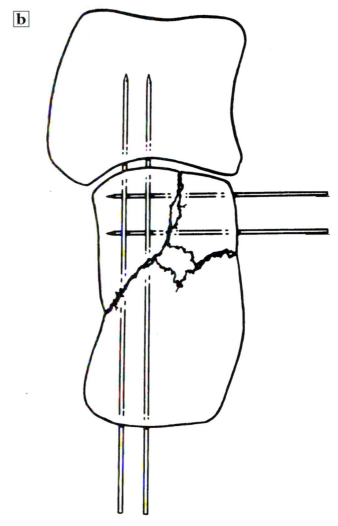

Figure 8

The posterior facet is held temporarily with two 0.045 inch Kirschner wires. (Reprinted by permission from Myerson & Multhopp-Stevens 1993)

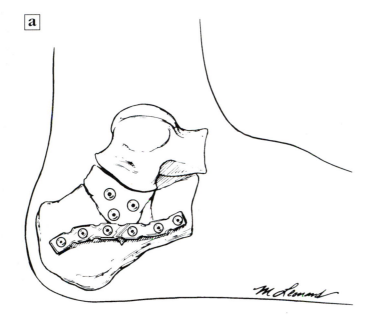

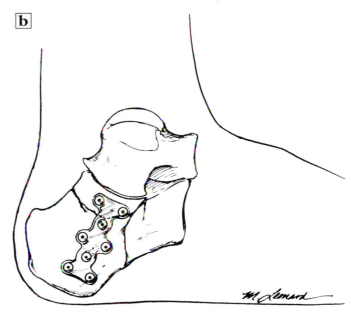

Figure 9

Alternative methods of plate fixation are presented, which depend on the size of the posterior facet fragment. (Reprinted by permission from Myerson & Multhopp-Stevens 1993)

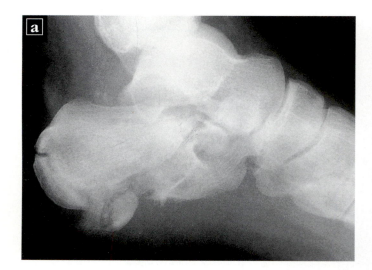

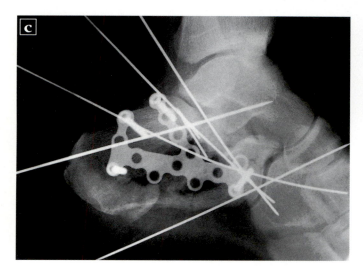

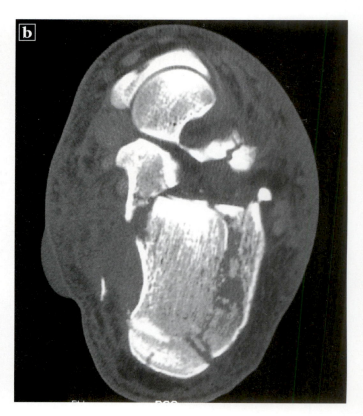

Figure 10

A lateral radiograph (a) and CT scan (b) document this patient's comminuted joint depression fracture. The intraoperative radiograph (c) shows the temporary Kirschner wires and a specially designed calcaneal plate

exercises. The patient is kept non-weight-bearing for 3 months, but toe-touch weight bearing and swimming pool exercises are commenced at 6–8 weeks.

Primary subtalar arthrodesis

In addition to severe comminution and loss of articular cartilage, arthrodesis is also of benefit if the sustentaculum is comminuted or if the entire tuberosity is dislocated (Fig. 12). In the fracture with dislocation of the entire tuberosity, it is unusual for the articular surface to be significantly disrupted. However, there is no bone medially to hold the fracture, and although it is easy to restore the alignment, short of transarticular Kirschner wires, arthrodesis is necessary.

In fractures with severe comminution and bone loss, a primary arthrodesis is often the procedure of choice. Although information about primary arthrodesis is sparse, Dick first described this technique in 1953, and a subse-

quent report by Noble & McQuillan (1979) confirmed its success. I have had excellent results with primary subtalar arthrodesis in selected patients (Myerson, 1992). Thompson & Friesen (1959) recommended a primary triple arthrodesis to address what they considered to be inevitable subsequent transverse tarsal arthritis, but Myerson & Quill (1993) found the need to fuse the talonavicular and calcaneocuboid joints to be quite rare. Furthermore, it is extremely difficult to restore the height and width of the hindfoot adequately with a primary triple arthrodesis. If the calcaneocuboid joint is involved in the acute fracture, then open reduction and internal fixation of this joint is performed, followed by subtalar arthrodesis if required.

Surgical technique
The goal of a primary subtalar arthrodesis is no different from that of open reduction and internal fixation: the anatomic restoration of the subtalar joint and the height and width of the calcaneus. The only difference between

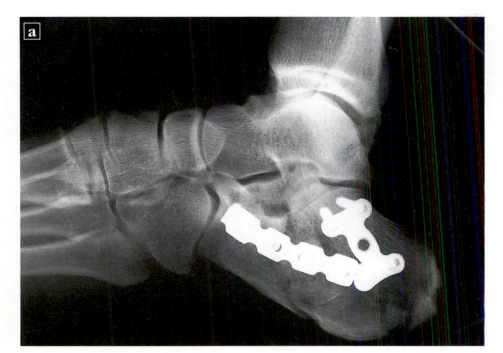

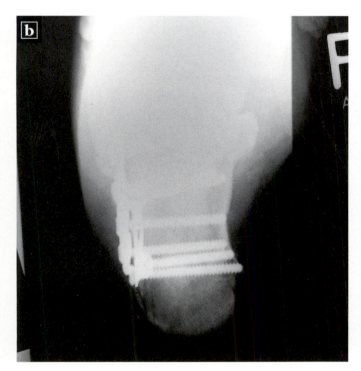

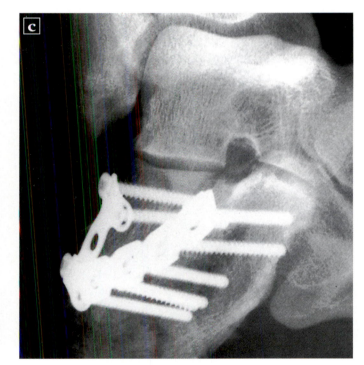

Figure 11

These postoperative radiographs show an alternative method of fixation using a short H-plate and a 3.5 mm reconstruction plate. Lateral (a), axial (b), and Broden's (c) views confirm reduction of the posterior facet and restoration of the width of the heel

this and the approach to the acute fracture described above is that the joint is completely denuded of articular cartilage. The surgical approach is similar, rigid fixation is used, and the articular cartilage is removed using either thin chisel blades or a burr (Myerson 1992).

Once the fracture has been reduced, bone graft is tamped into place and a compression screw is advanced across the subtalar joint. It is unusual to require a corticocancellous bone graft as described by Dick (1953), and I use copious amounts of cancellous bone harvested

from the ipsilateral iliac crest. Occasionally, there is such severe bone loss that a structural bone graft is required, and a tricortical block of iliac crest is used in addition to cancellous graft. It is useful to pack cancellous bone graft anteriorly into the sinus tarsi to achieve both intra- and extra-articular arthrodeses.

Depending on the amount of bone loss, one or more fully threaded cancellous screws can be used to avoid further compression of the joint. A cannulated screw is quite useful, since insertion of a large screw across the

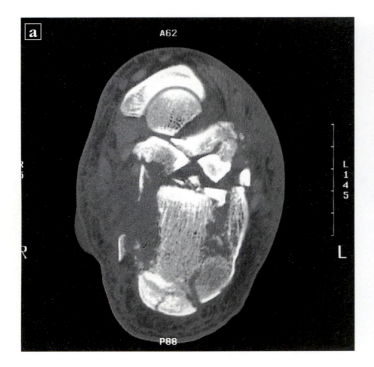
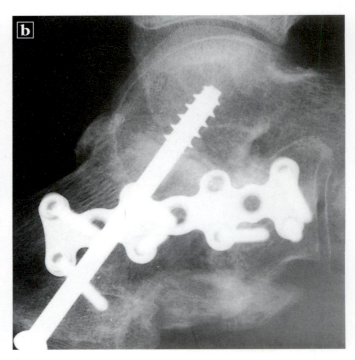

Figure 12

Severe comminution of the posterior facet with loss of the articular surface (a) is best treated with open reduction, internal fixation, and then primary arthrodesis with screw fixation and bone graft (b)

calcaneus into which multiple smaller screws have been placed can be difficult. Care is taken to align the subtalar joint in slight valgus prior to inserting the guide pin. The screws of the calcaneal fixation may interfere with placement of the cannulated screw guide pins, and one should be aware of the need for subsequent pin placement for the arthrodesis when performing the open reduction and internal fixation. One or two parallel large cannulated screws are used to fix the subtalar joint, and their positions are checked with intraoperative fluoroscopic imaging.

Results

Primary arthrodesis as described gives the best functional result with a minimal period of recuperation for severely comminuted fractures that cannot be fixed anatomically. The results with primary arthrodesis are encouraging, since the patients are able to resume active lifestyles. On average, patients can return to work and full activity approximately 8 months after injury. Patients are not allowed to bear weight on the affected extremity for 8 weeks after surgery. Once ambulation commences, the foot is protected in either a short leg cast or a prefabricated boot for an additional month. Usually 1–2 months of physical therapy and rehabilitation are required to maximize the strength and function of the limb. Despite the technical difficulties of performing a primary

arthrodesis, nonunion has not been a problem in patients treated with this method.

Reconstruction after old calcaneal fractures

Although persistent pain in the foot after a fracture of the calcaneus may result from inadequate or inappropriate primary treatment, fractures that are comminuted or intra-articular may not do well regardless of the initial treatment. Painful sequelae are common after calcaneal fractures, and their presentations vary. It is important to evaluate these patients carefully, since physical, economic, psychosocial, and medicolegal issues may all contribute to the patient's continued discomfort.

The most common physical modalities causing discomfort are soft tissue and tendon impingement, nerve-related pain, subtalar arthritis, calcaneofibular abutment, altered tibiotalar joint mechanics, pain from deformity due to unrecognized compartment syndromes, chronic pain syndromes, and the painful heel pad. These factors can be overwhelming when one considers that these injuries occur predominantly in young male workers in the prime of their productive lives. Many of these patients become unemployed, their incomes are drastically affected, and they and their families suffer from the physical and emotional consequences of unemployment. Owing to this chronic pain and, in some patients, the effects of nerve injury and the consequences of reflex sympathetic dystrophy (RSD), drug and alcohol abuse is a common problem. The therapeutic approaches for these conditions are therefore varied and range from judicious neglect, shoe modifications, physiotherapy, surgical reconstruction, sensory denervation of the heel, and even amputation. Obviously, there is much controversy regarding the most appropriate form of treatment and salvage, which stems from the relatively unsatisfactory results frequently reported.

The evaluation of these patients should therefore take these factors into consideration and include a complete social and medical history. Examination of the foot and ankle should include measurement of range of motion in dorsiflexion–plantarflexion and inversion–eversion of the ankle, hindfoot, and forefoot. Tenderness is evaluated by palpation of the soft tissues, and assessment of pain is determined on attempted range of motion of the ankle, subtalar, and transverse tarsal joints. Despite a careful physical and radiological examination, the exact source of pain may still be unclear. Pain on the lateral aspect of the foot and ankle may be the result of peroneal tendinitis, sural neuritis, calcaneofibular impingement, subtalar arthritis, or referred pain from tibial neuritis or heel pad disruption. For these patients, it is useful to supplement the physical examination with selective nerve, joint, and soft tissue blocks. This procedure may be particularly helpful, for example, in distinguishing the pain of subtalar arthritis from that of more simple calcaneofibular abutment. Small volumes of a local anesthetic are used to infiltrate either the sural nerve, the peroneal tendon sheath, the sinus tarsi, or the subtalar joint. These blocks can be administered at separate office visits if the exact source of pain is still unclear.

It is also important to differentiate between somatic and sympathetic pain. Diffuse burning pain, associated with sweating and increased warmth of the foot, is suggestive of RSD. Patients with this type of discomfort are often not helped by surgery, which is aimed at correcting sources of pain that are predominantly somatic in nature. In these patients, it is also helpful to block the tibial nerve to evaluate for sympathetically mediated pain or RSD.

Patients with diffuse, burning pain of the foot and ankle should be evaluated for tibial nerve entrapment with electrophysiologic testing of the tibial nerve and its branches. Pain referable to multiple nerves in a nonanatomic distribution, however, is suggestive of RSD. This diagnosis can be confirmed if a tibial nerve block using 10 cc of a combination of 1% xylocaine and 0.5% bupivacaine does not relieve pain, which is then felt to be suggestive of sympathetic origin. Technetium 99 scintigraphic studies have also been shown to be useful in the diagnosis of RSD (Holder et al 1992). If the

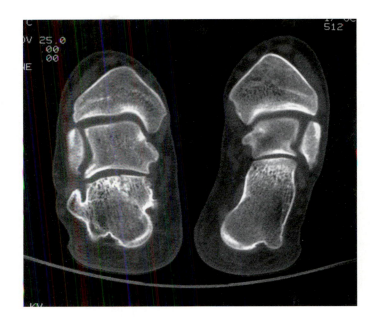

Figure 13

The CT scan demonstrates shortening and varus of the heel, with bone extrusion medially and laterally. The CT scan is useful but not necessary for preoperative planning

diagnosis of RSD is still in doubt, a lumbar sympathetic block can be used for both diagnostic and therapeutic purposes. I do not believe that patients with a confirmed diagnosis of RSD are suitable candidates for extensive surgical salvage, although the somatic focus of their pain, in addition to the sympathetic pain associated with RSD, may require treatment.

Radiographs of both feet are obtained, including anteroposterior and lateral weight bearing views, a 30° internal oblique view, Broden's views (Broden 1949), and a posterior tangential view of the calcaneus (Gamble & Yale 1975a, 1975b). These plain radiographs are most useful in delineating the existence and severity of subtalar or transverse tarsal arthritis and of calcaneofibular impingement. In some patients, calcaneofibular impingement or peroneal tendinitis is present without routine radiographic evidence of subtalar arthritis and may occur after more minor injuries, with lateral wall extrusion. In these patients, a CT is useful (Crosby & Fitzgibbons 1990) (Fig. 13).

The role of conservative treatment after these injuries is controversial. Once a patient experiences pain after a calcaneal fracture, it has been my experience that this pain seldom dissipates. Therefore, the following question arises: at what stage should reconstruction be performed? The answer probably depends on the extent and severity of the injury and deformity. If the fracture was anatomically reduced with open reduction and internal fixation, I would wait approximately 6–12 months before recommending reconstruction or arthrodesis. If, however,

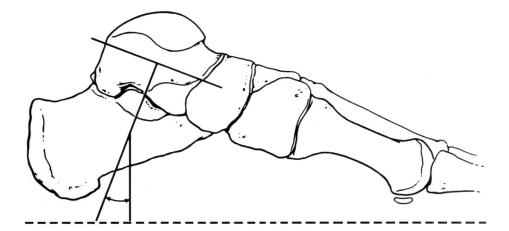

Figure 14

The talar declination angle is demonstrated (normal >20°)

severe deformity were present, or if the fracture had not been accurately repaired at surgery, then I would perform the reconstruction as soon as it were feasible. The problem with delaying treatment in these patients is that they are mostly young men involved in active manual labor. Delaying treatment may not be appropriate for these patients who are otherwise incapacitated with pain. I have found that the longer one waits to begin salvage, the less likely it is that these patients will ever return to gainful employment.

The recommended treatments after calcaneal fractures vary enormously. Those authors who recommend nonoperative treatment appear either to have adopted the philosophy of Bankart (1942), who wrote, 'the results of treatment of fractures of the os calcis are rotten . . .' or else to have embraced the view held by Barnard & Odegard (1955) that 'it appears hopeless as well as technically impossible to attempt to restore accurately a normal articular surface to a subtalar joint which has been disrupted'. I have been encouraged by the results of operative salvage of old painful calcaneal fractures and do not subscribe to the above philosophy of nihilistic neglect.

A subtalar distraction bone block arthrodesis is recommended for managing subtalar arthritis with or without anterior ankle pain and a significant loss of heel height. Carr et al (1988) have described the use of a bone block fusion for restoring the height of the hindfoot, modifying an earlier procedure described by Gallie in 1943. In a later study, Myerson & Quill (1993) reported similar success using this technique. The hindfoot collapse is easily demonstrated on bilateral standing lateral radiographs. Anterior tibiotalar impingement is best demonstrated by a talar declination angle of 20° or less on a standing lateral radiograph (Fig. 14). This angle is formed by the longitudinal axis of the talus and the plane of support on a weight bearing lateral radiograph and is a measure of the 'horizontal attitude' assumed by the talus (Gamble & Yale 1975a, 1975b, Carr et al 1988). An *in situ* subtalar arthrodesis is performed for subtalar arthri-

tis in the presence of more normal heel height and normal tibiotalar alignment. The subtalar bone block procedure is performed with the patient in the lateral decubitus position through a longitudinal incision posterior to the peroneal tendons. The sural nerve is identified and retracted. Although some authors recommend excision of the sural nerve with the incision, I find that this is not always necessary.

After exposure and distraction of the subtalar joint, the appropriately sized tricortical iliac crest bone graft is inserted. Insertion of the graft may cause the heel to tilt into varus. To prevent varus malunion, an external fixation construct using the femoral distractor (Synthes, Paoli, Pennsylvania, USA) may be applied medially with one pin in the calcaneus and one in the tibia. The subtalar joint is thereby distracted and simultaneously tilted into valgus while the graft is inserted. The size and shape of the bone graft may also affect the position of the hindfoot, and I have found that cutting a trapezoid graft 1–2 mm higher on the medial side may tilt the subtalar joint into slight valgus. Correct alignment can be difficult to judge with the patient in the lateral decubitus position but, nevertheless, I feel that the posterior distraction bone block arthrodesis technique is a better alternative to subtalar arthrodesis in appropriately selected patients because it restores the normal talocalcaneal and tibiotalar alignment and facilitates decompression of the peroneal tendons through the same incision (Figs 15 and 16).

Reich (1926, 1932) noted that subtalar arthrodesis in patients with old calcaneal fractures gave good results and shortened the period of disability. This has also been my experience, and I have found that patients treated with either an isolated subtalar arthrodesis or subtalar arthrodesis using the posterior bone block method have fared the best (Saxby et al 1992).

Thompson & Friesen (1959) reported on 56 fractures of the calcaneus all treated acutely by triple arthrodesis. My experience with triple arthrodesis as a primary or a late procedure is not so favorable, perhaps because it

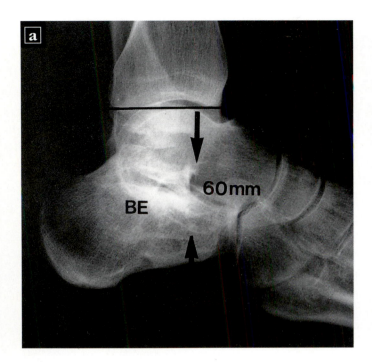
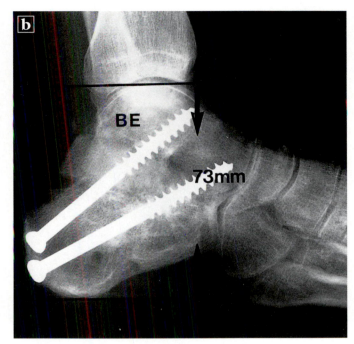

Figure 15

This patient had symptoms of subtalar arthritis and anterior ankle impingement 1 year after closed treatment of a calcaneal fracture. The preoperative height from the inferior calcaneus to the dorsal talus surface was 60 mm (a); it was corrected to 73 mm postoperatively with a bone block subtalar fusion (b)

fails to restore the height or width of the heel. A primary triple arthrodesis is extremely difficult to perform. Multiple small bone fragments are present, and it is difficult to restore the height and width of the hindfoot. In some patients, a triple arthrodesis is the only method of salvage, but these patients should be carefully selected. Although fusion of the subtalar joint limits motion, a triple arthrodesis restricts motion even further, and one should preserve as much motion of the hindfoot as possible. In the presence of arthritis of the subtalar and calcaneocuboid joints, I have performed arthrodesis of these joints alone, and have not found it necessary to fuse the talonavicular joint (Fig. 17). A triple arthrodesis is performed in the presence of arthritis of the subtalar as well as the transverse tarsal joint. Occasionally there is deformity of the midfoot that is not associated with arthritis but that cannot be corrected by a subtalar arthrodesis alone; a triple arthrodesis is performed in these patients.

Cotton (1921), Magnusson (1923), and Cabot & Binney (1907) recommended excision of the displaced calcaneus for management of calcaneofibular impingement. Cotton (1921) stated that in order for this ostectomy to succeed, one should remove a considerable amount of the lateral calcaneus, amounting to one-third to one-half of the width of the calcaneus. Resection of the distal end of the fibula, together with removal of the peroneal tendons from their sheath, was reported by Evans in 1968 and

Isbister in 1974 for this same condition. I have not experienced good results with a lateral wall ostectomy as the sole procedure for managing old calcaneal fractures. I found that, although some patients were improved, many continued to experience pain, some later requiring a subtalar fusion. In the other failures, there was recurrent calcaneofibular impingement, either with heterotopic bone formation or excessive subcutaneous fibrosis. I now recommend that patients should be carefully selected for the procedure of lateral ostectomy since it is unusual to find impingement in the absence of subtalar arthritis. This ostectomy is, however, an important adjustment to fusion procedures and is performed to restore a normal calcaneofibular recess.

Sallick & Blum (1948) reported on seven patients treated with tibial and sural neurectomy and sensory denervation of the heel to relieve intractable pain from calcaneal fractures; no harmful effects were observed, and no subsequent trophic changes were reported. I have no experience with this ablative procedure. Nerve compression syndromes do occur after calcaneal fractures, but they need not be treated with neurectomy (Byank et al 1989, Mann 1974). Reports of post-traumatic tarsal tunnel syndrome would indicate that if the nerve impingement is secondary to scarring, exostosis, or fracture, tarsal tunnel release is indicated (Byank et al 1989, Edwards et al 1969, Finkbeiner 1975, Meyer & Lagier 1977).

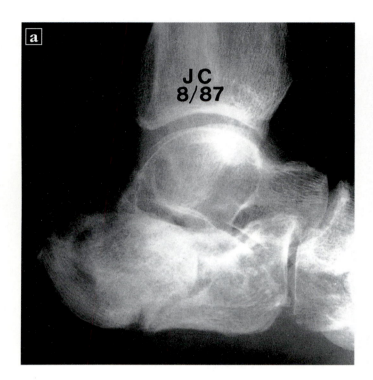

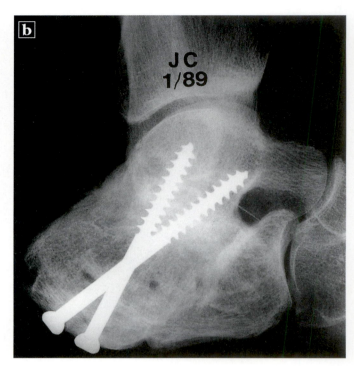

Figure 16

A posterior bone block arthrodesis of the subtalar joint (a) was performed in this patient. The postoperative appearance (b), with restoration of the height of the hindfoot

After the nerve decompression, most patients will benefit from physical therapy. I have attempted to maximize the recovery from the initial operative procedure by performing the tarsal tunnel release 2–3 months after the arthrodesis procedure. These reports, as well as the results in the patients, demonstrate that results from any of the operations on nerves after the fracture are unpredictable, and revision tarsal tunnel surgery was uniformly unsuccessful.

These patients need a critical evaluation of their diverse physical as well as social problems. The longer a patient remains out of work, the more difficult it is to return him to work and the normal activities of daily living. Although the salvage of patients who have had fractures of the calcaneus, with the complication of persistent pain, is technically demanding and diagnostically challenging, a standardized approach to determining the appropriate late salvage is ideal.

References

Bankart A S B 1942 Fractures of the os calcis. Lancet 2: 175

Barnard L, Odegard J K 1955 Conservative approach in the treatment of fractures of the calcaneus. J Bone Joint Surg 37A: 1231–1236

Bohler L 1931 Diagnosis, pathology, and treatment of fractures of the os calcis. J Bone Joint Surg 31: 75–89

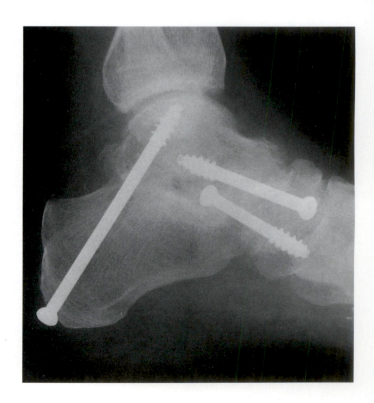

Figure 17

A triple arthrodesis was performed in this patient for treatment of both subtalar and transverse tarsal arthritis 2 years after closed treatment for a calcaneus fracture

Broden B 1949 Roentgen examination of the subtaloid joint in fracture of the calcaneus. Acta Radiol 31: 85–91

Burdeaux B D 1983 Reduction of calcaneal fractures by the McReynolds medial approach technique and its experimental basis. Clin Orthop 177: 87–103

Byank R P, Clarke H J, Bleecker M L 1989 Standardized neurometric evaluation in tarsal tunnel syndrome. Adv Orthop Surg 12: 249–253

Cabot H, Binney H 1907 Fractures of the os calcis and astragalus. Ann Surg 45: 51–68

Carr J B, Hansen S T, Benirschke S K 1988 Subtalar distraction bone block fusion for late complications of os calcis fractures. Foot Ankle 9: 81–86

Conn H R 1926 Fractures of the os calcis: diagnosis and treatment. Radiology 2: 228–235

Conn H R 1935 The treatment of fractures of the os calcis. J Bone Joint Surg 17: 392–404

Cotton F J 1921 Old os calcis fractures. Ann Surg 74: 294–303

Cotton F J, Wilson L T 1908 Fractures of the os calcis. Boston Med Surg J 159: 559–565

Crosby L A, Fitzgibbons T 1990 Computerized tomography scanning of acute intra-articular fractures of the calcaneus. A new classification system. J Bone Joint Surg 72A: 852–859

Dick I L 1953 Primary fusion of the posterior subtalar joint in the treatment of fractures of the calcaneum. J Bone Joint Surg 35B: 375–380

Eastwood D M, Langkamer V G, Atkins R M 1993 Intra-articular fractures of the calcaneum. Part II: Open reduction and internal fixation by the extended lateral transcalcaneal approach. J Bone Joint Surg 75B: 189–195

Edwards W G, Lincoln C R, Bassett F H III, et al 1969 The tarsal tunnel syndrome. Diagnosis and treatment. JAMA 207: 716–720

Essex-Lopresti P 1952 The mechanism, reduction technique, and results in fractures of the os calcis. Br J Surg 39: 395–419

Evans D 1968 Fractures of the calcaneus [abstr]. J Bone Joint Surg 50B: 884

Finkbeiner G, Stohr C, Leemreijze P 1975 [Tarsal tunnel syndrome and trauma. Case reports on the etiology and therapy]. Monatsschr Unfallheilkd 78: 269–274

Gallie W E 1943 Subastragalar arthrodesis in fractures of the os calcis. J Bone Joint Surg 25: 732–736

Gamble F O, Yale I 1975a Orthodigital problems. In: Clinical Foot Roentgenology, 2nd edn. Robert Kriger, Huntington, NY. pp. 248–270

Gamble F O, Yale I 1975b Traumatic effects. In: Clinical Foot Roentgenology, 2nd edn. Robert Krieger, Huntington, NY. pp 153–154, 252–254

Gissane W 1947 Comment on subtalar joint reduction. In: Proceedings of the British Orthopaedic Association. J Bone Joint Surg 29: 254–255

Hall M C, Pennal G F 1960 Primary subtalar arthrodesis in the treatment of severe fractures of the calcaneum. J Bone Joint Surg 42B: 336–343

Holder L E, Cole L A, Myerson M S 1992 Reflex sympathetic dystrophy in the foot: clinical and scintigraphic criteria. Radiology 184: 531–535

Isbister J F 1974 Calcaneo-fibular abutment following crush fracture of the calcaneus. J Bone Joint Surg 56B: 274–278

Lance E M, Carey E J, Wade P A 1964 Fractures of the os calcis: a follow-up study. J Trauma 4: 15–56

Leung K S, Chan W S, Shen W Y, et al 1989 Operative treatment of intraarticular fractures of the os calcis – the role of rigid internal fixation and primary bone grafting: preliminary reults. J Orthop Trauma 3: 232–240

Leung K S, Yuen K M, Chan W S 1993 Operative treatment of displaced intra-articular fractures of the calcaneum. Medium-term results. J Bone Joint Surg 75B: 196–201

Magnusson P B 1923 An operation for relief of disability in old fractures of the os calcis. JAMA 80: 1511–1513

Mann R A 1974 The tarsal tunnel syndrome. Orthop Clin North Am 5: 109–115

McReynolds I S 1982 The role for operative treatment of the os calcis. In: Leach R E, Hoaglund F T, Riseborough E J (eds) Controversies in Orthopedic Surgery. W B Saunders, Philadelphia. pp 232–254

Meyer J M, Lagier R 1977 Post-traumatic sinus tarsi syndrome. An anatomical and radiological study. Acta Orthop Scand 48: 121–128

Myerson M, Manoli A 1993 Compartment syndromes of the foot after calcaneal fractures. Clin Orthop 290: 142–150

Myerson M, Multhopp-Stevens H 1993 Fractures of the calcaneus. In: Myerson M (ed) Current Therapy in Foot and Ankle Surgery. Mosby–Year Book, St Louis. pp 249–257

Myerson M, Quill G E Jr 1993 Late complications of fractures of the calcaneus. J Bone Joint Surg 75A: 331–341

Myerson M S 1992 Open reduction and primary arthrodesis of a calcaneal fracture [commentary and interview by George E Quill Jr, MD]. Strategies Orthop Surg 11: 2–16

Myerson M S, Henderson M R 1993 Clinical applications of a pneumatic intermittent impulse compression device after trauma and major surgery to the foot and ankle. Foot Ankle 14: 198–203

Noble J, McQuillan W M 1979 Early posterior subtalar fusion in the treatment of fractures of the os calcis. J Bone Joint Surg 61B: 90–93

Paley D, Hall H 1993 Intra-articular fractures of the calcaneus. A critical analysis of results and prognostic factors. J Bone Joint Surg 75A: 342–354

Palmer I 1948 The mechanism and treatment of fractures of the calcaneus. Open reduction with the use of cancellous grafts. J Bone Joint Surg 39A: 2–8

Pozo J L, Kirwan E O, Jackson A M 1984 The long-term results of conservative management of severely displaced fractures of the calcaneus. J Bone Joint Surg 66B: 386–390

Reich R S 1926 Subastragaloid arthrodesis in the treatment of old fractures of the calcaneus. Surg Gynecol Obstet 42: 420–422

Reich R S 1932 End-results in fractures of the calcaneus. JAMA 99: 1909–1913

Romash M M 1988 Calcaneal fractures: three-dimensional treatment. Foot Ankle 8: 180–197

Rowe C R, Sakellarises H T, Freeman P A, et al 1963 Fractures of the os calcis: a long-term follow-up study of 146 patients. JAMA 184: 920–923

Sallick M A, Blum L 1948 Sensory denervation of the heel for persistent pain following fractures of the calcaneus. J Bone Joint Surg 30A: 209–212

Saxby T, Myerson M, Schon L 1992 Compartment syndrome of the foot following calcaneus fracture. Foot 2: 157–161

Soeur R, Remy R 1975 Fractures of the calcaneus with displacement of the thalamic portion. J Bone Joint Surg 57B: 413–421

Stephenson J R 1983 Displaced fractures of the os calcis involving the subtalar joint: the key role of the superomedial fragment. Foot Ankle 4: 91–101

Stephenson J R 1987 Treatment of displaced intra-articular fractures of the calcaneus using medial and lateral approaches, internal fixation, and early motion. J Bone Joint Surg 69A: 115–130

Thompson K R, Friesen C M 1959 Treatment of comminuted fractures of the calcaneus by primary triple arthrodesis. J Bone Joint Surg 41A: 1423–1436

IX.4 Midfoot and Navicular Injuries

John S Early and Sigvard T Hansen Jr

Injuries of the midfoot are uncommon and frequently overlooked in the care of the trauma patient. In the past, trauma to the midfoot has been viewed as being of little consequence to the patient's overall function. Follow-up of these patients has shown that, in fact, these injuries can cause significant disability, which compromises the patient's ambulatory function (Dewar & Evans 1968, Main & Jowett 1975, Sangeorzan et al 1993). Recent work by many individuals points to the need to address these injuries expeditiously in an attempt to avoid significant long-term pain and deformity.

Functional anatomy

The midfoot is an anatomic section of the foot between the boundaries of Chopart's and Lisfranc's joint lines (Fig. 1). Five bones make up the midfoot: the navicular and cuboid and the medial, middle (intermediate) and lateral cuneiforms. The midfoot has a unique role in foot function. First, it does not normally provide a primary weight bearing surface for ground contact. Secondly, the structure is relatively immobile compared to the subtalar joint of the hindfoot or the metatarsophalangeal joints of the forefoot despite the presence of many large articular surfaces.

The immobility between the bones of the midfoot is clearly related to its anatomic structure. Stability is due in large part to the numerous dense plantar ligaments, which tightly bind all the osseous structures in the midfoot together (Fig. 2). These ligaments also carry over to the hindfoot and medial forefoot to provide strong mechanical links between the three sections of the foot (Kapandji 1987, Sarrafian 1993). The inherent stability provided by these overlapping ligaments is seen in the maintenance of normal arch shape without the need for muscle action during standing (Basmajian & Stecko 1963, Mann & Inman 1964). This can be related mechanically to a multisegmented beam whose strength and stability is dependent on the tensile strength of the interseg-mental ties between the osseous structures on the under-surface (Hicks 1953, Hicks 1955). The multiple insertions of the tibialis posterior tendon are intertwined with the plantar ligamentous structures to provide dynamic support and mechanical overload protection (Perry 1992). It is significant that tibialis posterior is the only muscle that controls movement of the midfoot, attaching as it does to all five bones and moving them as a unit.

A second concept behind the function of the midfoot is in its participation in the medial and lateral support columns (Fig. 3). The medial column is composed of the talus, the navicular, and the three cuneiforms and their corresponding metatarsals. The lateral column consists of the calcaneus, cuboid and the lateral two rays. The inter-action between the talus and calcaneus, through the subtalar complex, serves as the proximal anchor to both columns. The resultant configuration is analogous to a three-legged stool. The stability of the stool is depen-dent on the relative length of each leg. The calcaneus, as the proximal weight bearing area in the foot, repre-sents one leg. The lateral two rays and the medial three rays are the ground contact points for the remaining two legs. The three-dimensional relationship of the cuboid to the navicular and cuneiforms will define the relative lengths of the lateral and medial columns and therefore the stability of the weight bearing platform. Shortening of the lateral column directly by trauma to the cuboid or by relative lengthening of the medial column through loss of ligamentous integrity can create significant malalignment between the forefoot and hindfoot (Fig. 4).

This inherent stability is important for two reasons. The medial arch provides a protective conduit and alcove for the neurovascular structures and intrinsic musculature of the plantar foot. These muscles are extremely important to the function and stability of the subtalar complex during propulsion. In its capacity as a beam, the midfoot solidly binds the forefoot to the hindfoot when the foot is supinated. Rotational changes in the hindfoot with ground contact are transmitted to the forefoot by the midfoot, which acts as a mechanical actuator. The midfoot also determines the weight bearing alignment of the hindfoot to the forefoot. Relative pronation or supina-tion of the forefoot to the hindfoot can significantly alter gait mechanics (Perry 1992, Sarrafian 1993).

Though stability is important, the midfoot is not totally without the potential to move, and cadaveric studies show that motion does occur between the individual midfoot structures (Ouzounian & Shereff 1989). This motion is small compared to the motion about the sub-talar complex or the metatarsophalangeal joints, but it plays a role in shock absorption during weight bearing. The functional description is that of a leaf spring which, within the confines of limited overall motion, performs elastic dampening and recoil of repetitive forces (Ker et al 1987, Hansen 1993). This is also associated with pronation, which takes place primarily through the subtalar and talonavicular joints.

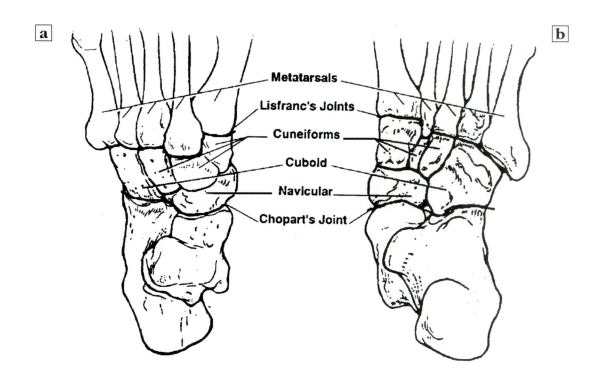

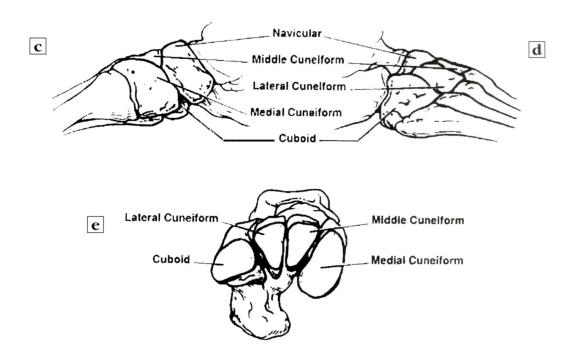

Figure 1

Bony anatomy of the midfoot: (a) dorsal view; (b) plantar view; (c) medial view; (d) lateral view; (e) coronal view at the tarsometatarsal (Lisfranc) joint line

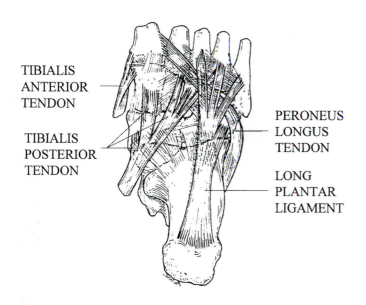

Figure 2

Plantar ligamentous structures of the midfoot. Note the multiple interlocking ligaments binding each osseous structure to its neighbor. The posterior tibialis tendon has a major role in the plantar support of the midfoot

Figure 3

Delineation of the medial and lateral columns in the foot

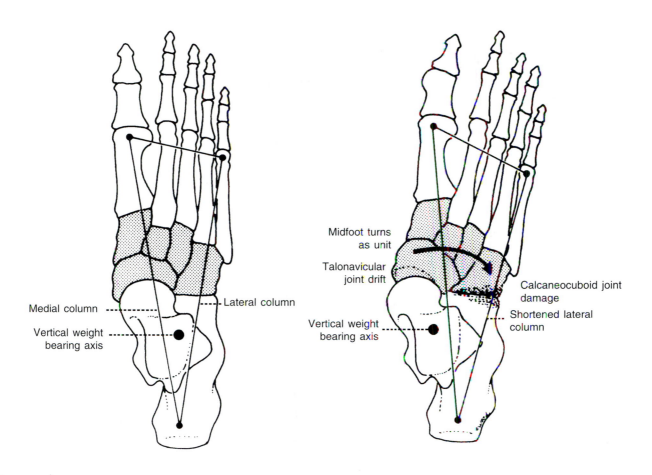

Figure 4

Disruption of column integrity. Change in the three-dimensional contour of either the medial or lateral column results in the distortion of the other. This adversely affects overall foot function. (Adapted with permission from Early & Hansen 1994)

When treating midfoot injuries the relative importance of the various functions of this section of the foot should be considered. Stability is of paramount importance. Secondly, maintenance of the relationship of the hindfoot to the forefoot weight bearing surfaces should be considered. The least important consideration is to maintain the articular integrity between the bones of the midfoot. Except for the talonavicular, calcaneocuboid and cuboid–fifth metatarsal joints, this can be done with little regard for maintaining joint motion, but rather with emphasis on stability and restoration of bony structure.

Assessment of the midfoot

Treatment of midfoot injuries depends on the structures involved and on the degree of injury. Patients with midfoot injuries usually are initially evaluated with anteroposterior, lateral, and oblique radiographs taken in a non-weight-bearing or unstressed position. This may or may not show the complete injury. Because of the possibility of significant ligamentous instability in the face of minor bony damage, it is also important to obtain stressed X-ray views to allow a complete assessment of the damage. These views should be weight bearing if possible. If necessary, after an initial neurovascular examination, a short-acting local anesthetic can be used for an ankle block. This will lessen the patient's discomfort and apprehension during the stress X-rays. Computed tomography (CT) can also be helpful in assessing bony damage. The significant amount of bony overlap in the midfoot makes clear viewing of each structure difficult with plain films.

Navicular injury

It is readily apparent in its bony architecture that the navicular is important not only for its position in the midfoot but also for its ability to transmit the motions generated by the subtalar complex to the forefoot. Injury to this bone is typically due to indirect forces. Most often, axial loading occurs through the forefoot, owing to a fall from a height or a motor vehicle accident. Different patterns are seen, depending on the direction and rate of loading of the axial force (Eichenholtz & Levine 1964, Main & Jowett 1975, Sangeorzan 1993).

Dislocation
Isolated dislocation of the navicular is extremely rare (Pathria et al 1988, Shelton & Pedowitz 1992). When this occurs, the navicular is found medial and dorsal to its normal position. The mechanism appears to be an initial hyperplantarflexion of the forefoot with subsequent axial loading. This tends to disrupt, firstly, the dorsal naviculo-

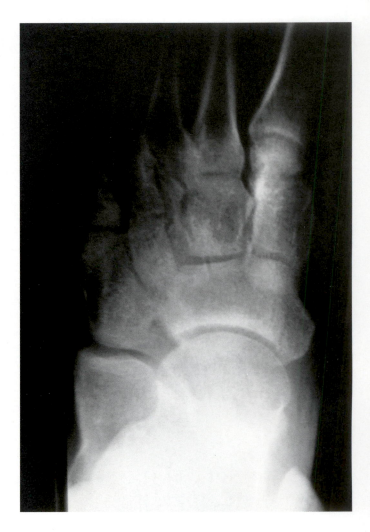

Figure 5

Navicular stress fracture in an adolescent tennis player. The X-ray was initially read as normal and reviewed only after 6 weeks of continued weight-bearing pain

cuneiform ligaments, followed next by the plantar naviculocuneiform ligaments, and finally the plantar talonavicular ligaments. It is important to obtain an anatomic reduction and stabilization of the navicular in order to preserve midfoot function. Open reduction of both the talonavicular and naviculocuneiform joints is necessary. This reduction should be maintained either by internal fixation screws across the naviculocuneiform and naviculocuboid joints or by smooth Steinman pins through the talonavicular joint. Non-weight-bearing casting should be undertaken for 8–10 weeks. The fixation screws should be removed at 6 months. This should allow sufficient time for ligamentous healing.

Fractures
There are four basic types of navicular fractures reported in the literature: stress fractures, cortical avulsion

fractures, tuberosity fractures and body fractures. Each represents the result of different stresses placed upon the navicular (Nyska et al 1989, Sangeorzan et al 1989, Sangeorzan et al 1993, Shelton & Pedowitz 1992).

Stress fractures

Stress fractures of the navicular appear most commonly in young athletes and military recruits (Khan et al 1992, Torg et al 1982). They are difficult to identify on X-ray and usually present as anterior or medial ankle pain, and they can therefore be misdiagnosed as anterior tibial tendinitis (Fig. 5). Because this population is highly competitive and active, the history can reflect more of a chronic discomfort which increases with weight bearing activity. Anteroposterior, lateral and oblique views of the foot should be obtained centered on the navicular to look for evidence of a fracture line. If the injury is suspected but not readily identifiable because it is incomplete or nondisplaced, it is best to initiate treatment with a non-weight-bearing short leg cast for a period of 4 weeks. Repeat films may be obtained at that time, and these may better show the extent of bony injury by the evidence of active remodeling. A bone scan can also be useful to help pinpoint the area of irritation, especially if the patient presents with chronic symptoms (see Chapter IX.6).

If the fracture is discernible on plain films, CT of the navicular should be obtained to judge displacement and direction. If talonavicular joint surface displacement is evident, these fractures should be treated as regular displaced fractures. Anatomic reduction of the joint surface can be undertaken, with stable fixation using 3.5 mm cortical screws placed across the fracture site with overdrilling of the near cortex to allow interfragmental compression (Fitch et al 1989, Khan et al 1992, Sangeorzan 1993). Exposure of the fracture is through a longitudinal dorsal incision at the fracture site. Fixation is introduced through stab wounds, and it is done such that the threads engage in the larger fragment.

Avulsion fractures

Avulsion or chip fractures can be found on the dorsal aspect of the proximal lip or the medial aspect of the navicular. They may appear minor on X-ray, and indeed they usually are if they are secondary to a direct blow. However, an avulsion fracture of the navicular may also be a marker for more significant ligamentous damage about Chopart's joint if the mechanism of injury is unclear (Fig. 6). Avulsion injuries caused by a fall from a height or a motor vehicle accident warrant further investigation of the midfoot. Fractures of the cuboid, anterior calcaneus and cuneiforms as well as marked instability of Chopart's joints have been reported in association with this injury (Davis et al 1993, Main & Jowett 1975, Shelton & Pedowitz 1992).

To evaluate the foot properly stress radiographs should be obtained of the midfoot. CT is also helpful in fully assessing the extent of bony and articular injury.

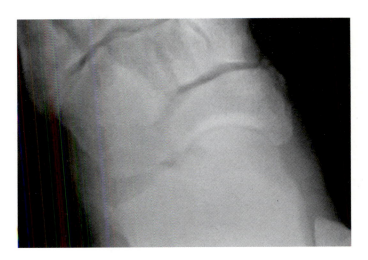

Figure 6

Avulsion fracture of the navicular; note disruption of calcaneocuboid joint

If there is no appreciable instability or associated fractures then treatment can begin in a short leg walking cast for 4 weeks. If other fractures are evident, they should be accurately reduced and stabilized to preserve normal bony relationships. Instability about Chopart's joints will require a significant period of rigid immobilization. These ligamentous injuries should be treated in a non-weight-bearing cast for 10–12 weeks. It is important to obtain radiographs in plaster after initial casting to ensure that the foot is immobilized in a reduced position.

A problem that occasionally arises from isolated dorsal lip fractures is the development of an osteophytic prominence on the dorsum of the mid-foot. This prominence can easily be excised if the patient becomes symptomatic because of wearing shoes.

Tuberosity fractures

Tuberosity fractures are usually the result of forced eversion of the foot resisted by the pull of the posterior tibialis. They are rarely due to a direct blow. These fractures rarely displace, owing to the thick ligamentous attachment about this area of the navicular, but they can cause significant pain because of the constant tension on the fracture site caused by the tibialis posterior. Two caveats: first, the literature shows a preponderance of associated injuries to the cuboid with this injury, and this should be ruled out before treatment begins (Main & Jowett 1975, Shelton & Pedowitz, 1992, Davis et al 1993); and secondly, there is a 10–12% incidence of accessory navicular (os tibiale) in the general population.

If the injury is seen acutely and is not displaced, treatment in a weight bearing short leg cast should be initiated for 6–8 weeks. Nonunion of this fracture is not

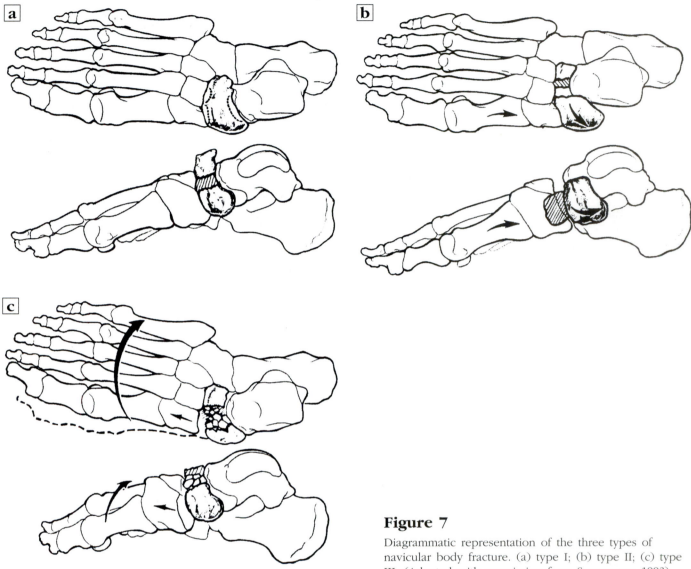

Figure 7

Diagrammatic representation of the three types of navicular body fracture. (a) type I; (b) type II; (c) type III. (Adapted with permission from Sangeorzan 1993)

uncommon and, if symptomatic, may require surgical intervention.

Fractures with significant displacement and fractures that are old or symptomatic usually require surgery. If the fragment is too small for compressive bony fixation, it should be excised, and the posterior tibial tendon firmly reattached to the navicular tuberosity. If the fracture fragment is of sufficient size, operative debridement of the fracture ends and compression fixation with a screw is recommended. Twelve weeks of casting should be anticipated, with the first 6 weeks being non-weight-bearing.

Body fractures

Acute navicular fractures that involve the body result from axial loading with the talar head and neck being driven into the navicular (Eichenholtz & Levine 1964). Of the four types of isolated navicular fractures

discussed, this is the most severe. It always involves the articular surface of the talonavicular joint, and it is usually displaced. This joint surface is the most important articular surface associated with the midfoot. It controls the ability of the forefoot to align itself with the hindfoot and the ground. Without the talonavicular joint, there is essentially no motion of the subtalar complex.

Fractures involving the body can be grouped into three types (Fig. 7). Type 1 fractures have a primary fracture line parallel to the sole of the foot, and the dorsal fragment usually involves less than half of the body. There is no medial column disruption noted on anteroposterior X-ray. Type 2 fractures are oblique, traveling from dorsolateral to plantomedial across the navicular body. The medial or dorsomedial fragment is the major fragment, and the smaller plantar lateral fragment is usually comminuted. The medial support column can appear disrupted, with adduction of the forefoot. Type 3 fractures involve central or lateral articular comminution. The medial column is usually disrupted with abduction of the forefoot (Sangeorzan et al 1993).

Open reduction and internal fixation of the navicular is recommended for any complete fracture of the body involving the talonavicular articular surface (Nyska et al 1989, Sangeorzan 1993, Shelton & Pedowitz 1992, Vaishya & Patrick 1991). Long-term results have been found to be poor when these fractures are not accurately stabilized. Surgery is done with the patient in supine position. If the fracture pattern is Type 2 with minimal comminution it may be readily handled through a single dorsal incision over the fracture line. Otherwise, two incisions are recommended in order to avoid excessive stripping, which may compromise navicular blood supply. Screws are placed through stab wounds either medially or laterally. The medial incision is located over the posterior tibial tendon. The lateral incision is on the dorsum of the foot just lateral to the navicular. Using the talar head as a template it is most important to reconstruct the talonavicular articular surface. To improve visualization, a small fragment distractor may be employed to temporarily lengthen the medial column of the foot.

Cancellous bone grafting may be necessary to fill any voids in the body which become apparent after reduction of the talonavicular articular surface. This is done to restore the bony contour to its normal size. If there is significant destruction of the naviculocuneiform joints, restoration of this articular surface should be sacrificed in favor of a stable fusion across these joints. These three joints normally exhibit minimal motion and can be a source of significant pain if they are not stable.

Reduction is maintained using two 3.5 mm cortical screws placed in a lag screw fashion. If there is insufficient bone stock in the lateral navicular fragment for screw fixation, the screws can be anchored into the cuboid or cuneiform bones without significantly affecting midfoot function (Fig. 8).

Postoperatively these fractures are treated non-weight-bearing in a short leg cast for 8 weeks. Thereafter, a removable brace should be employed along with progressive weight bearing and range of motion exercises. When painless full weight bearing is achieved the patient may return to normal shoe wear.

Nonunions or chronic stress fractures of the navicular should be addressed with open reduction and internal fixation. Autogenous iliac crest cancellous graft should be used to fill the void left after debridement of the nonunion site. Two lag-type fixation screws should be used to fix the fracture and obtain compression across the nonunion site.

Long-term problems of navicular fractures are related to either traumatic arthropathy of the articulating surfaces or avascular necrosis of the navicular body. Loss of the talonavicular articular surface will necessitate arthrodesis of the joint. If there is evidence of longitudinal collapse

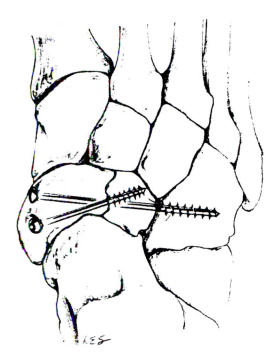

Figure 8

Fixation for displaced navicular fractures; one option for type II body fractures. Fixation into the cuboid is used to stabilize the small lateral fragment. (Adapted with permission from Sangeorzan 1993)

of the navicular, tricortical autogenous bone graft should be employed to restore length of the medial column with fusion of the adjacent articular surfaces.

Cuboid injury

There are reports in the literature of isolated subluxations and of complete dislocations of the cuboid. Painful subluxation, or cuboid syndrome, has a reported incidence of between 4% among high-performance athletes and 17% for professional ballet dancers (Newell and Woodie 1981, Marshall & Hamilton 1992). Symptoms include lateral foot pain, which can radiate to the anterior ankle, fourth ray, or plantar aspect of the midfoot; and complaints of weakness with forefoot pushoff. The typical findings are reported as a reduction in dorsoplantar mobility at the calcaneocuboid joint, peroneus longus spasm, and pain with plantarly applied pressure to the cuboid.

There is a suggestion in the literature that the entity is radiographically identifiable (Everson et al 1991). A subtle change in the normal 2 mm gap in the contour of the calcaneocuboid joint has been attributed to subluxation.

It is suggested that hyperpronated feet or those with forefoot abduction are susceptible to this injury. The mechanism appears to be forced pronation of the midfoot in relation to the hindfoot in the presence of axial loading. Anatomically, the cuboid has a proximal infero-medial beak, which normally fits within a corresponding depression in the inferomedial aspect of the calcaneus (Shelton & Pedowitz 1992). Studies of calcaneocuboid joint motion show that joint congruity is dependent on maintenance of rotational stability. A twisting force through this joint, with the cuboid moving in a pronated direction in relation to the calcaneus, will produce incongruity of the joint. The presence of the peroneus longus is its fibrous tunnel on the plantolateral aspect appears to assist in maintaining this incongruent posture.

Management

Several investigators have reported satisfactory results using closed reduction techniques to reduce the calcaneocuboid joint (Newell & Woodie 1981, Marshall & Hamilton 1992). The techniques described involve the need to relax the foot and then apply direct pressure. Relaxation of the dorsal long extensors and peronei is obtained with deep massage and gentle stretch. With the patient in the prone position and the foot fully plantarflexed, a direct pressure is placed on the plantar aspect of the cuboid. Maintenance of reduction is with firm to rigid orthoses supporting the dorsomedial arch. Marshall and Hamilton (1992) recommend postreduction taping, self mobilization techniques, or both, to maintain position.

Cuboid dislocation

Isolated dislocation of the cuboid is rare (Drummond & Hastings 1969, Jacobsen 1990). When this occurs, the cuboid displaces medially and inferiorly, disrupting the support of the lateral column of the foot. Dorsal or lateral displacement is prevented by bony prominences on the calcaneus and cuboid. The resulting deformity is best visualized with a lateral oblique radiograph. Open anatomic reduction and temporary stabilization of the cuboid should be carried out. Stable fixation can best be obtained with two 3.5 mm cortical fixation screws. One screw should stabilize the cuboid to the navicular, the other should traverse the calcaneocuboid joint. Owing to the pure ligamentous nature of this injury, immobilization in a cast should be for 3 months. Non-weight-bearing casting should be for the first 6–8 weeks. The calcaneocuboid screw should be removed at three months. This dislocation also occurs in the diabetic neuropathic foot. In this case reduction and calcaneocuboid fusion is recommended.

Cuboid fracture

A more frequent injury to the cuboid involves a compression fracture or fracture subluxation of the calcaneocuboid joint. This may occur as an isolated injury, but it usually is seen in association with injuries to the talonavicular joint, especially the tuberosity, or other structures in the midfoot (Hermel & Gershon-Cohen 1953, Sangeorzan & Swintkowski 1990, Koch & Rahimi 1991, Davis et al 1993). Without careful scrutiny, these injuries can be initially assessed as a lateral ankle sprain. Injury to the cuboid can be quite subtle but the long-term consequences to the lateral column can cause painful deformities. These structural changes include loss of bony arch support, shortening of the lateral column of the foot, and forefoot abduction (Dewar & Evans 1968).

Mechanism of injury

Fracture of the cuboid can occur from a direct blow to the lateral cortex without causing shortening or articular disruption. If after careful inspection no evidence of instability or deformity is noted, nonoperative care is recommended. Treatment involves non-weight-bearing short leg cast for 6–8 weeks. Weight bearing casting should be continued for a further 4 weeks.

Commonly the mechanism of injury is forced plantarflexion and abduction causing an indirect compressive load to be applied on the cuboid. This type of injury has been termed a nutcracker fracture (Hermel & Gershon-Cohen 1953, Koch & Rahimi 1991). The best visualization of the cuboid and the lateral midfoot structures is the lateral oblique radiograph. As discussed previously, if injury is suspected but not readily apparent, stress views should be obtained to assess the stability of the joint and the integrity of bony disruptions that are not visible on plain film. CT with longitudinal cuts along the axis of the foot can be extremely helpful in assessing the extent of bony damage (Fig. 9).

Management

Treatment of these injuries is controversial, and the results of individual series are difficult to evaluate because of their low patient numbers (Sangeorzan & Swintkowski 1990, Sangeorzan 1993, Sangeorzan et al 1993). Usually, significant depression and/or comminution of the articular surface of the cuboid is found. Nonoperative care with casting and non-weight-bearing appears to lead to poor results. With compression of the cuboid it is important to undertake open reduction of the fracture. Great care should be taken to restore the length and articular contour of the cuboid. The importance of maintaining lateral column length is integral to the proper functioning of the foot during weight bearing. Shortening can increase pronation and markedly destablize the forefoot lever arm during terminal stance.

Open treatment of cuboid fractures is easiest with the patient in the lateral decubitus position. The incision is made longitudinally along the lateral aspect of the cuboid. Care is taken to avoid the peroneal tendons and sural nerve. Complete exposure of the cuboid and its proximal and distal joints is done by sharp dissection. To

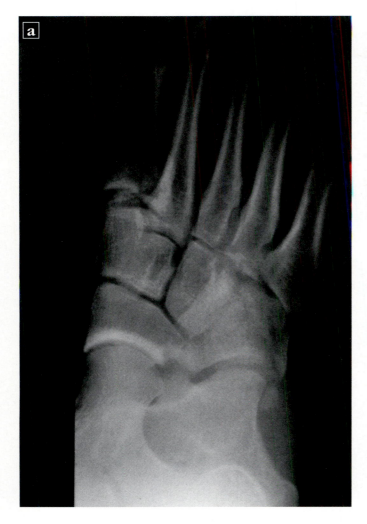

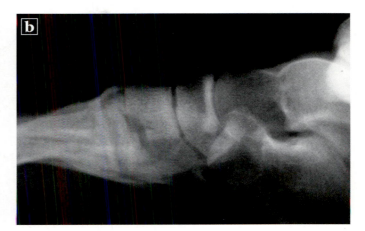

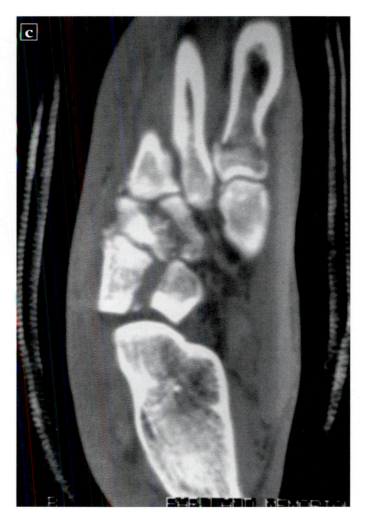

Figure 9

Closed cuboid fracture caused by indirect loading. (a&b) Lateral oblique and lateral radiographs showing displaced fracture of the cuboid; (c) longitudinal CT showing cuboid fracture and associated injury to the lateral cuneiform and the first metatarsal

assist in opening the fracture lines and restoring length, a small fragment distractor is used with pins placed in the calcaneus and fifth metatarsal base. This will allow neutralization of the normal compressive forces about the cuboid and permit easy exposure of the fracture lines and articular surface. The contour of the calcaneocuboid and or cubometatarsal articular surfaces are restored by using the calcaneus and metatarsal bases as templates. Usually, a corticocancellous defect is evident in the center of the

body once cuboid length and contours are restored. This is filled with iliac crest cancellous or corticocancellous graft. A small buttress plate is placed on the cuboid to help maintain length (Fig. 10). If there is severe comminution proximally, the plate can be extended to the anterior process of the calcaneus until healing is complete. An alternative to plating is the use of a laterally placed external fixator anchored into the calcaneus and the fifth metatarsal. The fixator should remain in

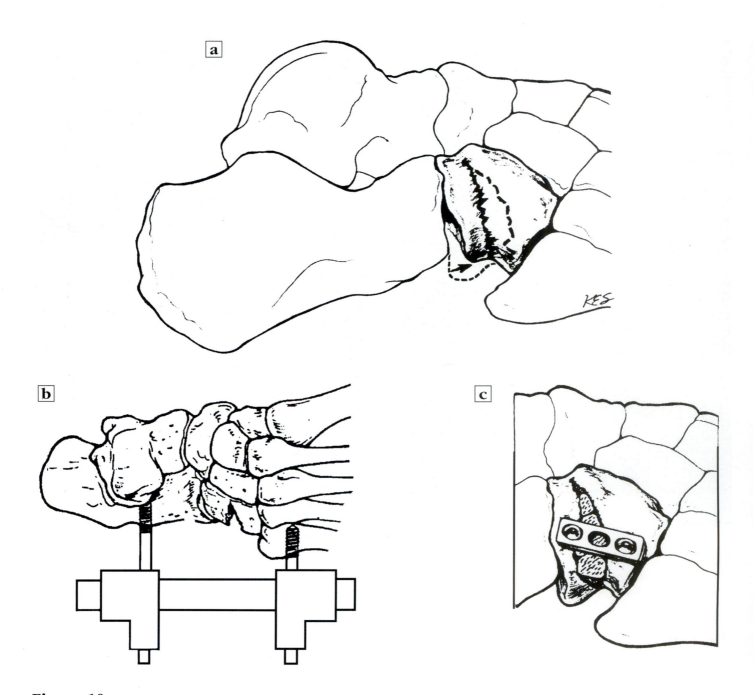

Figure 10
Treatment of displaced cuboid fractures: (a) impacted cuboid fracture with disruption of calcaneocuboid joint; (b) restoration of cuboid borders. Note the use of an external distraction device to restore the lateral column length; (c) corticocancellous graft is used to fill the defect. A lateral buttress plate is placed to stabilize the reconstruction. (Adapted with permission from Sangeorzan 1993)

place until bony union to prevent shortening. The patient is remanded to 3 months non-weight-bearing in a short leg cast. Internally placed hardware, if crossing the joint-line, is removed at 9 months.

Late presentation
Unfortunately, many cuboid injuries are diagnosed late, after initial healing has occurred. Isolated arthrodesis has been moderately successful in alleviating the pain. Many authors advocate a double or triple arthrodesis at this

stage because of the deformity of forefoot abduction and arch collapse that can be seen long term. Limited arthrodesis of the calcaneocuboid joint can be done with satisfactory results if there is no degenerative arthritis present in the remaining subtalar complex articulations and provided that care is taken to restore lateral column length with iliac crest bone graft at the site of fusion (Fig. 11). Restoration of length at the time of surgery is accomplished with a small fragment distractor as described previously.

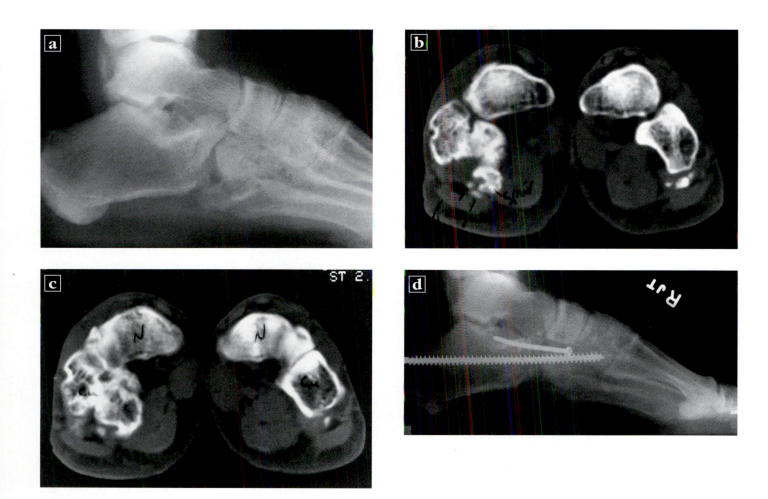

Figure 11

Long-term results of displaced cuboid fractures. (a) Lateral radiograph 5 years after initial injury. Note disruption of the calcaneocuboid joint and plantar prominence of the cuboid fracture fragment; (b,c) coronal CT views of the cuboid showing marked displacement of the plantar structures medially. The plantar prominence was palpable; (d) calcaneocuboid fusion with the removal of the plantar prominence and placement of interpositional bone graft to maintain lateral column length.

Cuneiform injury

Disruption of any or all three cuneiform bones is a rare injury of the foot. Isolated fractures have occurred from direct blows and there are reports of isolated dislocations but the majority of injuries appear to involve tarsometatarsal or cuboid disruptions. Injuries to the cuneiforms can be subtle and usually require CT and stress radiographs to discern the full extent of the injury.

It is the size and position of the cuneiforms and not their mobility that is important for proper foot function. Therefore accurate reduction and stabilization of dislocations is important to maximize results.

Dislocations

For truly isolated dislocations, closed reduction can be done as long as anatomic realignment can be achieved and maintained (McGlinche 1981). Irreducible dislocation of the medial cuneiform may be due to interposition of the tibialis anterior tendon (Compson 1992). An unstable cuneiform should be accurately stabilized with screw fixation into adjacent structures (Fig. 12). The patient should be casted for a period of 10–12 weeks, with non-weight-bearing through the forefoot for the first 6 weeks. Protective weight bearing may then progress as comfort allows. Internal fixation to stabilize these injuries can be removed after 6 months. The reason for this prolonged protection is the purely ligamentous nature of the injury. The vascular supply to the thick plantar ligaments is poor compared to other structures and this in turn hampers the reparative process.

Fractures

The mechanism of injury appears to involve indirect axial loading. The extent of damage is dependent on

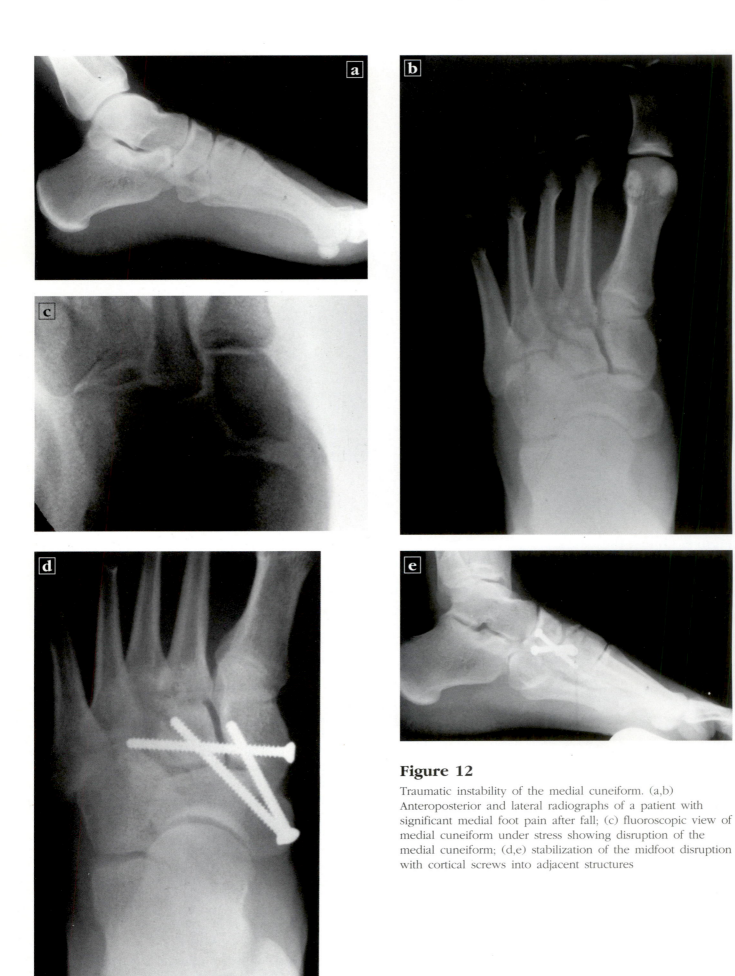

Figure 12

Traumatic instability of the medial cuneiform. (a,b)
Anteroposterior and lateral radiographs of a patient with
significant medial foot pain after fall; (c) fluoroscopic view of
medial cuneiform under stress showing disruption of the
medial cuneiform; (d,e) stabilization of the midfoot disruption
with cortical screws into adjacent structures

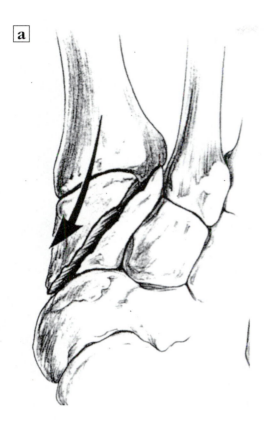 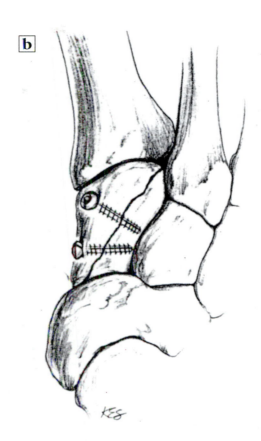

Figure 13

Fixation of a medial cuneiform fracture. (a) Medial cuneiform injuries are usually due to axial loading through the foot; (b) stabilization requires accurate reduction and stable fixation. (Adopted with permission from Sangeorzan 1993)

other simultaneous plantodorsally or mediolaterally directed forces (McGanity & Sanders 1990). Because of the close-packed nature of these bones and the numerous thick plantar ligaments, fractures usually require significant force and can signal significant ligamentous disruption analogous to a Lisfranc's injury. Compartment syndrome of the foot has been associated with injury to the cuneiforms.

Radiographic examination should include anteroposterior, lateral and lateral oblique views of the midfoot. Subtle plantar fractures can signal the presence of significant damage to the plantar ligamentous network that supports the normal bony architecture. These are difficult to discern on plain radiographs and should be ruled out with a CT scan. Missed fractures involving the articular surfaces can lead to late degenerative changes and pain in those joints.

Fractures, if not displaced, can be treated closed. Short leg casting should be used for 10–12 weeks with weight bearing through the forefoot beginning at 8 weeks and progressing as the patient can tolerate. Apart from injuries caused by a direct blow, these fractures are rarely isolated and nondisplaced. Usually, they are part of a more serious disruptive injury to the foot.

In treating these injuries, the goal is anatomic restoration of position (Patterson et al 1993, Sangeorzan 1993). Shortened cuneiforms should be fixed out to length (Fig. 13). Alignment of adjacent structures should be restored. An external fixator can be used to aid in the reduction. Stabilization should be achieved, if necessary, with screw fixation into adjacent structures to maintain position. If comminution does not permit direct fixation, corticocancellous graft should be used to fill any gaps that have been created by restoring the adjacent anatomy. Fusion of any joints sustaining severe comminution should also be undertaken when first recognized.

Postoperatively, these injuries require prolonged immobilization to allow healing. Non-weight-bearing casting should be done for four weeks. If satisfactory fixation was obtained initially to insure bony stability, partial to full weight bearing is then allowed in a cast for a further 8 weeks. If there is no bony stability, weight bearing should be avoided for 3 months. Internal hardware that has been used to stabilize and not to fuse joints can be removed at 6 months.

Long-term problems with cuneiform fractures can be related to either loss of anatomic position or degenerative arthritis (Jahn & Freund 1989). In either case,

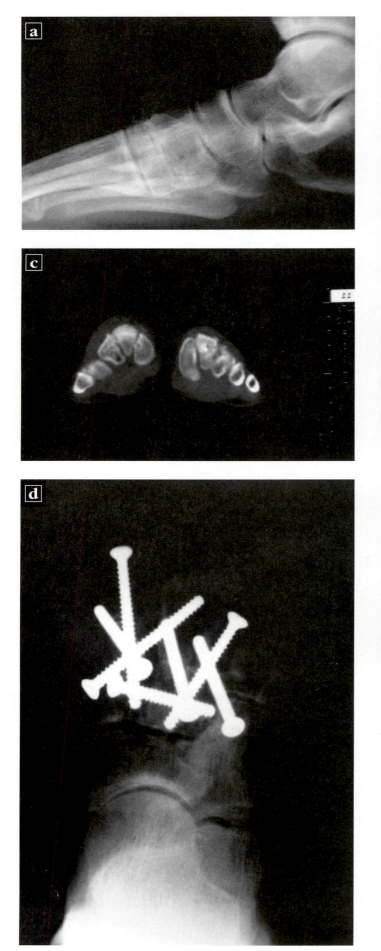

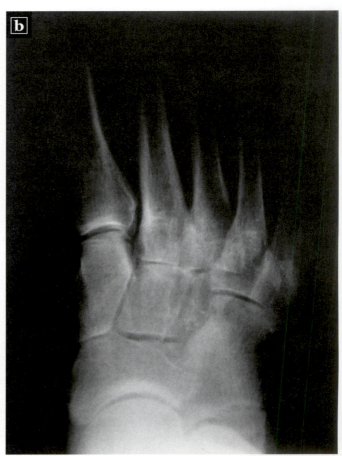

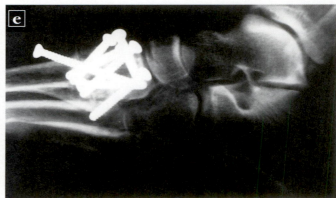

Figure 14

Middle cuneiform fracture. (a,b) Anteroposterior and lateral X-rays of foot now 2 years after initial injury; (c) coronal CT shows evidence of old fracture of middle cuneiform with subsequent arthropathy; (d,e) stabilization of the midfoot with fusion of the medial column at the tarsometatarsal joint line

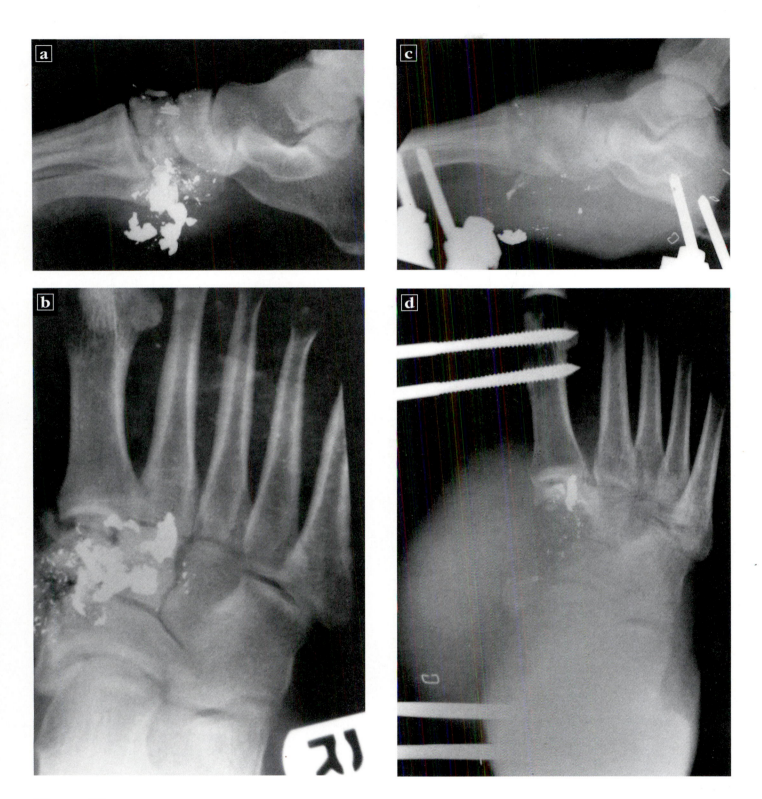

Figure 15

Gunshot wound to the midfoot. (a,b) Injury films show area of impact. This patient had a complete loss of soft tissue over the medial aspect of the arch due to the blast effect; (c,d) use of external fixation to stabilize bony anatomy while allowing soft tissue healing. This patient required a large free flap as can be seen in the large medial soft tissue shadow

arthrodesis in an anatomically reduced position is the preferred treatment. Corticocancellous graft may be used to fill any defects and regain length (Fig. 14).

Multiple midfoot injuries

The initial treatment of severe traumatic midfoot disruptions should be handled according to the well-established protocols for general musculoskeletal trauma care. Irrigation and debridement of open wounds as well as definitive treatment of compartment syndrome should receive top priority. Bony stability should be addressed next. In the face of open wounds or severe soft tissue trauma, external distraction and fixation should be used to restore length and position of the forefoot to the hindfoot. In the case where both medial and lateral columns sustain damage and loss of length, bilateral external distraction or ring fixation can be used to realign the foot. Once the soft tissues are stable, displaced structures involving the proximal metatarsals, cuboid or cuneiform fragments should be reduced by any means possible to preserve the integrity of the weight bearing lines of force. Internal screw fixation may be used once the soft tissue is closed and if the comminution of adjacent midfoot structures does not hamper fixation. Guidelines as previously established for individual fractures should be employed when trying to restore midfoot structure. In severe cases, arthrodesis can be done initially on any fractures involving articular surfaces except the talonavicular joint, the fourth and fifth tarsometatarsal joints and the calcaneocuboid joints. These four joint surfaces should be given every chance to recover, since their function is very important to overall foot function. External fixation can be replaced with internal buttress plates if the fracture pattern permits. Classic treatment of joint injury is of course anatomic interfragmental fixation and early non-weight-bearing motion.

Sometimes there appears to be no recognizable bony anatomy to restore; this is most often seen with gun shot wounds to the midfoot. In these cases, external fixation to maintain approximate forefoot–hindfoot alignment along with local wound care is best (Fig. 15). External fixation should be left in place 8 weeks or until soft tissue closure is obtained. This can require external fixation use for 3–4 months until all soft tissues have healed and radiographic consolidation is evident. A further month of protected weight bearing in a short leg cast is recommended to protect the healing foot while the patient begins weight bearing. The need for bone grafting or reconstruction can be decided at that time.

References

Basmajian J V, Stecko G 1963 The role of muscles in arch support of the foot. J Bone Joint Surg 45A: 1184–1190

Compson J P 1992 An irreducible medial cuneiform fracture dislocation. Injury 23: 501–502

Davis C A, Lubowite J, Thordarson D B 1993 Midtarsal fracture subluxation: case report and review of the literature. Clin Orthop 292: 264–268

Dewar F P, Evans D C 1968 Occult fracture–subluxation of the midtarsal joint. J Bone Joint Surg 50B: 386–388

Drummond D S, Hastings D E 1969 Total dislocation of the cuboid bone. J Bone Joint Surg 51B: 716–718

Early J S, Hansen S T 1994 Treatment of midfoot trauma. Int J Orthop Trauma 4: 11–15

Eichenholtz S N, Levine D B 1964 Fractures of the tarsal navicular bone. Clin Orthop 34: 142–157

Everson J I, Galloway H R, Suh J, Benninghoff K S, Griffiths H J. 1991 Cuboid subluxation. Orthopedics 14: 1044–1048

Fitch K D, Blackwell J B, Gilmour W N, 1989 Operation for non union of stress fracture of the tarsal navicular. J Bone Joint Surg 71B: 105–110

Hansen ST 1993 Biomechanical considerations in the hindfoot. In: Tscherne H, Schatzker J (eds) Major Fractures of the Pilon, the Talus, and the Calcaneus, Springer, New York

Hermel M B, Gershon-Cohen J 1953 Nutcracker fracture of the cuboid by indirect violence. Radiology 60: 850–854

Hicks J H 1953 The mechanics of the foot. J Anatomy 87: 235–357

Hicks J H 1955 The foot as a support. Acta Anat (Basel) 25: 34–45

Jacobsen FS 1990 Dislocation of the cuboid. Orthopedics 13: 1387–1389

Jahn H, Freund K 1989 Isolated fractures of the cuboid bone: two case reports with review of the literature. J Foot Surg 28: 512–515

Kapandji I A 1987 The Physiology of the Joints. Churchill Livingstone, New York, vol 2, 5th edn

Ker R F, Bennett M B, Bibby S R, Kester R C, Alexander R McN 1987 The spring in the arch of the human foot. Nature 325: 147–149

Khan K M, Fuller P J, Brunker P D, Kearney C, Burry H C 1992 Outcome of conservative and surgical management of navicular stress fracture in athletes. Am J Sports Med 20: 657–666

Koch J, Rahimi F. 1991 Nutcracker fractures of the cuboid. J Foot Surg 30: 336–339

Main B J, Jowett R L 1975 Injuries of the midtarsal joint. J Bone Joint Surg 57B: 89–97

Mann R, Inman V T 1964 Phasic activity of intrinsic muscles of the foot. J Bone Joint Surg 46A: 469–481

Marshall P, Hamilton W G 1992 Cuboid subluxation in ballet dancers. Am J Sports Med 20: 169–175

McGanity P, Sanders J O 1990 Intermediate cuneiform fracture– dislocation. J Orthop Trauma 4: 102–104

McGlinche J 1981 Dislocation of the intermediate cuneiform bone. Injury 12: 501–502

Newell S G, Woodie A 1981 Cuboid syndrome. Physician Sports Med 9: 71–76

Nyska M, Margulies J Y, Barbarawi M, Mutchler W, Dekel S, Segal D 1989 Fractures of the body of the tarsal navicular bone: case reports and literature review. J Trauma 29: 1448–1451

Ouzounian T J, Shereff M J 1989 In vitro determination of midfoot motion. Foot Ankle 10: 140–146

Pathria M P, Rosenstein A, Bjorkengren A, Gershuind D, Resnick D 1988 Isolated dislocation of the tarsal navicular: a case report. Foot Ankle 9: 146–149

Patterson R H, Peterson D, Cunningham R 1993 Isolated fracture of the medial cuneiform: a case report. J Orthop Trauma 7: 94–95

Perry J 1992 Gait Analysis: Normal and Pathologic Function. McGraw–Hill, New York

Sangeorzan B J 1993 Foot and ankle joint. In Hansen S T, Swintkowski M F (eds) Orthopedic Trauma Protocols. Raven Press, New York, pp 339–368

Sangeorzan B J, Benirschre S R, Mosca V, Mayo K, Hansen S T 1989 Displaced intra-articular fractures of the tarsal navicular. J Bone Joint Surg 71A: 1504–1510

Sangeorzan B J, Swintkowski M F 1990 Displaced fractures of the cuboid. J Bone Joint Surg 72B: 376–378

Sangeorzan B J, Mayo K A, Hansen S T 1993 Intra-articular fractures of the foot: talus and lesser tarsals. Clin Orthop 292: 135–141

Sarrafian S 1993 Anatomy of Foot and Ankle: Descriptive Topographic Functional. J B Lippincott, Philadelphia, 2nd edn

Shelton M L, Pedowitz W J 1992 Injuries to the talar dome, subtalar joint and midfoot. In Jahss MM (ed) Disorders of the Foot and Ankle, 2nd edn. W B Saunders; Philadelphia, pp 2274–2291

Torg J S, Pavlov H, Cooley L H, et al 1982 Stress fractures of the tarsal navicular: a retrospective review of twenty-one cases. J Bone Joint Surg 64A: 700–712

Vaishya R, Patrick J M 1991 Isolated dorsal fracture – dislocation of the tarsal navicular. Injury 22: 47–48

IX.5 Injuries to the Tarsometatarsal Joint Complex

Mark S Myerson

Introduction

The eponym 'Lisfranc dislocation' has been applied to injuries of the tarsometatarsal joint since the Napoleonic era, when cavalry troops quite commonly sustained these injuries. The fractures must have been associated with profound vascular deficits, necessitating amputation, because that was the only method of treatment used by Lisfranc, Napoleon's surgeon. He apparently performed the amputation with such speed that the term 'Lisfranc's joint' has remained. Since that period, equestrian activities have declined, and the stirrup has been modified, so that the more severe vascular complications from fracture–dislocations of the tarsometatarsal joint are less commonly seen today. In fact, these profound vascular disturbances occur rarely, and the only circumstances under which circulatory compromise is treated is in the presence of compartment syndromes.

Today, most of these fracture–dislocations occur secondary to motor vehicle, motorcycle, and (commonly) industrial accidents. One of the more interesting varieties of Lisfranc injuries that we have treated has been associated with wind-surfing. During surfing, the feet are firmly secured to the board by oblique straps across the dorsum of the midfoot. These straps serve to anchor the foot during pivoting motions, as do stirrups used in horseback riding. The injuries so caused may be associated with fracture patterns identical to those encountered in high-energy injuries. Although these injuries are typically associated with severe disruption of the tarsometatarsal joints, the injury can occur under any circumstances. Thus the clinician should always be alert for this problem, even after more minor twisting injuries, particularly in athletes and elderly patients.

There has been renewed interest in this injury over the past decade, and it is apparent that the concepts of treatment have changed. The recent trend in treatment has definitely been toward open reduction, utilizing more rigid forms of internal fixation. Although the goals of treatment are to provide an anatomic reduction and to maximize function, it is not always possible to achieve this with these injuries. Unfortunately, the true extent of the injury is often not appreciated or is misdiagnosed. Furthermore, it has been my experience that even when these injuries are correctly diagnosed, they are not always appropriately treated. Perhaps the biggest problem is in recognizing the more subtle forms of this injury and realizing that far greater injury may have occurred with partial spontaneous relocation. Since this injury is usually associated with fracture or dislocation of the cuneiform bones, cuboid, and navicular, I prefer to use the descriptive term 'tarsometatarsal joint complex,' which includes all the bones and joints that may be directly or indirectly injured in a tarsometatarsal fracture–dislocation (Myerson et al 1986).

Anatomy

In the coronal plane, the transverse plantar arch is an asymmetric arch at the level of the metatarsal bones as well as across the more proximal cuneiform and cuboid bones. The bases of the first, second, and third metatarsals are wedge-shaped, with the widest point dorsally, and they conform to a similar asymmetry of each cuneiform. Further structural rigidity is provided by the dovetailing of the second metatarsal base, which is surrounded by five adjacent bones, and the tight mortise created provides marked stability to the entire articulation.

The tarsometatarsal articulation consists of four separate parts. This partitioning of the tarsometatarsal joint has important implications in treatment, as segmental patterns of injury occur and recognition of these patterns enhances reduction and the approach to fixation. The medial articulation is formed by the base of the first metatarsal and the medial cuneiform; the adjacent second metatarsal and middle cuneiform form the second unit; the base of the third metatarsal and the lateral cuneiform form the third unit; and the lateral articulation is formed by the base of the fourth and fifth metatarsals with the cuboid.

The movements at each of these joints vary. The fourth and fifth metatarsals move more in both the sagittal and horizontal planes than the third metatarsal does. The second metatarsal is held rigidly in the mortise and moves minimally, whereas the first metatarsal is, again, more mobile. The medial ray, which includes the first metatarsal, medial cuneiform, and navicular, permits approximately 13° of dorsal plantar motion. Working as a functional unit, however, the movement at the tarsometatarsal joint is that of pronation and supination, in addition to movements of the sagittal plane. The movements at the articulation have been clarified by

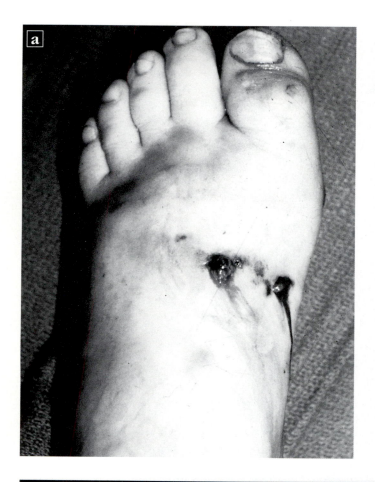

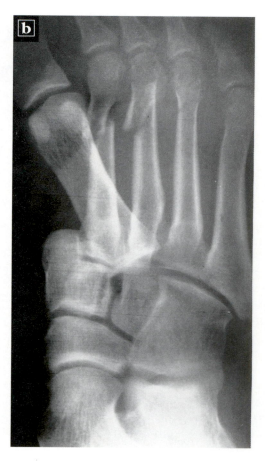

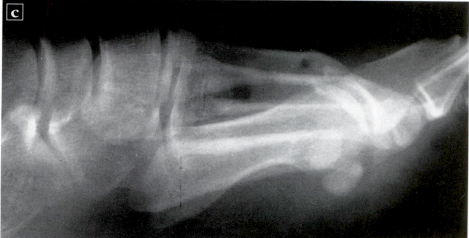

Figure 1

This patient sustained a crushing injury to the midfoot associated with a compartment syndrome and was treated with fasciotomy and ORIF of the fractures through the fasciotomy incisions (a). The displacement of the first metatarsal is well seen on the anteroposterior (b) and lateral (c) radiographs. The plantar dislocation of the metatarsals is typical of crushing injuries.

Ouzounian & Shereff (1989). In an excellent study using a digitizer in free space, they evaluated the relative total motion between the different segments of the tarsometatarsal joints. The total sagittal plane movement for each metatarsal was: first, 3.5 mm; second, 0.6 mm; third, 1.6 mm; fourth, 9.6 mm; and fifth, 10.2 mm. Inversion and eversion movement (pronation–supination) for each metatarsal was: first, 1.5 mm; second, 1.2 mm; third, 2.6 mm; fourth, 11.1 mm; and fifth, 9.0 mm.

The metatarsals are connected at their bases by strong transverse, oblique, and interosseous ligaments. The interosseous ligaments are located slightly more on the plantar aspect of the metatarsals. Each metatarsal base is connected by these ligaments, with the exception of the base of the first and second metatarsals, where none exists. Instead, a thick and extremely strong ligament extends from the medial base of the second metatarsal obliquely into the medial cuneiform. The Lisfranc ligament and the mortise effect created by the base of the second metatarsal are the main stabilizers of the entire tarsometatarsal articulation. The inherent stability of the second metatarsal base, as well as the arched effect of the entire articulation in the coronal plane, add to this stability. The secondary stabilizers of the tarsometatarsal joint are soft-tissue structures predominantly on the plantar aspect of the foot, including the plantar fascia, intrinsic muscles, and tendons. The insertions of the peroneal, anterior tibial, and posterior tibial tendons markedly reinforce the stability of the tarsometatarsal joint. These soft-tissue and bony stabilizers all combine to prevent dorsiflexion of the metatarsals and, hence, dislocation of the articulation.

Etiology and diagnosis

Etiology

Fracture–dislocations are produced by either direct or indirect forces. Direct forces, e.g. blows and crushing mechanisms of injury to the dorsum of the midfoot, produce a variety of dislocation patterns, depending on the exact point of application of the force (Wiley 1971, Myerson & Burgess 1991, Myerson 1991). In addition to obvious injury to the bones and joints, these direct mechanisms invariably cause marked damage to the skin and other soft-tissue structures, with an extended area of risk to the soft tissue distal to the point of impact (Fig. 1). This extended area of pathology is termed the zone of injury and is an important concept in managing all types of crush injuries to the foot (Myerson & Burgess 1991, Myerson & McGarvey 1993).

With indirect trauma, the forces produced are generally longitudinal and are applied to the foot with elements of torque, rotation, and compression. Since the foot is often plantarflexed at the time of impact, the additional flexion of the forefoot pushes the midfoot into a more cavus position, rupturing the far weaker dorsal soft-tissue structures of the tarsometatarsal joint. In order to subluxate, the dorsal capsules and ligaments tear; the dislocation is complete when the plantar surfaces of the metatarsal base fracture or the plantar joint capsular ligaments rupture. Uniplanar dislocation of the joints seldom occurs, as other forces shift the metatarsals on the tarsus, causing abduction and lateral displacements.

Although fractures and dislocations of the tarsometatarsal joint complex are commonly associated with dissipation of high energy in motor vehicle and motorcycle accidents and in the industrial setting, we have recently documented the occurrence of these injuries in athletes (Myerson 1993, Curtis et al 1993). Although they can be subtle and initially appear less severe than those incurred by other mechanisms, these injuries are associated with considerable morbidity (Fig. 2).

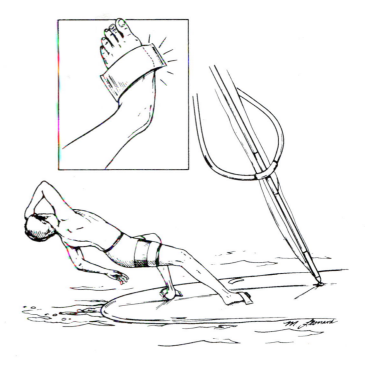

Figure 2

Injury to the tarsometatarsal joints may occur, owing to minor indirect forces such as depicted here in wind-surfing, where the limb externally rotates against a fixed foot that is firmly held in the stirrup.

Diagnosis

There are many classifications of tarsometatarsal joint injury; however, most emphasize the mechanism of injury. In 1986, we proposed an alternative classification based on joint incongruity and segmental instability, which we have since found to be useful in planning the initial treatment (Myerson et al 1986). Three basic types of incongruity are recognized (Table 1). The importance of this classification lies in its ability to help with preop-

Type	Description
A	Total incongruity of the joints in any plane or direction
B-1	Partial incongruity in which the displacement affects the medial articulation only
B-2	Partial incongruity in which the displacement affects one or more of the lateral metatarsals in any plane or direction
C	Divergent patterns with the first metatarsal displaced medially and the lateral group in any pattern of displacement with incongruity

Table 1 Classification of tarsometatarsal joint injury

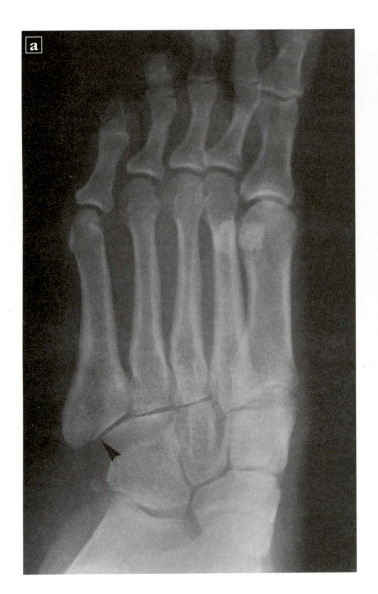

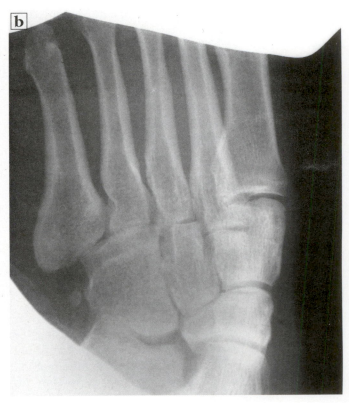

Figure 3

Lateral shift of the fifth metatarsal is evident (a, arrow). Intraoperative stress radiographs confirm significant instability (b).

erative planning and recognition of the forces involved in propagation of the fracture–dislocation.

Radiographic diagnosis

Major fracture–dislocations are easy to diagnose, but subluxations that appear more minor are often missed. The interpretation of anteroposterior and lateral radiographs and the identification of subtle deviations in the sagittal and horizontal planes may be difficult, owing to confusing overlapping of the bones and joints and to failure to demonstrate the fracture or dislocation. Certain points can be of some help with radiographic diagnosis: widening between the bases of the first and second metatarsals or between the middle and medial cuneiforms; a small fracture fragment off the base of the

second metatarsal or medial cuneiform; minor displacement of the lateral three metatarsal bases, best visualized on a 30° internal oblique radiograph; an overlap between the base of the fifth metatarsal and the cuboid; angulation of the shaft of the metatarsals associated with slight tilting of the base of the fourth or fifth metatarsal with subtle incongruity of the metatarsal cuboid joint; injury to the cuboid consisting of a small compression fracture of the distal lateral edge of the cuboid; stress radiographs performed under appropriate anesthesia with fluoroscopy (Fig. 3). In addition, reconstruction of the joint can be accomplished by lines drawn along the shaft of the metatarsals (Fig. 4); when these are extended proximally, they should not intersect the corresponding cuneiform bone. Rarely, tomography or computed tomography scanning of the foot is necessary to make the diagnosis; however, plain tomography may enhance the diagnosis of the extent of instability (Fig. 5).

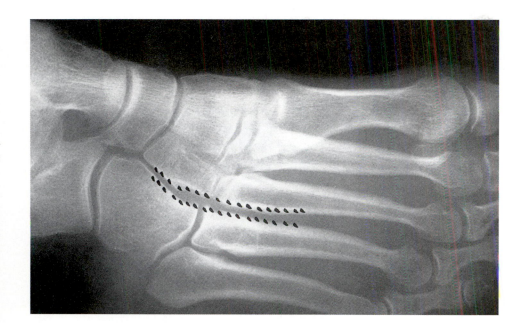

Figure 4

Projection of lines drawn along the metatarsals should not intersect the cuneiforms. These lines can be drawn along the third and fourth metatarsals on the 30° internal oblique view, or along the second metatarsal on the anteroposterior view.

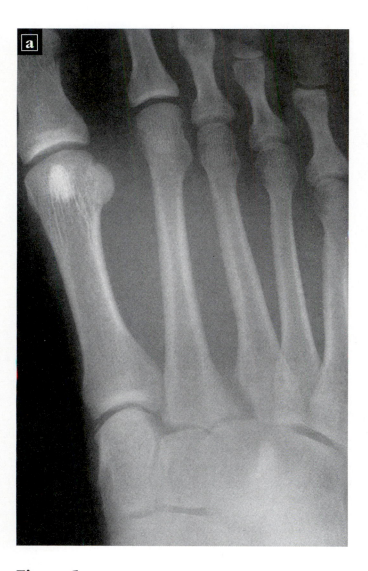

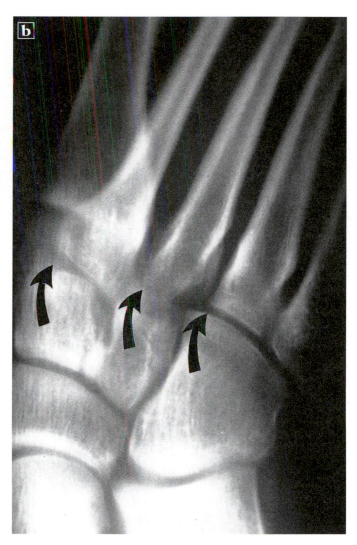

Figure 5

This oblique radiograph demonstrates a small avulsion fragment off the base of the third metatarsal (a). Tilting of the second metatarsal is evident, and lateral displacement of the third, fourth, and fifth metatarsals is clearly seen on the tomogram (b).

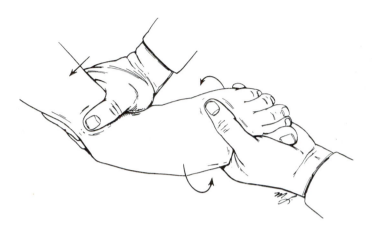

Figure 6

The diagnosis of tarsometatarsal injury or instability can be made with manipulation of the foot. Passive pronation and simultaneous abduction of the forefoot elicits severe pain, which appears to be specific for the tarsometatarsal joint.

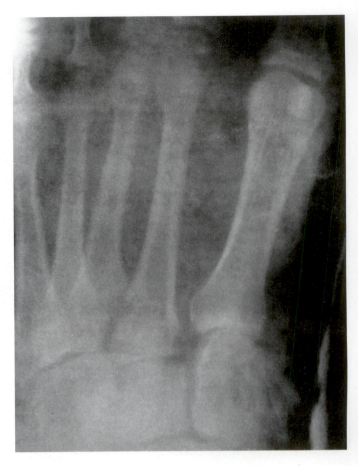

Figure 7

This fracture–dislocation was treated with cast immobilization. Note the diastasis between the first and second metatarsals. One year after injury, this patient experienced intractable pain, necessitating an arthrodesis.

Clinical diagnosis

Clinical diagnosis of these injuries can be difficult, as frequently there is no gross luxation or lateral deviation of the forefoot. In some instances, the diagnosis can be confirmed by a gentle manipulation of the foot. However, injuries associated with crushing typically present with massive swelling, and although the radiographic diagnosis may be difficult, the foot should not be manipulated in the emergency room to clarify displacement. Pain on passive pronation and abduction of the forefoot seems to be specific for injuries to the tarsometatarsal joint (Fig. 6).

Unfortunately, the true extent of the injury is often not appreciated. Spontaneous partial relocation of the joints may occur following injury, and the extent of the dislocation, particularly if subtle, is not always recognized.

ulation and thereby to maximize the function of the foot and prevent a deformity of the midfoot, but unfortunately this goal is not always realized (Myerson et al 1986, Myerson 1991).

Treatment

It is apparent that the concepts of treatment have changed quite drastically since the first recorded management of tarsometatarsal joint injury (Aitken & Poulson 1963, La Tourlette et al 1980, Hardcastle et al 1982, Goosens et al 1983, Myerson et al 1986, Myerson 1989, Ouzounian & Shereff 1989, Myerson 1991, Arntz et al 1988, Curtis et al 1993, Myerson 1993, Myerson & McGarvey 1993). The recent trend in treatment is toward open reduction, utilizing more rigid forms of internal fixation (Arntz et al 1988, Myerson 1989, Curtis et al 1993). The goal of treatment is to restore anatomic artic-

Conservative methods

There is little place for the conservative management of fractures and fracture–dislocations of the tarsometatarsal joint complex. Closed reduction and plaster immobilization do not provide optimal results since the advantages and adequate reduction that these methods can achieve are invariably lost when soft-tissue swelling decreases (Fig. 7). Although there have been reports of satisfactory results with conservative treatment associated with nonanatomic reduction (Aitken & Poulson 1963, Wiley 1971), this has not been my experience (Myerson et al 1986, Myerson 1989, Curtis et al 1993, Myerson 1993).

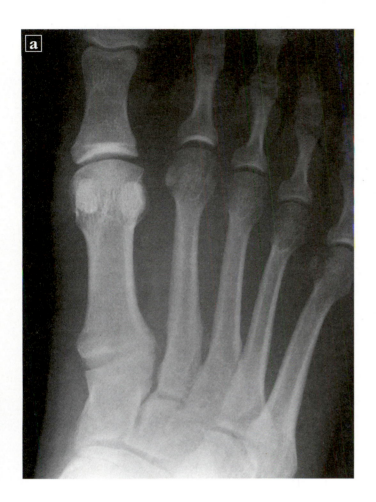

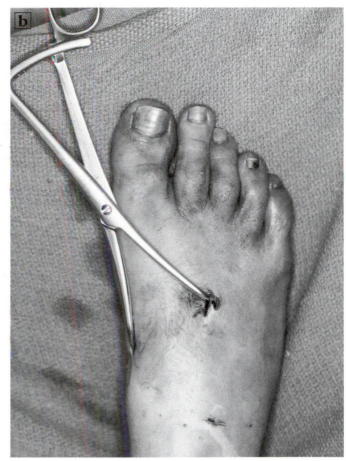

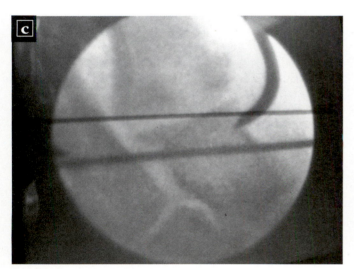

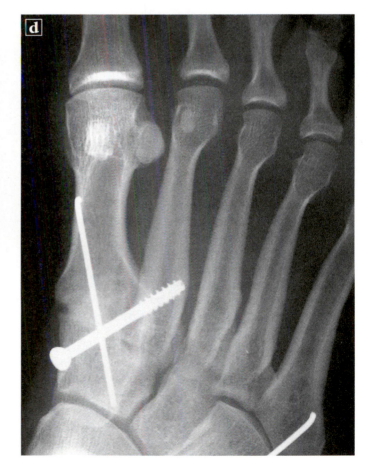

Figure 8

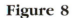

Although the instability in this patient does not appear significant (a), stress views obtained intraoperatively demonstrated marked displacement. Closed reduction was achieved with a percutaneously inserted large bone reduction clamp (b). The alignment was checked with fluoroscopy and the temporary pin fixation is shown. The image is reversed in the radiograph (c). Final fixation was achieved with reduction of the second metatarsal into the mortise with a partially threaded cancellous screw, and percutaneous pins for the first and fifth metatarsals (d).

Fractures of the tarsometatarsal joint complex are always associated with disruption of the dorsal capsule and ligaments, and this predisposes the once-reduced fracture to further displace and angulate in time. I have seen many instances of an excellent reduction, obtained through closed means, that has displaced while in a cast. Particular attention should be given to fractures asociated with elements of crushing. In these fractures, care of the soft tissues will determine the immediate success of treatment, and compartment pressures should be measured and fasciotomies performed if the pressure in either the central or interosseous compartment is greater than 40 mmHg (Myerson 1989, Myerson & Burgess 1991, Myerson 1993).

Operative methods

Reduction of the fracture–dislocation should be performed as soon as possible under appropriate anesthesia. We have been successful in managing these injuries using a regional ankle block (Myerson et al 1992). Occasionally the true extent of injury is unclear, and subtle radiographic displacements are therefore stressed intraoperatively under fluoroscopy. More significant instability patterns that require stabilization may then be clarified. It is my firm belief that these injuries should be treated with reduction and internal fixation.

Closed reduction

Certainly, closed reduction and percutaneous pin or screw fixation is an option. The manipulative maneuver involves longitudinal distal traction, which can be achieved with woven wire traps on the toes and counter-traction with weights suspended across the ankle. If the joints are dislocated without fracture, then closed reduction and internal fixation is an option. I initially manipulate the first metatarsal by pushing the distal metatarsal or hallux medially. While holding the hallux in varus, a pin is inserted into the metatarsocuneiform joint and a radiograph obtained. If the position obtained is anatomic, the second metatarsal is then reduced, also in a closed fashion. Two small puncture incisions are made, one over the dorsum of the second metatarsal and one over the medial surface of the medial cuneiform. A large bone reduction clamp reduces the second metatarsal into the mortise and a radiograph is obtained (Fig. 8). If reduced, a partially threaded screw is inserted obliquely from the medial cuneiform into the second metatarsal base; this can be easily accomplished using a cannulated screw under fluoroscopy. This procedure often realigns the entire articulation, since the second metatarsal pulls the third and fourth metatarsals with it. For a complete dislocation, the fifth metatarsal should be stabilized across the cuboid, and this, too, may be performed percutaneously

using either a wire or screw. If a Kirschner wire is to be used, it should measure at least 0.062 inch (1.57 mm) since a 0.045-inch (1.14 mm) Kirschner wire does not hold the metatarsals rigidly enough.

If a fracture fragment is present at the base of the second metatarsal, a closed reduction rarely succeeds. Although my preference is for an accurate open reduction, a closed reduction as described above should be carefully checked radiographically for any diastasis between the metatarsals and/or cuneiforms, in which case an open reduction and internal fixation is performed. Not infrequently, such a diastasis is caused by small bone fragments or soft tissue interposed between the small joints, which can prevent a stable anatomic closed reduction regardless of the means of fixation. Dislocation of the anterior tibial tendon into the medial tarsal metatarsal joint, blocking closed reduction, has been reported (Lenczner 1974, DeBenedetti et al 1978, Blair 1981).

Open reduction and internal fixation (ORIF)

In most instances, ORIF should be performed to obtain an anatomic reduction. Internal fixation can be performed with Kirschner wires or with screw fixation (Fig. 9). Whichever method of fixation is used, it is essential to incorporate the base of the second and occasionally the third metatarsal for all fracture patterns except the partial medial fracture (B-1 type).

The surgical approach depends on the fracture pattern, but a dorsal longitudinal incision centered over the second tarsometatarsal joint provides adequate exposure to most medial types of fracture–dislocation (B-1 and B-2 patterns).

The first (medial) incision is lateral to the neurovascular bundle, which is easy to locate as it lies deep to the extensor hallucis brevis tendon. Once the incision is deepened to the second metatarsal base, with careful subperiosteal dissection, the joint is identified. The entire periosteal and soft-tissue flap, including the neurovascular bundle, can now be raised over toward the first metatarsal. Small fracture fragments should be removed from the depth of the joint with a small rongeur or curette. Reduction of the second metatarsal bone into its mortise is often accompanied by spontaneous reduction of the laterally dislocated metatarsals. If the adjacent lateral metatarsals do not relocate, they also require an open reduction. The second (lateral) incision should be made over the fourth metatarsal to ensure a wide and viable skin bridge, although this has not proved to be a problem. The dorsal lateral cutaneous branch of the superficial peroneal nerve should be dissected free as it is in a vulnerable location with the lateral incision. These two incisions are generally all that are needed, as the remaining pins or screws can be inserted through small incisions or introduced percutaneously.

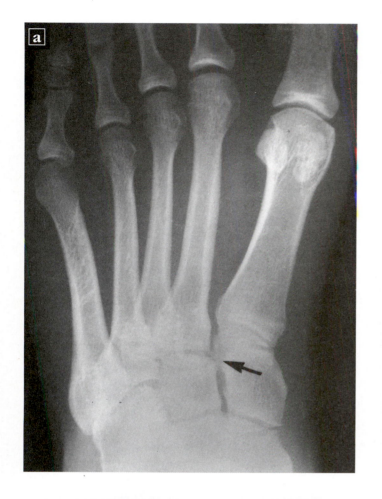

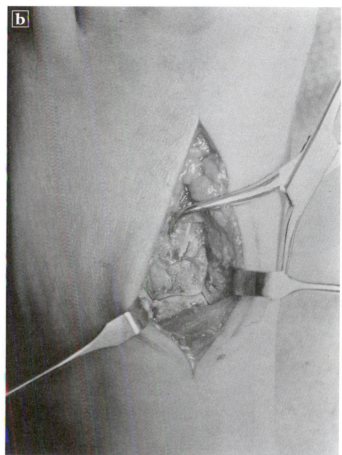

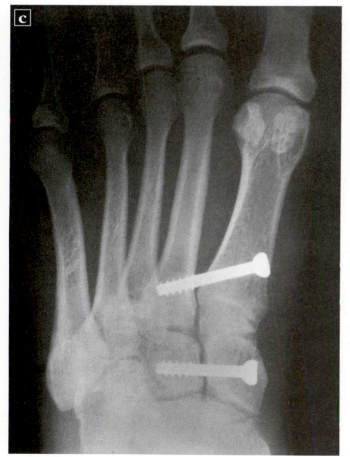

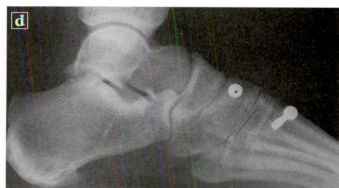

Figure 9

Diastasis of the entire medial column is evident in this patient, with widening (arrow) of the space between the first and second metatarsals and between the medial and middle cuneiforms (a). Note the anatomic restoration of the second metatarsal into the mortise, held reduced by the externally applied bone clamp (b). This was followed with percutaneous pin fixation with cannulated lag screws (c, d).

Generally, I use 3.5-mm cortical screws, placing them wherever they are needed, depending on the fracture pattern. One aspect of fixation has become quite clear: the second metatarsal has to be incorporated in the construct. Traditional techniques of fixation depended on cross Kirschner wires for stability, and if these are inserted diagonally across the first and fifth metatarsals, the second and third metatarsals are generally missed. This fixation does nothing to immobilize the middle segment, which is the primary stabilizer of the articulation.

When planning the screw fixation, remember the depth of each metatarsal base and the fact that, at the plantar surfaces, the bones are apical in shape. The entry point for the screw should be about 12 mm distal to the joint at an angle of 45° to the metatarsal shaft. It is essential to countersink the screw, as the proximal metatarsal has a tendency to fracture or split when this step is omitted. Occasionally, with gross instability patterns and marked displacements, the screw can be inserted percutaneously from the medial cuneiform obliquely and distally into the base of the second metatarsal. This technique is particularly useful in fusions of the same joints, where this will lock in the base of the second more rigidly. For partial medial instabilities or divergent patterns, the first metatarsal is included, but this screw can be inserted percutaneously into the medial cuneiform to avoid an additional incision. Once the second metatarsal is fixed, the third metatarsal usually follows, provided the interosseous ligaments are intact. If the third metatarsal is still unstable, then it should be secured with a screw inserted in a manner similar to that of the second metatarsal, but into the lateral cuneiform. The final point of fixation is across the fifth and fourth metatarsals, and this screw is directed percutaneously into either the cuboid or the lateral cuneiform across the metaphyseal flare of the fifth metatarsal.

Internal fixation is best accomplished using compression screws, the latter of which provide the most rigid form of internal fixation and facilitate earlier rehabilitation of the foot. There is still, however, some apprehension concerning the use of screws across a normal joint, despite the excellent results that have recently been reported with screw fixation (Arntz et al 1988). We have been using screws successfully for the past decade, and feel that the resulting stability far outweighs the potential for delayed degenerative arthrosis. Infection is always a possibility when using percutaneous pins, and the reduction can be compromised if the pins have to be removed prematurely. Therefore, if pins are used, it is a good idea to bury them subcutaneously so that they can be retrieved later before weight bearing begins. A combination of screws and 0.045-inch (1.14-mm) Kirschner wires for fragments too small for screws can be used.

Postoperative procedures

One of the problems with rehabilitation after these injuries is persistent postoperative swelling, which can be minimized by early range of motion exercises when fixation is accomplished with screws. We have successfully used an intermittent compression foot pump (AV Impulse System, Kendall, Mansfield MA, USA) to reduce postoperative foot swelling (Myerson & Henderson 1993). Patients are placed in a non-weight-bearing cast or splint for the first 2 weeks, followed by toe-touch weight bearing in a short leg cast or articulated brace for 6–10 weeks. Early range of motion of the foot is ideal and is enhanced by rigid skeletal fixation. These are primarily ligamentous injuries which take 3–5 months to heal fully, and rehabilitation with physical therapy modalities is encouraged. Prior to commencement of full activities, all hardware should be removed, usually at about 4 months. If patients are asymptomatic, we have occasionally left the screws in the middle column of the foot across which little motion occurs.

Complications

Vascular complications rarely accompany these injuries today (Jeffrey 1963, Wiley 1971, Lenczner et al 1974), and we have treated circulatory compromise only in the presence of associated compartment syndrome of the foot (Myerson 1990, Myerson & Burgess 1991, Myerson & Manoli 1993). There are, however, many other potential complications of treating fractures and dislocations of the tarsometatarsal joint complex (Myerson et al 1986, Arntz et al 1988).

Arthritis

Perhaps the most common and frustrating of these complications is the development of post-traumatic arthritis. As noted above, these are high-energy injuries associated with significant morbidity. If the articular surfaces are abraded or crushed during impact, the development of later arthritis is not surprising; later arthritis may develop even after a perfect reduction. Skeptics of ORIF have argued that arthritis may be the result of using screws across these joints. This is unlikely. Minimal motion occurs at these joints, and the joint that is most likely to be associated with later arthritis is the second tarsometatarsal joint, the one with the least motion. The fifth metatarsocuboid joint moves the most in both the sagittal and horizontal planes, but is the least likely to be involved in later symptomatic arthritis. Therefore, it is apparent that the rigidities of the second and third articulations are the least forgiving, and the use of screws is not likely to worsen the potential for arthritis.

Having noted this, however, it is uncommon for symptomatic arthritis to develop if anatomic reduction has been achieved. More likely, subtle deformity or incongruity still remains as the most likely cause of arthritis. As noted previously, arthritis occurs far more frequently if reduction is not anatomic; it is also associated with closed methods of treatment (Myerson et al 1986).

Neuritis

Perhaps the most common problem I treat after ORIF is a neuroma of the superficial or deep peroneal nerves. These nerves are small, particularly the dorsal middle cutaneous branch of the superficial peroneal nerve. For this reason, I advocate using loupe magnification during the initial dissection until the deeper tissue planes are reached and the nerve or nerves can be retracted. Transection of the deep peroneal nerve rarely occurs, provided the entire soft-tissue mass is retracted. Since the perforating branch of the dorsal pedis artery dives down between the first and second metatarsal approximately 1–2 cm distal to the tarsometatarsal joint, this artery occasionally has to be ligated to obtain sufficient soft-tissue exposure, and then the entire neurovascular bundle may be retracted.

A neuroma of these nerves must be treated promptly upon diagnosis since, if left untreated, it may be associated with the development of a reflex sympathetic dystrophy. Post-traumatic neuritis can be treated with various physical therapy modalities, including deep tissue massage, phonophoresis, and home use of a transcutaneous electrical nerve stimulator. If the nerve or nerves are extremely irritated, the temporary use of a neuroleptic medication such as amitriptyline is quite useful. If symptoms become chronic, neuritis may require surgical treatment (see below).

Infection

Wound problems and infection do occur after treatment, and they are usually associated with a crushing type of injury. If associated with a compartment syndrome, fasciotomy should be performed. I advocate the use of two dorsal incisions, one medial to the second metatarsal and the other lateral to the fourth metatarsal (Myerson 1990, Myerson & Manoli 1993, Myerson & McGarvey 1993). Provided this skin bridge is maintained, necrosis rarely occurs, and since the incisions are left open after fasciotomy, infection has not been a problem. Wound problems also occur as a result of excessive skin retraction and poor handling of the soft tissues. To some extent, these problems may be avoided by meticulous handling of the soft tissues, preserving full-thickness skin flaps, and releasing the retractors when full visualization of the area is not required.

Nonunion

Nonunion of fracture in this location is not a common problem, since the majority of these injuries are dislocations and the fractures occur in metaphyseal bone. However, malunion (usually of the second metatarsal) does occur. When malunion is present, the second metatarsal usually ends up slightly dorsal and laterally angulated, and, as noted above, it is associated with arthritis. In addition to symptoms of arthritis, there may be pain under the forefoot in the region of the third metatarsal, caused by transfer of weight from the dorsally displaced second metatarsal.

Cosmetic deformity

The dorsum of the midfoot has no subcutaneous muscles or fat, so any abnormality will produce a noticeable deformity. Patients also usually have an uninvolved opposite foot which appears normal and with which they can compare the injured foot. Even under ideal circumstances the normal postoperative healing will result in some abnormality of appearance, and it is important to advise the patient of this before treatment. To treat these injuries only by closed methods of reduction will almost certainly result in a midfoot deformity that most patients will find unacceptable. In some patients a foot with significant deformity always seems to give more discomfort. Moreover, such deformities cannot be fully corrected at a later stage by arthrodesis. This is also true if insufficient methods of internal fixation are used.

References

Aitken A P, Poulson D 1963 Dislocations of the tarsometatarsal joint. J Bone Joint Surg 45A: 246–260

Arntz C T, Veith R G, Hansen S T Jr 1988 Fractures and fracture–dislocations of the tarsometatarsal joint. J Bone Joint Surg 70A: 173–181

Blair W F 1981 Irreducible tarsometatarsal fracture–dislocation. J Trauma 21: 988–990

Curtis M J, Myerson M, Szura B 1993 Tarsometatarsal joint injuries in the athlete. Am J Sports Med 21: 497–502

DeBenedetti M J, Evanski P M, Waugh T R 1978 The unreducible Lisfranc fracture. Case report and literature review. Clin Orthop 136: 238–240

Goosens M, De Stoop N 1983 Lisfranc's fracture–dislocations: etiology, radiology, and results of treatment. A review of 20 cases. Clin Orthop 176: 154–162

Hardcastle P H, Reschauer R, Kutscha-Lissberg E et al 1982 Injuries to the tarsometatarsal joint. Incidence, classification and treatment. J Bone Joint Surg 64B: 349–356

Jeffreys T E 1963 Lisfranc's fracture–dislocation. Clinical and experimental study of tarso-metatarsal dislocations and fracture–dislocations. J Bone Joint Surg 45B: 546–555

La Tourlette G, Perry J, Patzakis M et al 1980 Fractures and dislocations of the tarsometatarsal joint. In: Bateman J E, Trott A W (eds)

The Foot and Ankle. Thieme–Stratton; New York. pp 40–51

Lenczner E M, Waddell J P, Graham J D 1974 Tarsal–metatarsal (Lisfranc) dislocation. J Trauma 14: 1012–1020

Myerson M S 1989 The diagnosis and treatment of injuries to the Lisfranc joint complex. Orthop Clin North Am 20: 655–664

Myerson M S 1990 Diagnosis and treatment of compartment syndromes of the foot. Orthopedics 13: 711–717

Myerson M S 1991 Injuries to the forefoot and toes. In: Jahss M H (ed) Disorders of the Foot and Ankle. Medical and Surgical Management, 2nd edn, vol 3. W. B. Saunders Co, Philadelphia. 2233–2273

Myerson M 1993 Tarsometatarsal joint injury. Phys Sports Med 21: 97–107

Myerson M S, Burgess A R 1991 The initial evaluation and treatment of the acutely traumatized foot and ankle. In: Jahss M H (ed) Disorders of the Foot and Ankle. Medical and Surgical Management, 2nd edn, vol 3. W. B. Saunders Co, Philadelphia. pp 2209–2232

Myerson M S, Henderson M R 1993 Clinical applications of a pneumatic intermittent impulse compression device after trauma and major surgery to the foot and ankle. Foot Ankle 14: 198–203

Myerson M S, Manoli A 1993 Compartment syndromes of the foot after calcaneal fractures. Clin Orthop 290: 142–150

Myerson M, McGarvey W C 1993 Crush injuries and compartment syndromes. In: Myerson M (ed) Current Therapy in Foot and Ankle Surgery. Mosby–Year Book, St. Louis. 264–273

Myerson M S, Fisher R T, Burgess A R, et al 1986 Fracture dislocations of the tarsometatarsal joints: end results correlated with pathology and treatment. Foot Ankle 6: 225–242

Myerson M S, Ruland C M, Allon S M 1992 Regional anesthesia for foot and ankle surgery. Foot Ankle 13: 282–288

Ouzounian T J, Shereff M J 1989 In vitro determination of midfoot motion. Foot Ankle 10: 140–146

Wiley J J 1971 The mechanism of tarso-metatarsal joint injuries. J Bone Joint Surg 53B: 474–482

IX.6 Stress Fractures

Michael Devas

This chapter deals with stress fractures in the foot, as well as those in the lower tibia and fibula, which may give rise to diagnostic problems because of referred pain.

Definition

A stress fracture occurs in the normal bone of a normal individual with normal activity and no history of a traumatic event. Because stress fractures are very common in the leg and foot of athletes, who are usually considered to be in peak condition, it is very unlikely that there can be any inherent abnormality in the bone that sustains a stress fracture, although there is some evidence that female athletes prone to stress fractures do have hormonal imbalance and poor dietary calcium intake (Myburgh et al 1990). Any form of rest or immobilization followed by intense activity may well produce a stress fracture, so that, for example, a person who has had a foot encased in plaster and then reverts to heavy exercise too rapidly is at risk of a stress fracture.

Patients with rheumatoid arthritis have a propensity to stress fractures. Although it cannot be said that a patient with rheumatoid arthritis has normal bones, their bones sometimes being osteoporotic, particularly if they have had steroid treatment, the stress fractures that they sustain are identical to those in the otherwise normal person.

A bone that is in any way diseased, such as by metastatic deposits from a carcinoma, cannot be considered to have a stress fracture, but rather a pathological fracture.

History

Stress fractures have been known for a long time, even before the advent of radiography. Other names are used to describe these fractures, mostly based in the activity that produces the fracture. The march fracture was the first to be described in 1855 by Breithaupt, a German military surgeon (though in 1733, Gooch had given a good description of a cough fracture of the rib). Probably the first radiograph of a stress fracture of a metatarsal bone was taken by Stechow in 1897. It must be recalled that in 1855, Lane described the effects of pressure on bony skeleton, but it was not until 1917 that Koch published his laws of bone architecture. Aleman in 1929 published an important work, which shows that he well understood how stress affected bone.

Types of stress fractures

The best way to classify stress fractures is radiologically: oblique, transverse, compression and longitudinal.

The oblique variety is the commonest type and is seen particularly in long bones and especially in the metatarsal bones. The transverse stress fracture carries with it a grim prognosis because often the bone will break completely and, having broken, displacement may be considerable and disability severe. It is seen in particular in the tibia and also occurs in the fifth metatarsal bone. The compression stress fracture can occur at any age, but is usually seen in children and older people,

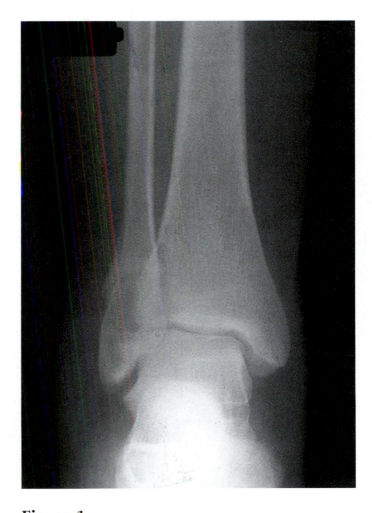

Figure 1

Typical runner's fracture of the fibula, above the external malleolus. Callus is already forming. (By courtesy of Mr A G Apley)

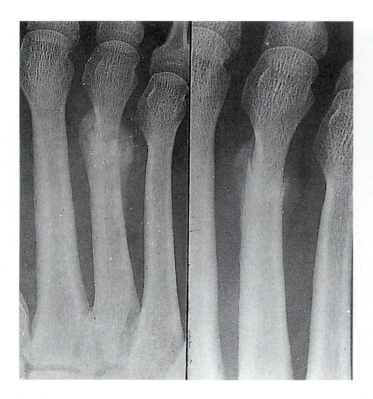

Figure 2

A young female athlete had pain in the left foot. The radiograph shows a well developed stress fracture of the neck of the third metatarsal

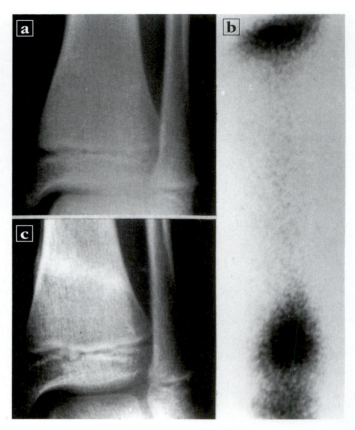

Figure 3

Immediately after the fracture occurs, a radiograph (a) may show nothing, whereas the technetium-99 scan (b) reveals a hot spot. Three weeks later the stress fracture is evident even on the radiograph (c). (By permission from Apley & Solomon 1984)

though it does occur in the first metatarsal bone in the young adult. The longitudinal variety is probably merely an extension along the length of a bone of an oblique stress fracture and is common as a variety of the march fracture.

Clinically, stress fractures can be considered in children, adolescents, young adults and athletes (Figs. 1, 2), the middle aged and the elderly.

Stress fractures in children develop very quickly, and the whole episode is over within a few weeks, whereas in adults it may take a few months for symptoms to subside completely. The situation in adolescents can be most interesting in that the fracture may be of the child's variety, but it may also be adult in type and this does not seem to bear any relationship to the activity of the youth concerned. The fracture is probably dependent on the extent of the development of the skeletal system. Thus, the upper tibia is a common site in children for a compression stress fracture, whereas the adolescent may have that type or the commoner oblique stress fracture, as seen in the adult. In children and adolescents, stress on apophyses and other parts of bone often gives rise to 'osteochondritis', which is a reaction of cartilage and bone to stress, giving rise to Sever's and Kienbock's diseases.

The middle-aged can sustain any form of stress fractures and it is often fairly slow in onset and equally slow to heal. Perhaps this is because activity in the middle-aged tends to be less and the fracture is often associated with one or another particular episode of normal but unusual activity, such as an intensive shopping expedition or an extrastrenuous round of golf. In the elderly, the pattern tends more to that of the child, but certain definite varieties predominate, such as the compression stress fracture of the lower end of the tibia. This gives rise to pain in the foot and ankle; a preliminary radiograph will show nothing and, as there is usually no follow-up radiography, the pain continues for many months as an undiagnosed chronic condition.

Radiology and scanning

The radiology of stress fractures is very important, because if too much faith is placed in the early radio-

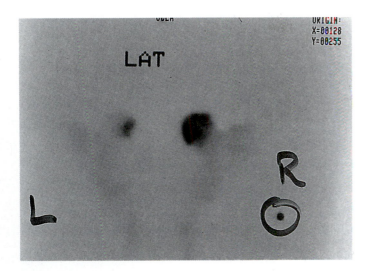

Figure 4

A 34-year-old male runner presented with persistent right heel pain. Plain radiographs were non-diagnostic. Technetium-99 bone scans were obtained and indicated a stress fracture of the calcaneum. The symptoms resolved with restriction of activities for 6 weeks. (By courtesy of Dr A Cracchiolo III)

graphs, the diagnosis may not be made. It must always be remembered that radiology lags far behind the clinical symptoms, thus pain in a forefoot may have been present for 3 weeks, but there may be no evidence of X-ray changes until 5 or 6 weeks. Stress fractures of the calcaneum are particularly difficult in this respect, at times taking 3 months to be seen radiologically. This can also apply to the stress fractures of the lower tibia, which again may take 2–3 months before radiographs confirm the lesion. Furthermore, it is important to have very good technique, so that the fine bone detail is shown, and to have the positioning accurate, so that, if necessary, not only the normal two anteroposterior and lateral views are taken, but also the necessary oblique or tangential views.

Technetium 99m (labelled diphosphonate) scanning is, however, a very much quicker method of diagnosing a bony lesion and, although an area of increased uptake of technetium is not diagnostic of a stress fracture, if it is combined with the proper history, then it may be taken as confirmatory evidence (Fig. 3). The use of the scan is not normally necessary if a clinical diagnosis can be made. However, there are occasions when the delay of normal radiography as confirmatory evidence has to be bypassed, such as in the case of an early lesion in an athlete to whom an immediate and firm diagnosis is essential (Fig. 4).

When scanning is not available, the patient must be treated on clinical grounds. Especially important is the enforcement of rest. The radiographic changes vary with age, not only in the type of stress fracture that may

occur, but also with the speed of confirmation; a stress fracture of the fibula in a child will develop so rapidly that within 1 week radiographic changes will be confirmatory. This is also useful should there be any doubt about the differential diagnosis in a child because within a few days the early changes will have developed into the full picture of a stress fracture.

Aetiology

The cause of a stress fracture is bending of the bone concerned. Whereas long bones are able to bend in all directions, it must be remembered that bones also will compress – this is what happens to the bones of the foot, such as the calcaneum, which in particular suffers from compression stress fractures.

With bending of a bone it might be considered that eventually the bone would break if the bending strains were continued long enough, like breaking a piece of wire, but the actual cause of the stress fracture is probably molecular change. Any force that is absorbed by the bone, such as a bending or a compression strain, produces a denaturing of the hydroxyapatite crystals that are present in bone to give rigidity to the otherwise elastic collagen ground substance. However, the structure has a degree of flexibility and so, with each periodic muscular activity of the part, the bones will bend to a greater or lesser extent. It is not the hitting of the heel on the ground that causes the bone to bend – it is the muscular activity that goes with it; thus, when a runner lands on his forefoot, the muscles contract at the moment of impact to maintain plantar flexion, for otherwise the foot would collapse. It is this pull of the muscles on their origins and insertions that causes the bone to bend and the stress fracture to occur.

If a forefoot is severely and violently dorsiflexed against the resistance of the calf muscles, a similar-shaped fracture to a stress fracture will occur. If, however, the compression is a result of jumping from a height and landing on the heels, the line of the fracture is transverse, parallel with the ground. Thus compression stress fractures are caused by muscular pull and not by rhythmic banging of the heel or foot on the ground.

It is the fundamental problem of bone strength that first gave rise to the march fracture, because it occurred in recruits. Often poorly fed and developed before they were enrolled into the Armed Forces, muscular strength and weight increased rapidly under their new conditions, but the intensive training produced fractures because muscle strength can be increased far more rapidly than the strength of bone can. Therefore, the overtraining of recruits or athletes may contribute considerably to stress fractures, particularly in the lower leg and particularly again in the foot (Fig. 5). A mechanical origin to stress fracture was confirmed using a mathematical model developed by Simkin and Leichter (1990).

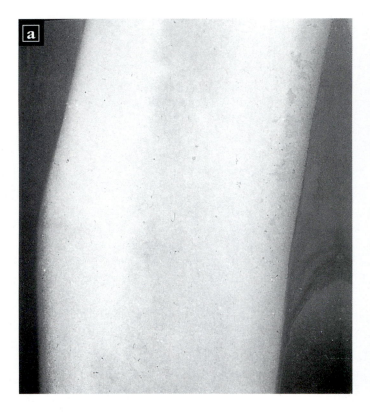

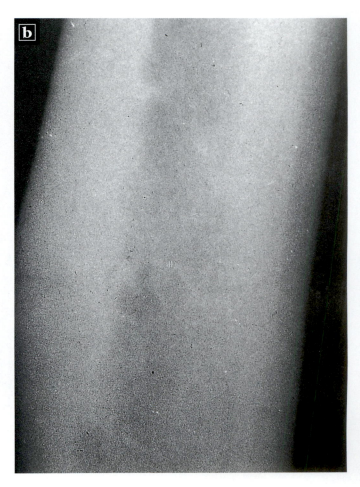

Figure 5

A marine suffered pain in his thigh after particularly heavy exercise. (a,b) There is a transverse stress fracture in the femur, which can be seen (c) going transversely across the cortex. These transverse stress fractures are dangerous and will cause a complete fracture if not treated

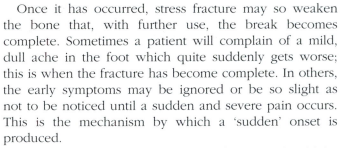

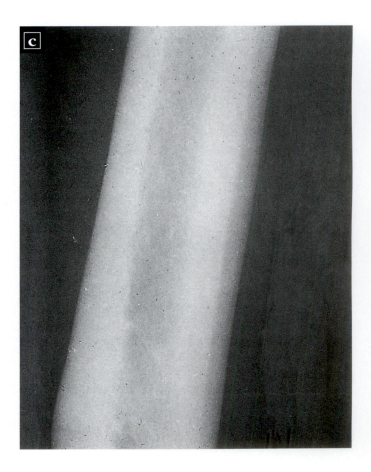

Once it has occurred, stress fracture may so weaken the bone that, with further use, the break becomes complete. Sometimes a patient will complain of a mild, dull ache in the foot which quite suddenly gets worse; this is when the fracture has become complete. In others, the early symptoms may be ignored or be so slight as not to be noticed until a sudden and severe pain occurs. This is the mechanism by which a 'sudden' onset is produced.

It would be expected that stress fractures should be bilateral and they often are. However, it is unlikely that in every person the fractures would develop at exactly the same rate, because as soon as symptoms on the worst side occur, activity lessens and the less advanced stress fracture can start to heal. Nevertheless, the opposite limb must always be carefully examined. In the foot, two or more march fractures are often found, sometimes with the fracture in one bone far further advanced than the other.

Stress fractures may also occur in sequence, perhaps with a year or more between them, and the runner may have a stress fracture of the lateral malleolus, only to be followed by another in a metatarsal bone.

Treatment

In general, rest from the activity causing the pain is sufficient. In the foot, this can often be aided by elastic adhesive strapping, foam inserts, or insoles. Usually, about 3 weeks is sufficient to allow healing to start, but restriction on activity must not be lifted for another 3 weeks and even then with caution. Any recurrence of the pain from the stress fracture indicates the need for further rest.

In particular, athletes and other energetic people must get back to training or activity with great care, for an overstrenuous session may not only restart symptoms in the original lesion, but may initiate a new stress fracture in the part already a little weaker (from disuse secondary to the rest) than it was before any symptoms were seen.

Prevention

The foot was developed for walking or running on earth; it was not designed to walk with hard leather sole, on hard concrete pavements. Therefore, it is wise to ensure that shoes, especially for sport, have thick, soft soles to absorb some of the impact and thereby lessen the muscle pull necessary to hold the foot correctly, whether at footfall or take off. McPoil and Cornwall (1992) have demonstrated in a single individual that soft materials alter the vertical forces exerted on the foot during exercise and will contribute to the prevention of injury.

The importance of training cannot be emphasized too much, particularly in the service recruit and the athlete, whether amateur or professional. It has been mentioned that the musculature in the service recruit will develop faster than the strength of bone, so initially, heavy and violent exercises should give way to general toughening up of muscles with exercise such as swimming. Linenger and Shwayhat (1992) were able to show an incidence of podiatric injuries in US army recruits of three per thousand recruit training days, with stress fractures of the foot having the highest incidence. Milgrom et al (1992), in a randomized trial, were able to reduce the incidence of stress fractures in army recruits by asking them to wear modified basketball boots rather than standard army issue footwear. They concluded such simple modifications would reduce the risks of stress fracture in all but vertically induced injuries. The athlete who has been out of sport for any length of time is at risk of stress fracture if resumption of training is not progressive and is especially at risk if the leg has been encased in plaster.

Stress fractures of the calcaneum

Stress fractures of the calcaneum occur at any age in adults, but are perhaps commonest in late middle age.

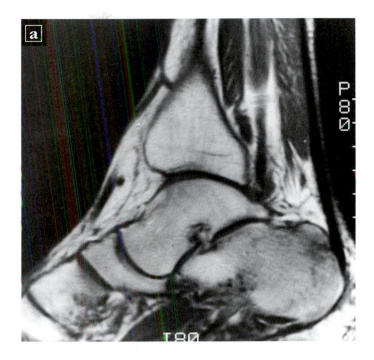

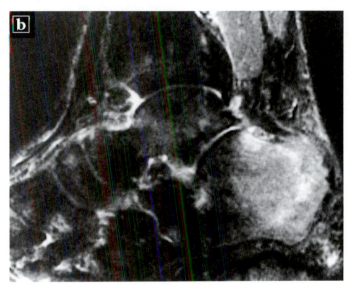

Figure 6

(a) T1-weighted MRI of the foot of a 34-year-old man with heel pain, whose plain radiographs showed no pathology. Because he was a runner and wished to continue with his sport, an MRI was performed. The stress fracture of the posterior tubercle can easily be seen using this study. (b) The T2-weighted image of this study delineated the fracture and the surrounding oedema of this cancellous portion of bone. (By courtesy of Dr A Cracchiolo III)

They also occur in children in the form of an apophysitis, or Sever's disease. This stress fracture often accounts for the painful heel that is slow to be diagnosed because of the vagueness of the symptoms and particularly because radiological confirmation is always lacking in the initial stages.

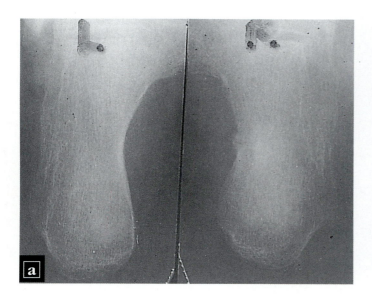
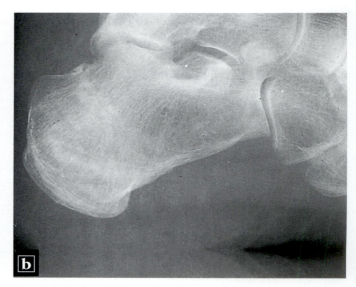

Figure 7

(a) A middle-aged woman had a painful heel and internal callus can be seen on the right. (b) The lateral view shows the line of callus at right angles to the trabeculae of the calcaneum

Symptoms and signs

The patient may indicate that there has been an increase in activity, an alteration in footwear, a different habit in walking or some similar alteration in the pattern of life. Sometimes symptoms start abruptly and the patient may complain that the foot, or particularly the heel, has become swollen. Tangential radiographs may also show the callus and be very helpful in diagnosis (Fig. 6).

Examination occasionally reveals some swelling of the hindfoot. There is always considerable tenderness in and around the heel, especially on the plantar surface, and this, because it is localized at the centre of the heel, may give rise to the mistaken diagnosis of a plantar fasciitis. However the greatest tenderness will be found on each side of the calcaneal tuberosity; otherwise movements of the foot and ankle are found to be free and full, but the patient may not be able to stand on the bare heel and will certainly not be able to stamp on the ground. Examination must be painstaking to exclude all other local lesions, including stress fractures at the lower end of the tibia or fibula, and to make sure that there is no lesion of the calcaneal tendon or its bursa or plantar fasciitis.

Other conditions that can mimic the symptoms are the medial or lateral nerve compression syndrome and tenosynovitis. It must be realized that the symptoms of a stress fracture can be very chronic and that sometimes they do not cause great disability. The patient will cut down activities to an acceptable level of discomfort, which both prevents healing and maintains the fracture – hence the length of the history that is often found.

Radiology

The confirmation of a stress fracture of the calcaneum may be very long delayed and this must always be borne in mind (Figs. 7, 8). Clear bone detail must be obtained in the lateral and tangential radiographs to ensure that the earliest disruption of the trabeculae and the earliest haze of internal callus are easily seen. In older patients, who are often osteoporotic, compression may actually show in the bone.

Sometimes the fracture appears to be double with two lines of callus visible, which may not be always concomitant in time. It makes no difference to the diagnosis or to the outlook, as both heal well in due course. If one heel is to be radiographed, the other heel should always be done also, because subclinical stress fractures often exist in the opposite limb.

Differential diagnosis

A stress fracture in the calcaneum may be difficult to confirm, but should not be misdiagnosed provided the condition is remembered when the patient is first seen, so that the radiographs may be repeated in due course, thus confirming the diagnosis. The history may not always give a period of increased or different activity. Swelling of the hindfoot is important, but is not usual by the time the patient seeks advice. However, if the patient is asked to stand on tip toe and to move in this position, pain is almost always reproduced in the heel

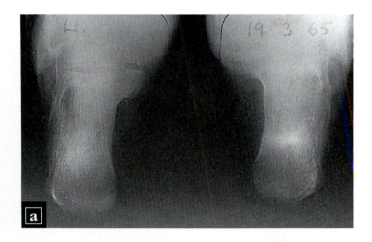

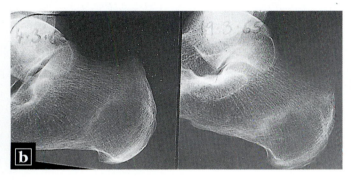

Figure 8

(a) A middle-aged woman had pain in both heels. (b) The lateral views show the line of internal callus in both bones very satisfactorily

because it is this action that has produced the stress fracture. Next in importance is the palpation of the tuberosity of the calcaneum and, if this is done with care and gentleness, the tenderness will be found to follow the line of the stress fracture down both sides of the bone as well as underneath on the plantar surface. If only the plantar surface is examined and pressed heavily the patient may be rather resistant to further examination because of the intense pain that can be produced and further (and perhaps lesser) tenderness may then be missed.

The differentiation between an acute plantar fasciitis and a compression stress fracture of the calcaneum may be difficult, but it is of tremendous importance because local injection of an insoluble steroid will have no effect on the stress fracture but may be curative for the plantar fasciitis. If there is still difficulty in the early stages, it is better to treat conservatively, because this will soon differentiate the two and will allow time for radiological (or scanning) confirmation. The tenderness of plantar fasciitis is very localized, whereas the tenderness of the stress fracture is much more general and goes round the sides of the bone.

The general conditions that may mimic the stress fracture of the calcaneum are gout, rheumatoid arthritis, Reiter's disease and ankylosing spondylitis. Early symptoms of a prolapsed intervertebral disc affecting the first sacral nerve root can also produce pain in the heel. In the differential diagnosis of the radiographs there is one condition that may confuse – calcification in the posterior tibial artery as it passes down the posteromedial side of the ankle. This is because, if calcified, the shadow may resemble that of a stress fracture. However, the tangential view will show no abnormality within the bone.

Treatment

The heel should be raised and padded: this both absorbs the impact of the footfall (which is resisted by muscular contraction causing the stress fracture) and relaxes the calf muscles and the long plantar ligament. Wearing such a pad within a shoe with a soft, rather than a leather, heel and a similar sole will give the patient immediate comfort, if not total relief. However, the treatment must be continued for several weeks and the patient must be warned that if the pad is removed too soon the symptoms will recur. In the older patient at least 2–3 months are needed.

Stress fractures of the calcaneum in children

The stress fracture that occurs in the apophysis of the tuberosity of the calcaneum is known as Sever's disease and characteristically it is described as an 'osteochondritis' or an 'apophysitis'. It is, in fact, identical in aetiology to Osgood–Schlatter's disease and other so-called osteochondritides; it is the reaction of the apophysis to stress. Instead of the compression stress fracture ocurring within the bone, the apophysis, which is buffered between itself and the calcaneum by its cartilaginous growth plate, becomes both compressed and distracted by the excess strength that has been imposed upon it. The pain of which the child complains is characteristic of a stress fracture. It comes on in the evening or after a bout of exercise, but rarely does it completely stop the child playing or give rise to a very severe complaint of pain. Examination will show that the tenderness is greater at the back of the heel than underneath. Treatment involves reassurance of the parents, the forbidding of those activities that cause pain, and wearing a soft pad under the heel in shoes that have soft heels themselves. With this regime, the symptoms should subside within two or three weeks.

The radiographs show fragmentation in one or other plane of the apophysis, but occasionally an actual fracture line can be seen through the apophysis.

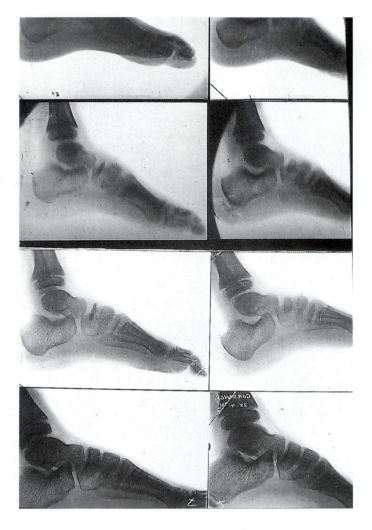

Figure 9
Köhler's disease of bone: all stages. (By courtesy of Mr B Helal)

Stress fractures of the navicular bone

These are very rare, but when they occur are very distinctive. So far they have been seen in early middle age in active people playing golf. The cause of a stress fracture of the navicular bone is the resistance to the pull of the muscles by the bone when the forefoot is flexed or when weight is taken on the ball of the foot. The form the fracture takes in adults is that of a transverse type of stress fracture. However, owing to the shape of the bone, the line of the fracture is, in fact, not transverse but longitudinal down the bone and is in the line of the first metatarsal bone. In children the condition known as Köhler's disease has the same causes and may be a compression stress fracture leading to avascularity (Fig. 9). Ultimately the bone will regenerate if the foot is treated correctly.

Symptoms and signs

Pain in the middle of the foot which is worse after exercise and towards the end of the day is the usual history, and a special activity may gradually have to stop earlier than would otherwise be the case. A history of pain in the foot is so common in middle age that the connection between a stress fracture and rather vague histories will be missed unless emphasis has always been placed on asking the relationship of pain to activity.

Differential diagnosis

The differential diagnosis includes all the usual conditions causing pain on the medial side of the foot; these must be eliminated. Careful and gentle palpation of the medial arch will show that the maximum tenderness is in the navicular bone. A stress fracture of the base of the first metatarsal will, of course, have to be considered, although this is usually seen at an earlier age.

Radiology

The fracture appears to run caudally through the centre of the navicular bone, almost as though the talus was trying to force its way through. The fracture line develops slowly and stops developing as soon as rest occurs and some internal callus can be seen around the crack. The initial lesion is difficult to see early and must be looked for with great care in good radiographs.

Treatment

It may be difficult to relieve pain if the patient continues to partake of normal activity, in which case a below-knee walking plaster may be applied for 3–4 weeks to start the healing process. Thereafter, firm support with elastic adhesive bandages is sufficient, and a stiff support in soft soled shoes will complete the cure.

Avascular necrosis of the navicular bone

The child presents with pain in the foot and limping. If the tenderness is looked for very carefully without frightening the child, it can be localized to the navicular bone. Usually by the time the child is seen, fragmentation has occurred radiologically. The opposite foot must also be examined carefully, for the condition is often bilateral, but the limp will be on the side where the condition is most developed. Provided the child is kept at rest so that pain does not occur and proper support given to the foot until radiological healing is apparent, the bone will develop apparently normally and hopefully give rise to no further problems in adult life.

Stress fractures have not been described in the cuboid bone, but rare though they are, they are possible, and this diagnosis should always be considered in a lesion that causes pain in the typical manner but that cannot be otherwise explained.

March fracture

This is the commonest stress fracture of all and those that occur in the second or third metatarsal shafts are the most frequent. It is not nowadays possible to give accurate statistics on the number of march fractures that occur except in closed communities such as an Armed Forces Camp, because the condition is so well known that many patients are treated for the condition without ever being referred to hospital or an orthopaedic surgeon. The symptoms of pain and arching in the forefoot are soon relieved by rest and support to the foot, usually in the form of elastic adhesive strapping. Many patients can give a history of having had a march fracture (or apparently such a condition) which responded to simple restriction of activity and avoidance of those conditions that caused pain without ever attending for treatment. Nevertheless, there are certain march fractures that can cause extreme trouble and even severe disability.

After the single march fracture, multiple forms are the commonest. Sometimes the outer three metatarsal bones will sustain stress fractures either together or in sequence. Bilateral march fractures occur, but are rare because (even if both feet sustain a march fracture at the same time) the slight limitation of activity with the more advanced side giving rise to symptoms first, allows the opposite lesion to heal before it becomes apparent clinically or radiologically. However, multiple march fractures involve the third metatarsal bone more often than not, followed closely by the fourth metatarsal bone.

The site of the stress fracture in the metatarsal bone may be at the base, the shaft, or the neck, and in children the actual metatarsal head may be involved, giving rise to avascular necrosis and the so-called Frieberg's infraction. Usually, however, there is an oblique stress fracture in the metatarsal neck and this may start either medially or laterally. No reason for the laterality has been found. In children the fracture tends to be more longitudinal in type, as shown by the length of callus up and down the bone, although this can also occur in adults.

Unless the X-ray beam passes directly through the plane of the fracture it is not easily seen and only the callus that occurs on the outside of the bone indicates that the lesion exists. This particular type of stress fracture occurs in the tibia and may cause aching in one or both feet (if it is bilateral).

It has been said that march fractures occur more commonly after operations, particularly those for hallux valgus, but this is not universally accepted. There seems to be no reason why a foot that has undergone some reconstructive or other procedure should develop stress fractures any more readily than a normal foot, provided the patient does not take too much excessive exercise too quickly after prolonged immobilization. However, it is well known that following even successful hallux valgus surgery there is lateral shift in loading and this may account for any increased incidence of subsequent stress fractures.

The march fracture is commonest in the middle-aged adult, but, of course, it was first diagnosed in and is still common in the Service recruit and the athlete, for which the explanation has been given above. The march fracture has also had many names applied to it, but it is considered that repetition of these names would only contribute to their unnecessary perpetuation. Even when standing apparently at rest, there is considerable muscle tone so that if, under these conditions, slight symptoms are present, active treatment is indicated.

Stress fractures of the first and fifth metatarsal bones are often different in pattern, the first showing the compression stress fracture and the fifth the transverse, which has a poor prognosis.

Stress fracture of the second, third and fourth metatarsal bones

The march fracture is well known and is extremely common at all ages. There appears to be no definite cause other than activity. There are many different varieties of stress fractures in the metatarsal bones, either when affected singly or together. The second and third metatarsal bones are probably affected equally commonly, with far fewer fractures being seen in the fourth.

Symptoms and signs

An ache or pain in the forefoot is the usual presenting feature, and it may have been related to some special activity (classically a 'march') such as a day's outing, an extra-long walk or a rather tiring game of golf. The pain gradually increases in intensity each day, but it is possible for the patient to continue walking, sometimes limping, sometimes flat-footed (taking all the weight on the heel) and sometimes hobbling on the inner or outer border of the foot. Running is the most painful activity.

In a few patients the pains comes on abruptly, sometimes as a severe exacerbation of a trivial ache. This indicates that the initial crack has become complete.

The child may complain that there is aching which produces a limp on a long walk although not on a short one. The older child usually takes longer to heal.

Inspection of the foot will show that swelling of the forefoot may or may not be present, but it is rare to find swelling only over the affected bone. In the old person the whole foot may swell.

Palpation will reveal tenderness localized in the metatarsal shaft. It is difficult to be sure which shaft is tender, so gentle palpation is essential. Pressure under the forefoot may cause pain and manipulating the bone by holding its head gives rise to pain. Standing on tiptoe is painful. Swelling at the fracture site may not be felt even at the start.

Radiology

The radiological confirmation may be late, and the appearances do not bear much relationship to the signs and symptoms. Sometimes the stress fracture will have a long fracture line running the length of the shaft, or it may show a haze of bone only.

Despite the differences in the radiological findings, it is not possible to correlate these findings with a clinical prognosis. Sometimes the early radiological changes show little callus, at other times a large amount, and this may relate to the level of movement that is allowed to occur at the fracture site early on, and in turn may be associated with the pain threshold. If the fracture line is seen in the callus it indicates that there is still movement at the fracture site during healing. There is some connection between the site of the fracture and the length of history, and the more proximal the fracture in the shaft, the longer severe symptoms are likely to have been present.

Stress fractures of the third metatarsal bone are common, but a little less so than those of the second metatarsal bone. They can occur at most ages and they are more commonly involved in multiple stress fractures of the metatarsal bones than those of the second. One out of every two patients with a stress fracture of the third metatarsal bone will have one or more other metatarsal stress fractures. This characteristic is shared to an even greater extent by the fourth metatarsal, which is more often involved with another metatarsal than it is singly. Usually the other metatarsals involved are either the second or the third. In other words, the first and the fifth metatarsal bones do not share in this multiplicity of fractures; furthermore, if the fifth metatarsal is implicated, it is not at its base but in the shaft that the fracture occurs.

The fourth metatarsal bone does not have nearly so many stress fractures as the second and third, but, apart from the symptoms and signs being more on the outer side of the foot, there is little difference in presentation.

Stress fractures of the first metatarsal bone

The base of this bone is affected by a compression stress fracture and, being in line with the navicular bone, this is to be expected.

Symptoms are slow to occur as are those of most compression stress fractures. The usual complaint is of the gradual onset of pain with activity, which comes on earlier and earlier and gets more and more severe until the patient seeks advice. Usually at this time the early haze of internal callus can be seen. The lesion can be localized by careful palpation and it may be possible to feel some local swelling because the anteromedial side of the first metatarsal base is subcutaneous. Treatment is either by restricting activity with or without strapping or, if symptoms are severe, a below-knee plaster cast for some time.

Stress fractures of the fifth metatarsal bone

This bone sustains a transverse stress fracture at its base as well as the more ordinary oblique type in its shaft. The former is dangerous to the extent that nonunion occurs even if properly treated, so it is important that any lesion of this particular nature should be treated immediately as an emergency.

It is considered that this transverse type of stress fracture is caused by the tremendous muscle pull that can occur at the base of the fifth metatarsal in activity, such as squash. Again, the opposite foot must be looked at carefully to make sure there is not a similar stress fracture on that side. The traumatic or muscular avulsion fracture of the base of the fifth metatarsal bone is also well known and must be differentiated, but the typical history of pain after sport or activity, gradually coming on earlier and earlier, is usual. Not infrequently there is an insidious history leading up to a sudden onset of severe pain, indicating that the whole of the metatarsal base has now been broken off. The period of immobilization must be sufficient to allow complete healing or symptoms will recur and may then lead again to nonunion.

Oblique fractures of the fifth metatarsal shaft are much the same as those of the neighbouring bones.

Stress fractures of the sesamoid bones of the hallux

Stress fractures are difficult to diagnose in the sesamoid bone, because at first the pain is mild and it may take a long time for the patient to attend for advice.

Furthermore, a bipartite sesamoid may have a bursitis or a form of inflammation, which may masquerade as a stress fracture. The counterpart in the patella is not uncommon in its various forms but in the sesamoid only the transverse stress fracture has been seen.

Diagnosis is made on clinical examination and history, confirmed by radiography. Scintillography may be difficult to interpret. The lesion, even if seen early, will show a separation of the two parts and this will develop further (see Chapter V.5).

Treatment is by the usual methods of rest and support, but a metatarsal bar may be advantageous. It can be discarded at leisure. A custom-made first metatarsal neck support may also be effective. It is not possible to secure union of the sesamoid, which should be allowed to remain bipartite. Gradually symptoms resolve and the foot becomes fully functional.

Stress fractures of the ankle and lower leg

Stress fractures in the lower leg are included because they can cause a difficulty in diagnosis when the symptoms are only slowly progressive and of a dull, aching nature. The dull ache is often referred to the foot, either in fact or because aching feet are so common that the patient is self-indoctrinated as to the site of the pain.

After the march fracture, the commonest site for a stress fracture is the lower third of the fibula just at or above the lateral malleolus. This is particularly common in athletes and has been termed 'the runner's fracture', but it also often occurs in middle aged people and following an unusual but not abnormal activity, such as a lengthy shopping expedition.

Symptoms and signs

At first there is a dull ache towards evening in the outer side of the ankle, often referred to the foot; if so it will be on the outer side of the foot. The pain will come on earlier and earlier with exercise and, in the case of an athlete, sport eventually has to be abandoned. Usually it takes about 2–3 weeks for the patient to attend for treatment. By then there is often a little swelling, pain is localized to the lower fibula above the lateral malleolus, and walking is painful.

Examination reveals a swelling in most patients. This is, of course, unusual, but the lower end of the fibula is subcutaneous and, therefore, like the base of the first metatarsal bone, swelling can be seen. The swelling will be tender to the touch and springing the fibula may cause pain at the site of the swelling. However, the radiograph may still show no abnormality unless it has been taken with extreme care and not overexposed. The

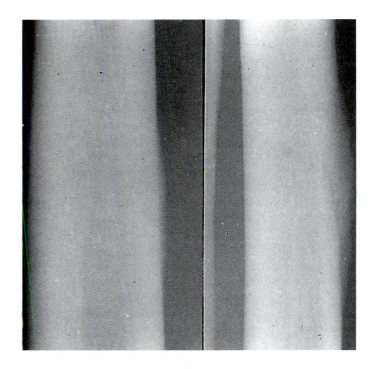

Figure 10
The radiological appearances of shin soreness. There is only some periosteal thickening of the medial side of the lower tibia

cause of the stress fracture in the fibula cannot be weight bearing, because it is not a weight-bearing bone, but it has been shown that during muscular contraction of the calf muscles the fibula is pulled towards the tibia and the maximum bend occurs at the site of maximum occurrence of stress fractures; that is about 1–2 cm above the lateral malleolus.

Radiology

The radiographs do not show any lesions for some 3 weeks in the usual course of events, but a scan will normally show a hot spot at the fracture within a week of the onset of symptoms. The oblique stress fracture may become complete and this is usually signalled by a sudden increase in the pain.

The treatment is the same as for stress fractures in the foot – that is cessation of the sport or activity that has caused the problem, and elastic adhesive bandaging. However, in the excessively keen sportsman it may be necessary to add a below-knee walking plaster to curb enthusiastic attempts at returning to excess activity too soon.

Any return to a painful activity means that the healing has been delayed and union will take longer to become solid.

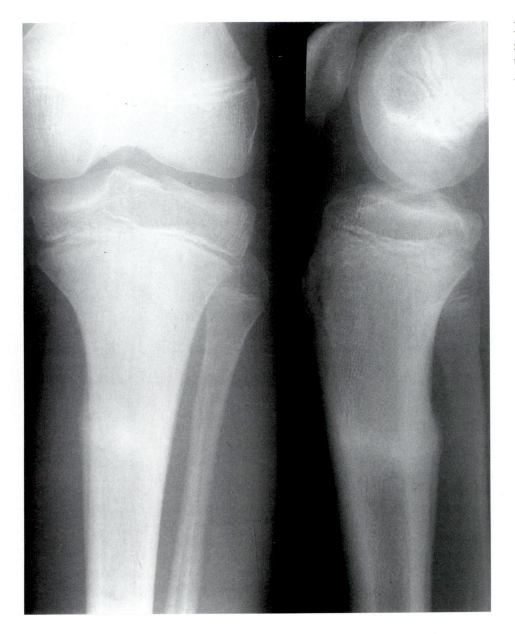

Figure 11
Stress fracture of the upper end of the tibia. (By courtesy of Mr A G Apley)

Stress fractures of the medial malleolus

These are extremely rare and have been seen in runners. The symptoms are very similar to those of a stress fracture of the fibula, but the symptoms are on the medial side of the ankle and the time lag between diagnosis and X-ray confirmation may be considerable. Local examination will reveal tenderness around the medial malleolus, but it may not be possible to see swelling.

Stress fractures of the lower tibia

Any lesion in the lowermost third of the tibia may give rise to pain in, or going down into, the foot. The very dangerous transverse stress fracture seen in ballet dancers and others who do much jumping, such as basketball players, may also give pain referred to the ankle and foot. The physical signs of tenderness and swelling are present, but they must be looked for carefully.

The shin soreness type of stress fracture of the athlete is very common in the lowermost third of the tibia and has been named 'shin splints' by athletes (Fig. 10). Suffering a chronic continuing pain in the ankle and foot, athletes may blame their running and foot placement. The longitudinal stress fracture of the lower tibia gives very similar symptoms to the oblique type, of which it may be a variant. The compression stress fracture, however, is commonest in the older person, and sometimes 'spreads' into the fibula. The history of these fractures is usually very long and it may take up to 3 months for the radiograph to show the first haze of internal callus.

Such a stress fracture may also occur at the upper end of the tibia (Fig. 11).

Conclusions

Stress fractures occur in healthy bone and, provided the sequence of events is remembered, the diagnosis should not be difficult, even though physical signs are limited and radiographical confirmation is late. Early confirmation of the diagnosis can be achieved by technetium scanning. Treatment is usually rest from painful activity combined with support.

References

Aleman O 1929 Omsk Marchschalst (syndesmites metatarsea). Tidskrift i Militar Halsovard 54: 191–208

Apley G, Solomon L 1984 Apley's System of Orphopaedics and Fractures, 6th edn. Butterworth Heinemann, London

Breithaupt 1855 Zur Pathologie des Menschlichen Fusses. Med Zeitung Berlin 24: 169

Koch J C 1917 The laws of bone architecture. Am J Anat 21: 177

Lane W A 1855 Some points in the physiology and pathology of the changes produced by pressure in the bony skeleton of the trunk and shoulder girdle. Guy's Hospital Report 43: 321

Linenger J M, Shwayhat A F 1992 Epidemiology of podiatric injuries in US marine recruits undergoing basic training. J Am Pod Med Assoc 82: 269–271

McPoil T G, Cornwall M W 1991 Rigid vs soft foot orthoses. J Am Med Pod Assoc 81: 638–642

Milgrom C, Finestone A, Shlamkovitch N, Wosk J, Laor A, Voloshin A, Eldad A 1992 Prevention of overuse injuries of the foot by improved shoe shock attenuation. A randomized prospective study. Clin Orthop 381: 189–192

Myburgh K H, Hutchins J, Fatar A B, Hough S F, Noakes T D 1990 Low density is an etiologic factor for stress fractures in athletes. Ann Int Med 113: 745–749

Simkin A, Leichter I 1990 Role of the calcaneal inclination in the energy storage capacity of the human foot – a biomechanical model. Med Biol Eng Comp 28: 149–152

Stechow 1897 Fussodem und Röntgenstrahlen. Deutsche Militärärtzliche Zeitschrift 26: 465

Further reading

Devas M 1975 Stress Fractures. Churchill Livingstone, Edinburgh

Eisele S A, Sammarco G J 1993 Fatigue fractures of the foot and ankle in the athlete. Instructional course lectures. American Academy of Orthopaedic Surgeons 42: 175–183

IX.7 Reflex Sympathetic Dystrophy

R M Atkins

Introduction

Reflex sympathetic dystrophy (RSD) is a curious condition characterized by excessive pain in an extremity associated with autonomic dysfunction and joint stiffness and contracture. In the past it has been viewed variously as an inevitable consequence of failure to mobilize a traumatized limb (Watson Jones 1952), as the result of inadequate fixation of a fracture (Müller et al 1979) or as an extremely rare complication of trauma which was difficult to treat (Plewes 1956). It is now emerging as a relatively frequent complication of trauma; it is normally transient and often sub-clinical, but it is responsible for significant morbidity in those affected (Atkins 1989, Atkins et al 1989, Atkins et al 1990, Bickerstaff 1990, Field et al 1992).

The syndrome has been given a number of names reflecting a variety of precipitating events, sites of involvement and modes of presentation. Mitchell (Mitchell et al 1864) coined the term 'causalgia', from the Greek, literally meaning burning pain, because of observations made on soldiers who had sustained peripheral nerve injuries following gunshot wounds in the American Civil War. Südeck (1900, 1901) investigated a number of conditions which were characterized by a severe osteoporosis, and the condition was given the name of Südeck's atrophy by Nonne in 1901. The term 'reflex dystrophy' or 'reflex sympathetic dystrophy' was introduced by De Takats in 1937. Homans (1940) used the term 'minor causalgia' in order to imply a relationship between Mitchell's causalgia, which was renamed major causalgia, and similar conditions arising without direct nerve injury. When it was subsequently shown that algodystrophy without nerve injury was more common, De Takats (1945) introduced the term 'causalgic state'. Patman et al (1973) used the term 'mimo causalgia' as a collective term for all causalgic disorders. Fortunately, today the term 'causalgia' has returned to its original connotation of Mitchell's major causalgia, in which an injury to a nerve produces severe RSD associated with burning pain.

In 1947, Steinbrocker introduced the term 'shoulder–hand syndrome' for a condition which is sometimes considered to be a separate disorder from true RSD.

The term 'algoneurodystrophy' was introduced by Glick & Helal in 1976, and 'algodystrophy' was introduced by French rheumatologists in the late 1960s. This seems a satisfactory name for the condition since it does not imply involvement of any particular tissue, aetiology or location, but reflects the clinical association of pain and disuse of the limb.

There is a related condition, 'sympathetically maintained pain', which is diagnosed by the finding of pain associated with hyperpathia (increased sensitivity to a noxious stimulus, also known as hyperalgesia) and allodynia (pain provoked by stimuli that are not usually considered painful, such as light touch) and relieved by selective sympathetic blockade. The exact association between RSD and sympathetically maintained pain is obscure. A simple way of looking at this problem is that in RSD a significant proportion of the pain is sympathetically maintained and therefore is relieved by sympathetic blockade. However in RSD there is also occurring a process that leads to initial tissue oedema followed by severe contracture. This tissue contracture does not appear an inevitable association of sympathetically maintained pain (Janig 1990).

Incidence and epidemiology

The incidence of RSD varies greatly between reported series. Full blown clinical RSD is fortunately uncommon (Louyot et al 1967); however, in a mild and often sub-clinical form it occurs following 30% of tibial fractures (Sarangi et al 1993). The incidence has been more fully investigated following upper limb fracture, where it used to be thought to be rare, being found in up to 2% of the population studied in retrospective series (Bacorn & Kurtz 1953, Green & Gay 1956, Plewes 1956, Lidström 1959, Frykman 1967, Poole 1973, Stewart et al 1985).

More recently, a number of series (Aubert 1980, Atkins et al 1989, Atkins et al 1990, Bickerstaff 1990) have shown that the true incidence following a distal radial fracture is of the order of 30%. It seems likely that appropriate studies will demonstrate a similar incidence following other fractures in the lower limb and that the incidence following more minor trauma such as ankle sprains may be higher than has been believed.

The condition is most common in adults between the ages of 40 and 60 years. However no age is exempt and it is becoming increasingly recognized in children, where the presentation and clinical course differ from that seen in adults (Wilder et al 1992). The condition is seen in both sexes and normally the sex distribution reflects the precipitating cause. It is, however, reported to occur more frequently in girls than boys (Wilder et al 1992). All races can be affected by the condition. There is some evidence that it may be more common in the winter months, possibly owing to the cold (Aubert 1980).

Aetiology

The aetiology of RSD is obscure. It seems that there is not one single cause but a variety of precipitating factors which, occurring in individuals with a particular predisposition, result in the disease. The features are almost certainly the result of an abnormal sympathetic reflex.

Langford (1982) has suggested that a persistent painful stimulus is necessary to initiate the condition. However in some cases no such factor can be identified (so called primary or idiopathic algodystrophy). In the majority of cases there is an obvious precipitating event. The most common is trauma, which varies from the very severe injuries of Mitchell's original description (1864) to minor knocks or bruises (Serre et al 1973). Some authors suggest that immobilization rather than the initial trauma may be the precipitating factor (Bernstein et al 1978, Serre et al 1973, Fam & Stein 1981), and untimely or overvigorous rehabilitation following injury has also been suggested as a cause (Savin 1974). It must be remembered that these observations are subjective, and properly controlled prospective studies of the role of immobilization and physiotherapy in the condition have not been undertaken.

The original description of RSD by Mitchell (1864) involved direct trauma to a peripheral nerve as the precipitating cause of the condition. There have also been a number of reports of RSD secondary to irritation of a spinal nerve, either by disc herniation or secondary to bony entrapment in the lateral recess (Oppenheimer 1938, Rosen & Graham 1957, Drucker et al 1959, Serre et al 1973, Karlson et al 1977, Bernini & Simeone 1981). Serre et al (1973) identified 12 cases of lower limb RSD from a series of 188 which were associated with sensory radiculopathy, and Karlson et al (1977) reported two cases in association with lumbar disc protrusion confirmed by radiculopathy. Moretton & Wilson (1970) reported two cases of lower limb RSD as a complication of myelography itself, and Druker et al (1959) reported algodystrophy caused by spinal anaesthesia. Herpes zoster infection may lead to subsequent development of RSD (Südeck 1901, Richardson 1954, Baer 1966), although the majority of these reports refer to the shoulder–hand syndrome.

Cerebrovascular accidents are associated with the subsequent development of RSD (Moskowitz et al 1958, Eto et al 1980). The condition has been reported in association with cervical cord injury, head injury and subarachnoid haemorrhage (Rosen & Graham 1957), brain tumours (Walker et al 1983) and disease of the spinal cord (De Takats 1945, Evans 1947).

Upper limb RSD has been classically described following angina (Steinbroker 1947), myocardial infarction (Froment et al 1956) and arterial or venous thrombosis (De Takets 1945).

Some patients with RSD exhibit a particular personality type, being apparently emotionally labile, insecure, fearful and having a low threshold for pain (De Takats 1943). This type of personality is sometimes termed 'Südecky'.

The combination of adverse emotional sequelae to RSD and the disparity between the appreciated severity of pain and findings on physical examination has led to the suggestion that the pain is psychogenic (Bergan and Conn 1968, Wirth & Rutherford 1971, Hill 1980, Pack et al 1970). Omer and Thomas (1971) found that 45% of their patients required psychiatric consultation and Bernstein (1978) reported similar findings in children suffering from RSD. In contrast, psychiatric problems were not a feature of the series reported by Wilder et al (1992), although in certain patients the symptoms of the condition were amplified by adverse psychological circumstances.

It is, of course, always difficult to know to what extent an apparent psychological abnormality predates RSD and to what extent it is the result of unremitting, severe, chronic pain.

Pelissier et al (1981) applied the Minnesota multi-phasic personality inventory (MMPI) to patients with RSD and noted a tendency towards hysterical or depressive neuroticism. Subbarao & Stillwell (1981) found similar results. In contrast Vincent et al (1982) found great difficulty in applying the MMPI, and using Rorscharch's test they were unable to pinpoint a single abnormality. No study has conclusively proved or disproved an association between a pre-existing abnormality of personality and the occurrence of RSD. It is, however, the common experience of clinicians that patients with the particular personality type outlined above and sometimes described as 'Südecky', tend to have a poor outcome when they develop the condition. This should lead the astute clinician to treat patients with RSD who present with this personality type more vigorously in an attempt to avoid a poor result.

Diabetes mellitus, hyperlipidaemia and hyperthyroidism have all been associated with RSD (Schiano et al 1976, Lequesne et al 1977, Pinals & Jabbs 1972, Doury et al 1981) as has pregnancy (Curtis & Kincaid 1959, Beaulieu et al 1976), although the reported cases almost exclusively involve the hip.

Several forms of drug treatment have been associated with RSD. These include barbiturates (van der Korst et al 1966) antituberculous therapy (Mackewsic & Soo 1961, Good 1970), phenytoin and radioactive iodine for hyperthyroidism (Schiano et al 1976). There is also an increased incidence in smokers (An et al 1988).

Pathogenesis

The pathogenesis of RSD has not been fully elucidated. Any acceptable theory must account for the presence of atypical and excessive pain which is frequently abolished by sympathetic blockade, and for the clinical findings of vasomotor instability, early swelling and late atrophy and contracture.

It seems likely that an initial painful distal stimulus is transferred to the spinal column by way of both somatic and sympathetic afferent fibres. This results in stimulation of the internuncial neurone pool, which induces prolonged overactivity. This is initially dependent on the peripheral stimulus but after a period becomes independent and is further modified by higher neural centres (Livingstone 1938, 1943, Lorente de No 1938, Melzack & Wall 1965).

Support for this theory comes from a number of recent experiments which have shown that patients with algodystrophy have an abnormal difference in cutaneous sensory threshold between the affected limb and the contralateral one in basal conditions, and an abnormal pattern of nerve activity in response to stimulation in both the affected and contralateral limbs. These abnormalities were reversed by sympathetic blockade (Francini et al 1979, Procacci et al 1979). The pathophysiology of the local tissue effects of algodystrophy have been difficult to investigate in the past because of a lack of a large homogeneous population of patients with early algodystrophy. It seems probable that there is a local imbalance in the capillary bed, which leads to capillary stasis, local increased pressure and exudation. These processes would lead to local tissue anoxia, which would cause further stimulation of afferent pain fibres and release of local mediators which maintain the abnormal state (Ficat et al 1971, 1973, Renier et al 1979).

Roberts (1986) has emphasized the role of both low threshold mechanoreceptors and central dorsal horn mechanisms in the pathogenesis of RSD. He suggests that the initial painful stimulus activates unmyelinated nociceptors, which leads to sensitization of wide dynamic range (WDR) neurones in the dorsal horn. The sensitized WDR neurones are now further activated by low-threshold mechanoreceptors, which explains allodynia. Low-threshold mechanoreceptors can also be activated by sympathetic efferent activity and so a vicious cycle incorporating the central nervous system is set up. More recently (Schwartzman 1992) the role of the WDR neurone has been questioned.

Peripherally, sensitization of receptors probably occurs in RSD. Sympathetic activity can activate not only mechanoreceptors but also peripheral nociceptors directly (Campbell et al 1988). It is suggested that α-adrenergic receptors may become expressed on nociceptors following soft tissue or nerve injury and that these receptors can be directly activated by sympathetic discharge through the release of adrenaline. Once again this will lead to a vicious cycle involving sympathetic activity.

It has also been suggested that trauma to a nerve distally causes an abnormal synapse to be set up at the site of the injury (Doupe et al 1944). However these 'ephapses' are found rarely and even then only late in the condition.

Clinical features

RSD generally affects the extremities; thus in the leg, the foot is most commonly involved, followed by the knee.

Typically, but not invariably, it will follow minor trauma such as a sprain. The cardinal features are pain and tenderness, vasomotor instability and abnormalities of sweating, and soft tissue oedema early in the condition, which later gives way to atrophy and loss of joint mobility. Vasomotor instability and swelling are most marked when the condition affects the foot, as opposed to the knee or hip.

The major clinical feature of RSD is persistent pain. This is often described as having a burning quality. Classically the pain of algodystrophy begins some time after the musculoskeletal pain of the precipitating trauma has subsided. The pain of reflex sympathetic dystrophy is of a different type and easily distinguished from the pain of the original trauma. The pain tends to begin distally and radiate more proximally as the condition continues and is normally out of proportion to the initiating cause. Allodynia and hyperpathia are often seen in the condition; however, their absence does not exclude RSD (Merskey 1979). The pain may be aggravated by emotional factors such as fear, anger or a sudden noise. Tenderness is a universal accompaniment of the pain and is associated with a lowering of the threshold to pain in response to applied pressure. This phenomenon has been exploited in the technique of dolorimetry.

Dolorimetry is a reproducible method of quantifying the severity of algodystrophy by comparing the pain threshold to pressure on the affected and unaffected side (Steinbrocker 1949, Hollander & Young 1963, McCarty et al 1965 and 1968, Kozin et al 1976a). This device has been shown to be useful in both upper and lower limb RSD (Atkins & Kanis 1989, Sarangi et al 1991).

Vasomotor changes and abnormalities of sweating are prominent when RSD affects the periphery. The changes are most marked early in the condition when swelling is a feature (Fig. 1) and tend to disappear as the atrophic phase of the condition begins. Classically the vasomotor instability has been described in three phases and these have been used to stage the condition:

Phase 1: In the first few weeks the affected limb is swollen, red, hot and dry (see Fig. 1). This appearance gives way after a few weeks, to

Phase 2: The limb is cold, blue mottled and clammy.

Phase 3: After a further few months, the vasomotor instability fades completely (Fig. 2). Soft tissue atrophy and contractures predominate (Steinbrocker & Argyros 1958, Doury et al 1981, Wilson 1990).

In practice, this classical evolution is rarely seen. It tends to occur in more severe cases, especially when the patient is a 'Südecky' type. In my experience, vasomotor instability is most frequently an abnormal temperature sensitivity and, although it is more prominent early in the condition, it is sometimes seen at a later stage as well.

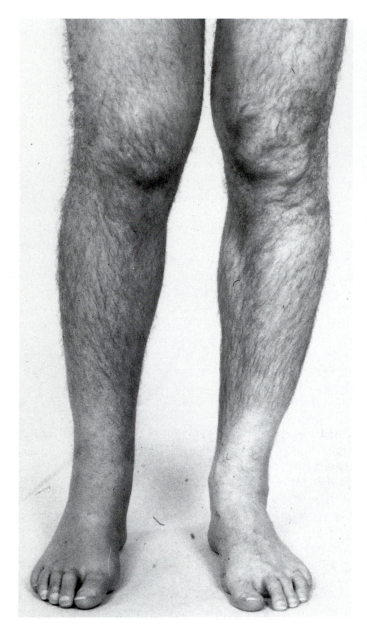

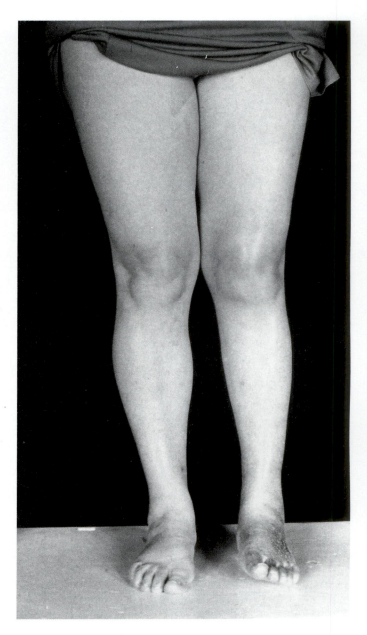

Figure 1

Early RSD affecting the right leg and foot. Swelling is obvious. The leg was hot and pink with no evidence of excessive sweating

Figure 2

Late RSD affecting the left foot and calf. Fixed varus of the foot is seen, with shiny discoloured and atrophic skin. Note the calf wasting

Swelling is an early feature of the condition. The oedema may be pitting. As the condition evolves, the oedema disappears and is replaced by atrophy of all of the soft tissues. At this late stage the skin is thinned with loss of the normal joint creases. Curiously, however, the skin of the plantar surface of the foot is relatively preserved, although the callus pattern is reduced by lack of load bearing. Permanent thinning of the plantar fat pad may cause local overpressure problems. Hair growth is normally diminished but occasionally it is increased. The hairs are often thin, curled and fragile. Nail growth is abnormal. In a mild case there will be some discoloration and pitting; however, in a severe case the nails may be ridged, brittle and sometimes grossly abnormal.

Early in the condition, the loss of joint movement appears to be due to a combination of the swelling and pain, which is made worse by joint movement. As the condition progresses, limitation of joint movement is due to soft tissue contractures. The contractures that affect the foot are usually equinus of the ankle with some varus of the hindfoot. The midfoot usually becomes rigid in a neutral position, although cavus is more common

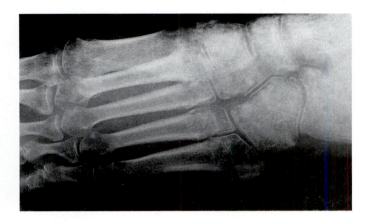

Figure 3

A plain radiograph of a patient suffering from RSD of the foot. The patchy osteoporosis that is characteristic of the early phase of the condition is seen particularly well in the tarsal bones

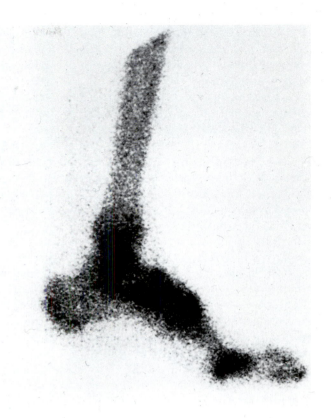

Figure 5

The bone scan in RSD of the foot. There is increased uptake throughout the affected region. The greatest increase in uptake occurs in the periarticular regions. This is a feature of the early stage of the condition

Stage 1: The early part of the condition, dominated by vasomotor instability and swelling. Loss of joint mobility at this stage is primarily due to swelling and pain. Treatment must be started during this stage of the condition if a good result is to be obtained (see Fig. 1).

Stage 2: The vasomotor instability is far less marked and the swelling has given way to severe atrophy. Loss of joint movement is due to contracture. If the patient reaches this stage, then treatment rarely succeeds. Joint mobility is normally lost permanently and it may not be possible to relieve the pain (see Fig. 2).

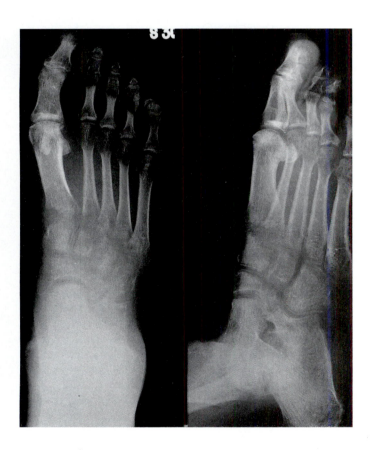

Figure 4

A plain radiograph of a patient suffering from RSD of the foot. Marked bone loss affecting particularly the juxta-articular regions of the tarsus is seen

than planus, perhaps as an association of the hindfoot varus. Intrinsic contracture leads to clawing of the toes.

Rather than dividing the condition into three phases, I prefer to recognise two stages.

Investigations

There is no diagnostic test for RSD. However X-rays, bone scanning, and magnetic resonance image (MRI) scanning may all be helpful.

The radiographic abnormalities are most completely described (Figs 3 and 4). Patchy osteoporosis is seen, and this is most marked in the juxta-intraarticular region. It may be so severe as to mimic erosive changes (Kozin et al 1976b). Late in the condition, there is severe diffuse osteoporosis. These features are those of rapid and excessive osteoclastic activity. They are not diagnostic of RSD.

Technetium-99 labelled diphosphonate bone scanning gives characteristic appearances early in the condition (Fig. 5). The delayed image shows increased uptake. This was originally thought to be confined to the peri-articular region (Kozin et al 1976b, Mackinnon & Holder 1984), but more recently, quantitative studies have shown that the abnormality is, in fact, a diffuse increase in uptake throughout the region affected (Demangeat et al 1988, Atkins et al 1993).

Reports of the appearances of RSD on MRI scanning are few and tend to be anecdotal. The changes seen early in the condition are those of bone and soft tissue oedema.

The degree of osteoporosis may be quantified using densitometry (Bickerstaff et al 1993), and changes in vasomotor function have been investigated using thermography (Perelman et al 1987). These two investi-gations are, however, of little diagnostic use, although in a research situation they may find application.

Algodystrophy does not cause arthritis and indeed maintenance of the joint space is an important finding to aid differentiation from early arthritis. Because the patients defunction their limbs so successfully in the condition, fractures are rare.

The full blood count, erythrocyte sedimentation rate, viscosity and C-reactive protein levels are normal, as is the remainder of the serum biochemistry.

Differential diagnosis

RSD presents with such a variety of clinical manifesta-tions that a wide variety of differential diagnoses may be considered. The most common is that of a swollen, tender foot. Trauma and fracture, cellulitis, arthritis and malignancy are the most common alternative diagnoses. The diagnosis of RSD is essentially a clinical one. A patient presenting with pain, vasomotor instability and sweating with swelling and loss of movement of a foot and refusing to bear weight, presents little difficulty. It is the marginal case where diagnosis can be difficult.

Kozin et al (1981) have suggested a classification into definite RSD (pain, tenderness, oedema, vasomotor and sudomotor changes), probable RSD (pain, tenderness, and either vasomotor and sudomotor changes or swelling), possible RSD (vasomotor or sudomotor changes), and doubtful RSD (unexplained pain and tenderness). Although this approach has attractions, in orthopaedic practice it is more important to exclude RSD than to categorize it in this way.

If there is clinical doubt concerning the presence of RSD, I find it useful to perform comparative radiographs, undertaking an anteroposterior radiograph of both feet side by side on the same X-ray film and, if indicated, similar anteroposterior radiographs of both ankles and a three-phase bone scan. If the radiographs do not show osteoporosis and the bone scan is normal, the patient is extremely unlikely to have RSD.

Management

RSD is an extremely difficult condition to treat and the patient may be difficult to cope with. From a surgical perspective there are several important considerations.

1. Not every patient who develops early RSD will go on to a chronic condition or to develop contractures. The condition is normally self-limiting and mild.
2. Most patients who develop RSD are sensible people who are extremely worried at the development of pain that they cannot understand.
3. A patient with RSD who is submitted to surgery may well become significantly worse.
4. The best results of treatment of RSD are obtained when the condition is treated early.

The key to successful management of RSD is therefore to make the diagnosis early, treat the patient sympa-thetically and avoid surgery where possible. It is thus necessary to keep a very high index of clinical suspicion concerning the diagnosis. RSD is emerging (as outlined above) as an extremely common consequence of trauma, including surgical trauma, which is normally self-limiting. It is not, therefore, necessarily reprehensible to have caused a case of RSD through one's surgery. It is, however, unfortunate if diagnosis and subsequent treat-ment are delayed, and such a delay may contribute to a poor outcome.

The first-line treatment of RSD is reassurance, sympa-thetic physiotherapy and simple analgesia. Nonsteroidal anti-inflammatory drugs appear to give better pain relief than opiates. The aim of these treatments is to maintain the range of joint movement so that when the condition has passed off there are no residual contractures.

For the patient in whom these simple measures are not effective, particularly if there is development of an equinus deformity and refusal to bear weight, it is sometimes useful to perform an examination under anaesthetic and place the patient in a below-knee weight bearing plaster with the foot in neutral. This presupposes that the condition has not progressed to fixed contrac-ture and that therefore the foot is correctable to neutral under anaesthetic. Caution must be employed in this approach, since the patient may find the plaster too painful.

Beyond these simple options, a multitude of different sorts of treatment have been suggested. These are often unsuccessful and many patients are left with pain and significant disability. There are very few well set up placebo-controlled trials of treatment of RSD, and the wide variation in symptoms and diagnostic criteria and outcome measures and the tendency for RSD to remit spontaneously mean that most of the recommendations for treatment are anecdotal. At this stage it is wise to involve a pain specialist and continue treatment on a shared basis.

Sympathetic blockade is the mainstay of treatment for the serious or intractable case. Some authorities would suggest that abolition of pain in response to a sympathetic block is a necessary diagnostic criterion for RSD. However, while this may be true (by definition) of sympathetically maintained pain, it is my view that RSD is a clinical diagnosis and I not infrequently find that in cases with clinically definite RSD, the response to sympathetic blockade may be disappointing. Where the first sympathetic block fails, repeated blocks may be successful. However, there is clearly little point in pursuing a painful form of treatment that is ineffective.

The exact form of sympathetic interruption varies. Lumbar paravertebral blockade has been shown to be an effective form of treatment compared to conservative management in a retrospective study (Wang et al 1985) and in the upper limb intravenous guanethidine blockade has been compared successfully to stellate ganglion blockade (Bonelli et al 1983). The advantage of guanethidine blockade is that, although it requires careful supervision, it is easier to administer than paravertebral sympathetic blockade. Recently, however, it has been suggested that a significant part of the effect of guanethidine blockade is due to placebo (Glynn et al 1981).

Epidural blockade has also been used, particularly in reflex sympathetic dystrophy of the knee. The combination of sympathetic blockade and analgesia allow mobilization using continuous passive motion. Recently, a randomized cross-over study of 15 patients with chronic lower limb RSD has found little difference between guanethidine blockade and epidural anaesthesia and has suggested that these treatments benefit only a minority of these patients whose mean duration of disease was nearly three years (Pountain et al 1993).

A number of other treatments have been suggested. Corticosteroids have been used (Kozin et al 1981, Christensen et al 1982); however, their benefit is not universally accepted. Calcitonin is, in my experience, sometimes effective. However, in recent studies, benefit has been marginal or not significant (Gobelet et al 1986, Bickerstaff & Kanis 1991).

Treatment with α-adrenergic blockade (Abram & Lightfoot 1981, Ghostine et al 1984) and a variety of other vasodilators (Prough et al 1985, Moesker et al 1985) have been recommended. Evidence for efficacy of these drugs, backed by well-constructed prospective randomized placebo-controlled studies, is lacking.

Transcutaneous nerve stimulation has been reported to be effective, particularly in children (Kesler et al 1988). Finally acupuncture may be efficacious (Fielka et al 1993).

The role of surgery in treatment of reflex sympathetic dystrophy is very limited. The use of surgery to correct fixed contractures is controversial and, in my experience, the need is rare. Surgery represents a painful stimulus and there is therefore a risk of exacerbating the RSD or precipitating a new attack, and this risk must be very carefully balanced against the proposed benefit. Contractures usually involve all of the soft tissues and therefore, where contemplated, surgical releases must be radical and include not merely tendon lengthening but capsulotomies.

This sort of surgery should be kept until the active phase of RSD has completely passed and probably there should be a gap of at least a year since the patient last experienced pain and swelling. The operation must be performed carefully and with minimal soft tissue trauma. Expectations must be limited and it is essential to provide adequate analgesia in the postoperative period. Thus the use of indwelling epidural catheters has been advocated. Some would suggest that any tendency to precipitate RSD can be minimized by a prophylactic lumbar sympathetic block or guanethidine. I have no direct experience of this.

References

Abram S E, Lightfoot R W 1981 Treatment of long-standing causalgia with prazosin. Reg Anaesth 6: 79–81

An H S, Hawthorne K B, Jackson W T 1988 Reflex sympathetic dystrophy and cigarette smoking. J Hand Surg 13A: 470–472

Atkins R M 1989 Algodystrophy. DM Thesis, Oxford

Atkins R M, Kanis J A 1989 The use of dolorimetry in the assessment of post traumatic algodystrophy of the hand. Br J Rheumatol 28: 404–409

Atkins R M, Duckworth T, Kanis J A 1989 Algodystrophy following Colles' fracture. J Hand Surg 14B: 161–164

Atkins R M, Duckworth T, Kanis J A 1990 Features of algodystrophy following Colles' fracture. J Bone Joint Surg 72B: 105–110

Atkins R M, Tindale W, Bickerstaff D, Kanis J A 1993 Quantitative bone scintigraphy in reflex sympathetic dystrophy. Br J Rheumatol 32: 41–45

Aubert P G 1980 Etude sur le risque algodystrophique. Thèse pour le doctorat en médecin diplome d'état. University of Paris, Val de Marne

Bacorn R W, Kurtz J F 1953 Colles' fracture: a study of 2000 cases from the New York State Workmen's Compensation Board. J Bone Joint Surg 35A: 643–658

Baer R D 1966 Shoulder hand syndrome. Its recognition and management. South Med J 59: 790–794

Beaulieu J G, Razzano C D, Levine R B 1976 Transient osteoporosis of the hip in pregnancy. Clin Orthop 115: 165–168

Bergan J J, Conn J 1968 Sympathectomy for pain relief. Med Clin North Am 52: 147–159

Bernini P M, Simeone F A 1981 Reflex sympathetic dystrophy associated with low lumbar disc herniation. Spine 6: 180–184

Bernstein B H, Singsen B H, Kent J J, et al 1978 Reflex neurovascular dystrophy in children. J Pediatr 93: 211–215

Bickerstaff D R 1990 The natural history of post traumatic algodystrophy. MD Thesis, University of Sheffield

Bickerstaff D R, Kanis J A 1991 The use of nasal calcitonin in the treatment of post traumatic algodystrophy. Br J Rheumatol 30: 291–294

Bickerstaff D R, Charlesworth D, Kanis J A 1993 Changes in cortical and trabecular bone in algodystrophy. Br J Rheumatol 32: 46–51

Bonelli S, Conoscente F, Movilia P G, Restelli L, Francucci B, Grossi E 1983 Regional intravenous guanethidine vs stellate ganglion block in reflex sympathetic dystrophies: a randomised trial. Pain 16: 297–307

Campbell J N, Raga S N, Meyer R A 1988 Painful sequelae of nerve injury. In: Dubner R, Gebhart GF, Bond MR (eds). Proceedings of the 5th World Congress on Pain. Elsevier Science Publishers, Amsterdam. pp. 135–143

Christensen K, Jensen E M, Noer I 1982 The reflex sympathetic dystrophy syndrome. Response to treatment with systemic cortico-steroids. Acta Chir Scand 148: 653–655

Curtis P H, Kincaid W E 1959 Transitory demineralisation of the hip in pregnancy. J Bone Joint Surg 41A: 1327–1332

Demangeat J, Constantinesco A, Brunot B, Foucher G, Farcot J. 1988 Three-phase bone scanning in reflex sympathetic dystrophy of the hand. J Nucl Med 29: 26–32

De Takats G 1937 Reflex dystrophy of the extremities. Arch Surg 34: 939–956

De Takats G 1943 The nature of painful vasodilatation in causalgic states. Arch Neurol 53: 318–326

De Takats G 1945 Causalgic states in peace and war. JAMA 128: 699–704

Doupe J, Cullin C H, Chance G Q 1944 Post traumatic pain in causalgic syndrome. J Neurosurg Psychiatry 733

Doury P, Dirheimer Y, Pattin S 1981 Algodystrophy: diagnosis and therapy of a frequent disease of the locomotor apparatus. Springer Verlag, Berlin

Drucker W R, Hubay C A, Holden W D, Bucknovic J A 1959 Pathogenesis of post traumatic sympathetic dystrophy. Am J Surg 97: 454–465

Eto F, Yoshikawa M, Ueda S, Hirai S 1980 Post hemiplegic shoulder hand syndrome with special reference to related cerebral localiza-tion. J Am Geriatr Soc 28: 13–17

Evans J A 1947 Reflex sympathetic dystrophy: report on 57 cases. Ann Intern Med 26: 417–426

Fam A G, Stein J 1981 Disappearance of chondrocalcinosis following reflex sympathetic dystrophy. Arthritis Rheum 24: 747–749

Ficat P, Allet J, Pujol M, Vidal R 1971 Traumatisme dystrophie reflexe et ostéonécrose de la tête femorale. Ann Chir 25: 911–917

Ficat P, Allet J, Lartigue G, Pujol M, Tramm A 1973 Algodystrophie reflexe post traumatique. Etude Hémodynamique et Anatomopathologique. Rev Chir Orthop 59: 401–414

Field J, Warwick D, Bannister G C 1992 The features of algodystro-phy 10 years after Colles' fracture. J Hand Surg 17B: 318–320

Fielka V, Resch K L, Ritter-Diuetrich D, et al 1993 Acupuncture for reflex sympathetic dystrophy. Arch Int Med 82: 728–732

Francini F, Zoppi M, Maresca M, Procacci P 1979 Skin potential and EMG changes induced by electrical stimulation. 1. Normal man in arousing a non-enrousing environment. Appl Neurophysiol 42: 113–124

Froment D, Perrin A, Goni N A, Jandet R 1956 Periarthrites scapulo-humérales et autres manifestations neurotrophiques d'origine coronar-ienne. Troisième Conference du Rhumatisme: Aix les Bains 1956

Frykman G 1967 Fracture of the distal radius and its complications including the shoulder hand syndrome. Acta Orthop Scand Suppl 108

Ghostine S Y, Comair Y G, Turner D M, Kassell N F, Azar C G 1984 Phenoxybenzamine in the treatment of causalgia. Report of 40 cases. J Neurosurg 60: 1263–1268

Glick E N, Helal B 1976 Post traumatic neurodystrophy. Treatment by corticosteroids. Hand 8: 45–47

Glynn C J, Baselow R W, Walsh J A 1981 Pain relief following post ganglionic sympathetic blockade with intravenous guanethidine. Br J Anaesth 53: 1297–1301

Gobelet C, Meier J, Schaffner W, Bischol-Delaloye A, Gerster J, Burckhardt P 1986 Calcitonin and reflex sympathetic dystrophy syndrome. Clin Rheumatol 5: 382–388

Good A E 1970 Rheumatism and chemotherapy of tuberculosis. Ann Intern Med 72: 752–753

Green J T, Gay F H 1956 Colles' fracture residual disability. Am J Surg 91: 636–642

Hill G J 1980 Outpatient surgery. W B Saunders, Philadelphia. p. 684

Hollander J L, Young D G 1963 The palpameter: an instrument for quantitation of joint tenderness. Arthritis Rheum 6: 277

Homans J 1940 Minor causalgia. A hyperaesthetic neurovascular syndrom. N Engl J Med 222: 870–874

Janig W 1990 The sympathetic nervous system in pain: Physiology and pathophysiology. In: Stanton-Hicks M (ed) Pain in the Sympathetic Nervous System. Kluwer Academic Publishers, Massachusetts. pp. 17–89

Karlson D H, Simon H, Wegner W 1977 Bone scanning in diagnosis of reflex sympathetic dystrophy secondary to herniated lumbar discs. Neurology 27: 791–793

Kesler R W, Saulsbury F T, Miller L T, Rowlingson J C 1988 Reflex sympathetic dystrophy in children: treatment with transcutaneous electric nerve stimulation. Pediatrics 82: 728–732

Kozin F, McCarty D J, Sims J, Genant H 1976a The reflex sympa-thetic dystrophy syndrome. I. Clinical and histological studies: evidence for bilaterality, response to corticosteroids, and articular involvement. Am J Med 60: 321–331

Kozin F, Genant H K, Bekerman C, McCarty D J 1976b The reflex sympathetic dystrophy syndrome. II. Roentgenographic and scinti-graphic evidence of bilaterality and of periarticular attenuation. Am J Med 60: 332–338

Kozin F, Ryan L M, Carerra G F, Soin J S, Wortmann R L 1981 The reflex sympathetic dystrophy syndrome (RSDS); III. Scintigraphic studies, further evidence for the therapeutic efficacy of systemic corticosteroids and proposed diagnostic criteria. Am J Med 70: 23–30

Langford L L 1982 Reflex sympathetic dystrophy. In: Green DP (ed) Operative Hand Surgery. Churchill Livingstone, New York. pp. 539–563

Lequesne M, Dang N, Benfasson M, Mery C 1977 Increased associa-tion of diabetes mellitus with capsulitis of the shoulder in shoul-der hand syndrome. Scand J Rheumatol 6: 53–56

Lidström A 1959 Fractures of the distal end of radius. A clinical and statistical study of end results. Acta Orthop Scand Suppl 41

Livingstone W K 1938 Post traumatic pain syndromes. Interpretation of underlying pathological physiology. West J Surg Obstet Gynecol 46: 341–426

Livingstone W K 1943 Pain Mechanisms: A Physiological Interpretation of Causalgia and its Related States. MacMillan, New York

Lorente de No R 1938 Analysis of the activity of the chain of inter-nuncial neurones. J Neurophysiol 1: 207–244

Louyot P, Gaucher A, Montet Y, Combebias J F 1967 Algodystrophie du membre inférieur. Rev Rhum Mal Osteoartic 34: 733–737

McCarty D J, Gatter R A, Phelps P 1965 A dolorimeter for the quantification of articular tenderness. Arthritis Rheum 8: 551–559

McCarty D J, Gatter R A, Steele A O 1968 A 20 lb dolorimeter for quantitation of articular tenderness. Arthritis Rheum 11: 696–698

Mackewsic A B, Soo J M 1961 Clinical and metabolic studies of the shoulder hand syndrome in tuberculosis patients. Arthritis Rheum 4: 4–6

Mackinnon S E, Holder L E 1984 The use of three phase radio nucleotide bone scanning in the diagnosis of reflex sympathetic dystrophy. J Hand Surg 9A: 556–563

Melzack R, Wall P D 1965 Pain mechanisms: new theory. Science 150: 971

Merskey H 1979 Pain terms: a list with definitions and notes on usage. Pain 6: 249–252

Mitchell S W, Morehouse G G, Keen W W 1864 Gunshot wounds and other injuries of nerves. JB Lippincott, Philadelphia

Moesker A, Boersma F T, Scheijgrond H W, Cortvriendt W 1985 Treatment of post traumatic sympathetic dystrophy (Südeck's atrophy) with guanethidine and ketanserin. Pain Clinic 1: 171–176

Moretton L B, Wilson M 1971 Severe reflex algodystrophy (Südek's atrophy) as a complication of mylography. Report of two cases. Am J Roentgenol 10: 156–158

Moskowitz E, Bishop H F, Pe H, Shibutlni K 1958 Post hemiplegic reflex sympathetic dystrophy. JAMA 167: 836–838

Müller M E, Allgower M, Schneider R, Willenegger H 1979 Manual of Internal Fixation. Techniques Recommended by the AO Group, 2nd edition. Springer-Verlag, Berlin

Nonne N 1901–1902 Über die radiolographisch Nachweisbare akute und kronische "Knochenatrophie" (Südeck bei Nerven-Erkrankungen). Fortschr Geb Rontgenstr 5: 293–297

Omer G, Thomas S 1971 Treatment of causalgia: review of cases at Brook General Hospital. Texas Med 67: 93–96

Oppenheimer A 1938 The swollen atrophic hand. Surg Gynecol Obstet 67: 446–454

Pack T J, Martin G M, Magnus J L, Kavanaugh G J 1970 Reflex sympathetic dystrophy: review of 140 cases. Minn Med 53: 507–512

Patman R D, Thompson J E, Persson A V 1973 Management of post traumatic pain syndromes. Report of 113 cases. Am Surg 177: 780–787

Perelman R B, Adler D, Hympreys M 1987 Reflex sympathetic dystrophy: electronic thermography as an aid to diagnosis. Orthop Rev 1987; 16: 53–58

Pelissier J, Touchon J, Besset A, Chartier J, Blotman F, Baldy Molinier M, Simon L 1981. La personnalite du sujet souvrant d'algodystrophie sympathique reflexe. Etudes Psychometriques par le test MMPI. Rheumatologie 1981; 23: 351–354

Pinals R S, Jabbs J M Type 4 hypolipoproteinaemia and transient osteoporosis (letter). Lancet 1972; 1: 929

Plewes L W 1956 Südeck's atrophy of the hand. J Bone Joint Surg 38B: 195–203

Poole C 1973 Colles' fracture. A prospective study of treatment. J Bone Joint Surg 55B: 540–544

Pountain G D, Chard M D, Smith E M, Hazleman B L, Jenner J R, Hughes D L 1993 Comparison of guanethidine blocks and epidural analgesia in longstanding algodystrophy of the lower limb. Br J Rheumatol 32 (suppl 2): 53

Procacci P, Francini F, Maresca M, Zoppi M 1979 Skin potential and EMG changes induced by cutaneous electrical stimulation. 2. Subjects with reflex sympathetic dystrophies. Appl Neuro Physiol 42: 125–134

Prough D S, McLeskey C H, Poehling C G et al 1985 Efficacy of oral nifedipine in the treatment of reflex sympathetic dystrophy. Anesthesiol 62: 796–799

Renier J C, Moreau R, Benat M, Basle M, Jallet P, Minier J F 1979 Apport des explorations isotopiques dynamiques dans l'étude des algodystrophies. Rev Rheum Mal Osteoartic 46: 235–241

Richardson A T 1954 Shoulder hand syndrome following herpes zoster. Am J Phys Med 2: 132–134

Roberts W J 1986 A hypothesis on the physiological basis for causalgia and related pains. Pain 24: 297–311

Rosen P S, Graham W 1957 The shoulder hand syndrome: historical review with observations on 73 patients. Can Med Assoc J 77: 86–91

Sarangi P, Ward A, Smith D J, Atkins R M 1991 The use of dolorimetry in the assessment of post traumatic algodystrophy of the foot. Foot 1: 157–163

Sarangi P, Smith E J, Ward A, Atkins R M 1993 Algodystrophy and osteoporosis following Colles' fracture. J Bone Joint Surg 75B: 450–452

Savin R 1974 La responsabilité de la ré-éducation fonctionnelle dans le declenchenent des algodystrophie reflexes post-traumatiques des membres. Memoirs CES Rheumatologies, University of Paris

Schiano A, Eisinger J, Aquaviva P C 1976 Les algodystrophies. Laboratoire Armour-Montagu, Paris

Schwartzman R J 1992 Reflex sympathetic dystrophy and causalgia. Neurol Clin 10: 953–973

Serre H, Simon L, Claustre J, Sany J 1973 Formes cliniques des algodystrophies sympathetiques des membres inférieurs. Rheumatologie 23: 43–54

Steinbrocker O 1947 Painful homolateral disability of the shoulder and hand with swelling and atrophy of the hand. Ann Rheum Dis 6: 80–84

Steinbrocker O 1949 A simple pressure gauge for measured palpation in physical diagnosis and therapy. Arch Phys Med 30: 289

Steinbrocker O, Argyros T G 1958 The shoulder hand syndrome: present status as a diagnostic and therapeutic entity. Med Clin North Am 42: 1533–1553

Stewart H D, Innes A R, Burke F D 1985 The hand complications of Colles' fractures. J Hand Surg 10B: 103–106

Subbarao J, Stillwell G K 1981 Reflex sympathetic dystrophy syndrome of the upper extremity: analysis of total outcome of management in 125 cases. Arch Phys Med Rehabil 62: 549–554

Südeck P 1900 Über die acute entzündliche Knochenatrophie. Arch Klin 762: 147–156

Südeck P 1901–1902 Uber die akute (reflektorische) Knockenatrophie nach Entzündungen und Verletzungen an den Extremitäten und ihre klinischen Erscheinungen. Fortschr Geb Rontgenstr 5: 277–293

van der Korst J K, Colenbrander H, Cats A 1962 Phenobarbitol and the shoulder hand syndrome. Ann Rheum Dis 25: 553–555

Vincent G, Ernst J, Henniaux M, Beaubigny M 1982 Essais d'aproche psychologique dans les algoneurodystrophies. Rev Rhum 49: 767–769

Walker J, Belsole R, Jermain B 1983 Shoulder hand syndrome in patients with intracranial neoplasms. Hand 15: 347–351

Wang J K, Johnson K A, Ilstrup D M 1985 Sympathetic blocks for reflex sympathetic dystrophy. Pain 23: 13–17

Watson Jones R 1952 Fractures in Joint Injuries, 4th Edition. E S Livingstone, Edinburgh and London

Wilder R T, Berde C B, Wolohan M, Vieyra M A, Masek B J, Micheli L J 1992 Reflex sympathetic dystrophy in children. J Bone Joint Surg 74A: 910–919

Wilson P R 1990 Sympathetically mediated pain: diagnosis, measurement, and efficacy of treatment. In: Staon-Hicks M (ed) Pain and the Sympathetic Nervous System. Kluwer Academic Publishers, Boston. pp. 90–123

Wirth F P, Rutherford R B 1971 A civilian experience with causalgia. Arch Surg 100: 633–638

IX.8 Osteochondritides

Pierce E Scranton Jr and David I Rowley

Osteochondroses have been described in over 50 anatomic sites. We are concerned here with the description of the occurrence and treatment of those osteochondritides in the foot. Table 1 illustrates the classification of common osteochondritides of the foot and their more common eponyms. This classification is based on anatomic location, because the aetiologies of these osteochondritides may vary and, as yet, the aetiologies have not been clearly defined. There has been little recent activity in taking forward the issues of aetiology or management of the osteochondritides around the foot.

Clearly, a combination of trauma or increased stress, coupled with vascular embarrassment, may be implicated in the aetiology of a majority of lower extremity osteochondroses. There is a very high incidence of trauma in association with osteochondritis dissecans of the talus, and a high association of increased mechanical stress seen in so-called 'Sever's disease', Freiberg's infraction, and in the osteochondritides of the sesamoids. The vascularity of these bones may be compromised, either because of increased venous pressure secondary to 'sludging' with resultant infarction, or because of frank transection of the blood supply, such as when a severe ankle inversion avulses a transchondral chip of talar dome. A consequence of tarsal or metatarsal avascular necrosis in growing children is the interruption of enchondral ossification with secondary deformity or later fragmentation of the bone. The hallmark of treatment, then, is the protection of the avascular bone from deforming forces until revascularization and structural stability return.

In considering the embryological and postnatal development of the human foot, certain development patterns are seen, which may later predispose to the occurrence of osteochondritides. Most obvious is the pattern of development of the longer second metatarsal beginning at 6 months. Excessive length certainly predisposes to increased stress and, possibly, Freiberg's infraction. The delay in ossification of the navicular in males correlates well with the increased incidence of Köhler's disease.

The talus (osteochondritis dissecans)

Patients with a history of ankle sprain who present with persistent ankle pain must be suspected of having osteochondritis dissecans of the talus (Biedert 1991). In fact, this represents a transchondral fracture of the medial or lateral aspect of the dome of the talus. A history of trauma is generally obtained in patients presenting with this lesion. Berndt & Harty (1959) were able to reproduce these fractures in cadaver specimens through two mechanisms: strong inversion of the foot with a dorsiflexed ankle produced a lateral dome fracture, and inversion with a plantar flexed foot and lateral rotation of the tibia produced medial dome fractures. Alexander & Lichtman (1980) found trauma associated with this lesion in 92% of their Armed Forces patients. Males predominate in presentation (70%).

Radiographic diagnosis of the transchondral fracture is sometimes difficult, owing to bony overlap in the talocrural joint, as well as to overlap produced by the dome of the talus itself. It has been most helpful in suspected cases to take mortise radiographs of the ankle with the foot at neutral, and at maximum plantar and dorsiflexion. These views assist not only in diagnosing the transchondral fracture, but in localizing it anteriorly or posteriorly. A fracture apparent only in the plantarflexed X-ray is posterior; if seen only in the dorsiflexion film it is anterior. Localization of anatomical site reduces the necessity of performing an unnecessary medial malleolar osteotomy in the surgical exposure of smaller, medial transchondral fractures.

MRI (Fig. 1) has proven itself a valuable way to obtain a visual impression of the ankle and may also be used to get a functional image of any pathology (Dipaolo et al 1991, Kabbani & Mayer 1994, Wester et al 1994, Cova et al 1995).

An anteromedial or posteromedial arthrotomy or arthroscopy will suffice to provide adequate visualization. An arthrogram can also be particularly helpful in determining both the size of the fragment and whether it has separated from the talus (Fig. 2). A classification (Stage I–IV) has been developed based on the degree of fragment separation, with Stage IV lesions having the fragment completely displaced in the joint. However, treatment is based on symptoms and the size of the fragment. 'Staging' a transchondral talar dome fracture is of descriptive value only.

Table 1 Common osteochondritides of the foot

Talus	Osteochondritis dissecans
Calcaneous	'Sever's disease', 'pump bumps' etc.
Navicular	Köhler's disease
Metatarsals	Hallux rigidus, Freiberg's infraction
Sesamoids	Stress fractures, osteochondritis dissecans

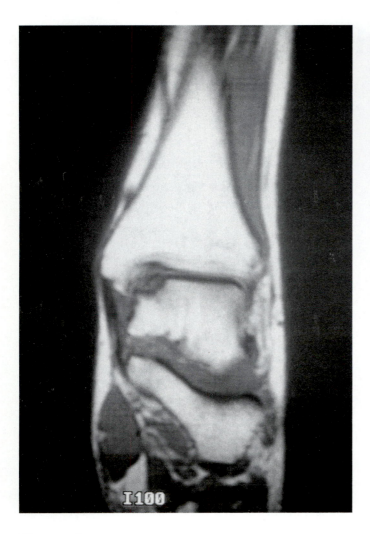

Figure 1

An anteroposterior MRI revealing a Berndt-Harty Grade III osteochondral defect

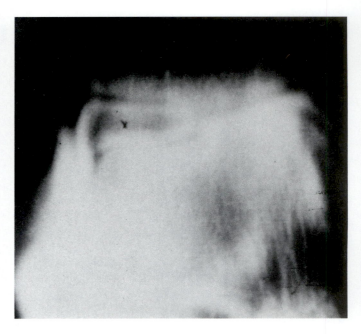

Figure 2

An arthrogram of a painful ankle revealing a large transchondral fracture with dye beneath the fragment, indicating that this fragment is loose

The treatment of transchondral fractures in children should initially be conservative. These fractures are generally not diagnosed at the time of injury, but later, when the symptom of an intermittent, sharp ankle pain with activity persists. In my experience, these talar dome fragments are small (less than 5 mm). Once the diagnosis is made, treatment should be by the application of a non-weight-bearing cast for six weeks, followed by a walking cast for a further six weeks.

Conservative treatment in older adolescents or adults is less likely to be helpful. Berndt & Harty (1959) have reported the results of nonsurgical treatment in 149 patients: 74% – poor, 9% – fair, and 17% – good. In contrast, operative results in adult patients are good 88% – good, 8% – fair, and 4% – poor. Operative treatment varies with the size of fragment and reported results of such treatment are variable (Bruns & Rosenbach 1992, Ly & Fallat 1993). Small transchondral fractures are treated by removing the fragment, curetting and drilling the talar bed; then non-weight-bearing, free ankle motion for 6 weeks. Large medial talar fractures may require a malleolar osteotomy for better exposure. To secure the medial malleolus after treating the talar fracture, the screw hole should be *predrilled* before the osteotomy is made. The talar fragment may be excised, followed by curettage and drilling of the talar bed. In my experience, several patients have presented with extremely large transchondral fractures (greater than one quarter of the articular surface), and these have been treated by curettage and drilling of the talar bed, followed by fixation of the fragment, using retrograde 0.62-mm diameter Kirschner wires. A non-weight-bearing cast is applied for 6 weeks. The wires are then removed in the clinic, followed by the application of a walking cast for a further 6 weeks.

The calcaneum

Previously, painful heels in children were misinterpreted as representing avascular necrosis of the calcaneal apophysis, or Sever's disease. The increased radiodensity of the calcaneal apophysis (Fig. 3) was finally recognized by Ferguson & Gingrich (1959) as representing the normal pattern of apophyseal ossification. Since this classic paper, many aetiologies of pain in the heels of children have been described. However, true avascular necrosis of the calcaneal apophysis has never been documented.

In the female, the ossification centre of the calcaneal apophysis appears at an average age of 5.6 years. In males, it appears at an average of 7.9 years. There is broad variation, with the male apophyseal ossification centre appearing anywhere between 6 and 10 years. From the time of appearance, it takes an average of 7.1 years for the apophysis fully to develop and fuse to the body of the calcaneus.

During apophyseal development, flecks of calcification are first seen, heralding the appearance of the ossific nucleus. Frequently, several ossification centres may form (see Fig. 3), developing independently, but coalescing to form the mature calcaneum. Variations in the development of the calcaneal apophysis can predispose to various pain syndromes in the heels of children, which were originally misinterpreted as avascular necrosis.

Athletically-oriented children between the ages of 9 and 12 years are often seen with painful heels. These children are frequently involved in sports, such as basketball or gymnastics, in which repetitive impact on the heel occurs. Symptoms of pain are gradual in onset, and generally not related to a specific traumatic event. Repetitive rebounding drills in basketball and practising 'dismounts' in gymnastics are most common, in my experience, in producing symptoms of heel pain.

Examination of the child reveals complaints of specific exquisite pain with deep pressure over a localized area of the calcaneal apophysis. The Achilles tendon, plantar fascia, and retrocalcaneal bursal area are entirely asymptomatic. Figure 3 illustrates such a patient who has the normal variation of multiple ossification centres of the calcaneal apophysis. However, on the right foot, the more superior fissure was exquisitely painful with deep pressure and this pressure reproduced the patient's symptoms, experienced when practising gymnastics. A technetium 99 bone scan with pinhole collimation revealed the predictable increased activity in both apophyses, but a substantial increase in activity at the right superior 'fissure'. Clearly, this represented an apophyseal stress fracture through the weaker cartilaginous junction between two separate ossification centres.

The treatment for apophyseal stress fractures is, of course, rest. Experience shows that cessation of repetitive impact on the heel for three weeks will generally eliminate the symptoms. A promising young athlete does not have to give up the sport completely, only modify the practice. Approximately 20 children have been seen in whom the diagnosis of calcaneal apophyseal stress fracture was certain, and only two had persistent symptoms which required 3 weeks' casting before symptoms subsided.

Patients may be seen with painful heels in association with a prominence of the posterior calcaneus. Chronic pressure of the shoe's heel counter over this bony prominence leads to symptoms of painful bursitis. This syndrome has been called 'pump bump', so named for women wearing fashionable 'pumps', presenting with

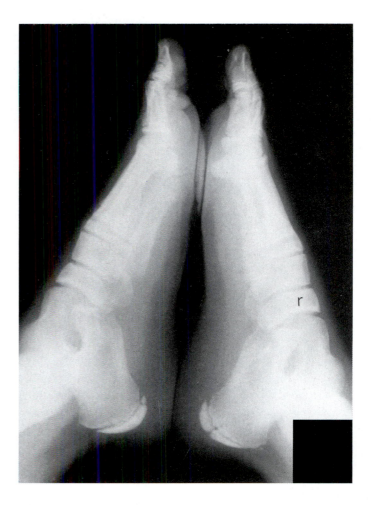

Figure 3

The lateral radiograph of a 10-year-old gymnast with separate calcaneal ossification centers and a painful right stress fracture. Note the relative increased radiodensity of the apophysis

chronic calcaneal bursitis in association with the constant heel counter pressure.

True bony protrusions of the posterior calcaneum do occur, however, and these will interfere substantially with shoe wear. Here again, careful examination of the Achilles tendon and plantar fascia is unremarkable. Symptoms are specifically located over the calcaneal prominence, with some radiation through the inflamed bursae, which may communicate with the retrocalcaneal bursae.

Radiographs of the calcaneus are helpful in determining the size of the prominence, utilizing the lateral, oblique, and Harris views when necessary. The symptoms are produced by mechanical irritation of the heel counter over the prominence, and treatment is therefore directed towards eliminating the mechanical irritant. An alteration in shoe wear is important, and protective 'doughnut padding' with felt or foam rubber can be helpful. When symptoms of bursitis are severe, a single bursal injection with cortisone and 1% lignocaine solution is helpful, and the lignocaine's immediate anaesthetic effect will help confirm the diagnosis. Care should be taken not to inject the Achilles tendon. The injection may be supplemented with twice daily ice cube massage for 10 minutes, and an anti-inflammatory medication.

When symptoms are chronic and secondary to a large posterior bony prominence, surgery is indicated (see further Chapter V.6). The operative incision should be made on either side, closest to the prominence. A posterior incision over the Achilles tendon should be avoided. Adequate bone should be resected with an oscillating saw or osteotome, removing the bursae as well. The Achilles tendon and its insertion distally should be protected. On the medial side, care should be taken to protect the calcaneal branch of the posterior tibial nerve. If a lateral approach is used, the sural nerve should be identified and protected. I prefer to use a *small* amount of bone wax to prevent excessive cancellous bone bleeding and the recurrence of a protruding spike. Antibiotic irrigation is used, and the patient immobilized in a short leg walking cast until the wound is healed. Early motion before the wound is healed should be discouraged, as an infection would be disastrous for both the Achilles tendon or calcaneus. Experience shows that operative intervention for 'pump bumps' is rarely indicated, and patients should be discouraged from surgical treatment, unless prolonged conservative therapy fails. It is far easier to fit shoes to the foot, than to cut the foot to fit shoes.

In children, heel pain from sources other than those mentioned above is uncommon. Plantar fasciitis is not seen in children, though traumatic plantar fascial ruptures do occur. Achilles tendinitis has been seen occasionally, and it is easily treated with rest, deep heat, and salicylate therapy. A tight heel cord may be seen in children experiencing rapid growth, but this generally will produce pes valgus, not Achilles tendinitis. Osteomyelitis occurs in the calcaneum, presenting as heel pain in children who previously stepped upon a foreign body. In the paediatric population, however, heel pain in association with stress fractures, or bursitis associated with calcaneal protuberances are the most common clinical entities.

The navicular

In 1923, Köhler described an osteochondritis of the tarsal navicular, now referred to as Köhler's disease. It has also been called Panner's disease, Köhler–Mouchet disease, naviculare pedis retardum, tarsal scaphoiditis and osteoarthrosis juvenilis. Its aetiology originally was thought to be tuberculosis, or some unknown inflammatory process. We now know that Köhler's disease represents avascular necrosis of the tarsal navicular.

Males predominate, at a ratio to females of about 6:1, in presentation of the disease. This is probably due to variations in ossification and vascularization of the navicular. In females, the ossific nucleus is seen between 18 and 24 months, whereas in males it is seen between 30 and 36 months. Approximately 37% will ossify from multiple centres, which then coalesce, while the remaining 63% ossify from a single centre. Overlapping multiple ossific centres may be misinterpreted as representing Köhler's disease, but in an asymptomatic foot, this tentative diagnosis should be abandoned.

It is quite possible that the aetiology of Köhler's disease is a combination of mechanical and vascular vulnerability. The tarsal navicular is the last bone of the foot to ossify, and therefore it is more susceptible than others to the arch compression forces of weight bearing. The fact that the male incidence of occurrence is substantially higher, in association with their average delay in ossification as compared to females, supports this theory. Further, most patients with Köhler's disease have a single ossific nucleus, and it is possible that this absence of a surrounding vascular arcade in combination with increased mechanical compression leads to the avascular necrosis. The normal navicular receives a branch from the dorsalis pedis and medial plantar artery forming an arcade around the tuberosity. Specimens have been seen, however, where a single penetrating artery nourishes the ossific nucleus. It seems, then, that a combination of mechanical and vascular vulnerability would predispose to the onset of avascular necrosis.

The diagnosis is made clinically, with pain on weight bearing, localized tenderness with palpation, and swelling being the hallmarks of presentation. Occasionally an increase in local temperature is apparent. The average age at onset in males is approximately 5 years, and in females, 3 years 10 months. Bilateral cases in eight of 24 patients were reported by Martinie-Dubousquet (1956). Rare cases have been reported in adults (Palamarchuk & Aronson 1995).

Radiographs show varying features, depending upon the state of the avascular process (Fig. 4). Increased radiodensity of the involved navicular is seen, with flattening of the involved bone as compared with the opposite side. In bilateral cases, this may be difficult to determine, and the diagnosis is made more on a clinical basis and confirmed by subsequent roentgenographic changes. The increased radiodensity may be due to three factors: a relative density compared to surrounding hypervascularity from synovitis, actual increased density due to mechanical crushing and compression of the ossific nucleus, and increased density secondary to neo-ossification superimposed on the dead ossific matrix.

The treatment of Köhler's disease is conservative, and consists of application of a short leg walking cast, with care taken to mould the arch. The cast should be applied for eight weeks. In Williams & Cowell's (1981) study, those not casted recovered in an average of 15 months, whereas those casted 8 weeks or longer recovered in an average of 10 weeks.

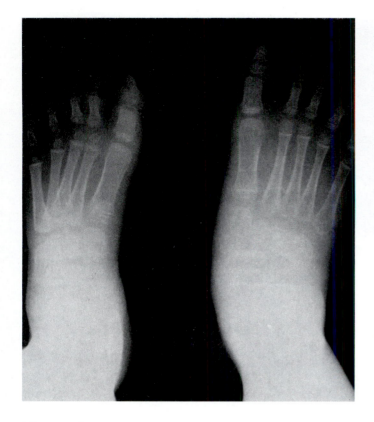

Figure 4

An anteroposterior radiograph of the feet of a 5-year-old male with Köhler's disease of the right tarsal navicular

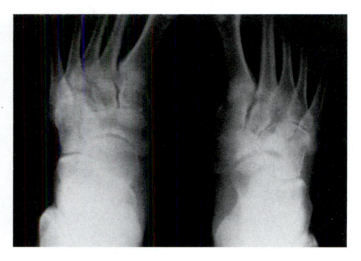

Figure 5a

The anteroposterior radiograph of a 46-year-old male who went untreated for a painful limp at age 5. Note the fragmentation of the right navicular

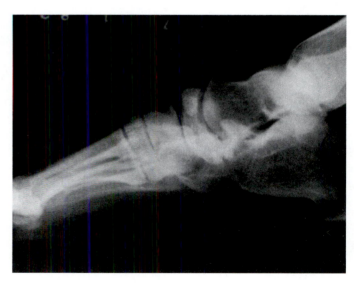

Figure 5b

The lateral radiograph of the same patient's foot, revealing navicular fragmentation and flattening of the longitudinal arch

Protecting the navicular from compression forces during the revascularization reossification process is of paramount importance. Figure 5 illustrates a 46-year-old individual's right foot, which was not treated at age 5 for an undiagnosed painful limp. The persistent fragmentation of the navicular with unilateral talonavicular sag, early degenerative arthritis, and a symptomatic unilateral flat foot are seen. Two such cases have been seen, both treated with a rigid orthotic and antiinflammatory medication.

The first metatarsal

Osteochondritis dissecans of the first metatarsal head appears to be traumatic in origin. It represents a cleavage lesion of the articular cartilage of the anteriorsuperior metatarsal head. Occasionally, the lesion may involve the avulsion of subchondral bone as well. In my experience, it is most commonly seen in athletic young adults. Soccer players frequently present with symptoms of pain with activity, and limited dorsiflexion at the great toe. It is less commonly seen in adolescents, though here too a history of antecedent trauma is common (Fig. 6). Later presenta-

tions are associated with prominent dorsal osteophytes and painfully restricted dorsiflexion. Medial or lateral osteophytes, or both, may also be apparent.

There has been some debate regarding the aetiology of this disorder. Dorsal hyperextension of the first metatarsal was suggested by Lambrinudi (1938) and by Jack (1940). In a similar vein, Jansen (1921) felt that pronation of the forefoot led to the disorder. An abnormally long first metatarsal has also been reported in association with the disorder. Though these variations in

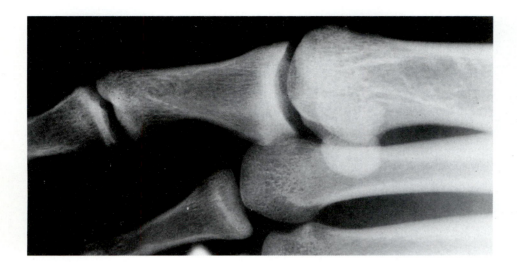

Figure 6

An oblique radiograph of a 24-year-old male with early pain and lucency at the metatarsal head after 'jamming' his foot on an athletic field. Symptoms of pain and synovitis resolved with rest and the use of a firm-soled shoe

forefoot anatomy may predispose to increased forefoot stress, repetitive microtrauma or a single traumatic event are probably primary in aetiology.

The treatment varies with the patient's age and stage of joint degeneration. For patients presenting early with symptoms of pain and radiographic evidence of a subchondral defect only (see Fig. 6), rest or casting are indicated. Application of a short leg walking cast for 3–6 weeks may unload the metatarsophalangeal joint enough to allow healing of the defect. The use of a rocker-bottom sole on the shoe is also helpful, both in resting early cases and in those patients with significant degenerative spurring and a painful restriction of dorsiflexion.

Patients with chronic symptoms and a persistent subchondral defect may benefit from an arthrotomy and excision of the defect. A concomitant debridement of restricting spurs may also be helpful (cheilectomy), but postoperative joint motion must be restored or the debridement will fail. Frequently, patients' main complaints are of the inability to dorsiflex. Hence, push-off or going up or down stairs is restricted. A proximal phalangeal or distal metatarsal dorsally based osteotomy can restore some dorsiflexion. Care should be taken to prevent excessive dorsal angulation, or a hallux elevatus will result.

Active patients with marked degenerative changes should be treated with an arthrodesis. Here again, the metatarsophalangeal angulation should be 10–20°, relative to the floor, or 30–40° dorsiflexion relative to the first metatarsal. I prefer 20° dorsiflexion in women to allow them to wear a higher heel, and 10° in men. I prefer to perform this operation with a micro-oscillating saw, using crossed, oblique, smooth Kirschner wires (0.62 mm) for fixation. The wires are placed in a retrograde fashion, bent and cut outside the skin, and removed 6 weeks after surgery. A short leg walking cast is applied for these 6 weeks. Given the current state of technology in metatarsophalangeal joint replacement, there does not appear to be a place for Silastic joint

replacement under the age of 50, depending upon the health and activity of the patient.

The second metatarsal

In 1914, Freiberg described an 'infraction' of the second metatarsal head. He noted an increased incidence of callus formation of the skin under the second metatarsal, and it was speculated that a longer second metatarsal might predispose to this disorder. It is unlikely that Freiberg's infraction represents a traumatic chondral avulsion as in osteochondritis dissecans of the first metatarsal. Rather, it represents partial or complete avascular necrosis of the second metatarsal head.

The infraction is seen more commonly in females. Symptoms consist of pain with weight bearing, and localized swelling and tenderness at the second metatarsal head. A roentgenogram will reveal relative increased radiodensity of the second metatarsal, and occasionally a subchondral fracture with flattening of the articular surface is seen as well (Fig. 7). With avascular necrosis of the subchondral bone, collapse and flattening of the head can occur, leading to later 'squaring' of the metatarsal head and spur formation.

Nonoperative management of cases diagnosed early may include simple rest, if symptoms demand, in plaster. However, the natural course of Freiberg's disease is incompletely understood and many cases may recover spontaneously, as may be evidenced by an incidental finding on a radiograph taken in later childhood (Helal 1987).

In more painful cases if there is fragmentation and infractal collapse then surgical intervention to remove the fragments and perform a synovial debridement is reasonable (Smillie 1957). If conservative treatment does fail and the infraction is severe Smith et al (1991) have reported a series of 16 feet managed by means of a shortening osteotomy held rigidly with a bone plate and

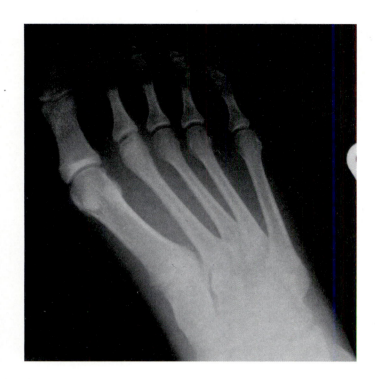

Figure 7

Avascular necrosis (Freiberg's infraction) in a 16-year-old girl. Protective casting for 6 weeks resulted in complete recovery without deformity

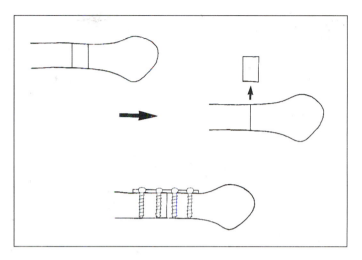

Figure 8

Shortening osteotomy and bone plate for Freiberg's infraction

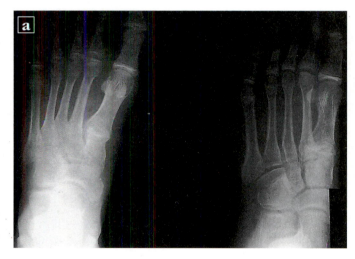

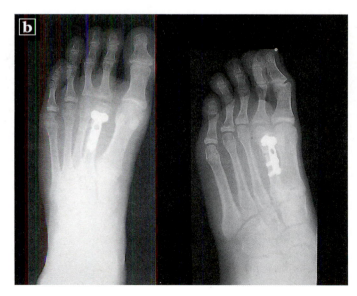

Figure 9

Patient (a) before and (b) after the shortening osteotomy and bone plate for Freiberg's infraction

screws (Figs 8, 9). They found that such an operation is associated with head remodelling not seen in the cases permitted to take a natural course. The major benefit reported was, however, a marked shortening of distressing symptoms in a frustrated group of otherwise active young adults.

It must be stated that excision of the whole of the second metatarsal head is not recommended, since this always leads to increase in local pressure and forefoot dysfunction.

The sesamoid bones

There is great variation in the sesamoid bones, and this can lead to a confusion in the diagnoses of various forefoot maladies. Inconsistencies in terminology have also led to diagnoses such as sesamoiditis, osteochondritis, osteomalacia, osteitis fibrosa, juvenile necrotic osteopathy, Köhler's or Schlatter's disease of the sesamoids, and sesamoid insufficiency.

The sesamoids become identifiable as undifferentiated connective tissue within the flexor hallucis brevis tendon by the eighth week of fetal life. Chondrification begins at the twelfth week, but ossification will not occur until approximately the eighth year of life. Single or multiple ossification centres may appear, and these may or may not coalesce. Bi-, tri-, and quadripartite sesamoids are commonly seen in the adult. In addition, up to 75% of the partite sesamoids can be unilateral. Thus, the absence of bilaterality does not necessarily delineate a possible fractured sesamoid from a partite sesamoid. Indeed, partite sesamoids will frequently split at the weaker fibrocartilaginous junction to produce symptoms of exquisite pain. A technetium 99 bone scan with pinhole collimation will frequently assist in differentiating a fractured sesamoid or split partite sesamoid from an otherwise normal partite sesamoid.

Sesamoids may be involved in diverse disease processes (Wülker et al 1991) but for purposes of discussion, disorders of the sesamoids may be grouped into two main categories. Chondromalacia and 'sesamoiditis' are regarded as synonomous, descriptive of a painful inflammation of the metatarsosesamoid articulation. Invariably, trauma or repetitive mechanical stress is associated with the production of symptoms. The second category consists of osteochondritis or true avascular necrosis of the sesamoid bone(s). Again, trauma or increased mechanical stress underlie the aetiology. True avascular necrosis of the sesamoid may occur in association with stress fractures, isolated traumatic fractures, prolonged running, or repetitive impact loading, such as in the marching of military recruits. Patients may present with partite sesamoids that have been split with chronic stress with one segment becoming avascular and fragmenting further. Conservative therapy is rarely helpful in true osteochondritis. Protective padding, a rocker-bottom sole on the shoe, or casting for up to six weeks should be attempted. However, those patients with avascular necrosis will require excision of the fragmented sesamoid. Care should be taken not to damage the insertion of the flexor hallucis brevis tendon, and the tendon's defect after sesamoid excision should be repaired. Removal of both sesamoids is to be avoided at all costs (Leventen 1991).

References

Alexander H, Lichtman D 1980 Surgical treatment of transchondral talar-dome fractures (osteochondritis dissecans). J Bone Joint Surg 62A: 646–651

Berndt A, Harty M 1959 Transchondral fractures (osteochondritis dissecans) of the talus. J Bone Joint Surg 41A: 988–1020

Biedert R 1991 Anterior ankle pain in sports medicine: aetiology and indications for arthroscopy. Arch Orthop Trauma Surg 110: 293–297

Bruns J, Rosenbach B 1992 Osteochondritis dissecans of the talus. Comparison of results of surgical treatment in adolescents ands adults. Arch Orthop Trauma Surg 112: 23–27

Cova M, Assante M, Frezza F et al 1995 Anatomia della risonanza magnetica delle articolazioni tibiotarsica e sottoastragalica. Radiol Med (Torino) 89: 203–210

Dipaola J D, Nelson D W, Colville M R 1991 Characterizing osteochondral lesions by magnetic resonance imaging. Arthroscopy 7: 101–104

Ferguson A, Gingrich R 1959 The normal and the abnormal calcaneal apophysis and tarsal navicular. Clin Orthop 10: 87–95

Jack E A 1940 The aetiology of hallux rigidus. Br J Surg 27: 492–497

Jansen M 1921 The aetiology of hallux rigidus and malleus. J Orthop Surg 3: 87–90

Kabbani Y M, Mayer D P 1994 Magnetic resonance imaging of osteochondral lesions of the talar dome. J Am Podiatr Med Assoc 84: 192–195

Lambrinudi E 1938 Metatarsus primus elevatus. Proc Roy Soc Med 31: 1273

Leventen E O 1991 Sesamoid disorders and treatment. An update. Clin Orthop Rel Res 269: 236–240

Ly P N, Fallat L M 1993 Trans-chondral fractures of the talus: a review of 64 surgical cases. J Foot Ankle Surg 32: 352–374

Martinie-Dubousquet J 1956 Scaphoidite tarsienne (premier maladie de Köhler). Ann Chir 32: C177–C194

Palamarchuk H J, Aronson S M 1995 Osteochondritis of the tarsal navicular in a female high school distance runner. J Am Podiatr Med Assoc 85: 226–229

Smillie I S 1957 Freiberg's infraction (Köhler's second disease). J Bone Joint Aurg (Br) 39: 580

Smith T W. Stanley D, Rowley D I 1991 Treatment of Freiberg's disease. A new operative technique. J Bone Joint Surg (Br) 73: 129–130

Wester J U, Jensen I E, Rasmussen F et al 1994 Osteochondral lesions of the talar dome in children. A 24 (7–36) year follow-up of 13 cases. Acta Orthop Scand 65: 110–112

Williams G, Cowell H 1981 Köhler's disease of the tarsal navicular. Clin Orthop 158: 53–58

Wülker N, Wirth C J, Massmann J 1991 Erkrankungen an den Sesambeinen der Grosszehe. Z Orthop Ihre Grenzgeb 129: 431–437

X ENVIRONMENTALLY RELATED DISORDERS

X.1 Injuries in the Athlete

Mark S Myerson

Acute ankle and subtalar sprains

Anatomy and biomechanics

The ligamentous support of the ankle consists of three ligaments: the anterior talofibular (ATF), the calcaneofibular (CF), and the posterior talofibular ligaments. The ligaments of the subtalar joint, including the CF ligament, the lateral talocalcaneal ligament, the interosseous talocalcaneal ligament, and the cervical ligament, also have an integral role when considering ankle injury. The extensor retinaculum also contributes to the support both of the ankle and of the subtalar joints, particularly the inferior margin of the extensor retinaculum where it divides into its three bundles.

The ATF ligament is short, blends with the fibers of the lateral capsule of the ankle, and inserts into the lateral aspect of the talus just anterior to the articular surface. It is relaxed when the ankle is dorsiflexed and tightens when the ankle is plantarflexed. The ATF is the first ligament to tear in a typical ankle sprain when the foot collapses into plantarflexion and inversion. The ATF has a lower load to failure than the other ankle ligaments (Siegler et al 1988, Attarian et al 1985). Patients with hindfoot varus are at significant risk of recurrent inversion sprain and gradual stretching and attenuation of both the ATF and CF ligaments (Myerson 1993). Rasmussen (1985) has demonstrated that one of the primary problems with recurrent ankle sprains is not inversion but rotation of the talus. Recurrent inversion instability does not cause a simple uniplanar deformity of the talus, rather it causes a rotatory instability of the talus in the ankle mortise.

The CF ligament originates from the anterior distal border of the fibula. It is generally directed posteriorly at an angle of 45° to insert on the calcaneus, just superior to the peroneal tubercle. This ligament is tight in dorsiflexion, is loose in plantarflexion, and inhibits adduction. In plantarflexion, this ligament acts with the ATF, but in dorsiflexion, when the ATF is loose, the CF ligament acts independently.

The extensor retinaculum provides major support both to the ankle and to the subtalar joints. The contribution of the extensor retinaculum to ankle and subtalar instability has been emphasized over the past decade since Gould et al (1980) published their modification of the Brostrom procedure.

The biomechanics of the subtalar joint ligamentous complex are less well understood. Many anatomic studies have attempted to reproduce subtalar instability through sequential sectioning but have failed to identify substantial rotatory instability, which occurs clinically. The cervical ligament is an extremely taut and strong ligament and with the interosseus talocalcaneal ligament supports the subtalar joint. It is likely that the cervical ligament limits inversion, but both the cervical and interosseous talocalcaneal ligaments are responsible for rotational control of the subtalar joint (Smith 1958).

Diagnosis

Clinical evaluation
Patients report a popping or tearing in the lateral aspect of the ankle associated with a plantarflexion inversion injury. Tenderness, swelling, and ecchymosis are usually present over the anterolateral aspect of the ankle. It is easy to reproduce the patient's pain by direct palpation over the affected ligaments and by gentle stress of the ankle, particularly in plantarflexion and inversion. It is important to examine the foot and ankle carefully for the associated injuries that often occur secondary to plantarflexion and inversion: injury to the peroneal tendons, the subtalar joint, the anterior process of the calcaneus, the talus, and the fifth metatarsal. Each of these areas should be carefully examined with particular attention to maximum tenderness over the lateral aspect of the foot.

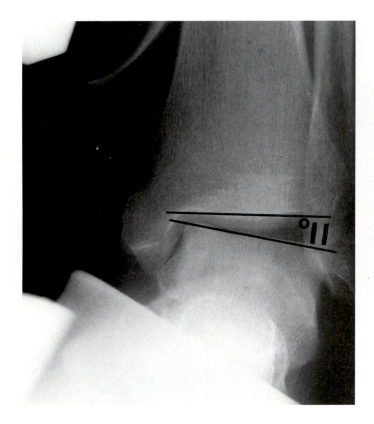

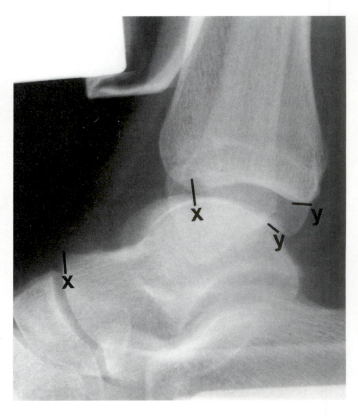

Figure 1

Inversion (varus) stress was applied to this ankle. There was 11° of talar tilt, but this should be compared with the opposite ankle to assess its clinical significance

Figure 2

The anterior drawer test. The amount of instability may be measured using points y–y or x–x and should be compared with the opposite ankle

Radiographic evaluation

Radiographic examination of an ankle sprain should include anteroposterior, lateral, and internal oblique views of the ankle and anteroposterior, lateral, and oblique views of the foot. In this manner, injuries to the anterior process to the calcaneus, the lateral process of the talus, the dome of the talus, and the base of the fifth metatarsal are less likely to be missed and can be evaluated. I am not in favor of performing stress views of the ankle after acute ligamentous injury. This examination is painful, adds no useful information, and does not affect the decision-making in treatment.

Radiographic evaluation for chronic recurrent ankle instability should focus on both the foot and ankle in the weight bearing position, as well as with stress. Recurrent ankle instability is often associated with fixed hindfoot varus or decreased motion in the subtalar joint. For this reason, an axial view of the calcaneus and weight bearing views of the foot should be obtained in addition to routine views of the ankle. The stress view or a talar tilt view of the ankle is an anteroposterior view of the ankle while inversion stress is applied. Although this force can be applied manually, a commercially avail-

able stress device is useful and accurate. I do not use any anesthesia to perform this stress manipulation of the ankle. When obtaining a stress view of the ankle, the opposite ankle should also be examined since significant variation in talar tilt occurs. Quite a wide range of 'normal' talar tilt exists (Berridge & Bonnin 1944, Bonnin 1949, Sedlin 1960). Despite this variation in both normal and abnormal ankles, the difference in the talar tilt between both ankles should be less than 5°. The inversion stress test should be performed with the foot in a consistent position. Since laxity increases with the foot in plantarflexion, it should be performed with the foot in a neutral position or in slight dorsiflexion. Since the inversion stress or talar tilt measures injury to the calcaneofibular ligament, it is highly likely that this ligament is disrupted if talar tilt is greater than 12°.

The anterior drawer test measures the integrity of the anterior talofibular ligament and is probably more reliable than the inversion or positive talar tilt test (Fig. 1). This stress test should also be performed with comparative views of the opposite ankle. There are two methods of evaluating the anterior drawer measurements, both of which are reliable (Fig. 2). I prefer to quantify the anterior subluxation according to the distance between the anterior edge of the distal tibia and the anterior dorsal surface of the talus.

Management

Although many classification systems of ankle sprains have been reported (Jackson et al 1974, Smith & Reischl 1988, Leach & Schepsis 1990), these are of clinical use only if they determine the course of treatment. Since I treat all acute ankle sprains nonoperatively, it is less important to stage the severity of this injury. If bone, joint, or tendon injuries are present, then an operative approach may be used, and the ankle ligaments are repaired primarily. No study exists demonstrating the advantage of an operative approach for severe ankle sprains whether in the athletic or nonathletic population. I therefore advocate using whatever modalities are necessary to rest the ankle and commence early functional rehabilitation. Eversion strengthening with the foot in plantarflexion is emphasized, as is proprioceptive training during rehabilitation.

Although Leach & Schepsis (1990) have advocated operative repair of the acute ankle sprain in the athlete, 90% of all athletes will recover after a nonoperative treatment program. Of the remaining 10% who experience recurrent ankle symptoms, most are able to be treated with a rehabilitation and taping program. Certainly the concept of 'down time' for the high-performance athlete is a valid one, so if the athlete has to remain 'off' for a specified length of time after the injury, he may as well be treated operatively. I do not advocate an operative approach for these injuries, regardless of the magnitude of the tear, unless it is associated with injuries that of themselves warrant surgical intervention.

Chronic ankle instability

Assessment

Patients with chronic ankle instability should be carefully evaluated, since recurrent instability of the ankle may involve the ligamentous supports of the ankle and subtalar joints as well as the articular surfaces and surrounding tendons. Hindfoot varus, cavovarus deformity of the foot, and decreased motion in the subtalar joint all predispose to recurrent ankle instability. It is important to assess for generalized ligamentous laxity, since this will have an impact on the choice of operative procedure if needed.

Conservative rehabilitation of the foot and ankle for recurrent instability is important regardless of the

decision to pursue operative or nonoperative treatment. There is value in improving proprioception and eversion strengthening of the foot in plantarflexion before surgery.

Surgical correction

I use only two operative procedures for reconstructing lateral ankle instability, the Brostrom (Brostrom 1966a, 1966b) and the Chrisman–Snook procedures (Chrisman & Snook 1969, Snook et al 1985), although numerous others are available (Elmslie 1934, Watson-Jones 1955, Evans et al 1984, Larsen 1988, Larsen & Lund 1991). The tenodesis procedures (Elmslie 1934, Watson-Jones 1955, Chrisman & Snook 1969, Evans et al 1984, Snook et al 1985, Larsen 1988, Larsen & Lund 1991) all require using all or part of the peroneus brevis tendon and routing it through various bone tunnels to reconstruct the anterior talofibular and, in some cases, the calcaneofibular ligaments. Although the reported results are satisfactory, the Watson-Jones (1955) and Evans (1953) procedures do not restore any stability to the subtalar joint.

The direct repair of the ATF and CF ligaments was originally described by Brostrom (1966a, 1966b) and recently modified by Gould et al (1980). This method of repair is particularly important in dancers, gymnasts, and other athletes in whom the peroneal tendons are extremely important for maximum performance and function. The modified Brostrom procedure is a direct repair of both the ATF and CF ligaments. It is not so easy to repair the CF ligament with this approach; however, redundancy in this ligament is easy to identify and with experience the same surgical repair can be used on the CF as on the ATF ligament. The addition of the extensor retinaculum imbrication not only reinforces both these repairs but, importantly also contributes to stabilizing the subtalar joint.

The Chrisman–Snook procedure is particularly useful in patients who are obese, in heavy football players, and in those with structural deformity of the hindfoot. The Chrisman–Snook procedure is also particularly useful where ankle instability is a result of neuromuscular peroneal weakness. In these patients, the entire peroneus brevis tendon may be used instead of a split tendon procedure as is more commonly performed. It is unlikely that the stability of the ankle can be restored in the presence of fixed hindfoot varus. In these patients, I simultaneously perform an osteotomy of the calcaneus to stabilize the mechanical axis of the hindfoot and ankle. It is particularly important to address any malalignment of the hindfoot mechanical axis simultaneously with a calcaneal osteotomy. The calcaneal tuberosity is shifted with a triplanar osteotomy, as previously described (Saxby & Myerson 1993).

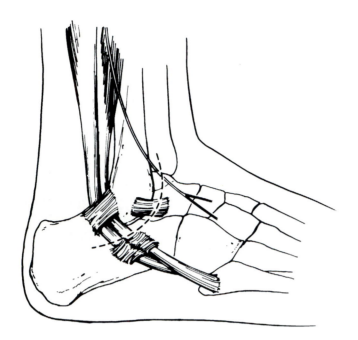

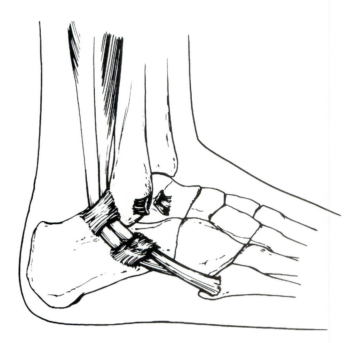

Figure 3

The skin incision for the modified Brostrom procedure is identified by the dotted lines

Figure 4

The anterior talofibular ligament and capsule are incised, leaving a small cuff of tissue attached to the fibula

Modified Brostrom procedure

The procedure is performed on an outpatient basis under local anesthesia: 30 cm³ of 0.5% bupivacaine with 1:200 000 epinephrine mixed is used for the regional block. The ankle and subtalar joints are blocked as are the tibial, superficial peroneal, and sural nerves.

The incision curves over the anterior aspect of the distal fibula inferiorly toward the peroneal tendons (Fig. 3) and is deepened through subcutaneous tissue, taking care to avoid injury to the lateral cutaneous branch of the superficial nerve, which crosses just medial to this incision. The sural nerve is not visualized since it is inferior to the peroneal tendons. It is important to identify the extensor retinaculum and to mobilize this off the anterior talofibular ligament and capsule. This retinaculum varies in thickness, but it is always present and easily identifiable. The incision is made through the anterior talofibular ligament and capsule without attempting to dissect the ligament off the capsule (Fig. 4). I leave a small cuff of capsule and ligament attached to the fibula approximately 3–4 mm in length. It is easy to recognize if the ATF ligament is redundant, in which case the incision is made directly in the substance of the ligament.

Occasionally, the ligament is avulsed off the fibula with a small bone fragment. If an avulsion off the fibula is present, then I prefer to harvest the ligament and capsule more proximally directly off the fibular and then to imbricate this up against the fibula with non-

absorbable sutures. This can be attached either with a suture anchor or through drill holes into the fibula.

More inferiorly, the CF ligament is identified lying underneath the peroneal tendons. The CF ligament blends inferiorly with the peroneal tendon sheath, which should be opened to examine the ligament. If no redundancy in the CF ligament is identified, it is left alone. Usually, however, the ligament needs to be tightened by excising a 2 mm segment. Both the ATF and CF ligaments are now repaired. The ATF ligament is imbricated in a vest-over-pants manner using nonabsorbable sutures (Fig. 5). Owing to the thickness of the combined ATF ligament and ankle capsule, this imbrication is not always possible and I sometimes excise an ellipse from the tissue and do a direct end-to-end repair.

Once the repair of both the ATF and CF ligaments is complete, the ankle is taken through a full range of motion, and an anterior drawer is performed to determine stability. The extensor retinaculum is now advanced up to the fibula and attached with absorbable 2/0 sutures (Fig. 6). It is important to tie the sutures in the ATF and CF ligaments as well as the imbrication with the ankle in dorsiflexion and slight eversion. Postoperatively, patients are immobilized in a posterior splint for 10 days, after which the dressing is changed and ambulation is begun in a short leg cast for an additional 2–3 weeks. Between 4 and 6 weeks, the cast is removed, a removable splint is applied to the ankle, and exercises and rehabilitation commence.

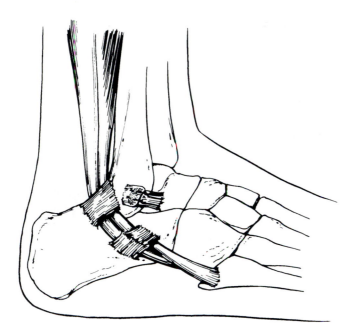

Figure 5

The anterior talofibular ligament and capsule are imbricated either by excising a segment or repairing the ligament with a 'vest-over-pants' method, as demonstrated here

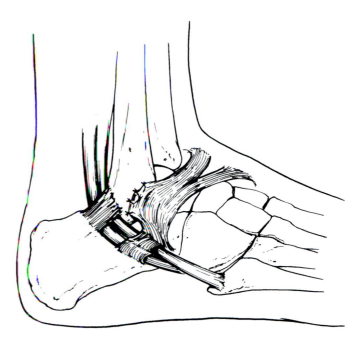

Figure 6

The extensor retinaculum is advanced proximally to the anterior edge of the fibula to tighten and reinforce the repair

Modified Chrisman–Snook procedure

This procedure is indicated in patients with generalized ligamentous laxity, in obesity, in the heavy athlete, and in patients with recurrent instability after prior surgical correction, where associated significant subtalar instability is present. In the presence of fixed deformity of the subtalar joint, particularly hindfoot varus, this procedure is also useful. As originally described by Chrisman & Snook (1969) and then by Snook et al (1985), half of the peroneus brevis tendon is harvested. Occasionally, tears of the peroneal tendons are present, and the split peroneus brevis tendon can be harvested through the torn portion; occasionally the entire tendon is used. This is also applicable to patients with neuromuscular deformity whose peroneal muscle is not functional; in these cases the entire peroneus brevis tendon is used.

The procedure is performed with the patient in the lateral decubitus position using local anesthesia with 30 cm³ of 0.5% bupivacaine with 1:200 000 epinephrine. No tourniquet is needed. The incision is made parallel to the peroneal tendons from 7.5 cm proximal to the ankle joint. It then crosses distally over the peroneal tendons towards the peroneal tubercle (Fig. 7). I have not found it necessary to extend the incision more proximally into the leg, since sufficient tendon can be harvested from this limited incision. The sheath is opened and both tendons are inspected. Tears of the peroneus brevis tendon should be treated. The peroneus brevis tendon is split using the anterior half of the

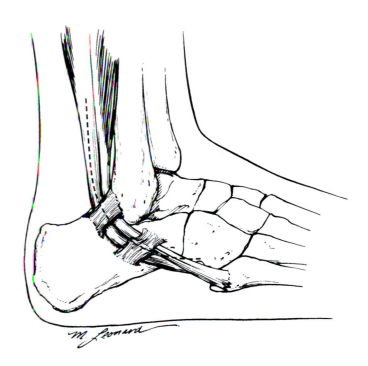

Figure 7

The incision for the modified Chrisman–Snook procedure is made parallel to the peroneal tendons and posterior to the fibula

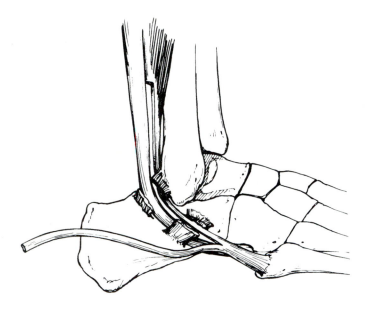

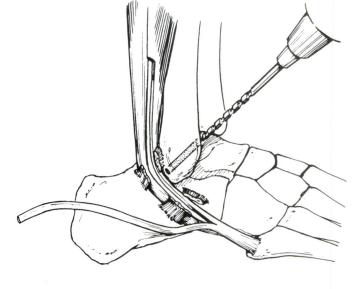

Figure 8

The anterior half of the peroneus brevis is harvested, leaving the posterior half attached to the muscle (reprinted by permission from Myerson 1993)

Figure 9

A 4.5 mm drill hole is made from anterior to posterior at the tip of the fibula (reprinted by permission from Myerson 1993)

tendon for the transfer, leaving the posterior half attached to the muscle (Fig. 8).

During the subcutaneous dissection, it is important to identify the sural nerve, which lies immediately posterior to the incision and can be visualized with the lesser saphenous vein. The nerve is retracted with the posterior skin flap. Care needs to be taken not to cut the nerve where it crosses distally, anterior and dorsal to the peroneal tendons. A subcutaneous soft-tissue flap is elevated anteriorly and the anterior talofibular ligament and anterior capsule are identified under the extensor retinaculum. To prevent dislocation of the peroneal tendons, a small 1 cm slip of the peroneal sheath may be left intact at the tip of the fibula. I have not found this step necessary, since the split peroneal transfer is brought anterior to the remaining peroneal tendons to restrain them from anterior dislocation. Although an imbrication of the anterior talofibular ligament and capsule may be performed simultaneously, I have not routinely performed this step.

The periosteum over the anterior distal fibula is elevated, leaving a small cuff to which the tendon transfer is sutured. The tendon is split just distal to the peroneal tubercle and then brought anteriorly for the transfer. A 4.5 mm drill hole is made from anterior to posterior perpendicular to the axis of the fibula (Fig. 9). The free tendon is passed from anterior to posterior through the osseous tunnel (Fig. 10). The lateral wall of the calcaneus is then prepared with subperiosteal dissection beneath the peroneus longus tendon. As originally

described by Chrisman & Snook (1969) and then by Snook et al (1985), a tunnel is made in the calcaneus. However, I find this cumbersome and prefer to attach the tendon using a screw with a small spiked ligament washer, as this is extremely stable and it allows early range of motion postoperatively.

With the tendon pulled through the fibular osseous tunnel, the ankle is held in the neutral position and two absorbable sutures are inserted in the anterior aspect of the fibula. The graft is passed over the peroneus longus and the remaining peroneus brevis tendon, and then, with the subtalar joint in the neutral position, the tendon is secured to the lateral wall of the calcaneus with a 4.0 mm partially threaded cancellous screw and a small spiked plastic ligament washer (Fig. 11). It is not necessary to use the remaining tendon to pull it up to the fibula with this technique (Fig. 12). The imbrication of the ATF and CF ligaments may then be performed. The peroneal retinaculum is closed with absorbable sutures and, after closure through subcutaneous tissue and skin, the foot is held in neutral position with a posterior plaster splint incorporated with a bandage.

The patient is allowed to commence weight bearing at 10 days in a short leg cast. In the athlete, I encourage early weight bearing with protection in a removable ankle brace. At 6 weeks, function rehabilitation is encouraged in a controled physical therapy program emphasizing dorsiflexion and eversion strengthening exercises.

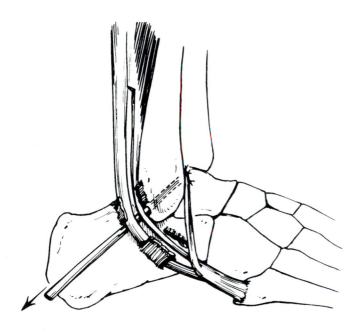

Figure 10

It is preferable to pass the split peroneus brevis tendon superficial to and not deep to the two tendons, as demonstrated here (reprinted by permission from Myerson 1993)

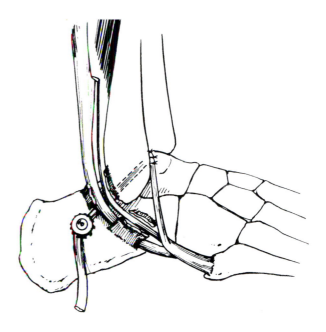

Figure 11

The tendon is secured to the calcaneus with a spiked ligament washer and a 4.0 mm cancellous screw (reprinted by permission from Myerson 1993)

I have been encouraged by the success of this procedure with one exception, and that is a tendency to overtighten the repair. It is extremely important to perform the tenodesis with the ankle in neutral and not in an everted position, to prevent overtightening of the repair, and, thereby limit inversion movement of the ankle. I would also caution the use of this procedure in patients with work-related injuries since my personal results in this group of patients have not paralleled those in the athletic population.

Subtalar instability

Only in the past decade have we begun to recognize the contribution of the subtalar joint to acute and chronic laxity to the hindfoot and ankle. Despite this recent enthusiasm, the diagnosis and treatment of subtalar instability is still unclear. We have learned much about the functional anatomy of the subtalar joint complex, but less about methods to diagnose instability.

Diagnosis

It is difficult to distinguish between symptoms of ankle and subtalar instability. Patient complaints are very similar, and the location of discomfort in both is in the

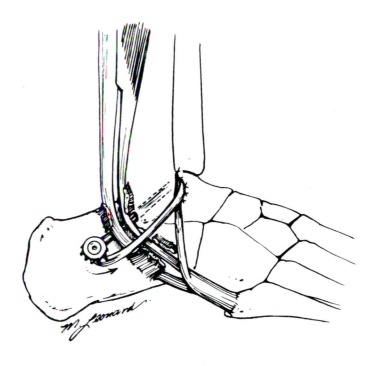

Figure 12

If sufficient tendon length is present, the stump may be advanced to the tip of the fibula. This step is not necessary with rigid screw fixation (reprinted by permission from Myerson 1993)

anterolateral ankle. Pain in the sinus tarsi is more diagnostic, particularly if one is able to localize isolated pain just interior and inferior to the fibula. This becomes more confusing when one realizes that ankle and subtalar joint instability can coexist.

The diagnosis of subtalar instability is made easier if a patient with symptoms of chronic instability does not have any significant talar tilt or drawer sign on stress testing. Stress radiographs of the subtalar joint have been previously described (Clanton 1989, Clanton et al 1990, Harper 1991). On the stress lateral view of the ankle, additional forward subluxation of the calcaneus on the talus can be demonstrated with anterior gliding of the undersurface of the posterior facet. Varus instability of the subtalar joint is more difficult to demonstrate and is probably not of functional significance, since subtalar instability is rotatory and not uniplanar. Nevertheless, stress Broden's views of the subtalar joint may be used to visualize the posterior facet of the subtalar joint (Fig. 13). Other methods of evaluating the joint, including stress tomography (Zollinger et al 1983) and arthrography (Meyer et al 1988a, 1988b), are less useful. I have never correctly diagnosed an acute subtalar sprain.

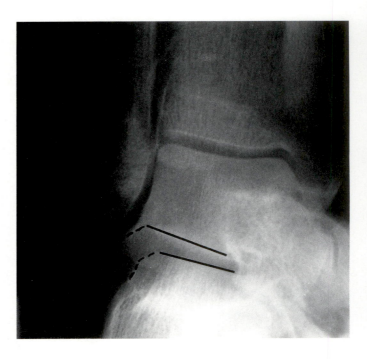

Figure 13

Inversion stress was applied to the ankle, which remained stable. On a 40° Broden's view, the subtalar joint is noted to subluxate forward and to rotate internally

Treatment

In 1988, Meyer et al (1988a) reported on a group of acute subtalar sprains and recommended surgical management based on subtalar arthrography. I find it hard to justify this form of treatment and would recommend managing these patients in the same manner as a patient with acute ankle sprain. However, the patient with symptoms of chronic instability and pain is different. Although eversion strengthening and proprioceptive training may suffice to improve symptoms in these patients, inflammation in the sinus tarsi is often present, requiring a more directed treatment approach. Delayed reconstruction for subtalar joint instability uses a tenodesis to reconstruct the torn ligaments. In the 1930s Elmslie (1934) described a procedure to reconstruct the ankle joint that simultaneously addresses the components of subtalar instability. Most procedures, including those described by Elmslie (1934), Larsen (1988), Larsen & Lund (1991), Chrisman & Snook (1969), and Snook et al (1985), address both the subtalar and ankle components of instability simultaneously.

I have used the Chrisman–Snook procedure, or modifications thereof, to address subtalar instability. Schon et al (1991), Clanton (1989), and Clanton et al (1990) have described a reconstructive procedure that is a modification of the Chrisman–Snook procedure. I have not specifically addressed the subtalar component of instability using the modified hole in the lateral calcaneus and talus as described by Schon et al (1991). In my experience, the modified Chrisman–Snook procedure, as described

above for ankle instability, suffices for treatment of combined ankle and subtalar instability or, in fact, subtalar instability. Certainly, the additional tunnels in the lateral calcaneus and talus are not too difficult to construct, but are probably unnecessary.

Peroneal tendon injury

Although dislocation of the peroneal tendons may occur spontaneously because of deficiency in the peroneal retinaculum and fibular groove and although congenital deficiencies of the fibular groove have been described (Edwards 1928), most peroneal tendon pathology, including tears and dislocations, occurs after trauma. I have identified complete dislocations of peroneal tendons after trauma where no fibular groove is present at all. It is likely that the groove was not sufficient to begin with, and that with the absence of the peroneal tendons in the retrofibular region, the groove 'filled in'. This has been identified after open reduction and internal fixation for calcaneus fractures in which the peroneal tendons are dislocated and the groove is palpated and noted to be present. If the tendons are not satisfactorily relocated, the groove may subsequently be totally deficient and absent. Retrofibular deficiency may therefore be the effect as well as the cause of peroneal tendon dislocation.

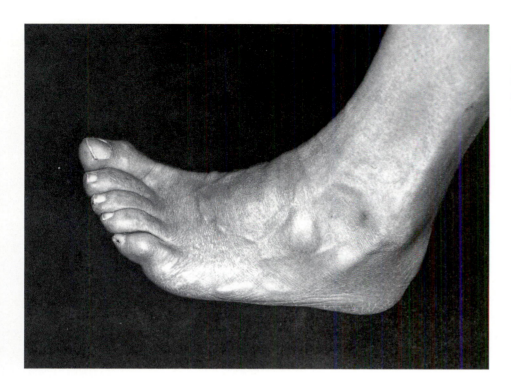

Figure 14

This patient reported a chronic popping behind the ankle and was able to actively dislocate the peroneal tendon(s). Note the tendon(s) lying anterior to the fibula

Anatomy

The peroneal tendons pass behind the fibula in a fibro-osseous tunnel. The anterior aspect of the retrofibular groove has a fibrocartilaginous rim analogous to the labrum in the shoulder. The depth of the retrofibular sulcus varies (Edwards 1928), and the height of the sulcus is increased by this fibrocartilaginous rim. In addition to the natural restraints formed by this groove, the superior peroneal retinaculum also maintains the tendons in their position behind the fibula. Division of the peroneal retinaculum, however, is not sufficient to cause dislocation of the tendons. I have seen this repeatedly after surgical correction when the tendons are relocated and the retinaculum is not yet repaired. Since these procedures are performed under local anesthesia, the patient is asked to attempt to dislocate the tendon voluntarily. The depth of the groove created is sufficient to prevent the tendons from dislocating.

Superiorly, the brevis and longus tendons pass through a single retinaculum that splits more distally, and the inferior retinaculum houses each tendon separately over the peroneal tubercle. However, the inferior peroneal retinaculum does not play a role in peroneal tendon pathology and dislocation. Although the peroneal retinaculum may be torn in the acute form of injury, some reports indicate that this tearing does not occur (Das De & Balasubramaniam 1985), a position originally supported by Eckert & Davis (1976). In a study of more than 70 cases of acute peroneal injury, Eckert & Davis (1976) showed that the peroneal retinaculum was not torn but stripped away from the edge of the fibula with or without involvement of the fibrocartilaginous rim.

Acute dislocation

Diagnosis

Clinicians often miss the acute form of dislocation of the peroneal tendon, which occurs after resisted dorsiflexion with or without eversion. Although the injury may occur after inversion stress on the foot, it is usually associated with resistance or contraction of the peroneals. Dislocation is reportedly common in skiing injuries, where vigorous contraction of the peroneals with the foot in dorsiflexion or eversion causes the tendons to dislocate. Diagnosis of the acute injury is based on pain posterior to the fibula associated with ecchymosis. Plantarflexion and inversion is not painful, but resisted eversion is most uncomfortable. Owing to swelling, it is difficult to appreciate the subluxation or dislocation of the tendons.

Treatment

Once the diagnosis of acute dislocation is made, I, as well as other clinicians (Earl et al 1972, Eckert & Davis 1976), advocate an operative approach in preference to

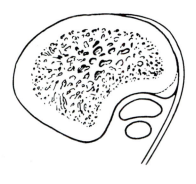
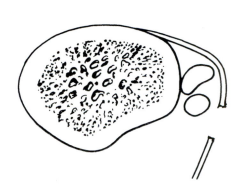

Figure 15

The peroneal tendons are well located in the groove on the left but, when associated with recurrent dislocation, the fibula groove becomes shallow, and the anterior fibrocartilaginous rim is avulsed with or without a tear of the retinaculum

conservative immobilization in a cast, since the latter has been associated with less than optimal results (McLennan 1980), with a high likelihood of recurrent problems, and with longer rehabilitation.

Acute repair involves direct approach to the retinaculum and fibrocartilaginous rim. The pathology is addressed directly by imbrication of the retinaculum in a vest-over-pants manner or reattachment of the fibrocartilaginous rim. I have not found it necessary to deepen the groove in these patients, although this can be performed if the groove is noted to be completely deficient. Postoperatively, the patients are allowed to ambulate after 1 week in a prefabricated boot or a cast for 3–4 weeks, when functional rehabilitation commences.

Chronic recurrent dislocation

Diagnosis

With chronic instability of the peroneal tendons, patients report varying symptoms of discomfort associated with clicking and popping in the posterolateral aspect of the ankle (Fig. 14). This vague sense of instability is often more diagnostic of recurrent dislocation than a demonstration by the patient of the dislocation. Inability to demonstrate a dislocation does not imply that chronic dislocation is not occurring. Although I routinely obtain radiographs of the ankle to rule out a small avulsion fracture of the tip of the fibula, this finding is not often present. I have rarely resorted to CT scans or MRI to make the diagnosis, which by and large is a clinical one.

Treatment

Treatment for chronic instability is varied and, again, may depend on the underlying pathology. Although numerous soft-tissue and bony procedures have been described (Kelly 1920, Jones 1932, Sarmiento & Wolf 1975, Pozo & Jackson 1984), I prefer to address the problem directly by deepening the fibular groove, as

reported by others (Edwards 1928, Jones 1932, Zoellner & Clancy 1979). This procedure is simple to perform, does not involve the sacrifice of any other adjacent structures, and avoids any bone block type procedure, which in my experience is associated with potential attritional tearing of the peroneal tendons.

I perform this procedure under local anesthesia as an outpatient procedure. The patient is turned to a lateral decubitus position and 20 cm³ of 0.5% bupivacaine with 1:200 000 epinephrine are administered. The superficial peroneal nerve and sural nerve are infiltrated through a field block, as is the peroneal tendon sheath. More distally, the ankle and subtalar joints are infiltrated with 5 cm³. An incision, commencing 7.5 cm proximal to the tip of the fibula and extending 2.5 cm distal to the tip of the fibula, is made directly over the peroneal tendons and is usually anterior to the sural nerve, which, however, needs to be identified. The incision is deepened through subcutaneous tissue, and the peroneal sheath is carefully identified. It is important at this stage to identify the underlying pathology (e.g. peroneal retinacular laxity or an avulsion of the fibrocartilaginous rim) (Fig. 15). If the rim is avulsed and a small bone or cartilaginous fragment is identified, then the incision in the retinaculum is made through this defect. If the rim is still attached, then the peroneal retinaculum is divided, leaving a 3 mm cuff attached to the edge of the fibula. The retinaculum is opened and the tendons are inspected. It is not uncommon to find elements of tenosynovitis with or without tearing of the tendon, usually the peroneus brevis. The tendon tears are repaired as described below.

Since the procedure is performed under local anesthesia, it is useful to instruct the patient to attempt to dislocate the tendons actively. In this manner, one can assess the need for further deepening of the groove, which can be accomplished with a combination of gouges, curettes, chisels, and burrs.

Deepening the groove in this manner can leave a rough cancellous bone surface to which the tendons could potentially adhere. In the past, I have tried to

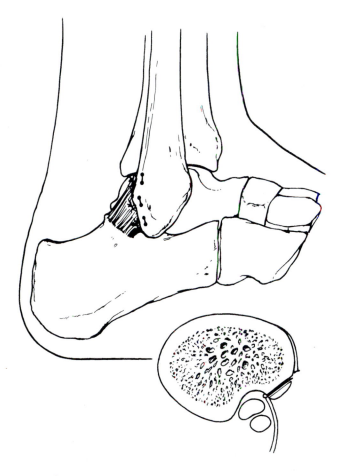

Figure 16

A groove is made posterior to the fibula, and the extensor retinaculum is advanced deep to the groove and attached through two or three pairs of drill holes

address this potential problem by the application of bone wax, but I have abandoned this method since the wax seldom remains adherent to the bone surface and can cause a foreign body reaction and further tenosynovitis. I have also attempted the alternative method described by Zoellner & Clancy (1979) for deepening the groove. This involves raising an osteoperiosteal flap, leaving it attached inferiorly, and following it with curettage of the underlying cancellous bone. I have discontinued using this procedure as well, because the osteoperiosteal flap has often broken off. I now use a high-speed 5 mm oval burr to round off and smooth the edges. This is particularly important distally at the tip of the fibula where the tendons pass at an acute angle and may be prone to attritional wear and tear.

Once the groove is sufficiently deepened, it is extremely unlikely that the tendons will redislocate. However, I reinforce this repair by suturing the peroneal retinaculum to the undersurface of the deepened groove (Fig. 16). Note that the retinaculum is sutured to the undersurface of the deepened groove and not to the

edge of the fibula. In this manner, a portion of the groove has a synovial layer.

Postoperatively, patients are kept non-weight-bearing for approximately 4 weeks. Early motion, however, is encouraged and commenced when the sutures are removed 5–7 days postoperatively. This early motion helps prevent adherence of the tendons to the rough cancellous bone surface. I have not encountered any recurrent dislocations or stenosing tenosynovitis with this method of repair. For salvage of recurrent dislocations, however, I recommend the method described by Martens et al (1986), which includes a bone block transposition of the calcaneofibular ligament.

Tendinitis and rupture

Tenosynovitis and degenerative tendinosis occur in an older patient population. Although acute rupture is rare, Thompson & Patterson (1989) have described acute rupture of the peroneus longus tendon, predominantly in elderly individuals who probably had underlying predisposing degenerative tendinosis. However, because this acute injury is difficult to diagnose, it is likely that rupture of the peroneus longus occurs far more frequently than is recognized.

Complete rupture of both the longus and brevis tendons does occur, as highlighted by Sammarco et al (1993) and Sobel et al (1990a, 1990b) in their reports on the attritional tearing of the peroneus brevis tendon that commonly occurs with recurrent instability of the ankle. However, longitudinal splits and fissures of the tendon, particularly the brevis tendon, are more common (Fig. 17). The biomechanics of peroneal tendon splits have also been highlighted, particularly in relation to recurrent ankle instability (Sobel et al 1990b).

Diagnosis
The patient will present with pain, warmth, and swelling over the peroneal tendon sheath, often associated with recurrent ankle instability. In this setting, I will often inject 2–3 cm³ of 1% lidocaine into the tendon sheath for diagnostic purposes. Radiographic examination of the foot is important since the os vesalianum, which is in the substance of the peroneus longus tendon, may be seen to retract more proximally. However, the sesamoid is occasionally absent and diagnosis should not rely on retraction. Acute ruptures of the peroneus longus tendon may occur either posterior to the fibula or more distally as the tendon passes under the cuboid. MRI may be required to diagnose this type of rupture.

Treatment
Acute tendinitis will respond to complete rest, nonsteroidal anti-inflammatory medication, and immobilization in either

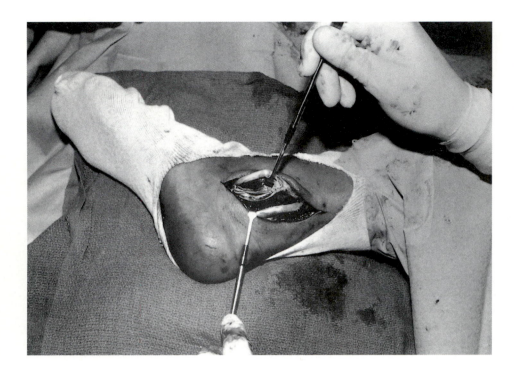

Figure 17

This patient sustained an acute partial tear of the peroneus brevis tendon, which was also dislocated anteriorly. This was treated by resection of the torn portion of the tendon and repair of the peroneal retinaculum

a cast or a removable brace. I have not had much success with the conservative treatment of chronic degenerative tenosynovitis in the athlete and, for these patients, I advocate surgery. Longitudinal fissures are often present and these are debrided. If the peroneus brevis tendon is extensively involved, that portion of the tendon may be excised and a side-to-side tenodesis to the peroneus longus tendon may be performed proximal and distal to the longitudinal rupture. An end-to-end repair is rarely feasible in these patients.

Postoperatively, patients are treated with early mobilization but should be non-weight-bearing for 2–4 weeks. Peroneal rehabilitation is encouraged and is the mainstay of treatment. Athletes are usually able to return to activity 2–3 months after repair.

Achilles tendon injury

Anatomy

The Achilles tendon insertion is on the posterior inferior one-third of the calcaneal tuberosity with insertional fibers extending to the plantar aspect of the calcaneus. The insertion of the Achilles tendon is broad, and detaching the medial or lateral edge of the tendon does not functionally weaken it. The Achilles tendon is surrounded by a loose matrix of tissue, referred to as mesotenon, paratenon, and pseudosheath (Booth 1987, Bradley & Tibone 1990, Garrett et al 1988), that functions similarly

to a tendon sheath. The vascularity of the Achilles tendon has been implicated in the pathogenesis of inflammation, degeneration, and ultimate rupture. Microvascular studies have demonstrated decreased blood flow in and to the Achilles tendon 2–6 cm proximal to its insertion into the calcaneus (Garrett et al 1987), which is in the same location as inflammation and rupture.

The retrocalcaneal bursa is a loose, fluid-filled sac that helps the Achilles tendon glide against the superior edge of the calcaneus. There also is a small bursal sac, referred to as the subcutaneous or precalcaneal bursa, between the skin and the Achilles tendon. Either of these bursae can become inflamed and painful.

Etiology

Achilles tendon dysfunction occurs in two separate groups of patients, determined largely by their age and activity levels. The first group is composed of individuals aged 35–50 years who are low-level competitive athletes and who typically sustain ruptures of the tendon. Of all Achilles tendon ruptures, 75% are sustained by predominantly male athletes between the ages of 30 and 40. The second group consists of a younger population of highly active athletes who develop inflammatory changes in the tendon and its lining paratenon. Athletes who participate in racquet sports and long distance running are particularly susceptible to these inflammatory changes. Approximately 15% of Achilles tendon ruptures are associated with symptoms of antecedent tendinitis. This has particular significance when treating patients with chronic retrocalcaneal pain.

Increased pronation during stance is likely to cause pathologic changes in the Achilles tendon. With functional hyperpronation, the accompanying contraction of the gastrocnemius soleus complex causes excessive stress along the medial aspect of the Achilles tendon. During the phase of gait when the foot is flat, particularly if pronation is present, there is internal rotation of the tibia, and this further adds to the stress along the medial aspect of the tendon. The combination of repetitive microtrauma associated with hyperpronation and presumed poor vascularity is the cause of most forms of Achilles tendon pathology. These factors cause repetitive microtrauma to the Achilles tendon with a cumulative effect leading to inflammation, degeneration, and potentially, rupture. Achilles tendinitis may present as acute peritendinitis and a more chronic tendinosis.

Diagnosis

Peritendinitis is an inflammatory condition of the tendon pseudosheath or the paratenon, whereas tendinosis is a degeneration of the substance of the Achilles tendon itself. In acute peritendinitis, the tendon is warm and inflamed. This is easy to diagnose by squeezing the tendon between the thumb and forefinger and gliding over the tendon, which may have a feeling of crepitus. In chronic Achilles tendinosis, the tendon is often thicker, resisted plantarflexion is weak. and posterior heel pain that worsens with activity is present. Retrocalcaneal bursitis and subcutaneous bursitis are common differential diagnoses of posterior heel pain in the runner and can be caused by enlargement of the superior tuberosity of the calcaneus, by improperly fitting shoes, or by impingement of the Achilles tendon on the calcaneus.

Retrocalcaneal bursitis presents with heel pain but localization of the pain can be elicited by squeezing the soft tissues in a medial and lateral direction just anterior to the Achilles tendon. Plain radiographs will demonstrate soft-tissue swelling and, occasionally, calcification within the tendon.

Treatment of Achilles tendinitis

If the tendinitis is severe and acute, a brief period of immobilization in a short leg cast is indicated and nonsteroidal anti-inflammatory medication is used. Once the acute inflammation has subsided, athletic activity is increased and gastrocnemius–soleus strengthening and stretching is begun. Custom orthotic devices or heel lifts are used to control hyperpronation. Local modalities, including ice massage, ultrasound, and iontophoreses,

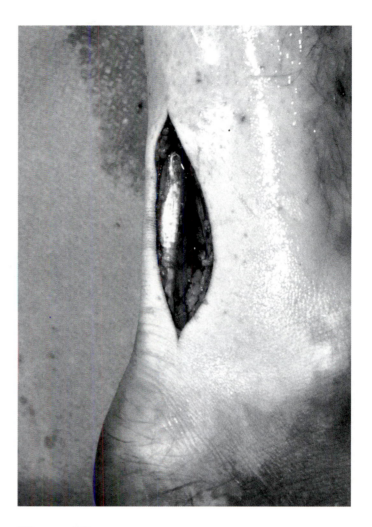

Figure 18

Chronic inflammatory Achilles paratendinitis is evident with thickening of the paratenon and an acute inflammatory infiltrate over the tendon

can be beneficial. Gradual resumption of physical activity can begin with swimming, cycling, and other low-impact activities. Steroid injection to treat inflammation of the Achilles tendon is contraindicated, although a short course of tapered doses of oral steroid is occasionally warranted.

Retrocalcaneal bursitis, which has been refractory to conservative measures, is treated by debridement of all bursal tissue and aggressive resection of the superior aspect of the calcaneal tuberosity. This is usually performed in conjunction with excision of a prominent posterior lateral calcaneal tuberosity. Refractory cases of Achilles tendinitis can be managed surgically with a posteromedial longitudinal incision and debridement of the inflammatory tissue surrounding the tendon. The granular thickened paratenon is easily identified and excised (Fig. 18). After this procedure, patients are able to gradually resume athletic activities within 1 month of the tendon stripping.

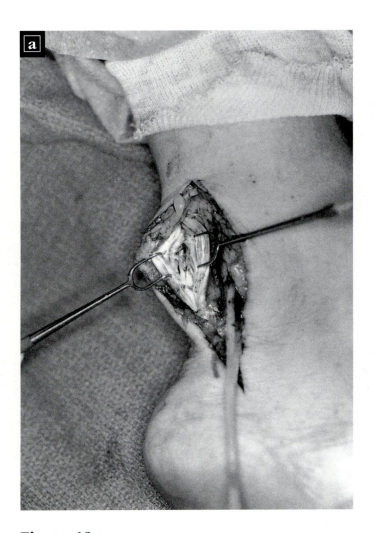 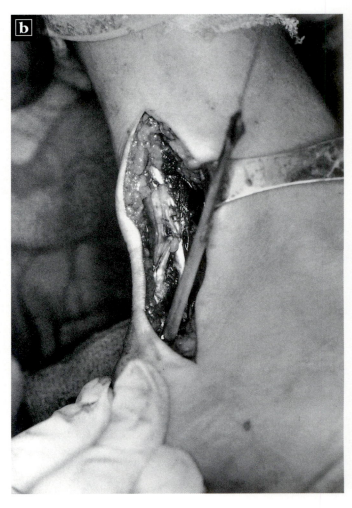

Figure 19

Chronic inflammatory Achilles tendinosis is demonstrated in this 54-year-old athlete (**a**). This was treated with excision of the degenerated portion of the tendon and transfer of the flexor hallucis longus muscle and tendon to reinforce the repair (**b**)

This inflammatory peritendinitis is far easier to treat surgically than chronic degenerative tendinosis. Although the diseased tendon is easy to visualize both clinically and on MRI as a fusiform thickening 2.5–5 cm proximal to the insertion, it is not always easy to identify the diseased portions of the tendon at surgery (Fig. 19a). These longitudinal fissures or degenerative tears may be excised, but I have never been certain as to the extent of tendon debridement required. For more extensive disease with weakness, the tendon is explored for necrotic or degenerated segments and, if severe, the repair is augmented with the flexor hallucis longus muscle (Wapner et al 1993). This muscle not only strengthens the repair, but also brings in needed blood supply to the poorly perfused Achilles tendon. The Achilles tendon is exposed along its length posteromedially, and an incision is made in the foot to harvest the flexor hallucis tendon, which is then transferred proximally through a drill hole in the calcaneus (Fig. 19b).

Achilles tendon rupture

Etiology and diagnosis

Approximately 75% of Achilles tendon ruptures occur in athletes (Fox et al 1975, Clancy et al 1976, Jozsa et al 1989, Bradley & Tibone 1990), predominantly in males between 30 and 40 years old (Inglis et al 1976). Injury is undoubtedly related to certain forms of activity and exercise, since the incidence of Achilles tendon rupture is more common in countries where work is generally sedentary and is markedly decreased in countries, such as China, where physical work is commonplace (Sun et al 1977). The etiology of Achilles tendon rupture is still unclear, but many theories have been proposed, including repetitive microtrauma (Soma & Mandelbaum 1994), inhibitor mechanism malfunction (Stephenson et al 1990), a correlation of rupture with blood type O (Soma & Mandelbaum 1994), hypoxic and mucoid degeneration, decreased perfusion that results in degenerative changes (Lagergren & Lindholm 1958), and systemic or locally infiltrated corticosteroids (Mahler & Fritschy 1992, Soma & Mandelbaum 1994).

A patient who sustains an acute rupture typically presents with a history of acute sharp pain and a sensation of a loud snap or pop commonly reported as being like being struck in the back of the leg. After rupture, patients are either completely incapacitated or can bear some weight on the extremity but lack the ability to plantarflex the foot forcibly. This ability to plantarflex the ankle actively and to walk, albeit with some weakness, can be confusing and leads to errors in diagnosis. The diagnosis of acute rupture is therefore occasionally missed, and the patient may be evaluated late with a chronic rupture, persistent weakness, and difficulty with push-off. Regardless of the etiology, this injury occurs in a wide range of individuals, from the recreational or weekend sports participant to the high-grade athlete.

Treatment options

Treatment goals are to minimize the morbidity of this injury and to optimize the rapid return to full function. Operative options include percutaneous repair (Ma & Griffith 1977, 1981), gastrocnemius flap (Lindholm 1959), simple suture (Nistor 1981), pullout wire (Ralston & Schmidt 1971), fascial reinforcement (Abraham & Pankovich 1975), and polyacetate implant (Clemow & Chen 1986). All treatment options – whether by non-operative closed methods (Haggmark et al 1987, Jacobs et al 1978), open surgical procedures, or percutaneous methods of repair (Ma & Griffith 1977, 1981, Bradley & Tibone 1990) – utilize a short or long leg cast as part of the recovery process.

The rationale for using a cast is that immobilization (for approximately 8 weeks) will achieve tendon healing through hematoma to collagen proliferation and maturation. Unfortunately, immobilization is associated with many complications, including muscle atrophy and long-term weakness, articular cartilage weakening and degeneration, skin necrosis, deep vein thrombosis, and joint stiffness. In addition, from a functional standpoint, cast immobilization never allows full rehabilitation of the extremity, regardless of what operative or nonoperative protocols are used. With a cast as part of the treatment, Nistor (1981) reported at least a 10% deficit regardless of protocol use, Bradley & Tibone (1990) demonstrated a 13–20% deficit, and Inglis and coworkers (Inglis & Sculco 1981, Inglis et al 1976) described a deficit of 12–15% as standard. Cumulatively, these studies indicate that there was never less than a 10% power or strength deficit with protocols utilizing immobilization. Thus, it can be concluded that immobilization, used in conjunction with reparative techniques, may cause increased morbidity.

Several studies demonstrated that mobilization is optimal for connective tissue. Booth (1982, 1987) showed that muscle atrophy can be minimized; Pepels

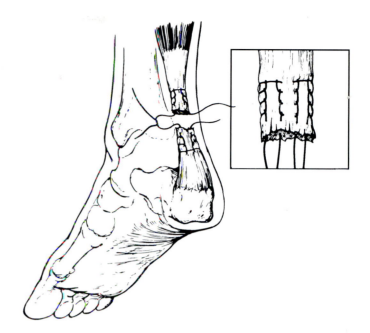

Figure 20

Achilles tendon repair, using locking sutures. One or more strands of suture may be used (reprinted with permission from Mandelbaum 1993)

et al (1983) demonstrated a decreased time of fibril polymerization to collagen; and Gelberman et al (1984) reported that mobilized extremities enhanced the orientation and organization of collagen. Many of these concepts of early mobilization and aggressive rehabilitation have been incorporated into a surgical protocol for management of Achilles tendon rupture.

Although many different methods of suture repair of the Achilles tendon are available, until recently none has been strong enough to allow early range of motion of the foot and ankle. Over the past 8 years, I have been using surgical repair of Achilles tendon rupture in athletes followed by early range of motion and aggressive rehabilitation. This protocol is based on the work of Garrett et al (1987, 1988) and Taylor et al (1990), which reports on collagen's response to loading. This has been extrapolated to repair after Achilles tendon rupture. This treatment emphasizes early and aggressive motion and weight bearing to enhance tendon healing and strength.

Using the technique described below, I have obtained a rigid and stable fixation that allows early range of motion, strengthening, and functional rehabilitation. Although the reported success rates of nonoperative treatment for Achilles tendon rupture emphasize low complication rates, I strongly recommend operative repair for Achilles tendon ruptures in active individuals and athletes. The rerupture rate is far higher with non-operative than with operative treatment, but to the athlete, early return to maximum function is far more important and cannot be realistically attained with conservative treatment (Booth 1982).

Surgical technique

Surgery is performed with the patient in the prone position using general or local anesthesia. I find it useful to prepare both limbs and drape both into the operative field. This permits the examination of the dynamic resting position and establishes the correct tension on the repair by comparison with the opposite limb.

The incision is made medially so that the plantaris tendon, if present, may be incorporated into the repair. The rupture is identified, and the tendon ends are debrided. It is important to establish the correct length of the tendon ends before the sutures are tied. This is not always easy, since the frayed and elongated ends of the tendon do not meet evenly. The bulk of the tendon ends are therefore approximated before the sutures are inserted. The repair is performed with a No. 2 non-absorbable polyfilament suture (Fig. 20). One or two strands of suture may be used, depending on the diameter of the tendon. When the sutures are approximated, the tendon ends should meet. It is important not to repair the tendon with any elongation since this will functionally weaken the muscle. If the plantaris tendon is present, it is cut proximally, and then it is opened up so that the tendon forms a thin sheet, which may be used to cover the repair. The peritenon is repaired using absorbable sutures of 4/0 vicryl, achieving a tight closure over the tendon. To accomplish this, a posterior release of the fascia between the superficial and deep compartments of the leg is often required. Skin closure is performed with a dermal mattress suture of 4/0 nylon, and the lower leg is immobilized with a below-the-knee posterior splint and the ankle in slight equinus.

Approximately 3 days after surgery, the bandages are changed to a removable posterior splint, and an early range of motion program is initiated. The patient is instructed to move the ankle passively and within the limits of comfort four to five times a day through 10–20° of plantarflexion and dorsiflexion. The splint is worn when passive exercises are not being performed.

At 2 weeks, the sutures are removed and, if the wound is fully healed, early weight-bearing, coupled with range-of-motion exercises, is initiated. Patients are fitted with hinged walking boots that permit full plantarflexion but block dorsiflexion at 10° of equinus. At 4 weeks, patients may continue to use the walker boot, which is adjusted to block dorsiflexion at neutral.

Ideally, the repair is performed between 1 and 7 days after injury, depending on the amount of swelling present. If one waits more than 2 weeks, the proximal tendon retracts, and it is not always easy to approximate the ends. If this occurs, it is helpful gently to pull on the proximal tendon with the suture attached for 5–10 minutes. This will always gain 1–2 cm of tendon length, particularly if the repair is performed late. If there is a sizeable defect

between the tendon ends that cannot be corrected by gradual stretch, then tendon transfers using the flexor hallucis longus or peroneus brevis can be used to augment the repair. Other methods, including a turn down of the proximal central portion of the tendon and a slide of the entire musculotendinous unit, have been described.

References

Abraham E, Pankovich A M 1975 Neglected rupture of the Achilles tendon. Treatment by V–Y tendinous flap. J Bone Joint Surg 57A: 253–255

Attarian D E, McCrackin H J, De Vito D P, et al 1985 Biomechanical characteristics of human ankle ligaments. Foot Ankle 6: 54–58

Berridge F R, Bonnin J G 1944 The radiographic examination of the ankle joint including arthrography. Surg Gynecol Obstet 79: 383–389

Bonnin J G 1949 Radiological diagnosis of recent lesions of the lateral ligament of the ankle [comment on paper of this title by JR Hughes]. J Bone Joint Surg 31B: 478

Booth F W 1982 Effect of limb immobilization on skeletal muscle. J Appl Physiol 52: 1113–1118

Booth F W 1987 Physiologic and biomechanical effects of immobilization on muscle. Clin Orthop 219: 15–20

Bradley J P, Tibone J E 1990 Percutaneous and open surgical repairs of Achilles tendon ruptures. A comparative study. Am J Sports Med 18: 188–195

Brostrom L 1966a Sprained ankles. V. Treatment and prognosis in recent ligament ruptures. Acta Chir Scand 132: 537–550

Brostrom L 1966b Sprained ankles. VI. Surgical treatment of chronic ligament ruptures. Acta Chir Scand 132: 551–565

Chrisman O D, Snook G A 1969 Reconstruction of lateral ligament tears of the ankle. An experimental study and clinical evaluation of seven patients treated by a new modification of the Elmslie procedure. J Bone Joint Surg 51A: 904–912

Clancy W G Jr, Neidhart D, Brand R L 1976 Achilles tendonitis in runners: a report of five cases. Am J Sports Med 4: 46–57

Clanton T O 1989 Instability of the subtalar joint. Orthop Clin North Am 20: 583–592

Clanton T O, Schon L C, Baxter D E 1990 An overview of subtalar instability and its treatment. Perspect Orthop Surg 1: 103–113

Clemow A J T, Chen E H 1986 Induction of neo-tendons using a resorbable polymeric scaffold. Presented at the 32nd Annual Meeting of the Orthopaedic Research Society, New Orleans, Louisiana, USA, 17–20 February 1986

Das De S, Balasubramaniam P 1985 A repair operation for recurrent dislocation of peroneal tendons. J Bone Joint Surg 67B: 585–587

Earle A S, Mortiz J R, Tapper E M 1972 Dislocation of the peroneal tendons at the ankle: an analysis of 25 ski injuries. Northwest Med 71: 108–110

Eckert W R, Davis E A Jr 1976 Acute rupture of the peroneal retinaculum. J Bone Joint Surg 58A: 670–672

Edwards M E 1928 The relations of the peroneal tendons to the fibula, calcaneus, and cuboideum. Am J Anat 42: 213–253

Elmslie R C 1934 Recurrent subluxation of the ankle-joint. Ann Surg 100: 364–367

Evans D 1953 Recurrent instability of the ankle – a method of surgical treatment. Proc R Soc Med 46: 343

Evans G A, Hardcastle P, Frenyo A D 1984 Acute rupture of the lateral ligament of the ankle. To suture or not to suture? J Bone Joint Surg 66A: 209–212

Fox J M, Blazina M E, Jobe F W et al 1975 Degeneration and rupture of the Achilles tendon. Clin Orthop 107: 221–224

Garrett W E Jr, Nikolaou P K, Ribbeck B M, et al 1988 The effect of muscle architecture on the biomechanical failure properties of skeletal muscle under passive extension. Am J Sports Med 16: 7–12

Garrett W E Jr, Safran M R, Seaber A V, et al 1987 Biomechanical comparison of stimulated and nonstimulated skeletal muscle pulled to failure. Am J Sports Med 15: 448–454

Gelberman R H, Manske P R, Van deBerg J S, et al 1984 Flexor tendon repair in vitro: a comparative histologic study of the rabbit, chicken, dog, and monkey. J Orthop Res 2: 39–48

Gould N, Seligson D, Gassman J 1980 Early and later repair of lateral ligament of the ankle. Foot Ankle 1: 84–89

Haggmark T, Liedberg H, Eriksson E et al 1987 Calf muscle atrophy and muscle function after non-operative vs operative treatment of Achilles tendon ruptures. Orthopaedics 9: 160–164

Harper M C 1991 The lateral ligamentous support of the subtalar joint. Foot Ankle 11: 354–358

Inglis A E, Scott W N Sculco T P, et al 1976 Ruptures of the tendo Achillis – an objective assessment of surgical and non-surgical treatment. J Bone Joint Surg 58A: 990–993

Inglis A E, Sculco T P 1981 The patient: surgical repair of ruptures of the tendo Achillis. Clin Orthop 156: 160–169

Jackson D W, Ashley R L, Powell J W 1974 Ankle sprains in young athletes. Relation of severity and disability. Clin Orthop 101: 201–215

Jacobs D, Martens M, Van Audekercke R V et al 1978 Comparison of conservative and operative treatment of Achilles tendon rupture. Am J Sports Med 6: 107–111

Jones E 1932 Operative treatment of chronic dislocation of the peroneal tendons. J Bone Joint Surg 14: 574–576

Jozsa L, Kuist M, Balint B J et al 1989 The role of recreational sport activity in Achilles tendon rupture. A clinical, pathoanatomical and sociological study of 292 cases. Am J Sports Med 17: 338–343

Kelly R E 1920 An operation for the chronic dislocation of the peroneal tendons. Br J Surg 7: 502–504

Lagergren C, Lindholm A 1958 Vascular distribution in the Achilles tendon. Acta Chir Scand 116: 491–495

Larsen E 1988 Tendon transfer for lateral ankle and subtalar joint instability. Acta Orthop Scand 59: 168–172

Larsen E, Lund P M 1991 Peroneal muscle function in chronically unstable ankles. A prospective preoperative and postoperative electromyographic study. Clin Orthop 272: 219–226

Leach R E, Schepsis A A 1990 Acute injuries to ligaments of the ankle. In: Evarts C M (ed) Surgery of the Musculoskeletal System. Churchill Livingstone, New York. pp 3887–3913

Lindholm A 1959 A new method of operation in subcutaneous rupture of the Achilles tendon. Acta Chir Scand 117: 261–270

Ma G W, Griffith T G 1977 Percutaneous repair of acute closed ruptured Achilles tendon: a new technique. Clin Orthop 128: 247–255

Ma G W C, Griffith T G 1981 Percutaneous repair of acute closed ruptured Achilles tendon: a new technique. In: Moore T M (ed) Symposium on Trauma to the Leg and Its Sequelae. Mosby Year Book, St. Louis. pp 358–370

Mahler F, Fritschy D 1992 Partial and complete ruptures of the Achilles tendon and local corticosteroid injections. Br J Sports Med 26: 7–14

Mandelbaum B 1993 Disorders of the Achilles tendon. In: Myerson M (ed) Current Therapy in Foot and Ankle Surgery. Mosby Year Book, St Louis, pp 142–145

Martens M A, Noyez J F, Mulier J C 1986 Recurrent dislocation of the peroneal tendons. Results of rerouting the tendons under the calcaneofibular ligament. Am J Sports Med 14: 148–150

McLennan J G 1980 Treatment of acute and chronic luxations of the peroneal tendons. Am J Sports Med 8: 432–436

Meyer J M, Garcia J, Hoffmeyer P, et al 1988a The subtalar sprain. A roentgenographic study. Clin Orthop 226: 169–173

Meyer J M, Hoffmeyer P, Savoy X 1988b High resolution computed tomography in the chronically painful ankle sprain. Foot Ankle 8: 291–296

Myerson M 1993 Cavovarus foot. In: Myerson M (ed) Current Therapy in Foot and Ankle Surgery. Mosby Year Book, St Louis, pp. 203–209

Nistor L 1981 Surgical and non-surgical treatment of Achilles tendon rupture. J Bone Joint Surg 63A: 394–399

Pepels W R J, Plasmans C M T, Sloof T J H 1983 The course of healing of tendons and ligaments. Acta Orthop Scand 54: 952

Pozo J L, Jackson A M 1984 A rerouting operation for dislocation of peroneal tendons: operative technique and case report. Foot Ankle 5: 42–44

Ralston E L, Schmidt E R Jr 1971 Repair of the ruptured Achilles tendon. J Trauma 11: 15–21

Rasmussen O 1985 Stability of the ankle joint. Analysis of the function and traumatology of the ankle ligaments. Acta Orthop Scand Suppl 211: 1–75

Sammarco G J, Chalk D E, Feibel J H 1993 Tarsal tunnel syndrome and additional nerve lesions in the same limb. Foot Ankle 14: 71–77

Sarmiento A, Wolf M 1975 Subluxation of peroneal tendons. Case treated by rerouting tendons under calcaneofibular ligament. J Bone Joint Surg 57A: 115–116

Saxby T, Myerson M 1993 Calcaneus osteotomy. In: Myerson M (ed) Current Therapy in Foot and Ankle Surgery. Mosby Year Book, St Louis, pp 159–162

Schon L C, Clanton T O, Baxter D E 1991 Reconstruction for subtalar instability: a review. Foot Ankle 11: 319–325

Sedlin E D 1960 A device for stress inversion or eversion roentgenograms of the ankle. J Bone Joint Surg 42A: 1184–1190

Siegler S, Block J, Schneck C D 1988 The mechanical characteristics of the collateral ligaments of the human ankle joint. Foot Ankle 8: 234–242

Smith J W 1958 The ligamentous structures in the canalis and sinus tarsi. J Anat 92: 616–620

Smith R W, Reischl S 1988 The influence of dorsiflexion in the treatment of severe ankle sprains: an anatomical study. Foot Ankle 9: 28–33

Snook G A, Chrisman O D, Wilson T C 1985 Long-term results of the Chrisman–Snook operation for reconstruction of the lateral ligaments of the ankle. J Bone Joint Surg 67A: 1–7

Sobel M, Bohne W H, Levy M E 1990a Longitudinal attrition of the peroneus brevis tendon in the fibular groove: an anatomic study [see comments]. Foot Ankle 11: 124–128

Sobel M, Warren R F, Brourman S 1990b Lateral ankle instability associated with dislocation of the peroneal tendons treated by the Chrisman–Snook procedure. A case report and literature review. Am J Sports Med 18: 539–543

Soma C A, Mandelbaum B R 1994 Achilles tendon disorders. Clin Sports Med 13: 811–823

Stephenson C A, Seibert J J, McAndrew M P et al 1990 Sonographic diagnosis of tenosynovitis of the posterior tibial tendon. J Clin Ultrasound 18: 114–116

Sun Y S, Yen T F, Chie L H 1977 Ruptured Achilles tendon: report of 40 cases, Zhonghua Yixue Zazhi 57: 94–98

Taylor D C, Dalton J D Jr, Seaber A V, et al 1990 Viscoelastic properties of muscle–tendon units. The biomechanical effects of stretching. Am J Sports Med 18: 300–309

Thompson F M, Patterson A H 1989 Rupture of the peroneus longus tendon. Report of three cases. J Bone Joint Surg 71A: 293–295

Wapner K L, Pavlock G S, Hecht P J et al 1993 Repair of chronic Achilles tendon rupture with flexor hallucis longus tendon transfer. Foot Ankle 14: 443–449

Watson-Jones R 1955 Fractures and Joint Injuries, 4th ed, vol. 2. Williams & Wilkins, Baltimore

Zoellner G, Clancy W Jr 1979 Recurrent dislocation of the peroneal tendon. J Bone Joint Surg 61A: 292–294

Zollinger H, Meier C H, Waldis M 1983 Diagnosis of subtalar instability utilizing stress tomography. In: Hefte zur Unfallbeilkunde Heft 165. Springer-Verlag; Heidelberg. pp 175–177

X.2 Thermal Injuries

Burns

James D Frame, Douglas H Harrison and Nicholas Parkhouse

Introduction

Each foot makes up approximately 2.5% of the total body surface area in adults and the tissues respond to thermal injury as elsewhere in the body.

A burn of the foot is not commonly seen in isolation and it is usually part of a more extensive thermal injury. The plantar surface of the foot in particular is rarely accidentally burned in a western civilization. This is presumably because of the upright stance with plantar contact, the wearing of adequate protective footwear and the brisk flexor withdrawal response of the foot to painful stimuli. Clearly, unconscious patients and those suffering from a neuropathic disorder do not possess this protective sensory mechanism and the burns tend to be deep. In countries with warmer climates footwear is often not worn and there is thus little protection to thermal injury. In some developing countries, burning of the feet is practised as a supposed therapeutic measure in some medical conditions (Ofodile & Oluwasanmi 1978).

Causes of burn in general

The types of thermal injury and their relative incidences are approximately as follows:

75%	Flame or flash burns	
12%	Scalds	
13%	Direct contact burns	i.e. Molten metal, bitumen, radiator
	Chemical burns	i.e. Concentrated acids and alkalis, phosphorus, hydrofluoric acid, cement
	Electrical burns	inc. Flash injury, arc injury, high voltage entry and exit injury

It has been shown that approximately 50% of burns occur in the home and that two-thirds of these are preventable (Lynch 1979). This is obviously alarming as the aesthetic, social and functional disabilities can remain for the lifespan of the patient.

The aetiology of the foot burn will indicate the depth of tissue damage. For example, scalds are associated with superficial burns of the skin. Flame contact and chemical burns are associated with full thickness injury; and electrical exit injuries, burns in epileptics, paralysed or unconscious patients are associated with deep structural damage. The burns with massive tissue destruction involving skin and deep structures are associated with prolonged thermal contact, especially flame injury, and high voltage electrical conduction injury.

The cause of thermal injury tends to vary with the age of the individual. From birth to 6 months of age burn injury is rare, and nonaccidental injury (NAI) must be excluded. As a baby starts to crawl and walk then scalds are a frequent mode of injury, often from hot beverages. Climbing or being put into a bath of hot water can be a more serious injury in children than in adults because the skin on a child's foot is thinner and consequently will burn to a greater depth. With the onset of adolescence thermal injury appears to be more commonly associated with experimenting or 'playing' with such dangerous materials as matches, petrol and electricity. Into adulthood, occupational burns of the foot are common, and include electrical burns and chemical burns.

Normal skin anatomy

The anatomical basis of the foot has already been described in Chapter I.1. Each individual structure burned is a potential reconstructive problem. The skin itself has considerable powers of regeneration after thermal injury provided that some epithelial elements survive in the wound. Fig. 1 shows the important structures and their position within the skin layers. The cutaneous blood supply is through axial pattern vessels that feed a rich subdermal plexus, and these are obviously important in the healing process. It should be noted that the sole skin is different to the other areas of skin in the foot because it has:

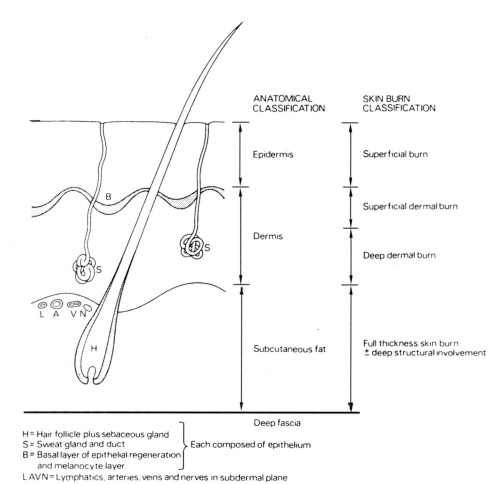

Figure 1

Positions of important structures
within skin layers

ANATOMICAL
CLASSIFICATION

SKIN BURN
CLASSIFICATION

Epidermis

Superficial burn

Superficial dermal burn

Dermis

Deep dermal burn

Subcutaneous fat

Full thickness skin burn
± deep structural involvement

Deep fascia

H = Hair follicle plus sebaceous gland
S = Sweat gland and duct   } Each composed of epithelium
B = Basal layer of epithelial regeneration
    and melanocyte layer
L A V N = Lymphatics, arteries, veins and nerves in subdermal plane

1. A thicker keratin layer
2. No hair follicles
3. Sweat glands deeper in the dermis and often
   adjacent to superficial fascia.

Both the skin and subcutaneous tissue of the sole are
highly adapted for weight bearing and functional repair
after a full thickness burn remains a reconstructive
challenge.

Pathology

The old classification of first degree, second degree and
third degree burns has been superseded. Excluding
simple erythema and superficial burns, skin burns are
classified as dermal (superficial or deep) or full thickness. A combination of all these types is usually present
in a significant thermal injury and it is well known that
burn depth can progress over up to 36 hours after the
burn (Lawrence 1974, deCamara et al 1982). Figure 2
shows that if the intermediate zone of stasis is at the
dermosubcutaneous junction and the deep hair follicle
epithelium has been included in this zone, then an

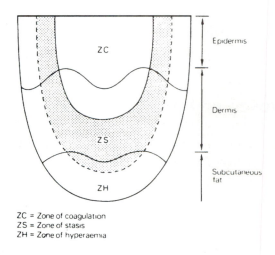

ZC = Zone of coagulation
ZS = Zone of stasis
ZH = Zone of hyperaemia

Figure 2

Burn depth progression

initially deep dermal burn may progress to a full thickness burn. Burn depth progression can be limited by
maintaining adequate hydration, preventing oedema and
controlling sepsis.

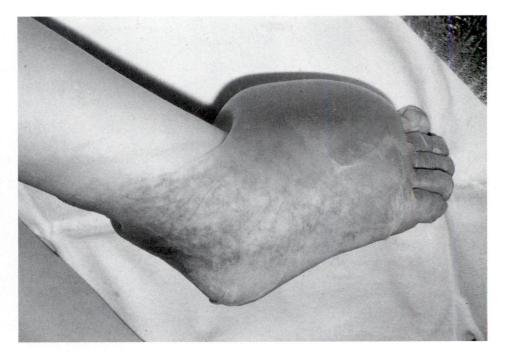

Figure 3
Superficial dermal burn caused by brief contact between skin and a chemical. Note that the blisters are thin walled

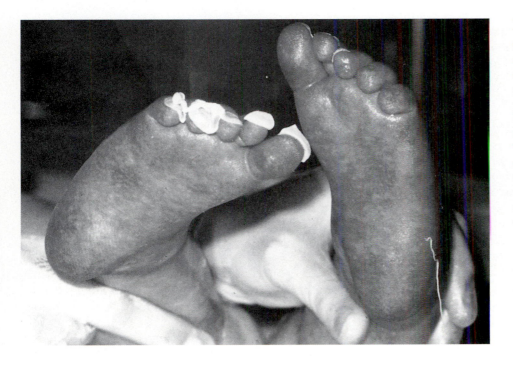

Figure 4
Contrast the injury in Fig. 3 with this deep dermal and full thickness injury on the plantar and dorsal surfaces of the feet, which was caused by prolonged immersion in very hot bath water. In this particular case a non-accident injury was identified. The blister roof is thick and the moist red base contains a few thrombosed veins. A child will tend to suffer a deeper burn than an adult in similar circumstances because a child's skin is thinner

A burn injury will heal by a process of epithelial regeneration based on intact basal epithelium and the epithelium related to the skin adnexae. The greater the density of viable epithelium at the base of the burn wound, the faster the burn will heal. Thus superficial burns heal very quickly, i.e. within 10 days, superficial dermal burns will heal within 3 weeks, deep dermal burns will heal in between 3 and 6 weeks and full thickness burns with no residual epithelial remnants may never heal. A full thickness burn can heal only by epithelial ingrowth from the healthy nonburned skin edges and there appears to be a finite gap over which epithelium can bridge. Clearly, therefore, a narrow band of full thickness burn may eventually heal but large areas will not heal without surgical intervention. A sterile moist environment enhances epithelialization but there must be a concomitant adequate nutritional intake. The thicker keratin layer on the sole helps to protect the area from thermal injury and the more deeply positioned sweat glands compensate for the lack of hair follicles with regard to available epithelium for healing purposes.

Deep structural burns essentially contain necrotic tissue, which can be life-threatening if left. Acute renal failure, disseminated intravascular coagulation, and deep seated sepsis (including clostridial) are all causes of burn mortality associated with deep burns.

Extensive damage from a high voltage electrical injury is a possible cause of such an injury where an early amputation may save the patient's life but a heroic attempt at salvage may cause the patient's death.

Inflammation causes oedema in and around the burned area, which may be severe for several days and then tends to subside. The degree of swelling can be controlled to some extent by leg elevation, bed rest and pressure dressing. It is important to control spreading cellulitis within the oedematous layer of the burned lower leg and foot, and of particular importance is careful daily toilet between the toes.

Clinical features

An adequate history will indicate burn depth even before viewing the injury. It is important to know the cause of burn, the duration of contact of the burning substance on the foot, the type of clothing and footwear worn at the time of burn and the immediate local management of the burned area. The exact time of injury, the percentage body surface area burned and the weight of the patient must be known to calculate an intravenous fluid resuscitation programme if appropriate.

A superficial burn presents rather similarly to simple erythema and the skin often appears intact, but if the burned area is gently rubbed with a gloved finger the superficial epidermis will 'peel' off to leave a raw, red, moist, tender bed. Blisters tend to develop some hours after the burn. The amount of burn oedema lost from such an injury is small and the area heals rapidly to leave a minimal scar. This type of thermal injury of the foot can often be managed on an out-patient basis.

A superficial dermal burn presents with a very painful area of early blistering (Fig. 3). The blisters are typically more thick walled than the superficial burns and are often burst by the time of presentation. The bed of the deroofed blister is very tender, is red–pink in colour and is rather moist in the acute phase. The area that is deroofed will blanche significantly if pressed with a gloved finger and rapidly return to its original colour on release.

A deep dermal burn may be blistered and the roof is composed of a relatively thick dead skin layer (Fig. 4). When deroofed, the bed is white, but still sensitive to pin prick. The healing time is rather prolonged in a deep dermal burn and the scars tend to become hypertrophic if allowed to heal without surgical intervention.

A full thickness skin burn often does not blister but appears as an area of thick leathery eschar (Figs. 5–6). If it includes the adjacent subcutaneous tissue, thrombosed vessels may be visible, confirming the diagnosis. As the cutaneous nerve ends have been destroyed, the burned area is insensitive except at the junction between

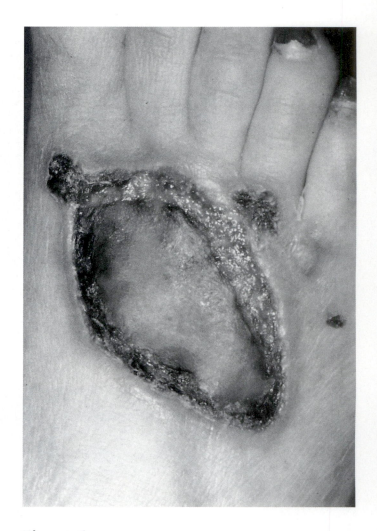

Figure 5
Full thickness skin burn caused by direct contact with molten metal

the burned and nonburned skin. In practice it is often difficult to distinguish accurately between a deep dermal burn and a burn that is just full thickness, but in theory pin prick sensation is present in the former. This investigation in an acutely burned and distressed patient is commonly inaccurate and may be superfluous as the clinical management does not alter. Perhaps the only indication for it is in the patient with a circumferential burn where an escharotomy is being considered.

In electrical burns where the foot has been an exit point, the heart should be checked for conduction defects. Surgery is deferred for 5 days to allow tissue necrosis to be completed. Excision and cover with a flap or skin graft if appropriate is then carried out. In high voltage electrical burns joints may be rigid, owing to severe muscle damage, which may lead to myoglobinuria and renal failure if not ruthlessly debrided. Venous and arterial thrombosis will intensify the volume of tissue damage. Amputation early in this process should be seriously considered to preserve life (Fig. 7).

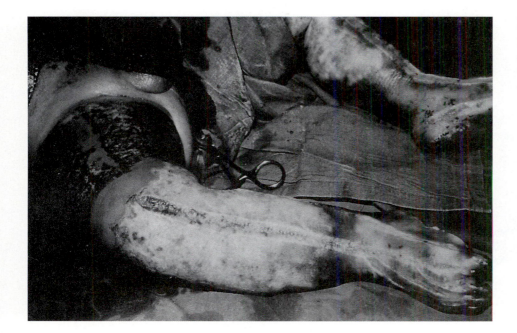

Figure 6

Full thickness flame burns of the feet and lower legs in a child. The burns were circumferential and escharotomies have been performed

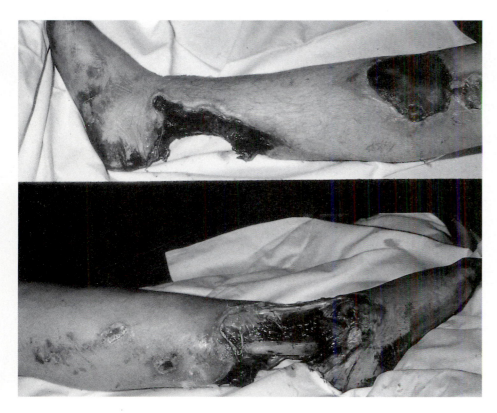

Figure 7

An extensive burn with considerable tissue destruction caused by high voltage electrical contact

Treatment

The primary aim of treating foot burns is to achieve healing in as short a time as possible. The secondary aim is to achieve a functional, cosmetically acceptable foot. In some respects the management to achieve these aims overlaps in that correct early treatment may prevent the need for further procedures.

Superficial burns of the feet should be managed conservatively with infrequent dressings as described later. They should heal within 10 days. Superficial dermal burns should be managed conservatively as above and they should heal within three weeks.

Deep burns on the sole of the foot often re-epithelialize through deep seated sweat gland epithelial proliferations. In such cases it is better to manage conservatively for a period of 3–4 weeks since both the quality and the

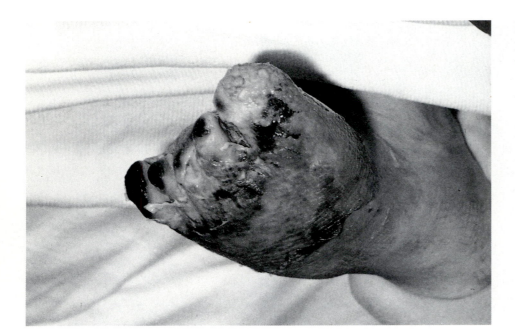

Figure 8

Autoamputation of the toes following a full thickness burn injury to the foot

innervation of the new surface epithelium are likely to be superior to those obtained with skin grafts. Full thickness skin burns should be treated surgically to obtain early skin cover and a better quality scar. The surgical management consists of tangential serial excision of the burn down to healthy tissue and covering the area with skin graft (either as a sheet, fenestrated, or meshed). It is sometimes difficult to identify burned tissue under a tourniquet and in this situation the clue to viability is bleeding of the tissues after release of the tourniquet. Under an exsanguinating tourniquet the phrase 'red is dead' is appropriate and excision down to a 'white is right' plane ensures a healthy base. Excision and grafting should be performed either before the fifth day after the burn or after the third week.

Intermediate grafting, i.e. between 5 days and 3 weeks, is not generally practised because of difficulty in assessing the depth of the tissue damage with no satisfactory plane of demarcation. Septicaemia due to bacterial spillage from the excised burn wound cannot be met by an adequate host immune response at this stage as this has not had time to develop. A circumferential full thickness skin burn of the leg or foot should have an escharotomy done as soon as diagnosed, and similarly a deep structural burn should have a fasciotomy.

By 3 weeks after the burn the eschar of a full thickness skin burn will have separated to leave a defect with a base of granulation tissue. A skin graft will take on such a surface but it is usual to rub the area with a gauze swab or even to shave the granulations down first. Recently, dermabrasion has been used effectively in deep dermal burns at 3 weeks to create a good bed on which to lay a skin graft and to produce cosmetically acceptable scars.

Full thickness skin burns with deeper structural damage should be excised before 5 days after the burn, as the necrotic zone may be easily assessed at this time. In the case of more widespread necrosis, either the dead tissue must be removed as soon as possible at a one-stage operation or as a series of debridement procedures, or the leg must be primarily amputated. If tendon, bone or joints are exposed then a decision must be made as to whether the foot is salvageable and if so then will the foot be of functional use to the patient or a major handicap. It is far easier if an amputation is done before embarking on a prolonged trail of failed reconstructive procedures. The toes may autoamputate (Fig. 8) following such a burn but occasionally surgical ablation in the acute phase may enhance mobilization.

Table 1 shows the general management appropriate to all depths of foot burn that is in general use. We have divided the post-burn period into the acute phase (0–36 hours), 36 hours to 5 days, 5 days to 3 weeks and a late phase (3 weeks onwards). It is assumed that the burning source has been removed, the burn size and severity warrants admission initially and the treatment chosen will be appropriate for the burn. The patient may be discharged from hospital and treated as an out-patient if appropriate.

Other burns

Strong acids and strong alkalis are initially different to scald or flame burns in that the burning agent is often still present on the burn. The immediate management should include irrigating or immersing the foot in a copious volume of water. If this fails to control the burn then irrigating the burn with a weak alkali (in the case of acid burns) or acid (in the case of alkali burns) may counter the burn. If these measures fail then there is an

Table 1 Patient management after a burn

Time after the burn	Local	General

0–36 hours	Medical
	  swab burn, nose, throat
	  photograph/chart burns
	  leg dressings
	Surgical
	  deroof blisters
	  escharotomy
	  fasciotomy
	  excision and graft
	  debridement dead muscle
	  amputation
	Beware: distal circulation
		Medical
		  assess patient generally
		  analgesia (intravenous)
		  correct hypovolaemia
		  — intravenous fluid resuscitation adults > 15% BSA
		                                             children > 10%
		  monitor urine output
		  — catheterize adults > 15%
		                      children > 15%
		  tetanus toxoid
		  ECG monitor electrical burns
		  blood tests: Hb, biochemistry, glucose, group and save
		  correct electrolyte imbalance
		  physiotherapy — chest and legs
		Beware: inhalation injury, stress ulcers, paralytic ileus

36 hours to 5 days	Medical
	  sepsis control
	  dressings every 2–3 days
	  footdrop splints
	  leg elevation
	Surgical
	  debridement
	  tangential excision and graft
	  excision and graft
	  excision and flap
		Medical
		  sepsis control
		  nutritional support
		Beware: hypostatic pneumonia, stress ulcers, pulmonary emboli

5 days to 3 weeks	Medical
	  sepsis control
	  dressings
	  footdrop prevention
	  mobilize nongrafted legs
	Surgical
	  avoid grafting
		Medical
		  sepsis control
		  nutritional support
		Beware: stress ulcers, pulmonary emboli

3 weeks onwards	Medical
	  sepsis control
	  dressings
	  mobilize
	  scar control
	Surgical
	  skin graft clean bed
	  shave and graft
	  dermabrade and graft
	  release contractures and graft
	  shave and overgraft
	  flap cover/tissue expansion
	  amputation
		Medical
		  mobilization and motivation
		  psychological adaptation
		  social and job review

indication for early surgery. Hydrofluoric acid occasionally burns the foot and this substance is renowned for its ability to remove calcium from the circulation. Calcium gluconate is the specific antagonist and is rubbed onto the burned area until the pain settles. The cream is applied topically as often as is necessary to relieve the pain. Some authorities inject 10% calcium gluconate into the subcutaneous tissues (except around the toes) but this is not a universal procedure. If the pain cannot be relieved by such measures then surgical excision of the burned area is indicated. The serum calcium may fall quite dramatically in such cases, and a patient with significant hydrofluoric acid burns should be admitted for close clinical and biochemical observation.

Phosphorus continues to ignite spontaneously if exposed to the air, therefore phosphorus burns should be immersed in water immediately. Copper sulphate solution turns the active phosphorus into recognizable black particles which can then be picked from the wound. A copper sulphate solution is potentially toxic with prolonged skin exposure, so total foot immersion for a prolonged period is not advised.

Control of sepsis

A burned patient is immunocompromised and as such is susceptible to a whole host of infections. The commonest organisms on a burn are *Pseudomonas aeruginosa* and *Staphylococcus aureus* (Lowbury 1979). These organisms often originate from the burned patient and therefore are of a relatively low virulence. Antibiotics are not routinely given to burn victims, even though a burn wound is an ideal culture medium, because it is better to be colonized with antibiotic-sensitive organisms than by rare or multiresistant organisms.

The only indications for the use of antibiotics are spreading cellulitis, septicaemia, and isolation of group A β-haemolytic streptococcus from the burn wound. Group A β-haemolytic streptococci rapidly destroy fresh skin grafts. It must be emphasized that pyrexia is the norm after a burn, and antibiotics should not be given for a low grade temperature in isolation.

It is, however, important to know the organisms on a burn wound in case an antibiotic is needed to control systemic sepsis. Swabs should be taken from the burn, the nose and the throat of the patient on admission and from the burn at each change of dressing. The surface colony counts on burned surfaces can be reduced by bathing or soaking the foot in a chlorhexidine bath regularly. It is very important to clean meticulously between the toes in a burned foot as it is often the harbouring site of bacteria.

Burn dressings

There are many types of commercial dressings available on the market, often with antibacterial action, but the usual dressings are:

1. For superficial and superficial dermal burns, vaseline impregnanted gauze (tulle gras) is the cheapest and most commonly used contact dressing. A foot with this type of burn can also be treated in a polythene bag containing chlorhexidine or silversulphadiazine.
2. For deep dermal and full thickness burns the decision must be made whether an early or a late grafting technique will be used. For early grafting the burn need only be dressed with tulle gras or a non-adherent silicone based dressing prior to surgery as previously described. In late grafting cases, frequent silversulphadiazine bags or dressings should be used. The silversulphadiazine is particularly effective in controlling pseudomonas species on the burn and also provides some pain relief to the patient.
3. Deep structural burns should be dressed with tulle gras as they will all be operated upon within 5 days.

Skin replacement

The ultimate aim in the management of the burned foot must be to obtain a cosmetically acceptable, functioning foot that will fit comfortably into a shoe and cause no long-term problems. In the first instance the priority is to gain complete wound healing and in the vast majority of cases the most superficial burns will heal on their own. Deep dermal and full thickness burns, however, are best treated by the early tangential excision and skin graft technique. A thin skin graft will take better than a thick skin graft but will also contract more. Thus a thicker skin graft should be preferred around a joint but a thinner graft should be preferred elsewhere. A thin skin graft donor site will also heal faster and be available for reharvest earlier. Obviously a skin graft on the weight-bearing area of the sole is not ideal but, if necessary, once the skin graft has matured it can be replaced by a flap. Flaps carried out early are often inset into an infected environment and are more likely to fail. Flaps on the foot are generally insensate, with certain exceptions. Insensate flaps are prone to the effects of pressure and shearing forces which frequently cause painless ulceration, which in turn is aggravated by hyperkeratosis (excessive callus) in the scars. Complications can be pre-empted by close follow-up, often in conjunction with a chiropodist or podiatrist, and by the use of custom made orthotic devices.

Skin grafts can be lost for a variety of reasons, including an unhealthy bed, colonization with group A β-haemolytic streptococci, an unsupported graft with leg dependency at an early stage, and haematoma under the graft. It is in order to minimize the last-named cause that a sheet of skin graft is often fenestrated or meshed. For a combination of an excellent chance of skin 'take' and good cosmesis a mesh of 1.5 : 1 is recommended. The most recent advance in skin graft technique is in the use of cultured autograft and homograft. At present, though, this method is not suitable in the coverage of the burned foot because not only is the 'take' poor but the skin that does take contracts by over 50% of its original surface area.

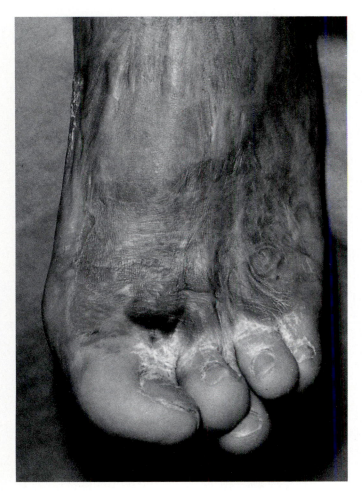

Figure 9

Contracture after a burn on the dorsum of the foot. The contracture is pulling the toes into a dorsal position and causing discomfort on wearing normal footwear

A skin graft will not take on exposed tendon or bare cortical bone and if these structures are to survive then they must be covered with a vascularized flap. After debriding the burned foot a local, regional, distal or free flap can be used. These are discussed in Chapter VII.4.

To preserve movement in exposed joints, flap cover is essential at an early stage and a vascularized tendon graft can be included in the free flap if indicated. Relatively early arthrodesis is recommended by some authors to obtain a stable pain-free limb if joint destruction is inevitable (Jackson 1976). To enable the foot to fit into a shoe a flap often needs to be thinned and this is done when the flap and scars have matured (Fig. 9).

Scar and contracture control

In general, the longer a burn takes to heal the deeper the burn and the greater the chance of developing an unsightly scar and problems with joint contractures. Superficial burns heal rapidly with minimal scar formation but deep dermal burns can take 3 weeks to heal and then form an unsightly scar with progressive contracture formation. A skin-grafted or a flap-covered burn tends not to become hypertrophic except at the margins. A normal scar can be expected to mature within 1 year, but a hypertrophic scar may take as long as 5 years to mature and a keloid scar can be present for decades. It is during the active phase that a scar is red, firm to hard, raised, unsightly and itchy, but the scar then becomes pale, soft and flat, and stops being itchy. During the active phase, the scar length tends to contract and if this is not countered then deformity will result. Thus at the earliest possible time (i.e. just before complete healing) patients with deep dermal and full thickness burns should be considered for pressure garment scar and contracture control. Custom-made elasticated garments are extremely useful in enhancing burn scar maturation and preventing contractures. In suitable cases, spacers can be fitted to prevent burn syndactyly. These garments can be used alone or in combination with silicone gel, which has recently been shown to have scar maturation properties of its own (Perkins et al 1982, Hirshowitz et al 1993). The burn scar should be regularly massaged with oily cream during the infrequent times that the pressure garment is not being worn.

For established hypertrophy, pressure therapy is still of use, but in addition triamcinolone injections, intra-lesional scar excision, or tangential shave and overgraft are useful alternatives.

Burn scar contractures will cause anatomical distortion of joints, which could lead to secondary irreversible joint changes. The deformity will vary with the site of the burn contracture:

1. *The dorsum of the foot*

Hyperextension of the metatarsophalangeal and ankle joints with impaired or abnormal growth pattern in children is not uncommon. Joint contractures such as these can sometimes be prevented by using pressure garments, splints, or custom-made moulded silicone shoes (Feldman et al 1974). Once established, however, a surgical release and skin graft or, in the case of a narrow linear contracture, a Z-plasty will correct the contracture. This is provided that the joints are not themselves irreversibly damaged. Occasionally, such as when tendons are exposed during the release of contracture, a skin graft will not take and flap cover is necessary. To assist in obtaining a good graft take, the joint over which the contracture was acting should be immobilized until the graft has consolidated, i.e. about 10 days. Fig. 9 shows a burn scar on the dorsum of the foot that is extending the metatarsophalangeal joints and preventing the wearing of reasonable footwear. The contracture was released and skin grafted, and the metatarsophalangeal joints were immobilized by using Kirschner wires.

2. *The sole of the foot*

Flexion deformity of the toes can cause problems with footwear. These contractures can be released and grafted as above but flap cover is more appropriate over the weight-bearing areas.

3. *Lateral and medial contractures around the ankle joint*

Burn scar contractures at these sites will tend to pull the forefoot into valgus and varus respectively. Although the deformity may be immediately correctable it will often recur if the release and skin graft technique alone is used. It is better to release the contracture and provide flap cover if possible.

4. *The heel and Achilles tendon region*

A contracture in this region will produce an equinus deformity, which is often difficult to correct. It is far better to avoid this problem by splinting and providing early flap cover if appropriate.

The problem with thick hypertrophic scars, areas of skin graft and noninnervated flaps is that they remain relatively insensitive and consequently trophic ulcers are not uncommon, especially on the sole. In these cases careful attention to foot hygiene and adequate protection are needed for the rest of the patient's life.

Other complications

Unstable scarring without contracture of any significance is a difficult problem. In the first instance, the scar should be managed conservatively with avoidance of pressure from footwear over the unstable area, keeping the area clean and then massaging the area with oily creams when healed. Adjacent hyperkeratotic areas should be pared down, preferably by a podiatrist. If these methods fail then the unstable scar will need reinforcing either by a shave and overgraft technique or by excising the area and introducing new tissue in the form of a flap. The overgraft method involves shaving the unstable epidermis and then covering the exposed dermis with a thick skin graft, thus providing a more stable base.

Syndactyly of the toes is not a functional problem unless there is a deformity due to differential growth patterns of the toes or due to concomitant dorsal or plantar contractures. In most instances, therefore, toe syndactyly is not operated upon. Toenail dystrophy is commonly associated with forefoot burns and can usually be managed satisfactorily by a podiatrist.

Acquired vertical talus deformity can follow some severe burns of the foot and leg in infancy (Jackson 1980). This is due to a shortening of the calf muscles, which pulls the talus and calcaneus into equinus, a scar contracture that pulls the forefoot into eversion, valgus and dorsiflexion, and an under-developed sustentaculum tali, which is a feature of the first year or two of life. It is the sustentaculum tali which normally prevents the downward dislocation of the head of the talus.

Septic arthritis has occasionally been reported in burned patients; often it is iatrogenic (Jackson 1980).

Cold injury

Michael Ward and Nicholas Parkhouse

Populations at risk

More than 100 million people worldwide may be at risk from cold injury, yet it is relatively uncommon in civilian life and is generally associated with illness, injury or unusually harsh climatic conditions.

In wartime, the position is different, as large numbers may be exposed to climatic extremes against which they cannot take normal precautions. Cold injury was of considerable significance in Napoleon's Russian campaign and in many previous wars. In World War II there were 90 000 casualties in the US Army due to cold, 87% from rifle companies, and in the winter of 1943 frostbite injuries among US heavy bomber crews were greater than all other casualties put together. In the British Army, because of vigorously enforced foot hygiene – a legacy from World War I when there were 115 000 cold injuries, cases were minimal. In the Korean Campaign, 1950–1952, 25% of all casualties were due to cold and in the Falklands in 1982, 15% were due to cold injury of the lower limbs. A small number of cases occur in polar travellers and mountaineers despite improvements in equipment, technique and knowledge (Washburn 1962, Schechter & Sarot 1968, Hanson & Goldman 1969, Ward 1974, Marsh 1983).

Temperature regulation

A useful but oversimplified concept is to imagine the body as consisting of a central core with a relatively uniform temperature of 37°C and an insulating shell with a temperature of 33°C. Heat transfer within the body occurs by convection through the circulation and conduction through peripheral tissue to skin surface.

As the maintenance of the central core temperature is essential to life this may occur at the expense of the peripheral 'expendable' structures such as toes and fingers. The control of body temperature depends on interaction between heat production and heat loss. The former depends on normal body metabolism, which at rest corresponds to an oxygen consumption of the order of 5 ml/kg/min. During heavy exercise and shivering, heat output may rise considerably; maximal oxygen consumption in athletes may be as high as 85 ml/kg/min, though this level cannot be maintained.

Heat loss in dry cold conditions is mainly by convection or transfer of heat by bulk movement when air adjacent to the body is heated. If air so heated remains trapped it will serve as insulation. If it is disturbed by external wind, considerable heat loss can occur; this is prevented by windproof clothing. Loss of heat by conduction occurs when clothes become wet from rain, sweat or melted snow. As water is a good conductor of heat, heat loss is increased.

Heat loss by radiation is independent of air movement. If the body heat is greater than the surroundings, heat is lost; if less, the body gains heat. In polar and high mountain environments heat gain by both direct and indirect radiation (the albedo) from snow may be of prime importance in survival (Chrenko & Pugh 1961). Heat gain at high altitude (5800 m and over) can be three times that occurring at sea level in desert regions (Pugh 1962).

Heat loss by evaporation may occur through perspiration or in expired air, and at the high ventilation rates of altitude the latter may be most important. Disordered lung function, or 'Eskimo-lung', caused by exposure for long periods at subzero temperatures, has been reported, and this depresses oxygen uptake and, therefore, heat production (Schaeffer et al 1980). Exhaustion may lead to reduced stroke volume, a falling peripheral resistance and shift in the distribution of blood to capacitance vessels. This failure of vasomotor regulation, with pooling of peripheral venous blood, will accelerate heat loss in cold conditions (Ekelund 1967), and low blood pressure states have been described following ascent to extreme altitude (Pugh & Ward 1956).

Perspiration occurs as a result of exercise and emotional stimulus, and the soles of the feet, palms of hands and axillae are particularly affected. On military operations emotional sweating may be increased when periods of great activity followed by immobility are common. Neglect in the designs of footwear can lead to serious cold injury. Varicose veins of the lower limbs may increase heat loss by convection, and cold phlebitis has been reported. Heat loss from the body is prevented by the insulation of tissues, air and clothes, and that provided by clothes is the most important. Insulation of the feet is by means of boots, which should be designed to keep the feet both dry and warm. Though less subject to cooling, the foot is less easy to rewarm than the hand as local metabolism and heat store are both poor. The part played by blood flow in heat input is relatively larger in the foot than in the hand.

Footwear in cold, underdeveloped countries often consists of animal skin packed with grass or leaves, and Eskimos use the mukluk, which operates on the same principle.

Modern ski boots with a plastic outer and moulded foam inners are remarkably warm, and this same principle is now used in the manufacture of mountaineering boots, which have a plastic outer shell and detachable inner boot of man-made fibre. This is much lighter and less clumsy than the double leather boot. Often a leather boot with a firm sole is worn with one or more pairs of socks and with an insole. Double leather boots with a detachable inner have been developed but are very heavy and clumsy. Vapour barrier boots suffer from the defect that feet remain constantly wet and liable to skin disorders.

A gaiter should be fixed to the boot and this should extend to the knee. Snow may easily enter the boot if only an ankle gaiter is used, and the snow will melt and cause cold injury.

For permanent shelter, huts, tents, snow-caves or individual snow slots should be used. In snow conditions, particularly if there is danger of avalanche, a snow hole or individual snow slot may be preferable to a tent. One accommodating four people takes about 3–4 hours to dig. It has the advantage of permanence, safety, warmth and relative· exclusion from wind noise. The entrance should be clearly marked.

High altitude and cold injury

Oxygen uptake falls with altitude. At extreme altitudes the margin between maximum oxygen consumption and that necessary for adequate heat production and work narrows, and cases of frostbite of the feet have been recorded in fully clad mountaineers. Both cold and high altitude raise the packed cell volume and viscosity and slow peripheral blood flow. Cold injury to capillary walls leads to plasma leakage and intravascular sludging. This local haemoconcentration will be increased at altitude, and impaired tissue nutrition and necrosis may occur more rapidly.

Dehydration, the result of abnormal water loss from the lungs caused by increased respiration, will also increase blood viscosity, and thrombosis may be encouraged by relative inactivity. Even at normal temperatures the blood flow in the skin is reduced at high altitude, the result of arteriolar vasoconstriction. Cardiac output is also decreased as may be basal metabolic rate and the ability to shiver. Hypoxia and cold blunt mental function and precautions taken against cold injury may be inadequate. Deterioration at altitude leading to poor appetite, which, with decreased calorie intake, results in diminution of the insulating layer of subcutaneous fat.

Cold injury to the feet often occurs during bivouacs. A snowcave must be dug, both crampons and boots removed and feet warmed in the companion's armpit or abdomen. Both fluid and food should be taken if available. With these precautions it has been possible to survive at night at 8600 m at −35°C without supplementary oxygen and without frostbite (Clarke 1976, Heath & Williams 1981, Ward et al 1995).

Cold injury complicating trauma

The risk of frostbite in exposed subdermal tissue is considerable. Devitalized tissue freezes in 1 minute at 0°C if wind speeds rise above 2 metres per second.

If hypotension or haemorrhagic hypovolaemia are present, the normal signs of hypothermia may be masked. The risk of hypothermia is also increased in victims with partially perfused exposed tissue at subzero temperatures. When warmed, these hypothermic patients may start to bleed profusely from injured tissue. In addition, the analgesic protection afforded by cold will be lost on rewarming. Wounds should be thermally protected as soon as possible by suture or wound dressing and a balance struck between thermal protection and the necessity for close observation (Pearn 1982).

Cold injury and renal failure

Incipient renal failure associated with rhabdomyolysis has been recorded following severe frostbite of both lower limbs and in nonfreezing cold injury of the feet in children. Severe exercise may also be a factor (Raifman et al 1978, Rosenthall et al 1981).

Cold injury and the elderly

The elderly are less active than younger people, and they have an inadequate diet and a sluggish metabolic and vasomotor response with progressive impairment of thermoregulatory mechanisms. The long-term conservative management, particularly that of freezing cold injury with the possible complications of hypostatic pneumonia, bedsores and urinary infection, has to be balanced against amputation and early mobility. Much depends on the mental status and physical activity of the patient (Emslie-Smith 1981, Ramstead et al 1980).

Physiopathology

Nonfreezing cold injury may progress to freezing cold injury and both may occur in the same lower limb and be associated with hypothermia. Nonfreezing cold injury usually occurs in wet and cold conditions between 0° and 15°C, though the upper limits have not been fixed and symptoms and signs of immersion injury have developed at higher temperatures (Mills & Mills 1993). Frostbite occurs at temperatures of 0°C and below in dry and cold conditions.

In nonfreezing cold injury the skin is less affected than deeper structures and probably the major damage is to the nerves, owing to the direct action of cold and indirectly to hypoxia, the result of vasospasm and haemagglutination. Nerve conduction may cease after 1–3 hours of prolonged cooling. Muscle is very sensitive to local cooling and the temperature of deep muscle after 2 hours immersion may be only 1–2°C above the fluid surrounding it. After 8 hours of such exposure the speed of muscle movement is greatly decreased. Cold-induced vasodilatation with hyperaemia follows the ischaemic phase. General body cooling can affect both the degree of vasodilatation and hyperaemia, which if suppressed results in the temperature of the affected part falling to that of the air or water surrounding it.

Tissues vary in their resistance to freezing cold injury; skin appears to freeze when its temperature reaches −0.53°C, and muscle, blood vessels and nerves are also highly susceptible. Connective tissue, tendons and bone are relatively resistant. Fat necrosis and atrophy occur.

Nerves

Decreasing temperature increases proportionally the clinical severity, which is matched in peripheral nerves by an increasingly severe morphological change. The main findings are primary axonal damage with an immediate increase in the mean diameter of myelinated and nonmyelinated fibres, marked oedema, and a delayed and selective axon degeneration. There is a selective vulnerability to cold based on nerve fibre diameter, myelinated fibres being more susceptible than nonmyelinated. Demyelination is confined to the regions just proximal to sites of axonal degeneration (Kennett & Gilliatt 1991a,b). Degeneration of nerve fibres is probably due to increased permeability of endoneurial vessels, which leads to diffuse oedema, the production of toxins, changes in osmolarity and increase in endoneural pressure. Whilst there is clear clinical and pathological evidence of ischaemia in freezing cold injury this is less clear in nonfreezing cold injury though some evidence suggests that a cyclical ischaemia reperfusion type of injury may be responsible (Irwin et al 1994).

Once the temperature falls below freezing for more than a few seconds, nerve degeneration occurs, affecting all nerve fibres equally. There is complete necrosis of all structures within the perineurium except the endothelial lining of blood vessels (Peyronnard et al 1977, Nukada et al 1981).

Skin

The freezing of skin at temperatures of −1.9°C for 7 minutes causes no lasting injury, whereas after 11½ minutes the skin is red and tender for several days. Repeated exposure for 20 minutes or more causes blistering.

Blood vessels

Damage to blood vessel walls depends on the period of contact and degree of cold, and plasma leaks into the tissues, forming blisters. These contain products of tissue breakdown associated with vasoconstriction, and increased leucocyte sticking and platelet aggregation occur.

Intravascular blood becomes more viscous and haemagglutination with blood vessel blockage and gangrene occurs. Owing to the actions of precapillary sphincters, arteriovenous shunts open and close in cycles and blood bypasses the frozen part. Complete closure of the arteriovenous shunts renders the part avascular and this mechanism protects the hypothalamic temperature-regulating centre from cooled blood and the patient from hypothermia.

Ice crystal formation in environmental freezing cold injury

Interstitial ice crystals form, and these enlarge at the expense of intracellular water: osmotic pressure rises and enzyme mechanisms are disturbed, with subsequent cell death.

Muscle

In freezing cold injury to muscles, the degree of injury depends on the degree of exposure. The superficial coldest layer shows coagulation necrosis, followed by slow necrosis with muscle atrophy alone in the deepest layer. Repair is by fibrous tissue.

Neither ice crystal formation nor ischaemia is necessary to produce these changes, which are due to cold alone (Lewis & Moen 1952).

Bone and joints

Bone cells are more sensitive than overlying skin and epiphyseal cartilage is more sensitive than bone. The direct action of cold on chondrocytosis or microvascular changes with end artery thrombosis or both may be the cause (McKendry 1981).

Oedema

Primary
Cold is normally associated with tissue dehydration; however the longer the limbs take to cool the more likely oedema is to occur, possibly because of changes in tissue pH.

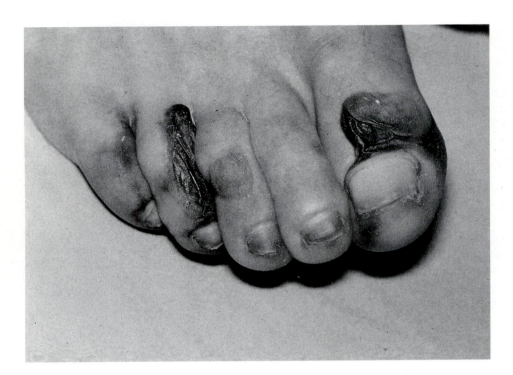

Figure 10
Superficial frostbite with blistering

Secondary

Secondary oedema is the result of rewarming and vaso-dilatation, and it forms within 12–24 hours. Plasma passes through the cold damaged capillaries into the interstitial tissue.

Exercise

Continuous submaximal exercise over several days produces an expansion of the extracellular compartment with either subclinical or overt (pitting) oedema of the ankles and feet, partly due to fluid retention and partly to shift from the intracellular compartment. This is independent of fluid balance and is affected by altitude. Compression of the tissues of the feet may occur as a result with increased susceptibility to cold injury (Williams et al 1979, Milledge et al 1982, Ross and Attwood 1984).

Figure 11

Physiopathology of the necrosis in (a) frostbite contrasted with (b) that of arteriosclerosis

Clinical features

Nonfreezing cold injury

Paraesthesia, numbness leading to loss of sensation and a feeling of 'walking on cotton wool' are usual. At night pain like an electric shock, together with swollen feet, makes sleep difficult. In the morning, weight bearing becomes almost unbearable for the first 10–15 minutes and this is then replaced by numbness. The affected area spreads proximally. Following the 'ischaemic' phase and after 2–5 hours in a warm environment, a high blood flow with full arterial pulses and hot, swollen and painful feet follows. Blistering may occur with partial return of sensation and power. Patchy gangrene with loss of tissue may be present. Sensory loss can persist and profuse sweating may be present. Loss of muscle power with resulting contraction can be serious. Freezing cold injury may intervene if the temperature falls further (Ungley et al 1945).

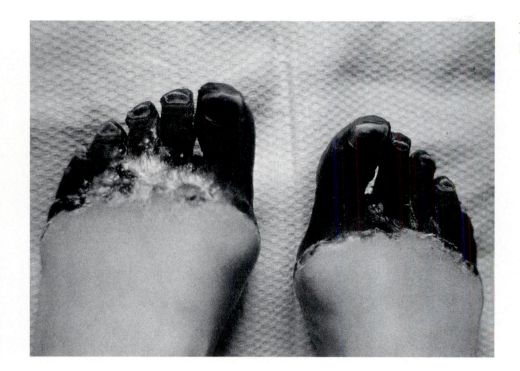

Figure 12
Deep frostbite of both feet

Freezing cold injury

Superficial

Only the skin and subcutaneous tissue are involved and the tissue, though white, is soft and pliable (Fig. 10). Blisters may occur within 24–48 hours – they are commoner on the dorsum of the foot and toes, where tissue is lax, than on the plantar surface. The blister fluid is absorbed, leaving a black insensitive carapace. There is associated oedema and within days a very definite line of demarcation occurs. If the contour of the black carapace corresponds to that of the original part, loss of tissue is unlikely, but if mummification and loss of contour occurs, tissue loss is likely. The gangrene is essentially superficial, only a few millimetres thick, and it peels off like a glove over the next few months, leaving shining red baby skin, which is abnormally sensitive to temperature and touch. Abnormal sweating may occur. In 2–3 months it will take on the general appearance of normal skin. The nail may be lost but is likely to grow again normally or only slightly deformed.

Figure 11 contrasts the physiopathology of frostbite with that of arteriosclerosis.

Deep

This involves the skin and subcutaneous tissue as well as muscle, tendons and bones (Figs 12 and 13). The affected part is cold, mottled, blue or grey and may remain swollen for months. Blistering, if it occurs, may take weeks to develop. Initially painless, shooting and throbbing pain may develop. Permanent tissue loss is almost inevitable and the loss of contour and form with a mummified appearance develops. Eventually a complete cast of toe or part of the foot separates.

As the muscles are at a distance from the most affected part and as tendons are resistant to cold, it will be possible to move the toes or the foot at the ankle.

Management

Prevention

It is extremely important to dress for the temperature with which the part will be in contact. The feet can be below freezing in deep powder snow or in near freezing water while the environmental temperatures may be many degrees above freezing. Feet must be kept as dry as possible. Tobacco smoking (but not race) is associated with a higher incidence of trench foot (Tek & MacKey 1993).

Principle

No form of violent therapy should ever be used. In a bivouac, boots should if possible be removed and feet warmed in the axillae, groin or on the abdomen of a companion. Crampons must be removed and extra clothing put on. At high altitude, use of supplementary oxygen will cause peripheral vasodilatation. Protection

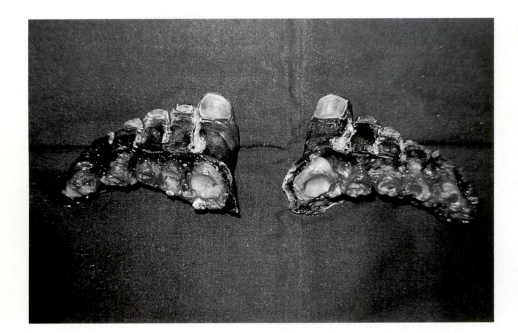

Figure 13
Deep frostbite after amputation

Treatment

Nonfreezing cold injury responds to conservative measures such as local and general warming, food and shelter. With frostbite, thawing in the field is contraindicated, since this will be followed by freezing, and the catastrophic freeze–thaw–freeze sequence precipitated. It is better to walk on frozen feet to a camp from which evacuation is possible, and only then start rapid rewarming, preferably using a water container, to 44°C, using a thermometer to check water temperature. Vasodilator drugs do not appear to improve tissue survival nor are the results of sympathectomy striking. Low molecular weight dextran and immediate sympathectomy using intra-arterial reserpine and intravenous blockade with guanethidine using the Bier technique have also been used, but with limited success. Hyperbaric oxygen seems to have been discarded. Dissolution of a blood clot by intra-arterial streptokinase has been used. Raised tissue compartment pressures may interfere with venous return and relief incisions may be considered. Rewarming in a pHisohex® whirlpool bath should last for 20 minutes at a time and a thermometer used to check water temperature.

The extent of tissue loss is hard to estimate. Tissue viability should be assessed by clinical examination and Doppler ultrasound, but tissue and bone scintigraphy are more accurate. Other methods include measurements of skin blood flow, ^{133}Xe muscle blood flow, muscle biopsy and thermography. Special probes may distinguish between superficial and deep frostbite, and ^{31}P NMR scans may be used daily to follow the state of the tissue (Kayser et al 1993).

Blisters should not be removed. Active movements must be encouraged using whirlpool baths and silicone oil. Unless infection has occurred antibiotics should not be given and the patient should be nursed in as sterile conditions as possible. Thrombolytic enzymes are being evaluated (Flora 1985) but there is a risk, especially if intracranial injuries are present. Fractures should be treated conservatively by closed rather than open methods; and dislocation reduced immediately to prevent tissue pressure.

Patients should be kept in pleasant surroundings, given a high calorie and high protein diet and antitetanus serum. Premature surgery is the most potent cause of morbidity, though relief of pressure by escharotomy and fasciotomy may be beneficial. Surgical intervention should be minimal. If amputation is necessary, as little tissue as possible should be removed, and it should be delayed for several weeks. Closure with viable skin is preferable to a skin graft. Further reconstruction can be considered in appropriate cases. Mental preparation is important for patients who may be emotionally labile (Ward 1983).

After effects

Both short-term and long-term effects of freezing and nonfreezing cold injury have been reported.

from the wind is essential. A snow hole should be dug if possible, as within it the environmental temperature will be higher than outside.

Skin may crack even at normal temperatures and cause painful fissures. Fungating and ulcerating squamous cell carcinoma of the heel have been reported in individuals frostbitten 40 years previously. The lesions were well differentiated, of low malignancy and with no evidence of spread. Treatment was by local excision and skin grafting. Block dissection of regional lymph glands was not carried out. Unstable scar tissue, chronic irritation and pressure were factors in aetiology (Rossis et al 1982).

Muscle may be replaced by fibrous tissue. Cold sensitization with an unusual degree of vasospastic response to cold and relative resistance to rewarming is well known. A high incidence of nonfreezing cold injury occurs in those with a history of local cold injury and this raises the question particularly in the Armed Forces of whether cold injured troops should be used again in a cold environment. Problems with rigidity of the feet and fallen arches have been reported, as has osteoporosis (Francis & Golden 1985).

There is histological evidence of axon regeneration in both myelinated and nonmyelinated fibres together with a gradual return of nerve function. Full return of function after nonfreezing cold injury may take nine months or longer. A burning sensation in the feet has been noted in 61% after apparent full recovery and intractable pain may occur for periods of up to 35 years. Other late sequelae include disturbance of autonomic function – both hyperhidrosis and anhidrosis have been reported (Suri et al 1978, Kumar 1982).

Changes in the epiphysis may occur in frostbitten children, and cartilage and bone abnormalities with deformity have been reported. Either the direct actions of cold on chondrocytes or microvascular change with end artery thrombosis or both may be implicated (McKendry 1981).

References

Chrenko F A, Pugh L G C E 1961 The contribution of solar radiation to the thermal environment of man in Antarctica. Proc R Soc Lond, Series B 155: 243–265

Clarke C R A 1976 On surviving a bivouac at high altitude. Letter Br Med J 1: 92

de Camara D L, Raine T J, London M D, Robson M C, Heggars J P 1982 Progression of thermal injury: A morphologic study. Plast Reconstr Surg 69: 491–499

Ekelund L G 1967 Circulatory and respiratory adaptation during prolonged exercise. Acta Physiol Scand 70 (Suppl) 292

Emslie-Smith D 1981 Hypothermia in the elderly. Br J Hosp Med 26: 442–453

Feldman A E, Thompson J T, MacMillan B G 1974 The moulded silicone shoe in the prevention of contractures involving the burn-injured foot. Burns Inc Therm Inj 1: 83–95

Flora G 1985 Secondary treatment of frost bite. In: Rivolier J, Cerretelli P, Foray F, Segantini (eds) High Altitude Deterioration. Karger, Basel. pp 159–169

Francis T J R, Golden F St C 1985 Non-freezing cold injury. The pathogenesis. J Roy Navy Med Serv 71: 31–38

Hanson H E, Goldman R F 1969 Cold injury in man. A review of its aetiology and discussion of its prediction. Milit Med 134: 1307–1316

Heath D A, Williams D R 1981 Man at High Altitude. The Pathophysiology of Acclimatisation and Adaption. Churchill Livingstone, Edinburgh

Hirschowitz B, Ullmann Y, Har-Shai Y, Vilenoki A, Peled I J 1993 Silicone occlusive sheeting (SOS) in the management of hypertrophic and keloid scarring, including the possible mode of action of silicone, by static electricity. Eur J Plast Surg 16: 5–9

Irwin M S, Thorniley M S, Green C J 1994 An investigation into the aetiology of non-freezing cold injury using near infrared spectroscopy. Biochem Soc Trans 24: 4185

Jackson D MacG 1976 Burns into joints. Burns Inc Therm Inj 2: 90–106

Jackson D MacG 1980 Destructive burns: Some orthopaedic complications. Burns Inc Therm Inj 7: 105–122

Kayser B, Binzoni T, Hoppeler H, et al 1993 A case of severe frostbite: a multi-technique approach. J Wilderness Med 4: 167–174

Kennett R P, Gilliatt R W 1991a Nerve conduction studies in experimental non-freezing cold injury. 1, Local nerve cooling. Muscle Nerve 14: 553–562

Kennett R P, Gilliatt R W 1991b Nerve conduction studies in experimental non-freezing cold injury. 2, Generalized nerve cooling by limb immersion. Muscle Nerve 14: 960–967

Kumar V N 1982 Intractable foot pain following frostbite. Arch Phys Med Rehabil 63: 284–285

Lawrence J C 1974 The perinecrotic zone in burns and its influence on healing. Burns Inc Therm Inj 1: 197–206

Lewis R B, Moen P W 1952 Further studies on the pathogenesis of cold induced muscle necrosis. Surg Gynecol Obstet 95: 543–551

Lowbury E J L 1979 Wits versus genes: The continuing battle against infection. J Trauma 19: 33–45

Lynch J B 1979 Thermal burns. In: Grabb W C, Smith J W (eds) Plastic Surgery, 3rd edn. Little, Brown & Company, Boston pp 453–483

McKendry R J R 1981 Frostbite arthritis. Can Med Assoc J 125: 1128–1132

Marsh A R 1983 A short but distant war – The Falklands Campaign. J R Soc Med 76: 972–982

Milledge J S, Bryson E I, Catley D M et al 1982 Sodium balance, fluid homeostasis and the renin-aldosterone system during the prolonged exercise of hill walking. Clin Sci 62: 595–604

Mills W J Jr, Mills W J III 1993 Peripheral non-freezing cold injury: immersion injury. Alaska Med 35: 117–128

Nukada H, Pollock M, Allpress S 1981 Experimental cold injury in peripheral nerves. Brain 104: 779–813

Ofodile F A, Oluwasanmi J O 1978 Burning the feet to treat convulsions. Br J Plast Surg 31: 356–357

Pearn J H 1982 Cold injury complicating trauma in sub-zero environments. Med J Aust 1: 505–507

Perkins K, Davey R B, Wallis K A 1982 Silicone gel: a new treatment for burn scars and contractures. Burns Inc Therm Inj 9: 201–204

Peyronnard J M, Pedneault M, Aguayo A J 1977 Neuropathies due to cold – quantitative studies of structural changes in human and animal nerves. In: Proceedings of 11th World Congress of Neurology, Amsterdam pp 303–329

Pugh L G C E 1962 Solar heat gain by man in the high Himalaya. UNESCO Symposium on Environmental Physiology and Psychology in Arid Conditions. Lucknow pp 325–329

Pugh L G C E, Ward M P 1956 Some effects of high altitude on man. Lancet 2: 1115–1121

Raifman M A, Berant M, Lenarsky C 1978 Cold weather and rhabdomyolysis. J Paediatrics 93: 970–971

Ramstead K D, Hughes R G, Webb A J 1980 Recent cases of trench foot. Postgrad Med J 56: 879–883

Rosenthall L, Kloiber R, Gagnon R, Damtew B, Lough J 1981 Frostbite with Rhabdomyolysis and renal failure. Am J Roentgenol 137: 387–390

Ross J H, Attwood E C 1984 Severe Repetitive Exercise and haematological status. Postgrad Med J 60: 454–457

Rossis C G, Yiacoumettis A M, Elemenoglou J 1982 Squamous cell carcinoma of the heel developing at site of previous frostbite. J R Soc Med 75: 715–720

Schaeffer O, Eaton R D P, Timmermans J, Hildes J A 1980 Respiratory function impairment and cardio-pulmonary consequences in long term residents of the Canadian Arctic. Can Med Assoc J 123: 997–1007

Schechter D C, Sarot I A 1968 Historical accounts of injuries due to cold. Surgery 63: 527–535

Suri M L, Vizayan G P, Puri H C, Barat A K, Singh N 1978 Neurological manifestations of frostbite. Indian J Med Res 67: 292–299

Tek D, MacKey S (1993) Non-freezing cold injury in a marine infantry battalion. J Wilderness Med 4: 353–357

Ungley C C, Channell G D, Richards R 1945 The immersion foot syndrome. Br J Surg 33: 17–31

Ward M P 1974 Frostbite. Br Med J 1: 67–70

Ward M P 1983 Thrombosis and frostbite. 'Man at altitude'. Seminars in Respiratory Medicine 5: 202–206

Ward M P, Milledge J S, West J B (1995) High Altitude Medicine and Physiology, second edition. Chapman & Hall, London

Washburn B 1962 Frostbite. What it is – how to prevent it – emergency treatment. N Eng J Med 266: 974–989

Williams E S, Ward M P, Milledge J S, Withey W R, Older M W J, Forsling M L 1979 Effect of the exercise of seven consecutive days hill-walking on fluid homeostasis. Clin Sci 56: 305–316

XI SHOES, NAILS AND SUPPORTS

XI.1 The Nails

George Rendall

Function

Toenails cover the major part of the dorsal surface of each distal phalanx. Their main function is to protect the dorsum and apices of the digits, though it may be argued that they are a remnant of an era when nails or claws were used for gripping, digging or defence. Protection is created by the hard inflexible plate, which directly resists focal trauma and assists in dispersing force through the subungual soft tissue, thereby reducing pressure.

Anatomy

Toenails consist of a keratinous plate curved around the distal portion of the distal phalanx both transversely and longitudinally. Normally, transverse curvature is somewhat greater than longitudinal. Most authors agree that the nail plate has three layers (Johnson et al 1991, Dawber 1980, Hashimoto 1971). The hard, thin dorsal nail plate is made up of flattened, densely packed keratinocytes, which are highly regularly arranged and tightly banded. Cells in the thicker intermediate layer (Achten 1982, Hashimoto 1971) and the ventral layer are less flat and progressively less densely packed toward the nail bed.

The three layers of the nail plate originate from three different matrical zones. The thin hard dorsal layer is produced in the dorsal nail matrix, which is entirely hidden by the proximal nail fold. The thicker intermediate plate receives most of its bulk from the distal portion of the matrix, much of which can be seen as the lunula, the whitish half moon that forms the most proximal part of the visible nail. Approximately 20% of the eventual bulk of the nail plate is derived from the nail bed beyond the lunula, or ventral matrix (Johnson

et al 1991). Achten (1982) suggests that the ventral nail plate consists of nail bed epidermis that is very strongly adhered to the intermediate nail plate. The nail bed has longitudinal grooves that are believed to enhance the adherence of the nail plate to the bed by producing a 'tongue-and-groove' effect (Zaias 1980).

Anteriorly, the solehorn, which also produces keratinous material, may provide a small tuft of nail in some cases. Toenail growth is approximately 1–2 cm per annum (Dawber & Baran 1992) with a peak in the second and third decades. Local and systemic health problems may lead to a reduction in growth rates or to an alteration in the synthesis of the nail.

Apart from the nail plate and matrix, a number of structures contribute to the gross anatomy of the nail (Fig. 1). The distal phalanx influences the shape of the nail and its matrix. The nail generally curves gently around the terminal phalanx. The proximal nail fold consists of modified skin devoid of hair follicles or fingerprint markings. It contains approximately one third of the length of the nail plate before extending anteriorly onto the dorsal aspect of the nail, where it forms the cuticle. The cuticle protects the soft matrical area from physical and microbial insult (Samman 1978). The lateral nail fold (nail sulcus) is continuous with the plantar skin. Distally the hyponychium marks the junction between the free edge of the nail plate and the soft tissue immediately distal to it. Immediately proximal to the free edge of the nail is a translucent band (Terry's onychodermal band) (Fig. 2).

Blood supply is by medial and lateral branches of the dorsal and plantar digital arteries, which form superficial, proximal and distal anastomoses in the subungual soft tissue (Fig. 3). Proximal innervation is by the dorsal digital nerves, small branches of the superficial and deep peroneal nerves and the sural nerve, and distal innervation is by the plantar digital nerves and small branches of the medial and lateral plantar nerves (Sarrafian 1983).

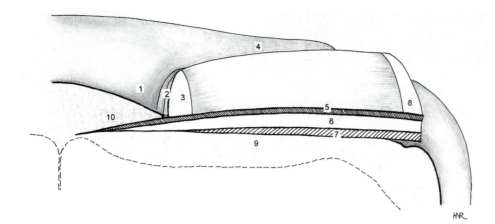

Figure 1

Lateral cross-section of the nail plate and periungual tissues

1 Proximal nail fold
2 Cuticle
3 Lunula
4 Lateral nail fold
5 Dorsal nail plate
6 Intermediate nail plate
7 Ventral nail plate
8 Free edge
9 Nail bed
10 Dorsal matrix

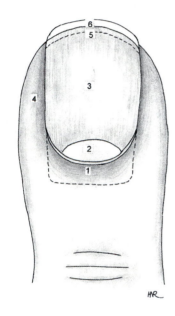

Figure 2

Nail plate, dorsal view

1 Dorsal matrix
2 Lunula
3 Nail plate
4 Lateral nail fold
5 Terry's onychodermal band
6 Free edge

Nail pathology

Ingrown toenails

Prevalence

Ingrown toenail or onychocryptosis is a painful condition in which the edge of the nail penetrates the epidermis of the lateral nail fold or sulcus. Prevalence is highly variable according to age, sex and footwear. It is usually accepted that it peaks amongst adolescent boys though quite why this should be so remains a matter for conjecture. Five per cent of all chiropody treatments under the National Health Service in the UK are for ingrown toenails (Widdicombe 1990).

Aetiology and classification

The most commonly accepted predisposing causes are abnormal nail shape (particularly involution), sulcus shape, sulcus condition, single major trauma and repeated microtrauma from footwear. One recent survey showed a very high prevalence (30%) in men wearing industrial footwear with restrictive steel toe caps (Marr & Quine 1992). It is also highly likely that the popular habit of picking or tearing toenails, instead of cutting them, is a common contributary cause, particularly in the young.

Involution is the most commonly acknowledged cause of ingrown toenail, though it may well produce symptoms other than those of classical onychocryptosis. In severely involuted nails, described by Baran (1974) as pincer nails, quite substantial pain can be experienced with no puncture and, in even mild involution, corn and callous formation in the lateral nail fold is common and can cause sufficient discomfort for the patient to seek treatment. Classification of involuted nails by shape has produced such terms as pincer, trumpet (Baran 1974) plicatured and tile shaped (Johnson 1993), but perhaps the simple definition of normal, abruptly curved, excessively curved and involuted, indicating greater than 180° of total curvature, is best (Middleton & Webb 1993). Pain is most likely in truly involuted and abruptly curved nails (Fig. 4).

Onychocryptosis, particularly in the young, often occurs with perfectly normal nails. In some cases this is attributable to trauma or poor nail management but often it is due to the shape or condition of the sulcus. An excessively fleshy nail fold may inhibit the lateral spread of the nail to such an extent that slight ragginess of the

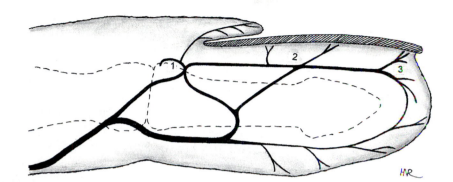

Figure 3

Blood supply to the periungual tissues

1   Superficial arcade
2   Proximal arcade
3   Distal arcade

nail edge produces penetration (see Fig. 4). In some cases a toe that looks perfectly normal on examination shows marked pulping on standing due to the extent to which it bears weight. This is particularly so where true or functional hallux limitus produces excessive distal loading of the first toe during the propulsive phase of gait.

A nail sulcus that is macerated, owing to hyperhidrosis, offers less resistance to penetration and is often held to be the reason for the high incidence amongst adolescent males (Johnson 1993). It seems unlikely, however, that this alone would create the conditions necessary for development of onychocryptosis, and only when combined with mechanical trauma can hyperidrosis be considered a causative agent.

Clinical features and pathology

Early signs are those of low-grade acute inflammation, mild pain, localized oedema, redness and heat, in the area where the epidermis is breached. Unless treated rapidly it is highly likely that infection will occur. With infection, the pain and swelling increase considerably and the sulcus and nail often become macerated either from the discharge or from localized sweating. This, combined with the colonizing bacteria, produces a characteristic warm, moist and unpleasant odour. If the offending spicule is not removed, a cycle of low-grade damage and repair is established, with the nail coming to be recognized as an inert foreign body. Initially this stimulates an excess of granulation tissue in the lateral nail fold, which may well extend over quite a substantial area of the surface of the nail. This tissue is prone to bleeding and forms a pocket around the nail which harbours bacteria. At this stage, infection may render the toe so exquisitely tender that the patient can hardly bear the bed clothes to rest on it. Alternatively, a reduction in pain may occur as a result of the spicule becoming so macerated that it softens and breaks off.

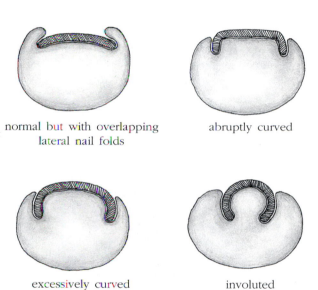

normal but with overlapping lateral nail folds

abruptly curved

excessively curved

involuted

Figure 4

Types of ingrown toenail

If the nail is left untreated or if there is no spontaneous resolution, epidermis grows over the hypergranulation tissue so that the lateral nail fold closes over the nail. This completely obscures the edges of the nail plate (Fig. 5) complicating both future treatment and the patient's ability to cut his or her own nails (Zaias 1980). Prolonged irritation may also produce chronic fibrosis, and a small fibroma may occur in the sulcus.

Differential diagnosis

In general, onychocryptosis is an easy diagnosis to make but this may have a drawback in that it compounds the difficulty of arriving at rare alternatives that occur around

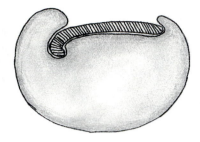

Figure 5

Epidermis may grow over the hypergranulation tissue so that the lateral nail fold closes over the nail. This completely obscures the edges of the nail plate, complicating both future treatment and the patient's ability to cut their own nails (Zaias 1980)

the sulcus. Practitioners should be particularly wary if there is pain without an obvious physical puncture. In true onychocryptosis there is always a puncture wound. Problems that may mimic onychocryptosis and fool the unwary practitioner include benign tumours such as pyogenic granuloma and fibroma. Both of these may have originated from the irritation caused by true onychocryptosis. Sepsis due to the entry of a foreign body such as a dog hair or an insect bite may also present with clinical features similar to ingrown toenails. Malignant tumours such as Kaposi's sarcoma may well develop around the site of nails and cases of amelanotic melanoma around nails are so potentially devastating that this very rare problem should always be borne in mind where hypergranulation tissue persists with no apparent cause (Thomson & Lang 1991). This diagnosis cannot be made without biopsy, but a useful clinical indicator is the possibility of faint trailing or leaking pigment around the periphery of the wound site.

Treatment

In the early stages most onychocryptosis can be treated conservatively. Treatment will in general consist of spicule removal with sharp sterile nippers, bathing with antiseptic solution packing under the edge of the nail with sterile gauze or cotton wool, and dressing. When trauma is the cause, or when a patient can be persuaded to change his or her footwear or habits (e.g. to stop picking the nails), conservative management may bring complete relief. Recurrent ingrowing toenail is, however, a troublesome and painful condition not helped by the fearful reputation that surrounds treatment. The primary aim of all treatment is to remove pain, heal the wound and reduce the likelihood of recurrence with the minimum of pain and disturbance to the patient. Good conservative management can generally achieve the dual objectives in the short term of eliminating pain and healing the wound. In older patients with involution, regular treatment can also give

good comfort in cases of painful involution and onychophosis.

If involution is a problem, curvature may be reduced by means of bracing the nails with orthodontic wire. This solution can bring substantial relief for the lifespan of the nail but it is more likely that the nail will regrow in its natural unbraced shape after 9 months to 1 year. A simpler means of reducing discomfort (at least from the practitioner's perspective) is to give sound advice on basic foot care. The patient should wear a shoe with room in the toebox, cut the toenails straight across, avoid digging down the sides of the nails and never pick or tear the nails. These simple guidelines should prevent recurrence in many cases of ingrown toenail, but a high number do not resolve or else recur periodically. These cases are likely to require surgical intervention. Surgery for ingrown toenail should be uncomplicated, should enable the patient to return quickly to normal activity, should heal quickly and should resist recurrence.

Operative procedures for nails vary from the very simple clearing of a sulcus to radical removal of tissue in the case of severe ingrowing nail. Foulston (1988) ranks surgical techniques according to the amount of tissue removed:

1. Amputation of the distal phalanx. DuVries (1959) reports that this procedure has been used in the past in order to avoid the possibility of regrowth of nail plate from undestroyed matrix and was simpler than plastic repair of the nail lip.
2. Total matrix removal was described by Zadik (1950). The whole nail plate is lifted and removed. A flap of tissue is lifted at the base of the nail and the nail matrix area at the proximal end is ablated down to the level of the distal phalanx and across the whole width of the toe. Sutures are used to close the incisions.
3. Partial matrix removal was described by Winograd (1929). A section of nail plate is lifted and removed. The associated nail matrix area is excised and the tissues sutured.
4. Antrum (1984) described a technique whereby the nailfold at the side of the nail plate is sliced away from proximal to distal ends and then removed by amputation at the proximal end. The lesion is dressed with topical antiseptic and allowed to heal.
5. Gabriel (1979) has described a careful method of surgical removal of a section of nail plate and the excision of a segment of germinal matrix without cutting the skin and with minimal interference to the nail wall.
6. Total and partial avulsions of nail plate have been carried out followed by chemical matricectomy using phenol or sodium hydroxide. This involves no incision and minimum disruption to the soft tissue. Dagnall (1981) has written an excellent review of the history and development of the phenolization techniques. The phenolization method is described

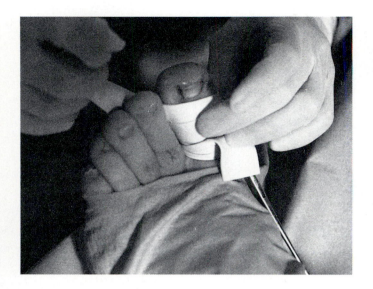

Figure 6

The toe is exsanguinated and a tourniquet applied by wrapping a bandage around the toe from distal to proximal and gripping proximally with locking forceps

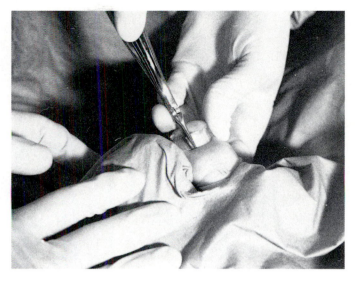

Figure 7

Nail thwaites are gently but firmly driven longitudinally under the nail

below. An alternative is the use of a metal probe and negative galvanic current to generate sodium hydroxide on site by hydrolysis of body fluids. Whichever surgical technique is used, postoperative management of the condition is to keep the wound drained and clean. Topical antiseptics are applied and antibiotic cover is maintained until any sepsis is reduced.

There are a number of reports that describe the effectiveness of the various techniques. Beaton et al (1990) compared two popular methods, wedge excision (after Gabriel 1979) and total or partial removal of nail followed by matrical phenolization (after Ross 1969) by surveying patients' attitudes and postoperative behaviour. The wedge excisions healed more quickly but were more painful, more likely to create difficulty in walking, more likely to leave the patient with persistent symptoms and less likely to leave a satisfactory result. Nearly 50% of the wedge excision group (19 of 41) had more than 3 days' absence from work after surgery compared to only 3% (1 of 35) after phenolization. Recurrence rates have also been shown to be better with matrical phenolization. Morkane et al (1984) described a controlled prospective study of 53 Winograd type wedge resections and 54 segmental phenolizations. There was no difference in discomfort after 1 week but over a 14-month follow-up there were 16 spikes of nail growth (30%) in the wedge resection group and only four (7%) in the phenol group. Palmer & Jones (1979) support these findings in a retrospective study of 245 operations on 208 patients at King's College Hospital in London. They report a recurrence rate for various techniques of 83% for avulsion of a strip of nail, 70% for total nail avulsion, 28% for Zadik's operation and 29% for wedge resection. They recommended

that immediate avulsion of toenails should not be a routine procedure. Recent work clearly supports matrical phenolization compared to other methods and this low-cost, low-pain procedure which allows instant loading has become the treatment of choice.

Method

1. Using a local anaesthetic (without epinephrine) a toe block is performed.
2. The side or sides to be avulsed are marked with a skin pen prior to initiating preoperative swabbing. The toe is likely to look quite different when exsanguinated after application of the tourniquet.
3. The toe and forefoot are swabbed with a surgical preparatory antiseptic such as 10% Povidone Iodine. This is ideal as it is fast acting, sporicidal, long lasting and colours the skin so that it is clear which areas have been prepared. Swabbing is always in the direction distal to proximal, and particular attention should be paid to the intertriginous areas, which are ideal harbours for pathogens.
4. The eponychium or cuticle at the front of the proximal nail fold should be gently separated from the nail. This will help to prevent tearing of this delicate tissue when the nail is removed.
5. The toe is exsanguinated and a tourniquet applied by wrapping a 2 cm bandage (1 cm if a lesser digit) around the toe from distal to proximal and gripping proximally with locking forceps (Fig. 6).
6. Nail thwaites (flat edged nippers for splitting nails) are gently but firmly driven longitudinally under the nail, flat side down. Conducting this with slow even pressure will minimize colateral separation, reducing

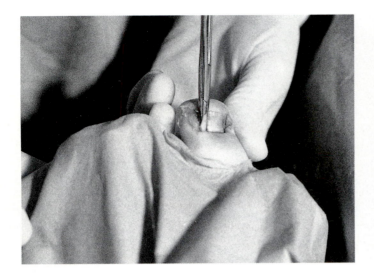

Figure 8

The nail to be removed is gripped with locking forceps and slowly twisted off. The twist should be in such a direction that the upper portion of the nail folds on top of itself

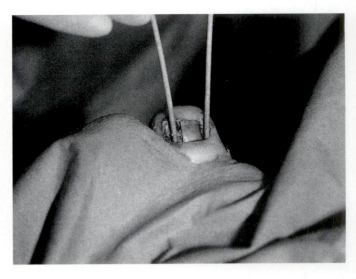

Figure 10

Phenolize the nail matrix with 80% liquified phenol. Simple orange sticks soaked in phenol are adequate for most nails. Many practitioners prefer to lightly abrade the matrix with a Black's file. The phenol is applied for 2 minutes, then swabbed dry, then applied for a further 1 minute

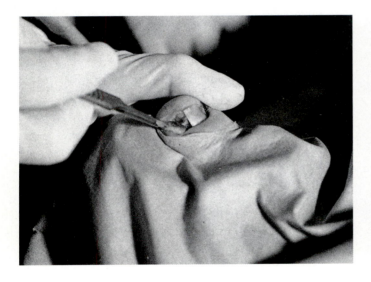

Figure 9

Removal of excessive granulation tissue minimizes risk of infection and reduces healing time

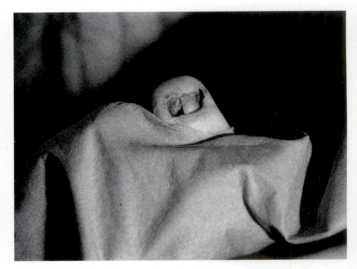

Figure 11

The toe is dried and a dressing applied

both immediate damage and the likelihood of phenol tracking under the nail and destroying tissue unnecessarily. When the thwaites reach the cuticle, split the nail (Fig. 7).

7. A small chisel or flat-ended Beaver blade is then used to split the nail under the proximal nail fold. Again, great care must be taken not to split the nail fold itself, so controlled firm pressure is used.

8. The nail to be removed is gripped with locking forceps and slowly twisted off. The twist should be in such a direction that the upper portion of the nail folds on top of itself (Fig. 8). After removal, check the sulcus and proximal nail fold for unwanted remnants of nail. These will perpetuate the problem and greatly increase the likelihood of postoperative infection. It may also be necessary to remove excessive granulation tissue (Fig. 9). Where previous surgery has been conducted remove any regrowth spicules. Swab the lateral nail fold to remove any debris or discharge.

9. Phenolize the nail matrix with 80% liquified phenol (Fig. 10). A wide range of methods have been used for applying the phenol but there is little evidence to indicate that any one method should prevail. Simple orange sticks, sterilized and soaked in phenol, are probably adequate for most nails. The addition of cotton wool to deliver a larger quantity of phenol is inadvisable, owing to the likelihood of stray fibres being left in the wound to complicate healing. Many practitioners prefer to lightly abrade the matrix with a Black's file and, although it is unnecessary for most cases, this may certainly help where previous regrowth has left a fibrous pocket which will be resistant to less vigorous treatment. Whichever method is used, the main focus should be in the corners of the matrix where the nail is firmly attached to the phalanx and regrowth is most likely to occur. The phenol is applied for 2 minutes, swabbed dry, then applied for a further 1 minute. At this stage the wound may be flushed with isopropyl alcohol, the intention being to dilute the phenol, thereby inhibiting its action. There is little evidence to support this or the opposite dogma of nonflushing (Dagnall, 1981). Goslin (1992), in a trial of 40 operations, showed that, with or without flushing, neither healing rates nor the period for which phenol remains in the tissue after application are significantly different.

10. The toe is dried and a dressing applied (Fig. 11). Moist dressings are preferable as they have been shown to significantly reduce healing times after nail avulsion when compared to dry dressings (Foley & Allen 1994).

11. A pressure bandage is applied by using several layers of size 12 tubular gauze bandage.

12. The patient should be seen within 1 week, with explicit instructions to contact the practitioner if there are problems.

13. Moist wound dressings at weekly intervals should bring about problem free healing in 4–6 weeks.

Where a nail is so involuted or disfigured that a good functional or cosmetic nail is not a likely outcome, total avulsion may be the treatment of choice. In such cases, the procedure is identical to that described above but either the whole nail is elevated with a MacKay's elevator and removed in one piece or it is split down the middle and removed as if it were two partial avulsions. Partial avulsion is often impractical on lesser toenails so that total removal is the usual treatment.

Onychomycosis

Prevalence

Fungal infection of toenails is a common problem with a prevalence estimated at 2–3% of the UK and US populations. It is commonest in those aged over 55 years and it occurs equally in men and women (Roberts 1992).

Classification

Fungal nail infection is classified into four types

Distal and lateral subungual onychomycosis
This is by far the commonest type seen in toenails. It begins at the free nail edge (distal or lateral) and affects the friable lower layers of the nail plate. It is usually a result of dermatophyte infection but it may, occasionally, be produced by yeasts (mostly *Candida albicans*) or by nondermatophytic moulds (e.g. *Hendersonula, Scopulariopsis*).

Superficial white onychomycosis
This is caused by *Tricophyton interdigitale* (also known as *T. mentagrophytes*) and is rarely seen.

Proximal subungual onychomycosis
This is a result of infection by yeasts. It is secondary to chronic paronychia, so it is more common in fingernails.

Total dystrophic onychomycosis
This can occur where onychomycosis of any type is unchecked and leads to destruction of the whole nail (Roberts et al 1990)

Aetiology

It is most likely that the source of the nail infection is from the patient's own dermatophyte skin infection. *Tinea pedis* has a high prevalence, generally estimated at between 10% and 15% of the population. This rises sharply in those whose habits or occupation necessitate regular communal showering, one study showing a prevalence of 80% skin infection in miners (Gotz & Hantschke 1965). Cross-infection from contaminated medical instruments or other family members is also a possible source.

Clinical features

There are rarely symptoms, but the nail is unsightly and surface roughness may tear hosiery. The nail in the early stages presents with a cloudy or yellow area at the front or side of the free edge, which is likely to have become detached from the nail bed. This will progress proximally, and in advanced onychomycosis the whole nail may be infected. In such cases the nail is grossly thickened, brownish yellow and has a crumbly, honeycombed texture. Clinical diagnosis is not usually difficult in advanced cases but early cases closely resemble primary or psoriatic onycholysis.

Confirmation is by isolation of fungi from nail clippings. This is a simple procedure providing enough material is taken from the infected margin (i.e. the most proximal section of infected nail), but culture may often fail, even when fungi are present. This is attributed to sampling insufficient nail from the infected site (Hay 1994). By far the commonest pathogen involved in fungal nail infection is *Tricophyton rubrum*, which is found in 85% of cases. *Tricophyton interdigitale* accounts for around 12% and *Epidermophyton floccosum* for around 2% of cases.

Treatment

Treatment is largely unsatisfactory, both for the patient and practitioner. The obsolete practice of drilling fungal nails to reduce thickness and roughness spreads huge numbers of fungal spores through the clinical environment (Harvey 1993). This is the most likely reason for approximately 30% of podiatrists having antibodies to *T. rubrum* compared to only 6.6% of controls (Abramson & Wilton 1985). Topical treatment of toenail infections with Phytex has occasionally produced good results in conscientious patients who diligently apply and file the nail with a clean emery board between applications. Similarly application of occlusive dressings (such as polythene or a rubber finger stool) over the top of antifungal ointments may work. These methods are, however, laborious, time consuming and unpredictable, so that the chances of achieving patient compliance, in the majority of cases, are slim. Amorfoline, an antimycotic nail lacquer, has recently been shown to produce cure in 50% of cases after 6 months, but mainly on fingernails and most effectively when the infection was mild and superficial (Rennel 1992).

Surgical removal of the nail plate followed by topical application of antifungals has been described by Hettinger & Velinsky (1991) who achieved 95% cure rate with 2% ketoconazole. Surgical removal has potential particularly in patients unsuited to oral therapy.

Systemic approaches to treatment of mycosis in toenails have, until recently, relied on griseofulvin, a weak fungostatic. A dosage of 1 mg is taken daily for 12–18 months. This produces a cure rate of around 30% and recurrence is common. Combined griseofulvin and topical therapy can improve this rate but makes further demands on patient compliance over a prolonged period.

Perhaps the main problem in treating toenails with fungostatics is that to clear the problem the infected nail must grow out (or be removed). Toenails grow slowly, particularly in the elderly population in whom nails may grow significantly less than their own length in a year. The recent introduction of terbinafine, a fungicide, has revolutionized fungal nail therapy. Terbinafine is an allylamine that inhibits cell membrane synthesis, killing the fungal cells. It is highly target-specific (Ryder 1992), safer than alternatives such as ketoconazole and itraconazole (Breckenridge 1992) and appears to be well tolerated (Villars & Jones 1992, van der Schroeff et al 1992, Goodfield 1992). It is available for oral administration and as an ointment. Villars & Jones (1992) indicate cure rates of 40% after 6 weeks and 70% after 3 months of oral therapy. Cure rates improve with longer term therapy. Baudraz-Rosselet et al (1992) indicate a cure rate of 77% after 6 months with further cures in resistant cases treated for longer. Recurrence after 1 year is 18% (compared to 40% or more for griseofulvin) though it is unclear whether this is attributable to recurrence or reinfection (van der Schroeff et al 1992, Goodfield 1992). All trials to date have excluded pregnant women and children. Terbinafine is expensive and relatively new, but current indications are that it will form the mainstay for management of onychomycosis for some time.

Thickened nails

Hypertrophy of nails probably occurs as a result of damage to the nail matrix. This may be caused by sudden or repeated high impact trauma or by chronic microtrauma such as stubbing due to foot hypermobility or compression in ill fitting footwear. Dermatophyte infection can also lead to thickening, as can poor peripheral circulation or systemic disease. The incidence of thick nails increases greatly in the elderly as longitudinal growth slows down. There is little evidence as to why this should be.

Onychauxis

Uniform nail thickening, onychauxis, may occur in all toenails and is very much commoner in the elderly. Microtrauma from ill-fitting footwear or abnormal foot function is the most likely cause, though poor peripheral circulation has also been blamed (Johnson 1993). Symptoms are rare and nail growth slow, but patients often seek treatment because the nails are too thick to be cut. Compression from footwear may lead to pain or the development of periungual corn and callous (onychophosis). Occasionally, a sterile ulcer develops beneath the nail, which may be painful.

Treatment usually consists of cutting with strong nail nippers and drilling to reduce thickness. Slow growth extends the period between treatments to several months.

Onychogryphosis

Irregular nail hypertrophy is described as onychogryphosis. After treatment this may be difficult to distinguish from onychauxis but in classical onychogryphosis, where long-term neglect leaves the nail well over normal length, a helical or circular twist is evident. This has led to the synonym 'ram's horn nail'. These nails are generally unevenly thickened and discoloured yellow–brown. Symptoms, if any, are the same as those of onychauxis, as are cause and treatment. High-impact trauma may well be more commonly a cause of distorted thickened nails than of onychauxis and the antiquated 'Ostler's toe' conjures up a vivid, if painful, picture of onychogryphosis as a rustic occupational hazard.

Other common nail problems

Subungual exostosis

Subungual exostoses may be painful and they sometimes create distortion of transverse and longitudinal curvature of nails. They are usually a result of trauma, though the trauma may be insidious (e.g. tight footwear or a hyper-extended distal phalanx) (Johnson 1993). The new bony growth tends to be central and distal. Certain diagnosis is by lateral X-ray, but palpation of the nail may reveal a blanched area directly above the exostosis. When it is problematic, the excess bone should be removed surgically.

Onycholysis

Separation of the nail from the nail bed is termed onycholysis. The separated portion is opaque and white, owing to air in and under the nail disrupting the passage of light. Onycholysis occurs as a result of trauma, infection (bacterial or fungal – see the sections on onychomycosis, paronychia and onychia), systemic or skin disease (especially psoriasis) or rarely from drug eruptions, or circulatory or nutritional disorders (Samman 1978, Johnson 1993). It is often idiopathic. There are rarely symptoms but where fingernails are involved it can be distressing and unsightly, and in toenails the free edge often snags hosiery. The area affected is highly variable, but in severe cases it can involve the whole nail. Treatment consists of cutting back the affected area to reduce nuisance.

Paronychia and onychia

Paronychia, a painful inflammation of the periungual soft tissues, particularly the proximal nail fold, is usually caused by bacterial infection. Onychia, inflammation of the nail bed, is much rarer. The infection is generally enabled by damage to the proximal nail fold. This damage may be: traumatic, caused by stubbing or jamming the toe; habitual, caused by constant or repeated wetting; or due to invasion of a foreign body such as a pet hair or splinter. Chronic paronychia is rare in toenails though *Candida albicans* may produce a chronic low-grade infection. Treatment is by removal of any obvious irritants, establishment and maintenance of drainage, and administration of antibiotics.

Subungual haematoma

This occurs as a result of trauma. A single blow is the most likely cause but repetitive stress, particularly during

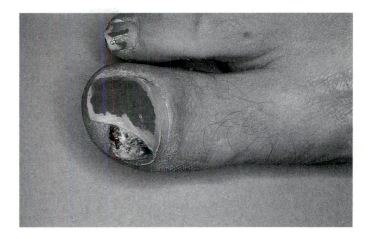

Figure 12

Subungual exostosis (courtesy of Mr G Hooper)

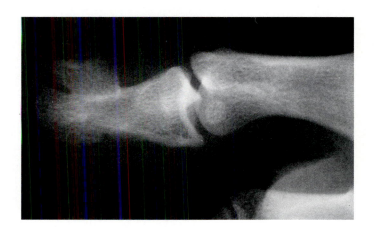

Figure 13

X-ray of subungual exostosis (courtesy of Mr G Hooper)

sporting activity, may be the presenting history. The appearance is or a purple or blue–black area underneath the nail plate. Pain may be severe in the early stages because of a rapid build up of subungual pressure. This can be effectively relieved by drilling an aperture in the nail plate. As blood coagulates and the clot desiccates under the nail, pain diminishes and the nail is best left to grow out. Where no history of trauma can be elicited, differential diagnosis includes pigmented naevi and vascular tumours, so that the nail above the blackened area should be removed for examination of the nail bed. Coagulated blood, indicative of haematoma, can be removed easily, but confirmation of alternative diagnoses is likely to necessitate biopsy.

Onychophosis

Corn or callous in the periungual epidermis is most likely to develop in the anterior part of the sulcus when an involuted nail or an overlapping sulcus combines with restrictive footwear. Visually it may be difficult to detect, but where pain persists after removal of a spicule or involuted edges, onychophosis is often the cause. Treatment is, firstly, softening the sulcus with water or hydrogen peroxide (10 volumes), then removing callous with a scalpel. If access is difficult, space may be cleared with a Black's file or needle bur.

Nail care

Care of toenails is the responsibility of the patient where the toenails are normal and the patient is able. The nails should be cut with nippers or sharp scissors, straight across and without digging into the corners. As patients grow older this may become increasingly difficult, owing to a wide range of factors such as inflexibility, loss of dexterity, diminished visual faculties or increased nail plate thickness. The elderly patient who complains that the 'feet seem to get further away' is in need of assistance with normal toenail care. Nurses or podiatry assistants with sound minimal training and good instruments can provide this.

Distorted or painful toenails may require further treatment. Patients at risk because of local, systemic, circulatory, sensory, dermatological or nutritional impairment require a cautious approach, even for care of normal nails. Determining who should deal with nail care must be based on informed judgement of risk rather than sweeping, categorical, disease-based criteria.

Diabetes is the most commonly acknowledged rationale for the professional taking charge of standard foot care. In many cases this is justified. Peripheral neuropathy may render a patient incapable of sensing an ingrown toenail or subungual callosity, whilst microvascular disease makes healing, even of minor injury, problematic. Severe ischaemia can create pains that can be misinterpreted by the inexperienced or poorly trained practitioner as nail symptoms, thereby causing a very high-risk toe to be subjected to unnecessary investigation and possibly damaging treatment. Other high-risk groups include those with compromised immunity, vascular impairment, rheumatoid arthritis, drug-induced risk (e.g. systemic corticosteroids) or a wide range of skin disorders.

Criteria that would merit professional intervention are:

1. Neuropathy.
2. Localized ischaemia. (In many diabetics of longstanding or mature diabetics, microangiopathy is difficult to establish in a clinical setting.)
3. Immunity compromised by systemic disease or drugs.
4. History of ulceration or ischaemic type pain.
5. Unstable or brittle diabetes.
6. Poor quality periungual tissues.

7. Loss of ability to undertake normal foot care.
8. Impairment of mental faculties.

If any of the above conditions exist, the patient must not take sole responsibility for care. If, however, the patient is dexterous, mobile, has good sight and normal nails, as is likely to be the case for many young diabetic patients, then the professional's role is to give guidance on good footcare practices. This does not preclude regular checks as part of routine diabetic care.

Acknowledgement

I would like to thank Hazel Newland-Ritchie for the illustrations.

References

Abramson C, Wilton J 1985 Nail dust aerosols from onychomycotic toenails: part II Clinical and serological aspects. J Am Podiatr Med Assoc 75: 631

Achten G 1982 Histopathology. In: Pierre M (ed) The Nail. Churchill Livingstone, Edinburgh, pp 1–4

Antrum R M 1984 Radical excision of the nailbed for ingrown nail. J Bone Joint Surg 66B: 63–65

Baran R 1974 Pincer and trumpet nails. Arch Dermatol 110: 639–640

Baudraz-Rosselet F, Rakosi T, Wili P B, Kenzelman R 1992 Treatment of onychomycosis with terbinafine. Br J Dermatol 126 (suppl 39): 40–46

Beaton D F, Kriss S M, Blacklay P F, Wood R F M, Skinner D 1990 Ingrowing toenails: a patient evaluation of phenolization versus wedge excision. Chiropodist (March): 62–64

Breckenridge A 1992 Clinical significance of interactions with antifungal agents. Br J Dermatol 126 (suppl 39): 19–22

Dagnall J C 1981 The history, development and current status of nail matrix phenolisation. Chiropodist 36: 315–324

Dawber R P R 1980 The ultrastructure and growth of human nails. Arch Dermatol Res 269: 197–204

Dawber R P R, Baran R 1992 Disorders of nails. In: Champion R H, Burton J L, Ebling F J G (eds) Textbook of Dermatology (5th edition). Blackwell Scientific, Oxford, pp 2497–2532

Du Vries H L 1959 Surgery of the Foot. C V Mosby, St Louis

Foley G B, Allen J 1994 Wound healing after toenail avulsion: a comparison of Kaltostat and melolin as post-operative dressings. Foot 4: 88–91

Foulston J 1988 Ingrowing toenail. In: Helal B, Wilson D W (eds) The Foot. Churchill Livingstone, Edinburgh, pp 858–867

Gabriel S S 1979 The ingrown toenail: a modified segmental matrix excision operation. Br J Surg 66: 285–286

Goodfield M J D 1992 Short-duration therapy with terbinafine for dermatophyte onychomycosis: a multicentre trial. Br J Dermatol 126 (suppl 39): 33–35

Goslin R W 1992 A comparison of the dilution and non-dilution of phenol with alcohol following nail avulsions. Foot 2: 225–228

Gotz H, Hantschke D 1965 Einblicke in die Epidemologie in Mykoses in Kohlenbergbau. Hautartz 16: 543, from Roberts D T 1992 Prevalence of dermatophyte onychomycosis in the United Kingdom: results of an omnibus survey. Br J Dermatol 126 (suppl 39): 23–27

Harvey C 1993 Comparison of the effectiveness of nail dust extractors. J Am Podiatr Med Assoc 83: 669–673

Hashimoto K 1971 Ultrastructure of the human nail. Ultrastruct Res 36: 391–410

Hay R J 1994 Fungal nail infections: topical or systemic therapy. Med Dialogue (Feb) 407a

Hettinger D F, Velinsky M S 1991 Treatment of onychomycosis with nail avulsion and topical ketoconazole. J Am Pod Med Assoc 81: 28–32

Johnson M 1993 The human nail and its disorders. In: Lorimer D L (ed) Neale's Common Foot Disorders (4th edition). Churchill Livingstone, Edinburgh. pp. 123–139

Johnson M, Comaish J S, Shuster S 1991 Nail is produced by the nail bed: a controversy resolved. Br J Dermatol 125: 27–29

Marr S J, Quine S Q 1992 Prevalence and type of foot problems amongst workers wearing safety footwear. J Br Podiatr Med 47: 239–240

Middleton A, Webb F 1993 Toenail surgery for diabetic patients. Foot 3: 109–113

Morkane A J, Robertson R W, Inglis G S 1984 Segmental phenolisation of ingrown toenails: a randomised controlled study. Br J Surg 71: 526–527

Rennel D 1992 Topical treatment in onychomycosis with Amorfiline 5% nail lacquer: comparative efficacy and tolerability of once and twice weekly use. Dermatology 184 (suppl 39): 21–24

Roberts D T 1992 Prevalence of dermatophyte onychomycosis in the United Kingdom: results of an omnibus survey. British Journal of Dermatology 126 (suppl 39): 23–27

Roberts D T, Evans E G V, Allen B R 1990 Fungal Nail Infection. Wolfe, London

Ross W R 1969 Treatment of the ingrown toenail. Surg Clin N Amer 49: 1499–1504

Ryder N S 1992 Terbinafine: mode of action and properties of squalene epoxidase inhibition. Br J Dermatol 126 (suppl 39): 2–7

Sarrafian S K 1983 Anatomy of the Foot and Ankle. J B Lippincott, Philadelphia, pp 317–358

Samman P D 1978 The Nails in Disease (3rd edition). William Heinemann, London

Thomson C, Lang S 1991 Clinical review of an atypical case of malignant melanoma. J Br Podiatr Med 46: 75–77

van der Schroeff J G, Cirkel P K S, Crijns M B, et al 1992 A randomized treatment duration-finding study of terbinafine in onychomycosis. Br J Dermatol 126 (suppl 39): 36–39

Villars V V, Jones T C 1992 Special features of the clinical use of oral terbinafine in the treatment of fungal diseases. Br J Dermatol 126 (suppl 39): 61–69

Widdicombe M J 1990 A comparative study of the public and private sectors in chiropodial care. (Socio-demographic determinants of the number and nature of lesions). Chiropodist, May: 97–104

Winograd A M 1929 A modification of the technique of operation for ingrown toenail. JAMA 92: 229–230

Zadik F R 1950 Obliteration of the nailbed of the great toe without shortening of the terminal phalanx. J Bone Joint Surg 32B: 66–67

Zaias N 1980 The Nail in Health and Disease. MTP Press, Lancaster

XI.2 Orthoses and footwear

General principles

David N Condie

Introduction

The normal functions of the ankle and foot are, like all elements of the locomotor system, dependent on an intact and mechanically adequate skeletal and ligamentous structure, a system of muscles capable of producing movement between the segments of this structure, a nervous system capable of controlling these movements and of providing sensory feedback relating to the status of the joints segments, and finally an adequate source of nutrition for all the involved tissues. Pathological conditions may arise as a result of an impairment to any one or all of these systems; pathology may occur congenitally or as a result of disease or trauma.

Whatever the cause of the impairment, the functional disorder may be considered as belonging to one of three types: deformity, instability or sensitivity.

Orthoses (and prescription footwear) are used in a number of pathological foot conditions to compensate for the disorder and so reduce the disability and handicap. These devices in the main achieve their aim by the application of forces, in a controlled manner, to the affected joints and segments. This concept may be amplified by stating that the forces that an orthosis applies to the body segments which it is in contact with, may be regarded as 'reactions'; that is, the forces arise as a result of the orthosis acting to prevent the abnormal movements or abnormal force distribution which is the consequence of the impairment and which occurs during physical activities.

This brief introduction to the uses of orthoses and footwear will describe the biomechanical principles underlying the design of successful prescriptions for each of the three previously defined categories of functional disorder.

Deformity

The term deformity is used here to refer to those situations where the foot or its constituent segments are fixed in an abnormal alignment and are not, therefore, capable of being restored to a normal plantigrade weight bearing configuration. Orthotic treatment of this situation is therefore based on the need to accommodate the deformity and to compensate for the resulting loss of normal foot and ankle function.

Typical causes of deformity include congenital talipes equinovarus, severe rheumatoid arthritis, and some chronic spastic conditions. This diversity of causes reinforces the point that the nature and the origin of the impairment are less important considerations than the type of functional disorder when planning orthotic treatment.

Planning orthotic treatment requires an understanding of the effect that the functional disorder will have on normal physical activities such as standing and walking. In the case of a deformity these may be summarized as follows.

1. The foot will be presented to the ground in an appropriate manner.
2. On the application of weight, the distribution of force on the plantar surface of the foot will be abnormal.
3. The movements between the foot and the leg at the ankle and the movements between the segments of the foot that are necessary for normal activities will be restricted.

The orthotic design should address each of these problems in a biomechanically acceptable manner as follows.

1. The outer surface of the device must be designed so as to establish initial foot contact with the heel of the shoe, progressing to overall contact at midstance (or when standing at rest), with terminal contact under the hallux. In very simple terms, the device must 'fill in' the space between the foot and the ground created by the deformity, thereby re-establishing normal foot and leg alignment. This will have the further beneficial effect of establishing a more normal pattern of external loading on the foot, which will in itself go some way towards overcoming the second problem
2. The inner surface of the device must create a more acceptable distribution of force on the plantar surface of the foot throughout the gait cycle. Once again, in simple terms, this will normally require the orthosis to be carefully moulded to the shape of the foot, taking proper account of pressure-sensitive and pressure-tolerant areas, thereby distributing these forces as widely as possible and so achieving minimal interface pressures.

3. The outer surface of the device will, in some instances, require further modification to attempt to compensate for the loss of joint function. In practice, however, the measures available to achieve this goal are rather limited.

These principles may be illustrated by the proposed design of a device to treat a fixed equinus position of the foot. The three elements of such a design may be listed as:

1. A built-up heel, and perhaps sole, which will re-establish a plantigrade position of the foot and result in a more normal pattern of ground reaction forces (Fig. 1a).
2. A moulded insole, which will relieve the pressure on the forefoot and redistribute it across the arch of the foot and the heel (Fig. 1b).
3. A cushioned heel to simulate ankle plantarflexion at heel contact and thus provide some shock absorption, and a rocker sole to compensate for the loss of normal dorsiflexion and hence assist rollover prior to final toe off (Fig. 1c).

Though this is a very simple example, it does illustrate very clearly the individual and the complementary nature of the three elements of the orthotic design, and it can be used as a model for the design of appropriate orthoses for other foot deformities.

Instability

The term instability is used here to refer to those situations in which the ranges of motion of the foot and its constituent segments are normal but where the control of their movements is impaired. Orthotic treatment of this situation is, therefore, based on the need first to correct and maintain the foot position, and secondly to compensate for any residual loss of normal ankle and foot function.

Typical causes of such a situation include lower motor neurone lesions resulting in muscle paralysis, some upper motor neurone lesions resulting in spastic behaviour and trauma, or joint disease which has destroyed normal joint integrity. The effect of this type of functional disorder on normal physical activities can be summarized as follows.

1. The foot may be presented to the ground in an abnormal and inappropriate manner.
2. Upon the application of weight the foot may adopt an inappropriate position or shape.
3. This will result in an abnormal and often unacceptable distribution of force on the plantar surface of the foot.
4. The movements between the foot and leg at the ankle and between the segments of the foot during

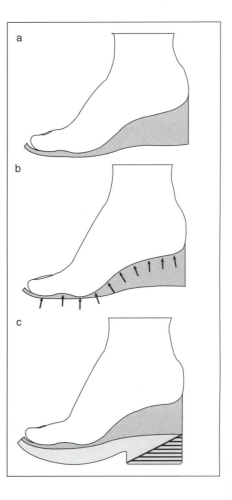

Figure 1

Design of a device to treat a fixed equinus position of the foot: (a) built up sole (to establish plantigrade attitude); (b) moulded insole (to redistribute plantar pressure); (c) cushion heel and rocker sole (to compensate for loss of normal ankle function)

physical activities will be impaired. This may take the form of excessive motion or a totally abnormal type of motion.

Once again it is possible to specify in general terms the biomechanical principles that should be used in the design of devices to address this type of disorder.

1. The device must correct (as far as possible) the position of the foot relative to the leg so that normal initial foot contact may occur.
2. The device must resist abnormal movement or deformity that arise on weight bearing. These two inter-related requirements may be achieved either by the direct application of force by the inner surface of the device to the appropriate leg and foot segments, or indirectly by modifying the outer surface of the device so that the pattern of external forces tends to achieve the required correction. This effect still

needs to be transmitted onto the limb segments through the inner surface of the device. (These two mechanisms will be clarified in the following clinical example.)

3. If full correction is achieved and maintained, the force distribution on the plantar surface of the foot will be made normal. If this is not the case, the inner and the outer surfaces of the device will need to be designed as described for the case of deformity in order to accommodate any remaining abnormality.

4. Similarly, the correction of the foot position and shape may allow normal joint movements to occur. However, if this is not the case, the device will need to replace or compensate for these functions. This may be achieved either by incorporating joint control mechanisms into the device or by further modifying the external surface of the device, as previously described.

These principles may be illustrated by reference to designs of device to treat an unstable pronating foot. The elements of such designs may be listed as follows:

1. The correction and maintenance of foot position and shape may be achieved **directly**. In rather mild cases, this requires the use of a moulded arch (valgus) support, which basically holds up the long arch of the foot, thereby resisting pronation on weight bearing. In more severe cases an ankle foot orthosis (AFO) will be required, which applies a three-point force system to the leg and foot to resist subtalar motion (Figs 2a,b).

   An alternative **indirect** approach which can be used in intermediate cases, comprises an externally floated and wedged shoe heel. This technique achieves the required function by effectively repositioning the point of application of the ground-reaction force at initial foot contact outside the medial aspect of the heel, where it will generate a corrective supinating moment about the subtalar joint axis. The effectiveness of this measure may be enhanced by the use of a moulded heel cup located inside the shoe, which will improve the efficiency with which the corrective moment is transmitted on to the foot (Figs 2c,d).

2. The foot orthosis and shoe adaptations just described basically leave the major ankle and foot articulations free to move in a relatively normal manner. An ankle foot orthosis, however, may inhibit or totally prevent any joint motion. Orthotic articulations or external shoe adaptations may be employed to allow free ankle motion; however no proprietary orthotic devices exist which will allow controlled subtalar motion. Alternatively, external shoe adaptations may be employed as previously described to compensate for loss of ankle function. However, once again no similar adaptations exist to compensate for loss of subtalar function.

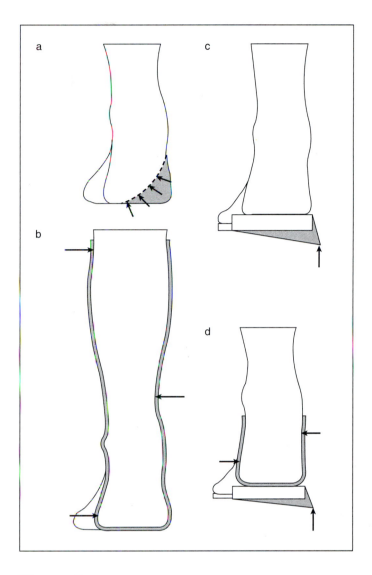

Figure 2

Design of a device to treat an unstable (but correctable) pronating foot: (a) moulded arch support; (b) ankle foot orthoses (applying 3 pt force system); (c) external wedged and floated heel; (d) external wedged and floated heel with moulded heel cup. (Posterior coronal plane view)

The orthotic measures applicable to the management of deformity and instability are very different and it is therefore vital in planning orthotic treatment to identify clearly whether the foot position is fixed (i.e. a deformity) and therefore requires accommodation, or mobile but unstable and should, therefore, be corrected. Once this basic consideration has been assessed, it is possible to move on to the specification of the detailed functions of the device design following the principles outlined for each of the two categories of disorder.

Sensitivity

The term 'sensitivity' is used here to refer to those situations in which the structure of the foot is intact and the range and control of foot movement is largely normal but the tissues of the foot are unable to tolerate the forces and pressures resulting from normal physical activity. Typical causes of this situation include diabetes mellitus, other neuropathies and, in developing countries, leprosy. The consequence of this form of functional disorder is obvious: any attempts to perform normal day-to-day physical activities is likely to result in tissue breakdown, often unknown to the patient, due to the frequently associated sensory deficit.

The design of a device to treat this situation requires the recognition of the three mechanical factors that contribute to the tissue breakdown, i.e. the absolute values of the pressure, the shear stress and the rate and duration of tissue loading. The principles and the techniques that are employed to address each of these factors may then be summarized.

1. The inner surface of the device must distribute the force acting on the plantar surface of the foot in such a manner as to avoid localized pressure concentrations. In practice, this requires the use of some form of moulded surface, which may be modified to provide specific relief for 'at risk' or previously damaged areas of tissue.
2. 'Shearing' of the tissues will arise inevitably during walking; however, it is unquestionably increased by flexion of the support surface particularly between heel off and toe off. This undesirable feature of the tissue loading can be avoided by stiffening the support surface to limit or eliminate flexion.
3. The unnatural foot contact pattern created by the stiffening of the sole already dictates some compensatory modification to the external surface of the footwear; however, this requirement is complemented by the need to reduce the shock of initial heel contact and to achieve a smooth transfer of the ground reaction forces during the entire walking cycle. The measures customarily adopted to achieve both these goals are some form of heel cushioning and a rocker bar modification to the sole of the shoe.

It is important to note that in addition to the mechanical factors that have been discussed, the avoidance of excessive temperature and humidity and the creation of a hygienic environment are critical to the successful management of this type of foot disorder.

General conditions

This discussion of the biomechanical principles applicable to the treatment of the differing types of foot disorder has inevitably concentrated on the means of transmitting the ground reaction forces to the plantar surface of the affected foot in order to avoid damaging or disabling consequences. It is also important, however, to consider the role of the shoe uppers. Firstly, the shoe upper must fit intimately to ensure that the relationship between the weight bearing aspects of the foot and the weight bearing aspects of the orthosis or footwear is maintained. Secondly, in those patients who exhibit deformities of the toes, it may be necessary to provide additional space to avoid pressure and subsequent pain and damage to these areas of the dorsum of the foot. This goal may be achieved alternatively by using extra depth or extra width stock footwear or by modifying the patient's shoes locally.

Conclusion

In conclusion, a general approach to the prescription and design of foot orthoses and special footwear is proposed, based on the classification of patients with pathological conditions of the foot as exhibiting deformity, instability or sensitivity. It should be remembered, however, that many patients will exhibit the characteristics of more than one type of disorder and that, as a consequence, the treatment objectives and the means adopted to achieve them will need to draw upon and combine elements of those described for the individual types of disorder.

Orthotic applications

David J Pratt

Introduction

The aim of this section is to describe the various orthoses relevant to the foot and to indicate some of their typical applications. Orthoses are rarely used on their own in the management of foot disorders, rather they form part of an overall treatment regime. Thus, they may be used to complement the effects of surgery, therapy or other noninvasive treatments such as taping (Whitney & Whitney 1990). In modern society, the use of shoes is the norm and as such must be an integral part of any orthotic prescription.

As described in the previous section, for orthoses to be effective they have to transmit their corrective forces to the skeletal structures via soft tissues. These have a tendency to be compressed by the applied force so that the skeletal effect of the force is delayed until after this compression has taken place. This 'lost motion' (Condie 1976) has to be taken into account, for as otherwise an orthosis may be rendered ineffective.

External shoe adaptations

These adaptations are used to help to accommodate noncorrectable deformities, to actively assist in maintaining correction of nonfixed deformities or to relieve discomfort. They should be as lightweight as possible so as not to have adverse effects on what might already be a poor quality, high energy-cost gait.

Wedges

These can be applied to either side of the heel, the whole length of the sole, a localized area of the sole (e.g. the fifth metatarsal area) or to any combination of these in order to achieve a tilting of the inside of the shoe relative to the ground (Fig. 3). It is unusual to have a wedge of more than 6 mm, with 4 mm being typical, as higher values than these tend to cause the foot to slide down the incline created without providing any additional correction or accommodation. It must be remembered that for wedges to work satisfactorily the foot should be flexible. Wedges can be of value in managing mild cases of pes planovalgus (medial heel wedge) and pes cavus (lateral heel and sole wedges) either on their own or in conjunction with other orthoses.

Heel flares

As with wedges, these can be applied to either side of the heel in order to provide a corrective moment at the heel during heel strike (Fig. 4). They can be used to help stabilize the subtalar joint in arthritic or unstable conditions, which often lead to recurrent ankle sprains.

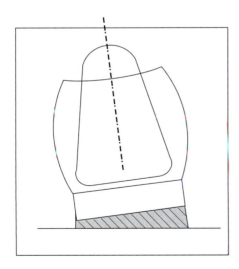

Figure 3

A heel wedge indicating the altered position of the calcaneus during weight bearing

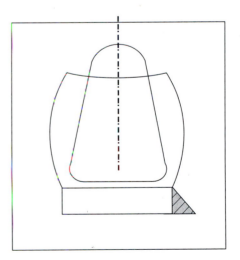

Figure 4

A heel flare does not change the position of the calcaneus during weight bearing but produces a correcting varus or valgus moment at heel strike

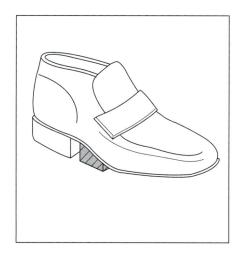

Figure 5

A metatarsal bar applied to the sole of a shoe

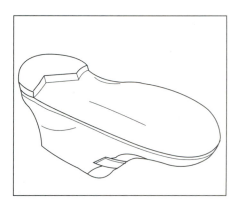

Figure 6

The medial extension of a Thomas heel

Metatarsal bars

These are added to the outside of the shoe proximal to the metatarsal head to encourage their off-loading (Fig. 5). Their effectiveness depends on the material and thickness of the sole, but they are generally less successful than metatarsal pads used inside the shoe.

Sole plates (shanks)

These stiffen the sole by the insertion of a spring steel shank. They are useful in the treatment of hallux rigidus or hallux limitus, because they prevent or limit extension at the metatarsophalangeal joint.

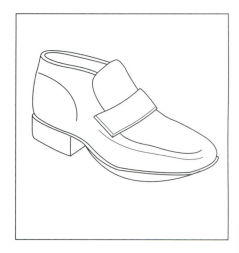

Figure 7

A rocker sole

Thomas heel

This is an anteromedial extension of the heel that can be used to provide additional support to the medial longitudinal arch of the foot, so increasing the efficiency of insoles in the heavier patient by reinforcing the shoe (Fig. 6). This may be used in conjunction with a medial heel flare or wedge in managing pes planovalgus, for example.

Heel and sole raises (lifts)

Leg length discrepancies have a number of proximal effects, including hip pain and, in extreme cases, scoliosis. Care is therefore needed when assessing and fitting shoe raises. Care should also be taken when adding raises to footwear, as flexibility of the sole is important for walking. If this cannot be maintained, an additional rocker should be considered. There is a relationship between increase in heel height and the requirements for increased dorsiflexion at the metatarsophalangeal joints, i.e. about 1° for each 5 mm of additional heel height. There is also an increase in forefoot loading as

heel height is increased (Gastwirth et al 1991). Common practice suggests that up to 12 mm may be added to the heel before it is necessary to raise the sole; this could be split, for example, by adding 6 mm inside the shoe and reducing the contralateral shoe outside by 6 mm.

Sole rockers (rocker-bottom soles)

These are used to alter the forward progression of the ground-reaction force so that loads, particularly shear, can be diminished about susceptible metatarsal heads. This is particularly relevant in the management of diabetic foot ulceration (Geary & Klenerman 1987) (Fig. 7). The reduction in toe dorsiflexion that rocker soles induce often helps to relieve metatarsal discomfort. They can also be used as described above to augment other orthotic devices and to compensate (e.g. through an arthrodesis of the ankle joint) for motion that has been lost elsewhere in the foot.

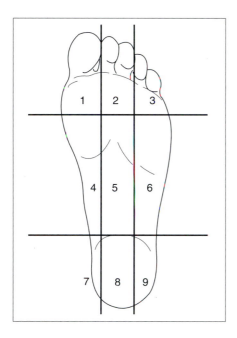

Figure 8

The nine areas of the foot used by Whitney & Whitney (1990) for insole prescription

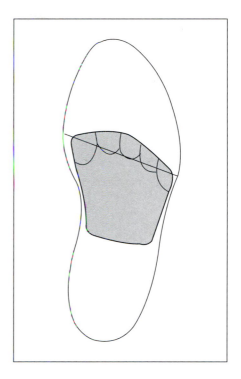

Figure 10

A metatarsal balance pad

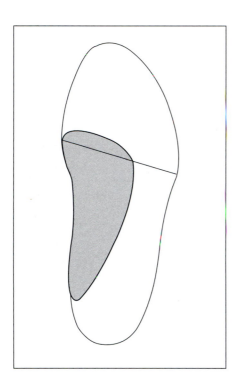

Figure 9

A valgus pad

Shoe inserts

Insoles

This group of orthoses includes all of the in-shoe devices made without taking a plaster cast of the foot, although impressions or footprints may be used to help in the placement of the corrective pads. The most satisfactory description of the use of pads is given by Whitney & Whitney (1990), who divide the foot into nine areas (Fig. 8) and assigned pads for specific purposes to each area. These pads can be used to provide relief of stress within the foot (and hence pain relief) to accommodate deformities or to test the likely outcome of the use of functional foot orthoses. This approach is often termed 'biomechanical footwear balancing'. Some examples of the types of pads and their location are presented here.

The valgus pad (Fig. 9) can be used for the relief of pronatory stress associated with compensated forefoot varus deformity or to accommodate a forefoot supinatus. To this basic design can be added features such as an extension under the first metatarsal head to manage, for example, metatarsus primus elevatus, or a medial flange to protect a bunion caused by hallux valgus.

One of the commonest devices used is the metatarsal balance pad (Fig. 10), used for the relief of focal or generalized metatarsal lesions and excess pressures. This pad has also been used for the pre-orthotic testing of a central forefoot post for the control of digital and

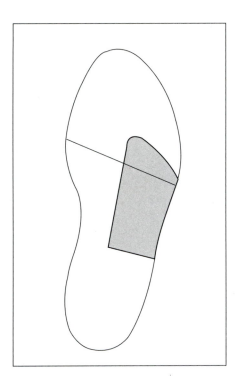

Figure 11

A varus pad

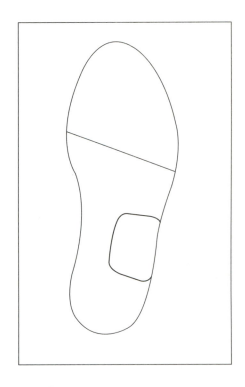

Figure 13

A calcaneocuboid pad

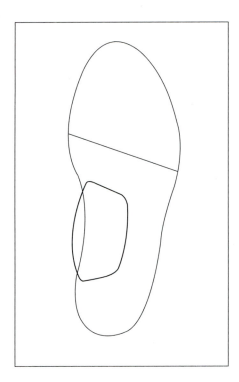

Figure 12

A talonavicular pad

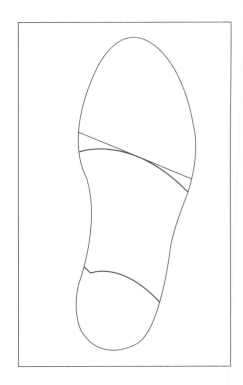

Figure 14

A cavus pad

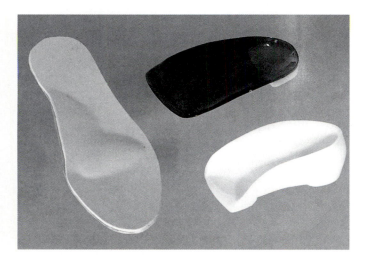

Figure 15

(a) A medial heel wedge; (b) a calcaneal spur pad; and (c) a lateral heel wedge

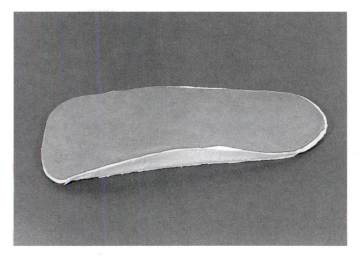

Figure 17

A total contact silicone insole

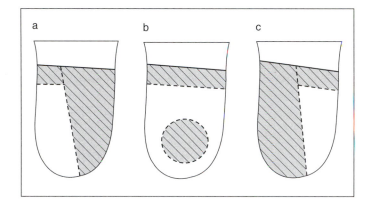

Figure 16

Illustration of three orthoses, moving clockwise from the left with an insole incorporating valgus and metatarsal balance pads, a rigid FFO with intrinsic rearfoot post and a UCBL orthosis or heel cup with both extrinsic rear and forefoot posts

metatarsal deformities. The pad can be modified by the addition of, for example, a first metatarsal extension to improve the weight bearing function of the first ray, or medial or lateral wedges for relief around first or fifth metatarsal bunions.

A varus pad (Fig. 11) is used to provide relief from lateral stress caused by a compensated forefoot valgus deformity, to accommodate a subtalar supination deformity, or for the pre-orthotic testing of a valgus post to control subtalar supination deformities. As with the pads discussed above, there are additions to this pad such as the lateral flange, which can assist with bunion relief, and the lateral extension, which can improve fourth and fifth metatarsal weight bearing.

Examples of some of the other possible inserts include the talonavicular pad (Fig. 12) to control subluxation of the talonavicular joint, the calcaneocuboid pad (Fig. 13) to control the calcaneocuboid joint, and the cavus pad (Fig. 14) used to provide stress relief associated with a cavus deformity. In addition, rearfoot pads can be used (Fig. 15) to provide medial or lateral wedges under the calcaneus, which have similar roles to the heel wedging already described, as well as the relief of pain due to calcaneal spurs. Fig. 16 shows an insole incorporating both valgus and forefoot balance pads.

A functional hallux rigidus device is described by Dannanberg (1988). Its use in rheumatoid arthritis is described by Clayton and Ries (1991), in which dorsiflexion of the hallux is prevented because of the weight bearing position of the foot and its forefoot to rearfoot relationship. It is claimed that slight plantarflexion of the first metatarsal shaft relative to the other shafts during forefoot loading enables the hallux to function correctly and relieves pain and compensation. The soft insert (placed inside an excavation in the shoe beneath the first metatarsal head) which allows this motion is the kinetic wedge.

The increase in sporting activities, particularly jogging, among the general public has raised the level and awareness of associated injuries, e.g. shin splints, plantar fasciitis and stress fractures. This has led to the rapid introduction of many 'shock absorbing' insoles to help reduce skeletal shocks transmitted through the foot to proximal structures. It was known that many pathological conditions, such as rheumatoid arthritis, also benefitted from the use of such insole materials. Insoles for shock attenuation have been tested to verify their performance under actual and simulated usage conditions (Pratt & Sanghera 1987) and the performance was found to vary considerably with temperature. In addition, long-term tests showed that their effectiveness diminished quickly with use (Pratt 1990), and this indicates that regular replacement is essential. The use of these insoles, it is claimed, leads to improvements in comfort for those who spend long hours on their feet (Basford & Smith 1988) and particularly to those with low back pain (Voloshin & Wosk 1982).

Moulded accommodating insoles

These orthoses are made from a plaster cast or impression of the foot taken whilst weight bearing. They are used to help reduce stress in the joints of the foot, especially when caused by fixed deformities. Many materials can be used for these insoles, e.g. silicone (Pratt et al 1984), polyurethane foamed *in situ*, and heat-formed foam sheets such as high-density Plastazote. They are total contact devices (Fig. 17) that spread the forces due to weight bearing over as large an area as possible, thus reducing focal pressures and relieving soft tissue stresses. It is possible to incorporate the principles of padding, as just described, to improve their efficacy, and these insoles are found to be useful for many conditions associated with degenerative processes.

Functional foot orthoses

This type of orthosis was pioneered by Dr Merton Root in the USA around 1960, and it was developed into an apparently sophisticated but much misunderstood device. The functional foot orthosis (FFO) is designed to control abnormal foot pressures caused by structural or functional deficits by three main processes. Firstly, the main FFO encourages the subtalar joint to function about its neutral position; secondly, it locks the midtarsal joints in full pronation to stabilize the forefoot on the rearfoot; and thirdly, it allows normal plantarflexion of the first metatarsal during the propulsive phase of gait.

These orthoses consist of a rigid plastic shell (often an acrylic-based material) which has a combination of rearfoot and forefoot posts (or wedges) used to realign and control the foot (see Fig. 16). The rearfoot post (or wedge) usually has its medial edge ground at an angle to allow the subtalar joint to pronate slightly during walking.

FFOs are produced usually from a non-weight-bearing cast of the foot taken with the foot held in subtalar neutral and the midtarsal joints fully pronated. This is necessary as the weight bearing foot adopts the compensated position, the very position requiring correction. The consequence of taking a non-weight-bearing cast is that alterations need to be made to the cast to accommodate the changes that naturally occur in the loaded foot, i.e. lowering of the medial arch and spread of the plantar tissues. These cast alterations have been the subject of much interest; they range from simple additions for the above changes through the inverted technique of Blake & Ferguson (1991) to the complex polysectional triplanar posting technique of Lundeen (1988).

Before the casts are taken for these orthoses, the patient has to be examined and the philosophy of the FFO requires that a full description of the interrelationships between the tibial orientation, rearfoot and forefoot planes and the ground should be established (Philps 1990). From this description, the posting angles and casting process that are most suitable can be selected (Anthony 1991). The degree of accuracy required for the measurements is claimed by many to be within 1°, a level that is difficult to support especially when 'tuning' of the first orthosis allows for the final posting angles to be adjusted by more than this.

This rigid process of biomechanical evaluation does ensure that a full mechanical description of the foot is obtained with as little inherent error as possible, a laudable aim for any orthotic prescription. The established techniques do seem to produce good therapeutic results and the validity of the approach is supported by many (Phillips et al 1985, Sanner 1989). There is evidence of good repeatability using these techniques in experienced hands (Freeman 1990) but a healthy scepticism still remains (Kidd 1991, Pratt et al 1993).

These devices have proved to be useful for a number of foot or leg problems resulting in foot compensation, including forefoot invertus and evertus, subtalar joint varus and valgus, internal/external limb rotations (in young children only), tibial varus and valgus, paralysis of tibialis anterior and peroneus longus (Root et al 1977, Anthony 1991), plantar fasciitis, calcaneal spurs, and diabetes (Novick et al 1991). Their use in treating pes planovalgus in children with cerebral palsy is limited but they can be used with care. With the increase in general sporting activity there has been an associated increase in foot problems and the value of FFOs in sports is well accepted (Subotnick 1979, Eggold 1981).

Heel cups

These are sometimes called UCBL foot orthoses and are based on a concept proposed by Helfet called the heel seat (Helfet 1956). Further modification by Rose (1962) produced the basis for the current designs (see Fig. 16) and apparently more sophisticated devices such as the negative anatomically modified foot orthosis or NAMFO (Marvin & Brownrigg 1983). Produced from casts of the foot they provide more effective control of the rear- and midfoot than FFOs, but they should nevertheless be based on similar assessments and posting principles. They are found to be effective for the same kinds of conditions listed above for FFOs but they are used in the more severe cases. In addition, it is claimed that they are helpful in the treatment of plantar fasciitis and calcaneal spurs (Campbell & Inman 1974).

Talus control foot orthoses

These devices are designed to control varus and valgus positions of the foot in such conditions as cerebral palsy.

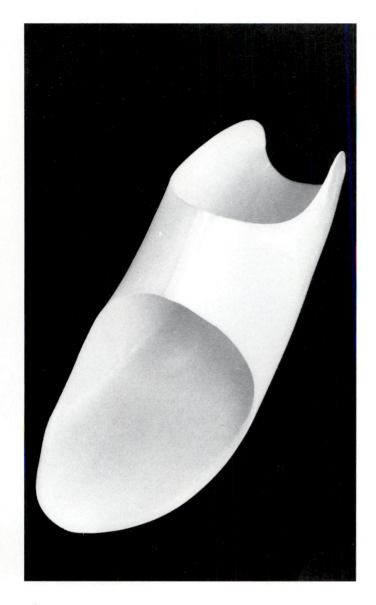

Figure 18
A talus control foot orthosis

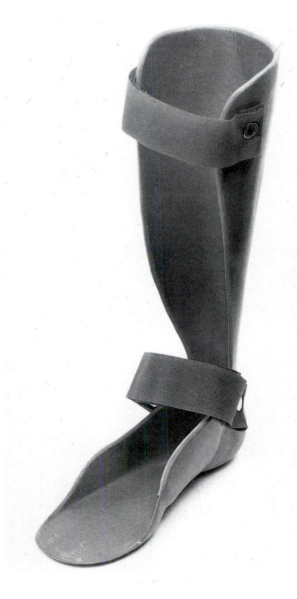

Figure 19
A rigid AFO

Their design is based on new concepts founded on dorsal control of the foot (Pratt et al 1994) (Fig. 18). It is felt that by moving the point of contact of the orthosis directly onto the talus, control is close to the joints that require stabilization, particularly the subtalar joint. The benefit of such devices is that ankle motion is not affected by extending orthotic control above the ankle joint, as occurs in ankle foot orthoses. They are produced from a cast of the foot. The basis of this design is to hold the talus dorsally, stabilize the calcaneus and provide a stable base from which to function. Unlike the orthoses previously described, little motion is allowed, other than that allowed by the distortion of the material. Plaster alterations to the cast centre around accommodation of the tendons of extensor hallucis longus and tibialis anterior, and the comfortable grip of the talus is more difficult to carry out than many plaster alterations.

Moulded ankle foot orthoses

These are possibly the most widely studied of all orthoses and there are many variations available. The rigid ankle foot orthosis (AFO) concept is used for a number of purposes not related to foot dysfunction, e.g. knee stabilization with the anterior ground reaction AFO (Glancy & Lindseth 1972). The primary use for the rigid AFO is the control of ankle plantarflexion in the child with cerebral palsy (Fig. 19), where it limits plantarflexion during the swing phase of gait and helps to control midfoot stability during stances (Meadows 1984). The use of rigid AFOs is advocated by some as the best way of assisting these patients (Butler et al 1992), but rigid AFOs do have some functional disadvantages associated with the inherent limitation of dorsiflexion. Alterations in material thickness,

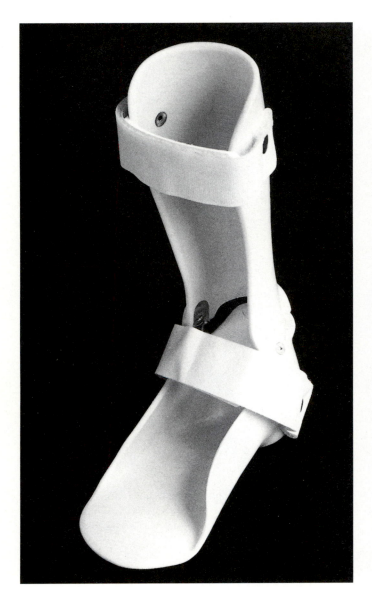

Figure 20

A hinged APO incorporating Gillette ankle hinges

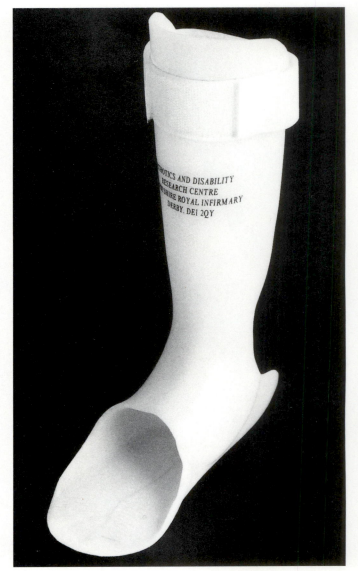

Figure 21

A talus control AFO

trim lines, and orthotic contour can help to alleviate this but a more useful solution is to use ankle hinges.

There are many types of hinge available in both metal and plastic (Fig. 20) and one study (Middleton et al 1988) has shown that hinged orthoses produce a more natural and symmetrical walking pattern, with a consequent reduction in energy usage and improved patient acceptability. However, care must be taken to ensure that the foot is correctly assessed, as midfoot stability is prerequisite for their success (Weber 1991). It must be remembered that for any AFO to work well the ankle must be capable of being held in the desired position with the knee fully extended to facilitate walking.

Improvements have been made in the ability of AFOs to control midfoot instability, particularly by the Carlson technique (Carlson & Berglund 1979). In addition, the

application of some of the posting principles used in FFOs can lead to considerable improvements in effectiveness of AFOs. The talus control principle has also been applied to AFOs with a mixture of benefits to the user (Brown et al 1987) (Fig. 21).

The application of the three point fixation principle is used in AFOs to help control the position of the calcaneus in particular. Care has to be exercised so that excessive pressure is not applied over sensitive areas such as the malleoli (Fig. 22).

Caution is required if using AFOs in treating patients with fixed deformity resulting from contractures of the soleus and gastrocnemius muscles. Serial casting or adjustable AFOs (Fig. 23) can be used to reduce the contracture, but if the knee is flexed during casting or use of the AFO, and if the gastrocnemius is tight when

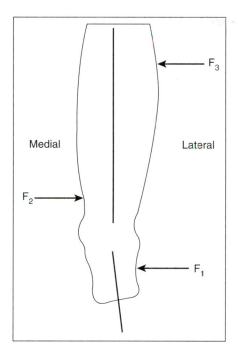

Figure 22

The three point force system (F1–F3) showing where these are applied to control a valgus calcaneus

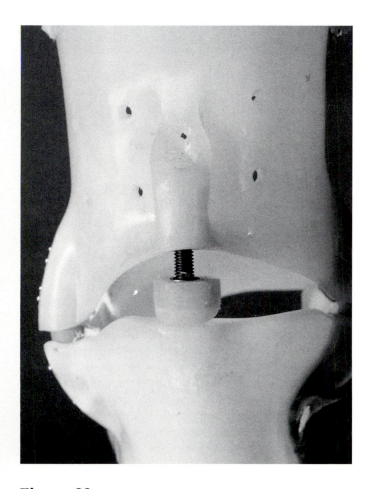

Figure 23

The screw adjuster sometimes used with hinged AFOs

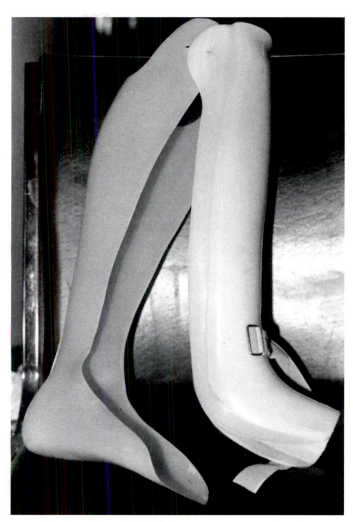

Figure 24

A patella tendon bearing (PTB) AFO with a hinged anterior section used to off-load the foot

the knee is extended, large forces are generated in the Achilles tendon, which result in a plantarflexed os calcis and forefoot dorsiflexion about the subtalar joint – a rocker bottom foot. In such cases surgery may be the treatment of choice.

Modified versions of the moulded AFO can be used to offload the foot, either to relieve pain or to help control excessive loads on areas of the foot. These modified versions consist of an AFO with a hinged anterior section that offloads the foot via the patella tendon, a principle often used in below-knee prosthetics (Fig. 24).

Conventional AFOs (calipers)

These orthoses have been used for many years and in some instances are still required. They consist of either

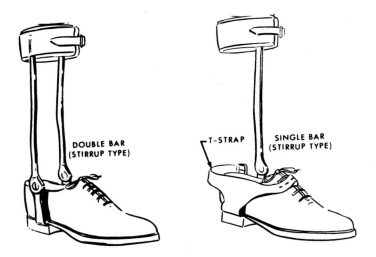

Figure 25

Conventional calipers showing on the left a double bar type with ankle hinges. On the right is a single bar with a T-strap to help control, in this case, a varus tendency of the ankle

one or two, usually metal, side bars that extend from the outside of the heel of the shoe to the top of the calf (Fig. 25). They come in many variations and perform tasks similar to the moulded plastic AFO, though they are generally used for the more difficult conditions. The use of plastic AFOs can present problems for the user in that the sweat developed under the plastic is unable to evaporate quickly and can cause skin irritation in those sensitive to this. In addition, diurnal changes in limb volume can cause the AFO to be too tight for part of the day which, in the presence of circulatory disorders and neuropathy, can lead to skin lesions. If orthotic treatment is still required for these patients then conventional devices are the only realistic choice.

Mediolateral corrective forces can be applied via straps that are used to pull the foot and ankle over in the required direction, called T or Y straps (see Fig. 25). Better functional results are obtained by having ankle joints in the side bars aligned as closely as possible to the anatomical joint rather than having the bars inserted into the heel (Condie 1976). These orthoses tend to be heavier and less cosmetically appealing than their plastic counterparts but they do tend to last longer than many plastic devices.

Ankle stabilizers

These orthoses are not generally bespoke items but stock products that are used to control mediolateral ligamen-

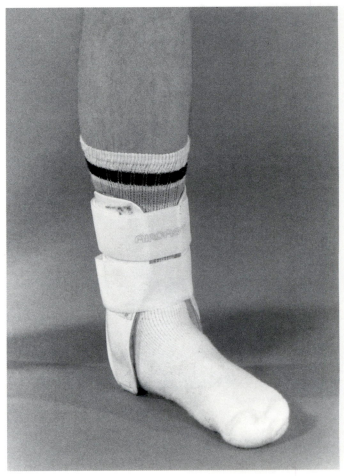

Figure 26

An ankle stabilizer (in this case by Aircast) which limits mediolateral motion but does not restrict plantar and dorsiflexion at the ankle

tous instability at the ankle regardless of the cause. They consist of two plastic sections that extend from the calcaneus to the mid-shank level on both sides of the leg. They are strapped to the leg with Velcro (or similar) and are held together under the heel by a flexible strap (Fig. 26). The inside surfaces of the shells have cells containing either air or gel which contour themselves to the ankle region when the orthosis is strapped to the leg. They provide reasonable control of mediolateral instability without unduly affecting ankle plantarflexion and dorsiflexion. Their value has been demonstrated not only for ligamentous injuries but also in patients suffering from a stroke (Stover & York 1980, Burdett et al 1988).

Footwear function and clinical requirements

Marilyn Lord

Introduction

The main purposes of normal footwear are to protect the soft tissues of the foot from external mechanical insult, to cushion the plantar surface and redistribute foot pressure and shearing stresses, to provide shock absorption and thermal insulation, and perhaps to give support to the bony structure. The aesthetic role of footwear is obvious.

Shoes affect the functioning of the foot in varying degrees depending on their construction. In general, the shod foot makes less adaptation for uneven ground than the bare foot. The ranges of motion encountered at the joints of the foot are reduced to a greater or lesser extent depending on the shoe construction. The shoe can be of a solid base construction like a clog and this feature precludes the flexing across the metatarsophalangeal joint which normally occurs at push-off. Footwear can also restrict the range of subtalar joint motion, relying on the stiffness of the heel counters and contours of the heel base. The contours of the shoe bed from the heel through the midfoot may offer support to the medial longitudinal arch of the foot, and restrict foot pronation under weight bearing conditions.

During walking, there are horizontal components of the ground reaction force in addition to the vertical anti-gravity component. The major horizontal component lies in the direction of the line of progress. This is an inertial force corresponding to the forward acceleration of the body at push-off and the deceleration at heel strike. In barefoot walking, the horizontal force is sustained between the floor and the sole of the shoe. In shod walking, it can be transmitted to the foot by a combination of shear at the plantar surface and direct pressure over other areas presenting a vertical projection onto the frontal plane. In particular, the forward acceleration forces can be opposed in the area of the shoe heel counter, and, in a high-fronted shoe, the deceleration forces which give the foot a tendency to slip forward can be opposed across a firmly-closed instep. Contoured shoe beds can also play a part in shear reduction, providing an analogue to a runner's starting block for the foot to push directly against (Snijders 1987); the net result is a reduction in the shear stresses on the plantar surface.

Shearing stresses and frictional effects at the skin surface are also affected by the wearing of hosiery. Without hosiery, relative movement between the foot surface and the shoe can rapidly result in frictional damage and blistering. The intervention of a well-fitting sock can ensure that any sliding friction occurs preferentially between the sock outer surface and the shoe. Also, some special socks with a double skin claim to allow limited sliding to occur freely between the two layers and thus minimize the shear transmitted to the skin. Although this may give reduced shearing stresses on the skin, the level of foot security and the underfoot stability are compromised (Wilson 1993).

Because the development of systems for measuring in-shoe plantar shear and pressure distribution is fairly recent, it is still true to say that determination of the relationship between footwear design and these factors remains a major challenge for the future.

Shoe requirements for clinical conditions

General requirements

The special nature of orthopaedic footwear can be described as either accommodative or corrective.

In the case of fixed deformities that cannot be contained within a normal shoe, orthopaedic shoes or boots may represent the only option to accommodate the foot. Special footwear may also be required to accommodate undeformed feet if deep shoe inserts are needed as described in the previous section.

For flexible feet with inherent joint instability or misalignment, the footwear requirements are corrective and are aimed at maintenance of appropriate orientation of the skeletal structure.

There are general requirements that all orthopaedic shoes should be comfortable, acceptable in appearance and weight, and effective in their role of accommodation and support. It is assumed that all orthopaedic shoes for everyday wear will be made of a good quality leather, primarily because of its ability to transmit sweat. Maintenance of a healthy dry climate around the foot is dependent on this ability to disperse perspiration. A perception of discomfort due to heat may be exacerbated by dampness even when the foot is within the normal comfortable range of temperature of approximately 18–32°C. Leather is far superior with regard to its hydrophytic and permeability properties than the PVC synthetic materials often used in cheaper fashion shoemaking. It has a thermal conductivity similar to that of synthetic materials.

Specific conditions requiring footwear

Diabetes mellitus

Foot complications occur in a significant number of patients with diabetes mellitus. The problems are

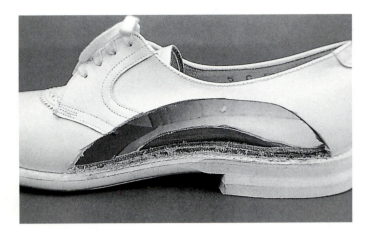

Figure 27

Diabetic shoe with contoured insole

typically described as being vascular or neuropathic or both in origin. The challenges for footwear for the two groups are quite distinct.

Diabetic patients with a history of neuropathic plantar ulceration have abnormally high pressures under the foot in walking (Stokes et al 1975, Cterctetko et al 1981, Boulton et al 1983) with peaks of pressure occurring most frequently under the metatarsal heads and correlated with the sites of ulceration. Control of plantar ulceration is a priority for footwear management of this group. Reduction of the pressure peaks can be achieved by the provision of special shoes with deep or moulded inserts (Cavanagh et al 1987, Lord & Hosein 1994) which form an important part of an effective management programme for the neuropathic foot (Fig. 27).

The specification of shoes for diabetic neuropathy includes provision of

- extra depth shoes to accommodate cushioning or moulded inserts for reduction of pressure peaks;
- extra depth in the toe box and soft uppers to prevent rubbing on claw toes;
- a good fit in the hindfoot and secure fastening to prevent any sliding action, which could result in plantar shear and pressures on the distal tip of the toes;
- in severe cases, rocker-bottom outer soles to reduce the loading under the metatarsal heads.

The problems of the ischaemic foot are quite different. The main requirement of any footwear provided for these patients is to prevent excessive pressure and rubbing of the shoe on the dorsum of the foot. The specification for these shoes includes

- light weight;
- soft uppers over the forefoot, with minimal or no toe puff; and
- soft foam liner.

Rheumatoid arthritis

A very high percentage of adult patients with rheumatoid arthritis experience problems with their feet (Vainio 1975). The five commonest features are hallux valgus, pronation of the foot, depression of the metatarsal heads, claw toes, and tendocalcaneal bursitis or spur formation (Soames et al 1982, Wilson 1993). The rheumatoid foot becomes deformed, hypersensitive and painful, and these are conditions that the footwear must address. In addition, the footwear must acknowledge the problems that may be experienced in gait. Weakness in particular in the calf muscles, restricted ranges of motion in the ankle, and involvement of the joints higher up the leg (Dimonte & Light 1982) all contribute to an abnormal flat foot gait pattern. The objectives of the footwear must be to reduce pain, to prevent or accommodate deformity and to assist in walking.

The primary requirements can be summarized as the provision of

- cushioning under the ball of the foot;
- adequate forefoot width to prevent compression of joints;
- accommodation of any fixed deformities, e.g. extra depth in the toebox to prevent rubbing on the dorsum of clawed toes;
- support and maintenance of flexible joints in hindfoot and midfoot with contoured shoe bed;
- in extreme cases, immobilization of the joints by rigid shoe;
- reduction of shock loading by resilient heels and viscoelastic inserts;
- lightweight construction in deference to sensitivity; and
- ease of donning and fastening in the presence of upper extremity involvement.

Orthopaedic conditions

A common orthopaedic condition linked to footwear requirements is that of hallux valgus. In extreme cases, the hallux will cross over the adjacent toes and may even cause adjacent metatarsophalangeal joints to sublux. Hallux valgus, most common in women, has hereditary tendencies, although it has also been suggested that there is a link between the wearing of tight shoes and the hallux deformity (Sim-Fook & Hodgson 1958, Frey et al 1993). Treatment is primarily surgical. Nevertheless it is recommended that the foot with hallux valgus should be fitted with a shoe that is made on a last with a straight medial border, so that no mediolateral pressure can be exerted to push the hallux further out of line.

Other less frequent deformities, such as congenital pes planus, congenital vertical talus, metatarsus adductus, and talipes equinovarus, also usually require surgery. Footwear may then be needed to accommodate fixed deformities resulting from fusion of impaired joints or misalignments that cannot be totally corrected.

The use of corrective footwear for minor orthopaedic conditions of children is a topic that arouses strong and contradictory opinions. Many observed 'deformities' will resolve in time without the need for treatment. For example, the efficacy of using corrective shoe as a treatment for flexible flatfoot in children has been brought into question in recent years (Wenger et al 1989). However for correction of metatarsus adductovarus the use of splinting followed by reverse-lasted shoes (out-flared foreparts) may assist in preventing persistent problems (Allen et al 1993).

Expectations of the patient

Satisfying the patient is a matter of achieving a good functional outcome whilst additionally meeting the patient's own expectations in appearance of shoes. There are differing opinions as to the extent to which a compromise should be made when the patient's expectations of style, weight, and materials are in conflict with the clinician's functional specifications. It must always be recognized that the patient may choose not to wear the shoes if he or she does not like them. This is a frequent outcome in neuropathic cases, where pain relief is not a factor and there may be a concomitant degree of denial. Lack of patient compliance in this respect can lead to a waste of funds and a serious deterioration in the condition of the patient's feet.

According to surveys of consumer satisfaction carried out in the UK (Fisher & McLellan 1989; Costigan et al 1989) patients were concerned with aspects of comfort, style, durability and delivery of special footwear provided through the National Health Service. There is still room for exploration and innovation to meet patients' expectations within tight cost constraints. Improvements will come from materials and manufacturing advances that can make better styled, better fitting, lighter shoes at realistic prices. Immediate measures open to the prescribing clinician to ensure the best customer response are:

- take the patient's expectations and lifestyle fully into consideration when making a prescription;
- discuss sympathetically with the patient the specification of the footwear and probability of compliance before proceeding: this can at best lead to improved acceptance, and at worse lead to the conclusion that the footwear prescription is futile;
- provide the maximum possible choice within the confines of a functional specification, and admit the possibility of a compromise in function;
- identify those orthopaedic suppliers who take positive steps to address issues of concern to the patient, such as quality measures to ensure better fit, fast delivery, genuine choice of styles via an up-to-date catalogue, prompt and effective response to

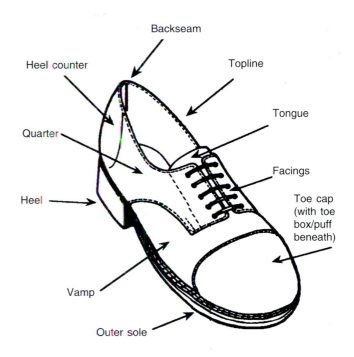

Figure 28
Shoe terminology

consumer requests, and attention to details, e.g. punch stitching, colour of laces and decorative features.

Basics of footwear construction

Structure of a shoe and boot

The discrete components that are obvious in inspection of a shoe or boot are the upper, sole, heel and linings (Fig. 28).

The upper usually consists of a number of leather pieces that are stitched together. Stiffeners of fibre, leather or synthetic materials are inserted between the upper and the linings to maintain shape particularly around the toe area – 'the toe puff' – and the heel area – 'the heel counter'. The main parts of the upper are the vamp in the front and the quarters at the rear. The edge around the opening for the foot is referred to as the topline, which may be padded around the heel area and is designed to pull tight for a snug fit of the hindfoot. The backseam at the rear of the heel is shaped over the heel counter and clipped in at the topline for heel grip.

The sole usually has a sandwich construction, with an outer sole of either leather or, preferably, a lightweight resilient synthetic material, an inner sole of leather and a compressible filler between the two. In order to prevent excessive flexing of the shoe in the midfoot area, a metal shank is also fitted into the sole, running from

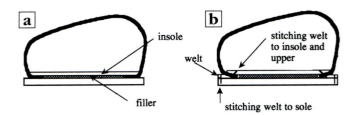

Figure 29

(a) Glued and (b) welted sole attachment

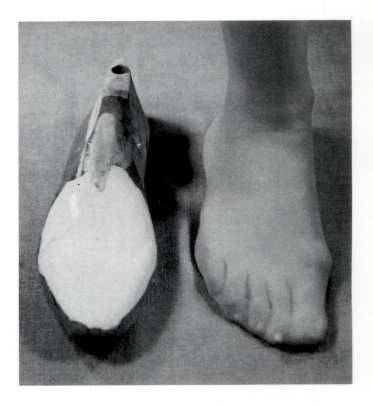

Figure 31

A shoe last made to measure for the foot beside it

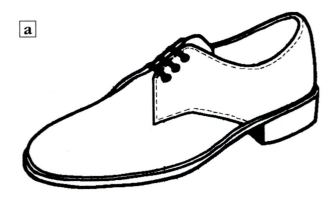

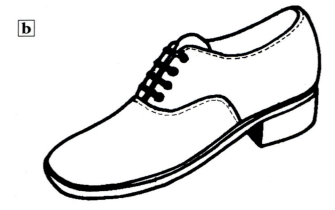

Figure 30

(a) The Gibson and (b) the Oxford styles

the heel area to the ball of the shoe. Sole and upper were traditionally attached together by stitching a 'welt', a strip of leather, to both the upper and the sole. The two components are now more often attached directly by a cement or stitch down process (Fig. 29). When viewing an unworn shoe placed on a flat surface from the side, the sole at the toe end is canted upwards to achieve 'toe-spring'. Flattening of the toe-spring in standing causes tension in the vamp area, which discourages the formation of creasing. For prescription footwear, the heel heights are generally about 25 mm for men and up to 35 mm for women. In cases where greater heel

heights are required for clinical reasons, there must also be adjustment of the inclination of the seat under the heel in order to avoid misalignment and pain in the foot. Suggested inclinations at sample heel heights are 10 mm, 4°; 25 mm 10°; 55 mm, 15°.

Shoe styles

Two very traditional shoe styles form the basis of most orthopaedic shoes, the Oxford and the Gibson (Fig. 30). The Gibson is often preferable because the lace panel can be folded completely back to afford good access for the foot, and this style is also used for boots. T-bar and trainer styles are also frequently supplied. Fastenings are traditionally by lace for the basic styles but buckles, velcro and zippers may be used as alternatives.

Shoemaking process and the importance of the shoe last

At the heart of the shoemaking process is the shoe last (Fig. 31). This is the form over which the shoe is constructed, and it determines the interior shape of the finished shoe. It is important to understand that shoe lasts are not and should not be identical to the shape of the foot that the shoe is destined to fit. Indeed that would be an impossibility, since a foot does not have a single shape, but changes considerably from loaded to off-loaded conditions and during articulation of the joints during walking. When comparing the plaster cast of a foot (see Fig. 31) and the matching shoe last, the last shape is found to be a compromise to ensure the best fit, taking into account the way in which the shoe construction restrains the distortion of the upper during weight bearing and the flexion of the shoe during walking. In the toe area, the last is shaped more for aesthetic appearance.

The design of shoe lasts has evolved over long periods of time, and in the fashion industry these are adjusted cautiously to adapt to the new season's appearances or else purchased from specialist companies. Small alterations in shaping of a last can dramatically affect the fit of a shoe.

A major dilemma in orthopaedic last-making for individualized shoes is whether to modify an existing last to fit the individual's measures, or to modify a cast of the foot into a new last. The first operation is more rapid and arguably provides better fitting shoes as long as the modifications are not too great.

Pattern pieces for the upper are designed by various traditional shoemaking craft processes to fit a specific last, and more recently by computer-aided design methods introduced later in this chapter. The upper is then closed, by sewing together all the flat parts, and pulled over the top surface of the last to shape the flat leather into a three-dimensional form.

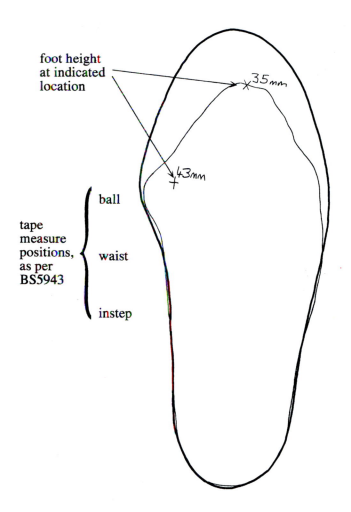

Figure 32

Comparison of the foot outline and the outline of a made-to-measure last for a well-fitting orthopaedic shoe

Shoe fit

Concept of good shoe fit

In the opinion of Cinderella's ugly sisters, shoes fit if the foot can possibly be crammed into them. Although most people apply a little more common sense, it is extremely difficult to put down any hard and fast rules concerning a good fit for either normal or for orthopaedic footwear. Both the orthotist's and the patient's preference for tightness, styles, etc, will inevitably introduce subjective variability. The following section is offered as a guideline to the principles and good practice despite its woeful lack of quantitative measures.

Orthopaedic criteria

As a general principle, prescription footwear should fit snugly in the heel and mid foot, where supportive and retentive forces are required. This is achieved by pulling the foot firmly back into the shoe by a secure closure over the instep, which demands a high cut shoe with an adjustable tightening. Across the ball, the foot should be located adequately to prevent slipping, but the fit must avoid any lateral squeezing across the metatarsophalangeal joint, a source of metatarsalgia. Forward of the ball, clearance is required on the toes at all points. This is to avoid sideways pressure causing deviation of the toes, to prevent lengthwise stubbing leading to interphalangeal and metatarsophalangeal joint damage, and to prevent skin lesions over the interphalangeal joints, particularly if there are hammer toes.

As a preliminary requirement for fit, the outline of the weight bearing foot and the insole of the shoe should correspond from heel to ball (Fig. 32). A shoe with a pointed toe will have to be longer than one with a rounded toe. In this respect, the notion of an 'effective length' of a shoe is useful. This represents the useable distance from the heel up to the furthest forward point in the toebox which is of sufficient height and width to accommodate the forefoot (Fig. 33). The three elements of toe room allowance are

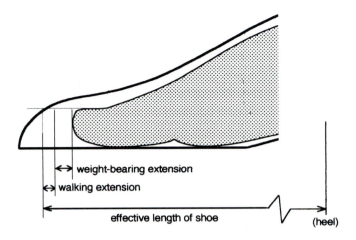

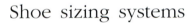

Figure 33

The shoe has toe room for extension of the foot due to weight-bearing, flexion during walking and, in the case of children, growth, plus the styling extension which is too narrow or low to accommodate the toes

1. foot extension on weight-bearing (0–12 mm for adults);
2. anterior motion of toes at push-off due to extension at the metatarsophalangeal joint (2–6 mm for adults); and
3. growth with children (5–8 mm).

Shoe sizing systems

The basis of shoe sizing is determined by two measures, overall length of the last and girth at the ball. The length measure is referred to generally as the 'size', and the girth measure as the 'width fitting'. Sizing systems are based on the dimensions of the shoe last, not the foot. The nominal last length for the size should correspond to the effective length, rather than the overall length.

From the very crude nature of defining a last by only the length and ball girth, it should be obvious that this information is insufficient to select a shoe that will fit. Shoe sizing was predominantly a system for volume manufacturers to maximize their coverage of the market with a minimum stock of shoes. There are three important shoe sizing systems in use today, namely the American, English and Continental systems.

Prescription footwear design

Footwear adaptations

Various adaptations of the patient's own footwear can be made (Fig. 34). A well-constructed shoe is a prerequisite for such modifications. Because many fashion shoes

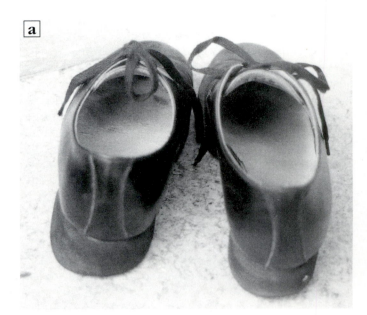

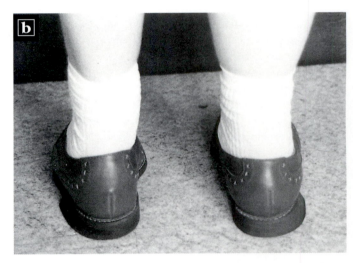

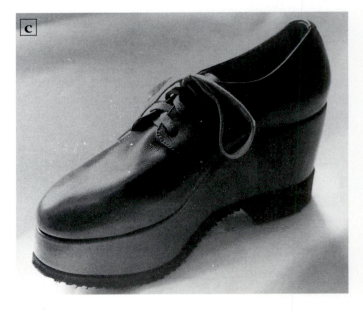

Figure 34

Adaptations which can be made to normal shoes: (a) external wedging; (b) sole flares; (c) external raises

would not meet this criterion, a stock prescription shoe (see below) might be considered as the basis for these modifications. The modifications are discussed earlier in the chapter.

Stock shoes

Ranges of stock prescription shoes are offered by various companies. The distinguishing features of these shoes are mostly that the last is of a foot-like shape with sufficient room in the toe box, and often a full-length extra depth is allowed to leave room for a thick insert. These shoes are also known as 'extra-width' or 'extra-depth'. Each manufacturer will use a limited range of basic last models, perhaps only between two and 10 in number. As with fashion shoes the lasts from one company might be a better overall fit for any individual than those of another, and for this reason using more than one range offers better fitting possibilities.

The use of stock shoes ordered from a catalogue is limited by the difficulty in specifying the correct size first time. Standard sizing of shoes by length and width cannot guarantee a fit. Attempts to provide better information include:

- qualitative descriptions of the last shapes which are used (Fig. 35);
- more detailed last dimensions; and
- provision of sets of insole templates for comparison with foot outline.

Semi-bespoke shoes

Some manufacturers offer a compromise system that lies in complexity and cost between that of stock and bespoke (individualized) shoes. A basic range of stock shoes is maintained for trial fitting. From the trial fit, the orthotist can request that certain modifications are made by the temporary addition of material to a stock last to provide the required shoes for this particular patient. This permits a degree of customization to accommodate minor deformities without incurring the costs of a fully bespoke shoe.

Bespoke shoes

A bespoke prescription shoe is one that is individually made for the patient. For fairly normal shaped or moderately deformed feet, the process begins with measurement of the feet individually. British Standard BS5943:1980 'A Method for Measuring and Casting for Orthopaedic Footwear' describes the basic process.

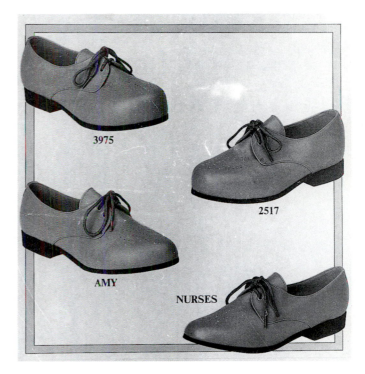

Figure 35

An example of visual descriptions of last shapes for stock shoes (courtesy of P R Cooper (Footline) Ltd))

Because the majority of the prescription footwear trade owes its origins to the skilled craftsmen of old Europe, very similar practices are found internationally.

The last-maker then crafts a last to match the corresponding foot measures or foot cast. There are no hard and fast guidelines for this process, although recent work in both the prescription and the volume shoe trades is aimed at a better understanding of these relationships (Rossi 1983, Salaman 1986, Browne 1993), since it is at this point that much of the variability in fit arises. A moulded insert may be formed against the last, or the last adjusted in depth to accommodate a proposed insert.

Most shoes on a new order are trial fitted. The shoes may be initially only 'rough finished', i.e. the upper is only temporarily tacked down, a temporary sole attached and the insole positioned, so that they can be sent for a fitting. On return, the last and uppers might be adjusted in response to the fitter's comments before the final soling is done.

An alternative practice widely observed in continental Europe utilizes plastic trial shoes to avoid costly reworking of the leather uppers. These shell shoes are vacuumformed over the last and trimmed to the lines of a shoe. The shoe lasts are modified on the basis of the shell shoe fitting, and then the final shoes can be cut and finished for delivery. Shell fitting has been found comparable in most respects to normal trial shoe fitting with respect to the evaluation made (van der Zande et al

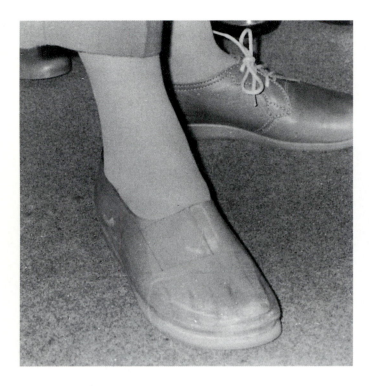

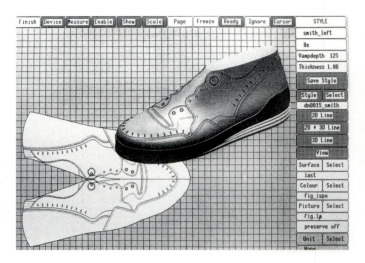

Figure 37

Computer-aided design of shoe styles over a 3-D representation of the last linked to automatic flattening to 2-D and pattern generation, using the Shoemaster system from C&J Clark International

Figure 36

A clear-plastic shell shoe is compared to the normal shoe made over the same last

1992, Lord et al 1992) (Fig. 36), but patients need to be mentally prepared for this process to avoid disappointment at being presented with a plastic shell instead of their new shoes to try on.

Advanced technology – the future for orthopaedic footwear

Background and example systems

Advanced technology is already widely used in the volume shoe trade (Flutter 1983) for style design and pattern generation. An example of computer-aided design of a style over a three-dimensional model of a last is shown in Fig. 37. The two-dimensional patterns are generated automatically by mathematical 'flattening' of the three-dimensional surface, which takes the stretch of the leather into account.

The initial foray into the use of advanced technology for prescription footwear was related to the problem of storage of lasts. It was envisaged that the vast banks of shoe lasts that are routinely stored for many years could be replaced by storage on computer disks (Vickers & Foort 1980). A number of developments into all aspects of footwear design have begun, with commercial

availability of first generation systems just beginning at this time. The visible part of the system in the clinic is anticipated to be a foot shape-scanner. Although improving the reliability of the measurement technique in this way is an important factor, it is only one of many which will determine the success of the whole system. There are many other reasons for introducing advanced technology; these are briefly explored in the following section.

The scope of an advanced technology system lies in three basic manufacturing elements, each making use of the input of digitized shape and load information to a computer, the storage and manipulation of shape in the computer, and finally fabrication of a physical component via a computer-numerically controlled (CNC) machine. These are:

1. design and manufacture of orthopaedic shoe lasts;
2. design and pattern cutting for the shoe uppers to fit to an individual last;
3. design of orthotic inserts from plantar shape and pressure measurements (Staats & Kriechbaum 1989).

Information handling and storage elements are just as important as the manufacturing elements. These include:

1. potential for large data-bases, or 'libraries' of last shapes with orthopaedic features, which can be used as a basis for customized design, giving rapid access to potentially large numbers of well-designed lasts for many conditions and style considerations;
2. surface modification packages to make systematic modifications to these basic lasts to meet the

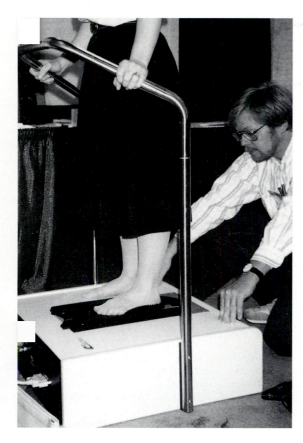

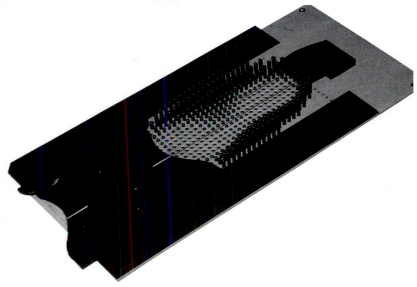

Figure 38

A novel plantar-shape measuring device from Amfit Inc. is part of a CAD insole-production system (photographed at ISPO World Congress exhibition, Chicago, 1992).

customer's individual needs, giving facilities, for example, to add localized bumps or to alter proportions of heel and forefoot widths;

3. customer last libraries stored in digital form, saving physical space and facilitating electronic transfer for patients to hold their own lasts.

4. style libraries with specific features for orthopaedic applications, giving facilities to map well-designed and up-to-date styles onto the customer's last;

5. integration of pressure and shape measurements for design of inserts (TIDE Project Inscad).

Potential service benefits of computer-aided design and manufacture

The key to realization of clinical benefits from advanced technology is the vertical integration of the system into service delivery. The new approaches provide a technological basis for development of features which can be of substantial clinical benefit. Quality of service is a more appropriate indicator of benefit than quality of the footwear per se, with number of patient visits required to achieve a result, time to delivery, prescriber and patient satisfaction with the end product, patient compliance and long-term outcome as potential quality measures.

Conclusion

Well-fitting functional orthopaedic footwear which is acceptable to the patient requires a sensitive prescription and a thorough knowledge of biomechanics, shoe construction and the fitting process. This is a time of service improvement. Major advances in in-shoe instrumentation will further the understanding of the foot–shoe biomechanics and interface leading to tighter prescription; advances in materials and manufacturing technology will permit better shoes to be made economically and delivered on time.

References

Allen W D, Weinder D S, Riley P M 1993 The treatment of rigid metatarsus adductovarus with the use of a new hinged adjustable shoe orthosis. Foot Ankle 14: 450–454

Anthony R J 1991 The manufacture and use of the functional foot orthosis. Karger, Basel

Basford J R, Smith M A 1988 Shoe inserts in the workplace. Orthopaedics 11: 285–288

Blake R L, Ferguson H 1991 Foot orthosis for severe flatfoot in sports. J Am Podiatr Med Assoc 81: 549–555

Boulton A J M, Hardisty C A, Betts R P, et al 1983 Dynamic foot pressure and other studies as diagnostic and management aids in diabetic neuropathy. Diabetes Care 6: 26–33

Brown R N, Byers-Hinkley K and Logan L 1987 The talus control ankle foot orthosis. Orthot Prosthet 41: 22–31

Browne R 1993 Better lasts, better fit. SATRA Bulletin, UK Shoe and Allied Trade Research Association April pp 57–58

Burdett R G, Borello-France D, Blatchly C, Potter C 1988 Gait comparison of subjects with hemiplegia walking unbraced, with ankle foot orthoses and with Air-Stirrup brace. Phys Ther 68: 1197–1203

Butler P B, Thompson N, Major R E 1992 Improvement in walking performance of children with cerebral palsy: preliminary results. Dev Med Child Neurol 34: 567–576

Campbell J W, Inman V T 1974 Treatment of plantar fasciitis and calcaneal spurs with UC-BL shoe inserts. Clin Orthop 103: 57–59

Carlson J M, Berglund G 1979 An effective design for controlling the unstable sub-talar joint. Orthot Prosthet 33: 39–49

Cavanagh P R, Sanders L J, Sims D S Jr 1987 The role of pressure distribution measurements in diabetic foot care. Rehabilitation Research and Development Progress Reports, Veterans Administration, p. 54

Chen C C 1993 An investigation into shoe last design in relation to foot measurement and shoe fitting for orthopaedic footwear. PhD Thesis, London University

Clayton M L, Ries M D 1991 Functional hallux rigidus in the rheumatoid foot. Clin Orthop 271: 233–238

Condie D N 1976 The mechanics of lower limb bracing. In: Murdoch G (ed) The Advances in Orthotics. Edward Arnold, London

Costigan P S, Miller G, Elliot C, Wallace W A 1989 Are surgical shoes providing value for money? BMJ 299–950

Cterctetko G C, Dhanendran M, Hutton W C, Le Quesne L P 1981 Vertical forces acting on the feet of diabetic patients with neuropathic ulceration. Br J Surg 68: 609–614

Dannanberg H J 1988 The kinetic wedge. J Am Podiatr Med Assoc 78: 98–99

Dimonte P, Light H 1982 Pathomechanics, gait deviations, and treatment of the rheumatoid foot. Phys Ther 8: 1148–1156

Eggold J 1981 Orthotics in the prevention of runners' overuse injuries. Physician Sports Med 9: 125

Fisher L R, McLellan D L 1989 Questionnaire assessment of patient satisfaction with lower limb orthoses from a district hospital. Prosthet Orthot Int 13: 29–35

Flutter A G 1983 Introducing CADCAM into the shoe industry. IMechE C171/83

Freeman A C 1990 A study of inter observer and intra observer reliability in the measurement of resting calcaneal stance position and neutral calcaneal stance position. J Podiatr Med Surg 2: 6–8

Frey C, Thompson F, Smith J, Sanders M, Horstman H 1993 American Orthopaedic Foot and Ankle Society Women's Shoe Survey. Foot Ankle 14: 78–81

Gastwirth B W, O'Brien T D, Nelson R M, Manger D C, Kindig S A 1991 An electrodynographic study of foot function in shoes of varying heel height. J Am Podiatr Med Assoc 81: 463–472

Geary N P J, Klenerman L 1987 The rocker soled shoe; a method of reduce peak forefoot pressure in the management of diabetic foot ulceration. In: Pratt D J, Johnson G R (eds) The Biomechanics and Orthotic Management of the Foot 1. Orthotics and Disability Research Centre, Derby. pp. 161–173

Glancy J, Lindseth R E 1972 The polypropylene solid ankle orthosis. Orthot Prosthet 26: 14–26

Helfet A J 1956 A new way of treating flat feet in children Lancet 1: 262–264

Kidd R 1991 An examination of the validity of some of the more questionable cornerstones of modern chiropodial diagnosis. J Br Podiatr Med 9: 172–173

Lord M, Hosein R 1994 Pressure redistribution by moulded inserts in diabetic footwear: a pilot study. J Rehabil Res Dev 31: 214–221

Lord M, Chen R, van der Zande M 1992 A comparison of two fitting procedures used for orthopaedic shoes. Abstracts ISPO World Congress, Chicago, p. 104

Lundeen R O 1988 Polysectional triaxial posting: a new process for incorporating correction in foot orthoses. J Am Podiatr Med Assoc 78: 55–59

Marvin R, Brownrigg P 1983 The negative anatomically modified foot orthosis (NAMFO) Orthot Prosthet 37: 24–31

Meadows C B 1984 The influence of polypropylene ankle foot orthoses on the gait of CP children. PhD Thesis, University of Strathclyde, Glasgow

Middleton E A, Hurley G R B, McIlwain J S 1988 The role of rigid and hinged polypropylene ankle foot orthoses in the management of cerebral palsy: a case study. Prosthet Orthot Int 12: 129–135

Novick A, Birke J A, Hoard A S, Brasseaux D M, Broussard J B, Hawkins E S 1991 Rigid orthoses for the insensitive foot: the rigid relief orthosis. J Prosthet Orthot 4: 31–40

Phillips R D, Christeck R, Phillips R L 1985 Clinical measurement of the axis of the sub-talar joint. J Am Podiatr Med Assoc 75: 119–131

Philps J W 1990 The functional foot orthosis. Churchill Livingston, Edinburgh

Pratt D J 1990 Long term comparison of some shock attenuating insoles. Prosthet Orthot Int 14: 59–62

Pratt D J, Sanghera K S 1987 The assessment of some shock attenuating insole materials at in-shoe temperatures and humidity. In: Pratt D J, Johnson G R (eds) The biomechanics and orthotic management of the foot 1. Orthotics and Disability Research Centre, Derby

Pratt D J, Rees P H, Butterworth R H H 1984 RTV silicone insoles. Prosthet Orthot Int 8: 54–55

Pratt D J, Tollafield D R, Johnson G R, Peacock J C 1993 Foot orthoses. In: Bowker P, Bader D L, Condie D N, Pratt D J, Wallace W A (eds) The biomechanical basis of orthotic management. Butterworth Heinemann, Oxford

Pratt D J, Iliff P M, Ward J B 1994 Talus control foot orthoses. Foot 4: 31–33

Root M L, Orien W, Weed J H 1977 Normal and Abnormal Function of the Foot. Clinical Biomechanics Corporation, Los Angeles

Rose G K 1962 Correction of the pronated foot. J Bone Joint Surg 44B: 642–647

Rossi W A 1983 Footwear and the podiatrist. The enigma of shoe sizes. J Am Podiatr Assoc 73: 272–274

Salaman R A 1986 Dictionary of Leather-Working Tools c. 1700–1950 and The Tools of Allied Trades. George Allen & Unwin, London

Sanner W H 1989 The functional foot orthosis prescription. In: Jay R (ed) Mechanical Therapy in Podiatric Medicine. Decker, Philadelphia

Sim-Fook L, Hodgson AR 1958 A comparison of foot forms among the non-shoe and shoe wearing Chinese population. J Bone Joint Surg 40A: 1058–1062

Snijders C H 1987 Biomechanics of footwear: clinics in podiatric medicine and surgery. Occup Med 629–643

Soames R W, Stott J R R, Goodbody A, Blake C D, Brewerton D A 1982 Measurement of pressure under the foot during function. Med Biol Comput 20: 489–495

Staats T B, Kriechbaum M P 1989 Computer aided design and computer aided manufacturing of foot orthoses. J Prosthet Orthot 1: 182–186

Stokes A F, Faris I B, Hutton W C 1975 The neuropathic ulcer and loads on the foot in diabetic patients. Acta Orthop Scand 46: 839–847

Stover C N, York J M 1980 Air stirrup management of ankle injuries in athletes. Am J Sports Med 8: 360–365

Subotnick S I 1979 Cures for common running disorders. Anderson World Inc: Mountain View, California

TIDE Project INSCAD 1991 European Economic Community Programme, Brussels

Vainio K 1975 Orthopaedic surgery in the treatment of rheumatoid arthritis. Ann Clin Res 7: 216–224

van der Zande M, Winkelmolen W, Lord M 1992 An investigation into the relationship between foot and last shape. Abstracts ISPO World Congress, Chicago, p. 105

Vickers G W, Foort J 1980 Shoe last duplication by automatic means. US Veterans Admin Contract Report V630P-1690

Voloshin A, Wosk J 1982 An in-vivo study of low back pain and shock absorption in the human locomotor system. J Biomech 15: 21–27

Weber D 1991 Use of the hinged AFO for children with spastic cerebral palsy and midfoot instability. J Assoc Child Prosthet Orthot Clin 25: 61–65

Wenger D R, Mauldin D, Speck G, Morgan D, Leiber R L 1989 Corrective shoes and inserts for treatment for flexible flatfoot in infants and children. J Bone Joint Surg 71A: 800–809

Whitney A K, Whitney K A 1990 Padding and taping therapy. In: Levy L A, Hetherington V J (eds) Principles and Practice of Podiatric Medicine. Churchill Livingston, New York

Wilson M 1993 Influence of instock friction on comfort and performance. SATRA Bulletin, UK Shoe and Allied Trades Research Ass., November, 148–150

XI.3 Conservative Treatment for the Foot in Sport

Steven I Subotnick

Introduction

The foot is a wonder of biomechanical engineering. It allows for conversion of rotations that begin in the pelvis and hip to be converted into meaningful forward or side-to-side movements. Subtalar joint pronation and supination is required by various unidirectional and multidirectional sports. Alterations of normal biomechanics of the foot affect the entire lower extremity as well as the pelvis and lower back. Uniplanar abnormalities of the lower extremity require triplane compensation in the foot at the subtalar joint. In order to understand the interplay between accommodation, balance and propulsion in the foot as it affects the lower extremity, an understanding of normal and abnormal biomechanics is necessary (Subotnick 1996) (Fig. 1).

Biomechanics of the foot in sports

Sports can be either unidirectional or multidirectional. Unidirectional sports are those, such as walking, race walking or running, in which there is chronic stress with the foot functioning in a repetitive way. Multidirectional sports involve cutting, twisting, moving from side to side, going forward and backwards; these include tennis, basketball and the various types of football. In addition, there are edge control sports, such as skating or skiing (where the foot gear has a blade or edge), and jumping sports, such as basketball, volleyball and ballet dancing (Fig. 2).

Unidirectional sports
In unidirectional sports the foot acts first as a mobile adapter during the first 25% of the stance phase of gait. The pronation that takes place allows the shock of impact to be dissipated, and furthermore allows the foot to adapt to weight-bearing surfaces. In mid-stance, the foot becomes a balancing and support organ that allows the rest of the body to be delicately balanced about it. When this occurs, there is maximum energy conservation and muscles are minimally used to maintain the center of gravity.

From the middle of mid-stance until heel off, the foot is becoming a rigid lever for the purpose of propulsion

at the end of the stance phase of gait. The foot moves through three basic functions, the first at contact being adaptation and dissipation of stress, the second at the middle phase being that of balance and stability and the last being that of rigidity and propulsion.

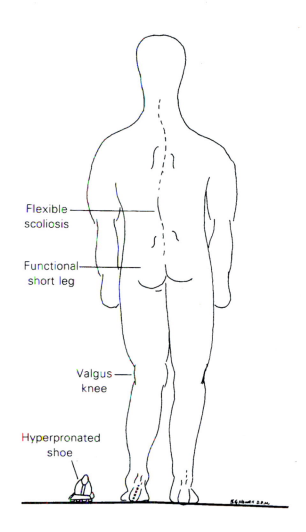

Figure 1

Compensation in forefoot and rearfoot varus on the left. The rear view of a patient with excessive pronation of the left foot is shown. There is hypermobility and pronation of the calcaneus with excessive calcaneal valgus, functional valgus at the knee, a functionally short right leg, and a flexible scoliosis. The right scapula is lower than the left scapula, and there is compensation at the cervical area

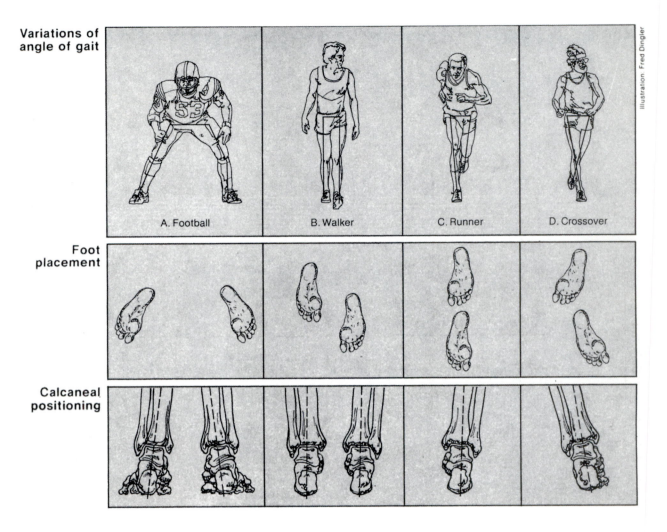

Variations of angle of gait — A. Football · B. Walker · C. Runner · D. Crossover

Foot placement

Calcaneal positioning

Illustration Fred Dingler

Figure 2

Comparison of the angle and base of gait. (A) Football players with a low center of gravity have a wide angle and base of gait and pronated rearfoot. (B) Exercise walkers with a narrow base of gait have a parallel angle of gait and a neutral rearfoot. (C) Runners with a high center of gravity have a zero base and angle of gait and a varus rearfoot. (D) Joggers usually have crossover and functional varus. (From Subotnick 1996 with permission)

Multidirectional sports

In multidirectional sports the center of gravity is lower and the feet are wider apart as well as being externally rotated. This allows for cutting from side to side, and lateral and backwards motion. Much twisting takes place and it is important for the feet to provide a stable base for the center of gravity to change rapidly. As such, there is more pronation of the subtalar joint to allow the foot to adapt to varying surfaces. Mid-stance and propulsion are usually initiated from a pronated position. During jumping, the foot maximally supinates at toe off and the foot may land in a supinated position, which is poor for dissipating shock. In golf, the foot must act as an adaptable organ to allow the golfer to have the feet firmly planted on surfaces that are often tilted and irregular.

Foot function

Understanding the specific biomechanical requirements for the foot in various sports activities, allows the practitioner to evaluate better footwear and various external treatment devices, ranging from taping and strapping to accommodating padding to semifunctional devices, and finally functional foot orthotics of a permanent nature. Permanent foot orthotics, which may be suitable for running, might over-correct for multidirectional sports such as soccer or tennis. Foot orthotics for walking, with a wider base of gait, may not have enough varus cant to control abnormal pronation in the long-distance runner.

Forces in sports

Exercise walker

The ground reactive force for walking is approximately twice body weight. The average exercise walker's foot is on the ground for three-quarters of a second. One foot (or both feet) are on the ground at all times. The base of gait is wide for stability, and feet may be externally rotated. The center of gravity is relatively high.

Jogger

The jogger running from 3–20 miles a week, may go at a rate of 9–12 minutes a mile. The jogger typically lands on the back of the heel or on the heel and the lateral aspect of the foot. The foot rapidly hits the support surface and the foot is generally on the ground for 300–350 milliseconds. Inexperienced joggers who tend to pronate excessively may have inefficient propulsion and bounce up and down, predisposing to injuries. The ground reactive force on level surfaces is at least three times body weight. One foot or no feet are on the ground and there is much more weight going through the support foot than in walking. Poor footwear (pronated shoes), poor runner's biomechanics, foot imbalances and weak muscles all lead to injury of the knee, leg, ankle and/or foot (Fig. 2).

Exercise runner

The exercise runner typically runs at 8–9 miles an hour and may cover 20–40 miles a week. The foot is on the ground for 250 milliseconds. Ground reactive force on level surfaces is three to three and a half times body weight, uphill two times body weight, and downhill four to five times body weight. The angle of gait is zero and one foot lands where the other foot was. There is a functional varus, which predisposes even runners with excellent biomechanics of the lower extremity, which would be termed as normal, to pronate as a function of the sport of running in itself. This excessive pronation may lead to abnormal biomechanics and subsequent overuse injury (see Fig. 3).

Long-distance runner

The long-distance runner covers from 40–70 miles a week at a pace of 6–8 minutes a mile. Marathons and marathon-style events are often the goal of long-distance runners. Their foot is typically on the ground for 200 milliseconds. The excessive running as well as increased speed predisposes them to a multitude of overuse injuries involving the foot, leg, knee, thigh, hip and low back.

'Ultra-marathoners' are highly competitive runners who train at 70–110 miles a week. They typically run slower than marathoners, at 9–10 miles an hour. They compete

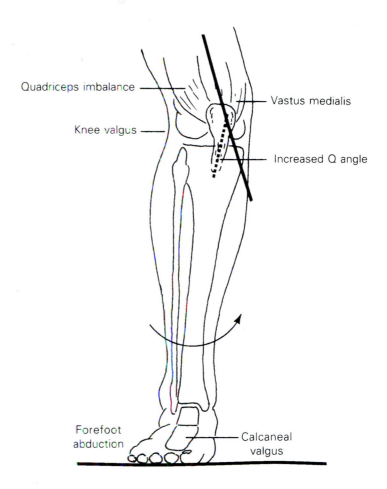

Figure 3

Effect of closed kinetic chain pronation on the foot and leg – miserable malalignment syndrome. The closed kinetic chain consists of internal rotation of the tibia. When the subtalar axis is close to 45° in the sagittal plane, there is approximately 1° of calcaneal eversion for each degree of tibial and talus internal rotation. Thus, in kinetic chain pronation, the calcaneus everts and the leg rotates internally. The forefoot abducts on the rearfoot as the talus rotates (adducts) internally. The medial longitudinal arch is lowered as the talus relatively plantarflexes and the foot relatively dorsiflexes. The center of gravity is therefore medial to the foot. This causes a relative functional valgus at the knee. There is excessive tension on the medial structures of the knee. A functional increased Q angle results, and the quadriceps, which are contracting to decrease abnormal flexion at the knee, pull the patella laterally. The so-called lateral override of the patella is created, with associated patellar femoral-related running symptomatology and pathology. The medial plantar fascia and abductor hallucis are stretched as the forefoot abducts on the rearfoot and the medial longitudinal arch is lowered. The tibialis posterior is overtaxed as it attempts to decelerate the rapid internal rotation of the leg and concomitant lowering of the medial longitudinal arch. The anterior tibial muscle is likewise overtaxed in its attempts to support the medial longitudinal arch

in ultra-marathons ranging from 35–50 miles. At times, hundred-mile races are attempted.

Jumping sports

In jumping sports, the landing (such as after a rebound in basketball) subjects the body to up to seven times the body weight.

Acceleration–deceleration sports

These types of sports, such as tennis, subject the foot to continual twisting, torque, counter-torque and acceleration–deceleration. This may lead to soft tissue injuries such as tendonitis, myositis, or a rupture of the plantar fascia.

Contact and collision sports

These sports include American football, rugby and basketball, and involve high-speed collision, with the foot often anchored to the support surface. This creates acute trauma, such as ruptured ankle ligaments.

Types of injuries

Injuries can be broadly divided into acute, subacute, chronic and overuse.

Acute injuries

Acute injuries are often known as sprains or strains. They happen suddenly and have a predictable healing course. These injuries typically involve partial ruptures of muscles and tendons, acute tenosynovitis and plantar fascial tears and strains. At times there may be a hyperextension injury of the great toe ('turf toe') or an avulsion fracture at the base of the fifth metatarsal, on the proximal aspect of the sesamoid, or of the lateral malleolus. Acute injuries are well known by sports physicians, and routine treatments for the various phases of healing are indicated. These include physical therapy, correction of any training errors, foot function or improper selection of footwear. It is important to emphasize strength, power, flexibility and balance.

Subacute injuries

Subacute injuries are those that linger between the acute and chronic phase and may not progress to normal healing. The commonest cause of this in athletes is returning to sports too early without adequate rehabilitation or healing of the original problem. Failure to correct improper foot function or to provide for maximum dynamic strength, flexibility and balance of the lower extremity may predispose to this problem.

Chronic injuries

Chronic injuries are those that have failed to proceed to complete recovery. They include chronic plantar fasciitis following an acute rupture or stretching incident, chronic medial shin (or anterior shin syndrome) and chronic lateral instability of the ankle following an acute grade 3 sprain with incomplete and/or inadequate healing of the lateral ligaments of the ankle. These injuries may require additional physical therapy, injection therapy to break up chronic abnormal fibrosis and scar tissue or, at times, surgery (e.g. in cases of chronic lateral instability of the ankle or chronic tenosynovitis with central necrosis of the tendo Achillis. Other chronic conditions that may require a surgical approach include retrocalcaneal bursitis and exostosis, heel spur syndrome that fails to respond to adequate and appropriate conservative treatment and Morton's neuroma.

Overuse injuries

Overuse injuries are caused by chronic, repetitive stress. They are commoner in the novice athlete with underdeveloped sensory feedback, proprioception, strength, flexibility, balance and skill. These athletes often have inadequate foot control or poor footwear and they lack knowledge of appropriate training techniques and procedures. The sports physician dealing with foot problems, intrinsic or as they relate to the rest of the body, must be aware of these training errors and help the athlete correct them for a full return to active sports.

Overuse injuries are commoner in unidirectional sports such as race walking and long-distance running. As the foot performs the same function over and over again it is essential to have sound, biodynamic foot orthotics with appropriate shoes. These shoes must fulfill the function of attenuating and dissipating impact shock, while providing stability against excessive pronation and/or supination. It is not uncommon for a modern running shoe to begin having material failure of the midsole material after 1000 miles of running. That being the case, shoes may need to be replaced often. In the novice athlete, improper selection of running shoes is one of the main causes of overuse injuries. The use of a treadmill with video and slow motion play-back clearly demonstrates improper selection of foot gear to the athlete, as excessive, prolonged pronation and/or eccentric foot patterns are easily seen. It is appropriate and important to have the athlete bring in prescribed shoes and recheck them on the treadmill to make sure that they are fulfilling their function (Fig. 4).

Another factor for overuse injuries is fatigue. It is well known by seasoned marathoners that the last 6 miles of the marathon is when they 'hit the wall'. At this time there is depletion of both glycogen and stored fatty acid, and the athletes are running on zero. Muscles are sore, tired, and inadequately oxygenated and fueled, and they fail to respond in a manner that allows them to absorb shock and to position the joints and the appendages in

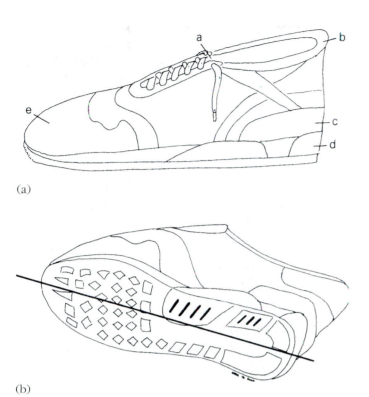

(a)

(b)

Figure 4

Qualities of good running shoes. (a) Side view. a, well-padded tongue; b, molded Achilles pad; c, firm heel counter; d, flared and beveled heel; e, high, rounded toebox. (b) Bottom view. Straight last and studded sole

appropriate biomechanical relationships in order to withstand impact shock and acceleration–deceleration forces. Fatigue is a major cause of injury in both unidirectional and multidirectional sports. Fatigue plays a factor in injuries of skiing which occur during the last run. Injuries in contact and collision sports are more frequent during the final minutes of the game, owing to fatigue and loss of normal, quick reflex response.

Treatment considerations

Fortunately most sports injuries involving the foot respond readily and satisfactorily to appropriate conservative treatment. Surgery is rarely indicated. It must be understood by the treating physician that sports are an important part of the athlete's life. A physician must listen to the athlete's careful description of the present and past injuries to ascertain training error or patterns of training that may need correction. If the injury is severe enough to warrant stopping the particular sport while healing is taking place, an alternative aerobic activity should be substituted. Running in water with a flotation device, using an exercise bike or walking if without

symptoms will often suffice. Seasoned athletes will usually complain that nothing takes the place of their chosen sport. This is true for the long-distance runner, the basketball player, tennis player, golfer or bowler. The fulfilment found in one sport is seldom replaced by another sport.

Treatments

Most foot deformities, injuries, ailments and/or imbalances of the foot which are affecting the ankle, leg, knee, hip and/or pelvis will respond to a variety of strapping, accommodating and bracing devices. Strapping or taping are well known to athletic trainers and provide a means of support and protection which allows for function. Accommodating uses various thicknesses of felt, foam or sponge rubber devices to shift the pressure from the painful bony protuberance or area of injury to asymptomatic areas while not adversely affecting foot function or functional biomechanics. Bracing can include everything from innersoles, soft temporary foot supports, accommodative foot devices, semifunctional devices to permanent functional sport foot orthotics. Bracing further involves inflated casts, ambulatory removable ankle–foot orthosis (AFO) braces, removable casts and well-formed plaster of Paris or synthetic fiberglass-type casts. Various external devices, such as postoperative shoes for stress fractures, negative heel postoperative shoes for forefoot problems, anterior heels for metatarsalgia and neuromas and lateral or medial wedges on heels for ankle and foot instability all may be helpful.

Shielding, supportive padding, strapping, bracing and mechanical methods of applying materials under, around or on the foot and ankle can be tried to eliminate or minimize extrinsic friction and pressure, to redistribute weight-bearing forces, and to replace or reinforce the stabilizing structure of the foot and leg.

Shields or appliances fashioned from natural or synthetic fibers are applied for the purpose of relieving pressure, friction or protect the tender part of the foot. Examples are felt pads for painful bunions (Fig. 5) or a sponge rubber 'doughnut' pad for painful, blistered 'pump bump' on the back of the heel (Fig. 6).

Supportive padding (accommodative padding) is used to re-establish weight-bearing forces or realign structural abnormalities. These pads may be applied directly to the skin of the foot (Figs 7,8). They may also be applied to the innersole of the shoe or standard innersoles may be modified and placed in the athlete's shoe. Examples are a felt first-ray padding to compensate for forefoot varus deformity or a felt varus heel wedge glued to the innersole of the shoe, to realign the calcaneus in a neutral varus attitude.

Strappings are made of various adhesive tapes or fabrics that are supportive and compressive. They are applied either alone or in conjunction with supportive

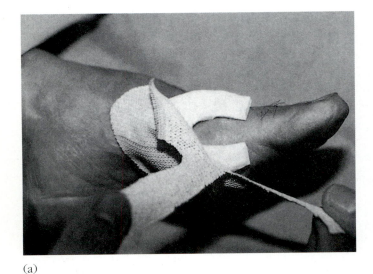

(a)

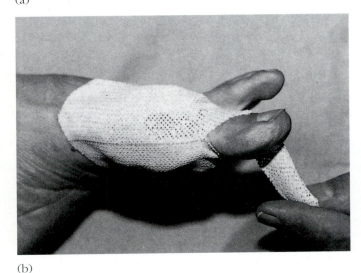

(b)

Figure 5

Bunion pads. (a) Accommodative horseshoe pad of adhesive-backed ⅛-inch felt has an elasticated cover. (b) Applying elasticated plaster cover over an accommodative felt horseshoe-shaped pad

pads in an attempt to realign the structural abnormalities of the foot. Examples are Campbell's rest strap for sprained arch, or the time-proven low-dye strapping for plantar fascial strain with or without heel spur padding (Fig. 9).

Braces are used to replace or reinforce an injured or lost ligament or tendon. The purpose is to provide external support and to stabilize unstable parts. An example of brace strapping is the classic ankle tape with or without heel lock for an acutely sprained ankle. Another is a double upright, lace-up brace for a chronic unstable ankle. A wide variety of supplies are available for the fabrication and application of shields, pads, straps and braces used in the treatment of athletic injuries. The materials most often used for shielding and accommodating padding are adhesive back moleskin and felt.

(a)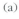

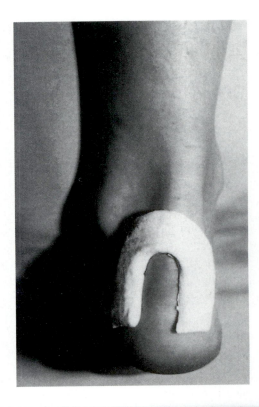

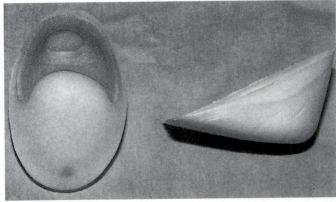

(b)

Figure 6

Pump bump. (a) A ¼-inch (6 mm) adhesive felt horseshoe-shaped pad is designed for painful retrocalcaneal exostosis or bursitis (pump bump). (b) The pad can be constructed of a variety of materials and applied directly to the foot orthotic device, or glued directly into the shoe

Foot orthotics

Orthotic foot devices

Orthoses of a temporary or permanent nature may be indicated for the recreational as well as the serious athlete. These devices serve biodynamically to guide the foot through various functions, encouraging it to be adaptable at heel and foot contact, supportive and balancing at mid-stance and a rigid lever at propulsion. Generally, the more rigid, the more biodynamic devices

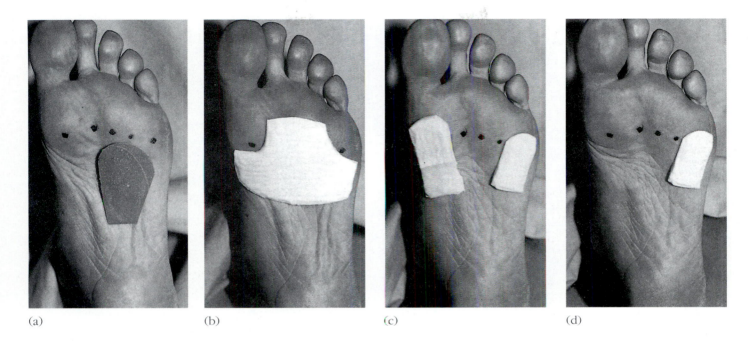

(a)   (b)   (c)   (d)

Figure 7

Metatarsal padding. (a) This dense rubber metatarsal pad is similar to the classic one. It is used to accommodate a neuroma and is placed just proximal to the fourth metatarsal head. (b) An accommodative first and fifth metatarsal adhesive felt ¼-inch (6 mm) cut-out pad may be used for painful calluses beneath the metatarsal heads or for a painful sesamoid and fifth metatarsal capsulitis. (c) Classic biplanar padding is often used to transfer weight to the first and fifth metatarsal heads to relieve painful calluses or capsulitis of the second, third, and fourth metatarsals. (d) A lateral balance pad accommodates forefoot valgus deformity. This pad will increase weight bearing under the fifth metatarsal head

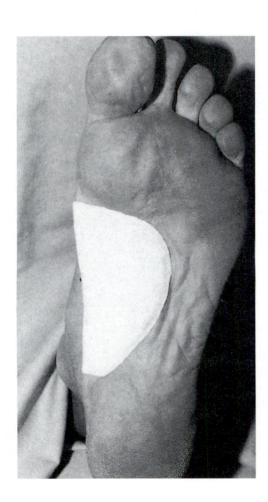

have greatest opportunity for maximum effectiveness as well as abuse. When in doubt, use softer, more flexible materials. If the optimal biomechanical mid-stance neutral position cannot be sustained with these materials, try more supportive and rigid materials.

Types of devices

It is often necessary to provide athletes with an on-the-spot, temporary type of orthotic foot device. The simplest of these is created simply by modifying the innersole of the shoe, or using preformed innersoles. These innersoles can be wedged, padded, or accommodated with felt or rubber materials to improve biomechanics, decrease shock, decrease the tendency for blister formation and abnormal shear forces, and disperse or attenuate abnormal shock. A helpful material is nitrogen foam rubber, such as that used with wet suit devices. This is excellent in decreasing twisting shear

Figure 8

Plantar fascial strain. A medial longitudinal arch pad can be fabricated from ¼-inch (6 mm) adhesive felt. This classic arch pad is used for plantar fascial strain or symptoms associated with flexible flatfoot. The pad can be applied directly to the bottom of the foot or incorporated into an arch support

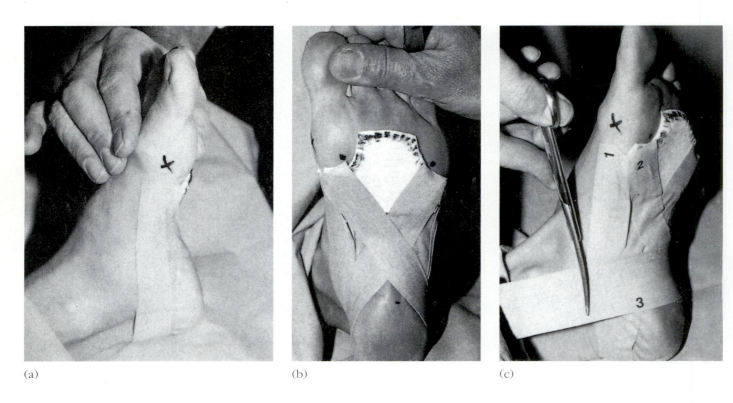

(a)   (b)   (c)

+Figure 9

Strapping. (a) With the foot held in neutral position, the first metatarsal should be slightly plantarflexed with the index finger. The tape is brought distal to just proximal to the first metatarsal head. This step is repeated two to three times, depending on the weight and degree of activity of the patient. (b) An additional two or three tapes may be criss-crossed on the plantar surface from the first and fifth metatarsal. (c) For stirrup strapping, tape number 3 extends from just inferior to the lateral malleolus across the plantar aspect of the foot, then extends superior to just beneath the medial malleolus to the level of the superior aspect of tape number 1

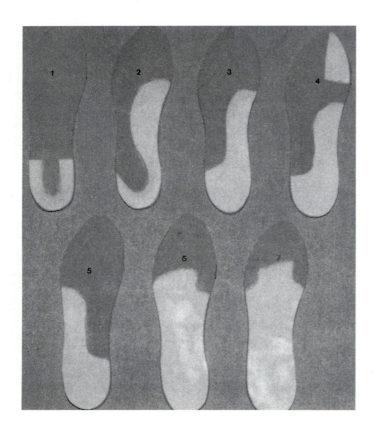

Figure 10

Uses of balance and accommodative paddings incorporated into temporary orthotics. (1) Plantar heel-spur accommodation used for plantar calcaneal spurs, plantar fasciitis, or painful lesions that occur plantar to the heel, such as bruises or apophysitis. (2) Cobra pad for rearfoot control and supporting a forefoot varus deformity. (3) Medial heel–medial sole. The lateral aspect of this pad is skived to create a varus attitude to the rearfoot. This is designed to compensate for a rearfoot varus–forefoot varus deformity and to support the medial arch. (4) Medial heel Morton's extension, created in a manner similar to the medial heel–medial sole insole with the same indications. Also, this enhances a great toe position and is mostly used in hallux limitus or hallux rigidus and Morton's foot. (5) Medial heel–lateral sole, designed to stimulate out-toe gait. (6) Medial heel–first-ray cutout, used to accommodate a plantarflexed first metatarsal, which is generally found with a high-arched cavus-type foot. The pad should be skived to create a 4–6° varus wedge on the rearfoot and to accommodate and allow the first metatarsal to sit in its neutral position. (7) Medial heel–fifth ray and first–fifth ray cutout, commonly used in a high-arched cavus foot with painful lesions below the first and fifth metatarsal heads

forces and reducing blisters. Surgical orthopedic splint wedged with felt is often useful. Additional shock absorbance is gained with nitrogen foam rubber.

The growing child with a foot imbalance, apophysitis, or plantar fasciitis often does well by modifying ready made Birkenstock orthotics. These are inexpensive and may be replaced as the child grows.

Elderly athletes with arthritis and fixed bony positions, often do well with softer materials such as used with the 'soft or on the spot orthoses'.

High-demand sports often require more sophisticated biodynamic devices made from a neutral foot cast. Full-length foot orthotics allow for increased proprioception and lend themselves well to various lateral- or medial-balance devices that protect athletes from abnormal landing forces in jumping sports. Unidirectional sports require semirigid to rigid orthotics with additional varus posting to correct for functional varus inherent to these sports. Multidirectional sports require a more flexible material with less rear foot control to allow for pronation and supination with rapid changes in speed and direction. Edge control sports require flexible, medial arch control with soft material under the ball of the foot and toes to improve proprioception and balance (Fig. 10).

Casting

Most feet can be casted non-weight-bearing in a prone position. The heel is placed neutral and there is pressure under the fourth and fifth metatarsal heads to lock and pronate the midtarsal joint. As with most orthopedic procedures it is always best to err in the direction of pronation and undercorrection. Deformed or arthritic feet will respond best to semi-weight-bearing casts. These devices hold the foot as it is and are useful in preventing further subluxation.

In-shoe casting

Orthoses for ski boots, skates and dancing shoes are often fashioned from a cast that is made with the foot in the athletic footwear. When fashioning any type of orthotic foot device, it is important to understand the sport-specific biomechanical demands and requirements.

Overall biomechanical goals

The overall goal of orthotic foot devices is to support, balance and align the foot and lower extremity. This improves function of the foot as well as the lower extremity, and provides for a level pelvis. A level pelvis is the foundation for the remainder of the spine. To that end, functional or anatomical limb length discrepancies from one-eighth to one-quarter of an inch or greater are treated appropriately with correction and/or heel lifts. An in shoe heel lift will suffice for a discrepancy up to ⅜-inch (10 mm). Beyond ⅜-inch (10 mm), with the exception of a high-top shoe or boot, the lift will not be tolerated within the shoe. In that case, part of the deformity

can be corrected up to ⅜-inch directly on the heel of the device and the rest of the deformity will need to be corrected on the heel and out sole of the shoe. In general, when using shoe corrections I prefer full correction in the heel, one-half correction mid-foot, with one-quarter to one-eighth correction in the ball and forefoot. With excessive deformity it is necessary to perforate the mid-sole of the shoe to allow for flexion between the ball of the foot and toes.

Common sports foot ailments

Plantar heel spur syndrome

Plantar heel spur syndrome has been called plantar fat pad syndrome, walkers' and runners' heel, plantar fasciitis and/or heel spur. I prefer to separate plantar fasciitis from heel spur syndrome. Heel spur syndrome in my experience is a post-traumatic condition of the medial plantar condyle of the calcaneous which involves the plantar fat pad, the insertion of the intrinsic musculature and medial plantar fascia to the medial plantar condyle of the calcaneous and the condyle and bone itself. Plantar heel syndrome is very common in the middle-aged and elderly walkers in my community. These patients began walking as a form of relaxation and to help reduce their weight. They have often been relatively inactive before taking up walking and have improper footwear. Many of them are obese or overweight and have abnormal biomechanics. They present with extreme pain and aching at the plantar medial aspect of the heel. X-rays will often show bilateral heel spurs though often only one is symptomatic. The presence of a spur, however, is not diagnostic or necessary to make the diagnosis. The spur is the result, not the cause, of the problem. In postmenopausal women, osteoporosis may lead to a softening of the bone and the patients may in fact have stress reaction of bone, or a stress fracture. Subclinical osteoporosis may allow for traction spurs and other bony problems. In middle-aged and elderly male patients, osteoporosis is usually not a problem.

The combination of increased activity and stress in this population of walkers appears to predispose the foot to calcaneal osteitis, fasciitis, myositis, and/or tendonitis. This is further complicated by a weakening of the plantar fat pad of the calcaneous as it loses its normal ability to absorb and attenuate shock as a result of the normal aging process, with collagen failure of the pad itself. The plantar fat pad tends to spread out and lose its normal columnar arrangement. The fat pad in a young healthy person is a major shock attenuator. As it flattens and loses its collagen elasticity, shock is transferred to the bone itself and transmitted more proximally, causing a multitude of symptoms. Viscoelastic polymeres are an external way of replacing the failing fat pad. Orthotics with a heel cup also hold the fat under the heel, where it belongs, allowing it to fulfil its function.

The presenting complaint is usually stiffness that is worse at first and improves with continued motion. Patients are usually worse in cold and damp weather and better when it is warm. After warming up the foot, they can usually walk, but as the problem progresses it is difficult to walk and exercise must be abandoned.

Medical conditions such as rheumatoid arthritis, gout or other collagen diseases should be ruled out. Initial treatment consists of strapping and padding the foot (see Figs 6 and 9). The patient then will progress to a soft temporary orthotic and/or a Birkenstock type orthotic (see Fig. 10). If problems persist and the foot cannot be controlled adequately in the temporary or semirigid devices, a more permanent orthosis is made over a neutral cast of the foot. Stretching of the calf muscle is essential. Stretching should be carried out with the leg extended and flexed. In addition, deep transverse friction massage is helpful. Patients can roll their foot over a tennis ball or wine bottle to help stretch out and dissipate fibrosis and the attachment of the plantar fascia.

Persistent problems may require injection therapy. Three to four injections, one to two weeks apart often will take care of the problem of a persistent, chronic heel spur syndrome. In those athletes objecting to the use of corticosteroids, I substitute a homeopathic and local anesthetic injection. When injecting a fluid lysis effect is desired. To this end, a 30 G needle is moved back and forth through the fibrous attachments at the intrinsic musculature and medial plantar fascia to the medial condyle of the calcaneus. Following these injections there may be a postinjection flare or pain and the patient is given a nonsteroidal anti-inflammatory to help with this. Soaking is helpful, as are contrast baths in which the patient places the foot in ice water for 30 seconds and then in warm water for 30 seconds, for a total of 5 minutes. The patient may resume exercise walking once normal ambulation is asymptomatic (Subotnick 1991).

Occasionally, patients will not respond in an acceptable period of time (8–12 weeks) with conservative treatment. In these cases they may be given a choice to wait one or two years, when most plantar heel spur syndromes resolve on their own or have a surgical release of the medial plantar fascia and rasping down of the spur. In my 25 years of practice, 18% of my patients have required heel spur surgery.

Heel spurs are not uncommon in competitive athletes involved in sports such as tennis, long-distance running, track, basketball, golf and bowling. In these instances, conservative treatment usually suffices, though occasionally surgery is necessary.

Plantar fasciitis

Plantar fasciitis is about as common in presentation as plantar heel spur syndrome. Plantar fasciitis is characterized by internal derangements of the collagen fibers of the plantar fascia proximally at the mid-aspect and even distally. This condition is treated in virtually the same way as heel spur syndrome. Taping is even more effective with plantar fasciitis and typically a low-dye strapping is utilized (see Fig. 9). Physical therapy can be helpful utilizing interferential or electrogalvanic stimulation (EGS) and ultrasound two to three times a week for 4–6 weeks. The same holds true for plantar heel spur syndrome. Injection therapy is indicated when conservative treatment with orthotics and strapping is not adequate. Three to four injections into the area of fibrosis, with or without corticosteroids based upon the physician's and athlete's preference, is carried out (Subotnick 1991). Fourteen per cent of those presenting with this problem have eventually required surgery in my clinic.

Peroneal cuboid syndrome

Peroneal cuboid syndrome is a poorly recognized condition which occurs at the calcaneocuboid articulation or the articulations of the cuboid with the fourth and fifth metatarsals. It involves the peroneal longus tendon as it passes underneath the cuboid. Typically, patients with plantar heel spur syndrome supinate their foot to take the pressure off the medial plantar heel. This causes an increased pressure on the lateral column of the foot, and the cuboid everts. When the cuboid everts, the fourth and fifth metatarsals, as well as calcaneocuboid articulations become unstable. The peroneal longus tendon is also unstable with lack of the normal fulcrum of the cuboid as it plantarflexes the first metatarsal during propulsion in gait. This condition can be appreciated by palpating the calcaneal cuboid and cuboid, fourth, fifth metatarsal articulations.

Treatment is that of initial strapping of the foot with lateral wedging and cuboid pads. Cuboid manipulation is necessary and usually achieved easily without the need for an anesthetic block (Subotnick 1996). In resistant or acute cases, with peroneal muscle spasm, which will not allow manipulation owing to pain, a local anesthetic block can be given at the dorsal lateral aspect of the calcaneocuboid joint. This relieves pain, eliminates peroneal spasm, and allows for the cuboid to be easily slipped back into place with an appropriate joint-specific adjustment. An audible click is often heard. Once the spasm is broken or the acute phase is over, the cuboid can be encouraged to maintain anatomical position with a cuboid pad, lateral wedging, or padding and strapping. Eventually, a biodynamic foot orthotic with a high lateral extension is necessary.

Peroneal cuboid syndrome is not uncommon after any medial plantar heel injury. It is common after heel spur surgery, as the patient walks on the outside of the heel to shift the weight away from the painful medial plantar aspect. This causes eversion forces to the cuboid and subsequent joint malposition. Peroneal cuboid syndrome may also be caused during an ankle sprain as the athlete lands on the lateral plantar aspect of the foot. This may be accompanied by an additional sprain of the lateral aspect of the subtalar joint. Patients with high arch cavus feet tend to be more prone to peroneal cuboid syndrome (Newell & Woodle, 1981). Jumping sports in which the athlete lands on the outside of the foot are also a cause.

Peroneal cuboid syndrome almost always responds to conservative treatment, although recurrent subluxations are not uncommon and may frustrate the athlete as well as the physician. These require repeated joint-specific adjustments or manipulations and strappings. Eventually, with a well-formed permanent orthosis, the condition stabilizes.

Retrocalcaneal exostosis and bursitis

Retrocalcaneal exostosis and bursitis is not uncommon in athletes. It may be caused by a high-pitched calcaneus, as seen in the cavus type foot. It is also more prevalent with hindfoot varus. Shoes with a firm counter aggravate any pressure points on the posterior or posterior lateral aspect of the calcaneus. Typically, patients present with an inflamed bursa and pain over the retrocalcaneal spur. This condition may be complicated with Achilles tendonitis insertional tendonopathy.

Initial treatment consists of altering footwear to take all pressure off of the posterior aspect of the calcaneus (see Fig. 6). Rigid or firm counters in shoes are removed or are broken down with a hammer, and elastic or softer material is substituted. This usually takes care of the etiology of the problem. Further care may be necessary, such as injections, physical therapy, or nonsteroidal anti-inflammatory drugs. Corticosteroids must be used with extreme caution, owing to the proximity of the retrocalcaneal bursa and exostosis to the Achilles tendon. Corticosteroids in and around tendons lead to necrosis and eventual failure. That being the case, I prefer to use local anesthetic and homeopathic remedies. For unresponsive hyperostosis of the calcaneus with chronic bursitis, surgical excision may be necessary. Less than 20% of the patients presenting with this problem have needed surgery in my experience.

Achilles tenosynovitis and insertional tendonitis

The Achilles tendon can be involved with tenosynovitis, peritendonitis, insertional tendonopathy and partial rupture with central necrosis. This can be caused by acute trauma or accumulative microtrauma.

Conservative treatment consists of physical therapy, deep transverse friction massage and stretching the posterior muscles with strengthening of the antigravity anterior muscles. Deep transverse friction after ultrasound is particularly helpful. Needling techniques (moving the needle back and forth) utilizing local anesthetic and homeopathic remedies have been most useful. Corticosteroids must be avoided. Ultrasound has been found to help regeneration of collagen. As vitamin C (5–6 g per day) and glycocyamine sulfate are important as precursors for collagen, nutritional supplements

can be added to the diet. When conservative treatment fails, an MRI or ultrasound may be useful in identifying the extent of damage or injury. Chronic, unresponsive cases may benefit from surgical decompression of the tendon, removal of necrotic tissue or central necrosis, and removal of insertional spurs. The level of activity the athlete returns to is dependent on the amount of pathology and results of surgery. Most athletes are able to return to some form of activity, but some may need to moderate the intensity of their involvement in sports because of stiffness or soreness.

Interdigital neuromas

Interdigital or Morton's neuromas normally occur in the second and third interspace. They are occasionally associated with fibular sesamoiditis in the first interspace, and very rarely a communicating branch from the third interspace to the fourth will cause pain. Bursitis or reactive fibrosis may complicate the condition. Diagnosis is easily made by placing some form of skin cream on the bottom of the foot and rubbing the fingers or thumb between the metatarsal heads until a clicking, painful mass is felt. The athlete complains of pain and numbness, which may shoot down toes or proximally or both.

Treatment consists of three to four injections of corticosteroids or a homeopathic preparation with local anesthetic. Stretching exercises and transverse friction to stretch the usually tight transverse metatarsal ligament are helpful. The patient may find relief in using orthotic foot devices to control abnormal pronation and accommodate the area of chief complaint. Metatarsal or neuroma pads and strapping are helpful in the acute phases (see Fig. 7). If problems persist, surgical excision is easily accomplished. Complications or regrowth occur after excision in 7% of cases, and a stump neuroma is usually more symptomatic than the original problem. Approximately 70% of those with neuromas respond to conservative treatment, and 30% need surgical excision. There is a failure rate of approximately 7%. When regrowth occurs, a secondary procedure excising the stump neuroma through a plantar approach will usually suffice. The use of electrocautery, laser or neuroclips after excision of the neuroma to inhibit any regrowth has not been successful. It is more useful to do a proximal excision of the nerve and then tuck the free branch into an interosseous muscle.

Plantar keratomas

Painful hyperkeratotic lesions or calluses usually occur under the metatarsal heads. They occasionally occur in the heel and are known as porokeratosis plantaris or plugged sweat gland syndrome.

The lesions under metatarsal heads will normally respond to padding and strapping (see Fig. 7). This shifts the weight from the prominent metatarsal heads to

Index

adjacent metatarsals. The lesions must be deeply debrided. If there is an adventitious bursa or neuroma associated with the lesion, a sublesional injection of local anesthetic and corticosteroid or a homeopathic remedy will alleviate the pain and problem. It will also allow for deep paring and debridement. Once the acute symptomatology is gone, a soft accommodative temporary orthosis can be made. A more permanent, semiflexible, accommodative orthosis can be made later and usually suffices. In long-distance runners, a biodynamic orthotic device with accommodation built into the forefoot of the runner's wedging is usually very helpful. (The runner's wedging is the 5° forefoot torus platform extending from behind the metatarsal heads to the base of the toe, being tapered distally.) Very occasionally, a plantarflexed metatarsal needs an osteotomy to resolve the problem of unresponsive, painful plantar keratosis. This procedure should be carried out with the utmost care, in as much as transfer lesions (plantar keratomas on an adjacent metatarsal head, resulting from the transfer of weight after surgery) are the rule rather than the exception, occurring in approximately 60% of cases. Plantar condylectomies are favored by some instead of osteotomies, but this procedure runs the risk of excessive fibrosis in the interspace or under the metatarsal head with disruption of intrinsic musculature. Fewer than 8% of athletes with plantar keratosis require surgery.

Bunions, hallux valgus with bunion, hallux limitus

Conditions of the first metatarsophalangeal joint, such as bunions, will often respond to modification of footwear and accommodative padding. Athletes with asymptomatic hallux valgus and bunions can be helped considerably by functional orthoses, with Morton's extensions in the case of a short metatarsal or accommodation for the first metatarsal in the case of a long first metatarsal. A short first metatarsal is predisposed to hallux valgus with bunion, whereas a long first metatarsal usually results in hallux limitus and/or rigidus with dorsal jamming of the joint.

Sprained ankle

A lateral or inversion sprain of the ankle is a common athletic injury involving the foot and ankle. Both the ankle and subtalar joint may be sprained and the sports physician must evaluate both these articulations. Conservative treatment consists of ice packs, physical therapy, anti-inflammatory medications, injection of the area with local anesthetic and homeopathic remedies and protective functional bracing devices that allow for motion within the physiological tolerance of the tissue. Casts and immobilization are to be discouraged because it causes weakness of tissue as well as narrowing of the joint space. Aircast or cast bracing is preferred, allowing the patient to have range of motion in the sagittal plane.

Grade 1 and 2 sprains respond well to conservative treatment. Grade 3 sprains usually heal without incidence following appropriate physical rehabilitation. Occasionally, grade 3 sprains will lead to chronic instability of an ankle in which case a lateral stabilization procedure or delayed primary repair of ruptured ligaments will be necessary. Orthotic foot devices to correct abnormal rearfoot varus or forefoot valgus are essential with chronic repetitive foot sprains.

Sinus tarsi syndrome

Sinus tarsi syndrome often follows acute sprains of the ankle. There is a pain in the sinus tarsi of the subtalar joint at the lateral aspect of the foot. The surface marking of the subtalar joint is one finger below and in front of the tip of the lateral malleolus. A fibrous fat pad develops from repeated sprains. Often an athlete who has apparently healed from an acute lateral sprain, will complain of annoying, aching discomfort in the sinus tarsi. A fibrous fat pad can be palpated. Elderly patients who pronate excessively may also form a sinus tarsi fat impingement secondary to compressive forces.

Treatment consists of injecting with local anesthetic and a corticosteroid. Homeopathic remedies may be substituted. Three to four injections will take care of the problem. Occasionally when there is significant fibrosis that is unresponsive to conservative treatment the fat pad needs to be excised. Joint-specific adjusting of the calcaneus and talus or manipulation are often very helpful. Orthoses to correct abnormal supination or pronation are essential.

Related problems

One of the commonest running problems related to the foot is that of runner's knee. Patellar compression syndrome, or patellar lateral mal-tracking is usually secondary to excessive pronation with valgus deformity at the knee. This causes a functional increase in the Q angle and lateral mal-tracking of the patella (see Fig. 3). Controlling abnormal foot pronation as well as strengthening the vastus medialis obliques takes care of this problem in almost all athletes. If there is a congenital deformity of the patella, bracing or orthopedic lateral releases may be necessary.

Shin splint syndrome

Shin splint syndromes of the anterior or posterior medial compartment of the leg are not uncommon with excessive pronation of the foot. They readily respond to corrective foot orthotic devices, physical therapy and anti-inflammatory modalities. Patients who present with shin splint syndrome and with point tenderness should be suspected of having a stress reaction of bone or a stress fracture. X-rays or bone scans may be indicated and the patient should rest until a definitive diagnosis is made.

Pelvic girdle and lower back

The pelvic girdle, the lower back and the hip are all affected by abnormal foot biomechanical function. Pronation causes a relative rotation of the pelvis with lowering of the anterior superior iliac spine and raising of the posterior superior iliac spine. Excessive pronation with valgus of the knee causes a functionally short limb with pelvic malrotation. The abnormally rotated pelvis causes compensation of the lumbar vertebra above, and compression of the intravertebral foramen or nerve roots may occur. As the pelvis rotates, the acetabulum of the hip changes in its pitch, causing the femoral head either to decline or raise. All of these subtle imbalances in the pelvic girdle may be helped significantly with appropriate correction of abnormal foot function (see Fig. 1).

be corrected and biomechanical foot abnormalities corrected and accounted for. Footwear must be properly chosen. Foot orthotic devices must be carefully prescribed or made. Physical therapy and rehabilitation are often helpful for foot injuries, as are injection and injection needling techniques. At times, corticosteroids and even anti-inflammatory medications can be replaced with homeopathic medications. When treating the athlete, the axiom 'first no harm' is helpful. The 'quick fix' with corticosteroids or pain killers, allowing the athlete to return to sports too soon before adequate rehabilitation, leads to chronic soft tissue and joint failure and predisposes the athlete to later years of pain and suffering. Fortunately, most foot problems respond well to non-invasive techniques.

Summary

Most sports related conditions of the foot respond readily to simple, conservative treatment modalities and measures. Understanding the sport-specific biomechanics of the foot is essential in treatment and allows for safe, functional and full return to sport. Training errors must

References

Newell S, Woodle A 1981 Cuboid syndrome. Physician and Sports Medicine, 9: 71–76

Subotnick S I 1991 Sports and Exercise Injuries. North Atlantic Press, Berkeley

Subotnick S I 1996 Sports Medicine of the Lower Extremity 2nd edn. Churchill Livingstone, New York

Index